DORLAND'S MEDICAL SPELLER

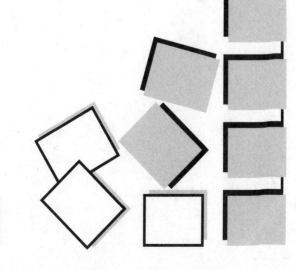

Consultant
ELLEN DRAKE, CMT

Consultant for Syllabication
CAROL A. STILLMAN, PhD

DORLAND'S MEDICAL SPELLER

W.B. SAUNDERS COMPANY
A Division of Harcourt Brace & Company
Philadelphia London Toronto Montreal Sydney Tokyo

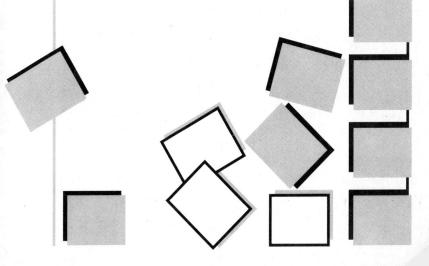

W. B. SAUNDERS COMPANY
A Division of
Harcourt Brace & Company

The Curtis Center
Independence Square West
Philadelphia, Pennsylvania 19106

Library of Congress Cataloging-in-Publication Data

Dorland's medical speller / consultant. Ellen Drake ; consultant for
syllabication. Carol A. Stillman.

    p. cm.

  ISBN 0-7216-3599-7

   1. Medicine—Nomenclature.   I. W. B. Saunders Company.

II. Title: Medical speller.

  [DNLM: 1. Nomenclature. W 15 D711]

R123.D67   1992

616'.014—dc20

DNLM/DLC

for Library of Congress   91-32838
                                                CIP

Editor: Margaret M. Biblis
Chief Lexicographer: Douglas Anderson
Lexicographic Coordinator: Michelle Elliott
Designer: Karen O'Keefe
Production Manager: Linda R. Garber
Cover Designer: Ellen Bodner-Zanolle

Dorland's Medical Speller   ISBN 0-7216-3599-7

Printed in the United States of America.

Last digit is the print number: 9   8   7   6   5

Preface

The large (and constantly growing) body of medical terminology presents a daunting prospect to those who deal with it. In fact, no book can attempt to present any more than a small fraction of it. For nearly one hundred years one of the most respected resources for those who use medical words has been *Dorland's Illustrated Medical Dictionary*. Recent editions of the Dictionary have been prepared from a continually updated electronic database. Since this database contains a large, authoritative, and readily available list of medical terms, it seemed only natural that it should be used as the foundation for a large and comprehensive general medical word book. The result is *Dorland's Medical Speller*.

The aim of *Dorland's Medical Speller* is to present as many medical terms as possible within the confines of a book of reasonable size. In order to increase the scope of this book, a large number of entries were added to the list derived from the database by our consultant Ellen Drake, CMT. Since many of the terms presented are used across a number of specialties, they are arranged in a single alphabetic list without division by specialty. In order to make the book as easy to use as possible, eponyms and hard to find terms are given multiple listings. An added feature is the provision of acceptable end of line syllable breaks, something that can be very difficult to find for specialized medical words.

Although no more than a small fraction of the biomedical vocabulary can be presented, no effort has been spared to make this book as complete as possible. It is our belief that *Dorland's Medical Speller* is the most comprehensive source of medical terms available today.

Thanks are owed to a number of people who have made this book possible: to Ellen Drake, for the task of reviewing and expanding the terms list from the dictionary database; to Carol Stillman, PhD, to whom goes the credit for the syllabication of the main words; and last but not least, to the many generations of users of and contributors to *Dorland's Illustrated Medical Dictionary*, from which this book is derived.

DOUGLAS M. ANDERSON
Chief Lexicographer

How This Book Is Arranged

Order of Entries

Dorland's Medical Speller follows the same scheme of arrangement as *Dorland's Illustrated Medical Dictionary*. Main entries follow one another in letter-by-letter alphabetical order regardless of spaces or hyphens that occur within them (see below for special rules for eponyms and chemical names); compound entries consisting of one or more adjectives and a noun will be found as subentries under the noun. In some cases where there might be a question about where to look to find an entry, entries have been given in more than one place, even under an adjective.

Eponymic Terms. Terms containing a proper name are listed twice, once after the thing named and once under the eponym; thus *Down syndrome* is listed at both *Down* and *syndrome*. For such terms, only the proper name is counted for alphabetical order. For the example just given, the term is alphabetized as if it were only the name *Down* both at the main entry at *D* and as a subentry under *syndrome*. Everything following the name is ignored (including *'s* if it occurs) unless there are a number of terms containing the same name, in which case the words after the name are counted. Thus the following terms occur in this order:

Hartmann's pouch
Hartmann's procedure
Hartmann's speculum
Hartmannella

If more than one proper name occurs in a term, only the first one determines alphabetical order, unless the first name in consecutive terms is the same. In this case the second name and, if necessary, subsequent names are counted for alphabetization. This is illustrated by the following list:

Babès' treatment
Babès' tubercles
Babès-Ernst bodies
Babès-Ernst granules

Umlauts are ignored for alphabetization:
Löwe's ring
Lowe's syndrome
Löwenberg's canal
Löwenthal's tract
Lower's rings
Proper names beginning *Mc* or *Mac* are alphabetized as though spelled *Mac.*

Chemical prefixes. Italicized chemical prefixes such as the letters *p*- and *o*- and *cis*- and *trans*-, together with numbers, Greek letters, and the small capitals L- and D-, do not count for alphabetization. When prefixes are written out in full, however, as *para*- instead of *p*-, they are counted for alphabetical order.

Subentries

Each subentry appears on a new line following the main entry and is indented. The main entry word in a subentry is represented only by the initial letter (as *blast c.* under *cell*), with two exceptions: regular English plurals, in which the abbreviation is the initial letter followed by *'s* (as *b's* for *bones*), and irregular or Greek or Latin plurals, in which case the entire plural form is written out (as *teeth* under *tooth* and *ligamenta* under *ligamentum*). In subentries the main entry word is ignored for alphabetization, as are prepositions, conjunctions, and articles.

Possessive Forms

The use of the possessive in eponyms is controversial. This book follows the example of *Dorland's Illustrated Medical Dictionary,* that is, the *'s* is favored where the sources for a term justify its appearance. Whether or not to use the possessive form is a matter left to the individual; owing to the present lack of consistency and consensus, no prescription can be given. There are of course some terms in which the possessive is never used, such as *Christmas disease* and *Down syndrome.*

Abbreviations and Acronyms

A number of abbreviations and acronyms are given, together with the words or phrases that they stand for. The selection is of course only a small fraction of the abbreviations and acronyms in actual use. If more than one word or phrase is listed with an abbreviation, the terms are given in alphabetical order and each additional term is placed on a new line and indented.

Word Divisions

Acceptable word divisions are given for main entries; syllabication is based on pronunciation. Not all syllable breaks are shown; for example, because single letters at the beginnings and ends of words may not be separated from the rest of the word, such divisions are not given. Likewise, single letters should not be separated from the word elements they belong to in compound words. Breaks that could confuse the reader as to the meaning of a word are to be avoided. In many cases, words may be broken at other places than the ones that appear in this book (for example, different pronunciations imply different word breaks); it is impossible to show every break that could occur for every word. What appears here is one possible system.

Alternative Spellings

A number of words have alternative spellings, ranging from the difference of a single letter to the use of variant forms of Greek and Latin stems. Although every effort has been made to ensure that the spellings included in this book are valid, no indications of preference are given; in some cases a spelling that is favored by one specialty is not the same as the spelling preferred by another specialty.

Brackets and Parentheses

In a few cases alternative spellings are enclosed by parentheses; these are mainly proper names, particularly proper names that have been transliterated from another alphabet. Some entries require a bit of explanation; these explanations are also enclosed in parentheses. Brackets are sometimes used as a part of Latin anatomical nomenclature to enclose an eponym in the genitive case; in this book such eponyms generally appear all lower case (as in *Dorland's Illustrated Medical Dictionary*) but an initial capital for the name is acceptable.

Brackets also are used in this book at the ends of entries for chemical names containing the symbols *o-*, *p-*, and *m-*; in these cases the brackets are not part of the term but enclose the full form of the prefix that may be used instead of the symbol, for example, *p-* aminobenzoic acid [para-] to indicate that it may also be written *para*-aminobenzoic acid.

Plurals

Plurals for foreign words, nearly all of them Greek and Latin, are given with the appropriate entries. In addition, they are given again as separate entries if they do not occur within a few lines of the singular form.

A — accommodation
adenine
adenosine
alveolar gas
ampere
anode
A. — L. annum (year)
A — absorbance
activity
admittance
area
mass number
A_2 — aortic second sound
Å — angstrom
a — accommodation
arterial blood
atto-
a. — L. annum (year)
L. aqua (water)
L. arteria (artery)
a — acceleration
activity (of a chemical species)
specific absorptivity
ā — L. ante (before)
α — Bunsen coefficient
heavy chain of IgA
AA — achievement age
Alcoholics Anonymous
amino acid
aminoacyl
aa. — L. arteriae (arteries)
A̅A̅ — of each (in prescription writing, following the names of two or more ingredients)
AAA — American Association of Anatomists
AAAS — American Association for the Advancement of Science
AABB — American Association of Blood Banks
AACN — American Association of Critical-Care Nurses

AACN — American Association of Colleges of Nursing
AACP — American Academy of Child Psychiatry
AAD — American Academy of Dermatology
AADP — American Academy of Denture Prosthetics
AADR — American Academy of Dental Radiology
AADS — American Association of Dental Schools
AAE — American Association of Endodontists
AAFP — American Academy of Family Practice
American Association of Family Physicians
AAGP — American Academy of General Practice
AAI — American Association of Immunologists
AAID — American Academy of Implant Dentistry
AAIN — American Association of Industrial Nurses
AAL — anterior axillary line
AAMA — American Association of Medical Assistants
AAMC — American Association of Medical Colleges
AAMD — American Association on Mental Deficiency
AAMT — American Association for Medical Transcription
AAN — American Academy of Neurology
American Academy of Nursing

1

AANN — American Association of Neurological Nurses

AANA — American Association of Nurse Anesthetists

AAO — American Academy of Ophthalmology
American Academy of Otolaryngology
American Association of Orthodontists

AAOP — American Academy of Oral Pathology

AAOS — American Academy of Orthopaedic Surgeons

AAP — American Academy of Pediatrics
American Academy of Pedodontics
American Academy of Periodontology
American Association of Pathologists

AAPA — American Academy of Physician Assistants

AAPB — American Association of Pathologists and Bacteriologists

AAPMR — American Academy of Physical Medicine and Rehabilitation

AARC — American Association for Respiratory Care

Aar·on's sign

Aar·skog syndrome

Aar·skog-Scott syndrome

AART — American Association of Respiratory Therapy

AAS — atomic absorption spectroscopy

Aase syndrome

aas·mus

AAV — adeno-associated virus

AB — L. Artium Baccalaureus (Bachelor of Arts)

Ab — antibody

ab — abortion

abac·te·ri·al

Aba·die's sign

abaisse·ment

aban·don·ment

ab·ap·i·cal

abap·tis·ton pl. abap·tis·ta

abar·og·nos·is

abar·thro·sis

ab·ar·tic·u·lar

ab·ar·tic·u·la·tion

aba·sia
a. astasia
a. atactica
choreic a.
paralytic a.
paroxysmal trepidant a.
spastic a.
trembling a.
a. trepidans

aba·sic

abate

abate·ment

abat·ic

ab·ax·i·al

ab·bau

Ab·bé's condenser

Ab·be's flap

Ab·be-Est·lan·der operation

Ab·bé-Zeiss counting cell

Ab·bo·cil·lin-DC

Ab·bo·ki·nase

Ab·bott's meth·od

Ab·bott-Mil·ler tube

Ab·bott-Raw·son tube

ABC — antigen-binding capacity
aspiration biopsy cytology

ABCD — Adriamycin (doxorubicin), bleomycin, CCNU (lomustine), and dacarbazine

ab·do·men
acute a.
boat-shaped a.

ab·do·men *(continued)*
    carinate a.
    navicular a.
    a. obstipum
    pendulous a.
    scaphoid a.
    surgical a.
ab·dom·i·nal
ab·dom·i·nal·gia
    periodic a.
ab·dom·i·no·an·te·ri·or
ab·dom·i·no·cen·te·sis
ab·dom·i·no·cys·tic
ab·dom·i·no·gen·i·tal
ab·dom·i·no·hys·ter·ec·to·my
ab·dom·i·no·hys·ter·ot·o·my
ab·dom·i·no·per·i·ne·al
ab·dom·i·no·plas·ty
ab·dom·i·no·pos·te·ri·or
ab·dom·i·nos·co·py
ab·dom·i·no·scro·tal
ab·dom·i·no·tho·rac·ic
ab·dom·i·no·uter·ot·o·my
ab·dom·i·no·vag·i·nal
ab·dom·i·no·ves·i·cal
ab·du·cens
    nervus a.
ab·du·cent
ab·duct
ab·duc·tion
ab·duc·tor
Abegg's rule
ab·em·bry·on·ic
ab·en·ter·ic
ab·ep·i·thy·mia
ab·e·quose
Abercrombie's degeneration
Abercrombie's syndrome
Ab·er·ne·thy's fascia
ab·er·rant
ab·er·ra·tio
    a. lactis
    a. testis
ab·er·ra·tion
    chromatic a.
    chromatic a., lateral
    chromatic a., longitudinal
    chromosome a.

ab·er·ra·tion *(continued)*
    dioptric a.
    distantial a.
    heterosomal a.
    homosomal a.
    intrachromosomal a.
    lateral a.
    longitudinal a.
    mental a.
    meridional a.
    monochromatic a.
    newtonian a.
    optical a.
    penta-X chromosomal a.
    spherical a.
    spherical a., negative
    spherical a., positive
    tetra-X chromosomal a.
    triple-X chromosomal a.
    zonal a.
ab·er·rom·e·ter
abeta·lipo·pro·tein·emia
ab·evac·u·a·tion
abey·ance
ABG — arterial blood gases
ab·i·a·tro·phy
ab·i·ent
abil·i·ty
    general a.
    impaired urinary
      concentrating a.
    primary mental a.
    template a.
    verbal a.
abio·gen·e·sis
abio·ge·net·ic
abi·og·e·nous
abio·log·ic
abi·ol·o·gy
abi·on·er·gy
abio·phys·i·ol·o·gy
abi·os·is
abi·ot·ic
abio·troph·ic
abi·ot·ro·phy
    retinal a.
ab·ir·ri·tant
ab·ir·ri·ta·tion

ab·ir·ri·ta·tive
abi·u·ret
abi·u·ret·ic
ab·lac·ta·tion
ablas·tem·ic
ablas·tin
ab·late
ab·la·tio
    a. placentae
    a. retinae
ab·la·tion
    electrical a.
ableph·ar·ia
ableph·a·ron
ableph·ar·ous
ableph·a·ry
ablep·sia
ablep·sy
ab·lu·ent
ab·lu·mi·nal
ab·lu·tion
ab·lu·to·ma·nia
ab·mor·tal
ab·ner·val
ab·nor·mal
ab·nor·mal·i·ty
    potential a. of glucose
      tolerance (pot AGT)
    previous a. of glucose
      tolerance (prev AGT)
ab·nor·mi·ty
ab·oc·clu·sion
ab·orad
ab·oral
ab·orig·i·nal
abort
abor·ti·cide
abor·tient
abor·ti·fa·cient
abor·ti·gen·ic
abor·tin
abor·tion
    accidental a.
    ampullar a.
    artificial a.
    cervical a.
    complete a.
    criminal a.

abor·tion *(continued)*
    elective a.
    habitual a.
    idiopathic a.
    imminent a.
    incomplete a.
    induced a.
    inevitable a.
    infected a.
    infectious a.
    justifiable a.
    late a.
    missed a.
    natural a.
    nontherapeutic a.
    partial a.
    a. in progress
    psychiatric a.
    recurrent a.
    septic a.
    spontaneous a.
    therapeutic a.
    threatened a.
    tubal a.
abor·tion·ist
abor·tive
abor·tus
abouche·ment
abou·lia
ABP — arterial blood pressure
ABR — auditory brain stem
  response
abra·chia
abra·chi·a·tism
abra·chio·ceph·a·lia
abra·chio·ceph·a·lus
abra·chio·ceph·a·ly
abra·chi·us
abrad·ant
abrade
Abra·hams' sign
Abra·mi's disease
Abrams' (heart) reflex
Abram·son catheter
abra·sio
    a. corneae
abra·sion
    dental a.

abra·sion *(continued)*
    dicing a's
    a. of gingiva
    marginal a.
abra·sive
abra·sor
ab·re·ac·tion
    motor a.
ab·reu·og·ra·phy
Abri·ko·sov's (Abri·kos·soff's)
    tumor
ab·rin
ab·rism
ab·ro·ta·num
abro·sia
ab·rup·tio
    a. placentae
ab·rup·tion
    a. of placenta
Abrus pre·ca·to·rius
abs — absolute
ab·scess
    acute a.
    acute dentoalveolar a.
    alveolar a.
    amebic a.
    anorectal a.
    apical a.
    apical a., acute
    apical a., chronic
    appendiceal a.
    appendicular a.
    arthrifluent a.
    atheromatous a.
    axillary a.
    bartholinian a.
    Bezold's a.
    bicameral a.
    bile duct a.
    bilharziasis a.
    biliary a.
    blind a.
    bone a.
    brain a.
    breast a.
    broad ligament a.
    Brodie's a.
    bursal a.

ab·scess *(continued)*
    canalicular a.
    caseous a.
    cerebellar a.
    cerebral a.
    cheesy a.
    cholangitic a.
    chronic a.
    circumscribed a.
    circumtonsillar a.
    cold a.
    collar-button a.
    crypt a.
    deep a.
    dental a.
    dentoalveolar a.
    diffuse a.
    Douglas' a.
    dry a.
    Dubois' a.
    embolic a.
    emphysematous a.
    encapsulated a.
    encysted a.
    entamebic a.
    epidural a.
    epiploic a.
    extradural a.
    fecal a.
    filarial a.
    follicular a.
    frontal a.
    fungal a.
    gangrenous a.
    gas a.
    gingival a.
    glandular a.
    gravitation a.
    gravity a.
    gummatous a.
    helminthic a.
    hematogenous a.
    hemorrhagic a.
    hepatic a.
    hot a.
    hypostatic a.
    idiopathic a.
    intracranial a.

ab·scess *(continued)*
    intradural a.
    intramastoid a.
    intramedullary a.
    ischiorectal a.
    kidney a.
    lacrimal a.
    lacunar a.
    lateral a.
    lateral alveolar a.
    lateral root a.
    liver a.
    lumbar a.
    lung a.
    lymphatic a.
    mammary a.
    marginal a.
    mastoid a.
    mediastinal a.
    metastatic a.
    metastatic tuberculous a.
    migrating a.
    miliary a.
    milk a.
    mother a.
    Munro a.
    mural a.
    nocardial a.
    orbital a.
    ossifluent a.
    otic cerebral a.
    otogenic a.
    palatal a.
    pancreatic a.
    parafrenal a.
    parametrial a.
    parametric a.
    parametritic a.
    paranephric a.
    parapancreatic a.
    parapharyngeal a.
    parietal a.
    parotid a.
    Pautrier's a.
    pelvic a.
    pelvirectal a.
    perianal a.
    periapical a.

ab·scess *(continued)*
    periarticular a.
    pericemental a.
    pericoronal a.
    peridental a.
    perinephric a.
    periodontal a.
    peripleuritic a.
    periproctic a.
    perirectal a.
    perirenal a.
    peritoneal a.
    peritonsillar a.
    periureteral a.
    periurethral a.
    perivesical a.
    phlegmonous a.
    phoenix a.
    pilonidal a.
    pneumococcic a.
    postcecal a.
    Pott's a.
    prelacrimal a.
    premammary a.
    preperitoneal a.
    primary a.
    prostatic a.
    protozoal a.
    psoas a.
    pulmonary a.
    pulp a.
    pulpal a.
    pyemic a.
    pylephlebitic a.
    renal a.
    residual a.
    retrocecal a.
    retromammary a.
    retroperitoneal a.
    retropharyngeal a.
    retrotonsillar a.
    retrovesical a.
    ring a.
    root a.
    sacrococcygeal a.
    satellite a.
    scrofulous a.
    secondary a.

ab·scess *(continued)*
  septal a.
  septicemic a.
  serous a.
  shirt-stud a.
  spermatic a.
  spirillar a.
  splenic a.
  stellate a.
  stercoraceous a.
  stercoral a.
  sterile a.
  stitch a.
  streptococcal a.
  strumous a.
  subacute a.
  subaponeurotic a.
  subarachnoid a.
  subareolar a.
  subdiaphragmatic a.
  subdural a.
  subepidermal a.
  subfascial a.
  subgaleal a.
  submammary a.
  subpectoral a.
  subperiosteal a.
  subperitoneal a.
  subphrenic a.
  subscapular a.
  subungual a.
  sudoriparous a.
  superficial a.
  suprahepatic a.
  supralevator a.
  sympathetic a.
  syphilitic a.
  temporal lobe a.
  thecal a.
  thymic a.
  tonsillar a.
  tooth a.
  Tornwaldt (Thornwaldt) a.
  traumatic a.
  tropical a.
  tuberculous a.
  tubo-ovarian a.
  tympanitic a.

ab·scess *(continued)*
  tympanocervical a.
  tympanomastoid a.
  urethral a.
  urinary a.
  urinous a.
  verminous a.
  vitreous a.
  von Bezold's a.
  walled off a.
  wandering a.
  warm a.
  Welch's a.
  worm a.
ab·sces·sus
ab·scise
ab·scis·sa
ab·scis·sion
  corneal a.
ab·scon·sio *pl.* ab·scon·si·o·nes
ab·scop·al
ab·sence
  atypical a.
  complex a.
  congenital ossicular a.
  enuretic a.
  myoclonic a.
  retrocursive a.
  retropulsive a.
  subclinical a.
ab·sen·tia ep·i·lep·ti·ca
abs. feb. — L. absente febre
  (while fever is absent)
Ab·sid·ia
ab·sinthe
ab·sinth·in
ab·sinth·ism
ab·sin·thi·um
ab·so·lute
ab·sorb
ab·sor·bance
ab·sor·be·fa·cient
ab·sor·ben·cy
ab·sor·bent
ab·sorb·er
ab·sorp·ti·om·e·ter

ab·sorp·ti·om·e·try
    dual photon a.
    photon a.
ab·sorp·tion
    agglutinin a.
    bone a.
    broad-beam a.
    cross a.
    cutaneous a.
    disjunctive a.
    enteral a.
    excrementitial a.
    external a.
    internal a.
    interstitial a.
    intestinal a.
    net a.
    parenteral a.
    pathologic a.
    pathological a.
    percutaneous a.
    protein a.
    wall a.
    x-ray a.
ab·sorp·tive
ab·sorp·tiv·i·ty
    molar a.
    specific a.
abst — abstract
ab·ster·gent
ab·sti·nence
    alimentary a.
abstr — abstract
ab·stract
ab·strac·tion
ab·ter·min·al
ab·tor·sion
ab·trop·fung
Abul·ca·sis
abu·lia
abu·lic
Abul·ka·sim
abun·dance
    isotropic a.
abuse
    child a.
    drug a.
    psychoactive substance a.

abuse *(continued)*
    spouse a.
    substance a.
abut
abut·ment
    auxiliary a.
    implant a.
    intermediate a.
    isolated a.
    multiple a.
    primary a.
    secondary a.
    terminal a.
ABVD — Adriamycin
    (doxorubicin), bleomycin,
    vinblastine, and dacarbazine
AC — acromioclavicular
    Adriamycin (doxorubicin)
      and CCNU (lomustine)
    adrenal cortex
    air conduction
    alternating current
    anodal closure
    aortic closure
    axiocervical
a.c. — L. ante cibum (before
    meals)
ACA — American College of
    Angiology
    American College of
      Apothecaries
Aca·cia
    A. catechu
    A. georginae
aca·cia
acal·cer·o·sis
acal·ci·co·sis
acal·cu·lia
acamp·sia
acan·tha
acan·tha·ceous
acan·tha·me·bi·a·sis
Acanth·amoe·ba
acan·thar·i·an
acan·thes·the·sia
Acan·thia lec·tu·la·ria
acan·thi·on
Acan·thob·del·lid·ea

Acan·tho·ceph·a·la
acan·tho·ceph·a·lan
acan·tho·ceph·a·li·as·is
acan·tho·ceph·a·lous
Acantho·ceph·a·lus
Acantho·chei·lo·ne·ma
    A. *perstans*
    A. *streptocerca*
acan·tho·chei·lo·ne·mi·a·sis
acan·tho·cyte
acan·tho·cy·to·sis
acan·thoid
acan·tho·ker·a·to·der·mia
acan·thol·y·sis
acan·tho·lyt·ic
ac·an·tho·ma *pl.* ac·an·tho·
  mas, ac·an·tho·ma·ta
    a. adenoides cysticum
    basal cell a.
acan·tho·pel·vis
acan·tho·pel·yx
Acanth·ophis
    A. *antarctica*
Acan·tho·po·di·na
ac·an·tho·sis
    congenital a.
    a. nigricans
    a. seborrheica
ac·an·thot·ic
acan·thro·cyte
acan·thro·cy·to·sis
a capite ad calcem
acap·nia
acap·ni·al
acap·nic
Aca·ra·pis
acar·bia
acar·dia
acar·di·ac
acar·di·a·cus
acar·dio·tro·phia
acar·di·us
    a. acephalus
    a. acormus
    a. amorphus
    a. anceps
acari
acar·i·an

ac·a·ri·a·sis
acar·i·cide
ac·a·rid
Acar·i·dae
acar·i·dan
acar·i·di·a·sis
Ac·a·ri·na
ac·a·rine
ac·a·ri·no·sis
acar·i·o·sis
ac·a·ro·der·ma·ti·tis
    a. urticarioides
ac·a·roid
ac·a·rol·o·gist
ac·a·rol·o·gy
ac·a·ro·pho·bia
ac·a·ro·tox·ic
Acar·to·myia
Ac·a·rus
    A. *folliculorum*
    A. *gallinae*
    A. *hordei*
    A. *rhyzoglypticus hyacinthi*
    A. *scabiei*
    A. *siro*
    A. *tritici*
ac·a·rus *pl.* ac·a·ri
acar·y·ote
ACAT
ACAT — automatic
  computerized axial
  tomography
acat·a·la·se·mia
acat·a·la·sia
acat·a·lep·sia
acat·a·lep·sy
acat·a·ma·the·sia
acat·a·pha·sia
acat·a·sta·sia
acat·a·stat·ic
ac·a·thec·tic
ac·a·thex·ia
ac·a·thex·is
ac·a·this·ia
acau·dal
acau·date
acau·li·no·sis

ACC — American College of
  Cardiology
    anodal closure contraction
Acc — accommodation
ac·cel·er·ant
ac·cel·er·a·tion
    angular a.
    central a.
    centripetal a.
    developmental a.
    linear a.
    negative a.
    positive a.
    standard a. of free fall
ac·cel·er·a·tor
    C3b inactivator a.
    serum prothrombin
      conversion a. (SPCA)
    serum thrombotic a.
    thromboplastin generation
      a.
    a. urinae
    Van de Graaff a.
ac·cel·er·in
ac·cel·er·om·e·ter
ac·cen·tu·a·tion
    presystolic a.
ac·cen·tu·a·tor
ac·cep·tor
    hydrogen a.
    oxygen a.
ac·cess
ac·cès per·ni·cieux
ac·ces·si·flex·or
ac·ces·so·ri·us
ac·ces·so·ry
ac·ci·dent
    cerebrovascular a.
ac·ci·den·tal·ism
ac·ci·dent prone
ac·cip·i·ter
ACCl — anodal closure clonus
ac·cli·ma·ta·tion
ac·cli·ma·tion
ac·cli·ma·ti·za·tion
ac·cli·ma·tize
ac·colé

ac·com·mo·da·tion
    absolute a.
    amplitude of a.
    binocular a.
    excessive a.
    histologic a.
    negative a.
    nerve a.
    obstetric a.
    positive a.
    range of a.
    reflex a.
    a. reflex
    relative a.
    subnormal a.
    synaptic a.
ac·com·mo·da·tive
ac·com·mo·dom·e·ter
ac·com·plice
ac·couche·ment
    a. forcé
ac·cou·cheur
ac·cou·cheuse
ACCP — American College of
  Chest Physicians
ac·cre·men·ti·tion
ac·cre·tio
    a. cordis
    a. pericardii
ac·cre·tion
ac·cro·chage
ac·cul·tur·a·tion
ac·cu·ra·cy
ACD — absolute cardiac
  dullness
    acid citrate dextrose
    allergic contact dermatitis
ACE — adrenocortical extract
    angiotensin converting
      enzyme
ac·e·bu·to·lol
Ace-Fisch·er fixator
ac·e·cai·nide hy·dro·chlo·ride
ace·cli·dine
ac·e·dap·sone
acel·lu·lar
ace·lo·mate

ace·lous
ace·nes·the·sia
acen·o·cou·ma·rin
acen·o·cou·ma·rol
acen·tric
ACEP
ACEP — American College of
  Emergency Physicians
ace·pha·lia
ace·phal·ic
Aceph·a·li·na
aceph·a·lism
aceph·a·lo·bra·chia
aceph·a·lo·bra·chi·us
aceph·a·lo·car·dia
aceph·a·lo·car·di·us
aceph·a·lo·chi·ria
aceph·a·lo·chi·rus
aceph·a·lo·cyst
aceph·a·lo·gas·ter
aceph·a·lo·gas·tria
aceph·a·lo·po·dia
aceph·a·lo·po·di·us
aceph·a·lo·rha·chia
aceph·a·lo·sto·mia
aceph·a·los·to·mus
aceph·a·lo·tho·ra·cia
aceph·a·lo·tho·rus
aceph·a·lous
aceph·a·lus *pl.* aceph·a·li
  a. athorus
  a. dibrachius
  a. dipus
  a. monobrachius
  a. monopus
  a. paracephalus
  a. sympus
aceph·a·ly
ac·e·pro·ma·zine maleate
Ac·e·ra·ria
  A. spiralis
acer·bi·ty
ac·er·ate
acer·e·bral
acer·in
ace·ro·la
acer·vu·li
acer·vu·line

acer·vu·lo·ma
acer·vu·lus *pl.* acer·vu·li
aces·cence
aces·cent
aces·o·dyne
ac·e·tab·u·la
ac·e·tab·u·lar
Ac·e·tab·u·la·ria
ac·e·tab·u·lec·to·my
ac·e·tab·u·lo·plas·ty
ac·e·tab·u·lum *pl.* ac·e·tab·u·li
  sunken a.
ac·e·tal
ac·et·al·de·hyde
ac·et·al·de·hyde de·hy·dro·gen·ase
ac·et·al·de·hyde re·duc·tase
acet·am·ide
ac·et·am·i·dine
acet·a·min·o·phen
ac·et·an·i·lid
ac·et·an·i·line
ac·et·an·i·si·dine
ac·e·tan·nin
ac·et·ar·sol
ac·et·ar·sone
ace·tas
ace·tate
  cellulose a.
ac·e·tate ki·nase
ac·et·a·zol·a·mide
  sodium a., sterile
ace·te·nyl
Ace·test
ac·et·eu·ge·nol
ace·tic
  a. aldehyde
ace·tic acid
  glacial a.a.
acet·i·co·cep·tor
acet·i·fy
ac·e·tim·e·ter
ac·e·tin
Aceti·vib·rio
ac·e·to·ac·e·tate de·car·box·y·lase
ac·e·to·ace·tic acid

ac·e·to·ac·e·tyl-CoA
ac·e·to·ac·e·tyl-CoA re·duc·
    tase
ac·e·to·ac·e·tyl-CoA thi·o·
    lase
ac·e·to·ac·e·tyl co·en·zyme A
ac·e·to·ac·e·tyl thi·ol·ase
Aceto·bac·ter
Ace·to·bac·te·ra·ceae
ac·e·to·car·mine
ace·to·form
ac·e·to·hex·a·mide
ac·e·to·hy·drox·am·ic acid
acet·o·in
ac·e·to·kin·ase
ac·e·to·lac·tic acid
ac·e·to·lase
ac·e·tol·y·sis
ac·e·tom·e·ter
ac·e·to·mor·phine
ac·e·to·naph·thone
ac·e·to·na·tion
ac·e·tone
ac·e·ton·emia
ac·e·ton·emic
ac·e·ton·gly·cos·uria
ac·e·to·ni·trile
ac·e·to·num
ac·e·to·nu·mer·a·tor
ac·e·ton·uria
ac·e·to·or·ce·in
ac·e·to·phen·a·zine ma·le·ate
ac·e·to·phe·net·i·din
ac·e·to·py·rine
acet·o·sal
ac·e·to·sol·uble
ac·e·to·sul·fone so·di·um
ace·tous
acet·phe·nar·sine
acet·phe·net·i·din
acet·py·ro·gall
ac·e·tri·zo·ate
ace·tum
ac·e·tu·rate
ac·e·tyl
    a. chloride
    a. peroxide
    a. sulfisoxazole

ac·e·tyl·a·mi·no·ben·zene
ac·e·tyl·ami·no·flu·o·rene
acet·y·lase
acet·y·la·tion
acet·y·la·tor
ac·e·tyl·car·bro·mal
ac·e·tyl·cho·line
    a. chloride
ac·e·tyl·cho·lin·es·ter·ase
ac·e·tyl-CoA
ac·e·tyl-CoA ac·e·tyl·trans·
    fer·ase
ac·e·tyl-CoA acyl·trans·fer·
    ase
ac·e·tyl-CoA car·box·yl·ase
ac·e·tyl-Coa: α-glu·cos·am·i·
    nide-*N*-ac·e·tyl·trans·fer·
    ase
ac·e·tyl-Coa: hep·a·ran-α-
    D-glu·cos·am·i·nide *N*- ac·e·
    tyl·trans·fer·ase
ac·e·tyl-CoA syn·the·tase
ac·e·tyl co·en·zyme A
ac·e·tyl·cys·te·ine
ac·e·tyl·dig·i·tox·in
acet·y·lene
N-ac·e·tyl·ga·lac·tos·
    amine-4-sul·fa·tase
N-ac·e·tyl·ga·lac·tos·
    amine-6-sul·fa·tase
α-*N*-ac·e·tyl·ga·lac·tos·a·
    min·i·dase
β-*N*-ac·e·tyl·ga·lac·tos·a·
    min·i·dase
N-ac·e·tyl·glu·cos·
    amine-6-sul·fa·tase
α-*N*-ac·e·tyl·glu·cos·a·min·i·
    dase
N-ac·e·tyl-α-D-glu·cos·am·i·
    nide-6-sul·fa·tase
N-ac·e·tyl·glu·cos·am·i·nyl·
    phos·pho·trans·fer·ase
N-ac·e·tyl-β-hex·os·a·min·i·
    dase
acet·y·li·za·tion
ac·e·tyl·meth·a·dol
N-ac·e·tyl·mu·ram·ic acid
N-ac·e·tyl·neu·ra·min·ic acid

ac·e·tyl·phen·yl·hy·dra·zine
ac·e·tyl phos·phate
ac·e·tyl·pro·ma·zine mal·e·ate
ac·e·tyl·sal·i·cyl·am·ide
ac·e·tyl·sal·i·cyl·ic acid
ac·e·tyl·stro·phan·thi·din
ac·e·tyl·sul·fa·di·a·zine
ac·e·tyl·sul·fa·guan·i·dine
ac·e·tyl·sul·fa·thi·a·zole
ac·e·tyl sul·fi·sox·a·zole
ac·e·tyl·tan·nic acid
ac·e·tyl·trans·fer·ase
ACG — American College of Gastroenterology
    angiocardiography
AcG — accelerator globulin (coagulation Factor V)
ACh — acetylcholine
ACHA — American College of Hospital Administrators
ach·a·la·sia
    pelvirectal a.
    sphincteral a.
Achard's syndrome
Achard-Thiers syndrome
Ach·a·ti·na
    A. fulica
AChE — acetylcholinesterase
ache
achei·lia
achei·lous
achei·ria
achei·ro·po·dia
achei·rus
Achil·les bur·sa
Achil·li·ni, Ales·san·dro
achil·lo·bur·si·tis
achil·lo·dy·nia
achil·lo·gram
ach·il·lor·rha·phy
achil·lo·te·not·o·my
    plastic a.
achil·lot·o·my
achlor·hy·dria
achlor·hy·dric
achlo·ride
achlor·op·sia

Ach·lya
Acho·le·plas·ma
    A. granularum
    A. laidlawii
Acho·le·plas·ma·ta·ceae
acho·lia
acho·lic
achol·uria
achol·uric
achon·dro·gen·e·sis
achon·dro·pla·sia
achon·dro·plas·tic
achon·dro·plas·ty
achor·dal
achor·date
ach·o·re·sis
AChRab — acetylcholine receptor antibody
achres·tic
achroa·cy·to·sis
achro·ma
    central a.
    consecutive a.
achro·ma·sia
achro·mat
achro·mate
achro·mat·ic
achro·ma·tin
achro·ma·tin·ic
achro·ma·tism
achro·ma·tize
achro·mato·cyte
achro·ma·to·cy·to·sis
achro·ma·tog·no·sia
achro·ma·tol·y·sis
achro·ma·to·phil
achro·ma·to·phil·ia
achro·ma·top·sia
achro·ma·to·sis
achro·ma·tous
achro·ma·tu·ria
achro·mia
    cortical a.
    a. parasitica
achro·mic
achro·min
Achro·mo·bac·ter
    A. lwoffi

achro·mo·cyte
achro·mo·der·ma
achro·mo·phil
achro·moph·i·lous
achro·mo·trich·ia
Achro·my·cin
ach·roo·am·y·loid
ach·roo·dex·trin
Ach·u·cár·ro's stain
achy·lia
achy·lo·sis
achy·mia
achy·mo·sis
acic·u·lar
acic·u·late
acic·u·lum
ac·id
   acetic a.
   acetoacetic a.
   acetylacetic a.
   acetylsalicylic a.
   aconitic a.
   actithiazic a.
   adenylic a.
   aldonic a.
   alginic a.
   allantoic a.
   amino a.
   aminoacetic a.
   aminobenzoic a.
   p-aminobenzoic a. (PABA)
    [para-]
   aminocaproic a.
   aminoglutaric a.
   aminolevulinic a.
   6-aminopenicillanic a.
    (6-APA)
   aminophenylstibinic a.
   aminosalicylic a.
   p-aminosalicylic a. [para-]
   aminosuccinic a.
   anacardic a.
   anthranilic a.
   antiteichoic a.
   apurinic a.
   apyrimidinic a.
   arachidonic a.
   arsonic a.

ac·id *(continued)*
   arylarsonic a.
   ascorbic a.
   aseptic a.
   aspartic a.
   atractylic a.
   aurintricarboxylic a.
   barbituric a.
   benzoic a.
   bile a's
   binary a.
   boric a.
   borosalicylic a.
   Brønsted a.
   butyric a.
   cahincic a.
   cantharic a.
   carbamoylaspartic a.
   carbolic a.
   carbonic a.
   γ-carboxyglutamic a.
   carboxylic a.
   cathartic a.
   chaulmoogric a.
   chloroacetic a.
   chlorogenic a.
   chlorosulfonic a.
   choleic a's
   cholic a.
   chorismic a.
   chromic a.
   cinchonic a.
   a. citrate dextrose (ACD)
   citric a.
   conjugate a.
   deoxyribonucleic a. (DNA)
   desoxyribonucleic a.
   diacetic a.
   diacetyltannic a.
   2,6-diaminopimelic a.
   dibasic a.
   dichloroacetic a.
   dihydrofolic a.
   dihydrolipoic a.
   dihydroxyphenylpyruvic a.
   2,3-dihydroxypropanoic a.
   diiodophenylamino-
    propionic a.

ac·id *(continued)*
- diiodosalicylic a.
- djenkolic a.
- ethanedioic a.
- ethanoic a.
- ethylenediaminetetraacetic a.
- fatty a.
- folic a.
- formic a.
- formiminoglutamic a.
- gallic a.
- glucuronic a.
- glutamic a.
- glyceric a.
- glycocholic a.
- glycuronic a.
- haloid a.
- hexadecanoic a.
- homogentisic a.
- hydriodic a.
- hydrochloric a.
- hydrocyanic a.
- hydrosuccinic a.
- hydroxy a.
- hydroxytoluic a.
- imino a.
- inorganic a.
- lactic a.
- Lewis a.
- linoleic a.
- linolenic a.
- linolic a.
- lysergic a.
- malic a.
- malonic a.   *methyl malonic*
- mandelic a.
- mersalyl a.
- methanoic a.
- mineral a.
- monobasic a.
- muriatic a.
- nicotinic a. amide
- nicotinic a.
- nitric a.
- noncarbonic a's
- nucleic a.
- 9-octadecenoic a.

ac·id *(continued)*
- oleic a.
- organic a.
- oxalic a.
- oxo a.
- oxygen a.
- palmitic a.
- pantothenic a.
- pectic a.
- pentanoic a.
- perchloric a.
- phenic a.
- phenylglycolic a.
- phosphoric a.
- phosphorous a.
- phosphotungstic a.
- picric a.
- polybasic a.
- polyene a's
- prussic a.
- pteroylglutamic a.
- pyruvic a.
- 13-*cis*-retinoic a.
- ribonucleic a. (RNA)
- salicylic a.
- saturated fatty a.
- silicic a.
- sodium *p*-aminohippuric (PAH) a. [para-]
- stearic a.
- succinic a.
- sulfo-a.
- sulfonic a.
- sulfosalicylic a.
- sulfuric a.
- sulfurous a.
- tannic a.
- tartaric a.
- taurocholic a.
- ternary a.
- thio a.
- thymidine diphosphoric a.
- thymidine triphosphoric a.
- titratable a.
- tribasic a.
- trichloroacetic a.
- 3,4,5-trihydroxybenzoic a.
- unsaturated fatty a.

ac·id *(continued)*
    uric a.
    valeric a.
ac·id·al·bu·min
Ac·id·ami·no·coc·cus
ac·id·am·in·uria
ac·id an·hy·dride
ac·id chlo·ride
ac·i·de·mia
    argininosuccinic a.
    glutaric a.
    isovaleric a.
    methylmalonic a.
    propionic a.
acid-fast
ac·id-form·ing
acid·ic
acid·i·fi·a·ble
acid·i·fi·ca·tion
acid·i·fi·er
acid·i·fy
ac·i·dim·e·ter
ac·i·dim·et·ry
ac·id·ism
ac·id·is·mus
acid·i·ty
acid·o·cyte
ac·i·do·cy·to·pe·nia
ac·i·do·cy·to·sis
ac·i·do·gen·ic
Aci·dol
acid·o·phil
    alpha a.
    epsilon a.
acid·o·phile
ac·i·do·phil·ia
ac·i·do·phil·ic
ac·i·doph·i·lism
ac·i·do·re·sis·tant
ac·i·do·sic
ac·i·do·sis
    bicarbonate wastage renal
        tubular a.
    carbon dioxide a.
    compensated a.
    diabetic a.
    hypercapnic a.
    hyperchloremic a.

ac·i·do·sis *(continued)*
    lactic a.
    metabolic a.
    metabolic a., compensated
    nonrespiratory a.
    renal hyperchloremia a.
    renal tubular a.
    respiratory a.
    respiratory a.,
        compensated
    starvation a.
    uremic a.
ac·i·dos·teo·phyte
ac·i·dot·ic
ac·id phos·pha·tase
ac·id-proof
ac·id sul·fate
acid·u·lat·ed
Acid·u·lin
acid·u·lous
ac·id·uria
    acetoacetic a.
    argininosuccinic a.
    beta-aminoisobutyric a.
    ethylmalonic-adipic a.
    glutamic a.
    glutaric a. (GA)
    L-glyceric a.
    glycolic a.
    methylmalonic a.
    orotic a.
    paradoxical a.
    pyroglutamic a.
    xanthurenic a.
ac·id·uric
ac·i·dyl
acid·y·la·tion
ac·in·ac·i·form
ac·i·nar
ac·i·ne·sia
ac·i·net·ic
Aci·ne·to·bac·ter
    A. anitratus
    A. calcoaceticus
    A. lwoffi
ac·i·ni
acin·ic
acin·i·form

acin·i·tis
acin·i·tra·zole
ac·i·nose
ac·i·no·tu·bu·lar
ac·i·nous
aci·nus *pl.* aci·ni
   liver a.
   pulmonary a.
   a. renalis [malpighii]
   a. renis [malpighii]
ac·i·pen·ser·in
ackee
ACL — anterior cruciate
  ligament
aclad·i·o·sis
Acla·di·um
Ac·land clip
acla·sia
acla·sis
   diaphyseal a.
   metaphyseal a.
   tarsoepiphyseal a.
aclas·tic
acleis·to·car·dia
ACLS — advanced cardiac life
  support
aclu·sion
ac·me
   a. of contraction
ac·mes·the·sia
ACMI Mar·tin endoscopy
  forceps
ac·ne
   adolescent a.
   a. agminata
   apocrine a.
   a. artificialis
   a. atrophica
   bromide a.
   a. cachecticorum
   chlorine a.
   a. ciliaris
   colloid a.
   common a.
   a. conglobata
   congoblate a.
   contact a.
   contagious a. of horses

ac·ne *(continued)*
   a. cosmetica
   cystic a.
   a. decalvans
   a. detergicans
   epidemic a.
   a. estivalis
   excoriated a.
   a. excoriée des jeunes filles
   a. frontalis
   a. fulminans
   halogen a.
   a. indurata
   infantile a.
   iodide a.
   a. keloid
   a. keratosa
   Mallorca a.
   a. mechanica
   mechanical a.
   a. medicamentosa
   a. necrotica miliaris
   neonatal a.
   a. neonatarum
   occupational a.
   oil a.
   a. papulosa
   petroleum a.
   picker's a.
   pomade a.
   premenstrual a.
   a. pustulosa
   a. rosacea
   a. scrofulosorum
   steroid a.
   summer a.
   a. syphilitica
   systemic a.
   a. tarsi
   a. telangiectodes
   tropical a.
   a. tropicalis
   a. urticata
   a. varioliformis
   a. venenata
   a. vulgaris
ac·ne·gen
ac·ne·gen·ic

ac·ne·iform
ac·ne·mia
ac·ni·tis
ACNM — American College of
    Nurse-Midwives
ac·o·as·ma
Aco·can·the·ra
ac·o·can·ther·in
acoe·lom·ate
ACOG — American College of
    Obstetricians and
    Gynecologists
ac·og·no·sia
acol·o·gy
ac·o·lous
aco·mia
acom·ple·men·te·mia
Acon
acon·a·tive
ac·o·nine
acon·i·tase
acon·i·tate hy·dra·tase
ac·o·nite
ac·o·nit·ic acid
acon·i·tine
Ac·o·ni·tum
ac·on·ure·sis
acop·ro·sis
acop·rous
aco·py·rine
acor
aco·rea
aco·ria
ac·o·rin
acor·mia
acor·tan
Aco·rus
ACOS — American College of
    Osteopathic Surgeons
Acos·ta's disease
aco·state
acou·asm
acous·ma *pl.* acousmata
acous·mat·am·ne·sia
acous·tic
acous·ti·co·fa·cial
acous·ti·co·mo·tor
acous·ti·co·pho·bia

acous·tics
acous·ti·gram
acous·to·gram
ACP — acid phosphatase
    American College of
        Physicians
ACPS — acrocephalopolysynda-
    ctyly
ac·quired
ac·qui·si·tion
ac·qui·si·tus
ACR — American College of
    Radiology
ac·rag·no·sis
ac·ral
acra·nia
acra·ni·al
Acra·ni·a·ta
acra·ni·us
acrat·ure·sis
Ac·rel's gan·gli·on
Ac·re·mo·ni·el·la
ac·re·mo·ni·o·sis
Ac·re·mo·ni·um
    A. kiliense
ac·rid
ac·ri·dine
    a. orange
ac·ri·fla·vine
ac·ri·mo·ny
ac·ri·sor·cin
acrit·i·cal
ac·ri·to·chro·ma·cy
ACRM — American Congress
    of Rehabilitation Medicine
ac·ro·ag·no·sis
ac·ro·an·es·the·sia
ac·ro·ar·thri·tis
ac·ro·a·tax·ia
ac·ro·blast
ac·ro·brachy·ceph·a·ly
ac·ro·bys·tia
ac·ro·bys·tio·lith
ac·ro·bys·ti·tis
ac·ro·cen·tric
ac·ro·ce·pha·lia
ac·ro·ce·phal·ic

ac·ro·ceph·a·lo·poly·syn·dac·
  ty·ly (ACPS)
ac·ro·ceph·a·lo·syn·dac·tyl·
  ia
ac·ro·ceph·a·lo·syn·dac·ty·
  lism
ac·ro·ceph·a·lo·syn·dac·ty·ly
ac·ro·ceph·a·lous
ac·ro·ceph·a·ly
    a.-syndactyly
ac·ro·chor·don
ac·ro·ci·ne·sis
ac·ro·ci·net·ic
ac·ro·con·trac·ture
ac·ro·cy·a·no·sis
ac·ro·der·ma·ti·tis
    a. chronica atrophicans
    a. continua
    a. enteropathica
    Hallopeau's a.
    a. hiemalis
    infantile a.
    papular a. of childhood
    a. papulosa infantum
    a. perstans
    pustular a.
    a. vesiculosa tropica
ac·ro·der·ma·to·sis *pl.* ac·ro·
  der·ma·to·ses
ac·ro·dol·i·cho·me·lia
ac·ro·dyn·ia
    rat a.
ac·ro·dys·es·the·sia
ac·ro·dys·pla·sia
ac·ro·es·the·sia
ac·ro·ger·ia
ac·rog·no·sis
ac·ro·hy·per·hi·dro·sis
ac·ro·hy·po·ther·my
ac·ro·ker·a·to·elas·toi·do·sis
ac·ro·ker·a·to·sis
    paraneoplastic a.
    a. verruciformis
ac·ro·kin·e·sia
acro·le·in
ac·ro·mac·ria
ac·ro·mas·ti·tis
ac·ro·me·ga·lia

ac·ro·me·gal·ic
ac·ro·meg·a·lo·gi·gan·tism
ac·ro·meg·a·loid·ism
ac·ro·meg·a·ly
ac·ro·mel·al·gia
ac·ro·me·lia
ac·ro·mel·ic
ac·ro·meta·gen·e·sis
acro·mi·al
ac·ro·mi·a·le
    a. os
    os a.
    a. os secundarium
ac·ro·mic·ria
ac·ro·mik·ria
acro·mio·cla·vic·u·lar
acro·mio·cor·a·coid
acro·mio·hu·mer·al
acro·mi·on
acro·mio·nec·to·my
acro·mio·plas·ty
acro·mio·scap·u·lar
acro·mio·tho·rac·ic
acrom·pha·lus
ac·ro·myo·to·nia
ac·ro·my·ot·o·nus
ac·ro·nar·cot·ic
ac·ro·neu·rop·a·thy
ac·ro·neu·ro·sis
ac·ro·nine
ac·ro·nym
ac·ro·nyx
ac·ro-os·te·ol·y·sis
ac·ro·pach·ia
ac·ro·pachy
ac·ro·pachy·der·ma
    a. with pachyperiostitis
ac·ro·pa·ral·y·sis
ac·ro·par·es·the·sia
    Nothnagel a.
    Schultze a.
ac·ro·pa·thol·o·gy
acrop·a·thy
    amyotropic a.
    ulcerative mutilating a.
ac·ro·pep·tide
acrop·e·tal
ac·ro·pho·bia

ac·ro·pig·men·ta·tio re·tic·u·
  lar·is
ac·ro·pos·thi·tis
ac·ro·pur·pu·ra
ac·ro·pus·tu·lo·sis
ac·ro·scle·ro·der·ma
ac·ro·scle·ro·sis
ac·ro·some
ac·ro·sphac·e·lus
ac·ro·sphe·no·syn·dac·tyl·ia
ac·ro·spi·ro·ma
    eccrine a.
ac·ro·ste·al·gia
ac·ro·syn·dac·ty·ly
ac·ro·ter·ic
Ac·ro·the·ca ped·ro·soi
Ac·ro·the·si·um floc·co·sum
acrot·ic
ac·ro·tism
ac·ro·tropho·dyn·ia
ac·ro·tropho·neu·ro·sis
acry·late
acryl·ic
acryl·ic acid
ac·ry·lo·ni·trile
ACS — American Cancer
  Society
    American Chemical
      Society
    American College of
      Surgeons
    anodal closing sound
    antireticular cytotoxic
      serum
ACSM — American College of
  Sports Medicine
act
    compulsive a.
    forced a.
    imperious a.
    impulsive a.
    reflex a.
Ac·taea
    A. odorata
    A. richardsoni
    A. spicata
ac·ta·pla·nin

ACTe — anodal closure
  tetanus
ACTH — adrenocorticotropic
  hormone
Ac·thar
ACTH-RF — corticotropin
  (adrenocorticotropic
  hormone) releasing factor
Ac·ti·dil
Ac·ti-Di·one
ac·tin
ac·ting out
ac·tin·ic
ac·ti·nic·i·ty
ac·tin·ide
ac·tin·i·form
α-ac·tin·in
ac·ti·nism
ac·tin·i·um
ac·ti·no·bac·il·lo·sis
Ac·tino·ba·cil·lus
    A. actinoides
    A. actinomycetemcomitans
    A. equuli
    A. lignieresii
    A. mallei
    A. pseudomallei
    A. suis
    A. whitmori
ac·ti·nob·o·lin
ac·ti·no·chem·is·try
ac·ti·no·con·ges·tin
ac·ti·no·der·ma·ti·tis
ac·tin·o·lyte
Ac·ti·no·ma·du·ra
    A. madurae
    A. pelletierii
ac·ti·nom·e·ter
ac·ti·nom·e·try
ac·ti·no·my·ce·li·al
Ac·ti·no·my·ces
    A. antibioticus
    A. asteroides
    A. bovis
    A. brasiliensis
    A. dentocariosus
    A. eppingeri
    A. eriksonii

Ac·ti·no·my·ces (continued)
  A. gonidiaformis
  A. israelii
  A. luteus
  A. muris
  A. muris-ratti
  A. naeslundii
  A. necrophorus
  A. odontolyticus
  A. pseudonecrophorus
  A. vinaceus
  A. viscosus
ac·ti·no·my·ces *pl.* ac·ti·no·my·ce·tes
Ac·ti·no·my·ce·ta·ceae
Ac·ti·no·my·ce·ta·les
ac·ti·no·my·cete
ac·ti·no·my·ce·tes
ac·ti·no·my·ce·tic
ac·ti·no·my·ce·tin
ac·ti·no·my·ce·to·ma
ac·ti·no·my·cin
ac·ti·no·my·co·ma
ac·ti·no·my·co·sis
  cervicofacial a.
ac·ti·no·my·cot·ic
ac·ti·no·my·co·tin
ac·tin·on
ac·ti·no·neu·ri·tis
ac·ti·no·phage
ac·ti·no·phy·to·sis
Ac·ti·no·pla·na·ceae
Ac·ti·no·pla·nes
  A. teichomyceticus
ac·tino·qui·nol so·di·um
ac·ti·no·ther·a·peu·tics
ac·ti·no·ther·a·py
ac·ti·no·tox·in
ac·tion
  adipokinetic a.
  antagonistic a.
  automatic a.
  bacteriocidal a.
  bacteriostatic a.
  ball-valve a.
  buffer a.
  calorigenic a.
  capillary a.

ac·tion *(continued)*
  compulsive a.
  contact a.
  cumulative a.
  diastatic a.
  disordered a. of heart
  electrocapillary a.
  nicotinic a.
  protein sparing a.
  reflex a.
  specific a.
  specific dynamic a.
  synergistic a.
  tampon a.
  thermogenic a.
  trigger a.
ac·ti·thi·az·ic acid
ac·ti·vate
ac·ti·va·tion
  epileptic a.
  lymphocyte a.
  macrophage a.
  spore a.
  stretch a.
  thermal neutron a.
ac·ti·va·tor
  active plate a.
  bow a.
  functional a.
  monoblock a.
  plasminogen a.
  polyclonal a.
  Schwarz a.
  tissue plasminogen a.
    (t-PA, TPA)
ac·tive
  optically a.
ac·tiv·i·ty
  asynchronous a.
  background a.
  blocking a.
  catalytic a.
  continuous muscle fiber a.
  cumulated a.
  a's of daily living
  elevation a's
  enzyme a.

ac·tiv·i·ty *(continued)*
    leukemia-associated
      inhibitory a. (LIA)
    nonsuppressible
      insulin-like a.
    optical a.
    plasma renin a.
    pseudomotor a.
    salaam a.
    specific a.
    spike and wave a.
    spontaneous a.
    surface a.
    synchronous a.
ac·to·dig·in
ac·to·my·o·sin
Ac·trap·id
Ac·u·a·ria spi·ra·lis
acu·clo·sure
Ac·u·fex forceps
Ac·u·fex instrument
Ac·u·fex punch
acu·fi·lo·pres·sure
acu·i·ty
    auditory a.
    Vernier a.
    visual a.
acu·la·lia
acu·le·ate
acu·mi·nate
acu·point
acu·pres·sure
acu·punc·ture
acus
acu·sec·tion
acu·sec·tor
Acu·son computed sonography
acus·ti·cus
acute
acu·te·nac·u·lum
acu·tor·sion
acy·a·no·blep·sia
acy·a·nop·sia
acy·a·not·ic
acy·clia
acy·clic
acy·clo·gua·no·sine
acy·clo·vir

ac·y·e·sis
acyl
Ac·yl·an·id
ac·yl·ase
ac·yl·a·tion
ac·yl car·ri·er pro·tein
ac·yl·cho·line ac·yl·hy·dro·lase
ac·yl-CoA
ac·yl-CoA de·sat·ur·ase
ac·yl-CoA syn·the·tase
ac·yl co·en·zyme A
ac·yl en·zyme
ac·yl·sphin·go·sine de·acyl·ase
ac·yl·trans·fer·ase
acys·tia
acys·ti·ner·via
acys·ti·neu·ria
AD — alcohol dehydrogenase
    anodal duration
A.D. — L. auris dextra (right
    ear)
ADA — adenosine deaminase
ADA — American Dental
  Association
    American Diabetes
      Association
    American Dietetic
      Association
ADAA — American Dental
  Assistants Association
adac·tyl·ia
adac·ty·lism
adac·ty·lous
adac·ty·ly
Adair-Digh·ton syn·drome
Ad·am's ap·ple
Ad·a·man·ti·a·des-Be·hçet
  syndrome
ad·a·man·tine
ad·a·man·ti·no·car·ci·no·ma
ad·a·man·ti·no·ma
    pituitary a.
    a. of long bones
    a. polycysticum
    tibial a.
ad·a·man·to·blast

ad·a·man·to·blas·to·ma
ad·a·man·to·ma
ad·a·mas
    a. dentis
Ad·ami's theory
Adam·kie·wicz demilunes
Ad·ams' dis·ease
Ad·ams' operation
Adams-Stokes disease
Adams-Stokes syncope
ad·ams·ite
Ad·an·so·nia
ad·an·so·ni·an
adap·ta·bil·i·ty
ad·ap·ta·tion
    auditory a.
    chromatic a.
    color a.
    dark a.
    enzymatic a.
    genetic a.
    light a.
    phenotypic a.
    photopic a.
    physiologic a.
    retinal a.
    scotopic a.
    sensory a.
    social a.
adap·ter
ad·ap·tom·e·ter
    color a.
ad·ar·tic·u·la·tion
ad·ax·i·al
ADC — anodal duration
  contraction
        axiodistocervical
ADCC — antibody-dependent
  cell-mediated cytotoxicity
ADD — attention deficit
  disorder
add. — L. adde (add)
    L. addetur (let there be
      added)
adde
ad·der
    death a.
    puff a.

ad·dict
ad·dic·tion
    alcohol a.
    drug a.
    polysurgical a.
Ad·dis count
ad·di·sin
Ad·di·son's anemia
Ad·di·son's planes
Ad·di·son-Bier·mer anemia
ad·di·so·ni·an
ad·di·son·ism
ad·di·tive
ad·du·cent
ad·duct
ad·duc·tion
ad·duc·tor
Ad·e·le·i·na
Adel·mann operation
adelo·mor·phic
adelo·mor·phous
adel·pho·tax·is
ad·e·nal·gia
ad·e·nase
aden·dric
aden·drit·ic
ad·e·nec·to·my
ad·en·ec·to·pia
ad·e·nem·phrax·is
ade·nia
aden·ic
aden·i·form
ad·e·nine
    a. arabinoside
    a. deoxyriboside
    a. hypoxanthine
    a. nucleotide
ad·e·nine phos·pho·ri·bo·syl
  trans·fer·ase
ad·e·ni·tis
    cervical a.
    acute infectious a.
    mesenteric a.
    phlegmonous a.
    syphilitic inguinal a.
    tuberculous a.
Ade·ni·um
ad·e·ni·za·tion

ad·e·no·ac·an·tho·ma
ad·e·no·am·e·lo·blas·to·ma
ad·e·no·a·myg·dal·ec·to·my
ad·e·no·blast
ad·e·no·can·croid
ad·e·no·car·ci·no·ma
   acinar a.
   acinous a.
   alveolar a.
   clear cell a.
   follicular a.
   a. of kidney
   mammary a.
   mucinous a.
   mucoid a.
   papillary a.
   polypoid a.
   renal a.
   scirrhous a.
   sebaceous a.
   testicular a. of infancy
ad·e·no·cele
ad·e·no·cel·lu·li·tis
ad·e·no·chon·dro·ma
ad·e·no·cyst
ad·e·no·cys·to·ma
   papillary a.
     lymphomatosum
ad·e·no·cyte
ad·e·no·dyn·ia
ad·e·no·ep·i·the·li·o·ma
ad·e·no·fi·bro·ma
   a. edematodes
   a. of ovary
   pseudomucinous a.
   serous a.
ad·e·no·fi·bro·sis
ad·e·no·gen·e·sis
ad·e·nog·e·nous
ad·e·no·graph·ic
ad·e·nog·ra·phy
ad·e·no·hy·poph·y·se·al
ad·e·no·hy·poph·y·sec·to·my
ad·e·no·hy·poph·y·si·al
ad·e·no·hy·poph·y·sis
ad·e·noid
ad·e·noid·ec·to·my
ad·e·noid·ism

ad·e·noid·i·tis
ad·e·no·leio·myo·fi·bro·ma
ad·e·no·li·po·ma
ad·e·no·li·po·ma·to·sis
ad·e·no·log·a·di·tis
ad·e·no·lym·phi·tis
ad·e·no·lym·pho·cele
ad·e·no·lym·pho·ma
ad·e·nol·y·sis
ad·e·no·ma
   acidophilic a.
   acinar a.
   a. adamantinum
   adnexal a.
   adrenocortical a.
   a. alveolare
   apocrine a.
   basophil a.
   basophilic a.
   bronchial a's
   carcinoid a. of bronchus
   ceruminous a.
   chief cell a.
   chromophobe a.
   chromophobic a.
   clear cell a.
   colloid a.
   cortical a's
   cystic a.
   duct a.
   embryonal a.
   endometrioid a.
   a. endometrioides ovarii
   eosinophil a.
   fetal a.
   fibroid a.
   a. fibrosum
   follicular a.
   a. gelatinosum
   hepatocellular a.
   a. hidradenoides
   Hürthle cell a.
   islet a.
   langerhansian a.
   liver cell a.
   macrofollicular a.
   malignant a.
   mesonephric a.

ad·e·no·ma *(continued)*
 microfollicular a.
 mucinous a.
 mucoid cell a.
 multiple endocrine a's
 oncocytic a.
 a. ovarii testiculare
 oxyphilic granular cell a.
 papillary cystic a.
 Pick's testicular a.
 Pick's tubular a.
 pituitary a.
 pleomorphic a.
 pseudomucinous a.
 racemose a.
 renal cortical a.
 sebaceous a.
 a. sebaceum
 a. simplex
 a. substantiae corticalis
  suprarenalis
 a. sudoriparum
 testicular a.
 toxic thyroid a.
 trabecular a.
 tubular a.
 tubular a. of Pick
 a. tubulare testiculare
  ovarii
 tubulovillous a.
 villous a.
 water-clear cell a.
 wolffian a.
ad·e·no·ma·la·cia
ad·e·no·ma·toid
ad·e·no·ma·tome
ad·e·no·ma·to·sis
 fibrosing a.
 multiple endocrine a.
 a. oris
 pancreatic-islet a.
 pluriglandular a.
 polyendocrine a.
 pulmonary a.
ad·e·no·ma·tous
ad·e·no·meg·a·ly
ad·e·no·mere
ad·e·no·myo·ep·i·the·li·o·ma

ad·e·no·myo·fi·bro·ma
ad·e·no·my·o·hy·per·pla·sia
ad·e·no·my·o·ma
 a. psammopapillare
ad·e·no·my·o·ma·to·sis
ad·e·no·my·o·ma·tous
ad·e·no·myo·me·tri·tis
ad·e·no·myo·sar·co·ma
 embryonal a.
ad·e·no·my·o·sis
 a. externa
 stromal a.
 a. subbasalis
 a. tubae
 a. uteri
ad·e·non·cus
ad·e·no·neu·ral
ad·e·nop·a·thy
 hilar a.
 tracheobronchial a.
ad·e·no·phar·yn·gi·tis
ad·e·no·phleg·mon
ad·e·noph·thal·mia
ad·e·no·pit·u·i·cyte
ad·e·no·sal·pin·gi·tis
ad·e·no·sar·co·ma
 embryonal a.
ad·e·no·scle·ro·sis
aden·o·sine
 a. arabinoside
 cyclic a. monophosphate
  (cyclic AMP, cAMP,
  3ʹ,5ʹ-AMP)
 a. diphosphate (ADP)
 a. monophosphate (AMP)
 a. phosphate
 a. 3ʹ-phosphate
 a. 5ʹ-phosphate
 a. triphosphate (ATP)
aden·o·sine de·am·i·nase
aden·o·sine ki·nase
aden·o·sine·tri·phos·pha·tase
ad·e·no·sis
 blunt duct a.
 florid a.
 mammary sclerosing a.
 sclerosing a.
 sclerosing a. of breast

ad·e·no·sis *(continued)*
   a. vaginae
ad·e·no·squa·mous
S-aden·o·syl·ho·mo·cys·teine
S -aden·o·syl·me·thi·o·nine
aden·o·syl·trans·fer·ase
   methionine a.
ad·e·no·tome
ad·e·not·o·my
ad·e·no·ton·sil·lec·to·my
ad·e·nous
ad·e·no·var·ix
ad·e·no·vi·ral
ad·e·no·vi·rus
ad·e·nyl
aden·yl·ate
aden·yl·ate cy·clase
aden·yl·ate de·am·i·nase
aden·yl·ate ki·nase
ad·e·nyl cy·clase
ad·e·nyl·ic acid
ad·e·nyl·ic ac·id de·am·i·nase
ad·e·nyl·o·suc·ci·nase
ad·e·nyl·o·suc·ci·nate ly·ase
ad·e·nyl·py·ro·phos·phate
ad·e·nyl·yl
ad·e·nyl·yl trans·fer·ase
ad·eps
   a. anserinus
   a. benzoinatus
   a. lanae
   a. lanae hydrosus
   a. ovillus
   a. porci
   a. renis
   a. suillus
ad·e·qua·cy
   velopharyngeal a.
ad·equal
ader·mia
ader·mine
ader·mo·gen·e·sis
Ad grat. acid. — L. ad gratum
   aciditatem (to an agreeable
   sourness)
ADH — alcohol
   dehydrogenase
     antidiuretic hormone

ADHA — American Dental
   Hygienists Association
Ad·ha·to·da
ad·her·ence
   bacterial a.
   graft a.
   immune a.
ad·he·si·ec·to·my
ad·he·sin
ad·he·sio *pl.* ad·he·si·o·nes
   a. interthalamica
ad·he·sion
   amniotic a's
   anomalous mesenteric a's
   banjo-string a.
   fibrinous a.
   filmy a's
   interthalamic a.
   preputal a.
   primary a.
   secondary a.
   serologic a.
   sublabial a.
   traumatic uterine a's
ad·he·si·o·to·my
ad·he·sive
   Biobrane a.
   cyanoacrylate a.
   dental a.
   denture a.
   ligand a.
   methylmethacrylate a.
ad·he·sive·ness
   platelet a.
adi·a·do·cho·ci·ne·sia
adi·a·do·cho·ci·ne·sis
adi·a·do·cho·ki·ne·sia
adi·a·do·cho·ki·ne·sis
adi·a·do·ko·ki·ne·sia
adi·a·do·ko·ki·ne·sis
Adi·an·tum
adi·a·pho·re·sis
adi·a·pho·ria
adi·ap·neu·stia
adi·a·spi·ro·my·co·sis
adi·a·spore
adi·as·to·le
adi·a·ther·man·cy

ad·i·cil·lin
Ad·ie's pupil
adi·emor·rhy·sis
ad·i·ent
adi·e·tet·ic
ad·i·pec·to·my
ad·i·phen·ine hy·dro·chlo·
   ride
adip·ic
adip·ic acid
ad·i·po·cele
ad·i·po·cel·lu·lar
ad·i·po·cer·a·tous
ad·i·po·cere
ad·i·po·cyte
ad·i·po·fi·bro·ma
ad·i·po·gen·e·sis
ad·i·po·gen·ic
ad·i·pog·e·nous
ad·i·po·he·pat·ic
ad·i·poid
ad·i·po·kin·e·sis
ad·i·po·kin·et·ic
ad·i·po·ki·nin
ad·i·pol·y·sis
ad·i·po·lyt·ic
ad·i·pom·e·ter
ad·i·po·ne·cro·sis
   a. subcutanea neonatorum
ad·i·po·pec·tic
ad·i·po·pex·ia
ad·i·po·pex·ic
ad·i·po·pex·is
ad·i·pos·al·gia
ad·i·pose
ad·i·po·sis
   a. cerebralis
   a. dolorosa
   a. hepatica
   a. orchia
   a. tuberosa simplex
   a. universalis
ad·i·pos·i·tas
   a. cerebralis
   a. cordis
   a. ex vacuo
ad·i·pos·i·tis

ad·i·pos·i·ty
   cerebral a.
   pituitary a.
ad·i·po·so·gen·i·tal dys·tro·
   phy
ad·i·po·su·ria
adip·sia
ad·i·tus *pl.* ad·i·tus
   a. ad antrum
   a. ad aquaeductum cerebri
   a. glottidis inferior
   a. glottidis superior
   a. ad infundibulum
   a. ad pelvem
   a. laryngis
   a. orbitae
   a. vaginae
ad·junct
ad·junc·tive
ad·just·er
   Negus ligature a.
ad·just·ment
   occlusal a.
ad·ju·vant
   A. 65
   antigen a.
   centrally acting a.
   depot-forming a.
   double emulsion a.
   Freund's a.
   immunologic a.
   mycobacterial a.
   oil emulsion a.
   pertussis a.
   solubilized water-in-oil a.
   water-in-oil-in-water
      emulsion a.
ad·ju·van·tic·i·ty
ADL — activities of daily
   living
Adler
Ad·ler's test
Ad·ler's theory
ad·ler·i·an psychoanalysis
ad·ler·i·an psychology
ad lib. — L. ad libitum (at
   pleasure)

ad·lu·mi·dine
ad·lu·mine
ad·max·il·lary
ad·me·di·al
ad·me·di·an
ad·min·ic·u·lum *pl.* ad·min·
    ic·u·la
        a. lineae albae
ad·mit·tance
ad·mix·ture
ad·mor·tal
admov. — L. admove (add)
        — L. admoveatur (let
        there be added)
ADN — Associate Degree in
    Nursing
ad·na·sal
ad·nate
ad nau·se·am
ad·ner·val
ad·neu·ral
ad·nexa
        fetal a.
        a. mastoidea
        a. oculi
        a. uteri
ad·nex·al
ad·nex·ec·to·my
ad·nex·i·tis
ad·nexo·pexy
ad·nex·or·ga·no·gen·ic
ad·o·les·cence
ad·o·les·cent
ad·or·al
ADP — adenosine
    diphosphate
ADP·glu·cose
Ad pond. om. — L. ad pondus
    omnium (to the weight of the
    whole)
ad·re·nal
        Marchand's a's
adre·nal·ec·to·mize
adre·nal·ec·to·my
Adren·a·lin
adren·a·line
        a. acid tartrate
adren·a·lin·emia

adren·a·lino·gen·e·sis
adren·a·lin·uria
ad·re·nal·ism
adren·a·li·tis
adren·a·lone
adre·nal·op·a·thy
adren·a·lo·trop·ic
ad·ren·ar·che
ad·re·ner·gic
adre·nic
adre·nin
adre·nine
ad·re·ni·tis
adre·no·cep·tive
adre·no·cep·tor
adre·no·chrome
adre·no·cor·ti·cal
adre·no·cor·ti·co·hy·per·pla·
    sia
adre·no·cor·ti·coid
adre·no·cor·ti·co·mi·met·ic
adre·no·cor·ti·co·ster·oid
adre·no·cor·ti·co·troph·ic
adre·no·cor·ti·co·troph·in
adre·no·cor·ti·co·trop·ic
adre·no·cor·ti·co·trop·in
adre·no·dox·in
ad·re·no·gen·ic
adre·no·gen·i·tal
ad·re·nog·e·nous
adre·no·glo·mer·u·lo·tro·pin
ad·re·no·gram
ad·re·no·ki·net·ic
adre·no·leu·ko·dys·tro·phy
adre·no·lu·tin
adre·no·lyt·ic
adre·no·med·ul·lary
adre·no·med·ul·lo·trop·ic
adre·no·meg·a·ly
adre·no·mi·met·ic
ad·ren·op·a·thy
adre·no·pause
adre·no·pri·val
adre·no·re·cep·tor
Adre·no·sem
adre·no·stat·ic
adre·no·ste·rone
adre·no·sym·pa·thet·ic

adre·no·tox·in
adre·no·troph·ic
adre·no·tro·phin
adre·no·trop·ic
adre·no·tro·pin
Adri·a·my·cin
Adri·an-Bronk law
adro·mia
Ad·royd
Adru·cil
ad·rue
ADS — antidiuretic substance
Ad·son's maneuver
Ad·son's rongeur
Ad·son's suction tube
Ad·son's syndrome
Ad·son's test
ad·sorb
ad·sor·bate
ad·sor·bent
ad·sorp·tion
    agglutinin a.
    immune a.
ad·sorp·tion-he·mag·glu·ti·
    na·tion
ad·ster·nal
adst. feb. — L. adstante febre
    (while fever is present)
ADT — anodal duration
    tetanus
ad·ter·mi·nal
ad·tor·sion
Ad 2 vic. — L. ad duas vices
    (at two times for two doses)
adult
adul·ter·ant
adul·te·ra·tion
adum·bra·tion
Adv. — L. adversum (against)
ad·vance
ad·vance·ment
    capsular a.
    maxillary a.
    tendon a.
ad·ven·ti·tia
ad·ven·ti·tial
ad·ven·ti·tious
ad·ver·sive

ad·vo·cate
    patient a.
ady·na·mia
    a. episodica hereditaria
ady·nam·ic
AE — above elbow
Aeb·li scissors
Ae·by's muscle
aeci·um *pl.* aecia
Aedes
    A. *aegypti*
    A. *africanus*
    A. *albopictus*
    A. *cinereus*
    A. *flavescens*
    A. *ingrami*
    A. *leucocelaenus*
    A. *polynesiensis*
    A. *pseudoscutellaris*
    A. *scapularis*
    A. *simpsoni*
    A. *sollicitans*
    A. *spencerii*
    A. *taeniorhynchus*
    A. *togoi*
    A. *varipalpus*
aed·oeo·ceph·a·lus
Aeg. — L. aeger, aegra (the
    patient)
Aegyp·ti·a·nel·la
    A. *pullorum*
aelu·ro·pho·bia
AEP — auditory evoked
    potential
aer·at·ed
aer·a·tion
aer·emia
aer·en·ter·ec·ta·sia
aer·i·al
aer·if·er·ous
aer·i·form
aero·al·ler·gen
Aero·bac·ter
    A. *aerogenes*
    A. *cloacae*
aer·obe
    facultative a's

aer·obe *(continued)*
    obligate a's
aer·o·bic
aero·bi·ol·o·gy
aero·bi·on
aero·bi·o·sis
aero·bi·ot·ic
aero·bul·lo·sis
aero·cele
    epidural a.
    intracranial a.
Aero·coc·cus
    A. *viridans*
aero·col·pos
aero·cys·tog·ra·phy
aero·cys·to·scope
aero·cys·tos·co·py
aero·der·mec·ta·sia
aer·odon·tal·gia
aer·odon·tics
aero·em·bo·lism
aero·em·phy·se·ma
aero·gas·tria
    blocked a.
aero·gel
aero·gen
aero·gen·e·sis
aero·gen·ic
aer·og·e·nous
aero·gram
aero·mam·mog·ra·phy
aero·med·i·cine
aero·mo·nad
Aero·mo·nas
    A. *caviae*
    A. *hydrophila*
    A. *sobia*
aero-odon·tal·gia
aero-odon·to·dy·nia
aer·op·a·thy
aero·peri·to·ne·um
aero·peri·to·nia
aero·pha·gia
aer·oph·a·gy
aero·phil
aero·phil·ic
aer·oph·i·lous
aero·pho·bia

aero·phore
aero·pi·eso·ther·a·py
aero·plank·ton
Aero·plast
aero·ple·thys·mo·graph
Aero·seb-Dex
aero·si·a·loph·a·gy
aero·si·nu·si·tis
aer·o·sis
aer·o·sol
    mainstream a.
    sidestream a.
aero·sol·i·za·tion
Aero·spo·rin
aero·stat·ics
aero·tax·is
aero·thor·ax
aer·oti·tis
aero·tol·er·ant
aero·to·nom·e·ter
aer·ot·ro·pism
aero·tym·pa·nal
aero·ure·thro·scope
aero·ure·thros·co·py
aes·cu·la·pi·an
Aescu·la·pi·us
    staff of A.
aes·cu·lin
Aes·cu·lus
aes·tus
aet. — L. aetas (age)
aeti·on·y·mous
Aëti·us (Aeti·os) of Am·i·da
AFB — acid-fast bacillus
AFBG — aortofemoral bypass
    graft
AFCR — American
    Federation for Clinical
    Research
afe·brile
afe·tal
af·fect
    blunted a.
    flat a.
af·fec·tion
    celiac a.
af·fec·tive
af·fec·tiv·i·ty

af·fec·to·mo·tor
af·fen·spalte
af·fer·ent
    flexor reflex a's
    Ib a.
    pressoreceptor a.
    primary a.
    somatic a.
af·fer·en·tia
    tendon organ a.
    visceral a.
af·fer·en·ti·a·tion
af·fin·i·ty
    chemical a.
    elective a.
    genetic a.
    selective a.
af·fin·ous
af·flux
af·flux·ion
afi·brin·o·gen·emia
    congenital a.
af·la·tox·i·co·sis
af·la·tox·in
AFO — ankle-foot orthosis
AFP — alpha-fetoprotein
Af·rin
AFS — American Fertility
  Society
af·ter·ac·tion
af·ter·birth
af·ter·brain
af·ter·care
af·ter·cat·a·ract
af·ter·con·trac·tion
af·ter·cur·rent
af·ter·damp
af·ter·dis·charge
af·ter·ef·fect
af·ter·gil·ding
af·ter·glow
af·ter·hear·ing
af·ter·hy·per·po·lar·i·za·tion
af·ter·im·age
    Purkinje a.
af·ter·im·pres·sion
    ventricular a.
af·ter·move·ment

af·ter·pains
af·ter·per·cep·tion
af·ter·po·ten·tial
af·ter·pres·sure
af·ter·sen·sa·tion
af·ter·taste
af·ter·treat·ment
af·ter·vi·sion
af·to·sa
afunc·tion
AG — atrial gallop
AGA — American
  Gastroenterological
  Association
    appropriate for gestational
    age
aga·lac·tia
    contagious a.
aga·lac·to·sis
aga·lac·tos·uria
aga·lac·tous
ag·a·lor·rhea
agam·ete
aga·met·ic
agam·ic
agam·ma·glob·u·lin·emia
    Bruton's a.
    common variable a.
    lymphopenic a.
    Swiss type a.
    X-linked infantile a.
Ag·a·mo·coc·ci·di·i·da
aga·mo·cy·tog·e·ny
Ag·a·mo·di·sto·mum
Ag·a·mo·fi·la·ria
    A. streptocerca
aga·mo·gen·e·sis
aga·mo·ge·net·ic
aga·mog·o·ny
Ag·a·mo·mer·mis cu·li·cis
Ag·a·mo·ne·ma
aga·mont
aga·mous
agan·gli·on·ic
agan·gli·on·o·sis
agar
    bacteriostasis a.
    bismuth sulfite a.

agar *(continued)*
    blood a.
    Bordet-Gengou a.
    brain-heart infusion a.
    Brucella a.
    Campylobacter selective a.
    cetrimide a.
    charcoal yeast extract a.
    chocolate a.
    clostrisel a.
    Czapek-Dox a.
    deoxycholate-citrate a.
    dextrose a.
    egg-yolk a.
    Endo a.
    eosin-methylene blue
      (EMB) a.
    GC a.
    gelatin a.
    heart infusion a.
    Kligler's a.
    Kligler iron a.
    Krumwiede a.
    Krumwiede triple sugar a.
    Levine's EMB
      (eosin-ethylene blue) a.
    Löffler serum a.
    Löwenstein-Jensen a.
    MacConkey a.
    modified TM a.
    Mueller-Hinton a.
    Mycoplasma a.
    neomycin assay a.
    nystatin assay a.
    phenylalanine a.
    polymyxin test a's
    potato-blood a.
    potato dextrose a.
    Pseudomonas-selective a.
    Russell's double sugar a.
    Sabouraud a.
    saccharose-mannitol a.
    Salmonella-Shigella a.
    seed a.
    standard methods a.
    streptomycin assay a. with
      yeast extract
    sulfite a.

agar *(continued)*
    tellurite a.
    tellurite glycine a.
    Thayer-Martin (TM) a.
    triple sugar iron a.
    urea a.
    Zein a.
agar-agar
agar·ic
    fly a.
    larch a.
    purging a.
    surgeons'a.
    white a.
agar·ic acid
Agar·i·ca·les
ag·a·ri·cic acid
Aga·ri·cus
    A. campestris
    A. muscarius
agar·ose
agas·tria
agas·tric
aga·tha·nasia
Ag·a·thi·nus of Spar·ta
Aga·ve
AGCT — Army General
  Classification Test
age
    achievement a.
    anatomical a.
    Binet a.
    bone a.
    childbearing a.
    chronological a.
    a. of consent
    coital a.
    developmental a.
    emotional a.
    fertilization a.
    fetal a.
    functional a.
    gestational a.
    a. of menarche
    menarcheal a.
    menstrual a.
    mental a.
    ovulational a.

age *(continued)*
    physical a.
    physiological a.
    postovulatory a.
    reproductive a.
    skeletal a.
agen·e·sia
    a. corticalis
agen·e·sis
    anorectal a.
    callosal a.
    gonadal a.
    nuclear a.
    ovarian a.
    renal a.
    sacral a.
agen·i·tal·ism
ageno·so·mia
ageno·so·mus
agent
    activating a.
    adrenergic blocking a.
    adrenergic neuron blocking
     a.
    afterload reducing a.
    alkylating a.
    alpha-adrenergic blocking
     a.
    antibacterial a.
    antifoaming a.
    beta-adrenergic blocking a.
    Bittner a.
    blocking a.
    caudalizing a.
    chelating a.
    chemotherapeutic a.
    chimpanzee coryza a.
    cholinergic blocking a.
    clearing a.
    delta a.
    desensitizing a.
    disclosing a.
    dorsalizing a.
    Eaton a.
    embedding a.
    F a.
    fixing a's
    ganglionic blocking a.

agent *(continued)*
    inducing a.
    levigating a.
    lissive a.
    luting a.
    Marcy a.
    mesodermalizing a.
    metal complexing a.
    milk a.
    mouse mammary tumor a.
    myoneural blocking a.
    Norwalk a.
    oncotic a.
    A. Orange
    oxidizing a.
    Pittsburgh pneumonia a.
    progestational a's
    reducing a.
    sequestering a.
    transforming a.
    uncoupling a.
    vacuolating a.
    virus-inactivating a.
    wetting a's
AGEPC — acetyl glyceryl
  ether phosphoryl choline
ager·a·sia
ageu·sia
    central a.
    conduction a.
    peripheral a.
ageu·sic
ageus·tia
ag·ger *pl.* ag·ge·res
    a. nasi
    a. perpendicularis
    a. valvae venae
ag·ger·es
agglom·er·at·ed
ag·glu·ti·na·ble
ag·glu·ti·nant
ag·glu·ti·na·tion
    acid a.
    bacteriogenic a.
    cold a.
    cross a.
    group a.
    H a.

ag·glu·ti·na·tion *(continued)*
   heterophil a.
   intravascular a.
   O a.
   passive a.
   platelet a.
   salt a.
   spontaneous a.
   Vi a.
ag·glu·ti·na·tive
ag·glu·ti·na·tor
ag·glu·ti·nin
   anti-A a.
   anti-B a.
   anti-M a.
   anti-N a.
   anti-P a.
   anti-Rh a.
   anti-S a.
   chief a.
   cold a.
   complete a.
   cross a.
   cross-reacting a.
   flagellar a.
   group a.
   H a.
   immune a.
   incomplete a.
   leukocyte a.
   major a.
   MG a.
   minor a.
   natural a.
   O a.
   partial a.
   plant a.
   platelet a.
   saline a.
   serum a.
   somatic a.
   T a.
   warm a.
ag·glu·tin·o·gen
ag·glu·ti·no·gen·ic
ag·glu·ti·no·phil·ic
ag·glu·ti·no·phore
ag·glu·to·gen·ic

ag·glu·tom·e·ter
aggred. feb. — L. aggrediente
   febre (while the fever is
   coming on)
Ag·gre·ga·ta
ag·gre·gate
   tubular a.
ag·gre·gat·ed hu·man IgG
   (AHuG)
ag·gre·ga·tion
   cell a.
   familial a.
   platelet a.
ag·gre·gom·e·ter
ag·gre·gom·e·try
ag·gres·sin
ag·gres·sion
   displaced a.
ag·ing
ag·i·ta·tion
ag·i·to·graph·ia
ag·i·to·la·lia
ag·i·to·pha·sia
Agit. vas. — L. agitato vase
   (the vial being shaken)
Ag·kis·tro·don
aglan·du·lar
aglau·cop·sia
aglo·mer·u·lar
aglos·sia
aglos·so·sto·mia
aglu·con
aglu·ti·tion
agly·ce·mia
agly·con
agly·cos·uric
ag·min·at·ed
ag·mi·na·tion
ag·na·thia
ag·na·thous
ag·na·thus
ag·nea
ag·no·gen·ic
ag·no·sia
   acoustic a.
   auditory a.
   apraxic a.
   body-image a.

ag·no·sia *(continued)*
    chromatic a.
    developmental a.
    digital a.
    a. for faces
    finger a.
    geometrical a.
    ideational a.
    localization a.
    nonsymbolic visual a.
    position a.
    spatial a.
    symbolic visual a.
    tactile a.
    time a.
    topographical a.
    visual a.
    visuospatial a.
ag·nos·ic
agof·ol·lin
ag·om·phi·a·sis
agom·phi·ous
ag·om·pho·sis
ago·nad
agon·a·dal
ago·na·dism
ag·o·nal
ag·o·nist
ag·on·ist·ic
ag·o·ny
ag·o·ra·pho·bia
agou·ti
agraffe
agram·ma·pha·sia
ag·ram·ma·ti·ca
agram·ma·tism
agram·ma·to·lo·gia
agran·u·lar
agran·u·lo·cyte
agran·u·lo·cyt·ic
agran·u·lo·cy·to·sis
    infantile genetic a.
    infantile lethal a.
    infectious feline a.
agran·u·lo·plas·tic
agraph·es·the·sia
agraph·ia
    absolute a.

agraph·ia *(continued)*
    acoustic a.
    a. amnemonica
    a. atactica
    cerebral a.
    jargon a.
    literal a.
    mental a.
    motor a.
    musical a.
    optic a.
    sensory a.
    verbal a.
agraph·ic
agrav·ic
Ag·rio·li·max
    A. laevis
Ag·ro·bac·te·ri·um
    A. radiobacter
    A. tumefaciens
ag·ro·ma·nia
Ag·ros·tem·ma gi·tha·go
agryp·nia
agryp·no·co·ma
agryp·node
agryp·not·ic
AGS — American Geriatrics
  Society
AGT — antiglobulin test
AGTH — adrenoglomerulotrop-
  in
ague
    brass-founders'a.
    shaking a.
    smelter-worker' a.
    welders' a.
    zinc-smelters' a.
AGV — aniline gentian violet
agy·ria
agy·ric
ah — hyperopic astigmatism
AHA — American Heart
  Association
    autoimmune hemolytic
      anemia
ahap·to·glo·bin·emia
AHF — antihemophilic factor

AHG — antihemophilic globulin
Ahl·feld sign
AHP — Assistant House Physician
AHS — Assistant House Surgeon
AHuG — aggregated human IgG
AI — anaphylatoxin inhibitor
 aortic incompetence
 aortic insufficiency
 apical impulse
 artificial insemination
 axioincisal
AIC — Association des Infirmières Canadiennes
Ai·car·di syndrome
aich·mo·pho·bia
aid
 air conduction hearing a.
 binaural hearing a.
 body-worn hearing a.
 bone conduction hearing a.
 contralateral routing of signals (CROS) a.
 electric hearing a.
 first a.
 hearing a.
 in-the-ear hearing a.
 mechanical hearing a.
 pharmaceutic a.
 pharmaceutical a.
 speech a.
 ultrasonic mobility a.
AID — artificial insemination by donor (heterologous insemination)
AIDS — acquired immunodeficiency syndrome
AIH — American Institute of Homeopathy
 artificial insemination by husband (homologous insemination)
AIHA — American Industrial Hygiene Association

AIHA — American Industrial Hygiene Association
 autoimmune hemolytic anemia
AILD — angioimmunoblastic lymphadenopathy with dysproteinemia
ail·ment
ai·lu·ro·pho·bia
AIM — acute intermittent porphyria
ain·hum
air
 alkaline a.
 alveolar a.
 ambient a.
 complemental a.
 complementary a.
 dead space a.
 functional residual a.
 liquid a.
 reserve a.
 residual a.
 stationary a.
 supplemental a.
 a. swallowing
 tidal a.
 venous alveolar a.
 vitiated a.
air·borne
Air·bra·sive
air·sick·ness
air·way
 anatomical a.
 artificial a.
 conducting a.
 endotracheal a.
 esophageal obturator a.
 nasopharyngeal a.
 oropharyngeal a.
 respiratory a.
AIUM — American Institute of Ultrasound in Medicine
Ajel·lo·my·ces
AK — above knee
 above-the-knee
akaryo·cyte
akaryo·mas·ti·gont

akar·y·o·ta
akar·y·ote
akat·a·ma
akata·ma·the·sia
akat·a·no·e·sis
ak·a·this·ia
 psychic a.
akee
ạkem·be
Åker·lund deformity
ak·i·ne·sia
 a. algera
 a. amnestica
 cerebral a.
 Nadbath a.
 O'Brien a.
 reflex a.
 spinal a.
ak·i·ne·sis
akin·es·the·sia
ak·i·net·ic
Aki·ne·ton
aki·ya·mi
ak·lo·mide
ako·ria
Ak·rin·ol
Aku·rey·ri disease
ALA — α-aminolevulinic acid
Ala — alanine
ala *pl.* alae
 a. alba medialis
 a. auris
 a. cerebelli
 a. cinerea
 a. cristae galli
 a. ilii
 alae lingulae cerebelli
 a. lobuli centralis cerebelli
 a. major ossis sphenoidalis
 a. minor ossis sphenoidalis
 a. nasi
 a. orbitalis
 a. ossis ilii
 a. parva ossis sphenoidalis
 a. pontis
 a. sacralis
 a. sacri
 a. of sacrum

ala *(continued)*
 a. temporalis ossis
  sphenoidalis
 a. vespertilionis
 a. of vomer
 a. vomeris
alac·ri·ma
alac·ta·sia
alae
Al·a·jou·a·nine's syndrome
ala·lia
 a. cophica
 developmental a.
 a. organica
 a. physiologica
 a. prolongata
alal·ic
al·a·me·cin
Alan·gi·um la·mar·ckii
al·a·nine
al·a·nine ami·no·trans·fer·
 ase
β-al·a·nin·emia
al·a·nine ra·ce·mase
al·a·nine trans·am·i·nase
β-al·a·nine trans·am·i·nase
Al·an·son's amputation
alan·tin
al·a·nyl
alar
alas·trim
alas·trim·ic
alate
ala·tus
Al·ba·lon
Al·ba·my·cin
Al·bar·rán's disease
al·be·do
 a. retinae
 a. unguium
Al·bee's operation
al·ben·da·zole
Al·bers-Schön·berg disease
Al·bert's diphtheria stain
Al·bert's operation
al·bi·cans
al·bi·du·ria
al·bi·dus

Al·bi·ni's nodules
al·bi·nism
    acquired a.
    Amish a.
    autosomal dominant
      oculocutaneous a.
    brown a.
    complete imperfect a.
    complete perfect a.
    cutaneous a.
    a. I
    a. II
    localized a.
    ocular a.
    ocular a., autosomal
      recessive (AROA)
    ocular a., Forsius-Eriksson
      type
    ocular a., Nettleship-Falls
      type
    ocular a., X-linked
      (Nettleship) (XOAN)
    oculocutaneous a. (OCA)
    partial a.
    piebald a.
    red a.
    rufous a.
    tyrosinase-negative
      (ty-neg) oculocutaneous a.
    tyrosinase-positive (ty-pos)
      oculocutaneous a.
    xanthous a.
    yellow mutant (ym)
      oculocutaneous a.
al·bi·nis·mus
    a. circumscriptus
al·bi·no
al·bi·noid·ism
    oculocutaneous a.
    punctate oculocutaneous a.
al·bi·not·ic
al·bin·uria
Al·bi·nus' muscle
Al·brecht's bone
Al·bright's syndrome
Al·bu·cas·is
al·bu·gin·ea
    a. oculi

al·bu·gin·ea *(continued)*
    a. ovarii
    a. penis
    a. testis
al·bu·gin·e·ot·o·my
al·bu·gin·e·ous
al·bu·gi·ni·tis
al·bu·go
al·bu·ka·lin
al·bu·men
al·bu·mim·e·ter
al·bu·min
    a. A
    acid a.
    alkali a.
    blood a.
    derived a.
    egg a.
    a. human
    iodinated I 125 serum a.
    iodinated I 131 serum a.
    macroaggregated a.
    native a.
    radioiodinated (^{125}I) serum
      a. (human)
    radioiodinated (^{131}I) serum
      a. (human)
    serum a.
    technetium Tc 99m
      aggregated a.
    vegetable a.
Al·bu·mi·nar
al·bu·mi·nate
al·bu·min·a·tu·ria
al·bu·min·emia
al·bu·mi·nif·er·ous
al·bu·mi·nim·e·ter
al·bu·mi·nim·e·try
al·bu·mi·nip·a·rous
al·bu·mi·no·cho·lia
al·bu·mi·no·cy·to·log·i·cal
al·bu·mi·nog·e·nous
al·bu·mi·noid
al·bu·mi·nol·y·sis
al·bu·mi·nom·e·ter
al·bu·mi·nop·ty·sis
al·bu·mi·no·re·ac·tion
al·bu·mi·nor·rhea

al·bu·mi·no·sis
al·bu·mi·nous
al·bu·min·uret·ic
al·bu·min·uria
    Bamberger's hematogenic
     a.
al·bu·min·uric
al·bu·mo·scope
al·bu·mose
al·bu·mo·se·mia
al·bu·mos·uria
al·bus
Al·bu·span
Al·bu·stix
Al·bu·tein
al·bu·ter·ol
    a. sulfate
Al·caine
Al·ca·lig·e·nes
    A. *dentrificans*
    A. *faecalis*
    A. *odorans*
al·cap·ton
al·cap·ton·uria
al·cap·ton·uric
Al·ci·an blue
al·clo·fen·ac
Al·cock's canal
al·co·gel
al·co·hol
    absolute a.
    acid a.
    amyl a.
    amyl a., tertiary
    anisyl a.
    aromatic a.
    azeotropic isopropyl a.
    benzyl a.
    bornyl a.
    butyl a.
    camphyl a.
    carnaubyl a.
    ceryl a.
    cetyl a.
    cinnamyl a.
    dehydrated a.
    denatured a.
    deodorized a.

al·co·hol *(continued)*
    dihydric a.
    diluted a.
    ethyl a.
    fatty a.
    fetal a. syndrome
    grain a.
    isoamyl a.
    isobutyl a.
    isopropyl a.
    isopropyl rubbing a.
    ketone a.
    lanolin a's
    methyl a.
    monohydric a.
    nicotinyl a.
    palmityl a.
    pantothenyl a.
    phenylethyl a.
    polyglucosic a.
    polyvinyl a.
    primary a.
    n-propyl a.
    rubbing a.
    secondary a.
    stearyl a.
    sugar a.
    tertiary a.
    tribromoethyl a.
    trihydric a.
    unsaturated a.
    wood a.
    wool a.
al·co·hol·ate
al·co·hol de·hy·dro·gen·ase
Al·co·hol, Drug Abuse, and
    Men·tal Health Ad·min·i·
    stra·tion
al·co·hol·emia
al·co·hol-ether
al·co·hol·ic
al·co·hol·i·ca
Al·co·hol·ics Anon·y·mous
al·co·hol·ism
    acute a.
    chronic a.
    epsilon a.
    paroxysmal a.

al·co·hol·i·za·tion
al·co·hol·ize
al·co·holo·ma·nia
al·co·hol·om·e·ter
al·co·holo·phil·ia
al·co·hol·uria
al·co·hol·y·sis
al·co·sol
al·cu·ro·ni·um chlo·ride
Al·dac·ta·zide
Al·dac·tone
al·de·hyde
    cinnamic a.
    cumic a.
    glycolic a.
    keto a.
    salicylic a.
    trichloroacetic a.
al·de·hyde de·hy·dro·gen·ase
  (NAD$^+$)
al·de·hyde fuch·sin
al·de·hyde-ly·ase
al·de·hyde ox·i·dase
Al·der's anomaly
al·di·mine
Al·din·a·mide
al·do·bi·on·ic acid
Al·do·chlor
al·do·hex·ose
al·dol
al·do·lase
Al·do·met
al·do·pen·tose
Al·do·ril
al·dose
al·dose 1-epim·er·ase
al·do·side
al·do·ster·one
al·do·ster·on·ism
    idiopathic a.
    primary a.
    pseudoprimary a.
    secondary a.
al·do·ster·on·o·gen·e·sis
al·do·ster·o·no·ma
al·do·ster·o·no·pe·nia
al·do·ster·on·uria
al·do·tet·rose

al·dox·ime
Al·dridge operation
Al·drich syndrome
Al·drich-Mees lines
al·drin
alec·i·thal
Alec·to·ro·bi·us ta·la·je
alem·bic
Alep·po boil
aleu·ke·mia
aleu·ke·mic
aleu·kia
    alimentary toxic a.
    congenital a.
    a. hemorrhagica
aleu·ko·cyt·ic
aleu·ko·cy·to·sis
aleu·rio·spore
Aleu·ro·bi·us fa·ri·nae
Aleu·ro·nat
al·eu·rone
al·eu·ro·noid
Al·ex·an·der of Tral·les
Al·ex·an·der's operation
Al·ex·an·der's disease
Al·ex·an·der-Ad·ams
  operation
alex·ia
    aphasic a.
    cortical a.
    Dejerine's a.
    developmental a.
    geometric a.
    isolated a.
    motor a.
    musical a.
    occipital a.
    optical a.
    parietal a.
    pure a.
    semantic a.
    sensory a.
    subcortical a.
    symbolic a.
    tactile a.
    verbal a.
alex·ic
alex·i·dine

alex·i·phar·mac
alex·i·thy·mia
aley·dig·ism
Al·ez·zan·dri·ni's syndrome
Alfenta
alfentanil hydrochloride
Al·flo·rone
ALG — antilymphocyte
  globulin
al·ga
al·gae
    blue-green a.
al·gal
al·gan·es·the·sia
al·ga·ro·ba
al·ge·don·ic
al·ge·fa·cient
al·gel·drate
al·ge·sia
al·ge·sic
al·ge·si·chro·nom·e·ter
al·ge·sim·e·ter
    Björnström's a.
    Boas'a.
al·ge·sim·e·try
al·ge·sio·gen·ic
al·ges·the·sia
al·ges·the·sis
al·ges·tone ace·to·phen·ide
al·get·ic
al·gi·cide
al·gid
al·gin
al·gi·nate
al·gin·ic acid
al·gin·ure·sis
al·gio·glan·du·lar
al·gio·met·a·bol·ic
al·gio·mo·tor
al·gio·mus·cu·lar
al·gio·vas·cu·lar
al·go·cep·tor
al·go·dys·tro·phy
al·go·gen·e·sia
al·go·gen·e·sis
al·go·gen·ic
al·go·lag·nia
    active a.

al·go·lag·nia *(continued)*
    passive a.
al·go·lag·nist
al·gom·e·ter
    pressure a.
al·gom·e·try
al·go·pho·bia
al·go·psy·cha·lia
al·gor
    a. mortis
al·go·rithm
al·go·spasm
al·go·vas·cu·lar
Ali Ab·bas
Al·i·bert's keloid
al·i·ble
al·i·cy·clic
Al·i·dase
alien·a·tion
ali·enia
alien·ist
ali-es·ter·ase
al·i·flu·rane
ali·form
align
align·ment
al·i·ment
al·i·men·ta·ry
al·i·men·ta·tion
    artificial a.
    forced a.
    parenteral a.
    rectal a.
    total parenteral a.
al·i·men·to·ther·a·py
ali·na·sal
al·i·phat·ic
alipo·gen·ic
ali·poi·dic
alipo·trop·ic
alip·tic
ali·quor·rhea
al·i·quot
ali·sphe·noid
aliz·a·rin
    a. monosulfonate
    a. No. 6
    a. red

aliz·a·rin *(continued)*
   a. yellow
al·i·zar·i·no·pur·pu·rin
al·ka·le·mia
al·ka·les·cence
al·ka·les·cens-dis·par
al·ka·les·cent
al·ka·li
   caustic a.
   fixed a.
   volatile a.
al·kal·i·fy
al·ka·lig·e·nous
al·ka·lim·e·ter
al·ka·lim·e·try
   Engel's a.
al·ka·line
al·ka·line phos·pha·tase
   leucocyte a.p.
al·ka·lin·i·ty
al·ka·lin·i·za·tion
al·ka·lin·ize
al·ka·lin·uria
al·ka·li·ther·a·py
al·ka·li·za·tion
al·ka·lize
al·ka·liz·er
al·ka·lo·gen·ic
al·ka·loid
   vinca a's
al·ka·lom·e·try
al·ka·lo·sis
   acapnial a.
   altitude a.
   carbon dioxide a.
   compensated a.
   congenital gastrointestinal
    a.
   hypochloremic a.
   hypokalemic a.
   metabolic a.
   metabolic a., compensated
   respiratory a.
   respiratory a.,
    compensated
al·ka·lo·ther·a·py
al·ka·lot·ic
al·kal·uria

al·ka·mine
al·kane
al·ka·net
al·kan·nin
al·kap·ton
al·kap·ton·uria
   spontaneous a.
al·kap·ton·uric
al·ka·tri·ene
al·ka·ver·vir
al·kene
Al·ker·an
alk·ox·ide
alk·oxy
alk·ox·yl
al·kyl
al·kyl·amine
al·kyl·ate
al·kyl·a·tion
al·kyl·o·gen
al·kyne
ALL — acute lymphoblastic
  leukemia
   acute lymphocytic
    leukemia
al·la·ches·the·sia
   optical a.
al·lan·ti·a·sis
al·lan·to·am·ni·on
al·lan·to·cho·ri·on
al·lan·to·en·ter·ic
al·lan·to·gen·e·sis
al·lan·to·ic
al·lan·to·ic·ase
al·lan·toid
al·lan·toi·de·an
al·lan·toi·do·an·gi·op·a·gous
al·lan·toi·do·an·gi·op·a·gus
al·lan·to·in
al·lan·to·in·uria
al·lan·to·is
Al·lar·ton's operation
al·lel
al·lele
   dominant a.
   leaky a.
   lethal a.
   modification a.

al·lele *(continued)*
    multiple a's
    recessive a.
    silent a.
    sublethal a.
al·le·lic
al·le·lism
al·le·lo·chem·ics
al·le·lo·tax·is
al·le·lo·taxy
al·le·lo·type
Al·le·mann's syndrome
Al·len's paradoxic law
Al·len's test
Al·len-Doi·sy test
al·ler·gen
    pollen a.
al·ler·gen·ic
al·ler·gic
al·ler·gid
al·ler·gist
al·ler·gi·za·tion
al·ler·gize
al·ler·goid
al·ler·go·log·i·cal
al·ler·gol·o·gist
al·ler·gol·o·gy
al·ler·go·sis *pl.* al·ler·go·ses
al·ler·gy
    atopic a.
    bacterial a.
    bronchial a.
    cold a.
    contact a.
    delayed a.
    drug a.
    food a.
    gastrointestinal a.
    hereditary a.
    humoral a.
    immediate a.
    intrinsic a.
    latent a.
    nasal a.
    physical a.
    pollen a.
    polyvalent a.
    seasonal a.

al·ler·gy *(continued)*
    spontaneous a.
Al·les·che·ria
    A. boydii
al·les·the·sia
    alleviant a.
    visual a.
al·le·thrin
al·li·ance
    therapeutic a.
    working a.
al·li·cin
al·li·ga·tion
All·ing·ham's fissure
All·ing·ham's ulcer
Al·lis's inhaler
al·lit·er·a·tion
al·li·thi·a·mine
Al·li·um
al·lo·al·bu·min
al·lo·an·ti·body
al·lo·an·ti·gen
al·lo·ar·thro·plas·ty
al·lo·bar
al·lo·bar·bi·tal
al·lo·bi·o·sis
al·lo·cen·tric
al·lo·chei·ria
al·lo·ches·the·sia
al·lo·che·zia
al·lo·chi·ral
al·lo·chi·ria
al·lo·chro·ic
al·lo·chro·ism
al·lo·chro·ma·cy
al·lo·chro·ma·sia
al·lo·ci·ne·sia
al·lo·col·loid
al·lo·cor·tex
Al·lo·der·ma·nys·sus
    A. sanguineus
al·lo·des·mism
al·lo·dip·loid
al·lo·dyn·ia
al·lo·erot·i·cism
al·lo·er·o·tism
al·lo·es·the·sia
al·log·a·my

al·lo·ge·ne·ic
al·lo·gen·ic
al·lo·go·tro·phia
al·lo·graft
    nerve a.
Al·lo·gro·mi·i·na
al·lo·group
al·lo·im·mune
al·lo·isom·er·ism
al·lo·ker·a·to·plas·ty
al·lo·ki·ne·sis
al·lo·ki·net·ic
al·lo·lac·tose
al·lo·la·lia
al·lom·er·ism
al·lo·met·ric
al·lo·met·ron
al·lom·e·try
Al·lo·mo·nas
al·lo·mor·phism
al·lon·o·mous
al·lo·path
al·lo·path·ic
al·lop·a·thist
al·lop·a·thy
al·lo·phan·amide
al·lo·phan·ate
al·lo·phan·ic acid
al·loph·a·sis
al·lo·phene
al·lo·phe·nic
al·lo·phore
al·loph·thal·mia
al·lo·pla·sia
al·lo·plas·mat·ic
al·lo·plast
al·lo·plas·tic
al·lo·plas·ty
al·lo·ploid
al·lo·poly·ploid
al·lo·preg·nane
al·lo·preg·nane·di·ol
al·lo·psy·chic
al·lo·pur·i·nol
al·lo·rhyth·mia
al·lo·rhyth·mic
all or none
al·lor·phine

al·lose
al·lo·sen·si·ti·za·tion
al·lo·some
    paired a.
    unpaired a.
al·lo·ster·ic
al·lo·ster·ism
al·lo·ste·ry
al·lo·sy·nap·sis
al·lo·syn·de·sis
al·lo·tet·ra·ploid
al·lo·therm
al·lo·thre·o·nine
al·lo·tope
al·lo·to·pia
al·lo·top·ic
al·lo·tox·in
al·lo·trans·plan·ta·tion
al·lot·ri·odon·tia
al·lot·rio·geu·stia
al·lo·trio·lith
al·lo·tri·oph·a·gy
al·lo·tri·os·mia
al·lot·ri·uria
al·lo·trope
al·lo·troph·ic
al·lo·trop·ic
al·lot·ro·pism
al·lot·ro·py
al·lo·type
    Am a's
    Gm a's
    Inv a's
    Km a's
    Oz a.
al·lo·typ·ic
al·lo·ty·py
al·low·ance
    recommended daily a.
    (RDA)
al·lox·an
al·lox·an·tin
al·lox·a·zine
al·lox·ure·mia
al·lox·uria
al·lox·uric
al·loy
    amalgam a.

al·loy *(continued)*
    chrome-cobalt a.
    dental a.
    Newton's a.
al·loy·age
al·lo·zy·gote
al·lo·zyme
all-*trans* retinal
al·lyl
    a. chloride
    a. isothiocyanate
al·lyl·am·ine
al·lyl·gua·ia·col
al·ly·sine
al·ma·drate sul·fate
Al·me·ida's disease
Al·mén's test
al·mond
    bitter a.
al·mo·ner
    hospital a.
alo·chia
Aloe
al·oe
al·oe-em·o·din
alo·et·ic
alo·gia
alo·gog·no·sia
al·o·in
al·o·pe·cia
    a. acquisita
    androgenetic a.
    a. areata
    a. capitis totalis
    cicatricial a.
    a. cicatrisata
    a. circumscripta
    congenital a.
    a. congenitalis
    congenital sutural a.
    congenital triangular a.
    drug a.
    drug-induced a.
    favic a.
    a. leprotica
    a. liminaris
    male pattern a.
    marginal a.

al·o·pe·cia *(continued)*
    mechanical a.
    moth-eaten a.
    a. mucinosa
    ophiasic a. areata
    pityriasic a.
    postpartum a.
    a. prematura
    premature a.
    pressure a.
    psychogenic a.
    radiation a.
    radiation-induced a.
    a. seborrheica
    senile a.
    stress a.
    syphilitic a.
    a. syphilitica
    a. totalis
    traction a.
    traumatic a.
    traumatic marginal a.
    a. universalis
    x-ray a.
al·o·pe·cic
al·ox·i·prin
ALP — alkaline phosphatase
Alpers' disease
Al·per's polioencephalopathy
al·pha
al·pha-am·y·lose
al·pha$_1$-an·ti·tryp·sin
Al·pha Chy·mar
al·pha-chy·mo·tryp·sin
al·pha·di·one
Al·pha·drol
al·pha-es·tra·di·ol
al·pha-fe·to·pro·tein
al·pha glob·u·lin
al·pha-lipo·pro·tein
al·pha-lo·be·line
al·pha·lyt·ic
al·pha$_2$-mac·ro·glob·u·lin
al·pha·mi·met·ic
al·pha·nu·mer·ic
al·pha·pro·dine hy·dro·chlo·ride
al·pha-to·coph·er·ol

al·pha·vi·rus
Al·port syn·drome
al·pra·zo·lam
al·pren·o·lol hy·dro·chlo·ride
al·pros·ta·dil
ALS — advanced life support
    amyotrophic lateral
        sclerosis
    antilymphocyte serum
Als·berg's angle
al·ser·ox·y·lon
Al·sev·er solution
Al·ström's syndrome
al·sto·nine
Alt. dieb. — L. alternis diebus
    (every other day)
al·te·plase
al·ter
al·ter·a·tive
al·ter·ego·ism
al·ter·nans
    auditory a.
    auscultatory a.
    electrical a.
    a. of the heart
    mechanical a.
    pulsus a.
Al·ter·na·ria
al·ter·nar·ia·tox·i·co·sis
al·ter·nat·ing
al·ter·na·tion
    cardiac a.
al·ter·no·bar·ic
Al·te·ro·mo·nas pu·tre·fa·ci·
    ens
al·thi·a·zide
Alt. hor. — L. alternis horis
    (every other hour)
Alt·mann's fluid
Alt·mann-Gersh method
al·to·fre·quent
al·trose
Alu-Cap
Alu·drine
Alu·drox
al·um
    ammonium a.

al·um (continued)
    burnt a.
    chrome a.
    concentrated a.
    dried a.
    exsiccated a.
    a. hematoxylin
    iron a.
    potassium a.
alu·men
    a. exsiccatum
alu·mi·na
    a. and magnesia
alu·mi·nat·ed
al·u·min·i·um
Alu·mi·noid
alu·mi·no·sis
alu·mi·num
    a. acetate
    a. aminoacetate
    a. ammonium sulfate
    a. carbonate, basic
    a. chlorhydrex
    a. chloride
    a. glycinate
    a. hydrate
    a. hydroxide
    a. hydroxide, colloidal
    a. monostearate
    a. nicotinate
    a. oxide
    a. penicillin
    a. phosphate
    a. potassium sulfate
    a. subacetate
    a. sulfate
alun·dum
Al·u·pent
Al·ur·ate
al·ve·at·ed
al·vei
al·veo·bron·chi·ol·i·tis
al·veo·lal·gia
al·ve·o·lar
al·ve·o·late
al·ve·o·lec·to·my
    transeptal a.
al·ve·o·li

al·ve·o·li·tis
   allergic a.
   extrinsic allergic a.
   fibrosing a.
   a. with honeycombing
   a. sicca dolorosa
al·ve·o·lo·ba·sal
al·ve·o·lo·cap·il·la·ry
al·ve·o·lo·cla·sia
al·ve·o·lo·den·tal
al·ve·o·lo·la·bi·al
al·ve·o·lo·la·bi·a·lis
al·ve·o·lo·lin·gual
al·ve·o·lo·me·rot·o·my
al·ve·o·lo·na·sal
al·ve·o·lo·pal·a·tal
al·ve·o·lo·plas·ty
   interradicular a.
   intraseptal a.
al·ve·o·lot·o·my
al·ve·o·lus *pl.* al·ve·o·li
   dental a.
   alveoli dentales
     mandibulae
   alveoli dentales maxillae
   alveoli pulmonis
   alveoli pulmonum
al·ve·rine citrate
al·ve·us *pl.* al·vei
   a. communis
   a. hippocampi
   a. of hippocampus
Al·vo·dine
al·vus
alym·phia
alym·pho·cy·to·sis
alym·pho·pla·sia
   thymic a.
Alzheimer's dementia
Alzheimer's disease
AM — L. Artium Magister
  (Master of Arts)
Am — americium
am — meterangle ametropia
  myopic astigmatism
a.m. — L. ante meridiem
  (before noon)

AMA — Aerospace Medical
  Association
  against medical advice
  American Medical
    Association
  Australian Medical
    Association
am·a·cri·nal
am·a·crine
amad·i·none ac·e·tate
Am·a·dori re·ar·range·ment
amal·gam
   copper a.
   dental a.
   retrograde a.
   silver a.
amal·gam·able
amal·ga·mate
amal·ga·ma·tion
amal·ga·ma·tor
Am·a·ni·ta
   A. virosa
ama·ni·tine
aman·i·to·tox·in
aman·ta·dine hy·dro·chlo·ride
ama·ra
Am·a·ran·thus
am·a·ranth
am·a·rine
am·a·roid
am·a·roi·dal
am·a·se·sis
amas·tia
amas·ti·gote
amatho·pho·bia
am·a·tol
am·au·ro·sis
   cat's eye a.
   central a.
   a. centralis
   cerebral a.
   a. congenita
   congenital a.
   a. congenita of Leber
   compression a.
   diabetic a.

am·au·ro·sis *(continued)*
    a. fugax
    intoxication a.
    Leber's congenital a.
    a. partialis fugax
    reflex a.
    saburral a.
    toxic a.
    uremic a.
am·au·rot·ic
ama·zia
am·be·no·ni·um chlo·ride
Am·berg's line
Am·ber·lite
am·bi·dex·ter·i·ty
am·bi·dex·trism
am·bi·dex·trous
am·bi·ent
am·bi·gu·i·ty
    ribosomal a.
am·bi·lat·er·al
am·bi·le·vos·i·ty
am·bi·le·vous
Am·bil·har
am·bi·oc·u·lar·i·ty
am·bi·o·pia
am·bi·sex·u·al
am·bi·sex·u·al·i·ty
am·bi·sin·is·ter
am·bi·si·nis·trous
am·biv·a·lence
am·bi·va·lent
am·bi·ver·sion
am·bi·vert
am·bly·acu·sis
am·bly·a·phia
am·bly·chro·ma·sia
am·bly·chro·mat·ic
am·bly·geu·stia
Am·bly·om·ma
    A. americanum
    A. cajennense
    A. hebraeum
    A. maculatum
    A. ovale
    A. tuberculatum
    A. variegatum
am·bly·ope

am·bly·o·pia
    alcoholic a.
    arsenic a.
    color a.
    crossed a.
    a. cruciata
    eclipse a.
    a.   ex anopsia
    nocturnal a.
    nutritional a.
    quinine a.
    receptor a.
    reflex a.
    strabismic a.
    suppression a.
    tobacco a.
    toxic a.
    traumatic a.
    uremic a.
    West Indian a.
am·blyo·scope
    major a.
am·bo
am·bo·cep·tor
Am·bo·dryl
am·bo·my·cin
am·bon
am·bo·sex·u·al
Am·bro·sia
am·bros·te·rol
am·bru·ti·cin
Am·bu bag
am·bu·lance
am·bu·lant
am·bu·la·tion
am·bu·la·to·ry
am·bu·phyl·line
am·bus·tion
am·bu·tox·ate hy·dro·chlo·ride
Am·bys·to·ma
am·cin·a·fal
am·cin·a·fide
am·cin·o·nide
am·di·no·cil·lin
ame·ba *pl.* ame·bae, ame·bas
ame·ban

ame·bi·a·sis
    a. cutis
    hepatic a.
    intestinal a.
    pulmonary a.
ame·bic
ame·bi·ci·dal
ame·bi·cide
ame·bi·form
ame·bi·o·sis
am·e·bism
ame·bo·cyte
ame·bo·flag·el·late
ame·boid
ame·boid·ism
am·e·bo·ma
ame·bu·la
ame·bu·ria
ame·da·lin hy·dro·chlo·ride
amei·o·sis
amel·a·no·sis
amel·a·not·ic
ame·lia
    brachial a.
    complete a.
    unilateral a.
amel·i·fi·ca·tion
amel·io·ra·tion
amelo·blast
amelo·blas·to·ma
    melanotic a.
    malignant a.
    pigmented a.
    pituitary a.
am·e·lo·blas·to·sar·co·ma
amelo·den·ti·nal
amelo·gen·e·sis
    a. imperfecta
am·e·lo·gen·ic
am·e·lo·gen·in
am·e·lus
ame·nia
amen·or·rhea
    dietary a.
    dysponderal a.
    functional a.
    hypothalamic a.
    lactation a.

amen·or·rhea *(continued)*
    nutritional a.
    ovarian a.
    physiologic a.
    pituitary a.
    premenopausal a.
    primary a.
    relative a.
    secondary a.
    traumatic a.
amen·or·rhe·al
amen·sal·ism
amen·tia
    nevoid a.
Amer·i·caine
Amer·i·can Type Cul·ture
    Col·lec·tion (ATCC)
am·er·ic·i·um
am·er·ism
am·er·is·tic
Ames test
ame·tab·o·lon
ame·tab·o·lous
ameta·chro·mo·phil
ameta·neu·tro·phil
ameth·o·caine hy·dro·chlo·
    ride
ameth·op·ter·in
ame·tria
am·e·trom·e·ter
am·e·tro·pia
    axial a.
    curvature a.
    index a.
    position a.
    refractive a.
am·e·trop·ic
am·fe·nac so·di·um
am·fo·ne·lic acid
Amh — mixed astigmatism
    with myopia predominating
AMI — acute myocardial
    infarction
am·i·an·thoid
am·i·bi·ar·son
Am·i·car
am·i·chlor·al
Am·i·ci's disk

ami·cro·bic
ami·cro·scop·ic
amic·u·la
amic·u·lum *pl.* amic·u·la
    a. olivare
    a. of olive
ami·dap·sone
am·i·dase
am·ide
    niacin a.
    nicotinic acid a.
am·ide syn·the·tase
am·i·din
am·i·dine
    insoluble a.
    tegumentary a.
am·i·dine-ly·ase
am·i·dino·trans·fer·ase
am·i·do·azo·tol·u·ene
am·i·do·ben·zene
am·i·do·gen
am·i·do·hex·ose
am·i·do·hy·dro·lase
am·i·do·li·gase
am·i·dox·ime
amid·u·lin
Am·i·gen
am·i·ka·cin sul·fate
Am·i·kin
amil·o·ride
amim·ia
    amnesic a.
am·in·a·crine hy·dro·chlo·
  ride
am·in·ar·sone
amine
    adrenergic a.
    biogenic a's
    catechol a.
    methyl dimethoxy methyl
      phenyl ethyl a.
    vasoactive a.'s
amine ox·i·dase
  (copper-containing)
amine ox·i·dase
  (flavin-containing)
am·i·ni·tro·zole
ami·no

ami·no·ace·tic acid
ami·no acid
    α-a. a.
    ω-a. a.
    aromatic a. a.
    basic a. a's
    essential a. a's
    ketogenic a. a.
    nonessential a.a's
    sulfur-containing a. a's
    uncoded a. a.
ami·no·ac·id·emia
ami·no·ac·i·dop·a·thy
D-ami·no-ac·id ox·i·dase
L-ami·no-ac·id ox·i·dase
ami·no·ac·id·uria
    imidazole a.
    overflow a.
    renal a.
    transport a.
ami·no·ac·ri·dine hy·dro·
  chlo·ride
ami·no·acyl
    a.-tRNA
ami·no·ac·yl aden·y·late
ami·no·acy·lase
ami·no·acyl his·ti·dine di·
  pep·ti·dase
ami·no·acyl·trans·fer·ase
ami·no·acyl-tRNA syn·the·
  tase
o-ami·no·azo·tol·u·ene
ami·no·ben·zene
p-ami·no·ben·zo·ic acid [para-]
γ-ami·no·bu·ty·rate
ami·no·bu·ty·rate ami·no·
  trans·fer·ase
γ-ami·no·bu·tyr·ic acid
ε-ami·no·ca·pro·ic acid
ami·no·cy·cli·tol
ami·no·di·ni·tro·phe·nol
2-ami·no·eth·a·nol
ami·no·gly·co·side
ami·no·hip·pu·rate
    a. sodium
ami·no·hip·pu·ric acid
p-ami·no·hip·pu·ric ac·id
  syn·the·tase [para-]

ami·no·hy·dro·lase
ami·no·hy·droxy·ben·zo·ic
   acid
ami·no·lev·u·lin·ate
ami·no·lev·u·lin·ate de·hy·
   dra·tase
5-ami·no·lev·u·lin·ate syn·
   thase
δ-ami·no·lev·u·lin·ic acid
ami·no·lip·id
ami·no·lip·in
am·i·nol·y·sis
2-ami·no-6-mer·cap·to·pu·
   rine
ami·no·met·ra·dine
ami·no·met·ra·mide
ami·no·ni·tro·thi·a·zole
6-ami·no·pen·i·cil·lan·ic acid
   (6-APA)
ami·no·pen·ta·mide sul·fate
ami·no·pep·ti·dase
ami·no·pep·ti·dase (cytosol)
p-aminophenol
ami·no·phen·yl·stib·in·ic acid
am·i·noph·er·ase
am·i·noph·yl·line
ami·no·po·ly·pep·ti·dase
am·i·nop·ter·in
ami·no·pu·rine
ami·no·py·rine
ami·no·quin·o·line
amin·o·rex
ami·no·sac·cha·ride
ami·no·sa·lic·y·late
p-ami·no·sal·i·cyl·ic ac·id
ami·no·si·dine sul·fate
am·i·no·sis
Ami·no·sol
ami·no·sug·ar
ami·nos·uria
Ami·no·syn
ami·no-ter·mi·nal
ami·no·trans·fer·ase
am·in·uria
ami·o·da·rone
Am·i·paque
am·i·phen·a·zole hy·dro·
   chlo·ride

am·i·quin·sin hy·dro·chlo·
   ride
am·iso·met·ra·dine
am·i·thi·o·zone
ami·to·sis
ami·tot·ic
am·i·trip·ty·line hy·dro·chlo·
   ride
AML — acute myeloblastic
   leukemia
am·me·ter
Am·mi
   A. majus
am·mine
am·mo·ac·id·uria
AMMOL — acute
   myelomonoblastic leukemia
Am·mon's filaments
Am·mon's horn
am·mo·ne·mia
am·mo·nia
   a. hemate
am·mo·ni·a·cal
am·mo·nia ly·ase
am·mo·ni·ate
am·mo·ni·emia
am·mon·i·fi·ca·tion
am·mo·ni·um
   a. acetate
   a. alum
   a. bromide
   a. carbonate
   a. chloride
   ferric a. citrate
   ferric a. sulfate
   a. mandelate
   a. muriate
   a. oxalate
   a. phosphate
   a. purpurate
   a. sulfate
   a. tungstate
am·mo·ni·uria
am·mo·nol·y·sis
am·mo·no·tel·ic
Am·mo·sper·moph·i·lus
   A. leucurus
am·mo·ther·a·py

am·ne·sia
  affective a.
  anterograde a.
  auditory a.
  Broca's a.
  circumscribed a.
  continuous a.
  elective a.
  emotional a.
  episodic a.
  generalized a.
  graphokinetic a.
  hysterical a.
  immunologic a.
  incomplete a.
  infantile a.
  lacunar a.
  localized a.
  mimokinetic a.
  olfactory a.
  organic a.
  patchy a.
  postconcussional a.
  posthypnotic a.
  post-traumatic a.
  psychogenic a.
  retroactive a.
  retrograde a.
  selective a.
  systematic a.
  tactile a.
  transient global a.
  traumatic a.
  verbal a.
  visual a.
am·ne·si·ac
am·ne·sic
am·nes·tic
Am·nes·tro·gen
am·nio·car·di·ac
am·nio·cele
am·nio·cen·te·sis
am·nio·cho·ri·al
am·nio·clep·sis
am·nio·cyte
am·nio·gen·e·sis
am·ni·og·ra·phy
am·ni·o·ma

am·ni·on
  anterior cul-de-sac a.
  caudal cul-de-sac a.
  ectoplacental a.
  a. nodosum
am·ni·on·ic
am·ni·o·ni·tis
Am·ni·o·plas·tin
am·ni·or·rhea
am·ni·or·rhex·is
am·nio·scope
am·ni·os·co·py
Am·ni·o·ta
am·ni·ote
am·ni·ot·ic
Am·ni·o·tin
am·ni·o·tome
am·ni·ot·o·my
amo·bar·bi·tal
  a. sodium
am·o·di·a·quine di·hy·dro·
  chlo·ride di·hy·drate
am·o·di·a·quine hy·dro·chlo·
  ride
Amoe·ba
  A. buccalis
  A. coli
  A. dentalis
  A. dysenteriae
  A. histolytica
  A. proteus
  A. urinae granulata
  A. verrucosa
Amoe·bi·da
amoe·bu·la
amok
AMOL — acute monoblastic
  leukemia
am·o·py·ro·quin hy·dro·chlo·
  ride
amorph
amor·pha
amor·phia
amor·phic
amor·phin·ism
amor·phism
amor·pho·gno·sia

amor·pho·syn·the·sis
amor·phous
amor·phus
Amoss' sign
amo·tio
    a. retinae
amox·a·pine
amox·i·cil·lin
Amox·il
AMP — adenosine
  monophosphate
3′,5′-AMP — cyclic adenosine
  monophosphate
amp
amp — ampere
AMP de·am·i·nase
am·per·age
am·pere
am·pere-sec·ond (A-s)
am·per·om·e·try
Am·phe·drox·yn
am·phet·a·mine
    a. phosphate
    a. sulfate
am·phi·ar·kyo·chrome
am·phi·ar·thro·di·al
am·phi·ar·thro·sis
am·phi·as·ter
am·phi·blas·tic
am·phi·blas·tu·la
am·phi·bol·ic
am·phib·o·lous
am·phi·car·ci·no·gen·ic
am·phi·cen·tric
am·phi·chro·ic
am·phi·chro·mat·ic
am·phi·cre·a·tine
am·phi·cre·at·i·nine
am·phi·cro·ic
am·phi·cyte
am·phi·cyt·u·la
am·phi·des·mic
am·phi·des·mous
am·phi·di·ar·thro·sis
am·phi·dip·loid
am·phi·gas·tru·la
am·phi·gen·e·sis
am·phi·ge·net·ic

am·phi·go·nad·ism
am·phig·o·ny
am·phi·kar·y·on
am·phi·leu·ke·mic
Am·phim·e·rus
am·phi·mix·is
am·phi·mor·u·la
am·phi·nu·cle·us
am·phi·path
am·phi·path·ic
am·phi·py·re·nin
Am·phis·to·ma
    A. conicum
    A. hominis
    A. watsoni
am·phis·tome
am·phi·sto·mi·a·sis
am·phi·tene
am·phi·the·a·ter
am·phit·ri·chous
am·phit·y·py
am·pho·chro·ma·to·phil
am·pho·chro·mo·phil
am·pho·cyte
am·pho·di·plo·pia
am·pho·gen·ic
Am·pho·jel
am·pho·lyte
am·pho·my·cin
am·pho·phil
am·pho·phile
am·pho·phil·ic
    a.-basophils
    gram-a.
    a.-oxyphil
am·phoph·i·lous
am·phor·ic
am·pho·ric·i·ty
am·pho·ril·o·quy
am·pho·roph·o·ny
am·pho·ter·ic
am·pho·ter·i·cin B
am·pho·ter·ic·i·ty
am·pho·ter·ism
am·phot·ero·di·plo·pia
am·phot·er·ous
am·phot·o·ny
amp·i·cil·lin

amp·i·cil·lin
   a. sodium
AMP ki·nase
Am·platz cardiac catheter
am·plex·a·tion
am·plex·us
am·pli·fi·ca·tion
   compression a.
   image a.
am·pli·fi·er
am·pli·tude
   a. of accommodation
   a. of convergence
am·poule
am·pul
am·pule
ampulla *pl.* am·pul·lae
   anterior membranaceous a.
   a. canaliculi lacrimalis
   a. chyli
   a. ductus deferentis
   a. ductus lacrimalis
   duodenal a.
   a. duodeni
   a. of gallbladder
   Henle's a.
   hepatopancreatic a.
   a. hepatopancreatica
   a. of lacrimal canaliculus
   ampullae lactiferae
   lateral membranaceous a.
   Lieberkühn's a.
   a. of Mascagni
   ampullae membranaceae
   a. membranacea   anterior
   a. membranacea lateralis
   a. membranacea posterior
   ampullae osseae
   a. ossea anterior
   a. ossea lateralis
   a. ossea posterior
   phrenic a.
   posterior membranaceous
      a.
   rectal a.
   a. recti
   a. of Thoma
   a. of thoracic duct

ampulla *(continued)*
   a. tubae uterinae [NA]
   a. of uterine tube
   a. of vas deferens
   a. of Vater
am·pul·lae
am·pul·lar
Am·pul·la·ri·el·la reg·u·la·ris
am·pul·la·ry
am·pul·late
am·pul·lif·u·gal
am·pul·lip·e·tal
am·pul·li·tis
am·pul·lu·la
am·pu·tate
am·pu·ta·tion
   above-knee (A-K) a.
   Alanson's a.
   Alouette's a.
   Anderson's a.
   aperiosteal a.
   Béclard's a.
   below-knee (B-K) a.
   Berger's a.
   Bier's a.
   bloodless a.
   Bunge's a.
   Callander's a.
   Carden's a.
   central a.
   cervix a.
   chop a.
   Chopart's a.
   cinematic a.
   cineplastic a.
   circular a.
   closed a.
   coat-sleeve a.
   a. in contiguity
   a. in continuity
   cutaneous a.
   definitive a.
   Dieffenbach's a.
   double-flap a.
   Dupuytren's a.
   eccentric a.
   elliptic a.

am·pu·ta·tion *(continued)*
   end-bearing a.
   Farabeuf's a.
   flap a.
   flapless a.
   Forbes a.
   forequarter a.
   Gritti's a.
   Gritti-Stokes a.
   guillotine a.
   Guyon's a.
   Hancock's a.
   Hey's a.
   hindquarter a.
   interilioabdominal a.
   interinnominoabdominal a.
   intermediary a.
   interpelviabdominal a.
   interscapulothoracic a.
   intrapyretic a.
   intrauterine a.
   Jaboulay's a.
   kineplastic a.
   Kirk's a.
   Langenbeck's a.
   Larrey's a.
   Le Fort's a.
   linear a.
   Lisfranc's a.
   Mackenzie's a.
   Maisonneuve's a.
   major a.
   Malgaigne's a.
   mediotarsal a.
   metacarpal a.
   minor a.
   mixed a.
   musculocutaneous a.
   oblique a.
   open a.
   osteoplastic a.
   oval a.
   pathological a.
   periosteoplastic a.
   phalangophalangeal a.
   Pirogoff's a.
   primary a.
   provisional a.

am·pu·ta·tion *(continued)*
   pulp a.
   racket a.
   ray a.
   rectangular a.
   Ricard's a.
   root a.
   secondary a.
   semicircular flap a.
   spontaneous a.
   Stokes's a.
   subastragalar a.
   submalleolar a.
   subperiosteal a.
   supracondylar a.
   Syme's a.
   Teale's a.
   tertiary a.
   through-knee a.
   a. by transfixion
   transmetatarsal a.
   traumatic a.
   traverse a.
   Tripier's a.
   Vladimiroff-Mikulicz a.
am·pu·tee
AMRA — American Medical
   Record Association
am·ri·none
AMRL — Aerospace Medical
   Research Laboratories
AMS — American
   Meteorological Society
ams — amount of a substance
AMSA — American Medical
   Student Association
Am·sler's chart
Am·sus·tain
amu — atomic mass unit
amuck
amu·sia
   amnesic a.
   instrumental a.
   motor a.
   receptive a.
   sensory a.
   tonal a.
   vocal motor a.

Amus·sat's operation
AMWA — American Medical
  Women's Association
    American Medical Writers'
    Association
amy·cho·pho·bia
amyc·tic
amy·dri·a·sis
amyd·ri·caine
amy·el·en·ce·pha·lia
amy·el·en·ceph·a·lus
amy·e·lia
amy·el·ic
amy·eli·nat·ed
amy·eli·na·tion
amy·e·lin·ic
amy·e·lon·ic
amy·e·lot·ro·phy
amy·e·lus
amyg·da·la
    a. accessoria
    accessory a.
    a. amara
    a. of cerebellum
    a. dulcis
amyg·da·lase
amyg·da·lic acid
amyg·da·lin
amyg·da·line
amyg·da·loid
amyg·da·loid·ec·to·my
amyg·da·loid·ot·o·my
amyg·da·lose
am·yl
    a. acetate
    a. nitrite
am·y·la·ceous
am·y·lase
    α-a.
    β-a.
    γ-a.
    endo-a.
    exo-a.
    pancreatic a.
    salivary a.
    serum a.
    urinary a.
am·y·las·uria

Am·yl·caine Hy·dro·chlo·ride
am·yl·emia
am·y·lene
    a. hydrate
amyl·ic
am·y·lin
am·y·lism
am·yl ni·trate
am·y·lo·bar·bi·tone
am·y·lo·cel·lu·lose
am·y·lo·clas·tic
am·y·lo·co·ag·u·lase
am·y·lo·dex·trin
am·y·lo·dys·pep·sia
am·y·lo·gen
am·y·lo·gen·e·sis
am·y·lo·gen·ic
am·y·lo-1,6-glu·co·si·dase
    deficiency
am·y·lo·hemi·cel·lu·lose
am·y·lo·hy·drol·y·sis
am·y·loid
am·y·loid·emia
am·y·loi·do·sis
    AA a.
    a. of aging
    AL a.
    Andrade type a.
    cutaneous a.
    familial a.
    hereditary a.
    heredofamilial a.
    idiopathic a.
    immunocyte-derived a.
    immunocytic a.
    Indiana type a.
    Iowa type a.
    kidney a.
    lichen a.
    light chain–related a.
    macular a.
    nodular a.
    Portuguese type a.
    primary a.
    reactive systemic a.
    renal a.
    secondary a.
    senile a.

am·y·lol·y·sis
am·y·lo·lyt·ic
am·y·lo·pec·tin
am·y·lo·pec·ti·no·sis
am·y·lo·pha·gia
am·y·lo·plast
am·y·lo·plas·tic
am·y·lor·rhea
am·y·lor·rhex·is
am·y·lose
    alpha-a.
am·y·lo·sis
am·y·lo·su·ria
am·y·lo·syn·the·sis
am·y·lo-1:4,1:6-trans·glu·co·
   si·dase deficiency
am·yl·pen·i·cil·lin sodium
Am·yl·sine Hy·dro·chlo·ride
am·y·lu·ria
amyo·es·the·sia
amyo·es·the·sis
amyo·pla·sia
   a. congenita
amyo·sta·sia
amyo·stat·ic
amy·os·the·nia
amy·os·then·ic
amyo·tax·ia
amyo·taxy
amyo·to·nia
   Oppenheim's a.
amyo·tro·phia
   neuralgic a.
   a. spinalis progressiva
amyo·troph·ic
amy·ot·ro·phy
   Aran-Duchenne a.
   diabetic a.
   neuralgic a.
   neuritic a.
   primary progressive a.
   progressive nuclear a.
   syphilitic a.
am·y·ous
Am·y·tal
amyx·ia
amyx·or·rhea
   a. gastrica

An — anodal
   anode
ANA — American Nurses'
   Association
ANA — antinuclear
   antibodies
ana
anab·a·sine
an·a·bat·ic
ana·bi·o·sis
ana·bi·ot·ic
an·a·bol·ic
anab·o·lism
anab·o·lite
an·a·camp·sis
an·a·camp·tic
an·a·camp·tom·e·ter
an·a·car·dic acid
Ana·car·di·um
an·a·car·dol
ana·cata·did·y·mus
ana·cat·es·the·sia
ana·cho·re·sis
ana·cho·ret·ic
ana·chor·ic
anach·ro·nism
an·acid·i·ty
   gastric a.
anac·la·sis
an·a·cli·sis
an·a·clit·ic
an·ac·me·sis
ana·co·bra
an·acou·sia
an·a·crot·ic
anac·ro·tism
an·acu·sis
an·a·di·crot·ic
an·a·di·cro·tism
an·a·did·y·mus
an·a·dip·sia
an·ad·re·nal·ism
an·ad·re·nia
An·a·drol
an·aer·obe
   facultative a's
   obligate a's

an·aer·obe *(continued)*
  spore-forming a.
an·aer·o·bi·an
an·aer·o·bic
an·aero·bi·o·sis
an·aero·gen·ic
an·aero·plas·ty
an·aer·o·sis
an·a·gen
Anag·nos·ta·kis' operation
an·a·go·ge
an·a·gog·ic
an·a·go·gy
an·a·go·tox·ic
ana·kata·did·y·mus
ana·kat·es·the·sia
an·akh·re
an·ak·me·sis
an·aku·sis
anal
an·al·bu·min·emia
an·a·lep·tic
an·al·ge·sia
  a. algera
  audio a.
  conduction a.
  congenital a.
  continuous caudal a.
  a. dolorosa
  electrical a.
  epidural a.
  hysterical a.
  infiltration a.
  narcolocal a.
  obstetrical a.
  paretic a.
  perineural a.
  permeation a.
  relative a.
  serial caudal a.
  spinal a.
  surface a.
an·al·ge·sic
an·al·get·ic
an·al·gia
an·al·gic
anal·i·ty
an·al·ler·gic

an·a·log
anal·o·gous
an·a·logue
  folic acid a.
  homologous a.
  metabolic a.
  purine a.
  pyrimidine a.
  substrate a.
anal·o·gy
an·al·pha·li·po·pro·tein·emia
anal·y·sand
anal·y·sis *pl.* anal·y·ses
  acoustic a. of speech
  activation a.
  antigenic a.
  bite a.
  blood gas a.
  bradycinetic a.
  cephalometric a.
  character a.
  chromatographic a.
  cluster a.
  colorimetric a.
  densimetric a.
  discriminant a.
  displacement a.
  distributive a.
  Downs' a.
  ego a.
  end-group a.
  Feather's a.
  fluctuation a.
  Fourier a.
  gasometric a.
  gastric a.
  gravimetric a.
  group a.
  isotope dilution a.
  multivariate a.
  nearest neighbor base
    frequency a.
  nearest neighbor sequence
    a.
  occlusal a.
  organic a.
  orthodox a.
  path coefficient a.

anal·y·sis *(continued)*
    pentagastrin stimulated a.
    probit a.
    proximate a.
    qualitative a.
    quantitative a.
    radiochemical a.
    regression a.
    ridit a.
    saturation a.
    sequential a.
    Simkin a.
    spectroscopic a.
    stop-flow a.
    structural a.
    tetrad a.
    transactional a.
    tubeless gastric a.
    ultimate a.
    a. of variance (ANOVA)
    vector a.
    volumetric a.
an·a·ly·sor
an·a·lyst
an·a·lyte
an·a·lyt·ic
an·a·ly·zer
    amino acid a.
    amino acid sequence a.
    auditory a.
    blood gas a.
    breath a.
    centrifugal fast a.
    frequency a.
    image a.
    kinetic a.
    oxygen gas a.
    pulse height a.
    sensory a.
    sequential multiple a.
      (SMA)
    visual a.
    voice a.
    wave a.
an·am·ne·sis
    associative a.
an·am·nes·tic
ana·mor·pho·sis

ana·mor·pho·sis
    dioptric a.
an·an·a·bol·ic
an·an·a·phy·lax·is
An·a·nase
an·an·as·ta·sia
an·an·casm
an·an·cas·tic
an·an·gi·oid
an·an·gio·pla·sia
an·a·pep·sia
ana·phase
    flabby a.
an·a·phia
an·a·pho·re·sis
an·a·pho·ret·ic
an·a·pho·ria
an·aph·ro·dis·iac
ana·phy·lac·tic
ana·phy·lac·tin
ana·phy·lac·to·gen
ana·phy·lac·to·gen·e·sis
ana·phy·lac·to·gen·ic
ana·phy·lac·toid
an·a·phy·lac·to·tox·in
ana·phy·la·tox·in
ana·phy·lax·is
    active a.
    aggregate a.
    antiserum a.
    generalized a.
    heterocytotropic a.
    homocytotropic a.
    inverse a.
    local a.
    passive a.
    passive cutaneous a. (PCA)
    reverse a.
    systemic a.
ana·phy·lo·tox·in
an·a·pla·sia
    monophasic a.
    polyphasic a.
an·a·plas·tic
an·a·ple·ro·sis
an·a·ple·rot·ic
an·ap·nea
an·ap·no·ther·a·py

an·apoph·y·sis
An·a·prox
an·ap·tic
an·a·rith·mia
an·ar·rhex·is
an·ar·thria
    a. literalis
an·a·sar·ca
an·a·sar·cous
an·a·schis·tic
an·a·scit·ic
an·a·stal·sis
an·a·stal·tic
an·a·stig·mat·ic
anas·to·le
anas·to·mose
an·as·to·mo·sis *pl.* an·as·to·mo·ses
    antiperistaltic a.
    aorticopulmonary a.
    a. arteriolovenularis
    a. arteriolovenularis
      simplex
    a. arteriovenosa
    a. arteriovenosa
      glomeriformis
    a. arteriovenosa simplex
    arteriovenous a.
    arteriovenous a.,
      glomeriform
    arteriovenous a., simple
    arteriovenular a.,
      glomeriform
    arteriovenular a., simple
    Baffe's a.
    Billroth's a.
    Brackin's a.
    Braun's a.
    Clado's a.
    Coffey's a.
    crucial a.
    direct transperitoneal
      uterocolic a.
    end-to-end a.
    end-to-side a.
    esophagojejunal a.
    faciohypoglossal a.
    Galen's a.

an·as·to·mo·sis *(continued)*
    genicular a.
    Haight's a.
    heterocladic a.
    homocladic a.
    hypoglossal-facial nerve a.
    Hyrtl's a.
    ileorectal a.
    intermesenteric arterial a.
    intersubcardinal a.
    intestinal a.
    isoperistaltic a.
    lymphaticovenous a.
    meningeal arterial a's
    nerve a.
    portacaval a.
    portosystemic a.
    postcostal a.
    post-transverse a.
    precapillary a.
    precostal a.
    pyeloileocutaneous a.
    rectosigmoid a.
    a. of Riolan
    Roux's a.
    Roux-en-Y a.
    Schmiedel's a.
    side-to-end a.
    side-to-side a.
    splenorenal a.
    stirrup a.
    Sucquet-Hoyer a.
    sutureless a.
    terminoterminal a.
    transureteroureteral a.
    triple a.
    ureteroileocutaneous a.
    ureterotubal a.
    ureteroureteral a.
    ventriculocisternal a.
an·as·to·mot·ic
an·as·tral
an·a·stroph·ic
anat. — anatomical
    anatomy
an·a·tom·ic
an·a·tom·i·cal
an·a·tom·i·co·med·i·cal

an·a·tom·i·co·path·o·log·i·
cal
an·a·tom·i·co·phys·i·o·log·i·
cal
an·a·tom·i·co·sur·gi·cal
anat·o·mism
anat·o·mist
anat·o·mist's snuff-box
an·a·to·mo·pa·thol·o·gy
anat·o·my
    applied a.
    artificial a.
    artistic a.
    clastic a.
    comparative a.
    corrosion a.
    cross-sectional a.
    dental a.
    descriptive a.
    developmental a.
    general a.
    gross a.
    histologic a.
    homologic a.
    macroscopic a.
    medical a.
    microscopic a.
    minute a.
    morbid a.
    pathological a.
    physiognomonic a.
    physiological a.
    plastic a.
    practical a.
    radiological a.
    regional a.
    special a.
    surface a.
    surgical a.
    systematic a.
    topographic a.
    transcendental a.
    veterinary a.
    x-ray a.
ana·tox·ic
ana·tox·in
    diphtheria a.
    a.-Ramon

ana·toxi·re·ac·tion
ana·tri·crot·ic
ana·troph·ic
ana·tro·pia
ana·trop·ic
ana·ven·in
an·az·o·lene so·di·um
ANC — absolute neutrophil
count
AnCC — anodal closure
contraction
An·cef
an·chor
    endosteal implant a.
an·chor·age
    cervical a.
    compound a.
    extramaxillary a.
    extraoral a.
    intermaxillary a.
    intraoral a.
    maxillomandibular a.
    multiple a.
    occipital a.
    reciprocal a.
    reinforced a.
    simple a.
    stationary a.
an·cil·la·ry
an·cip·i·tal
an·cis·troid
An·co·bon
an·con
an·co·nad
an·con·ag·ra
an·co·nal
an·co·ne·al
an·co·ne·us
an·co·ni·tis
an·co·noid
an·crod
An·cy·los·to·ma
    A. americanum
    A. braziliense
    A. caninum
    A. ceylonicum
    A. duodenale
an·cy·lo·sto·mat·ic

an·cylo·stome
an·cy·los·to·mi·a·sis
 a. cutis
 cutaneous a.
 a. dermatitis
An·cy·lo·sto·mi·dae
an·cy·roid
An·der·nach's ossicles
An·ders' disease
An·dersch's ganglion
An·der·sen's disease
An·der·son splint
An·der·son and Gold·ber·ger
 test
An·di·ra
An·dra·de's indicator
An·dral's decubitus
An·dral's sign
An·dré Tho·mas sign
an·drei·o·ma
an·dreo·blas·to·ma
An·dre·sen appliance
An·drews disease
an·dro·blas·to·ma
an·dro·cyte
an·dro·de·do·tox·in
an·droe·ci·um
an·dro·ga·lac·to·ze·mia
an·dro·gam·one
an·dro·gen
 adrenal a.
an·dro·gen·e·sis
an·dro·gen·ic
an·dro·ge·nic·i·ty
an·dro·gen·i·za·tion
an·drog·e·nized
an·drog·e·nous
an·dro·gone
an·dro·gyne
an·drog·y·nism
an·drog·y·noid
an·drog·y·nous
an·drog·y·ny
an·droid
an·droi·dal
an·drol·o·gy
an·dro·ma
An·drom·e·da

an·drom·e·do·tox·in
an·dro·mer·o·gon
an·dro·mer·o·gone
an·dro·me·rog·o·ny
an·dro·mi·met·ic
an·dro·mor·phous
an·drop·a·thy
an·dro·phile
an·droph·i·lous
an·dro·stane
an·dro·stane·di·ol
 a. glucuronide
an·dro·stane·di·one
an·dro·stan·o·lone
an·dro·stene
an·dro·stene·di·ol
an·dro·stene·di·one
an·dros·ter·one
AnDTe — anodal duration
 tetanus
an·ec·do·tal
an·ec·dy·sis
an·echo·ic
an·ec·ta·sis
An·ec·tine
An·el's operation
an·elec·tro·ton·ic
an·elec·trot·o·nus
ane·mia
 achlorhydric a.
 achrestic a.
 achylic a.
 a. achylica
 acquired sideroachrestic a.
 acquired sideroblastic a.
 acute a.
 Addison's a.
 Addison-Biermer a.
 addisonian a.
 aplastic a.
 arctic a.
 aregenerative a.
 aregenerative a., chronic
  congenital
 asiderotic a.
 atrophic a.
 autoimmune hemolytic a.
  (AIHA)

ane·mia *(continued)*
Bagdad Spring a.
Banti's a.
Bartonella a.
Blackfan-Diamond a.
cameloid a.
cattle a.
chlorotic a.
a. of chronic disease
congenital
  dyserythropoietic a.
congenital hypoplastic a.
congenital a. of newborn
congenital nonspherocytic
  hemolytic a.
constitutional aplastic a.
Cooley's a.
Coombs-negative immune
  hemolytic a.
cow's milk a.
crescent cell a.
cytogenic a.
deficiency a.
Diamond-Blackfan a.
dilution a.
dimorphic a.
Dresbach's a.
drug-induced immune
  hemolytic a.
Edelmann's a.
elliptocytary a.
elliptocytotic a.
enzyme deficiency
  hemolytic a.
equine infectious a.
erythroblastic a. of
  childhood
essential a.
Faber's a.
familial erythroblastic a.
Fanconi's a.
febrile pleiochromic a.
fish tapeworm a.
folic acid deficiency a.
fragmentation hemolytic a.
globe cell a.

ane·mia *(continued)*
glucose-6-phosphate
  dehydrogenase deficiency
  a.
goat's milk a.
ground itch a.
Heinz-body a's
hemolytic a.
hemolytic a., acquired
hemolytic a., acute
hemolytic a., congenital
hemolytic a., congenital
  nonspherocytic
hemolytic a., hereditary
  nonspherocytic
hemolytic a., immune
hemolytic a., infectious
hemolytic a.,
  microangiopathic
hemolytic a., toxic
hemorrhagic a.
Herrick's a.
hookworm a.
hyperchromic a.
hypochromic a.
hypochromic a., idiopathic
hypochromic microcytic a.
a. hypochromica sidero-
  chrestica hereditaria
hypoplastic a.
hypoplastic a., congenital
idiopathic a.
immunohemolytic a.
infectious a. of horses
intertropical a.
iron deficiency a.
Israels-Wilkinson a.
lead a.
Lederer's a.
Leishman's a.
leukoerythroblastic a.
lysolecithin hemolytic a.
macrocytic a.
macrocytic a., nutritional
macrocytic a., tropical
malignant a.
Mediterranean a.
megaloblastic a.

ane·mia *(continued)*
  megaloblastic a., familial
  megalocytic a.
  meniscocytic a.
  microangiopathic a.
  microcytic a.
  microdrepanocytic a.
  microelliptopoikilocytic a.
    of Rietti, Greppi, and
    Micheli
  milk a.
  miners'a.
  mountain a.
  myelopathic a.
  myelophthisic a.
  myelosclerotic a.
  a. neonatorum
  normochromic a.
  normocytic a.
  nutritional a.
  osteosclerotic a.
  ovalocytary a.
  pernicious a.
  pernicious a., juvenile
  physiologic a.
  polar a.
  posthemorrhagic a., acute
  posthemorrhagic a. of
    newborn
  primaquine-sensitive a.
  primary a.
  pure red cell a.
  pyridoxine-responsive a.
  pyruvate-kinase deficiency
    a.
  radiation a.
  a. refractoria sideroblastica
  refractory a.
  refractory sideroblastic a.
  Rietti, Greppi, and
    Micheli's a.
  Rundles-Falls a.
  Runeberg's a.
  scorbutic a.
  secondary a.
  sex-linked hypochromatic
    a. of Rundles and Falls
  sickle cell a.

ane·mia *(continued)*
  sideremic a.
  sideroachrestic a.
  sideroblastic a.
  sideropenic a.
  slaty a.
  spherocytic a.
  a. splenetica
  splenic a.
  spur-cell a.
  target cell a.
  thrombotic
    microangiopathic
    hemolytic a.
  toxic a.
  traumatic a.
  triose-phosphate isomerase
    deficiency a.
  tropical a.
  tunnel a.
  unstable hemoglobin
    hemolytic a.
  Wills' a.
  Witts' a.
ane·mic
Anem·o·ne
anem·o·nin
anem·o·nism
anem·o·nol
an·e·mop·a·thy
an·e·mo·pho·bia
an·en·ce·pha·lia
an·en·ceph·a·lic
an·en·ceph·a·lous
an·en·ceph·a·lus
an·en·ceph·a·ly
an·en·ter·ous
aneph·ric
aneph·ro·gen·e·sis
an·ep·i·plo·ic
an·ep·i·thym·ia
an·er·e·thi·sia
an·er·gia
an·er·gic
an·er·gy
  negative a.
  positive a.
an·er·oid

an·eryth·ro·pla·sia
an·eryth·ro·plas·tic
an·eryth·ro·poi·e·sis
an·eryth·rop·sia
an·eryth·ro·re·gen·er·a·tive
anes·the·ci·ne·sia
anes·the·ki·ne·sia
an·es·the·sia
  angiospastic a.
  balanced a.
  basal a.
  Bier's local a.
  block a.
  bulbar a.
  carbon dioxide absorption
   a.
  caudal a.
  central a.
  cerebral a.
  closed a.
  closed-circuit a.
  colonic a.
  compression a.
  conduction a.
  continuous caudal a.
  Corning's a.
  crossed a.
  dissociated a.
  dissociation a.
  doll's head a.
  a. dolorosa
  electric a.
  endobronchial a.
  endotracheal a.
  epidural a.
  facial a.
  field block a.
  frost a.
  gas-oxygen-ether a.
  gauntlet a.
  general a.
  girdle a.
  glove a.
  glove and stocking a.
  gustatory a.
  Gwathmey's oil-ether a.
  high pressure a.
  hyperbaric spinal a.

an·es·the·sia *(continued)*
  hypnosis a.
  hypobaric spinal a.
  hypotensive a.
  hypothermic a.
  hysterical a.
  infiltration a.
  inhalation a.
  insufflation a.
  intercostal a.
  intranasal a.
  intraoral a.
  intraosseous a.
  intrapulpal a.
  intraspinal a.
  intravenous a.
  isobaric spinal a.
  Kulenkampff's a.
  local a.
  lumbar epidural a.
  Meltzer's a.
  mental a.
  mixed a.
  muscular a.
  nasotracheal a.
  nausea a.
  nerve blocking a.
  olfactory a.
  one-lung a.
  open a.
  orotracheal a.
  paracervical block a.
  paraneural a.
  parasacral a.
  paravertebral a.
  partial a.
  peridural a.
  perineural a.
  peripheral a.
  permeation a.
  plexus a.
  pressure a.
  pudendal block a.
  rectal a.
  refrigeration a.
  regional a.
  sacral a.
  saddle block a.

an·es·the·sia *(continued)*
   segmental a.
   semiclosed a.
   semiopen a.
   sexual a.
   spinal a.
   splanchnic a.
   stocking a.
   subarachnoid a.
   surface a.
   surgical a.
   tactile a.
   thalamic hyperesthetic a.
   thermal a.
   thermic a.
   topical a.
   total a.
   transsacral a.
   traumatic a.
   twilight a.
   unilateral a.
   vein a.
   visceral a.
anes·the·sim·e·ter
Anes·the·sin
an·es·the·si·ol·o·gist
an·es·the·si·ol·o·gy
an·es·the·si·o·phore
anes·the·sog·no·sia
an·es·thet·ic
   general a.
   local a.
   topical a.
   volatile a.
anes·the·tist
anes·the·ti·za·tion
anes·the·tize
anes·the·tom·e·ter
an·es·theto·spasm
an·es·trum
an·es·trus
an·e·thene
an·e·thole
aneth·o·path
Ane·thum
anet·ic
an·etio·log·i·cal

an·e·to·der·ma
   Jadassohn's a.
   Jadassohn-Pellizari a.
   perifollicular a.
   postinflammatory a.
   Schweninger-Buzzi a.
an·eu·ga·my
an·eu·ploid
an·eu·ploi·dy
aneu·ri·lem·mic
aneu·rin
an·eu·rine hy·dro·chlo·ride
Aneu·ro·form
aneu·ro·gen·ic
an·eu·rysm
   abdominal a.
   ampullary a.
   aortic a.
   aortic sinusal a.
   arteriovenous a.
   arteriovenous pulmonary
     a.
   atherosclerotic a.
   axillary a.
   bacterial a.
   berry a.
   brain a.
   cardiac a.
   caroticocavernous a.
   cerebral a.
   Charcot-Bouchard a.
   cirsoid a.
   compound a.
   congenital cerebral a.
   cylindroid a.
   dissecting a.
   ectatic a.
   embolic a.
   false a.
   fusiform a.
   hernial a.
   infected a.
   innominate a.
   intracavernous a.
   intracranial a.
   intrathoracic a.
   lateral a.

an·eu·rysm *(continued)*
   miliary a.
   mycotic a.
   orbital a.
   Park's a.
   pelvic a.
   phantom a.
   peripheral a.
   Pott's a.
   racemose a.
   Rasmussen's a.
   renal a.
   Richet's a.
   Rodrigues' a.
   saccular a.
   sacculated a.
   serpentine a.
   Shekelton's a.
   silent a.
   subclinoid a.
   suprasellar a.
   syphilitic a.
   thoracic a.
   thoracoabdominal aortic a.
   traumatic a.
   true a.
   tubular a.
   varicose a.
   venous a.
   ventricular a.
   verminous a.
   worm a.
an·eu·rys·mal
an·eu·rys·mat·ic
an·eu·rys·mec·to·my
an·eu·rys·mog·ra·phy
an·eu·rys·mo·plas·ty
an·eu·rys·mor·rha·phy
an·eu·rys·mot·o·my
ANF — antinuclear factor
an·gei·al
An·gel·chick prosthesis
an·gi·ec·ta·sia
An·gel·i·ca
An·ge·luc·ci's syndrome
An·ger camera
Ang·he·les·cu's sign
an·gi·al·gia

an·gi·as·the·nia
an·gi·ec·ta·sis
an·gi·ec·ta·tic
an·gi·ec·to·my
an·gi·ec·to·pia
ang·i·itis *pl.* an·gi·it·i·des
   allergic granulomatous a.
   consecutive a.
   leukocytoclastic a.
   necrotizing a.
   visceral a.
an·gi·na
   abdominal a.
   a. abdominalis
   a. abdominis
   a. acuta
   agranulocytic a.
   benign croupous a.
   Bretonneau's a.
   a. catarrhalis
   a. cordis
   a. cruris
   a. decubitus
   a. diphtheritica
   a. dyspeptica
   a. epiglottidea
   exertional a.
   exudative a.
   a. follicularis
   fusospirochetal a.
   a. gangrenosa
   hippocratic a.
   hypercyanotic a.
   hysteric a.
   intestinal a.
   a. inversa
   lacunar a.
   a. laryngea
   Ludwig's a.
   malignant a.
   a. membranacea
   neutropenic a.
   a. nosocomii
   a. pectoris
   a. pectoris vasomotoria
   a. phlegmonosa
   Plaut's a.
   preinfarction a.

an·gi·na *(continued)*
    Prinzmetal's a.
    pseudomembranous a.
    a. rheumatica
    a. scarlatinosa
    Schultz's a.
    a. simplex
    a. sine dolore
    a. tonsillaris
    a. trachealis
    ulceromembranous a.
    a. ulcerosa
    unstable a.
    variant a. pectoris
    vasomotor a.
    Vincent's a.
an·gi·nal
an·gin·i·form
an·gi·noid
an·gino·pho·bia
an·gi·nose
an·gi·no·sis
an·gi·nous
an·gio·ac·cess
an·gio·ar·chi·tec·ture
an·gio·as·the·nia
an·gio·atax·ia
an·gio·blast
an·gio·blas·tic
an·gio·blas·te·ma
an·gio·blas·to·ma
an·gio·car·dio·gram
an·gio·car·di·og·ra·phy
    gas a.
    rapid biplane a.
    retrograde a.
    right-sided a.
    selective a.
an·gio·car·dio·ki·net·ic
an·gio·car·di·op·a·thy
an·gio·car·di·tis
an·gio·cath·e·ter
    Ependorf a.
an·gio·cav·er·nous
an·gio·chei·lo·scope
an·gio·chon·dro·ma
an·gio·cine·ma·tog·ra·phy
An·gio-Con·ray

an·gio·crine
an·gio·cri·no·sis
an·gio·cyst
an·gio·derm
an·gio·der·ma·ti·tis
    disseminated pruritic a.
an·gio·di·as·co·py
an·gi·odyn·ia
an·gio·dys·pla·sia
an·gio·dys·tro·phia
    a. ovarii
an·gio·dys·tro·phy
an·gio·ec·tat·ic
an·gio·ede·ma
    hereditary a.
    vibratory a.
an·gio·ede·ma·tous
an·gio·el·e·phan·ti·a·sis
an·gio·en·do·the·li·o·ma
an·gio·en·do·the·li·o·ma·to·sis
    a. proliferans
an·gio·fi·bro·ma
    a. contagiosum tropicum
    intranasal a.
    juvenile a.
    nasopharyngeal a.
an·gio·fol·lic·u·lar
an·gio·gen·e·sis
    tumor a.
an·gio·gen·ic
an·gio·gli·o·ma
an·gio·gli·o·ma·to·sis
an·gio·gram
an·gio·gran·u·lo·ma
an·gio·graph
an·gi·og·ra·phy
    aortic arch a.
    carotid a.
    cerebral a.
    coronary a.
    digital subtraction a.
    emission a.
    fluorescein a.
    intravenous digital
      subtraction a.
    intravenous renal a.
    orbital a.

an·gi·og·ra·phy *(continued)*
   pulmonary a.
   radionuclide a.
   spinal cord a.
   vertebral a.
an·gio·he·mo·phil·ia
an·gio·hy·a·li·no·sis
   a. hemorrhagica
an·gi·oid
an·gio·in·va·sive
an·gio·ker·a·to·ma
   a. circumscriptum
   a. corporis diffusum
   diffuse a.
   a. of Fordyce
   a. of Mibelli
   a. of scrotum
   solitary a.
an·gio·ker·a·to·sis
an·gio·ki·ne·sis
an·gio·ki·net·ic
an·gio·leio·my·o·ma
an·gio·leu·ci·tis
an·gio·leu·ki·tis
an·gio·li·po·leio·my·o·ma
an·gio·li·po·ma
an·gio·lo·gia
an·gi·ol·o·gy
an·gio·lu·poid
an·gio·lym·phan·gi·o·ma
an·gio·lym·phi·tis
an·gi·ol·y·sis
an·gi·o·ma
   a. arteriale racemosum
   arteriovenous a. of brain
   capillary a's
   a. cavernosum
   cavernous a.
   cerebral a.
   cherry a's
   a. cutis
   fissural a.
   hereditary hemorrhagic a.
   hypertrophic a.
   infectious a.
   a. lymphaticum
   plane a.
   plexiform a.

an·gi·o·ma *(continued)*
   sclerosing a.
   senile a's
   a. serpiginosum
   simple a.
   spider a.
   spinal a.
   stellate a.
   strawberry a.
   telangiectatic a.
   tuberous a.
   a. venosum racemosum
   venous a. of brain
an·gi·o·ma·toid
an·gi·o·ma·to·sis
   cerebroretinal a.
   congenital dysplastic a.
   diffuse corticomeningeal a.
   encephalofacial a.
   encephalotrigeminal a.
   hemorrhagic familial a.
   hepatic a.
   oculoencephalic a.
   a. of retina
   retinocerebral a.
   Sturge-Weber a.
an·gi·om·a·tous
an·gio·meg·a·ly
an·gio·myo·li·po·ma
an·gio·my·o·ma
an·gio·myo·neu·ro·ma
an·gio·myo·sar·co·ma
an·gio·myx·o·ma
an·gio·ne·cro·sis
an·gio·neo·plasm
an·gio·neu·ral·gia
an·gio·neu·rec·to·my
an·gio·neu·ro·path·ic
an·gio·neu·rop·a·thy
an·gio·neu·rot·ic
an·gio·neu·rot·o·my
an·gio·no·ma
an·gio-os·teo·hy·per·tro·phy
an·gio·pa·ral·y·sis
an·gio·pa·re·sis
an·gio·path·ol·o·gy
an·gi·op·a·thy
an·gio·phak·o·ma·to·sis

an·gio·plas·ty
   patch a.
   percutaneous transluminal
    a.
an·gio·poi·e·sis
an·gio·poi·et·ic
an·gio·pres·sure
an·gio·re·tic·u·lo·en·do·the·
  li·o·ma
an·gio·re·tic·u·lo·ma
an·gi·or·rha·phy
   arteriovenous a.
an·gio·sar·co·ma
an·gio·scle·ro·sis
an·gio·scle·rot·ic
an·gio·scope
an·gi·os·co·py
an·gio·sco·to·ma
an·gio·sco·tom·e·try
an·gio·spasm
an·gio·spas·tic
an·gio·sperm
an·gio·ste·no·sis
an·gi·os·te·o·sis
an·gi·o·sthe·nia
an·gi·os·to·my
an·gio·stron·gy·li·a·sis
An·gio·stron·gy·lus
   A. cantonensis
   A. costaricensis
   A. vasorum
an·gi·os·tro·phe
an·gi·os·tro·phy
an·gio·te·lec·ta·sis *pl.* an·gio·
  te·lec·ta·ses
an·gio·ten·sin
   a. I
   a. II
   a. amide
an·gio·ten·sin·ase
an·gio·ten·sin-I con·vert·ing
  en·zyme
an·gio·ten·sin·o·gen
an·gio·tome
an·gio·to·mog·ra·phy
an·gi·ot·o·my
an·gio·to·nase
an·gio·to·nia

an·gio·ton·ic
an·gio·to·nin
an·gio·tribe
an·gio·trip·sy
an·gio·troph·ic
an·gi·tis
an·gle
   a. of aberration
   acromial a.
   acromial a. of scapula
   alpha a.
   Alsberg's a.
   alveolar a.
   antegonial a.
   anterior a. of petrous
    portion of temporal bone
   anterior inferior a. of
    parietal bone
   a. of anterior chamber of
    eye
   a. of aperture
   auriculo-occipital a.
   axial a.
   axial line a.
   basal a.
   Bauman's a.
   Bennett a.
   beta a.
   biorbital a.
   Böhler's a.
   Boogaard's a.
   Broca's a.
   buccal a's
   Bull's a.
   cardiodiaphragmatic a.
   cardiohepatic a.
   cardiophrenic a.
   carrying a.
   cavity a's
   cavosurface a.
   cephalic a.
   cephalic-medullary a.
   cephalometric a.
   cerebellopontile a.
   chi a.
   collodiaphyseal a.
   condylar a.
   a. of convergence

an·gle *(continued)*
a. of convexity
coronary a.
costal a.
costophrenic a.
costosternal a.
costovertebral a.
craniofacial a.
critical a.
cusp a.
cusp plane a.
Daubenton's a.
a. of declination
a. of deviation
a. of direction
distal a's
duodenojejunal a.
Ebstein's a.
elevation a.
epigastric a.
ethmocranial a.
ethmoid a.
external a. of border of
  tibia
external a. of scapula
facial a.
a. of femoral torsion
filtration a.
Frankfort-mandibular
  plane a.
frontal a. of parietal bone
gamma a.
gonial a.
horizontal a.
ileocolic a.
a. of incidence
incisal a.
incisal guide a.
incisal mandibular plane a.
a. of inclination
inferior a. of duodenum
inferior a. of parietal bone,
  anterior
inferior a. of parietal bone,
  posterior
inferior a. of scapula
infrasternal a. of thorax
inner a. of eye

an·gle *(continued)*
inner a. of humerus
internal a. of tibia
iridial a.
iridocorneal a.
a. of iris
Jacquart's a.
a. of jaw
kappa a.
kyphotic a.
labial a's
lambda a.
lateral a. of border of tibia
lateral a. of cerebellum
lateral a. of eye
lateral a. of humerus
lateral a. of scapula
limiting a.
line a.
lingual a's
Louis' a.
Ludwig's a.
lumbosacral a.
a. of mandible
mandibular a.
manubriosternal a.
mastoid a. of parietal bone
maxillary a.
medial a. of eye
medial a. of humerus
medial a. of scapula
medial a. of tibia
mesial a's
metafacial a.
meter a.
Mikulicz's a.
a. of minimum deviation
minimum separabile a.
minimum separable a.
minimum visible a.
minimum visual a.
a. of mouth
a. of Mulder
nasal a. of eye
neck shaft a.
nu a.
occipital a.
occipital a. of parietal bone

an·gle *(continued)*
  ocular a's
  olfactive a.
  olfactory a.
  ophryospinal a.
  optic a.
  orifacial a.
  outer a. of eye
  parietal a.
  parietal a. of sphenoid bone
  a. of pelvis
  pelvivertebral a.
  phrenopericardial a.
  Pirogoff's a.
  point a.
  a. of polarization
  posterior inferior a. of
    parietal bone
  posterior a. of petrous
    portion of temporal bone
  principal a.
  prism a.
  a. of pubis
  QRS-T a.
  Quatrefage's a.
  Ranke's a.
  a. of reflection
  refracting a.
  a. of refraction
  a. of rib
  rolandic a.
  a. of Rolando
  sacrovertebral a.
  scattering a.
  Serres' a.
  sigma a.
  sinodural a.
  solid a.
  somatosplanchnic a.
  sphenoid a.
  sphenoidal a.
  sphenoidal a. of parietal
    bone
  squint a.
  sternal a.
  sternoclavicular a.
  a. of sternum
  subcostal a.

an·gle *(continued)*
  subpubic a.
  subscapular a.
  substernal a.
  superior a. of duodenum
  superior a. of parietal bone,
    anterior
  superior a. of parietal bone,
    posterior
  superior a. of petrous
    portion of temporal bone
  superior a. of scapula
  a. of supination
  a. of Sylvius
  temporal a.
  tentorial a.
  tooth a's
  Topinard's a.
  a. of torsion
  tuber a.
  uterine a.
  venous a.
  vertical a.
  vesicourethral a.
  vesicourethral a., anterior
  vesicourethral a., posterior
  a. of Virchow
  visual a.
  Vogt's a.
  Weisbach's a.
  Welcher's a.
  xiphoid a's
  Y a.
An·gle's classification
An·gle's splint
an·gle-form·er
ang·li·cus su·dor
an·go·phra·sia
an·gor
  a. animi
  a. nocturnus
  a. ocularis
  a. pectoris
ang·strom
  reciprocal a.
Ang·ström's law
Ang·ström's unit

An·guil·lu·la
  A. *aceti*
  A. *intestinalis*
  A. *stercoralis*
an·gu·lar
an·gu·la·tion
an·gu·li
an·gu·lus *pl.* an·gu·li
  a. acromialis
  a. costae
  a. infectiosus
  a. inferior scapulae
  a. infrasternalis thoracis
  a. iridis
  a. iridocornealis
  a. lateralis scapulae
  a. lateralis tibiae
  a. Ludovici
  a. mandibulae
  a. medialis scapulae
  a. medialis tibiae
  a. oculi lateralis
  a. oculi medialis
  a. oris
  a. pubis
  a. sternalis
  a. sterni
  a. subpubicus
  a. superior scapulae
  a. venosus
an·hal·o·nine
An·ha·lo·ni·um le·wi·nii
an·ha·phia
an·hap·to·glo·bin·emia
an·he·do·nia
an·he·mo·poi·e·sis
an·hi·dro·sis
  postmiliarial a.
  thermogenic a.
an·hi·drot·ic
an·his·tic
an·hy·drase
an·hy·dra·tion
an·hy·dre·mia
an·hy·dride
  acetic a.
  arsenous a.
  chromic a.

an·hy·dride *(continued)*
  perosmic a.
  silicic a.
  sorbitol a.
  sulfurous a.
  trimellitic a.
an·hy·dro·chlo·ric
an·hy·dro·hy·droxy·pro·ges·ter·one
An·hy·dron
an·hy·dro·sug·ar
an·hy·drous
ani·a·cin·am·i·do·sis
ani·a·ci·no·sis
Anich·kov's (Anitsch·kow's) cell
Anich·kov's (Anitsch·kow's) myocyte
an·ic·ter·ic
anid·e·an
anid·e·us
  embryonic a.
an·i·dox·ime
an·idro·sis
an·idrot·ic
an·ile
an·i·ler·i·dine
  a. hydrochloride
an·i·lid
an·i·lide
an·i·line
ani·lin·gus
an·i·lin·ism
an·i·lism
anil·i·ty
an·il·o·pam hy·dro·chlo·ride
an·il-quin·o·line
an·i·ma
  a. mundi
an·i·mal
  bulbopontine a.
  control a.
  conventional a.
  decerebrate a.
  decorticate a.
  experimental a.
  Houssay a.
  hyperphagic a.

an·i·mal *(continued)*
 Long-Lukens a.
 spinal a.
 thalamic a.
an·i·mal·cu·list
an·i·ma·tion
 suspended a.
an·i·mism
an·i·mus
an·ion
an·ion·ic
an·ion·ot·ro·py
an·irid·ia
an·i·sa·ki·a·sis
An·i·sa·kis
 A. marina
an·i·sate
an·is·chu·ria
an·ise
 Chinese a.
 Indian a.
 star a.
an·is·ei·ko·nia
an·is·ei·kon·ic
an·is·er·gy
anis·ic acid
an·is·in·di·one
an·iso·ac·com·mo·da·tion
an·iso·chro·ma·sia
an·iso·chro·mat·ic
an·iso·chro·mia
an·iso·co·ria
an·iso·cy·to·sis
an·iso·dac·ty·lous
an·iso·dac·ty·ly
an·iso·di·a·met·ric
an·iso·dont
an·iso·gam·ete
an·iso·ga·met·ic
an·isog·a·mous
an·isog·a·my
an·iso·ico·nia
an·iso·kary·o·sis
An·iso·lo·bis
an·iso·mas·tia
an·iso·me·lia
an·iso·mer·ic
an·iso·met·rope

an·iso·me·tro·pia
an·iso·me·trop·ic
An·iso·mor·pha
 A. buprestoides
an·iso·mor·phous
an·iso·pho·ria
an·iso·pia
an·iso·pi·esis
an·iso·poi·ki·lo·cy·to·sis
an·i·sos·mot·ic
an·iso·spore
an·isos·po·rous
an·iso·sthen·ic
an·iso·ton·ic
an·iso·tro·pal
an·iso·trop·ic
an·i·so·tro·pine meth·yl·bro·mide
an·isot·ro·py
an·i·su·ria
ani·trog·e·nous
an·kle
 cocked a.
 deck a's
 a. mortise
 tailors'a.
an·ky·lo·bleph·a·ron
 a. filiforme adnatum
an·ky·lo·chei·lia
an·ky·lo·col·pos
an·ky·lo·dac·ty·ly
an·ky·lo·glos·sia
 complete a.
 partial a.
 a. superior
an·ky·lo·poi·et·ic
an·ky·losed
an·ky·lo·ses
an·ky·lo·sis *pl.* an·ky·lo·ses
 artificial a.
 bony a.
 capsular a.
 cricoarytenoid joint a.
 dental a.
 extra-articular a.
 extracapsular a.
 false a.
 fibrous a.

an·ky·lo·sis *(continued)*
    intracapsular a.
    ligamentous a.
    operative a.
    partial a.
    spurious a.
    stapedial a.
    a. of stapes
    true a.
    unsound a.
an·ky·lo·sto·mi·a·sis
an·ky·lot·ic
an·ky·lot·o·my
an·kyl·ure·thria
an·ky·rin
an·kyr·ism
an·ky·roid
an·lage *pl.* an·la·gen
ANLL — acute
  nonlymphocytic leukemia
An·nan·dale's operation
an·neal
an·nec·tent
an·ne·lid
An·ne·li·da
An·no·na
an·not·to
an·nu·lar
an·nu·late
an·nu·let
an·nu·li
an·nu·lo·plas·ty
an·nu·lor·rha·phy
an·nu·lo·spi·ral
an·nu·lot·o·my
an·nu·lus *pl.* an·nu·li
    a. abdominalis
    a. ciliaris
    a. of conjunctiva
    a. conjunctivae
    a. femorais
    annuli fibrosi cordis
    a. inguinalis profundus
    a. inguinalis subcutaneus
    a. inguinalis superficialis
    a. iridis major
    a. iridis minor
    a. lymphaticus cardiae

an·nu·lus *(continued)*
    a. of nuclear pore
    a. ovalis
    a. of spermatozoon
    a. tendineus communis
    a. tracheae
    tympanic a.
    a. tympanicus
    a. umbilicalis
    a. urethralis
    Vieussens'a.
    a. of Zinn
AnOC — anodal opening
  contraction
ano·chro·ma·sia
ano·ci·as·so·ci·a·tion
ano·ci·ated
ano·ci·a·tion
ano·ci·the·sia
ano·coc·cy·ge·al
ano·cu·ta·ne·ous
an·o·dal
an·ode
    hooded a.
    rotating a.
ano·derm
an·od·mia
an·odon·tia
    partial a.
    total a.
    true a.
    a. vera
an·odon·tism
an·o·dyne
ano·gen·i·tal
anol
anom·a·lad
    amniotic band a.
    Robin's a.
anom·a·lo·scope
anom·al·ot·ro·phy
anom·a·lous
anom·a·ly
    Alder's a.
    Alder's constitutional
      granulation a.
    Alder-Reilly a.
    Alius-Grignaschi a.

anom·a·ly *(continued)*
    Aristotle's a.
    Axenfeld's a.
    Chédiak-Higashi a.
    Chédiak-Steinbrinck-
      Higashi a.
    Chiari's a.
    chromosomal a.
    chromosome a.
    congenital a.
    cor triatratum a.
    craniovertebral a's
    developmental a.
    Ebstein's a.
    fetal a.
    Freund's a.
    Hegglin's a.
    Jordan's a.
    May-Hegglin a.
    morning glory a.
    Pelger's nuclear a.
    Pelger-Huët a.
    Pelger-Huët nuclear a.
    Peters' a.
    Pierre Robin a.
    Poland's a.
    Rieger's a.
    Shone's a.
    Steinbrinck's a.
    Taussig-Bing a.
    Uhl's a.
    Undritz a.
an·o·mer
an·o·mer·ic
ano·mia
an·onych·ia
anon·y·ma
anon·y·mous
ano·pel·vic
ano·per·i·ne·al
Anoph·e·les
    A. albimanus
    A. balabacensis
    A. culicifacies
    A. darlingi
    A. dirus
    A. freeborni
    A. funestus

Anoph·e·les (continued)
    A. gambiae
    A. labranchiae
    A. maculipennis
    A. pseudopunctipennis
    A. quadrimaculatus
    A. superpictus
anoph·e·li·cide
anoph·e·li·fuge
anoph·e·line
Anoph·e·li·ni
anoph·e·lism
an·o·pho·ria
an·oph·thal·mia
an·oph·thal·mos
an·o·pia
an·op·sia
ano·plas·ty
An·op·lo·ce·phal·i·dae
An·o·plu·ra
an·or·chia
an·or·chid
an·or·chid·ic
an·or·chi·dism
an·or·chism
ano·rec·tal
ano·rec·tic
ano·rec·ti·tis
ano·rec·to·co·lon·ic
ano·rec·to·plas·ty
    Laird-McMahon a.
ano·rec·tum
ano·ret·ic
an·orex·ia
    hysterical a.
    a. nervosa
ano·rex·i·ant
ano·rex·ic
ano·rex·i·gen·ic
an·or·gan·ic
an·or·gas·my
an·or·thog·ra·phy
an·or·tho·pia
an·or·tho·scope
ano·scope
anos·co·py
ano·sig·moi·do·scop·ic
ano·sig·moi·dos·co·py

an·os·mat·ic
an·os·mia
    a. gustatoria
    preferential a.
    a. respiratoria
an·os·mic
ano·sog·no·sia
an·os·phra·sia
ano·spi·nal
an·os·teo·pla·sia
an·os·to·sis
an·otia
ano·tro·pia
an·otus
ANOVA — analysis of
  variance
ano·vag·i·nal
an·ovar·ia
an·ovar·i·an·ism
an·ovar·ism
ano·ves·i·cal
an·ov·u·lar
an·ov·u·la·tion
an·ov·u·la·to·ry
an·ov·u·lo·men·or·rhea
an·ox·emia
an·ox·emic
anox·ia
    altitude a.
    anemic a.
    anoxic a.
    diffuse cerebral a.
    fetal a.
    fulminating a.
    histotoxic a.
    myocardial a.
    a. neonatorum
    stagnant a.
anox·i·ate
anox·ic
ANS — anterior nasal spine
  autonomic nervous system
an·sa *pl.* an·sae
    a. cervicalis
    a. of Galen
    a. of Haller
    Henle's a.
    a. hypoglossi

an·sa *(continued)*
    a. lenticularis
    ansae nervorum spinalium
    a. peduncularis
    a. sacralis
    a. subclavia
    a. of Vieussens
    a. vitellina
    a. of Wrisberg
an·sae
an·sa·my·cin
an·sate
Ans·bach·er unit
an·ser·ine
anserinus
an·si·form
An·so·ly·sen
an·sot·o·my
An·spor
An·stie's limit
An·stie's rule
ant. — anterior
An·ta·buse
ant·ac·id
an·tag·glu·ti·nin
an·tag·o·nism
    bacterial a.
    metabolic a.
    salt a.
an·tag·o·nist
    adrenergic a.
    aldosterone a.
    alpha-adrenergic a.
    associated a's
    beta-adrenergic a.
    calcium a.
    competitive a.
    direct a's
    enzyme a.
    folic acid a.
    insulin a.
    metabolic a.
    narcotic a.
    sulfonamide a.
an·tal·ge·sia
ant·al·ge·sic
ant·al·gic
ant·al·ka·line

ant·aph·ro·di·si·ac
ant·ap·o·plec·tic
ant·arth·ri·tic
ant·as·then·ic
ant·asth·mat·ic
ant·atroph·ic
an·taz·o·line
    a. hydrochloride
    a. phosphate
an·te·bra·chi·al
an·te·bra·chi·um
an·te·car·di·um
an·te·ce·dent
    plasma thromboplastin a.
    (PTA)
an·te ci·bum
an·te·col·ic
an·te·cu·bi·tal
an·te·cur·va·ture
an·te·flect
an·te·flexed
an·te·flex·io
    a. uteri
an·te·flex·ion
an·te·go·ni·al
an·te·grade
an·te·lo·ca·tion
an·te mor·tem
an·te·mor·tem
an·te·na·tal
an·ten·na *pl.* an·ten·nae
An·te·par
an·te·par·tal
an·te par·tum
an·te·par·tum
an·te·phase
an·te·phi·al·tic
an·te·po·si·tion
an·te pran·di·um
an·te·pros·tate
an·te·pros·tat·ic
an·te·pros·ta·ti·tis
an·te·py·ret·ic
an·ter·eth·ic
An·ter·gan
an·te·ri·ad
an·ter·i·or
an·tero·clu·sion

an·tero·ex·ter·nal
an·tero·grade
an·tero·in·fer·i·or
an·tero·in·ter·i·or
an·tero·in·ter·nal
an·tero·lat·er·al
an·tero·lis·the·sis
an·tero·me·di·al
an·tero·me·di·an
an·tero·pa·ri·e·tal
an·tero·pos·ter·i·or
an·tero·pul·sion
an·tero·sep·tal
an·tero·su·per·i·or
ant·erot·ic
an·tero·trans·verse
an·tero·ven·tral
an·te·ver·sion
ant·he·lix
ant·hel·min·thic
ant·hel·min·tic
an·thel·my·cin
an·the·lot·ic
An·the·mis
ant·hem·or·rhag·ic
an·ther
an·ther·id·i·um *pl.* an·ther·
    id·ia
an·thero·zoid
ant·her·pet·ic
an·tho·cy·an·i·din
an·tho·cy·an·in
an·tho·cy·a·nin·emia
an·tho·cy·a·nin·uria
An·tho·my·ia
An·tho·my·ii·dae
An·tho·zoa
an·thra·cene
an·thrac·ic
an·thra·coid
an·thra·co·ma
an·thra·com·e·ter
an·thra·co·ne·cro·sis
an·thra·co·sil·i·co·sis
an·thra·co·sis
    a. linguae
an·thra·co·ther·a·py
an·thra·cot·ic

an·thra·cy·cline
An·thra-Derm
an·thra·lin
an·thra·my·cin
an·thra·nil·ic acid
an·thra·quin·one
an·thra·ro·bin
an·thrax
    agricultural a.
    cerebral a.
    cutaneous a.
    gastrointestinal a.
    industrial a.
    inhalational a.
    intestinal a.
    malignant a.
    meningeal a.
    pulmonary a.
    symptomatic a.
an·throne
an·thro·po·bi·ol·o·gy
an·thro·po·cen·tric
an·throp·ogen·ic
an·thro·pog·e·nous
an·thro·pog·e·ny
an·thro·pog·ra·phy
an·thro·poid
An·thro·poi·dea
an·thro·po·ki·net·ics
an·thro·pol·o·gy
    criminal a.
    cultural a.
    forensic a.
    hematological a.
    pathological a.
    physical a.
    social a.
    zoological a.
an·thro·pom·e·ter
an·thro·po·met·ric
an·thro·pom·e·trist
an·thro·pom·e·try
    forensic a.
    nutritional a.
an·thro·po·mor·phic
an·thro·po·mor·phism
an·thro·pon·o·my
an·thro·po·no·sis

an·thro·pop·a·thy
an·thro·po·phil·ic
an·thro·po·pho·bia
an·thro·pos·co·py
an·thro·po·zoo·no·sis
an·thro·po·zoo·phil·ic
ant·hys·ter·ic
an·ti·abor·ti·fa·cient
an·ti·ad·re·ner·gic
an·ti·ag·glu·ti·nin
an·ti·al·bu·min
an·ti·ame·bic
an·ti·am·y·lase
an·ti·ana·phy·lax·is
an·ti·an·dro·gen
an·ti·ane·mic
an·ti·an·gi·nal
an·ti·anoph·e·line
an·ti·an·ti·bo·dy
an·ti·an·ti·dote
an·ti·an·ti·tox·in
an·ti·an·xi·e·ty
an·ti·ap·o·plec·tic
an·ti·ar·ach·nol·y·sin
an·ti·a·rin
An·ti·a·ris
an·ti·ar·rhyth·mic
an·ti·ar·thrit·ic
an·ti·asth·mat·ic
an·ti·ath·ero·gen·ic
an·ti·au·tol·y·sin
an·ti·bac·te·ri·al
an·ti·bech·ic
an·ti·bi·o·sis
an·ti·bi·ot·ic
    broad-spectrum a.
    β-lactam a.
    macrolide a.
    polyene a.
an·ti·blas·tic
an·ti·blen·nor·rha·gic
an·ti·body
    acetylcholine receptor a's
    anaphylactic a.
    anti–acetylcholine receptor
      (anti-AChR) a's
    anti-D a.
    anti-DNA a.

an·ti·body *(continued)*
anti–glomerular basement
  membrane (anti-GEM) a's
anti-idiotype a.
antireceptor a's
antimicrosomal a's
antimitochondrial a's
antinuclear a's (ANA)
antithyroglobulin a's
antithyroid a's
auto-anti-idiotypic a's
autologous a.
bispecific a.
blocking a.
cell-bound a.
cell-fixed a.
cold a.
cold-reactive a.
complement-fixing a.
complete a.
cross-reacting a.
cytophilic a.
cytotoxic a.
cytotropic a.
duck virus hepatitis yolk a.
Forssman a.
heteroclitic a.
heterocytotropic a.
heterogenetic a.
heterophil a., heterophile
  a.
homocytotropic a.
hybrid a.
immune a.
incomplete a.
isophil a.
mitochondrial a's
monoclonal a's
natural a's
neutralizing a.
P-K a's
polyclonal a.,
Prausnitz-Küstner a's
protective a.
reaginic a.
Rh a's
saline a.
sensitizing a.

an·ti·body *(continued)*
TSH-displacing a. (TDA)
warm a.
warm-reactive a.
an·ti·bro·mic
an·ti·bu·bon·ic
an·ti·ca·chec·tic
an·ti·cal·cu·lous
an·ti·car·cin·o·gen
an·ti·car·ci·no·gen·ic
an·ti·car·di·um
an·ti·car·io·gen·ic
an·ti·car·i·ous
an·ti·cat·a·lyst
an·ti·cat·a·lyz·er
an·ti·ca·thex·is
an·ti·ceph·a·lal·gic
an·ti·chei·rot·o·nus
an·ti·chlo·rot·ic
an·ti·cho·le·litho·gen·ic
an·ti·cho·les·ter·emic
an·ti·cho·les·te·rol·emic
an·ti·cho·lin·er·gic
an·ti·cho·lin·es·ter·ase
an·ti·chy·mo·sin
an·ti·ci·pate
an·ti·ci·pa·tion
an·ti·clin·al
an·tic·ne·mi·on
an·ti·co·ag·u·lant
  circulating a.
  lupus a.
an·ti·co·ag·u·la·tive
an·ti·co·ag·u·lin
an·ti·co·don
an·ti·col·la·gen·ase
an·ti·com·ple·ment
an·ti·com·ple·men·ta·ry
an·ti·con·cep·tive
an·ti·con·vul·sant
an·ti·con·vul·sive
an·ti·cro·tin
an·ti·cu·ra·re
an·ti·cus
an·ti·cy·tol·y·sin
an·ti·cy·to·tox·in
an·ti-D
an·ti·de·pres·sant

an·ti·de·pres·sant
    tricyclic a's
an·ti·di·a·bet·ic
an·ti·di·a·be·to·gen·ic
an·ti·di·ar·rhe·al
an·ti·di·ar·rhe·ic
an·ti·di·u·re·sis
an·ti·di·uret·ic
an·ti·dot·al
an·ti·dote
    chemical a.
    Hall a.
    mechanical a.
    physiologic a.
    "universal" a.
an·ti·dot·ic
an·ti·drom·ic
an·ti·dys·en·ter·ic
an·ti·ec·ze·mat·ic
an·ti·ec·zem·a·tous
an·ti·edem·a·tous
an·ti·edem·ic
an·ti·emet·ic
an·ti·en·zyme
an·ti·ep·i·lep·tic
an·ti·ep·i·the·li·al
an·ti·er·ot·i·ca
an·ti·eryth·ro·cyte
an·ti·es·ter·ase
an·ti·es·tro·gen
an·ti·es·tro·gen·ic
an·ti·fe·brile
an·ti·fe·brin
an·ti·fib·ril·la·tory
an·ti·fi·bri·nol·y·sin
an·ti·fi·bri·no·lyt·ic
an·ti·fi·lar·i·al
an·ti·flat·u·lent
an·ti·flux
an·ti·fol
an·ti·fo·late
an·ti·fun·gal
an·ti·ga·lac·tic
an·ti·ga·me·to·cyte
an·ti·ge·lat·i·nase
an·ti·gen
    accessible a.
    allogeneic a.

an·ti·gen *(continued)*
    Am a's
    Au (Australia) a.
    autologous a.
    ayr a.
    ayw1 a.
    ayw2 a.
    ayw3 a.
    ayw4 a.
    B a.
    blood-group a's
    Boivin a.
    C a.
    capsular a.
    carbohydrate a's
    carcinoembryonic a. (CEA)
    chick embryo a.
    class I a's
    class II a's
    class III a's
    common a.
    common acute
      lymphoblastic leukemia
      a. (CALLA)
    common enterobacterial a.
    common leukocyte a's
    complement-fixing a.
    complete a.
    conjugated a.
    cross-reacting a.
    D a.
    delta a.
    E a.
    extractable nuclear a's
      (ENA)
    F a.
    febrile a's
    fetal a's
    flagellar a.
    Forssman a.
    Frei a.
    Gm a's
    group-specific a.
    H a.
    H-2 a's
    hepatitis a.
    hepatitis-associated a.
      (HAA)

an·ti·gen *(continued)*
    hepatitis B core a. (HBcAg)
    hepatitis B e a. (HBeAg)
    hepatitis B surface a.
      (HBsAg)
    heterogeneic a.
    heterogenetic a.
    heterologous a.
    heterophil a.
    Hikojima a.
    histocompatibility a's
    histocompatibility a's,
      major
    histocompatibility a's,
      minor
    HLA a's
    homologous a.
    H-Y a.
    Ia a.
    Inaba a.
    incomplete a.
    Inv group a.
    isogeneic a.
    isophile a.
    K a.
    Km a's
    Kunin a.
    Kveim a.
    LD a's
    lens a's
    Ly a's
    Lyb a's
    Lyt a's
    lymphocyte-defined (LD)
      a's
    lymphogranuloma
      venereum a.
    M a.
    Mitsuda a.
    mumps skin test a.
    NP a.
    nuclear a's
    O a.
    oncofetal a.
    organ-specific a.
    Oz a.
    pancreatic oncofetal a.
      (POA)

an·ti·gen *(continued)*
    partial a.
    pollen a.
    Pr a.
    private a's
    protective a.
    public a's
    recall a.
    SD a's
    self-a.
    sequestered a's
    sero-defined (SD) a's
    serologically defined (SD)
      a's
    serum hepatitis (SH) a.
    shock a.
    Sm a.
    somatic a's
    species-specific a's
    SS-A a.
    SS-B a.
    surface a.
    T a.
    Tac a.
    T-dependent a.
    theta (θ) a.
    Thy 1 a.
    thymus-dependent a.
    thymus-independent a.
    T-independent a.
    tissue-specific a.
    TL (thymus leukemia) a.
    transplantation a's
    tumor-associated a.
    tumor-specific a. (TSA)
    tumor-specific
      transplantation a. (TSTA)
    VDRL a.
    Vi a.
    viral capsid a.
    xenogeneic a.
an·ti·gen·emia
an·ti·gen·emic
an·ti·gen·ic
an·ti·ge·nic·i·ty
an·ti·ger·mi·nal
an·ti·glob·u·lin
an·ti·gly·ox·a·lase

an·ti·goit·ro·gen·ic
an·ti·go·nado·trop·ic
an·ti·growth
an·ti·hal·lu·cin·a·to·ry
an·ti-HBc
an·ti-HBs
an·ti·he·lix
an·ti·hel·min·tic
an·ti·he·mag·glu·ti·nin
an·ti·he·mol·y·sin
an·ti·he·mo·lyt·ic
an·ti·he·mo·phil·ic
an·ti·hem·or·rhag·ic
an·ti·het·er·ol·y·sin
an·ti·hi·drot·ic
an·ti·his·ta·mine
an·ti·his·ta·min·ic
an·ti·hor·mone
an·ti·hy·a·lu·ron·i·dase
an·ti·hy·drop·ic
an·ti·hy·per·cho·les·ter·ol·emic
an·ti·hy·per·gly·ce·mic
an·ti·hy·per·lipo·pro·tein·emic
an·ti·hy·per·ten·sive
an·ti·hyp·not·ic
an·ti·hy·po·ten·sive
an·ti·hy·ster·ic
an·ti-ic·ter·ic
an·ti-id·io·type
an·ti-in·fec·tious
an·ti-in·fec·tive
an·ti-in·flam·ma·to·ry
an·ti-in·su·lin
an·ti-isol·y·sin
an·ti·keno·tox·in
an·ti·ke·to·gen
an·ti·ke·to·gen·e·sis
an·ti·ke·to·ge·net·ic
an·ti·ke·to·gen·ic
an·ti·ke·to·plas·tic
an·ti·leish·ma·ni·al
an·ti·lep·rot·ic
an·ti·leu·ke·mic
an·ti·leu·ko·ci·din
an·ti·leu·ko·cyt·ic
an·ti·leu·ko·pro·te·ase

an·ti·leu·ko·tox·in
an·ti·lew·is·ite
    British a. (BAL)
an·ti·li·pe·mic
an·ti·lipo·trop·ic
an·ti·lipo·trop·ism
An·ti·lir·i·um
an·ti·lith·ic
an·ti·lu·et·ic
an·ti·lym·pho·cyt·ic
an·ti·ly·sin
an·ti·ly·sis
an·ti·lyt·ic
an·ti·ma·lar·i·al
an·ti·me·nin·go·coc·cic
an·ti·men·or·rha·gic
an·ti·me·phit·ic
an·ti·mere
an·ti·mes·en·ter·ic
an·ti·me·tab·o·lite
an·ti·met·he·mo·glo·bin·emic
an·ti·me·tro·pia
an·ti·mi·cro·bi·al
an·ti·min·er·alo·cor·ti·coid
An·ti·minth
an·ti·mi·to·chon·dri·al
an·ti·mi·tot·ic
an·ti·mon·gol·ism
an·ti·mon·go·loid
an·ti·mo·ni·al
an·ti·mo·nic
    a. acid
an·ti·mo·nid
    lithium a.
an·ti·mo·ni·ous
an·ti·mo·ni·um
an·ti·mo·ny
    a. pentoxide
    a. potassium tartrate
    a. sodium
       dimercaptosuccinate
    a. sodium tartrate
    tartrated a.
    a. trioxide
an·ti·mo·nyl
an·ti·morph
an·ti·mor·phic
an·ti·mus·ca·rin·ic

an·ti·mu·ta·gen
an·ti·my·as·then·ic
an·ti·my·co·bac·te·ri·al
an·ti·my·cot·ic
an·ti·nar·cot·ic
an·ti·na·tri·ure·sis
an·ti·nau·se·ant
an·ti·neo·plas·tic
an·ti·neo·plas·ton
an·ti·ne·phrit·ic
an·ti·neu·ral·gic
an·ti·neu·rit·ic
an·ti·neu·ro·tox·in
an·ti·neu·tri·no
an·ti·neu·tron
an·tin·i·ad
an·tin·i·al
an·tin·ion
an·ti·nu·cle·ar
an·ti·odon·tal·gic
an·ti·on·cot·ic
an·ti·ophid·i·ca
an·ti·op·so·nin
an·ti·ov·u·la·to·ry
an·ti·ox·i·dant
an·ti·ox·i·dase
an·ti·ox·i·da·tion
an·ti·oxy·gen
an·ti·par·al·lel
an·ti·par·a·lyt·ic
an·ti·par·a·sit·ic
an·ti·pa·ras·ta·ta
an·ti·para·sym·patho·mi·
   met·ic
an·ti·par·kin·so·ni·an
an·ti·par·ti·cle
an·ti·path·o·gen·ic
an·ti·pe·dic·u·lar
an·ti·ped·i·cu·lot·ic
an·ti·pep·sin
an·ti·pe·ri·od·ic
an·ti·per·i·stal·sis
an·ti·per·i·stal·tic
an·ti·per·spir·ant
an·ti·pha·go·cyt·ic
an·ti·phlo·gis·tic
an·ti·phry·nol·y·sin
an·ti·phthi·ri·ac

an·ti·phthis·ic
an·ti·plas·min
   α_2-a.
an·ti·plas·mo·di·al
an·ti·plas·tic
an·ti·plate·let
an·ti·pneu·mo·coc·cal
an·ti·pneu·mo·coc·cic
an·ti·po·dag·ric
an·tip·o·dal
an·ti·pode
an·ti·poly·cy·the·mic
an·ti·port
an·ti·po·sia
an·ti·prax·ia
an·ti·praxy
an·ti·pre·ci·pi·tin
an·ti·pros·tate
an·ti·pro·te·ase
an·ti·pro·throm·bin
an·ti·pro·to·zo·al
an·ti·pro·to·zo·an
an·ti·pru·ri·tic
an·ti·pso·ri·at·ic
an·ti·psy·cho·mo·tor
an·ti·psy·chot·ic
an·ti·pu·tre·fac·tive
an·ti·pyo·gen·ic
an·ti·py·re·sis
an·ti·py·ret·ic
an·ti·py·rine
an·ti·py·rot·ic
an·ti·ra·chit·ic
an·ti·ra·di·a·tion
an·ti·ren·nin
an·ti·re·tic·u·lar
an·ti·rheu·mat·ic
an·ti·ric·in
an·ti·rick·ett·si·al
an·ti·ro·bin
an·ti·sal·ure·sis
an·ti·sca·bi·et·ic
an·ti·sca·bi·ous
an·ti·schis·to·so·mal
an·ti·scor·bu·tic
an·ti·seb·or·rhe·ic
an·ti·sec·re·to·ry
an·ti·self

an·ti·sense
an·ti·sep·sis
    physiologic a.
an·ti·sep·tic
    Dakin's a.
an·ti·se·rum
    Erysipelothrix
      rhusiopathiae a.
    heterologous a.
    homologous a.
    monospecific a.
    monovalent a.
    nerve growth factor a.
    polyvalent a.
    rabies a.
    Rh (rhesus) a.
    therapeutic a.
an·ti·si·al·a·gogue
an·ti·si·al·ic
an·ti·sid·er·ic
an·ti·so·cial
an·ti·spas·mod·ic
    biliary a.
    bronchial a.
an·ti·spas·tic
an·ti·sper·mo·tox·in
an·ti·staph·y·lo·coc·cic
an·ti·staph·y·lo·he·mol·y·sin
an·ti·staph·y·lol·y·sin
an·ti·ste ·ril·i·ty
an·ti·ster·num
An·tis·tine
an·ti·strep·to·coc·cic
an·ti·strep·to·ki·nase
an·ti·strep·tol·y·sin
an·ti·su·do·ral
an·ti·su·dor·if·ic
an·ti·sym·pa·thet·ic
an·ti·syph·i·lit·ic
an·ti·tei·cho·ic acid
an·ti·tem·plate
an·ti·te·tan·ic
an·ti·te·ta·nol·y·sin
an·ti·the·nar
an·ti·ther·mic
an·ti·throm·bin
    a. I
    a. III

an·ti·throm·bo·plas·tin
an·ti·throm·bot·ic
an·ti·thy·mo·cyte
an·ti·thy·roid
an·ti·thy·ro·tox·ic
an·ti·thy·ro·trop·ic
an·ti·ton·ic
an·ti·tox·ic
an·ti·tox·i·gen
an·ti·tox·in
    botulism a.
    bovine a.
    Clostridium perfringens
      types C and D a.
    Crotalus a.
    diphtheria a.
    gas gangrene a.
    perfringens a.
    Staphylococcus a.
    tetanus a.
    tetanus and gas gangrene
      a's
    tetanus perfringens a.
an·ti·tox·in·o·gen
an·ti·trag·i·cus
an·ti·tra·gus
an·ti·trep·o·ne·mal
an·ti·trich·o·mo·nal
an·ti·tris·mus
an·ti·trope
an·ti·trop·ic
an·ti·trop·in
an·ti·try·pan·o·so·mal
an·ti·tryp·sic
α_1-an·ti·tryp·sin
an·ti·tryp·tase
an·ti·tryp·tic
an·ti·tu·ber·cu·lin
an·ti·tu·ber·cu·lot·ic
an·ti·tu·ber·cu·lous
an·ti·tu·bu·lin
an·ti·tu·mor
an·ti·tu·mor·i·gen·ic
an·ti·tus·sive
an·ti·ty·phoid
an·ti·ty·ro·sin·ase
an·ti·ul·cer·a·tive
an·ti·urat·ic

an·ti·vac·ci·na·tion·ist
an·ti·ven·ene
an·ti·ve·ne·re·al
an·ti·ven·in
    black widow spider a.
    a. (Crotalidae) polyvalent
    Latrodectus mactans a.
    a. *(Micrurus fulvius)*
    polyvalent crotaline a.
an·ti·ven·om
an·ti·ven·om·ous
an·ti·vi·ral
an·ti·vi·rot·ic
an·ti·vi·ta·mer
an·ti·vi·ta·min
an·ti·vivi·sec·tion
an·ti·vivi·sec·tion·ist
an·ti·xen·ic
an·ti·xe·roph·thal·mic
an·ti·xe·rot·ic
an·ti·zyme
an·ti·zy·mo·hex·ase
an·ti·zy·mot·ic
ant·odon·tal·gic
Anton's symptom
Anton's syndrome
An·ton-Ba·bin·ski syn·drome
An·to·ni neu·ri·lem·mo·ma
ant·oph·thal·mic
ant·or·phine
an·tra
an·tra·cele
an·tral
an·trec·to·my
An·tre·nyl
an·tri·tis
an·tro·at·ti·cot·o·my
an·tro·buc·cal
an·tro·cele
an·tro·du·o·de·nec·to·my
an·tro·dyn·ia
an·tro·my·co·sis
an·tro·nal·gia
an·tro·na·sal
an·tro·neu·rol·y·sis
an·tro·phore
an·tro·phose
an·tro·py·lo·ric

an·trorse
an·tro·scope
an·tros·co·py
an·tros·tome
an·tros·to·my
    intranasal a.
    radical maxillary a.
an·tro·tome
an·trot·o·my
    sublabial a.
an·tro·tym·pan·ic
an·tro·tym·pan·i·tis
an·trum *pl.* an·tra
    a. auris
    a. folliculare
    cardiac a.
    a. cardiacum
    duodenal a.
    ethmoid a.
    a. ethmoidale
    frontal a.
    gastric a.
    a. of Highmore
    a. highmori
    mastoid a.
    a. mastoideum
    a. maxillare
    maxillary a.
    a. pylori
    pyloric a.
    a. pyloricum
    tympanic a.
    a. tympanicum
    Valsalva's a.
    a. of Willis
An·try·pol
An·tu·rane
An·tyl·lus
a·nu·cle·ar
a·nu·cle·at·ed
anu·cle·o·lar
ANUG — acute necrotizing
  ulcerative gingivitis
an·u·ran
an·ure·sis
an·uret·ic
an·uria
    angioneurotic a.

an·uria *(continued)*
  calculous a.
  compression a.
  obstructive a.
  postrenal a.
  prerenal a.
  renal a.
  suppressive a.
an·uric
an·u·rous
anus
  artificial a.
  ectopic a.
  imperforate a.
  preternatural a.
  a. of Rusconi
  a. vesicalis
  a. vestibularis
  vulvovaginal a.
anus·i·tis
an·vil
an·xi·e·tas
  a. tibiarum
an·xi·e·ty
  castration a.
  existential a.
  free-floating a.
  neurotic a.
  separation a.
  signal a.
anx·io·lyt·ic
an·y·dre·mia
AO — anodal opening
  opening of the
    atrioventricular valves
AOA — American Optometric
  Association
  American Orthopsychiatric
    Association
  American Osteopathic
    Association
AOC — anodal opening
  contraction
AOCl — anodal opening
  clonus
AOMA — American
  Occupational Medical
  Association

AOO — anodal opening odor
AOP — anodal opening
  picture
aor·ta *pl.* aor·tae, aor·tas
  abdominal a.
  ascending a.
  bicuspal a.
  buckled a.
  descending a.
  descending thoracic a.
  dextropositioned a.
  dorsal embryonic a.
  double a.
  dynamic a.
  kinked a.
  overriding a.
  palpable a.
  pericardial a.
  primitive a.
  root of a.
  a. sacrococcygea
  thoracic a.
  ventral a.
aor·tae
aor·tal
aor·tal·gia
aor·tec·to·my
aor·tic
aor·ti·co·pul·mo·nary
aor·ti·co·re·nal
aor·ti·tis
  Döhle-Heller a.
  luetic a.
  nummular a.
  rheumatic a.
  syphilitic a.
  a. syphilitica
  ulcerative a.
aor·to·ar·te·ri·tis
aor·to·bi·fem·o·ral
aor·to·ca·val
aor·to·cor·o·nary
aor·to·du·o·de·nal
aor·to·en·ter·ic
aor·to·esoph·a·ge·al
aor·to·fem·o·ral
aor·to·gas·tric

aor·to·gram
    flush a.
aor·tog·ra·phy
    abdominal a.
    intravenous a.
    retrograde a.
    thoracic a.
    translumbar a.
aor·to·il·i·ac
aor·top·a·thy
aor·top·to·sis
aor·to·pul·mo·nary
aor·tor·rha·phy
aor·to·scle·ro·sis
aor·tot·o·my
AOS — anodal opening sound
AOTA — American
    Occupational Therapy
    Association
AOTe — anodal opening
    tetanus
AP — action potential
    angina pectoris
    anterior pituitary (gland)
    anteroposterior
    arterial pressure
APA — American
    Pharmaceutical Association
    American Podiatric
        Association
    American Psychiatric
        Association
    American Psychological
        Association
6-APA — 6-aminopenicillanic
    acid
ap·a·con·i·tine
apal·les·the·sia
Ap·a·mide
apan·crea
apan·cre·at·ic
Apan·sporo·blas·ti·na
apar·a·lyt·ic
apar·a·thy·re·o·sis
apar·a·thy·roid·ism
apar·a·thy·ro·sis
ap·ar·thro·sis
apas·tia

apas·tic
ap·a·thet·ic
ap·a·thy
ap·a·tite
ap·a·zone
APC — acetylsalicylic acid,
    phenacetin, and caffeine
    atrial premature
        contraction
APE — anterior pituitary
    extract
ap·ei·do·sis
apel·lous
ape·ri·ent
ape·ri·od·ic
aperi·os·te·al
aper·i·stal·sis
aper·i·tive
Apert's disease
Apert's syndrome
Ap·ert-Crou·zon disease
ap·er·tog·na·thia
    LeFort I a. repair
ap·er·tom·e·ter
aper·tu·ra pl. aper·tu·rae
    a. externa aqueductus
        vestibuli
    a. externa canaliculi
        cochleae
    a. inferior canaliculi
        tympanici
    a. inferior fossae axillaris
    a. lateralis ventriculi
        quarti
    a. medialis ventriculi
        quarti
    a. mediana ventriculi
        quarti
    a. nasalis anterior
    a. pelvis inferior
    a. pelvis superior
    a. piriformis
    a. sinus frontalis
    a. sinus sphenoidalis
    a. superior canaliculi
        tympanici
    a. superior fossae axillaris
    a. thoracis inferior

aper·tu·ra *(continued)*
   a. thoracis superior
   a. tympanica canaliculi
     chordae tympani
ap·er·tu·rae
ap·er·ture
   angle of a.
   angular a.
   bony anterior nasal a.
   cloacal a.
   coded-image a.
   external a. of aqueduct of
     vestibule
   external a. of canaliculus
     of cochlea
   external a. of tympanic
     canaliculus
   a. of frontal sinus
   a. of glottis
   inferior a. of axillary fossa
   inferior a. of minor pelvis
   inferior a. of thorax
   inferior a. of tympanic
     canaliculus
   internal a. of tympanic
     canaliculus
   a. of larynx
   lateral a. of fourth
     ventricle
   a. of lens
   median a. of fourth
     ventricle
   nasal a., anterior
   numerical a.
   orbital a.
   piriform a.
   posterior nasal a.
   a. of sphenoid sinus
   spinal a.
   spurious a. of facial canal
   spurious a. of fallopian
     canal
   superior a. of axillary fossa
   superior a. of minor pelvis
   superior a. of thorax
   superior a. of tympanic
     canaliculus
   thoracic a., inferior

ap·er·ture *(continued)*
   thoracic a., superior
   tympanic a. of canaliculus
     of chorda tympani
apex *pl.* apex·es, api·ces
   a. of arytenoid cartilage
   a. auriculae
   a. of bladder
   a. capitis fibulae
   a. cartilaginis arytenoideae
   a. cordis
   a. cuspidis
   darwinian a.
   a. of head of fibula
   a. of heart
   a. linguae
   a. of lung
   a. nasi
   a. ossis sacri
   a. of patella
   a. patellae
   a. pulmonis
   a. of sacrum
   a. of tongue
   a. vesicae urinariae
apex·car·dio·gram
apex·car·di·og·ra·phy
APF — animal protein factor
APGAR — adaptability,
  partnership, growth,
  affection, resolve
Apgar scale
Apgar score
APH — adenohypophyseal
  hormone
    anterior pituitary hormone
APHA — American Public
  Health Association
APhA — American
  Pharmaceutical Association
apha·gia
   a. algera
apha·go·prax·ia
apha·ke
apha·kia
apha·kic
apha·lan·gia

apha·sia
    acoustic a.
    ageusic a.
    amnemonic a.
    amnestic a.
    anomic a.
    anosmic a.
    apractic a.
    association a.
    associative a.
    ataxic a.
    auditory a.
    Broca's a.
    central a.
    color name a.
    combined a.
    commissural a.
    complete a.
    conduction a.
    cortical a.
    crossed a.
    efferent motor a.
    expressive a.
    expressive-receptive a.
    finger a.
    fluent a.
    frontocortical a.
    frontolenticular a.
    functional a.
    gestural a.
    gibberish a.
    global a.
    graphomotor a.
    Grashey's a.
    impressive a.
    intellectual a.
    jargon a.
    kinetic motor a.
    lenticular a.
    a. lethica
    Lichtheim's a.
    mixed a.
    monoglot a.
    motor a.
    musical a.
    nominal a.
    nonfluent a.

apha·sia *(continued)*
    optic a.
    parieto-occipital a.
    paroxysmal a.
    pathematic a.
    pictorial a.
    psychosensory a.
    pure motor a.
    receptive a.
    semantic a.
    sensory a.
    subcortical a.
    syntactical a.
    tactile a.
    temporoparietal a.
    total a.
    transcortical a.
    true a.
    verbal a.
    visual a.
    Wernicke's a.
apha·si·ac
apha·sic
apha·si·ol·o·gist
apha·si·ol·o·gy
aphas·mid
Aphas·mid·ia
ap·he·li·ot·ro·pism
aphe·mes·the·sia
aphe·mia
aphe·mic
aphe·pho·bia
aph·e·re·sis
apho·nia
    a. clericorum
    hysteric a.
    a. paralytica
    spastic a.
aphon·ic
apho·no·ge·lia
aphose
aphos·pha·gen·ic
aphos·pho·ro·sis
aphot·es·the·sia
aphot·ic
aphra·sia
aph·ro·dis·ia
aph·ro·dis·iac

aph·tha *pl.* aph·thae
    Bednar's aphthae
    Behçet's aphthae
    cachectic aphthae
    epizootic aphthae
    aphthae febriles
    Mikulicz's aphthae
    recurring scarring aphthae
    aphthae tropicae
aph·thae
aph·thoid
aph·thon·gia
aph·tho·sa
aph·tho·sis
    Touraine's a.
aph·thous
aph·to·vi·rus
aphy·lac·tic
aphy·lax·is
ap·i·cal
api·cec·to·my
ap·i·ces
ap·i·cil·ar
ap·i·ci·tis
    orbital a.
Ap·i·co·com·plexa
ap·i·co·com·plex·an
ap·i·co·ec·to·my
ap·i·col·y·sis
ap·i·cos·to·my
ap·i·cot·o·my
APIM — Association
    Professionnelle
    Internationale des Médecins
Apio·chae·ta fer·ru·gi·nea
apio·ther·a·py
api·pho·bia
api·tox·in
api·tu·i·tar·ism
apla·cen·tal
ap·la·nat·ic
aplan·a·tism
apla·sia
    a. axialis extracorticalis
      congenita
    a. cutis congenita
    germinal cell a.
    hereditary retinal a.

apla·sia *(continued)*
    lobular a.
    Mondin's a.
    nuclear a.
    a. of ovary
    pure red cell a.
    retinal a.
    thymic a.
    thymic-parathyroid a.
aplas·tic
apleu·ria
Ap·ley sign
ap·nea
    chemoreceptor a.
    deglutition a.
    hypersomnia sleep a.
    induced a.
    initial a.
    late a.
    a. neonatorum
    obstructive sleep a.
    postanesthesia a.
    sleep a.
    traumatic a.
ap·ne·ic
ap·neu·ma·to·sis
ap·neu·mia
ap·neu·sis
ap·neus·tic
apo·at·ro·pine
ap·o·cam·no·sis
ap·o·ce·no·sis
apo·chro·mat
apo·chro·mat·ic
apoc·o·pe
ap·o·cop·tic
apo·crine
apo·crin·i·tis
ap·o·crus·tic
apoc·y·nin
Apo·cy·num
ap·o·dal
Apod·e·mus
    A. sylvaticus
apo·dia
apo·en·zyme
ap·o·fer·ri·tin
apo·gam·ia

apog·a·my
ap·o·gee
ap·o·kam·no·sis
apo·lar
ap·o·le·gam·ic
ap·o·leg·a·my
apo·lipo·pro·tein
Ap·ol·lo·nia
apo·mor·phine
    a. hydrochloride
ap·o·neu·rec·to·my
ap·o·neu·rol·o·gy
ap·o·neu·ror·rha·phy
apo·neu·ro·sis *pl.* apo·neu·ro·
  ses
    abdominal a.
    bicipital a.
    a. bicipitalis
    clavicoracoaxillary a.
    crural a.
    Denonvilliers'a.
    epicranial a.
    extensor a.
    femoral a.
    a. of insertion
    intercostal aponeuroses,
      external
    intercostal aponeuroses,
      internal
    ischiorectal a.
    a. linguae
    lingual a.
    lumbar a.
    a. musculi bicipitis brachii
    a. of origin
    a. palatina
    palatine a.
    palmar a.
    a. palmaris
    perineal a.
    pharyngeal a.
    a. pharyngis
    pharyngobasilar a.
    a. pharyngobasilaris
    plantar a.
    a. plantaris
    Sibson's a.
    subscapular a.

apo·neu·ro·sis *(continued)*
    superficial perineal a.
    a. of vasti muscles
    supraspinous a.
    temporal a.
    vertebral a.
    a. of Zinn
ap·o·neu·ro·si·tis
ap·o·neu·rot·ic
ap·o·neu·ro·tome
ap·o·neu·rot·o·my
ap·o·phleg·mat·ic
apoph·y·sa·ry
ap·oph·y·sate
apoph·y·se·al
apoph·y·se·op·a·thy
apoph·y·ses
apoph·y·si·al
ap·o·phys·i·ary
apoph·y·sis *pl.* apoph·y·ses
    basilar a.
    calcaneal a.
    cerebral a.
    a. cerebri
    genial a.
    a. helicis
    a. of Ingrassias
    a. lenticularis incudis
    odontoid a.
    a. ossium
    pterygoid a.
    a. of Rau
    a. raviana
    a. rawii
apoph·y·si·tis
    a. tibialis adolescentium
ap·o·plas·mat·ic
ap·o·plec·tic
ap·o·plec·ti·form
ap·o·plec·toid
ap·o·plex·ia
    a. uteri
ap·o·plexy
    abdominal a.
    adrenal a.
    asthenic a.
    bulbar a.
    capillary a.

ap·o·plexy *(continued)*
  cerebellar a.
  cerebral a.
  delayed a.
  embolic a.
  fulminating a.
  heat a.
  ingravescent a.
  neonatal a.
  ovarian a.
  pancreatic a.
  parturient a.
  pituitary a.
  placental a.
  pontile a.
  pontine a.
  Raymond's a.
  renal a.
  spinal a.
  splenic a.
  thrombotic a.
  traumatic late a.
  urethral a.
  uterine a.
  uteroplacental a.
ap·o·pro·tein
ap·op·to·sis
ap·o·re·pres·sor
ap·o·some
apos·ta·sis
apos·thia
ap·o·tha·na·sia
apoth·e·cary
ap·o·the·ci·um
ap·o·them
ap·o·zem
ap·pa·rat·us *pl.* ap·pa·rat·us,
  ap·pa·rat·us·es
  Abbe-Zeiss a.
  absorption a.
  acoustic a.
  attachment a.
  auditory a.
  Barcroft's a.
  Beckmann's a.
  Benedict-Knipping a.
  Benedict-Roth a.
  biliary a.

ap·pa·rat·us *(continued)*
  Calandruccio compression
    a.
  central a.
  cerebellovestibular a.
  Charnley's a.
  chromidial a.
  chromatic a.
  ciliary a.
  cytopharyngeal a.
  a. derivatorius
  Desault's a.
  digestive a.
  a. digestorius
  electro-oculogram a.
  Finsen's a.
  genital a. of the female
  genitourinary a.
  Golgi a.
  a. of Goormaghtigh
  Haldane a.
  Hodgen's a.
  Horsley-Clarke a.
  hyoid a.
  ICLH (Imperial College,
    London Hospital) a.
  inhalation anesthesia a.
  inhalation therapy a.
  Jaquet's a.
  Junker a.
  juxtaglomerular a.
  Kirschner's a.
  Knipping's a.
  Krogh's a.
  lacrimal a.
  a. lacrimalis
  a. ligamentosus colli
  locomotor a.
  masticatory a.
  mytotic a.
  parabasal a.
  a. of Perroncito
  pilosebaceous a.
  reproductive a.
  a. respiratorius
  respiratory a.
  rocking a.
  Sayre's a.

ap·pa·rat·us *(continued)*
    Scholander's a.
    sound-conducting a.
    Soxhlet's a.
    spindle a.
    spine a.
    steadiness a.
    stereotaxic a.
    subneural a.
    sucker a.
    a. suspensorius lentis
    suspensory a. of pleura
    Taylor's a.
    a. of Timofeew
    Tiselius a.
    urogenital a.
    a. urogenitalis
    vasomotor a.
    vestibular a.
    vocal a.
    Waldenberg's a.
    Wangensteen's a.
    Warburg a.
ap·pen·dage
    atrial a.
    auricular a.
    caudal a.
    cecal a.
    cutaneous a's
    drumstick a.
    a. of epididymis
    epiploic a's
    a's of the eye
    a's of the fetus
    fibrous a. of liver
    ovarian a.
    preauricular a.
    a's of the skin
    testicular a.
    a. of the testis
    uterine a's
    a. of ventricle of larynx
    vermicular a.
    vesicular a's of epoöphoron
ap·pen·da·gi·tis
    epiploic a.
ap·pen·dec·to·my
    auricular a.

ap·pen·di·cal
ap·pen·dic·e·al
ap·pen·di·cec·to·my
ap·pen·di·ces
ap·pen·di·ci·tis
    actinomycotic a.
    acute a.
    amebic a.
    chronic a.
    a. by contiguity
    foreign-body a.
    fulminating a.
    gangrenous a.
    helminthic a.
    left-sided a.
    lumbar a.
    nonobstructive a.
    a. obliterans
    obstructive a.
    perforating a.
    perforative a.
    protective a.
    purulent a.
    recurrent a.
    relapsing a.
    segmental a.
    skip a.
    stercoral a.
    subperitoneal a.
    suppurative a.
    traumatic a.
    verminous a.
ap·pen·di·co·ce·cos·to·my
ap·pen·di·co·cele
ap·pen·di·co·en·ter·os·to·my
ap·pen·di·co·li·thi·a·sis
ap·pen·di·co·ly·sis
ap·pen·di·cop·a·thy
ap·pen·di·cos·to·my
ap·pen·dic·u·lar
ap·pen·dix *pl.* ap·pen·di·ces,
  ap·pen·dix·es
    auricular a.
    cecal a.
    ensiform a.
    a. epididymidis
    a. of epididymis
    epiploic appendices

ap·pen·dix *(continued)*
 appendices epiploicae
 a. fibrosa hepatis
 fibrous a. of liver
 Morgagni's a.
 omental appendices
 appendices omentales
 pelvic a.
 a. testis
 a. of ventricle of larynx
 a. ventriculilaryngis
 a. vermicularis
 vermiform a.
 a. vermiformis
 appendices vesiculosae
  epoöphori
 appendices vesiculosae
  epoöphorontis
 xiphoid a.
ap·pen·do·li·thi·a·sis
ap·per·cep·tion
ap·per·cep·tive
ap·per·son·a·tion
ap·per·son·i·fi·ca·tion
ap·pe·stat
ap·pe·tite
ap·pe·ti·tion
ap·pe·ti·tive
ap·pla·nate
ap·pla·na·tion
ap·pla·nom·e·ter
ap·ple
 Adam's a.
 bitter a.
 devil's a.
 Indian a.
 May a.
 a. of Peru
 thorn a.
ap·pli·ance
 Andresen a.
 Begg a.
 Bimler a.
 craniofacial a.
 crown of thorns a.
 Crozat a.
 Denholz a.
 edgewise a.

ap·pli·ance *(continued)*
 expansion plate a.
 extraoral a.
 fixed a.
 Frankel a.
 functional a.
 habit-breaking a.
 Hawley a.
 Jackson a.
 Johnson twin wire a.
 jumping-the-bite a.
 Kesling a.
 Kingsley a.
 labiolingual a.
 light round-wire a.
 monoblock a.
 multibanded a.
 occlusal overlay a.
 orthodontic a.
 permanent a.
 pin and tube a.
 prosthetic a.
 regulating a.
 removable a.
 retaining a.
 ribbon arch a.
 Roger Anderson pin
  fixation a.
 Schwarz a.
 speech a.
 split plate a.
 twin wire a.
 universal a.
 Walker a.
ap·pli·ca·tion
ap·pli·ca·tor
 beam-therapy a.
 Fletcher-Suit a.
 sandwich-mold a.
 sonic a.
 surface a.
ap·pli·qué
ap·pose
ap·po·si·tion
ap·prai·sal
 health risk a.
ap·pre·hen·sion

ap·proach
    idiographic a.
    Kocher-McFarland a.
    nomothetic a.
    Risdon a.
    transcranial a.
    transnasal a.
    transseptal a.
    transthoracic a.
ap·prox·i·mal
ap·prox·i·mate
ap·prox·i·ma·tion
    successive a.
ap·prox·i·ma·tor
    rib a.
    skin-edge a.
APR — anterior pituitary
  reaction
aprac·tic
aprac·tog·no·sia
    geometric a.
ap·ra·my·cin
aprax·ia
    agnosic a.
    akinetic a.
    amnestic a.
    Bruns'a. of gait
    classic a.
    congenital a.
    constructional a.
    cortical a.
    developmental a.
    geometric a.
    ideational a.
    ideokinetic a.
    ideomotor a.
    innervation a.
    Liepmann's a.
    limb-kinetic a.
    motor a.
    oculomotor a.
    optic a.
    sensory a.
    tongue a.
    transcortical a.
    trunk a.
    visual a.
aprax·ic

Apres·a·zide
Apres·o·line
aprin·dine
ap·ro·bar·bi·tal
aproc·tia
apron
    pudendal a.
    lead-rubber a.
apros·o·dy
apro·so·pia
apro·so·pus
apro·tic
apro·ti·nin
APRT — adenine
  phosphoribosyl transferase
APS — American
  Physiological Society
ap·sel·a·phe·sia
APT — alum precipitated
  toxoid
APTA — American Physical
  Therapy Association
ap·ter·ous
ap·ti·tude
APTT, aPTT — activated
  partial thromboplastin time
ap·ty·a·lia
ap·ty·a·lism
APUD — amine precursor
  uptake and decarboxylation
apud·o·ma
apul·mo·nism
apu·lo·sis
apu·lot·ic
apu·rin·ic acid
apus
apy·e·tous
apyk·no·morph
apyk·no·mor·phous
apy·og·e·nous
apy·ous
apy·rene
apy·ret·ic
apy·rex·ia
apy·rex·i·al
apyr·im·i·din·ic acid
apy·ro·gen·ic
AQ — achievement quotient

Aq. — L. aqua (water)
Aq. dest. — L. aqua destillata
(distilled water)
Aq. pur. — L. aqua pura (pure
water)
Aq. tep. — L. aqua tepida
(tepid water)
aq·ua *pl.* aq·uae
   a. amnii
   a. aromatica
   a. cinnamomi
   a. destillata
   a. fortis
   a. hamamelidis
   a. menthae piperitae
   a. oculi
   a. pericardii
   a. regia
   a. rosae
   a. rosae fortior
Aq·ua·care
aq·uae
aq·uae·duc·tus *pl.* aq·uae·
duc·tus
Aq·ua·MEPH·Y·TON
aq·ua·pho·bia
aq·ua·punc·ture
Aq·ua·tag
Aq·ua·ten·sen
aquat·ic
aq·ue·duct
   cerebral a.,
   a. of cochlea
   a. of Cotunnius
   fallopian a.
   a. of Fallopius
   a. of mesencephalon
   a. of midbrain
   a. of Sylvius
   ventricular a.
   a. of vestibule
aq·ue·duc·tus
   a. cerebri
   a. cochleae
   a. endolymphaticus
   a. mesencephali
   a. vestibuli

aque·ous
Aq·uex
aq·ui·par·ous
AR — alarm reaction
   aortic regurgitation
   artificial respiration
ara-A
ar·a·ban
ar·a·bate
ar·a·bic ac·id
ar·a·bin
arab·i·nose
ar·a·bin·o·sis
arab·i·no·su·ria
arab·i·no·syl·cy·to·sine
ar·a·bite
arab·i·tol
2-ara·bo·ke·tose
ar·a·bo·py·ra·nose
ara-C
ara·chic acid
arach·i·date
ar·a·chid·ic
ar·a·chid·ic acid
arach·i·don·ate 5-lip·oxy·gen·
ase
arach·i·don·ate 12-lip·oxy·
gen·ase
arach·i·don·ic acid
arach·ne·pho·bia
Arach·nia
   A. propionica
arach·nid
Arach·ni·da
arach·nid·ism
arach·ni·tis
arach·no·dac·tyl·ia
arach·no·dac·ty·ly
   contractural a., congenital,
   (CCA)
arach·no·gas·tria
arach·noid
   a. of brain
   cranial a.
   spinal a.
   a. of spinal cord
arach·noi·dal

arach·noi·dea *pl.* arach·noi·
   deae
   a. encephali
   a. mater encephali
   a. spinalis
arach·noi·deae
arach·noid·ism
arach·noid·i·tis
   basal a.
   a. of cerebral hemispheres
   chronic adhesive a.
   cisternal a.
   opticochiasmatic a.
   a. of posterior cerebral
      fossa
   spinal a.
arach·nol·y·sin
arach·no·pho·bia
aral·de·hyde-tanned
Ar·a·len
aral·kyl
Ar·a·mine
Ar·an's law
Ar·an-Du·chenne disease
Ar·an-Du·chenne muscular
   atrophy
Aran·e·ae
Ar·a·ne·i·da
ara·ne·ism
ara·ne·ous
Aran·ti·us' bodies
Aran·ti·us' canal
Aran·ti·us' duct
Aran·ti·us' ligament
Aran·ti·us' nodule
Aran·ti·us' ventricle
Aran·zi
ara·phia
ar·a·ro·ba
ar·ba·pros·til
Ar·ber, Werner
ar·bor *pl.* ar·bo·res
   a. bronchialis
   a. medullaris vermis
   a. vitae
   a. vitae cerebelli
   a. vitae uteri
   a. vitae of vermis

ar·bo·re·al
ar·bo·res
ar·bo·res·cent
ar·bo·ri·za·tion
   cervical mucus a.
ar·bo·roid
ar·bo·vi·ral
ar·bo·vi·rus
ARC — AIDS-related complex
   American Red Cross
   anomalous retinal
      correspondence
arc
   auricular a.
   autonomic reflex a.
   binauricular a.
   bregmatolambdoid a.
   carbon a.
   dorsal venous a.
   epiploic a. of Haller and
      Barkow
   external marginal a. of
      Zuckerkandl
   mercury a.
   nasobregmatic a.
   naso-occipital a.
   neural a.
   nuclear a.
   reflex a.
   retruded a. of closure
   Riolan's a.
   sensorimotor a.
ar·cade
   anomalous mitral a.
   arterial a's
   Flint's a.
   Riolan's a.
   temporal a.
ar·cate
Ar·cel·la
Ar·ce·lin's views
Ar·cel·lin·i·da
ar·ce·sis
arch
   abdominothoracic a.
   alveolar a.
   anastomotic a.
   anterior a. of atlas

arch *(continued)*
    a. of aorta
    aortic a's
    arterial a's
    axillary a.
    a. of azygos vein
    basal a.
    branchial a's
    carpal a's
    cervical a.
    cervical aortic a.
    a's of Corti
    cortical a's of kidney
    costal a.
    a. of cricoid cartilage
    crural a.
    dental a.
    diaphragmatic a., external
    diaphragmatic a., internal
    digital venous a's
    dorsal venous a.
    dorsal a. of wrist
    double aortic a.
    epiphyseal a.
    fallen a's
    femoral a., superficial
    fibrous a. of soleus muscle
    a's of foot
    gill a.
    glossopalatine a.
    Haller's a's
    hemal a.
    hyoid a.
    hyothyroid a.
    iliopectineal a.
    inferior palpebral a.
    inguinal a.
    intermesenteric arterial a.
    ischiopubic a.
    jugular venous a.
    Langer's axillary a.
    lingual a.
    longitudinal a. of foot
    lumbocostal a.
    malar a.
    mandibular a.
    marginal a. of eyelid
    maxillary a.

arch *(continued)*
    nasal a.
    neural a.
    open pubic a.
    oral a.
    palatal a.
    palatine a., anterior
    palatine a., posterior
    palatoglossal a.
    palatomaxillary a.
    palatopharyngeal a.
    palmar arterial a.
    palmar carpal a.
    palmar venous a.
    palpebral a.
    paraphyseal a.
    parieto-occipital a.
    a. of pelvis
    persistent right aortic a.
    pharyngeal a's
    pharyngoepiglottic a.
    pharyngopalatine a.
    plantar a.
    plantar venous a.
    popliteal a.
    postaural a's
    posterior a. of atlas
    prepancreatic a.
    primitive costal a's
    pubic a.
    a. of pubis
    pulmonary a's
    Reichert's a.
    residual a.
    residual dental a.
    rhinencephalic a.
    ribbon a.
    right aortic a.
    Riolan's a.
    saddle a.
    Salus a.
    Shenton's a.
    subpubic a.
    superciliary a.
    supraorbital a. of frontal
      bone
    systemic a.
    tarsal a's

arch *(continued)*
    tendinous a.
    a. of thoracic duct
    thyrohyoid a.
    transverse a. of foot
    trapezoidal a.
    Treitz's a.
    U-shaped a.
    venous a's of kidney
    a. of vertebra
    vertebral a.
    visceral a's
    volar venous a.
    V-shaped a.
    Zimmermann's a.
    zygomatic a.
Ar·chaeo·bac·te·ria
ar·chaeo·cer·e·bel·lum
ar·chaeo·cor·tex
ar·chae·us
Arch·ag·a·thus
ar·cha·ic
arch·am·phi·as·ter
Arch·an·gel·i·ca
ar·che·go·nium
arch·en·ceph·a·lon
arch·en·ter·on
ar·cheo·cer·e·bel·lum
ar·cheo·ci·net·ic
ar·cheo·cor·tex
ar·cheo·ki·net·ic
ar·che·spore
ar·che·spo·ri·um
ar·che·type
ar·chi·blast
ar·chi·blas·tic
ar·chi·carp
ar·chi·cer·e·bel·lum
ar·chi·cyte
ar·chi·gas·tru·la
ar·chi·gon·o·cyte
ar·chi·kary·on
ar·chil
ar·chi·mor·u·la
ar·chi·neph·ron
arch·i·pal·li·al
ar·chi·pal·li·um
ar·chi·spore

ar·chi·stome
ar·chi·stri·a·tum
ar·chi·tec·ton·ic
ar·ci·form
arc·ta·tion
ar·cu·al
ar·cu·al·ia
ar·cu·ate
ar·cu·a·tion
ar·cus *pl.* ar·cus
    a. adiposus
    a. alveolaris mandibulae
    a. alveolaris maxillae
    a. anterior atlantis
    a. aortae
    a. aorticus
    a. cartilaginis cricoideae
    a. corneae
    a. cornealis
    a. costalis
    a. costarum
    a. dentalis inferior
    a. dentalis superior
    a. dorsalis pedis
    a. ductus thoracici
    a. glossopalatinus
    a. iliopectineus
    a. inguinalis
    a. juvenilis
    a. lipoides corneae
    a. lipoides myringis
    a. lumbocostalis lateralis
    a. lumbocostalis medialis
    a. palatini
    a. palatoglossus
    a. palatopharyngeus
    a. palmaris profundus
    a. palmaris superficialis
    a. palpebrales
    a. palpebralis inferior
    a. palpebralis superior
    a. parieto-occipitalis
    a. pedis longitudinalis
    a. pedis transversalis
    a. pharyngopalatinus
    a. plantaris
    a. plantaris profundus
    a. plantaris superficialis

ar·cus *(continued)*
  a. posterior atlantis
  a. presenilis
  a. pubicus
  a. pubis
  a. senilis
  a. superciliaris
  a. tarseus inferior
  a. tarseus superior
  a. tendineus
  a. venae azygou
  a. venosi digitales
  a. venosus dorsalis pedis
  a. venosus juguli
  a. venosus palmaris
    profundus
  a. venosus palmaris
    superficialis
  a. venosus plantaris
  a. vertebrae
  a. vertebralis
  a. zygomaticus
ARD — acute respiratory
  disease
ard·an·es·the·sia
ar·dor
  a. urinae
ARDS — adult respiratory
  distress syndrome
area *pl.* areae, areas
  acoustic a.
  a. acustica
  alisphenoid a.
  anterior amygdaloid a.
  aortic a.
  apical a.
  arterial baroreceptor a.
  association a's
  asthmagenic a.
  auditory a.
  autonomic a.
  axial a.
  Bamberger's a.
  bare a. of liver
  basal seat a.
  B-dependent a.
  Betz cell a.
  body surface a.

area *(continued)*
  Broca's motor speech a.
  Broca's parolfactory a.
  Brodmann's a's
  buccopharyngeal a.
  cardiogenic a.
  catchment a.
  a. centralis
  central speech a.
  a. choroidea
  cingulate a.
  a. cochleae
  Cohnheim's a's
  contact a.
  cortical 4S a.
  cortical gustatory a.
  cortical oculomotor a.
  cortical speech a.
  cortical tactile a.
  cortico-oculocephalogyric
    a.
  cribriform a. of renal
    papilla
  a. cribrosa media
  a. cribrosa papillae renalis
  a. cribrosa superior
  a. of critical definition
  denture-bearing a.
  denture foundation a.
  denture-supporting a.
  depressor a.
  dermatomic a.
  donor a.
  dorsal hypothalamic a.
  effective reflecting a.
  embryonic a.
  entorhinal a.
  excitable a.
  excitomotor a.
  extrapyramidal motor a.
  eye a.
  a. of facial nerve
  first motor speech a.
  a's of Forel
  frontal a.
  fronto-orbital a.
  fusion a.
  gastric a's

area *(continued)*
areae gastricae
genital a's
glove a.
gustatory a.
Hines strip a.
hinge a.
hypoglossal a.
a. hypoglossi
hypothalamic a., lateral
impression a.
insular a.
intercondylar a's of tibia
interglobular a's
Kiesselbach's a.
Laimer-Haeckerman a.
language a.
Little's a.
a. martegiani
a. medullovasculosa
mesobranchial a.
mirror a.
mitral valve a.
motor a.
a. nervi facialis
a. nuda hepatis
olfactory a.
optic a.
Panum's a's
parastriate a.
a. paraterminalis
parolfactory a. of Broca
Patrick's trigger a's
a. pellucida
a. perforata
pericruciate a.
peristriate a.
piriform a.
portal a.
postcentral a.
post dam a.
posterior hypothalamic a.
posterior palatal seal a.
a. postrema
postrolandic a.
precentral a.
precommissural a.
prefrontal a.

area *(continued)*
premotor a.
preoptic a.
a. preoptica
pressor a.
pressoreceptive a's
pressure a.
pretectal a.
a. pretectalis
primary a's
primary receptive a.
projection a's
psychomotor a.
pulmonary a.
pulmonary valve a.
pyriform a.
receptive a.
relief a.
rest a.
rolandic a.
rugae a.
saddle a.
self-cleansing a.
sensorimotor a.
sensory a.
septal a.
silent a.
somatosensory a.
somesthetic a.
stress-bearing a.
a. striata
strip a.
a. subcallosa
subcallosal a.
supplementary a's
supporting a.
suppressor a's
T-dependent a.
temporal a.
thenar a.
thymus-dependent a.
thymus-independent a.
T-independent a.
traffic a.
triangular a.
tricuspid valve a.
trigger a.
vagus a.

area *(continued)*
    ventral tegmental a. of Tsai
    vestibular a.
    visual a.
    visuopsychic a.
    visuosensory a.
    vocal a.
    Wernicke's a.
ar·e·a·ta, ar·e·a·tus
Are·ca
ar·e·ca
arec·o·line
    a. hydrobromide
are·flex·ia
are·gen·er·a·tive
ar·e·na·ceous
Are·na·vi·ri·dae
ar·e·na·vi·rus
ar·e·noid
are·o·la *pl.* are·o·lae
    Chaussier's a.
    a. mammae
    a. of mammary gland
    a. of nipple
    a. papillaris
    primary a.
    second a.
    umbilical a.
are·o·lae
are·o·lar
are·o·late
are·o·li·tis
ar·e·om·e·ter
ar·eo·met·ric
ar·e·om·e·try
Ar·ey's rule
ARF — acute respiratory failure
Ar·fon·ad
Arg — arginine
arg. — L. argentum (silver)
ar·gam·bly·opia
Ar·gand burner
Ar·gas
    A. *americanus*
    A. *brumpti*
    A. *miniatus*

Ar·gas (continued)
    A. *persicus*
    A. *reflexus*
ar·gas·id
Ar·gas·i·dae
ar·ge·ma
Ar·ge·mo·na mex·i·ca·na
ar·gen·taf·fin
ar·gen·taf·fi·no·ma
    a. of bronchus
ar·gen·ta·tion
ar·gen·tic
ar·gen·to·phil·ic
ar·gil·la
ar·gil·la·ceous
ar·gi·nase
ar·gi·nine
    a. glutamate
    a. hydrochloride
    a. monohydrochloride
    suberyl a.
ar·gi·nine car·boxy·pep·ti·dase
ar·gin·i·ne·mia
ar·gi·ni·no·suc·cin·ase
ar·gi·ni·no·suc·cin·ate
ar·gi·ni·no·suc·cin·ate ly·ase
ar·gi·ni·no·suc·cin·ate ly·ase (ASAL, ASL) deficiency
ar·gi·ni·no·suc·cin·ate syn·the·tase
ar·gi·ni·no·suc·cin·ate (ASA) syn·the·tase (ASAS, ASS) deficiency
ar·gi·ni·no·suc·cin·ic·ac·i·de·mia
ar·gi·ni·no·suc·cin·ic·ac·id·uria
ar·gi·nyl
ar·gi·pres·sin
ar·gon
Ar·gonz-del Cas·til·lo syn·drome
Ar·gyle-Sa·lem sump tube
Ar·gyll Rob·ert·son pupil
Ar·gyll Rob·ert·son sign
ar·gyr·emia

ar·gyr·ia
    a. nasalis
ar·gyr·i·a·sis
ar·gyr·ic
ar·gyr·ism
Ar·gyr·ol
ar·gy·ro·phil
ar·gy·ro·sis
arhi·go·sis
arhin·en·ceph·a·lia
arhin·ia
arhyth·mia
Ar·i·as-Stel·la reaction
ari·bo·fla·vin·o·sis
Ar·ies-Pi·tan·guy procedure
ar·il
ar·il·done
ar·il·lode
aris·tin
Aris·to·cort
Aris·to·gel
Aris·to·lo·chia
aris·to·lo·chic acid
aris·to·lo·chine
Aris·to·span
Ar·is·tot·le's anomaly
arith·mo·ma·nia
ar·kyo·chrome
ar·kyo·sticho·chrome
Ar·la·cel A
Ar·li·din
Arlt's recess
Arlt's sinus
Arlt's trachoma
arm
    bar clasp a.
    bird a.
    chromosome a.
    circumferential clasp a.
    glass a.
    golf a.
    Krukenberg's a.
    prolapsed a.
    reciprocal a.
    retention a.
    retentive a.
    scanning a.
    stabilizing a.

ARM — artificial rupture of
  membranes
ar·ma·men·tar·i·um
Ar·man·ni-Eb·stein cells
ar·ma·ri·um
ar·ma·ture
Ar·mig·e·res
    A. obturbans
Ar·mil·li·fer
    A. armillatus
    A. moniliformis
arm·pit
Arm·strong's disease
Ar·my-Na·vy retractor
Ar·nal·dus de Vil·la·no·va
Arndt's law
Arndt-Schulz law
Ar·neth classification
Ar·neth count
Ar·neth formula
Ar·neth index
Ar·ni·ca
ar·ni·ca
Ar·nold of Vil·la·no·va
Ar·nold's bodies
Ar·nold's canal
Ar·nold's fold
Ar·nold's ligament
Ar·nold's nerve
Ar·nold's substance
Ar·nold's syndrome
Ar·nold-Chi·ari deformity
Ar·nold-Chi·ari malformation
Ar·nold-Chi·ari syndrome
ar·not·to
AROA — autosomal recessive
  ocular albinism
aro·ma
aro·ma·tase
ar·o·mat·ic
ar·o·ma·ti·za·tion
aro·mine
arous·al
ar·pri·no·cid
ar·rache·ment
ar·range·ment
    anterior tooth a.
    tooth a.

ar·ray
    annular a.
    linear switched a.
    phase steered a.
    transducer a.
ar·rec·tor *pl.* ar·rec·to·res
    a. pili (*pl.* arrectores
      pilorum)
ar·rest
    cardiac a.
    circulatory a.
    deep transverse a.
    developmental a.
    epiphyseal a.
    heart a.
    a. of labor
    maturation a.
    metaphase a.
    pelvic a.
    sinus a.
ar·rest·ed
ar·rha·phia
Ar·rhen·i·us' doctrine
Ar·rhen·i·us' equation
Ar·rhen·i·us' formula
Ar·rhen·i·us' theory
ar·rhe·no·blas·to·ma
ar·rhe·no·gen·ic
ar·rhe·no·kary·on
ar·rhe·no·ma
ar·rhe·no·plasm
ar·rhe·no·to·cia
ar·rhe·not·o·ky
ar·rhi·go·sis
ar·rhin·en·ce·pha·lia
ar·rhin·en·ceph·a·ly
ar·rhin·ia
ar·rhyth·mia
    continuous a.
    juvenile a.
    nodal a.
    perpetual a.
    phasic a.
    respiratory a.
    sinus a.
    vagal a.
ar·rhyth·mic
ar·rhyth·mo·gen·ic

ar·rhyth·mo·ki·ne·sis
ar·row·root
Ar·ro·yo's sign
ARRS — American Roentgen
    Ray Society
ar·sam·bide
ar·se·nate
ar·se·ni·a·sis
ar·se·nic
    a. chloride
    a. disulfide
    fuming liquid a.
    red a. sulfide
    a. trichloride
    a. trioxide
    a. trisulfide
    white a.
    a. yellow
ar·se·nic acid
ar·sen·i·cal
ar·sen·i·cal·ism
ar·sen·i·coph·a·gy
ar·sen·i·cum
ar·se·nide
    hydrogen a.
ar·sen·i·ous
ar·se·nism
ar·se·nite
ar·sen·iza·tion
ar·se·no·ben·zene
ar·seno·blast
ar·se·nol·y·sis
ar·se·no·re·sis·tant
ar·se·no·ther·a·py
ar·se·nous
ar·se·nous acid
ar·se·nous hy·dride
ar·se·num
ar·sine
ar·sin·ic acid
ar·son·ic acid
ar·so·ni·um
ars·phen·a·mine
ars·thi·nol
ART — Accredited Record
    Technician
    automated reagin test
Ar·tane

ar·te·fact
Ar·te·mi·sia
ar·te·ral·gia
ar·ter·ec·to·my
ar·te·re·nol
ar·te·ria *pl.* ar·te·riae
  a. acetabuli
  a. alveolaris
  a. anastomotica
  a. angularis
  a. anonyma
  a. appendicularis
  arteriae arciformes renis
  a. arcuata
  a. ascendens ileocolica
  a. auditiva interna
  arteriae auriculares
  a. axillaris
  arteriae azygoi vaginae
  a. basilaris
  a. brachialis
  arteriae bronchiales
  a. buccalis
  a. bulbi penis
  a. bulbi vestibuli vaginae
  a. caecalis anterior
  a. caecalis posterior
  a. callosomarginalis
  a. canalis pterygoidei
  arteriae
    caroticotympanicae
  a. carotis communis
  a. carotis externa
  a. carotis interna
  a. caudae pancreatis
  arteriae centrales
  a. cervicalis ascendens
  a. chorioidea
  arteriae ciliares
  a. circumflexa
  a. clitoridis
  a. colica
  a. collateralis
  a. comitans
  a. communicans
  arteriae conjunctivales
    anteriores

ar·te·ria *(continued)*
  arteriae conjunctivales
    posteriores
  a. coronaria dextra
  a. coronaria sinistra
  a. cremasterica
  a. cystica
  a. deferentialis
  a. dorsalis
  a. ductus deferentis
  a. epigastrica
  arteriae episclerales
  a. ethmoidalis
  a. facialis
  a. femoralis
  a. fibularis
  a. frontalis
  a. frontobasalis lateralis
  a. frontobasalis medialis
  arteriae gastricae
  a. gastroduodenalis
  a. gastroepiploica
  a. gastro-omentalis
  a. glutea inferior
  a. glutea superior
  a. gyri angularis
  arteriae helicinae penis
  a. hepatica
  a. hyaloidea
  a. hypogastrica
  a. hypophysialis inferior
  a. hypophysialis superior
  arteriae ilei
  a. ileocolica
  a. iliaca communis
  a. iliaca externa
  a. iliaca interna
  a. iliolumbalis
  a. infraorbitalis
  a. innominata
  arteriae insulares
  arteriae interlobulares
  a. interossea
  arteriae intestinales
  arteriae jejunales
  a. labyrinthi
  a. lacrimalis
  a. laryngea inferior

ar·te·ria *(continued)*
- a. laryngea superior
- a. lienalis
- a. lingualis
- a. lobi caudati
- arteriae lumbales
- a. lusoria
- a. mammaria interna
- a. masseterica
- a. maxillaris
- a. maxima Galeni
- a. media genus
- a. meningea media
- a. meningea posterior
- a. mentalis
- arteriae mesencephalicae
- a. musculophrenica
- arteriae nasales
- a. nutricia
- a. nutriens
- a. obturatoria
- a. occipitalis
- a. ophthalmica
- a. ovarica
- a. palatina
- arteriae palpebrales
- a. pancreatica
- arteriae
    pancreaticoduodenales
- a. paracentralis
- arteriae parietales
- a. parieto-occipitalis
- arteriae perforantes
- a. pericardiacophrenica
- a. perinealis
- a. peronea
- a. pharyngea ascendens
- arteriae phrenicae
- a. plantaris lateralis
- a. plantaris medialis
- a. plantaris profundus
- arteriae pontis
- a. poplitea
- a. precunealis
- a. profunda femoris
- a. pulmonalis
- a. pulmonalis dextra
- a. pulmonalis sinistra

ar·te·ria *(continued)*
- a. radialis
- a. recurrens
- arteriae renales
- a. renalis
- arteriae renis
- arteriae retroduodenales
- arteriae sacrales
- arteriae sigmoideae
- a. spermatica externa
- a. sphenopalatina
- a. spinalis anterior
- a. spinalis posterior
- a. splenica
- a. sternocleidomastoidea
- a. stylomastoidea
- a. subclavia
- a. subcostalis
- a. sublingualis
- a. submentalis
- a. subscapularis
- a. sulci centralis
- a. sulci postcentralis
- a. sulci precentralis
- a. supraduodenalis
- a. suprascapularis
- a. supratrochlearis
- arteriae surales
- a. temporalis anterior
- a. temporalis posterior
- a. temporalis profunda
    anterior
- a. temporalis profunda
    posterior
- a. temporalis superficialis
- a. testicularis
- a. thoracica interna
- a. thoracica lateralis
- a. thoracica suprema
- a. thoracoacromialis
- a. thoracodorsalis
- arteriae thymicae
- a. thyroidea ima
- a. thyroidea inferior
- a. thyroidea superior
- a. tibialis anterior
- a. tibialis posterior
- a. transversa faciei

ar·te·ria *(continued)*
  a. transversa scapulae
  a. tympanica
  a. ulnaris
  a. umbilicalis
  a. urethralis
  a. uterina
  a. vaginalis
  a. vertebralis
  a. zygomatico-orbitalis
ar·te·ri·al
ar·te·ri·al·iza·tion
ar·te·ri·ec·ta·sia
ar·te·ri·ec·ta·sis
ar·te·ri·ec·to·my
ar·te·ri·ec·to·pia
ar·te·rio·cap·il·lary
ar·te·rio·di·lat·ing
ar·te·rio·gen·e·sis
ar·te·rio·gram
ar·te·rio·graph
ar·te·ri·og·ra·phy
  axillary a.
  carotid a.
  catheter a.
  cerebral a.
  cine coronary a.
  completion a.
  femoral a.
  operative a.
  renal a.
  selective a.
  spinal a.
  vertebral a.
ar·te·ri·o·la *pl.* ar·te·ri·o·lae
  arteriolae ellipsoideae
  a. glomerularis afferens
  a. glomerularis efferens
  a. macularis inferior
  a. macularis superior
  a. medialis retinae
  a. nasalis retinae inferior
  a. nasalis retinae superior
  a. precapillaris
  arteriolae rectae renis
  arteriolae rectae spuriae
  arteriolae rectae vera

ar·te·ri·o·la *(continued)*
  a. temporalis retinae
   inferior
  a. temporalis retinae
   superior
  a. vaginatae
ar·te·ri·o·lae
ar·te·ri·o·lar
ar·te·ri·ole
  afferent a. of glomerulus
  central a.
  efferent a. of glomerulus
  ellipsoid a's
  Isaacs-Ludwig a.
  macular a., inferior
  macular a., superior
  medial a. of retina
  nasal a. of retina, inferior
  nasal a. of retina, superior
  postglomerular a.
  precapillary a's
  preglomerular a.
  sheathed a's
  straight a's of kidney
  straight a's of kidney, false
  straight a's of kidney, true
  temporal a. of retina,
   inferior
  temporal a. of retina,
   superior
ar·te·rio·lith
ar·te·rio·li·tis
ar·te·ri·ol·o·gy
ar·te·rio·lo·ne·cro·sis
ar·te·rio·lo·scle·ro·sis
ar·te·rio·lo·scle·rot·ic
ar·te·ri·o·lo·ve·nous
ar·te·ri·o·lo·ven·u·lar
ar·te·rio·mo·tor
ar·te·rio·myo·ma·to·sis
ar·te·rio·ne·cro·sis
ar·te·rio·neph·ro·scle·ro·sis
ar·te·ri·op·a·thy
  hypertensive a.
  idiopathic medial a.
  Takayasu's a.
ar·te·rio·plas·ty
ar·te·rio·pres·sor

ar·te·rio·re·nal
ar·te·ri·or·rha·phy
ar·te·ri·or·rhex·is
ar·te·rio·scle·ro·sis
    cerebral a.
    coronary a.
    hyaline a.
    hypertensive a.
    infantile a.
    intimal a.
    medial a.
    Mönckeberg's a.
    a. obliterans
    peripheral a.
    presenile a.
    retinal a.
    senile a.
ar·te·rio·scle·rot·ic
ar·te·ri·os·i·ty
ar·te·rio·spasm
ar·te·rio·spas·tic
ar·te·rio·ste·no·sis
ar·te·ri·os·teo·gen·e·sis
ar·te·ri·os·to·sis
ar·te·rio·strep·sis
ar·te·rio·sym·pa·thec·to·my
ar·te·ri·ot·o·my
ar·te·ri·ot·o·ny
ar·te·rio·trep·sis
ar·te·ri·ous
ar·te·rio·ve·nous
ar·te·rit·i·des
ar·ter·itis *pl.* ar·ter·it·i·des
    brachiocephalic a.
    a. brachiocephalica
    coronary a.
    cranial a.
    equine viral a.
    giant cell a.
    granulomatous a.
    Horton's a.
    infantile a.
    localized visceral a.
    necrotizing a.
    a. nodosa
    a. obliterans
    rheumatic a.
    syphilitic a.

ar·ter·itis *(continued)*
    Takayasu's a.
    temporal a.
    tuberculous a.
    a. umbilicalis
ar·te·ry
    accompanying a. of
      ischiadic nerve
    accompanying a. of median
      nerve
    accompanying a. of vein of
      Marshall
    acetabular a.
    acromial a.
    a. of Adamkiewicz
    adipose a's of kidney
    afferent a. of glomerulus
    alveolar a., inferior
    alveolar a's, superior,
      anterior
    alveolar a., superior,
      posterior
    anastomotic atrial a.
    anastomotica magna a.
    angular a.
    a. of angular gyrus
    anonymous a.
    appendicular a.
    arcuate a. of foot
    arcuate a's of kidney
    ascending cervical a.
    atrial anastomotic a.
    atrioventricular nodal a.
    auditory a., internal
    auricular a's, anterior
    auricular a., deep
    auricular a., left
    auricular a., posterior
    auricular a., right
    axial a.
    axillary a.
    azygos a's of vagina
    basilar a.
    brachial a.
    brachial a., deep
    brachial a., superficial
    brachiocephalic a.
    bronchial a's

ar·te·ry *(continued)*

bronchial a's, anterior
buccal a.
buccinator a.
bulbourethral a.
a. of bulb of penis
a. of bulb of vestibule of
  vagina
calcarine a.
callosomarginal a.
capsular a., inferior
capsular a., middle
caroticotympanic a's
carotid a., common
carotid a., external
carotid a., internal
caudal a.
caudal pancreatic a.
a. of caudate lobe
cecal a., anterior
cecal a., posterior
central a's, anterolateral
central a's, anteromedial
central a's, posterolateral
central a. of retina
central a's of spleen
a. of central sulcus
cephalic a.
cerebellar a., inferior,
  anterior
cerebellar a., inferior,
  posterior
cerebellar a., superior
cerebral a's
cerebral a., anterior
cerebral a., middle
cerebral a., posterior
cervical a., ascending
cervical a., deep
cervical a., descending,
  deep
cervical a., superficial
cervical a., transverse
cervicovaginal a's
a. of Charcot
a. of Charpy
choroid a.,anterior
ciliary a's, anterior

ar·te·ry *(continued)*

ciliary a's, long
ciliary a's, posterior, long
ciliary a's, posterior, short
ciliary a's, short
circumflex a., deep,
  internal
circumflex a., femoral,
  lateral
circumflex a., femoral,
  medial
circumflex a., humeral,
  anterior
circumflex a., humeral,
  posterior
circumflex a., iliac, deep
circumflex a., iliac,
  superficial
circumflex a. of scapula
a. of clitoris, deep
a. of clitoris, dorsal
coccygeal a.
cochlear a.
Cohnheim's a.
coiled a's
colic a., left
colic a., middle
colic a., right
colic a., right, inferior
colic a., superior, accessory
collateral digital a's
collateral a., middle
collateral a., radial
collateral a., ulnar, inferior
collateral a., ulnar,
  superior
a. to colliculi
communicating a.,
  anterior, of cerebrum
communicating a.,
  posterior, of cerebrum
companion a. to sciatic
  nerve
conal a.
conducting a's
conjunctival a's, anterior
conjunctival a's, posterior
conus a., left

ar·te·ry *(continued)*
  conus a., right
  conus a., third
  copper-wire a's
  cork-screw a's
  cornual a.
  coronary a., descending,
    posterior
  coronary a., left, of heart
  coronary a., left, of
    stomach
  coronary a., right, of heart
  coronary a., right, of
    stomach
  a. to corpus cavernosum
  cortical a's
  costocervical a.
  cremasteric a.
  cricothyroid a.
  crural a.
  cystic a.
  deep palmar a.
  deferential a.
  deltoid a.
  dental a's, anterior
  dental a., inferior
  dental a., posterior
  a. of dentate nucleus
  diaphragmatic a's
  diaphragmatic a's, superior
  digital a's, collateral
  digital a's of foot, dorsal
  digital a's of hand, dorsal
  digital a's, palmar,
    common
  digital a's, palmar, proper
  digital a's, plantar,
    common
  digital a's, plantar, proper
  digital a's, volar, common
  digital a's, volar, proper
  distributing a's
  dorsal carpal a.
  dorsal a. of clitoris
  dorsal a. of foot
  dorsal a. of nose
  dorsal a. of penis
  dorsalis pedis a.

ar·te·ry *(continued)*
  a. of Drummond
  a. of ductus deferens
  duodenal a's
  efferent a. of glomerulus
  elastic a's
  emulgent a.
  end a.
  a. of epididymis
  epigastric a., external
  epigastric a., inferior
  epigastric a., superficial
  epigastric a., superior
  episcleral a's
  esophageal a's, inferior
  ethmoidal a., anterior
  ethmoidal a., posterior
  facial a.
  facial a., deep
  facial a., transverse
  fallopian a.
  femoral a.
  femoral a., common
  femoral a., deep
  femoral a., superficial
  fetal umbilical a's
  fibular a.
  fifth lumbar a.
  a. of foot, dorsal
  frontal a.
  frontobasal a., lateral
  funicular a.
  gastric a., left
  gastric a., left inferior
  gastric a., posterior
  gastric a., right
  gastric a., right inferior
  gastric a's, short
  gastroduodenal a.
  gastroepiploic a., left
  gastroepiploic a., right
  gastro-omental a., left
  gastro-omental a., right
  genicular a., descending
  genicular a., inferior,
    lateral
  genicular a., inferior,
    medial

ar·te·ry *(continued)*

genicular a., middle
genicular a., superior, lateral
genicular a., superior, medial
glaserian a.
a. of glomerulus
gluteal a., inferior
gluteal a., superior
hardening of a's
helicine a's
helicine a's of penis
hemorrhoidal a., inferior
hemorrhoidal a., middle
hemorrhoidal a., superior
hepatic a., common
hepatic a., proper
Heubner's a.
humeral a.
hyaloid a.
a's of hybrid type
hyoid a.
hypogastric a.
hypophysial a., inferior
hypophysial a., superior
ileal a's
ileocolic a.
ileocolic a., ascending
iliac a., anterior
iliac a., common
iliac a., external
iliac a., internal
iliac a., small
iliolumbar a.
incisor a.
inferior profunda a.
infracostal a.
infraorbital a.
infrascapular a.
inguinal a's
innominate a.
insular a's
intercostal a's, anterior
intercostal a., first posterior
intercostal a., highest
intercostal a's, posterior

ar·te·ry *(continued)*

intercostal a., second posterior
intercostal a., superior
interlobar a's of kidney
interlobular a's of kidney
interlobular a's of liver
intermediate atrial a., left
intermediate atrial a., right
intermetacarpal a's, palmar
internal pudic a.
interosseous a., anterior
interosseous a., common
interosseous a., dorsal, of forearm
interosseous a., posterior, of forearm
interosseous a., recurrent
interosseous a., volar
intersegmental a's
interventricular a., anterior
interventricular septal a's, anterior
interventricular septal a's, posterior
intestinal a's
jejunal a's
Kugel's a.
labial a's, anterior, of vulva
labial a., inferior
labial a's, posterior, of vulva
labial a., superior
a. of labyrinth, labyrinthine a.
lacrimal a.
laryngeal a., inferior
laryngeal a., superior
left ventral paramedian a.
lenticulostriate a.
lingual a.
lingual a., deep
lumbar a's
lumbar a., fifth
lumbar a., lowest

ar·te·ry *(continued)*
  malleolar a., anterior,
    lateral
  malleolar a., anterior,
    medial
  malleolar a., posterior,
    lateral
  malleolar a., posterior,
    medial
  mammary a., external
  mammary a., internal
  mandibular a.
  marginal a. (of Drummond)
  marginal a., left
  marginal a., right
  masseteric a.
  mastoid a's
  maxillary a.
  maxillary a., external
  maxillary a., internal
  medial calcaneal a.
  medial a. of foot,
    superficial
  medial frontobasal a.
  median a.
  mediastinal a's, anterior
  mediastinal a's, posterior
  medullary a.
  meningeal a., accessory
  meningeal a., anterior
  meningeal a., middle
  meningeal a., posterior
  mental a.
  mesencephalic a's
  mesenteric a., inferior
  mesenteric a., superior
  metacarpal a's, dorsal
  metacarpal a's, palmar
  metacarpal a's, ulnar
  metacarpal a., volar, deep
  metatarsal a's, dorsal
  metatarsal a's, plantar
  a's of mixed type
  a's of Mueller
  muscular a's
  musculophrenic a.
  mylohyoid a.
  myomastoid a.

ar·te·ry *(continued)*
  nasal a., dorsal
  nasal a., external
  nasal a's, lateral posterior
  nasopalatine a.
  Neubauer's a.
  nodal a.
  a. of nose, dorsal
  nutrient a.
  nutrient a's of femur
  nutrient a. of fibula
  nutrient a's of humerus
  nutrient a's of kidney
  nutrient a. of tibia
  obliterated hypogastric a.
  obturator a.
  obturator a., accessory
  obtuse marginal (OM)
    coronary a.
  occipital a.
  occipital a., lateral
  occipital a., middle
  omphalomesenteric a.
  ophthalmic a.
  a. of optic chiasma
  a's to orbital muscles
  ovarian a.
  palatine a., ascending
  palatine a., descending
  palatine a., greater
  palatine a's, lesser
  palmar carpal a.
  palmar intermetacarpal a's
  palpebral a's, lateral
  palpebral a's, medial
  pancreatic a., dorsal
  pancreatic a., great
  pancreatic a., inferior
  pancreaticoduodenal a.,
    anterior superior
  pancreaticoduodenal a's,
    inferior
  pancreaticoduodenal a.,
    posterior superior
  paracentral a.
  paramedian a's
  parietal a's, anterior and
    posterior

ar·te·ry *(continued)*

parotid a.
pelvic a., posterior
penicilli a's
a. of penis, deep
a. of penis, dorsal
perforating a's
pericallosal a.
pericardiac a's, posterior
pericardiacophrenic a.
perineal a.
peroneal a.
peroneal a., perforating
pharyngeal a., ascending
phrenic a's, great
phrenic a's, inferior
phrenic a., superior
phrenicopericardial a.
plantar a., deep
plantar a., external
plantar a., lateral
plantar a., medial
pontine a's
popliteal a.
a. of postcentral sulcus
posterior intercostal a's
   I-XI
a. of precentral sulcus
precuneal a.
princeps pollicis a.
principal a. of thumb
profunda brachii a.
profunda femoris a.
pterygoid a's
a. of pterygoid canal
pubic a.
pudendal a's, external
pudendal a., internal
pulmonary a.
pulmonary a., left
pulmonary a., right
a. of the pulp
pyloric a.
quadriceps a. of femur
radial a.
radial a., collateral
radial a. of index finger

ar·te·ry *(continued)*

radial a., volar, of index
   finger
radiate a's of kidney
radicular a's
ranine a.
rectal a., inferior
rectal a., middle
rectal a., superior
rectosigmoid a.
recurrent a.
recurrent a., radial
recurrent a., tibial,
   anterior
recurrent a., tibial,
   posterior
recurrent a., ulnar
renal a.
renal a's
retrocostal a.
retroduodenal a's
revehent a.
right dorsocaudal a.
right ventral paramedian
   a.
Riolan's a.
a. of round ligament of
   uterus
sacral a's, lateral
sacral a., median
sacrococcygeal a.
scapular a., descending
scapular a., dorsal
scapular a., transverse
sciatic a.
screw a's
scrotal a's, anterior
scrotal a's, posterior
segmental a., anterior
segmental a., anterior
   inferior
segmental a., anterior
   superior
segmental a., inferior
segmental a., lateral
segmental a., medial
segmental a., posterior
segmental a., superior

ar·te·ry *(continued)*
  septal a's, anterior
  septal a's, posterior
  sheathed a's
  short central a.
  sigmoid a's
  silver-wire a's
  sinoatrial nodal a.
  sinuatrial nodal a.
  sinus node a.
  somatic a's
  spermatic a., external
  spermatic a., internal
  sphenopalatine a.
  spigelian a.
  spinal a's
  spinal a., anterior
  spinal a., posterior
  spiral a's
  splenic a.
  sternal a's, posterior
  sternocleidomastoid a.
  sternocleidomastoid a.,
    superior
  straight a's of kidney
  striate a's
  striate a's, lateral
  striate a's, medial
  stylomastoid a.
  subclavian a.
  subcostal a.
  sublingual a.
  submental a.
  subscapular a.
  sulcal a's
  superficial antebrachial a.
  superficial volar a.
  supraduodenal a.
  supraorbital a.
  suprarenal a., aortic
  suprarenal a., inferior
  suprarenal a., middle
  suprarenal a's, superior
  suprascapular a.
  supratrochlear a.
  sural a's
  sylvian a.
  tarsal a., lateral

ar·te·ry *(continued)*
  tarsal a's, medial
  temporal a., anterior
  temporal a's, deep
  temporal a., deep, anterior
  temporal a., deep, posterior
  temporal a., middle
  temporal a., posterior
  temporal a., superficial
  terminal a.
  testicular a.
  thalamogeniculate a.
  thalamoperforate a.
  thalamostriate a's,
    anterolateral
  thalmostriate a's,
    anteromedial
  thoracic a., highest
  thoracic a., internal
  thoracic a., lateral
  thoracicoacromial a.
  thoracodorsal a.
  thymic a's
  thyroid a., inferior
  thyroid a., inferior, of
    Cruveilhier
  thyroid a., lowest
  thyroid a., superior
  thyroidea ima a.
  tibial a., anterior
  tibial a., posterior
  a. of tongue, dorsal
  tonsillar a.
  transverse cervical a.
  transverse a. of face
  transverse a. of neck
  tubo-ovarian a.
  tympanic a., anterior
  tympanic a., inferior
  tympanic a., posterior
  tympanic a., superior
  ulnar a.
  ulnar collateral a., inferior
  ulnar collateral a., superior
  umbilical a.
  urethral a.
  uterine a.
  uterine a., aortic

ar·te·ry *(continued)*
vaginal a.
venous a's
ventral splanchnic a's
ventromedian a's
vermiform a.
vertebral a.
vesical a., inferior
vesical a's, superior
vestibular a's
vidian a.
vitelline a.
volar interosseous a.
a. of Zinn
zygomatico-orbital a.
ar·thrag·ra
ar·thral
ar·thral·gia
acromegalic a.
nonspecific a.
periodic a.
a. saturnina
ar·thral·gic
ar·threc·to·my
ar·threm·py·e·sis
ar·thres·the·sia
ar·thri·fuge
ar·thrit·ic
ar·thri·tide
ar·thri·tis *pl.* ar·thrit·i·des
acromegalic a.
acute a.
acute gouty a.
acute rheumatic a.
acute suppurative a.
atrophic a.
bacterial a.
Bekhterev's a.
blennorrhagic a.
chronic inflammatory a.
chronic villous a.
chylous a.
climactic a.
colitic a.
cricoarytenoid a.
crystal-induced a.
a. deformans
degenerative a.

ar·thri·tis *(continued)*
dysenteric a.
enteropathic reactive a.
exudative a.
fungal a.
a. fungosa
gonococcal a.
gonorrheal a.
gouty a.
hemophilic a.
hemorrhagic a.
hypertrophic a.
infectious a.
juvenile a.
juvenile chronic a.
juvenile rheumatoid a.
Lyme a.
Marie-Strümpell a.
menopausal a.
a. mutilans
mycotic a.
navicular a.
neurogenic a.
neuropathic a.
a. nodosa
nondeforming a.
noninflammatory a.
ochronotic a.
palindromic a.
a. pauperum
periosteal a.
postinfectious a.
proliferative a.
psoriatic a.
purulent a.
pyogenic a.
rheumatoid a.
rheumatoid a., juvenile
rheumatoid a. of spine
senescent a.
septic a.
a. sicca
suppurative a.
syphilitic a.
tuberculous a.
uratic a.
urethral a.
a. urethritica

ar·thri·tis *(continued)*
   venereal a.
   vertebral a.
   villous a.
   viral a.
ar·thro·cele
ar·thro·cen·te·sis
ar·thro·cha·la·sis
   a. multiplex congenita
ar·thro·chon·dri·tis
ar·thro·cla·sia
ar·thro·cli·sis
Arth·ro·der·ma
ar·thro·de·sia
ar·thro·de·sis
   extra-articular a.
   Moberg a.
   triple a.
ar·thro·dia
ar·thro·di·al
ar·thro·dyn·ia
ar·thro·dys·pla·sia
   hereditary a.
ar·thro·em·py·e·sis
ar·thro·en·dos·co·py
ar·thro·erei·sis
ar·throg·e·nous
ar·thro·gram
ar·throg·ra·phy
   air a.
ar·thro·gry·po·sis
   congenital multiple a.
   a. multiplex congenita
ar·thro·hy·al
ar·thro·ka·tad·y·sis
ar·thro·klei·sis
ar·thro·lith
ar·thro·li·thi·a·sis
ar·thro·lo·gia
ar·thro·log·ic
ar·throl·o·gy
ar·throl·y·sis
ar·thro·men·in·gi·tis
ar·throm·e·ter
ar·throm·e·try
ar·thron·cus
ar·thro·neu·ral·gia
ar·thro·ony·cho·dys·pla·sia

ar·thro-oph·thal·mop·a·thy
   hereditary progressive a.
ar·thro·os·teo·on·y·cho·dys·pla·sia
Ar·thro·pan
ar·thro·path·ia
   a. ovaripriva
   a. psoriatica
ar·thro·path·ic
ar·throp·a·thol·o·gy
ar·throp·a·thy
   Charcot's a.
   chondrocalcific a.
   degenerative vertebral a.
   diabetic a.
   dislocating a.
   disuse a.
   gonococcal a.
   Heberden's a.
   hemophilic a.
   inflammatory a.
   neurogenic a.
   neuropathic a.
   ochronotic a.
   osteopulmonary a.
   palindromic a.
   psoriatic a.
   pyrophosphate a.
   static a.
   stationary a.
   syphilitic a.
   tabetic a.
ar·thro·phy·ma
ar·thro·phyte
ar·thro·plas·tic
ar·thro·plas·ty
   Aufranc-Turner a.
   Austin Moore a.
   cementless a.
   Charnley 's hip a.
   Crawford-Adams a.
   interposition a.
   intracapsular
    temporomandibular joint a.
   Keller a.
   Lacey rotating hinge a.

Ashworth-Blatt

ar·thro·plas·ty *(continued)*
   McAtee-Tharias-Blazina a.
   McKee-Farrar a.
   Magnuson-Stack a.
   New England Baptist a.
   Putti-Platt a.
   Schlein-type elbow a.
   Stanmore shoulder a.
   Thompson a.
   total hip a.
   total knee a.
ar·thro·pneu·mog·ra·phy
ar·thro·pneu·mo·roent·ge·
   nog·ra·phy
ar·thro·pod
Ar·throp·o·da
ar·throp·o·dan
ar·thro·pod·ic
ar·throp·o·dous
ar·thro·py·o·sis
ar·thro·rheu·ma·tism
ar·thro·ri·sis
ar·thro·scin·ti·gram
ar·thro·scin·tig·ra·phy
ar·thro·scle·ro·sis
ar·thro·scope
ar·thros·copy
ar·thro·sis
   a. deformans
   temporomandibular a.
ar·thro·spore
ar·thros·te·i·tis
ar·thros·to·my
ar·thro·syn·o·vi·tis
ar·thro·tome
ar·throt·o·my
   Magnuson-Stack shoulder
   a.
ar·thro·tro·pia
ar·thro·trop·ic
ar·thro·xe·ro·sis
ar·throx·e·sis
Ar·thus phenomenon
Ar·thus reaction
Ar·thus-type reaction
ar·ti·cle
ar·tic·u·lar
ar·tic·u·la·re

ar·tic·u·lar·is cu·bi·ti
ar·tic·u·late
ar·tic·u·lat·ed
ar·tic·u·la·tio *pl.* ar·tic·u·la·
   ti·o·nes
   a. acromioclavicularis
   a. atlanto-axia′lis
   a. atlanto-occipitalis
   a. bicondylaris
   a. calcaneocuboidea
   a. capitis costae
   a. capitis humeri
   a. cochlearis
   a. condylaris
   articulationes
      costochondrales
   a. costotransversaria
   articulationes
      costovertebrales
   a. coxae
   a. cricoarytenoidea
   a. cricothyroidea
   a. cubiti
   a. cuneocuboidea
   a. cuneonavicularis
   a. dentoalveolaris
   a. genus
   a. humeri
   a. humeroradialis
   a. humero-ulnaris
   a. incudomallearis
   a.   incudostapedia
   articulationes
      interchondrales
   a. lumbosacralis
   a. radio-ulnaris
   a. sacrococcygea
   a. sacroiliaca
   a. sternoclavicularis
   articulationes
      sternocostales
   a.   subtalaris
   a. talocalcanea
   a. talocruralis
   a. talonavicularis
   a. tarsi transversa
   a. temporomandibularis
   a. tibiofibularis

ar·tic·u·la·tio *(continued)*
   articulationes vertebrales
   articulationes
      zygapophysiales
ar·tic·u·la·tion
   acromioclavicular a.
   articulator a.
   atlantoaxial a., lateral
   atlantoaxial a., medial
   atlantoepistrophic a.
   atlanto-occipital a.
   atloid a.
   a's of auditory ossicles
   balanced a.
   ball-and-socket a.
   bicondylar a.
   brachiocarpal a.
   brachioradial a.
   brachioulnar a.
   calcaneoastragaloid a.
   calcaneocuboid a.
   capitular a.
   carpal a's
   carpometacarpal a's
   carpometacarpal a., first
   carpometacarpal a. of
      thumb
   chondrosternal a's
   Chopart's a.
   cochlear a.
   composite a.
   compound a.
   condylar a.
   confluent a.
   congruent a.
   costocentral a.
   costochondral a's
   costosternal a's
   costotransverse a.
   costovertebral a's
   coxal a.
   coxofemoral a. of Buisson
   craniovertebral a.
   cricoarytenoid a.
   cricothyroid a.
   crurotalar a.
   cubital a.
   cubitoradial a., inferior

ar·tic·u·la·tion *(continued)*
   cubitoradial a., superior
   cuneocuboid a.
   cuneonavicular a.
   dentoalveolar a.
   a. of elbow
   ellipsoidal a.
   false a.
   femoral a.
   fibrous a's
   freely movable a.
   gliding a.
   a. of head of humerus
   a. of head of rib
   hinge a.
   a. of hip
   humeroradial a.
   humeroulnar a.
   a. of humerus
   iliosacral a.
   immovable a.
   incongruent a.
   incudomalleolar a.
   incudostapedial a.
   intercarpal a's
   interchondral a's
   intercostal a's
   intercuneiform a's
   intermetacarpal a's
   intermetatarsal a's
   intertarsal a's
   a. of knee
   lumbosacral a.
   mandibular a.
   manubriosternal a.
   maxillary a.
   mediocarpal a.
   metacarpocarpal a's
   metacarpophalangeal a's
   metatarsophalangeal a's
   occipital a.
   occipito-atlantal a.
   ovoid a.
   patellofemoral a.
   petrooccipital a.
   phalangeal a's
   a. of pisiform bone
   pisocuneiform a.

ar·tic·u·la·tion *(continued)*
    pivot a.
    plane a.
    a. of pubis
    radiocarpal a.
    radioulnar a.
    radioulnar a., distal
    radioulnar a., inferior
    radioulnar a., proximal
    radioulnar a., superior
    reciprocal a.
    sacrococcygeal a.
    sacroiliac a.
    saddle a.
    scapuloclavicular a.
    sellar a.
    a. of shoulder
    simple a.
    slightly movable a.
    spheroidal a.
    sternochondral a's
    sternoclavicular a.
    sternocostal a's
    subtalar a.
    synovial a's
    synovial a's of cranium
    talocalcaneonavicular a.
    talocrural a.
    talonavicular a.
    tarsometatarsal a's
    temporomandibular a.
    temporomaxillary a.
    a's of toes
    transverse tarsal a.
    trochoidal a.
    a. of tubercle of rib
    zygapophyseal a's
ar·tic·u·la·ti·o·nes
ar·tic·u·la·tor
    adjustable a.
    anatomic a.
    dental a.
    plain-line a.
ar·tic·u·la·to·ry
ar·tic·u·lo
    a. mortis
ar·tic·u·lus *pl.* ar·tic·u·li

ar·ti·fact
    mosaic a.
    pessary ring a.
ar·ti·fac·ti·tious
ar·ti·fi·cial
Ar·tio·dac·ty·la
ar·tio·dac·ty·lous
aru·case
Arum
Ar·vin
ARVO — Association for
    Research in Vision and
    Ophthalmology
ary·ep·i·glot·tic
ary·ep·i·glot·ti·cus
ary·ep·i·glot·tid·e·an
ar·yl·amine
ar·yl·ami·no·pep·ti·dase
ar·yl·ar·son·ic acid
ar·yl·es·ter·ase
ar·yl·es·ter hy·dro·lase
ar·yl·form·am·i·dase
ar·yl 4-hy·droxy·lase
ar·yl·sul·fa·tase
ar·y·te·na
ar·y·te·no·ep·i·glot·tic
ar·y·te·noid
ar·y·te·noid·ec·to·my
ar·y·te·noi·de·us
ar·y·te·noi·di·tis
ar·y·te·noi·do·pexy
ar·y·vo·ca·lis
AS — aortic stenosis
    arteriosclerosis
A.S. — L. auris sinistra (left
    ear)
As. — astigmatism
A-s — ampere-second
ASA — acetylsalicylic acid
    American Society of
        Anesthesiologists
    American Standards
        Association
    American Surgical
        Association
    argininosuccinic acid
asa·cria

as·a·fet·i·da
asa·phia
as·a·ron
As·a·rum
ASAS — American Society of
  Abdominal Surgeons
    argininosuccinic acid
      synthetase
ASAT — aspartate
  aminotransferase
ASB — American Society of
  Bacteriologists
as·bes·ti·form
as·bes·tos
  amphibole a.
  blue a.
  chrysotile a.
  crocidolite a.
  serpentine a.
  white a.
as·bes·to·sis
A-scan
as·ca·ri·a·sis
as·car·i·cid·al
as·car·i·cide
as·ca·rid
as·car·i·des
as·ca·ri·di·a·sis
As·ca·ri·di·dae
As·ca·ri·doi·dea
as·ca·ri·do·sis
as·ca·ri·o·sis
As·ca·ris
  A. lumbricoides
as·ca·ris *pl.* as·car·i·des
as·cen·dens
as·cend·ing
as·cen·sus
as·cer·tain·ment
  complete a.
  incomplete a.
  multiple a.
  single a.
  truncate a.
ASCH — American Society of
  Clinical Hypnosis
Asch's operation
Asch's splint

asc·hel·minth
Asc·hel·min·thes
Asch·er's negative glass-rod
  phenomenon
Asch·er's positive glass-rod
  phenomenon
Asch·er's syndrome
Asch·er·son's membrane
Asch·er·son's vesicles
Asch·heim-Zon·dek hormone
Asch·heim-Zon·dek test
Asch·ner's phenomenon
Asch·ner's reflex
Asch·ner's sign
Asch·ner's test
Asch·off's bodies
Asch·off's cell
Asch·off's node
Asch·off-Ta·wara node
ASCI — American Society for
  Clinical Investigation
as·ci
as·cia
as·ci·tes
  a. adiposus
  bile a.
  bloody a.
  chyliform a.
  a. chylosus
  a. chylosus
  chylous a.
  dialysis a.
  exudative a.
  fatty a.
  gelatinous a.
  hemorrhagic a.
  hydremic a.
  milky a.
  nephrogenic a.
  a. praecox
  preagonal a.
  pseudochylous a.
  transudative a.
as·cit·ic
as·ci·tog·e·nous
As·cle·pi·a·des
As·cle·pi·as
As·clep·i·os

ASCLT — American Society of
    Clinical Laboratory
    Technicians
ASCO — American Society of
    Clinical Oncology
        American Society of
        Contemporary
        Ophthalmology
As·cob·o·lus
as·co·carp
as·co·go·ni·um
As·co·li's reaction
As·co·li's test
As·co·li's treatment
As·co·my·ce·tae
as·co·my·cete
As·co·my·ce·tes
as·co·my·ce·tous
as·cor·bate
as·cor·be·mia
as·cor·bic acid
as·corb·uria
as·cor·byl pal·mi·tate
as·co·sin
as·co·spore
ASCP — American Society of
    Clinical Pathologists
as·cus *pl.* as·ci
ASD — atrial septal defect
ase·cre·to·ry
Asel·li's glands
Asel·li's pancreas
as·e·ma·sia
ase·mia
    a. graphica
    a. mimica
    a. verbalis
ase·mog·no·sia
asep·sis
asep·tate
asep·tic
    a.-antiseptic
asep·ti·cism
as·e·take
asex·u·al
asex·u·al·i·ty
ASF — aniline, formaldehyde,
    and sulfur

ASGE — American Society for
    Gastrointestinal Endoscopy
ASH — American Society of
    Hematology
AsH — hyperopic astigmatism
ash
ASHA — American School
    Health Association
        American Speech and
        Hearing Association
Ash·er·man syndrome
Ash·er·son's syndrome
ash·ing
ASHP — American Society of
    Hospital Pharmacists
asi·a·lia
asi·a·lo
asi·at·i·co·side
asid·er·o·sis
ASII — American Science
    Information Institute
ASIM — American Society of
    Internal Medicine
Asi·mi·na
asim·i·nine
ASIS — anterior superior iliac
    spine
asit·ia
as·ji·ke
As·ka·na·zy cell
As·kle·pi·os
ASL — antistreptolysin
        argininosuccinate lyase
As·lan·vi·tol
ASM — American Society for
    Microbiology
AsM — myopic astigmatism
Asn — asparagine
ASO — antistreptolysin O
        arteriosclerosis obliterans
aso·ma *pl.* aso·ma·ta
aso·ma·tog·no·sia
aso·ma·to·phyte
aso·nia
Aso·pia
ASP — American Society of
    Parasitologists
Asp — aspartic acid

as·pal·a·so·ma
as·par·a·gin·ase
as·par·a·gine
as·par·a·gi·nyl
as·par·tame
as·par·tate
as·par·tate ami·no·trans·fer·
ase
as·par·tate car·bam·o·yl
trans·fer·ase
as·par·tate trans·am·i·nase
as·par·thi·one
as·par·tic acid
as·par·tic pro·tein·ase
as·par·to·cin
as·par·tyl
β-as·par·tyl-*N*-ac·e·tyl·glu·
cos·amin·i·dase
as·par·tyl·gly·cos·amin·i·
dase
as·par·tyl·gly·cos·a·mi·nu·
ria
aspe·cif·ic
as·pect
    dorsal a.
    ventral a.
as·per
as·per·gil·lar
as·per·gil·li
as·per·gil·lic acid
as·per·gil·lin
as·per·gil·lo·ma
as·per·gil·lo·my·co·sis
as·per·gil·lo·sis
    aural a.
    bronchopneumonic a.
    pulmonary a.
as·per·gil·lo·tox·i·co·sis
As·per·gil·lus
    A. *auricularis*
    A. *barbae*
    A. *clavatus*
    A. *cookei*
    A. *fisherii*
    A. *flavus*
    A. *fumigatus*
    A. *giganteus*

As·per·gil·lus (continued)
    A. *glaucus*
    A. *gliocladium*
    A. *mucoroides*
    A. *nidulans*
    A. *niger*
    A. *ochraceus*
    A. *parasiticus*
    A. *repens*
    A. *terreus*
    A. *versicolor*
as·per·gil·lus *pl.* as·per·gil·li
as·per·gil·lus·tox·i·co·sis
as·per·ki·nase
asper·ma·tism
as·per·ma·to·gen·e·sis
asper·mia
ASPET — American Society
    for Pharmacology and
    Experimental Therapeutics
as·phyc·tic
as·phyc·tous
as·phyg·mia
as·phyx·ia
    autoerotic a.
    blue a.
    a. cyanotica
    fetal a.
    intrauterine a.
    a. livida
    local a.
    a. neonatorum
    a. pallida
    secondary a.
    sexual a.
    symmetric a.
    traumatic a.
    white a.
as·phyx·i·al
as·phyx·i·ant
as·phyx·i·ate
as·phyx·i·a·tion
As·pid·i·um
as·pid·i·um
as·pi·do·sper·mine
as·pi·rate
as·pi·ra·tion
    Cavitron a. unit

as·pi·ra·tion *(continued)*
 endometrial a.
 meconium a.
 vacuum a.
as·pi·ra·tor
 Dieulafoy's a.
as·pi·rin
 aluminum a.
asple·nia
 functional a.
asplen·ic
aspo·ro·gen·ic
as·po·rog·e·nous
aspor·ous
ASRT — American Society of Radiologic Technologists
ASS — anterior superior spine argininosuccinate synthetase
as·sault
 felonious a.
as·say
 biological a.
 blastogenesis a.
 cell-mediated lympholysis (CML) a.
 CH$_{50}$ a.
 complement a., hemolytic
 complement a., total
 complement a., whole
 C-terminal a.
 E rosette a.
 EAC rosette a.
 enzyme-linked immunosorbent a.
 Factor III multimer a.
 fluorescent a.
 four-point a.
 glycosylated hemoglobin a.
 hemagglutination inhibition (HI, HAI) a.
 hemolytic plaque a.
 immune a.
 immune adherence hemagglutination a. (IAHA)
 immunoradiometric a.
 Jerne plaque a.

as·say *(continued)*
 lymphocyte proliferation a.
 microbiological a.
 microcytotoxicity a.
 microhemagglutination a.—Treponema pallidum (MHA-TP)
 mixed lymphocyte culture (MLC) a.
 radioligand a.
 radiometric a.
 radioreceptor a.
 Raji cell a.
 stem cell a.
 thyroxine radioisotope a.
 Treponema pallidum hemagglutination a. (TPHA)
as·sess·ment
 Ballard gestational a.
 psychological a.
As·sé·zat's triangle
as·si·dent
as·sim·i·la·ble
as·sim·i·la·tion
 genetic a.
as·sis·tant
 physician's a.
Ass·mann's focus
as·so·ci·a·tion
 clang a.
 controlled a. test
 dream a's
 free a.
 individual practice a.
as·so·ci·us
as·sort·ment
as·sump·tion of risk
Ast. — astigmatism
as·ta·cin
asta·sia
 a.-abasia
 atonia-a.
astat·ic
as·ta·tine
as·ta·xan·thin
aste·a·to·des
aste·a·to·sis

as·ter
    sperm a.
aste·reo·cog·no·sy
aste·re·og·no·sis
as·te·ri·on pl. as·te·ria
as·ter·ix·is
aster·nal
aster·nia
as·ter·oid
As·ter·ol
Asth. — asthenopia
as·the·nia
    muscle a.
    myalgic a.
    neurocirculatory a.
    neurotic a.
    periodic a.
    tropical anhidrotic a.
as·then·ic
as·the·no·bi·o·sis
as·the·no·co·ria
as·the·nope
as·the·no·pia
    accommodative a.
    hysterical a.
    muscular a.
    nervous a.
    tarsal a.
as·the·nop·ic
as·the·no·sper·mia
as·the·nox·ia
as·thma
    abdominal a.
    allergic a.
    alveolar a.
    atopic a.
    bacterial a.
    bronchial a.
    bronchitic a.
    carders' a.
    cardiac a.
    cat a.
    catarrhal a.
    Cheyne-Stokes a.
    a. convulsivum
    cotton-dust a.
    cutaneous a.
    diisocyanate a.

as·thma (continued)
    dust a.
    Elsner's a.
    emphysematous a.
    essential a.
    extrinsic a.
    food a.
    grinders' a.
    Heberden's a.
    horse a.
    humid a.
    infective a.
    intrinsic a.
    isocyanate a.
    Kopp's a.
    Millar's a.
    millers' a.
    miners' a.
    nasal a.
    nervous a.
    platinum a.
    pollen a.
    potters' a.
    printers' a.
    reflex a.
    Rostan's a.
    silo workers' a.
    spasmodic a.
    steam-fitters' a.
    stone a.
    stripper's a.
    symptomatic a.
    thymic a.
    true a.
    Wichmann's a.
asth·mat·ic
asth·mat·i·form
asth·ma·toid
asth·mo·gen·ic
As·ti·ban
astig·ma·graph
astig·mat·ic
astig·ma·tism
    acquired a.
    a. against the rule
    compound a.
    congenital a.
    corneal a.

astig·ma·tism *(continued)*
   direct a.
   hypermetropic a.
   hypermetropic a.,
     compound
   hyperopic a.
   hyperopic a., compound
   hyperopic a., simple
   inverse a.
   irregular a.
   lenticular a.
   mixed a.
   myopic a.
   myopic a., compound
   myopic a., simple
   oblique a.
   physiological a.
   regular a.
   retinal a.
   a. with the rule
astig·ma·tom·e·ter
astig·ma·tom·e·try
as·tig·mato·scope
as·tig·ma·tos·co·py
astig·mia
as·tig·mic
as·tig·mom·e·ter
as·tig·mom·e·try
as·tig·mo·scope
as·tig·mos·co·py
Ast·ler-Col·ler classification
astom·a·tous
asto·mia
asto·mus
As·ton's rule
As·tra-8
As·tra·fer
as·trag·a·lar
as·trag·a·lec·to·my
as·trag·a·lo·cal·ca·ne·an
as·trag·a·lo·cru·ral
as·trag·a·lo·scaph·oid
as·trag·a·lo·tib·i·al
as·trag·a·lus
as·tral
as·tra·pho·bia
as·tra·po·pho·bia
astric·tion

astringe
astrin·gent
as·tro·blast
as·tro·blas·to·ma
as·tro·cele
as·tro·ci·net·ic
as·tro·coele
as·tro·cyte
   atypical a.
   fibrous a's
   gemistocytic a.
   plasmatofibrous a's
   protoplasmic a's
as·tro·cy·to·blast
as·tro·cy·to·ma
   anaplastic a.
   a. diffusum
   a. fibrillare
   gemistocytic a.
   pilocytic a.
   a. protoplasmaticum
as·tro·cy·to·ma·to·sis
  ce·re·bri
as·tro·cy·to·sis
as·trog·lia
as·tro·gli·o·ma
as·tro·gli·o·sis
as·tro·ki·net·ic
as·tro·pho·bia
as·tro·phor·ous
as·tro·pyle
as·tro·sphere
as·tro·stat·ic
As·trup method
asul·fu·ro·sis
asyl·la·bia
asy·lum
asym·bo·lia
   pain a.
   tactile a.
asym·bo·ly
asym·met·ri·cal
asym·me·try
   chromatic a.
   encephalic a.
asym·phy·tous
asymp·to·mat·ic
asyn·ap·sis

asyn·chro·nism
asyn·chro·nous
asyn·chro·ny
asyn·cli·tism
    anterior a.
    posterior a.
asyn·de·sis
asyn·ech·ia
asyn·er·gia
asyn·er·gia ma·jor
asyn·er·gic
asyn·er·gy
    axial a.
    axioappendicular a.
    progressive cerebellar a.
    progressive locomotor a.
    truncal a.
    verbal a.
asy·no·via
asyn·tax·ia
    a. dorsalis
asys·tem·ic
asys·to·le
asys·to·lia
asys·tol·ic
ATA — alimentary toxic
  aleukia
Ata·brine
atac·tic
atac·ti·form
atac·til·ia
at·a·rac·tic
at·ar·al·ge·sia
Ata·rax
at·a·rax·ia
at·a·rax·ic
at·a·raxy
at·a·vic
at·a·vism
at·a·vis·tic
atax·apha·sia
atax·ia
    acute a.
    acute cerebellar a.
    acute tabetic a.
    alcoholic a.
    appendicular a.
    autonomic a.

atax·ia *(continued)*
    Briquet's a.
    Bruns frontal a.
    bulbar a.
    central a.
    cerebellar a.
    cerebellofugal
      degeneration a.
    cerebral a.
    cervical a.
    dentate cerebellar a.
    diphtheric a.
    dynamic a.
    enzootic a.
    equilibratory a.
    family a.
    Fergusson and Critchley's
      a.
    Friedreich's a.
    frontal a.
    hereditary a.
    Holmes a.
    hysterical a.
    intrapsychic a.
    kinetic a.
    labyrinthic a.
    Leyden's a.
    limb kinetic a.
    locomotor a.
    Marie's a.
    motor a.
    nonequilibratory a.
    nutritional spinal a.
    ocular a.
    polyneuritic
      spinocerebellar a.
    postural a.
    professional a.
    pseudotabetic a.
    psychomotor a.
    Sanger Brown a.
    sensory a.
    spinal a.
    spinocerebellar a.
    static a.
    a.-telangiectasia
    thermal a.
    truncal a.

atax·ia *(continued)*
   vestibular a.
atax·ia·gram
atax·ia·graph
atax·i·am·e·ter
atax·i·am·ne·sic
ataxi·apha·sia
atax·ic
atax·io·phe·mia
atax·io·pho·bia
ataxo·phe·mia
ataxo·pho·bia
ataxy
ATCC — American Type
  Culture Collection
at·e·lec·ta·sis
   absorption a.
   acquired a.
   compression a.
   congenital a.
   congestion a.
   discoid a.
   initial a.
   lobar a.
   lobular a.
   obstructive a.
   patchy a.
   platelike a.
   postnatal asphyxia a.
   primary a.
   relaxation a.
   resorption a.
   secondary a.
   segmental a.
at·e·lec·tat·ic
atel·en·ce·pha·lia
atel·en·ceph·aly
ate·lia
ate·li·ot·ic
at·e·lo·car·dia
at·e·lo·ceph·a·lous
at·e·lo·ceph·a·ly
at·e·lo·chei·lia
at·e·lo·chei·ria
at·e·lo·en·ce·pha·lia
at·e·lo·en·ceph·a·ly
at·e·lo·glos·sia
at·e·log·na·thia

at·e·lo·my·e·lia
atel·op·id·tox·in
at·e·lo·po·dia
at·e·lo·pro·so·pia
at·e·lo·ra·chid·ia
at·e·lo·sto·mia
aten·o·lol
ATG — antithymocyte
  globulin
athal·po·sis
athe·lia
Ath·e·nae·us
ather·man·cy
ather·ma·nous
ather·mic
ather·mo·sys·tal·tic
ath·ero·em·bo·lism
ath·ero·em·bo·lus *pl.* ath·ero·
  em·bo·li
ath·ero·gen·e·sis
ath·ero·gen·ic
ath·er·o·ma
  cerebral a.
ath·er·o·ma·to·sis
ath·er·o·ma·tous
ath·ero·scle·ro·sis
  coronary a.
  a. obliterans
ath·ero·scle·rot·ic
ath·e·toid
ath·e·to·sis
  bilateral a.
  double a.
  double congenital a.
  posthemiplegic a.
  pupillary a.
  unilateral a.
ath·e·tot·ic
athi·a·mi·no·sis
ath·o·min
athrep·sia
ath·rep·sy
athrep·tic
ath·ro·cy·to·sis
ath·ro·phago·cy·to·sis
athym·ia
athym·ism
athy·mis·mus

athy·rea
athy·re·o·sis
athy·re·ot·ic
athy·ria
athy·roid·emia
athy·roid·ism
athy·roi·do·sis
athy·ro·sis
athy·rot·ic
Ath·y·sa·nus
At·kin·son-type lid block
ATL — adult T-cell
  leukemia/lymphoma
at·lan·tad
at·lan·tal
at·lan·to·ax·i·al
at·lan·to·bas·i·lar·is in·ter·
  nus
at·lan·to·did·y·mus
at·lan·toid
at·lan·to·mas·toid
at·lan·to-odon·toid
at·las
at·lo·ax·oid
at·lo·did·y·mus
at·loi·do-oc·cip·i·tal
atm — atmosphere
at·mi·at·rics
at·mo·graph
at·mol·y·sis
at·mom·e·ter
at·mos·phere
  standard a.
at·mos·pher·ic
at·mos·pher·iza·tion
at·mo·ther·a·py
ATN — acute tubular necrosis
  tyrosinase-negative
    (ty-neg) oculocutaneous
    albinism
ato·cia
ato·lide
at·om
  activated a.
  asymmetric carbon a.
  Bohr a.
  excited a.

at·om *(continued)*
  gram a.
  ionized a.
  nuclear a.
  radiating a.
  recoil a.
  rest a.
  Rutherford a.
  stripped a.
  tagged a.
atom·ic
at·om·i·za·tion
at·om·iz·er
ato·nia
  a.-astasia
  choreatic a.
aton·ic
at·o·nic·i·ty
at·o·ny
  chronic intestinal a.
  muscle a.
  primary ureteral a.
  uterine a.
at·o·pen
atop·ic
atop·og·no·sia
atop·og·no·sis
at·o·py
atox·ic
atox·i·gen·ic
ATP — adenosine
  triphosphate
ATPase — adenosinetriphospha-
  tase
ATP-co·bal·a·min aden·o·syl·
  trans·fer·ase
Atrac·tas·pis
atrac·toid
atrac·tyl·ic acid
atrac·tyl·i·gen·in
atrac·tylo·side
atra·cu·rium bes·y·late
atrans·fer·ri·ne·mia
atrau·mat·ic
A·trax
atre·mia
at·rep·sy
atrep·tic

atre·sia
  acquired a. of external
    auditory meatus
  anal a.
  a. ani
  aortic a.
  aural a.
  biliary a.
  choanal a.
  congenital a.
  duodenal a.
  esophageal a.
  a. of external auditory
    canal
  follicular a.
  a. folliculi
  intestinal a.
  a. iridis
  meatal a.
  mitral a.
  prepyloric a.
  pulmonary a.
  tricuspid a.
  vaginal a.
atre·sic
atret·ic
atre·to·ble·pha·ria
atre·to·ce·pha·lia
atre·to·ceph·a·lus
atre·to·cor·mia
atre·to·cor·mus
atre·to·cys·tia
atre·to·gas·tria
atre·to·le·mia
atre·to·me·tria
atre·top·sia
atre·tor·rhin·ia
atre·to·sto·mia
atre·ture·thria
atria
atri·al
atri·al·ized
atrich·ia
at·ri·cho·sis
atrich·ous
atrio·com·mis·su·ro·pexy
atrio·meg·a·ly
atrio·nec·tor

atrio·pep·ti·gen
atrio·pep·tin
atrio·sep·to·pexy
atrio·sep·to·plas·ty
atri·ot·o·my
atrio·ven·tric·u·la·ris com·
  mu·nis
atrip·li·cism
atri·um *pl.* atria
  a. alveolare
  common a.
  a. cordis
  a. dextrum
  a. glottidis
  a. of glottis
  a. of infection
  a. laryngis
  a. of larynx
  left a.
  a. mea′tus me′dii
  primitive a.
  a. pulmonale
  pulmonary a.
  right a.
  single a.
  a. sinistrum
  a. vaginae
At·ro·mid·S
At·ro·pa
atroph·e·de·ma
atro·phia
  a. bulborum hereditaria
  a. cerebri senilis simplex
  a. choroideae et retinae
  a. cutis
  a. cutis senilis
  a. dolorosa
  a. maculosa
  a. musculorum lipomatosa
  a. senilis
  a. striata et maculosa
  a. testiculi
  a. unguinum
atroph·ic
atro·phie
  a. blanche
  a. noire
at·ro·phied

at·ro·pho·der·ma
  a. biotripticum
  follicular a.
  idiopathic a. of Pasini and
    Pierini
  macular a.
  a. maculatum
  neuritic a.
  a. neuriticum
  a. of Pasini and Pierini
  a. reticulatum
    symmetricum faciei
  a. senile
  a. striatum et maculatum
  a. vermicularis
  vermiculate a. of cheeks
at·ro·pho·der·ma·to·sis
at·ro·pho·der·mia
  a. vermiculata
at·ro·phy
  acute yellow a.
  alveolar a.
  Aran-Duchenne muscular
    a.
  arthritic a.
  black a.
  blue a.
  bone a.
  brown a.
  cardiac a.
  cerebellar a.
  Charcot-Marie a.
  Charcot-Marie-Tooth a.
  circumpapillary
    chorioretinal a.
  circumscribed cerebral a.
  compensatory a.
  compression a.
  concentric a.
  convolutional a.
  correlated a.
  corticostriatospinal a.
  Cruveilhier's a.
  cutaneous a.
  cyanotic a.
  degenerative a.
  Dejerine-Sottas type of a.
  Dejerine-Thomas a.

at·ro·phy *(continued)*
  denervated muscle a.
  a. of disuse
  Duchenne-Aran muscular
    a.
  eccentric a.
  Eichhorst's a.
  endocrine a.
  endometrial a.
  Erb's a.
  exhaustion a.
  facial a.
  facioscapulohumeral
    muscular a.
  familial spinal muscular a.
  fat replacement a.
  fatty a.
  Fazio-Londe a.
  gastric a.
  gauntlet a.
  gingival a.
  granular a. of kidney
  gray a.
  gyrate a. of choroid and
    retina
  healed yellow a.
  hemifacial a.
  hemilingual a.
  hereditary optic a.
  Hoffmann's a.
  Hunt's a.
  hypoglossal a.
  idiopathic muscular a.
  inactivity a.
  infantile a.
  inflammatory a.
  interstitial a.
  a. of iris, essential
  ischemic muscular a.
  Jadassohn's macular a.
  juvenile muscular a.
  lactation a.
  lamellar cerebellar a.
  Landouzy-Dejerine a.
  leaping a.
  Leber's optic a.
  linear a.
  lobar a.

at·ro·phy *(continued)*
  macular a.
  muscular a.
  myelopathic muscular a.
  myopathic a.
  myotonic a.
  neural a.
  neuritic muscular a.
  neurogenic a.
  neuropathic a.
  neurotic a.
  neurotrophic a.
  numeric a.
  olivopontocerebellar a.
  olivoubrocerebellar a.
  optic a.
  optic a., primary
  optic a., secondary
  pallidal a.
  paraneoplastic cerebellar a.
  Parrot's a. of the newborn
  pathologic a.
  periodontal a.
  peroneal a.
  physiologic a.
  pigmentary a.
  postmenopausal a.
  post-traumatic a. of bone
  pressure a.
  progressive choroidal a.
  progressive diffuse cerebrocortical a.
  progressive muscular a.
  progressive neural muscular
  progressive neuromuscular a.
  progressive neuropathic (peroneal) muscular a.
  progressive spinal muscular a.
  progressive unilateral facial a.
  pseudohypertrophic muscular a.
  pseudomyopathic spinal muscular a.

at·ro·phy *(continued)*
  pulp a.
  red a.
  renal a.
  reversionary a.
  rheumatic a.
  scapuloperoneal muscular a.
  Schweninger-Buzzi macular a.
  segmental dissociation with brachial muscular a.
  senile a.
  senile a. of skin
  serous a.
  simple a.
  spinal muscular a.
  spinopontine a.
  striate a. of skin
  subacute a. of liver
  subchronic a. of liver
  Sudeck's a.
  syphilitic spinal muscular a.
  testicular a.
  Tooth's a.
  toxic a.
  traction a.
  traumatic a.
  trophoneurotic a.
  tubular a.
  unilateral facial a.
  vascular a.
  von Leber's a.
  Vulpian's a.
  Werdnig-Hoffmann a.
  Werdnig-Hoffmann spinal muscular a.
  white a.
  yellow a.
  Zimmerlin's a.
at·ro·pine
  fungal a.
  a. methonitrate
  a. methylbromide
  a. methylnitrate
  a. oxide hydrochloride
  a. salicylate

at·ro·pine *(continued)*
   a. sulfate
at·ro·pin·ic
at·ro·pin·ism
at·ro·pin·i·za·tion
at·ro·pism
At·ro·pi·sol
ATS — American Thoracic
  Society
   antitetanic serum
ATT — arginine tolerance test
at·tach·ment
   bar a.
   edgewise a.
   epithelial a. (of Gottlieb)
   extracoronal a.
   friction a.
   internal a.
   intracoronal a.
   key-and-keyway a.
   parallel a.
   muscle-tendon a.
   orthodontic a.
   precision a.
   semiprecision a.
   slotted a.
at·tack
   adversive a.
   anxiety a.
   apoplectiform a.
   cataplectic a.
   centrencephalic a.
   cerebellar a.
   cyclical epileptic a.
   decerebrate a.
   drop a.
   epileptic a.
   epileptiform a.
   focal a.
   heart a.
   myoclonic a.
   panic a.
   posterior a.
   tonic cerebellar a.
   transient ischemic a. (TIA)
   uncinate a.
   vagal a.
   vasovagal a.

at·tar
   a. of roses
at·ten·tion
at·ten·u·ant
at·ten·u·ate
at·ten·u·a·tion
at·ten·u·a·tor
At·ten·u·vax
at·tic
   tympanic a.
at·ti·ci·tis
at·ti·co·an·tral
at·ti·co·an·trot·o·my
at·ti·co·mas·toid
at·ti·cot·o·my
   transmeatal a.
at·ti·tude
   abstract a.
   a. of combat
   deflexion a.
   Devergie's a.
   discobolus a.
   fetal a.
   forced a.
   pugilistic a.
at·trac·tant
at·trac·tion
   a. of affinity
   capillary a.
   chemical a.
   electric a.
   magnetic a.
at·tri·bute
at·tri·tion
At·wat·er's chamber
At·wa·ter-Ben·e·dict
  calorimeter
At·wa·ter-Ben·e·dict chamber
at vol — atomic volume
At wt — atomic weight
atyp·ia
atyp·i·cal
atyp·ism
AU — Angström unit
   L. aures unitas (both ears
    together)
   L. auris uterque (each ear)

Au — gold (L. aurum)
Australian antigen
AUA — American Urological
Association
Au-an·ti·gen·emia
Aub-Du·bois table
Au·ber·ger·blood group
Au·bert's phenomenon
Auch·in·closs operation
Auch·mero·my·ia
a. luteola
au·dile
au·dio·an·al·ge·sia
au·dio·gen·ic
au·dio·gram
Békésy a.
cortical a.
pure tone a.
self-recording a.
serial a.
speech a.
au·di·ol·o·gist
au·di·ol·o·gy
au·di·om·e·ter
Békésy a.
evoked response a.
Langenbeck's noise a.
pure tone a.
semiautomatic pure tone a.
au·dio·met·ric
au·dio·me·tri·cian
au·di·om·e·try
air-conduction a.
Békésy a.
bone-conduction a.
brainstem-evoked response
a.
cortical a.
electrocochleographic a.
electrodermal a.
impedance a.
industrial a.
localization a.
psychogalvanic skin
response a.
pure tone a.
speech a.
au·dio·vis·u·al

au·di·tion
chromatic a.
a. colorée
gustatory a.
thought a.
au·di·tive
au·di·tog·no·sis
au·di·to·ri·us
au·di·to·ry
au·di·to·sen·so·ry
Au·dou·in's microsporon
Au·en·brug·ger's sign
Au·er's bodies
Au·er·bach's ganglion
Au·er·bach's plexus
Au·franc-Tur·ner cup
Au·franc-Tur·ner operation
Au·franc-Tur·ner prosthesis
Auf·recht's sign
Auf·richt elevator
Auf·richt retractor
Auf·richt speculum
AUG — acute ulcerative
gingivitis
au·gen·blick
Au·ger's effect
Au·ger's electron
aug·men·tor
aug·na·thus
Au·jesz·ky's disease
au·la
au·ra *pl.* au·rae
a. asthmatica
auditory a.
autonomic a.
dysmnesic a.
electric a.
epigastric a.
epileptic a.
generalized somatic a.
a. hysterica
illusional a.
intellectual a.
kinesthetic a.
motor a.
myoclonic a.
neuralgic a.

au·ra *(continued)*
  paramnesic a.
  a. procursiva
  reminiscent a.
  sensory a.
  somatosensory a.
  a. vertiginosa
  vertiginous a.
  visceral a.
  visual a.
au·ral
au·ra·mine O
au·ran·o·fin
au·ran·tia
au·ran·ti·a·sis
au·ran·tio·gli·oc·la·din
Au·re·lia
Au·reo·ba·sid·i·um
  a. pullulans
au·re·o·lin
Au·reo·my·cin
au·res
au·ri·a·sis
au·ric
au·ri·cle
  accessory a.
  cervical a.
  left a. of heart
  right a. of heart
au·ric·u·la *pl.* au·ric·u·lae
  a. atrii
  a. atrii dextri
  a. atrii sinistri
  a. cordis
  a. dextra cordis
  a. sinistra cordis
au·ric·u·lae
au·ric·u·lar
au·ric·u·la·re
au·ric·u·la·ris
au·ric·u·lec·to·my
au·ric·u·lo·cra·ni·al
au·ric·u·lo·tem·po·ral
au·ric·u·lo·ther·a·py
au·ric·u·lo·ven·tric·u·lar
au·rid
au·ri·form
au·rin

au·ri·na·ri·um
au·ri·na·sal
au·rin·tri·car·box·yl·ic acid
au·ri·pig·ment
au·ris *pl.* au·res
  a. externa
  a. interna
  a. media
au·ri·scope
au·rist
au·ris·tics
au·ro·chro·mo·der·ma
au·ro·ther·a·py
au·ro·thio·glu·cose
au·ro·thio·gly·ca·nide
au·ro·thio·ma·late di·so·di·um
au·ro·thio·sul·fate
au·rum
aus·cult
aus·cul·tate
aus·cul·ta·tion
  direct a.
  immediate a.
  Korányi's a.
  mediate a.
  obstetric a.
aus·cul·ta·to·ry
aus·cul·to·plec·trum
aus·cul·to·scope
Aus·tin Flint murmur
Aus·tin Flint respiration
Aus·tin Moore arthroplasty
Aus·tin Moore prosthesis
Aus·tra·lo·bil·har·zia
au·ta·coid
au·techo·scope
au·te·cic
au·te·cious
au·te·col·o·gy
au·te·me·sia
au·tism
  akinetic a.
  early infantile a.
  infantile a.
au·tis·tic
au·to·ac·ti·va·tion
au·to·ag·glu·ti·na·tion

au·to·ag·glu·ti·nin
au·to·al·ler·gic
au·to·al·ler·gi·za·tion
au·to·al·ler·gy
au·to·am·pu·ta·tion
au·to·anal·y·sis
au·to·an·am·ne·sis
au·to·an·ti·bo·dy
au·to·an·ti·com·ple·ment
au·to·an·ti·gen
au·to·an·ti·sep·sis
au·to·an·ti·tox·in
au·to·au·di·ble
au·to·bac·te·rio·phage
au·to·bi·ot·ic
au·to·body
au·to·ca·tal·y·sis
au·to·cat·a·lyst
au·to·cat·a·lyt·ic
au·to·ca·thar·sis
au·to·cath·e·ter·ism
au·to·cho·le·cys·tec·to·my
au·toch·tho·nous
au·to·ci·ne·sis
au·toc·la·sis
au·to·clave
Au·to·clip
au·to·crine
au·to·cys·to·plas·ty
au·to·cy·tol·y·sin
au·to·cy·tol·y·sis
au·to·cy·to·lyt·ic
au·to·cy·to·tox·in
au·to·der·mic
au·to·de·struc·tion
au·to·di·ges·tion
au·to·dip·loid
au·to·drain·age
au·to·echo·la·lia
au·to·echo·prax·ia
au·toe·cic
au·toe·cious
au·to·ec·zem·a·ti·za·tion
au·to·ep·i·la·tion
au·to·erot·ic
au·to·erot·i·cism
au·to·er·o·tism

au·to·eryth·ro·phago·cy·to·sis
au·to·flu·o·res·cence
au·to·flu·o·ro·scope
au·to·fun·do·scope
au·to·fun·dos·co·py
au·tog·a·mous
au·tog·a·my
au·to·gen·e·ic
au·to·gen·e·sis
au·to·ge·net·ic
au·tog·e·nous
au·tog·e·ny
au·to·graft
au·to·graft·ing
au·to·gram
au·to·he·mag·glu·ti·na·tion
au·to·he·mag·glu·ti·nin
au·to·he·mic
au·to·he·mol·y·sin
au·to·he·mol·y·sis
au·to·he·mo·lyt·ic
au·to·he·mo·ther·a·py
au·to·he·mo·trans·fu·sion
au·to·his·to·ra·dio·graph
au·to·hyp·no·sis
au·to·hyp·not·ic
au·to·im·mune
au·to·im·mu·ni·ty
au·to·im·mu·ni·za·tion
au·to·in·fec·tion
au·to·in·fla·tion
au·to·in·fu·sion
au·to·in·oc·u·la·ble
au·to·in·oc·u·la·tion
au·to·in·ter·fer·ence
au·to·isol·y·sin
au·to·ker·a·to·plas·ty
au·to·ki·ne·sia
au·to·ki·ne·sis
    visible light a.
au·to·ki·net·ic
au·to·la·vage
au·to·le·sion
au·to·leu·ko·ag·glu·ti·nin
au·tol·o·gous
au·tol·o·gy
au·tol·y·sate

au·tol·y·sin
au·tol·y·sis
    postmortem a.
au·to·ly·so·some
au·to·lyt·ic
au·to·lyze
au·to·mat·ic
Au·to·mat·ic Clin·i·cal An·a·
    lyz·er
au·tom·a·tism
    alcohol a.
    ambulatory a.
    command a.
    epileptic a.
    postepileptic a.
    postictal a.
    vigil ambulatory a.
au·to·mato·graph
au·tom·a·ton
Au·tom·e·ris io
au·to·mix·is
au·to·my·so·pho·bia
au·to·ne·phrec·to·my
au·to·neph·ro·tox·in
au·to·nom·ic
au·to·nomo·trop·ic
au·ton·o·mous
au·ton·o·my
au·to-oph·thal·mo·scope
au·to-oph·thal·mos·co·py
au·to-ox·i·da·tion
au·to·path
au·to·path·ic
au·to·pa·thog·ra·phy
au·top·a·thy
au·to·pha·gia
au·to·phago·some
au·toph·a·gy
au·to·phar·ma·co·log·ic
au·to·phar·ma·col·o·gy
au·to·phene
au·to·phil
au·to·phil·ia
au·to·pho·bia
au·to·pho·nom·e·try
au·toph·o·ny
au·toph·thal·mo·scope
au·to·phyte

au·to·plast
au·to·plas·tic
au·to·plas·ty
    peritoneal a.
au·to·ploid
au·to·po·di·um
au·to·poi·son·ous
au·to·pol·y·mer
au·to·pol·y·mer·i·za·tion
au·to·poly·ploid
au·to·pro·te·ol·y·sis
au·to·pro·throm·bin
    a. I
    a. II
    a. IIa
    a. C
au·to·pro·tol·y·sis
au·top·sia
au·top·sy
    forensic a.
    medicolegal a.
    psychological a.
au·to·psy·chic
au·to·psy·cho·rhyth·mia
au·to·ra·dio·gram
au·to·ra·dio·graph
au·to·ra·di·og·ra·phy
au·to·reg·u·la·tion
    heterometric a.
    homeometric a.
au·to·re·in·fec·tion
au·to·re·in·fu·sion
au·tos·co·py
au·to·sen·si·tive
au·to·sen·si·ti·za·tion
    erythrocyte a.
au·to·sen·si·tized
au·to·sep·ti·ce·mia
au·to·se·rous
au·to·se·rum
au·to·sex·ing
au·to·site
au·to·sit·ic
au·tos·mia
au·to·so·mal
au·to·so·ma·tog·no·sis
au·to·so·ma·tog·nos·tic
au·to·some

au·to·sper·mo·tox·in
au·to·sple·nec·to·my
au·to·spray
au·to·stim·u·la·tion
au·to·sug·ges·ti·bil·i·ty
au·to·sug·ges·tion
au·to·sym·pa·thec·to·my
au·to·syn·the·sis
au·to·tech·ni·con
au·to·tem·nous
au·to·ther·a·py
au·to·throm·bo·ag·glu·ti·nin
au·to·tomo·graph·ic
au·to·to·mog·ra·phy
au·tot·o·my
au·to·top·ag·no·sia
au·to·trans·fu·sion
    intraoperative a.
    postoperative a.
au·to·trans·plant
au·to·trans·plan·ta·tion
au·to·trep·a·na·tion
au·to·troph
    facultative a.
    obligate a.
au·to·troph·ic
au·tot·ro·phy
au·to·tu·ber·cu·lin
au·to·tu·ber·cu·lin·iza·tion
au·to·vac·ci·na·tion
au·to·vac·cine
au·to·vac·cin·ia
au·to·vac·ci·no·ther·a·py
au·tox·i·da·tion
au·tox·i·diz·a·ble
au·to·zy·gous
aux·ano·dif·fer·en·ti·a·tion
aux·ano·gram
aux·ano·graph·ic
aux·an·og·ra·phy
aux·e·sis
aux·et·ic
aux·il·i·a·ry
    torquing a.
aux·il·io·mo·tor
aux·i·lyt·ic
aux·in
aux·i·om·e·ter

auxo·ac·tion
auxo·car·dia
auxo·chrome
auxo·chro·mous
auxo·cyte
auxo·drome
auxo·flore
auxo·flur
auxo·gluc
aux·om·e·ter
auxo·met·ric
aux·om·e·try
auxo·neu·ro·trop·ic
auxo·spi·reme
auxo·spore
auxo·ton·ic
auxo·tox
auxo·troph
auxo·troph·ic
auxo·type
AV — arteriovenous
    atrioventricular
A-V — atrioventricular
avail·a·bil·i·ty
    biologic a.
    physiologic a.
av·a·lanche
    Townsend a.
aval·vu·lar
avas·cu·lar
avas·cu·lar·i·za·tion
avdp. — avoirdupois
Avel·lis' paralysis
Avel·lis' syndrome
Avel·lis-Lon·ghi syndrome
Ave·na
ave·nin
ave·no·lith
Aven·tyl
Av·en·zo·ar
av·er·age
    moving a.
    spatial a. temporal a.
      (SATA)
    spatial peak temporal a.
      (SPTA)
    time-weighted a.

averaging
   signal a.
   spike-triggered a.
av·er·mec·tin
Av·er·ro·es
aver·sive
Aver·tin
avi·ad·e·no·vi·rus
avi·an
Av·i·cen·na
av·i·din
avid·i·ty
avir·u·lence
avir·u·lent
avi·ta·min·o·sis
   conditioned a.
   a. D
avi·ta·min·ot·ic
avive·ment
Av·lo·sul·fon
AVM — arteriovenous
   malformation
      atrioventricular
      malformation
AVMA — American
   Veterinary Medical
   Association
Av·o·gad·ro's law
Av·o·gad·ro's constant
Av·o·gad·ro's number
avo·gram
avoid·ance
   phobic a.
avoid·ant
av·oir·du·pois
avo·par·cin
AVP — arginine vasopressin
avul·sion
   nerve a.
   phrenic a.
   scalp a.
   tooth a.
awa·ken·ing
   delayed a.
awu — atomic weight unit
ax. — axillary
   axis
Ax·el·rod, Julius

Ax·en·feld's anomaly
Ax·en·feld's syndrome
Ax·en·feld-Kruk·en·berg
   spindle
axen·ic
ax·es
ax·i·al
ax·i·a·tion
ax·if·u·gal
ax·i·lem·ma
ax·il·la *pl.* ax·il·lae
ax·il·lary
ax·il·lo·bi·fem·o·ral
ax·il·lo·fem·o·ral
ax·il·lo·pop·lit·e·al
ax·io·buc·cal
ax·io·buc·co·cer·vi·cal
ax·io·buc·co·gin·gi·val
ax·io·buc·co·lin·gual
ax·io·cer·vi·cal
ax·io·dis·tal
ax·io·dis·to·cer·vi·cal
ax·io·dis·to·gin·gi·val
ax·io·dis·to·in·ci·sal
ax·io·dis·to-oc·clu·sal
ax·io·gin·gi·val
ax·io·in·ci·sal
ax·io·la·bi·al
ax·io·la·bio·gin·gi·val
ax·io·la·bio·lin·gual
ax·io·lin·gual
ax·io·lin·guo·cer·vi·cal
ax·io·lin·guo·gin·gi·val
ax·io·lin·guo-oc·clu·sal
ax·io·me·si·al
ax·io·me·sio·cer·vi·cal
ax·io·me·sio·dis·tal
ax·io·me·sio·gin·gi·val
ax·io·me·sio·in·ci·sal
ax·io·me·sio-oc·clu·sal
ax·io-oc·clu·sal
ax·io·po·di·um
ax·io·pul·pal
ax·ip·e·tal
ax·is *pl.* ax·es
   anteroposterior a.
   arterial a., costocervical
   basibregmatic a.

ax·is *(continued)*
    basicranial a.
    basifacial a.
    binauricular a.
    a. bulbi externus
    a. bulbi internus
    celiac a.
    cell a.
    cephalocaudal a.
    condylar a.
    craniocaudal a.
    craniofacial a.
    dorsoventral a.
    Downs Y a.
    electrical a. of heart
    embryonic a.
    external a. of eye
    facial a.
    frontal a.
    group Ia a.
    a. of heart
    hinge a.
    horizontal a.
    HPA
        (hypothalamic-pituitary-adrenal) a.
    internal a. of eye
    a. of lens
    a. lentis
    long a. of body
    longitudinal a.
    mandibular a.
    normal a.
    a. oculi externa
    a. oculi interna
    opening a.
    optic a.
    a. optica
    optical a.
    a. opticus
    a. pelvis
    a. of pelvis
    pituitary-adrenocortical a.
    pituitary-gonadal a.
    pituitary-thyroid a.
    a. of preparation
    principal a.
    pupillary a.

ax·is *(continued)*
    renal a.
    renin-aldosterone a.
    renin-angiotensin a.
    right a.
    sagittal a. of eye
    secondary a.
    T a.
    thoracic a.
    thyroid a.
    uterine a.
    vertical a. of eye
    visual a.
    Y a.
ax·is cyl·in·der
axo·ax·on·ic
axo·den·drite
axo·den·drit·ic
axo·fu·gal
ax·o·graph
ax·oid
ax·oi·de·an
axo·lem·ma
ax·o·lotl
ax·ol·ysis
ax·om·e·ter
ax·on
    giant a.
    naked a.
    unmyelinated a.
ax·o·nal
ax·on·aprax·ia
ax·one
ax·o·neme
ax·o·nom·e·ter
ax·on·ot·me·sis
axo·not·o·my
ax·op·e·tal
axo·phage
axo·plasm
axo·plas·mic
axo·po·dia
axo·po·di·um *pl.* axo·po·dia
axo·so·mat·ic
axo·spon·gi·um
axo·style
Aya·la's equation
Aya·la's index

Aya·la's quotient
aya·pa·na
Ayer's test
Ayer-To·bey test
Ayer·za's disease
Ayer·za's syndrome
Ayre's brush
Ayre's tube
aza·bon
aza·clor·zine hy·dro·chlo·ride
aza·cos·ter·ol hy·dro·chlo·ride
aza·cy·clo·nol
5-aza·cy·ti·dine
az·a·guan·ine
aza·meth·o·ni·um bro·mide
aza·na·tor ma·le·ate
aza·nid·a·zole
aza·pet·ine phos·phate
aza·pro·pa·zone
aza·ri·bine
aza·ser·ine
aza·stene
azat·a·dine mal·e·ate
aza·thio·prine
    a. sodium
6-aza·uri·dine
azed·a·rach
az·e·la·ic acid
azeo·trop·ic
aze·ot·ro·py
aze·pin·amide
aze·te·pa
azide
az·i·do·thy·mi·dine (AZT)
azip·ra·mine
az·lo·cil·lin
azo·ben·zene
azo·bil·i·ru·bin
azo·car·mine
azo·ic
az·ole
Az·o·lid
azo·lit·min
azo·meth·ine

Azo·mo·nas
azo·my·cin
azoo·sper·ma·tism
azoo·sper·mia
azo·pig·ment
azo·pro·tein
Azor·e·an disease
azo·sul·fa·mide
az·ote
az·o·te·mia
    extrarenal a.
    postrenal a.
    prerenal a.
    renal a.
az·o·te·mic
Azo·to·bac·ter
Azo·to·bac·te·ra·ceae
az·o·tom·e·ter
azo·to·my·cin
az·o·tor·rhea
az·o·tu·ria
az·o·tu·ric
az·oxy·ben·zene
az·oxy compound
AZT — azidothymidine
az·tre·o·nam
az·ul
az·u·lene
Azul·fi·dine
az·ure
    a. I
    a. II
    a. A
    a. B
    a. C
    methylene a.
az·u·res·in
az·ur·in
az·u·ro·phil
az·u·ro·phile
az·u·ro·phil·ia
az·u·ro·phil·ic
az·y·ges
az·y·go·gram
az·y·gog·raphy

az·y·gos
azy·go·sperm
azy·go·spore

az·y·gous
azym·ia
azy·mic

B

B — bacillus
  bel
  boron
B — magnetic flux density
b — barn
  base (in nucleic acid
    sequencing)
β — *β* chain of hemoglobin
BA — Bachelor of Arts
Baas·trup's disease
Baas·trup's syndrome
Bab·bitt metal
Bab·cock's operation
Bab·cock sentence
Ba·bès' treatment
Ba·bès' tubercles
Babès-Ernst bodies
Babès-Ernst granules
Ba·be·sia
ba·be·si·a·sis
ba·be·si·o·sis
Ba·bin·ski's law
Ba·bin·ski's phenomenon
Ba·bin·ski's reflex
Ba·bin·ski's sign
Ba·bin·ski's syndrome
Ba·bin·ski-Fröh·lich syndrome
Ba·bin·ski-Na·geotte
  syndrome
Ba·bin·ski-Va·quez syndrome
ba·by
  blue b.
  collodion b.
  test-tube b.
ba·cam·pi·cil·lin hy·dro·chlo·
  ride

bac·cate
Bac·cel·li's mixture
Bac·cel·li's sign
bac·ci·form
Bach·man's reaction
Bach·man's test
Bach·mann's bundle
Bac·i·guent
Bac·il·la·ceae
bac·il·la·ry
bacille
  b. Calmette-Guérin (BCG)
bac·il·le·mia
ba·cil·li
ba·cil·lif·er·ous
ba·cil·li·form
ba·cil·lin
bac·il·lo·sis
ba·cil·lu·ria
Ba·cil·lus
  B. brevis
  B. cereus
  B. polymyxa
  B. stearothermophilus
  B. subtilis
ba·cil·lus *pl.* ba·cil·li
  acid-fast b. (AFB)
  Battey b.
  Boas-Oppler b.
  Bordet-Gengou b.
  Calmette-Guérin b.
  Chauveau's b.
  coliform bacilli
  DF-2 b.
  diphtheria b.
  Döderlein's b.

ba·cil·lus *(continued)*
  Ducrey's b.
  dysentery bacilli
  Escherich's b.
  Flexner's b.
  Friedländer's b.
  Frisch b.
  fusiform b.
  Gärtner's b.
  Ghon-Sachs b.
  Hansen's b.
  Hofmann's b.
  Johne's b.
  Klebs-Löffler b.
  Koch-Weeks b.
  lepra b.
  Morax-Axenfeld b.
  Morgan's b.
  Newcastle-Manchester b.
  paracolon bacilli
  Pfeiffer's b.
  Preisz-Nocard b.
  rhinoscleroma b.
  Schmitz's b.
  Schmorl's b.
  Shiga b.
  Sonne-Duval b.
  Stanley b.
  Strong's b.
  tubercle b.
  Vincent's b.
  Weeks' b.
  Welch's b.
  Whitmore's b.
bac·i·tra·cin
  b. zinc
back
  flat b.
  functional b.
  hollow b.
  hump b.
  hunch b.
  old man's b.
  poker b.
  saddle b.
  static b.
  sway b.
back·al·gia

back·bleed·ing
back·bone
back·cross
  double b.
back·flow
  pyelolymphatic b.
  pyelorenal b.
  pyelosinus b.
  pyelotubular b.
  pyelovenous b.
back·knee
back-rak·ing
back·scat·ter
bac·lo·fen
Bact. — Bacterium
bac·ter·e·mia
  puerperal b.
bac·te·re·mic
Bac·te·ria
bac·te·ria
Bac·te·ri·a·ceae
bac·te·ri·al
bac·te·ri·ci·dal
bac·te·ri·cide
  specific b.
bac·te·ri·cid·in
bac·ter·id
  pustular b.
bac·te·ri·emia
bac·ter·i·form
bac·te·rio·chlo·ro·phyll
bac·te·rio·ci·din
bac·te·rio·cin
bac·te·ri·o·cin·o·gen
bac·te·ri·o·cin·o·gen·ic
bac·te·rio·cla·sis
bac·te·rio·flu·o·res·cin
bac·te·ri·o·gen·ic
bac·te·ri·og·e·nous
bac·te·ri·oid
bac·te·rio·log·ic
bac·te·rio·log·i·cal
bac·te·ri·ol·o·gist
bac·te·ri·ol·o·gy
  clinical diagnostic b.
  medical b.
  pathological b.
  public health b.

bac·te·ri·ol·o·gy *(continued)*
    sanitary b.
    systematic b.
bac·te·ri·ol·y·sin
bac·te·ri·ol·y·sis
    immune b.
bac·te·rio·lyt·ic
Bac·te·rio·ne·ma
    B. matruchotii
bac·te·ri·o-op·so·nin
bac·te·rio·phage
    mature b.
    temperate b.
    vegetative b.
    virulent b.
bac·te·rio·pha·gia
bac·te·rio·phag·ic
bac·te·rio·pha·gol·o·gy
bac·te·rio·phy·to·ma
bac·te·rio·plas·min
bac·te·rio·pre·cip·i·tin
bac·te·rio·pro·tein
bac·te·ri·op·son·ic
bac·te·ri·op·so·nin
bac·te·rio·pur·pu·rin
bac·te·rio·rho·dop·sin
bac·te·ri·o·sis
bac·te·rio·sper·mia
bac·te·rio·sta·sis
bac·te·rio·stat
bac·te·rio·stat·ic
bac·te·rio·ther·a·py
bac·te·rio·tox·emia
bac·te·rio·tox·ic
bac·te·rio·tox·in
bac·te·ri·o·trop·ic
bac·te·ri·ot·ro·pin
bac·ter·it·ic
bac·te·ri·um
    acid-fast b.
    autotrophic b.
    beaded b.
    bifid b.
    blue-green b.
    Chauveau's b.
    chemoautotrophic b.
    chemoheterotrophic b.
    chromogenic b.

bac·te·ri·um *(continued)*
    coliform b.
    coryneform bacteria
    Dar es Salaam b.
    denitrifying b.
    gram-negative b.
    gram-postive b.
    hemophilic b.
    heterotrophic b.
    higher bacteria
    hydrogen b.
    iron b.
    lactic acid b.
    lysogenic b.
    mesophilic b.
    nitrifying b.
    nodule bacteria
    nonsulfur b., purple
    parasitic b.
    pathogenic b.
    photoautotrophic b.
    photoheterotrophic b.
    photosynthetic b.
    phototrophic bacteria
    propionic acid b.
    psychrophilic b.
    purple b.
    pyogenic b.
    pyrogenetic b.
    resistant b.
    rough b.
    saprophytic b.
    smooth b.
    sulfur b.
    thermophilic b.
    toxigenic b.
    toxinogenic b.
    water b.
bac·te·ri·uria
bac·te·ri·uric
bac·ter·oid
Bac·te·roi·da·ceae
Bac·te·roi·deae
Bac·te·roi·des
    B. asaccharolyticus
    B. bivius
    B. capillosus
    B. corrodens

Bac·te·roi·des (continued)
    B. disiens
    B. distasonis
    B. eggerthii
    B. fragilis
    B. fusiformis
    B. gingivalis
    B. intermedius
    B. melaninogenicus
    B. ochraceus
    B. oralis
    B. ovatus
    B. pneumosintes
    B. praeacutus
    B. putredinis
    B. splanchnicus
    B. thetaiotaomicron
    B. uniformis
    B. ureolyticus
    B. vulgatus
bac·te·roi·des
bac·te·roi·do·sis
bac·ter·uria
Bac·to·cill
bac·tro·pre·nol
bac·u·lo·vi·rus
bac·u·lum
Ba·dal's operation
badge
    film b.
Baelz's disease
BAEP — brainstem auditory
  evoked potential
Baer's cavity
Baer's law
Baer's method
Baer's vesicle
Baer·en·sprung's er·y·thras·
  ma
Bä·fver·stedts syndrome
baf·fle
    intra-atrial b.
    pericardial b.
    Senning type intra-atrial b.
bag
    Ambu b.
    Barnes' b.
    bolus b's

bag *(continued)*
    Bunyan b.
    Champetier de Ribes' b.
    colostomy b.
    Douglas b.
    Hagner b.
    ice b.
    ileostomy b.
    micturition b.
    nuclear b.
    Perry b.
    Petersen's b.
    Pilcher b.
    Politzer's b.
    reservoir b.
    testicular b.
    Tucker dilatable b.
    b. of waters
    Whitmore b.
bag·as·so·sis
Bag·gish hysteroscope
Ba·go·li·ni lens
Bail·lar·ger's bands
Bail·lar·ger's lines
Bail·lar·ger's sign
Bail·lar·ger's striae
Bail·lar·ger's stripe
Bain·bridge reflex
Ba·ker's cyst
Ba·ker's velum
Bakes dilator
BAL — bronchoalveolar
  lavage
    dimercaprol (British
      antilewisite)
bal·ance
    acid-base b.
    analytical b.
    calcium b.
    carbon b.
    electrolyte b.
    energy b.
    fluid b.
    genic b.
    glomerulotubular b.
    heat b.
    metabolic b.
    microchemical b.

bal·ance *(continued)*
   mineral b.
   nitrogen b.
   occlusal b.
   protein b.
   semimicro b.
   thermal b.
   torsion b.
   water b.
ba·lan·ic
bal·a·ni·tis
   amebic b.
   b. circinata
   b. circumscripta
     plasmacellularis
   b. diabetica
   erosive b.
   Follmann's b.
   b. gangraenosa
   gangrenous b.
   phagedenic b.
   plasma cell b.
   b. plasmacellularis
   b. xerotica obliterans
bal·a·no·blen·nor·rhea
bal·a·no·cele
bal·a·no·chlam·y·di·tis
bal·a·no·plas·ty
bal·a·no·pos·thi·tis
   b. chronica circumscripta
     plasmocellularis
   specific gangrenous and
     ulcerative b.
bal·a·no·pos·tho·my·co·sis
bal·a·no·pre·pu·ti·al
bal·a·nor·rha·gia
bal·an·tid·i·al
bal·an·ti·di·a·sis
bal·an·tid·i·o·sis
Bal·an·tid·i·um
   B. coli
bal·an·ti·do·sis
bal·a·nus
Bal·bi·ani's body
Bal·bi·ani's nucleus
Bal·bi·an·ia
bald·ness
   common male b.

bald·ness *(continued)*
   male pattern b.
Bal·dy's operation
Bal·dy-Web·ster operation
Bal·kan frame
Bal·kan splint
Bal·ke protocol
ball
   chondrin b.
   fatty b. of Bichat
   food b.
   b. of foot
   fungus b.
   hair b.
   Marchi b's
   oat hair b.
   pleural fibrin b's
   wool b.
Ball's valve
Bal·lance's sign
Bal·len·tine forceps
Bal·lan·tyne syndrome
Bal·lard gestational
   assessment
Bal·ler-Ger·old syndrome
Bal·let's sign
ball·ing
Bal·lin·gall's dis·ease
bal·lism
bal·lis·mus
bal·lis·tic
bal·lis·tics
   drug b.
   forensic b.
   wound b.
bal·lis·to·car·dio·gram
bal·lis·to·car·di·o·graph
bal·lis·to·car·di·og·ra·phy
bal·loon
   ACS b.
   Fogarty b.
   Grüntzig b.
   Honan b.
   Hunter b.
   Hunter-Sessions b.
   pilot b.
   Shea-Anthony antral b.
   sinus b.

bal·lot·a·ble
bal·lotte·ment
    abdominal b.
    indirect b.
    kidney b.
    renal b.
balm
    b. of Gilead
Balme's cough
bal·ne·ol·o·gy
bal·neo·ther·a·peu·tics
bal·neo·ther·a·py
Ba·ló's concentric encephalitis
Ba·ló's concentric sclerosis
Ba·ló's syndrome
Ba·los·er hysteroscope
bal·sam
    Canada b.
    friars' b.
    b. of Gilead
    Holland b.
    Mecca b.
    b. of Peru
    peruvian b.
    St. Thomas' b.
    silver b.
    tolu b.
    Turlington's b.
    Wade's b.
bal·sam·ic
Bal·sa·mo·den·dron
bal·sa·mum
    b. peruvianum
Bal·ser's fatty necrosis
bal·te·um ve·ne·re·um
Bal·ti·more, David
Bam·ber·ger's albuminuria
Bam·ber·ger's disease
Bam·ber·ger's sign
Bam·ber·ger-Ma·rie disease
bam·ber·my·cins
bam·nid·a·zole
Ban·croft's filariasis
ban·crof·ti·a·sis
ban·crof·to·sis
band
    A b.
    absorption b's

band *(continued)*
    amniotic b.
    anchor b.
    angiomesenteric b.
    Angle b.
    anisotropic b.
    anogenital b.
    anterior b. of colon
    atrioventricular b.
    auriculoventricular b.
    axis b.
    b's of Baillarger
    BB b's
    Bekhterev's b.
    b. of Broca
    Broca's diagonal b.
    Büngner's b's
    C b.
    chromosome b.
    cholecystoduodenal b.
    Clado's b.
    clamp b.
    contoured b.
    contraction b.
    coronary b.
    dentate b.
    diagonal b. of Broca
    elastic b.
    episternal b.
    Essick cell b.
    forbidden b.
    furrowed b.
    G b.
    genitomesenteric b.
    b's of Gennari
    Giacomini's b.
    H b.
    Hall b.
    Harris' b.
    Henle's b.
    His' b.
    b's of Hunter-Schreger
    I b.
    iliotibial b.
    Ladd's b's
    Lane's b's
    Leonardo's b.
    limbic b's

band *(continued)*
    lip furrow b.
    M b.
    Maissiat's b.
    Matas' b.
    matrix b.
    MB b.
    Meckel's b.
    mesocolic b.
    MM b.
    moderator b.
    molar b.
    omental b.
    omphalomesenteric b.
    orthodontic b.
    Parham b.
    perioplic b.
    periosteal b.
    phonatory b's
    Q b.
    R b.
    b. of Reil
    retention b.
    b's of Schreger
    Simonart's b's
    Soret b.
    sternal b.
    Tarin's b.
    valence b.
    Vicq d'Azyr's b.
    Z b.
    zonular b.
ban·dage
    Ace b.
    adhesive b.
    barrel b.
    Barton's b.
    Baynton's b.
    Borsch's b.
    Buller's b.
    butterfly b.
    capeline b.
    Champ elastic b.
    circular b.
    compression b.
    crucial b.
    demigauntlet b.
    Desault's b.

ban·dage *(continued)*
    E cotton b.
    elastic b.
    Elastomull b.
    Esmarch's b.
    figure-of-8 b.
    Flexilite b.
    four-tailed b.
    Fricke's b.
    gauntlet b.
    gauze b.
    Gibney b.
    hammock b.
    Hydron Burn B.
    immobilizing b.
    Kerlix b.
    many-tailed b.
    Martin's b.
    oblique b.
    plaster b.
    POP (plaster of Paris) b.
    pressure b.
    recurrent b.
    reversed b.
    roller b.
    Sayre's b.
    scultetus b.
    spica b.
    spiral b.
    spiral reverse b.
    suspensory b.
    T b.
    triangular b.
    Velpeau's b.
    Y b.
ban·da·let·ta
    b. diagonalis (Broca)
ban·deau
bandelette
ban·di·coot
band·ing
    chromosome b.
    high-resolution b.
    prophase b.
    pulmonary artery b.
    tooth b.
Ban·dl's ring
bane

bane·wort
Bang's method
Ban·ger·ter's method
ban·is·ter·ine
bank
Ban·nis·ter's disease
Ban·thine
Ban·ti's disease
Ban·ti's syndrome
Ban·ting, Sir Frederick Grant
BAO — basal acid output
Bap·ti·sia
    B. leucantha
bar
    arch b.
    b. of bladder
    chromatoid b.
    connector b.
    Dolder b.
    Erich arch b.
    House b.
    hyoid b's
    interureteric b.
    Kazanjian T b.
    Kennedy b.
    labial b.
    lingual b.
    lumbar b.
    median b.
    Mercier's b.
    metatarsal b.
    occlusal rest b.
    palatal b.
    Passavant's b.
    sternal b.
    sublingual b.
    tarsal b.
    terminal b's
    thyroid b.
    Winters arch b.
Bar's incision
bar·ag·no·sia
bar·ag·no·sis
bar·a·lyme
Bárány, Robert
Bá·rá·ny's pointing test
Bá·rá·ny's sign
Bá·rá·ny's symptom

Bá·rá·ny's test
bar·ba
bar·ba·loin
bar·bar·a·la·lia
Bar·ber's psoriasis
bar·ber·ry
bar·bi·tal
bar·bi·tone
bar·bi·tur·ate
bar·bi·tur·ic acid
bar·bo·tage
bar·bu·la
    b. hirci
Bar·clay's niche
Bar·coo disease
Bar·coo rot
Bar·croft's apparatus
Bard's sign
Bar·det-Biedl syndrome
bar·es·the·sia
bar·es·the·si·om·e·ter
Bar·gen streptococcus
bar·hyp·es·the·sia
bar·iat·rics
bar·i·to·sis
barium
    b. cyanoplatinate
    b. hydrate
    b. hydroxide
    b. oxide
    b. platinocyanide
    b. sulfate
    b. sulfide
    b. titanate
bark
    bearberry b.
    bitter b.
    buck-thorn b.
    calisaya b.
    casca b.
    chittem b.
    cinchona b.
    cramp b.
    dita b.
    dogwood b.
    druggists' b.
    eleuthera b.
    elm b.

bark *(continued)*
  grape b.
  Jesuits' b.
  Mancona b.
  Persian b.
  Peruvian b.
  Purshiana b.
  quillay b.
  sacred b.
  white oak b.
  wild black cherry b.
Bar·kan's operation
Bar·ker's point
Bark·man's reflex
Bar·kow's ligament
Bar·low's disease
Bar·low syndrome
barn
Barnes' bag
Barnes' curve
Barnes' dilator
baro·ag·no·sis
baro·cep·tor
bar·odon·tal·gia
baro·elec·tro·es·the·si·om·e·ter
bar·og·no·sis
baro·ma·crom·e·ter
baro·pac·er
baro·phil·ic
baro·re·cep·tor
baro·scope
baro·sen·si·tive
baro·si·nus·itis
baro·spi·ra·tor
bar·o·stat
bar·otal·gia
baro·tax·is
bar·oti·tis
  b. media
baro·trau·ma
  odontalgia b.
  otitic b.
  sinus b.
bar·ot·ro·pism
Barr body
Bar·ra·quer's disease
Bar·ra·quer's method

Bar·ra·quer's operation
Bar·ra·quer-Kru·meich-Swin·ger refractive set
Bar·ra·quer-Si·mons syn·drome
Barré's sign
Bar·ré-Guil·lain syndrome
Bar·rett's epithelium
Bar·rett's esophagus
Bar·rett's syndrome
Bar·rett's ulcer
bar·ri·er
  architectural b.
  blood-air b.
  blood-aqueous b.
  blood-brain b.
  blood–cerebrospinal fluid b.
  blood–gas b.
  blood-ocular fluid b.
  blood-testis b.
  blood-thymus b.
  energy b.
  filtration b.
  gastric mucosal b.
  hematoencephalic b.
  histohematic connective tissue b.
  Mercier's b.
  placental b.
  protective b.
  radiation b.
bar·sati
Bár·so·ny-Tesch·en·dorf syndrome
Bart's syndrome
Barth's hernia
Bar·tho·lin's duct
Bar·tho·lin's gland
bar·tho·lin·itis
Bar·thol·o·mew's rule
Bar·ton's bandage
Bar·ton's fracture
Bar·ton's operation
Bar·to·nel·la
  B. bacilliformis
Bar·to·nel·la·ceae
bar·to·nel·le·mia

bar·to·nel·li·a·sis
bar·to·nel·lo·sis
Bart·ter's syndrome
Bart·ter-Schwartz syndrome
Ba·ruch's law
Ba·ruch's sign
ba·ru·ria
Bar·well's operation
bar·ye
bary·es·the·sia
bary·glos·sia
bary·la·lia
bary·ma·zia
bary·pho·nia
ba·ry·ta
    synthetic b.
bar·y·to·sis
ba·sad
ba·sal
Ba·sal·jel
ba·sa·loid
ba·sa·lo·ma
base
    acidifiable b.
    acrylic resin b.
    Brønsted b.
    buffer b.
    cement b.
    conjugate b.
    data b., database
    denture b.
    denture b., tinted
    b. excess
    extension b.
    film b.
    free-end b.
    hexone b's
    histone b's
    b. of iris
    Lewis b.
    metal b.
    b. of nail
    nitrogenous b.
    ointment b.
    b. pair
    plastic b.
    purine b's
    pyrimidine b's

base *(continued)*
    rare b's
    record b.
    b. of renal pyramid
    Schiff b.
    Schreiner's b.
    shellac b's
    temporary b.
    time b.
    tinted denture b.
    tooth-borne b.
    trial b.
    xanthine b's
    whole blood buffer b.
    whole body buffer b.
    wobble b.
bas·e·doid
Bas·e·dow's disease
Bas·e·dow's triad
bas·e·dow·i·form
base·line
    Reid's b.
base·plate
    gutta-percha b.
    stabilized b.
ba·ses
bas-fond
Ba·sham's mixture
Ba·sham's solution
ba·si·al
ba·si·a·lis
ba·si·al·ve·o·lar
ba·si·ar·ach·ni·tis
ba·si·arach·noid·itis
ba·si·bran·chi·al
ba·si·caryo·plas·tin
ba·si·chro·ma·tin
ba·si·chro·mi·ole
ba·sic·i·ty
ba·si·cra·ni·al
ba·si·cy·to·para·plas·tin
ba·sid·ia
Ba·sid·i·ob·o·lus
    B. haptosporus
    B. meristosporus
ba·sid·io·carp
Ba·sid·io·my·ce·tes
ba·sid·io·my·ce·tous

ba·sid·io·spore
ba·sid·i·um pl. ba·sid·ia
ba·si·fa·cial
ba·sig·e·nous
ba·si·hy·al
ba·si·hy·oid
bas·i·lad
bas·i·lar
bas·i·la·ris
    b. cranii
ba·si·lat·er·al
ba·si·lem·ma
ba·sil·ic
bas·i·lo·ma
bas·i·lo·men·tal
bas·i·lo·pha·ryn·ge·al
ba·sin
    kidney b.
ba·si·na·si·al
ba·si·oc·cip·i·tal
ba·sio·glos·sus
ba·si·on
ba·si·ot·ic
ba·si·para·chro·ma·tin
ba·si·para·plas·tin
ba·sip·e·tal
ba·si·pha·ryn·ge·al
ba·si·phil·ic
ba·si·pre·sphe·noid
ba·si·rhi·nal
ba·sis pl. ba·ses
    b. capituli
    b. cartilaginis arytenoideae
    b. cerebri
    b. cochleae
    b. cordis
    b. cranii externa
    b. cranii interna
    b. encephali
    b. glandulae suprarenalis
    b. mandibulae
    b. metacarpalis
    b. metatarsalis
    b. modioli
    b. nasi
    b. ossis metacarpalis
    b. ossis metatarsalis
    b. ossis sacri

ba·sis *(continued)*
    b. patellae
    b. pedunculi cerebri
    b. phalangis digitorum
      manus
    b. phalangis digitorum
      pedis
    b. prostatae
    b. pulmonis
    b. pyramidis renalis
    b. scapulae
    b. stapedis
ba·si·sphe·noid
ba·sis pon·tis
ba·si·syl·vi·an
ba·si·tem·po·ral
ba·si·ver·te·bral
bas·ket
    cytopharyngeal b.
    fiber b's
    stone b.
Basle No·mi·na An·a·tom·i·ca
ba·so·cy·to·sis
ba·so·graph
ba·so·lat·er·al
ba·so·meta·chro·mo·phil
Ba·som·ma·toph·o·ra
ba·so·phil
    beta b.
    Crooke-Russell b's
    delta b.
ba·so·phile
ba·so·phil·ia
    pituitary b.
    punctate b.
ba·so·phil·ic
ba·soph·i·lism
    Cushing's b.
    pituitary b.
ba·soph·i·lous
ba·so·plasm
ba·so·squa·mous
Bass-Wat·kins test
Bas·sen-Korn·zweig disease
Bas·sen-Korn·zweig syndrome
Bas·set's operation
Bas·si·ni's operation

bas·so·rin
Bas·te·do's rule
Bas·ti·an syndrome
Bastian-Bruns law
Bastian-Bruns sign
Bate·man's disease
bath
- acid b.
- air b.
- alcohol b.
- alkaline b.
- alternant-contrast b.
- alum b.
- antipyretic b.
- antiseptic b.
- aromatic b.
- astringent b.
- borax b.
- bran b.
- Brand b.
- bubble b.
- cabinet b.
- camphor b.
- carbon dioxide b.
- cold b.
- colloid b.
- continuous b.
- contrast b.
- cool b.
- creosote b.
- douche b.
- drip-sheet b.
- earth b.
- emollient b.
- Finnish b.
- Finsen b.
- foam b.
- full b.
- gas-bubble b.
- gelatin b.
- glycerin b.
- graduated b.
- grease b.
- half b.
- herb b.
- hip b.
- hot b.
- hot-air b.

bath *(continued)*
- hyperthermal b.
- immersion b.
- infrared b.
- iron b.
- kinetotherapeutic b.
- light b.
- linseed b.
- lukewarm b.
- medicated b.
- milk b.
- moor b.
- mud b.
- Nauheim b.
- needle b.
- oatmeal b.
- oil b.
- oxygen b.
- pack b.
- paraffin b.
- peat b.
- sand b.
- sauna b.
- Schott b.
- sedative b.
- sheet b.
- sitz b.
- sponge b.
- stimulating b.
- sweat b.
- tepid b.
- transcutan b.
- vapor b.
- warm b.
- water b.
- wax b.
- whirlpool b.

bath·es·the·sia
bath·mo·trop·ic
- negatively b.
- positively b.

bath·mot·ro·pism
batho·chrome
batho·chro·mic
batho·chro·my
batho·flore
batho·mor·phic
batho·rhod·op·sin

bath·ro·ceph·a·ly
bathy·an·es·the·sia
bathy·car·dia
bathy·es·the·sia
bathy·hy·per·es·the·sia
bathy·hyp·es·the·sia
bathy·pnea
ba·to·net
Bat·son's plexus
Bat·son's system
Bat·ten's disease
Bat·tey ba·cil·li
bat·tey·in
Bat·tle's operation
Bat·tle's sign
Bat·tle-Ja·la·guier-Kam·mer·er incision
Batt·ley sedative
Bau·de·locque's diameter
Bau·de·locque's line
Bau·hin's gland
Bau·hin's valve
Bau·man's angle
Bau·mé's scale
Baum·gar·ten's glands
Baum·gar·ten's murmur
Baum·gar·ten's syndrome
bay
    lacrimal b.
Bayes' theorem
Bayle's disease
Bayle's granulations
Bay·ley Scales of Infant Development
Bayn·ton's bandage
Baz·ett's formula
Ba·zin's disease
BBA — born before arrival (of doctor, midwife)
BBB — blood-brain barrier
    bundle branch block
BBT — basal body temperature
BCAA — branched chain amino acid
BCAF — basophil chemotaxis augmentation factor

BCDF — B cell differentiation factors
BCF — basophil chemotactic factor
BCG — bacille Calmette-Guérin
    ballistocardiogram
    bicolor guaiac test
BCGF — B cell growth factors
b.d. — L. bis die (twice a day)
BDA — British Dental Association
Bdel·la
    B. cardinalis
Bdel·lo·vib·rio
bdel·lo·vib·rio
BDS — Bachelor of Dental Surgery
BDSc — Bachelor of Dental Science
    bacterial endocarditis
BE — barium enema
    base excess
bead
    rachitic b's
bead·ing
    b. of ribs
Bea·dle, George Wells
beak
    b. of sphenoid bone
    parrot's b.
beak·er
Beale's ganglion cells
beam
    broad b.
    cantilever b.
    continuous b.
    electron b.
    narrow b.
    neutron b.
    primary b.
    restrained b.
    simple b.
    useful b.
beam·ther·a·py
bean
    broad b.
    Calabar b.

bean *(continued)*
    castor b.
    jequirity b.
    ordeal b.
    soja b.
    St. Ignatius' b.
bear·ber·ry, bear ber·ry
beard
bear·ing
    central b.
bear·ing down
Bearn-Kun·kel-Sla·ter syndrome
bear·wood
beat
    apex b.
    atrial b.
    automatic b.
    capture b's
    ciliary b.
    combination b.
    coupled b's
    dependent b.
    dropped b.
    echo b.
    ectopic b.
    escaped b's
    forced b.
    fusion b.
    idioventricular b.
    interference b.
    mixed b.
    paired b's
    premature b.
    reciprocal b's
    retrograde b.
    summation b.
    ventricular fusion b.
    ventricular premature b.
Beau's disease
Beau's lines
Beau's syndrome
be·can·thone hy·dro·chlo·ride
Bec·ca·ri process
Bec·car·ia sign
bech·ic
Bech·te·rew
Bech·tol hip prosthesis

Beck's gastrostomy
Beck's triad
Beck·er's nevus
Beck·er's phenomenon
Beck·er's sign
Beck·er's test
Beck·mann's apparatus
Beck·with-Wie·de·mann syndrome
Bé·clard's amputation
Bé·clard's hernia
Bé·clard's nucleus
Bé·clard's triangle
bec·lo·meth·a·sone di·pro·pi·o·nate
bec·que·rel
Bec·que·rel's rays
bed
    air b.
    air-fluidized b.
    capillary b.
    circle b.
    CircOlectric b.
    Clinitron b.
    collateral vascular b.
    fracture b.
    Gatch b.
    hydrostatic b.
    Klondike b.
    metabolic b.
    mud b.
    nail b.
    placental b.
    plaster b.
    rocking b.
    Roto-Rest b.
    Sanders b.
    sawdust b.
    stomach b.
    vascular b.
    water b.
bed·bug
    Mexican b.
    Oriental b.
    Texas b.
be·dew·ing
bed·fast
Bed·nar's aphtha

bed·pan
bed·rest, bed rest
bed·rid·den
Bed·so·nia
bed·sore
bed·wet·ting
Beer's collyrium
Beer's knife
Beer's operation
Beer-Lam·bert law
beer·wort
bees·wax
    bleached b.
    unbleached b.
bee·tle
    blister b.
Bee·vor's sign
Beg·bie's disease
Begg's appliance
Begg's technique
Beg·gi·a·toa
Beg·gi·a·to·a·ceae
beg·ma
Bé·guez Cé·sar disease
be·hav·ior
    adaptive b.
    attachment b.
    automatic b.
    avoidance b.
    collective b.
    displacement b.
    impulsive b.
    instinctive b.
    invariable b.
    operant b.
    respondent b.
    species-specific b.
    variable b.
be·hav·ior·ism
be·hav·ior·ist
be·hen·ic acid
Beh·çet's syndrome (disease)
Bé·hier-Har·dy sign
Bé·hier-Har·dy symptom
Beh·la's bodies
Beh·ring, Emil Adolf von
Beh·ring's law

BEI — butanol-extractable
    iodine
Bei·gel's disease
bei·kost
bej·el
Békésy, Georg von
Bé·ké·sy audiometry
Bé·ké·sy calibration
Bekhterev's (Bechterew's)
    arthritis
Bekh·te·rev-Men·del reflex
bel
Bel·as·ca·ris
belch·ing
be·lem·noid
Bel·field's operation
Bell's law
Bell's nerve
Bell's palsy
Bell's paralysis
Bell's phenomenon
Bell's muscle
Bell's treatment
Bell-Ma·gen·die law
bel·la·don·na
bel·la·don·nine
Bel·li·ni's ducts
Bel·li·ni's ligament
Bel·li·ni's tubules
Bel·locq's cannula
Bel·locq's sound
Bel·locq's tube
bel·lows
bel·ly
    anterior b. of digastric
        muscle
    Delhi b.
    drum b.
    frontal b. of occipitofrontal
        muscle
    inferior b. of omohyoid
        muscle
    occipital b. of
        occipitofrontal muscle
    posterior b. of digastric
        muscle
    prune b.
    spider b.

bel·ly *(continued)*
    swollen b.
    wooden b.
bel·ly·but·ton
bel·o·ne·pho·bia
bel·o·noid
bel·o·no·ski·as·co·py
bel·ox·a·mide
Bel·sey Mark IV operation
bem·e·gride
Be·na·cer·raf, Baruj
ben·ac·ty·zine hy·dro·chlo·ride
Ben·a·dryl
ben·an·ser·in hy·dro·chlo·ride
ben·a·pry·zine hy·dro·chlo·ride
Bence Jones cylinder
Bence Jones protein
Bence Jones proteinuria
Bence Jones reaction
bend
    first order b's
    head b.
    iliac b. of ureter
    labyrinthine b's
    neck b.
    second order b's
    third order b's
    V b's
    varolian b.
ben·da·zac
Ben·der's test
Ben·der's Visual-Motor Gestalt Test
ben·dro·flu·a·zide
ben·dro·flu·me·thi·a·zide
bends
Ben·dy·late
be·ne
bene·cep·tor
Ben·e·deck's reflex
Ben·e·dict's test
Ben·e·dikt's syndrome
be·nef·i·cence
ben·e·fi·cial
ben·e·fi·ci·a·ry

ben·e·fit
    indemnity b.
    service b.
Ben·e·mid
be·nign
be·nig·nant
Bé·ni·qué's sound
Ben·i·sone
Ben·net's corpuscles
Ben·nett's angle
Ben·nett's disease
Ben·nett's fracture
Ben·o·quin
be·nor·ter·one
ben·ox·a·pro·fen
ben·ox·i·nate hy·dro·chlo·ride
Ben·ox·yl
ben·per·i·dol
ben·ser·a·zide
Bens·ley specific granules
Ben·son's disease
ben·taz·e·pam
ben·tir·o·mide
ben·ton·ite
    b. magma
Ben·tyl
ben·zal·de·hyde
ben·za·lin
ben·zal·ko·ni·um chlo·ride
ben·za·mine
ben·zan·thra·cene
benz·az·o·line hy·dro·chlo·ride
benz·bro·ma·rone
benz·cu·rine io·dide
Ben·ze·drex
Ben·ze·drine
ben·zene
    dimethyl b.
    b. hexachloride
    methyl b.
ben·ze·noid
ben·zes·tro·fol
ben·zes·trol
ben·ze·tho·ni·um chlo·ride
benz·hex·ol hy·dro·chlo·ride

benz·hy·dra·mine hy·dro·
  chlo·ride
ben·zi·dine
benz·il·o·ni·um bro·mide
ben·zim·i·da·zole
ben·zine
    petroleum b., purified b.
ben·zo·ate
ben·zo·at·ed
ben·zo·caine
benz·oc·ta·mine
ben·zo·depa
ben·zo·di·az·e·pine
ben·zo·di·ox·an
ben·zo·gy·nes·tryl
ben·zo·ic acid
ben·zo·ic al·de·hyde
ben·zo·in
ben·zol
ben·zol·ism
ben·zo·na·tate
ben·zo·no·na·tine
ben·zo·pur·pu·rine
    b. B
1,2-ben·zo·pyr·an
ben·zo[*a*]py·rene
ben·zo·pyr·ro·ni·um bro·mide
ben·zo·qui·none
ben·zo·qui·no·ni·um chlo·ride
ben·zo·ther·a·py
benz·ox·i·quine
ben·zo·yl
    b. ecgonine
    b. peroxide
    b. peroxide, hydrous
ben·zo·yl·gly·cine
ben·zo·yl·meth·yl·ec·go·nine
ben·zo·yl·pas cal·ci·um
ben·zo·yl·phen·yl·car·bi·nol
benz·phet·amine hy·dro·chlo·
  ride
benz·pi·per·y·lon
3,4-benz·py·rene
benz·py·rin·i·um bro·mide
benz·pyr·role
benz·quin·amide
benz·thi·a·zide
benz·tro·pine mes·y·late

ben·zur·e·stat
ben·zyd·amine hy·dro·chlo·
  ride
ben·zyd·ro·flu·me·thi·a·zide
ben·zyl
    b. benzoate
    b. bromide
    b. carbinol
ben·zyl·i·dene
ben·zyl·oxy·car·bon·yl
p-ben·zyl·oxy·phe·nol
ben·zyl·pen·i·cil·lin
    b. potassium
    b. procaine
    b. sodium
be·pas·cum
be·phe·ni·um
Ber·ar·di·nel·li syndrome
Bé·ra·neck's tuberculum
Bé·rard's ligament
Bé·raud's valve
ber·ber·ine
    b. bisulfate
Ber·ber·is
be·reave·ment
Ber·ens 3-character test
Ber·ens lid everter
Ber·ens muscle clamp
ber·ga·mot
Ber·ger's disease
Ber·ger's method
Ber·ger's operation
Ber·ger's paresthesia
Ber·ger rhythm
Ber·ger's sign
Ber·ger's symptom
Ber·ge·ron's chorea
Ber·ge·ron's disease
Ber·gey's classification
Berg·man's sign
Berg·mann's cells
Berg·mann's cords
Berg·mann's fibers
Berg·meis·ter papilla
Ber·go·nie method
Ber·go·nie treatment
Ber·go·nié-Tri·bon·deau law
Berg·ström, Sune

beri·beri
    atrophic b.
    cerebral b.
    dry b.
    infantile b.
    paralytic b.
    ship b.
    wet b.
beri·ber·ic
Berke operation
Ber·ke·feld filter
berke·li·um
Ber·kow scale
Berk·son bias
Ber·lin's disease
Ber·lin's edema
Ber·nard's canal
Ber·nard's duct
Ber·nard's layer
Ber·nard's puncture
Ber·nard's syndrome
Ber·nard-Hor·ner syndrome
Ber·nard-Sou·lier disease
Ber·nard-Sou·lier syndrome
Ber·nays' sponge
Bern·hardt's disease
Bern·hardt's paresthesia
Bern·hardt-Roth disease
Bern·hardt-Roth syndrome
Bern·heim syndrome
Bern·heim therapy
Bern·hei·mer's fibers
Ber·noul·li distribution
Ber·noul·li trial
ber·ry
    bear b.
    buckthorn b.
    fish b.
    horse nettle b.
    Indian b.
Ber·ry's ligament
Ber·the·lot reaction
Ber·the·lot reagent
Ber·ti·el·la
    B. satyri
    B. studeri
ber·ti·el·li·a·sis
Ber·tin's bones

Ber·tin's column
Ber·tin's ligament
Ber·tin's ossicles
Ber·to·lot·ti syn·drome
Be·ru·bi·gen
ber·yl·li·o·sis
ber·yl·li·um
be·ryth·ro·my·cin
bes·i·clom·e·ter
Bes·nier's prurigo
Bes·nier-Boeck disease
Best, Charles Herbert
bes·y·late
be·ta
Be·ta·bac·te·ri·um
Be·ta-Chlor
be·ta-cho·les·ta·nol
be·ta·cism
Be·ta·dine
be·ta-en·dor·phin
be·ta-es·tra·di·ol
be·ta glob·u·lin
    pregnancy-specific b.
be·ta·his·tine hy·dro·chlo·ride
be·ta-hy·droxy·bu·tyr·ic acid
be·ta·ine
    b. hydrochloride
be·ta-ke·to·bu·tyr·ic acid
be·ta-lac·ta·mase
be·ta-lac·tose
Be·ta·lin
be·ta-lipo·pro·tein
be·ta-ly·sin
be·ta·meth·a·sone
    b. acetate
    b. benzoate
    b. dipropionate
    b. sodium phosphate
    b. valerate
be·ta·mi·cin sul·fate
be·ta$_2$-mi·cro·glob·u·lin
be·ta·naph·thol
be·ta-naph·thol·sul·fon·ic acid
be·ta·naph·thyl
    b. benzoate
    b. salicylate

be·ta·nin
be·ta-oxy·bu·tyr·ic acid
Be·ta·par
Be·ta·pen-VK
Be·ta·prone
be·ta·pro·pio·lac·tone
be·ta·quin·ine
be·ta·tron
Be·tax·in
be·ta·zole hy·dro·chlo·ride
be·tel
    b. nut
be·thane·chol
be·thane·chol chlo·ride
be·than·i·dine sul·fate
Be·thea's method
Be·thea's sign
Bet·u·la
    B. alba
    B. lenta
be·tween·brain
Betz's cells
Betz's cell area
Bev·an's incision
Bev·an's operation
Bev·an Lew·is cells
Bev·i·dox
bex con·vul·si·va
bex·ia
Be·zie·hungs·wahn
    sensitiver B.
be·zoar
Be·zold's abscess
Be·zold's mastoiditis
Be·zold's perforation
Be·zold's sign
Be·zold's triad
Be·zold's ganglion
BF — blastogenic factor
BFP — biologic false-positive
Bi·al's reagent
Bi·al's test
bi·a·lam·i·col hy·dro·chlo·ride
bi·al·lyl·am·i·col
Bi·an·chi's nodules
Bi·an·chi's syndrome
Bi·an·chi's valve

bi·ar·tic·u·lar
bi·ar·tic·u·late
bi·as
    Berkson's b.
    Neyman's b.
bi·as·ter·ic
bi·au·ric·u·lar
bi·ax·i·al
bi·ball·ism
bi·ba·sal·ly
bi·ba·sic
Bi·ber-Haab-Dim·mer
    dystrophy
bi·bev·eled
Bib·lio·film
bib·lio·ther·a·py
bib·u·lous
bi·cam·er·al
bi·cap·su·lar
bi·car·bo·nate
    blood b.
    plasma b.
    b. of soda
bi·car·bo·nat·e·mia
bi·cau·dal
bi·cau·date
bi·cel·lu·lar
bi·ceph·a·lus
bi·ceps
    b. brachii
    b. femoris
Bi·chat's canal
Bi·chat's fissure
Bi·chat's foramen
Bi·chat's ligament
Bi·chat's membrane
Bi·chat's tunic
bi·chlo·ride
bi·chro·mate
Bi·cil·lin
bi·cip·i·tal
Bick·el's ring
bi·col·lis
bi·con·cave
bi·con·vex
bi·cor·nate
bi·cor·nis
bi·cor·nu·ate

bi·co·ro·ni·al
bi·cor·po·rate
bi·cou·date
bi·cus·pid
bi·cus·pi·dal
bi·cus·pi·date
bi·cus·pid·iza·tion
bi·cus·poid
b.i.d. — L. bis in die (twice a day)
bi·dac·ty·ly
Bid·der's ganglia
Bid·der's organ
bi·den·tal
bi·den·tate
bi·der·mo·ma
bi·duo·ter·tian
bid·u·ous
Bie·der·man's sign
Bie·dert's cream mixture
Biedl's disease
Biedl's syndrome
Biel·schow·sky's method
Biel·schow·sky-Jan·sky disease
Bie·mond syndrome
Bier's amputation
Bier's anesthesia
Bier·mer's anemia
Bier·mer's disease
Bier·mer's sign
Bier·nac·ki's sign
Bie·sia·dec·ki's fossa
Bi·ett's collar
bi·fas·cic·u·lar
bi·fid, bif·i·dus
Bi·fi·do·bac·te·ri·um
    B. adolescentis
    B. bifidum
    B. cornutum
    B. eriksonii
    B. infantis
bi·fi·do·bac·te·ri·um *pl.* bi·fi·do·bac·te·ria
bi·fix·ate
bi·fo·cal
bi·fo·rate
bi·for·myl

bi·fur·cate
bi·fur·ca·tio *pl.* bi·fur·ca·ti·o·nes
    b. aortae
    b. aortica
    b. carotidis
    b. tracheae
    b. trunci pulmonalis
bi·fur·ca·tion
    b. of aorta
    b. of bundle of His
    carotid b.
    b. of pulmonary trunk
    b. of trachea
bi·fur·ca·ti·o·nes
Big·e·low's ligament
Big·e·low's operation
Big·e·low's septum
bi·gem·i·na
bi·gem·i·nal
bi·gem·i·num *pl.* bi·gem·i·na
bi·gem·i·ny
    atrial b.
    atrioventricular nodal b.
    escape-capture b.
    nodal b.
    reciprocal b.
    ventricular b.
bi·ger·mi·nal
bi·go·ni·al
bi·is·chi·al
bi·labe
bi·lam·i·nar
Bil·ar·cil
bi·lat·er·al
bi·lat·er·al·ism
bi·lay·er
    lipid b.
bile
    A b.
    B b.
    C b.
    cystic b.
    gallbladder b.
    hepatic b.
    limy b.
    milk of calcium b.
    ox b.

bile *(continued)*
    white b.
Bil·har·zia
bil·har·zi·al
bil·har·zi·a·sis
bil·har·zic
bil·har·zi·o·ma
bil·har·zi·o·sis
bil·i·a·ry
bil·i·a·tion
bil·i·cy·a·nin
bil·i·di·ges·tive
bil·i·fac·tion
bil·i·fla·vin
bil·i·ful·vin
bil·i·fus·cin
bil·i·gen·e·sis
bil·i·ge·net·ic
bil·i·gen·ic
bi·lig·u·late
bil·i·hu·min
Bili-Lab·stix
Bili mask
bi·lin
bil·ious
bil·ious·ness
bil·i·pra·sin
bil·i·pur·pu·rin
bil·i·ra·chia
bil·i·ru·bin
    conjugated b.
    direct b.
    indirect b.
    unconjugated b.
bil·i·ru·bi·nate
bil·i·ru·bin·emia
bil·i·ru·bin·ic
bil·i·ru·bin UDP-glu·cu·ron·
   yl·trans·fer·ase
bil·i·ru·bin·uria
bi·lis
bil·i·uria
bil·i·ver·din
bil·i·ver·di·nate
bil·i·xan·thine
Bill·roth's cords
Bill·roth's disease
Bill·roth's operation

Bill·roth's strand
bi·lo·bate
bi·lob·u·lar
bi·lob·u·late
bi·loc·u·lar
bi·loc·u·late
bi·loc·u·la·tion
bi·lo·ma
Bil·opaque
bi·loph·odont
Bil·tri·cide
bi·ma·lar
bi·mal·le·o·lar
Bim·a·na
bi·man·u·al
bi·mas·toid
bi·max·il·lary
bi·me·thoxy·caine lac·tate
Bim·ler's appliance
bi·mo·dal
bi·mo·lec·u·lar
bin·an·gle
bi·na·ry
bi·na·sal
bin·au·ral
bin·au·ric·ular
bind
    bipolar double b.
    double b.
    unipolar double b.
bind·er
bi·neg·a·tive
Bi·net's test
Bi·net-Si·mon test
Bing's test
binge·ing
bin·ir·a·my·cin
bin·oc·u·lar
bi·no·mi·al
bin·oph·thal·mo·scope
bino·scope
bin·ot·ic
bin·ov·u·lar
Bins·wang·er's dementia
Bins·wang·er's encephalitis
bi·nu·cle·ar
bi·nu·cle·ate
bi·nu·cle·a·tion

bi·nu·cleo·late
bio·ac·cu·mu·la·tion
bio·acous·tics
bio·ac·tive
bio·aer·a·tion
bio·amine
bio·am·in·er·gic
bio·as·say
bio·avail·a·bil·i·ty
Bi·o·brane adhesive
Bi·o·brane glove
Bi·o·brane synthetic skin
   substitute
bio·chem·is·try
bio·che·mor·phic
bio·che·mor·phol·o·gy
bio·ci·dal
bio·col·loid
bio·com·pat·i·ble
bio·com·pat·i·bil·i·ty
bio·cy·cle
bio·de·grad·able
bio·deg·ra·da·tion
bio·di·al·y·sis
bio·dy·nam·ics
bio·elec·tric·i·ty
bio·elec·tron·ics
bio·en·er·get·ics
bio·en·gi·neer·ing
bio·equiv·a·lence
bio·equiv·a·lent
bio·eth·ics
bio·feed·back
   alpha b.
bio·fla·vo·noid
bio·gen·e·sis
bio·ge·net·ic
bi·o·gen·ic
bi·og·e·nous
bio·glass
Bio·graft
bio·graph
bio·haz·ard
bio·hy·drau·lic
bio·im·plant
bio·ki·net·ics
bi·o·log·ic, bi·o·log·i·cal
bi·o·log·i·cals

bi·o·log·i·cals
   lyophilized b.
bi·ol·o·gist
bi·ol·o·gy
   cell b.
   descriptive b.
   mathematical b.
   molecular b.
   population b.
   radiation b.
bio·lu·mi·nes·cence
bio·ma·te·ri·al
bio·math·e·mat·ics
bio·me·chan·ics
   dental b.
bio·med·i·cal
bio·med·i·cine
bio·mem·brane
bio·mem·bra·nous
bio·me·te·or·ol·o·gist
bio·me·te·or·ol·o·gy
bi·om·e·ter
bio·me·tri·cian
bio·met·rics
bi·om·e·try
bio·mi·cro·scope
   slit-lamp b.
bio·mi·cros·co·py
   slit-lamp b.
bio·mol·e·cule
bio·mo·tor
Bi·om·pha·la·ria
   B. alexandrina
   B. glabrata
bio·ne·cro·sis
bi·on·ics
bio·nu·cle·on·ics
bio·os·mot·ic
bio·phar·ma·ceu·ti·cals
bio·pho·tom·e·ter
bio·phy·lax·is
bio·phys·i·cal
bio·phys·ics
bio·phys·i·og·ra·phy
bio·phys·i·ol·o·gy
bio·pla·sia
bio·plasm
bio·plas·mic

bio·poly·mer
bio·po·ten·tial
bio·pros·the·sis
bi·op·sy
    aspiration b.
    biochemical b.
    bite b.
    brush b.
    chorionic villus b.
    cold cone b.
    cone b.
    cytological b.
    endoscopic b.
    excisional b.
    exploratory b.
    incisional b.
    needle b.
    nerve b.
    open b.
    percutaneous b.
    punch b.
    ring b.
    shave b.
    sponge b.
    sternal b.
    surface b.
    total b.
    trephine b.
    wound b.
bio·psy·chol·o·gy
bi·op·ter·in
bi·op·tic
bi·op·tome
bio·pyo·cul·ture
bio·ra·tio·nal
bi·or·bi·tal
Bi·örck syndrome
Bi·örck-Thor·son syndrome
bio·re·ver·si·ble
bi·or·gan
bio·rhe·ol·o·gy
bio·rhythm
bio·roent·gen·og·ra·phy
bi·os
    b. I
    b. II
bio·sci·ence
bi·o·sis

bi·os·mo·sis
bio·spec·trom·e·try
bio·spec·tros·co·py
bio·stat·ics
bio·stat·is·ti·cian
bio·sta·tis·tics
bio·ste·reo·met·rics
bio·syn·the·sis
bio·syn·thet·ic
Bi·ot's breathing
Bi·ot's respiration
Bi·ot's sign
bi·o·ta
bio·tax·is
bio·taxy
bio·tech·nol·o·gy
bio·tel·em·e·try
bio·the·si·om·e·ter
bio·tic
bio·tics
bio·tin
bi·o·tin·yl
bi·ot·o·my
bio·tox·i·ca·tion
bio·tox·i·col·o·gy
bio·tox·in
bio·trans·for·ma·tion
bio·type
bio·ty·pol·o·gy
bi·ov·u·lar
bi·pal·a·ti·noid
bi·para·sit·ic
bi·para·sit·ism
bi·par·en·tal
bi·pa·ri·e·tal
bip·a·rous
bi·par·tite
bi·ped
bip·e·dal
bi·pen·nate
bi·pen·ni·form
bi·per·fo·rate
bi·per·i·den
    b. hydrochloride
    b. lactate
bi·phas·ic
bi·phen·amine hy·dro·chlo·ride

bi·phe·nyl
    polychlorinated b. (PCB)
bi·phet·amine
bi·po·lar
Bi·po·la·ri·na
bi·po·lar·i·ty
bi·pos·i·tive
bi·po·ten·tial
bi·po·ten·ti·al·i·ty
    b. of the gonad
bi·pus
bi·ra·mous
Bir·beck granule
Bird's formula
Bird's treatment
Bird's sign
bird-arm
bird-leg
bi·re·frac·tive
bi·re·frin·gence
    crystalline b.
    flow b.
    form b.
    intrinsic b.
    strain b.
    streaming b.
bi·re·frin·gent
bi·rhin·ia
Bir·kett's hernia
Birn·berg bow
birth
    breech b.
    complete b.
    cross b.
    dead b.
    head b.
    immature b.
    live b.
    multiple b.
    partial b.
    post-term b.
    premature b.
    spontaneous breech b.
birth·ing
    alternative b.
birth·mark
    port wine stain b.
    strawberry b.

birth·weight
bis·ac·o·dyl
    b. tannex
bis·acro·mi·al
bis·al·bu·min·emia
bis·ax·il·lary
bis·chlo·ro·meth·yl ether
Bisch·of's myelotomy
Bisch·off's crown
Bisch·off's test
bis·cuit
    hard b.
    medium b.
    soft b.
bis·cuit·ing
bi·sec·tion
bi·sep·tate
bi·sex·u·al
bi·sex·u·al·i·ty
bis·fe·ri·ous
Bish·op's sphygmoscope
bis·hy·droxy·cou·ma·rin
bi·sil·i·ac
bis in die
bis·muth
    b. aluminate
    b. carbonate, basic
    b. glycoloylarsanilate
    b. magma
    milk of b.
    b. oxyiodide
    b. oxysalicylate
    precipitated b.
    b. subcarbonate
    b. subgallate
    b. subnitrate
    b. subsalicylate
bis·muth·ism
bis·mu·tho·sis
bis·o·brin lac·tate
bis·ox·a·tin acetate
2,3-bis·phos·pho·glyc·er·ate
bis·phos·pho·glyc·er·ate mu·
    tase
bis·phos·pho·glyc·er·ate
    phos·pha·tase
bis·phos·pho·glyc·ero·mu·
    tase

bi·spore
bisque
 high b.
 low b.
 medium b.
bi·stable
bi·ste·phan·ic
Bis·ton be·tu·la·ria
bis·tou·ry
bi·stra·tal
bi·sul·fate
bi·sul·fide
bi·sul·fite
bi·tar·trate
bite
 balanced b.
 check b.
 closed b.
 convenience b.
 cross b.
 deep b.
 edge-to-edge b.
 end-to-end b.
 locked b.
 open b.
 over b.
 raised b.
 rest b.
 scissors b.
 stork b.
 underhung b.
 wax b.
 X-b.
bite-block
bite·gage
bite·lock
bi·tem·po·ral
bite·plane
bite·plate
bi·ter·mi·nal
bi·thi·no·late sodium
bite-wing
bi·thi·o·nol
 b. sulfoxide
Bi·thyn·ia
 B. fuchsiana
Bi·tis
bi·tol·ter·ol

Bi·tot's patches
Bi·tot's spots
bi·tro·chan·ter·ic
bi·trop·ic
bit·ter
 aromatic b's
bit·ter·ling
bit·ters
Bitt·ner milk factor
Bitt·ner virus
Bit·torf's reaction
bi·tu·ber·al
bi·tu·men
bi·tu·mi·no·sis
bi·urate
bi·u·ret
biv·a·lence
bi·va·lent
bi·valve
bi·ven·ter
 b. cervicis
bi·ven·tral
bi·ven·tric·u·lar
bi·vi·tel·line
bix·in
bi·zy·go·mat·ic
Biz·zo·ze·ro cells
Biz·zo·ze·ro corpuscles
Biz·zo·ze·ro platelets
Bjer·rum's scotoma
Bjer·rum's screen
Bjer·rum's sign
Björk-Shi·ley aortic valve
 prosthesis
Björn·stad syndrome
black
 fat b. HB
 indulin b.
 ivory b.
 lamp b.
 Paris b.
 solvent b. 3
 Sudan b. B
Black·fan-Di·a·mond anemia
Black·fan-Di·a·mond
 syndrome
Black's classification
Black's formula

Black·berg and Wan·ger's test
black·fly
black haw
black·head
black·out
black·snake
blad·der
    allantoic b.
    atonic b.
    atonic neurogenic b.
    automatic b.
    autonomic b.
    autonomous b.
    chyle b.
    cord b.
    denervated b.
    double b.
    encysted b.
    fasciculated b.
    gall b.
    hypertonic b.
    irritable b.
    motor paralytic b.
    nervous b.
    neurogenic b.
    nonreflex b.
    paralytic b.
    reflex b.
    sacculated b.
    sensory paralytic b.
    spastic b.
    spinal shock b.
    string b.
    tabetic b.
    trabeculated b.
    uninhibited neurogenic b.
    urinary b.
blad·der·worm
blade
    banana b.
    Bard-Parker b.
    Beaver DeBakey b.
    Foregger b.
    Macintosh b.
    shoulder b.
    Superblade b.
blade·vent
Blain·ville's ear

Blake's disk
Blake·more-Seng·sta·ken tube
Bla·lock-Han·lon operation
Bla·lock-Taus·sig operation
Blanc·o·phor
Blan·din's glands
Blan·din and Nuhn's glands
blan·ket
    hypothermic b.
    mucus b.
blank·o·phore
Bla·si·us' duct
Blas·ko·vics operation
blast
blas·te·ma
    metanephric b.
blas·tem·ic
blas·tid
blas·tide
blas·tin
blas·to·chyle
blas·to·coele
blas·to·coel·ic
blas·to·cyst
Blas·to·cys·tis
    B. hominis
blas·to·cyte
blas·to·cy·to·ma
blas·to·derm
    bilaminar b.
    embryonic b.
    extraembryonic b.
    trilaminar b.
blas·to·der·mal
blas·to·der·mic
blas·to·disc
blas·to·gen·e·sis
blas·to·ge·net·ic
blas·to·gen·ic
blas·tog·e·ny
blas·to·ki·nin
blas·tol·y·sis
blas·to·lyt·ic
blas·to·ma *pl.* blas·to·mas,
  blas·to·ma·ta
    pluricentric b.
    pulmonary b.
    unicentric b.

blas·to·ma·toid
blas·to·ma·to·sis
blas·to·ma·tous
blas·to·mere
    formative b.
blas·to·mer·ot·o·my
blas·to·mo·gen·ic
blas·to·mog·e·nous
Blas·to·my·ces
    B. brasiliensis
    B. dermatitidis
blas·to·my·ces *pl.* blas·to·my·
    ce·tes
blas·to·my·cete
blas·to·my·ce·tes
blas·to·my·cin
blas·to·my·co·sis
    Brazilian b.
    cutaneous b.
    European b.
    keloidal b.
    North American b.
    South American b.
    systemic b.
blas·to·my·cot·ic
blas·to·neu·ro·pore
blas·toph·tho·ria
blas·toph·tho·ric
blas·to·phyl·lum
blas·toph·y·ly
blas·to·pore
blas·to·sphere
blas·to·spore
blas·to·stro·ma
blas·tot·o·my
blas·to·zo·oid
blas·tu·la *pl.* blas·tu·lae
blas·tu·lar
blas·tu·la·tion
Blatin's sign
Blat·ta
Blat·tel·la ger·man·i·ca
Blat·tidae
BLB mask
bleach·ing
    coronal b.
bleb
    filtering b.

bleb *(continued)*
    nuclear b.
bleed·er
bleed·ing
    dysfunctional uterine b.
    functional b.
    implantation b.
    midcyclical b.
    occult b.
    placentation b.
    postmenopausal b.
    punctate b.
    summer b.
blen·nad·e·ni·tis
blen·nem·e·sis
blen·no·gen·ic
blen·nog·e·nous
blen·noid
blen·nor·rha·gia
blen·nor·rhag·ic
blen·nor·rhea
    inclusion b.
    b. neonatorum
    Stoerk's b.
blen·nor·rhe·al
blen·no·sta·sis
blen·no·stat·ic
blen·no·tho·rax
blen·nu·ria
Blen·ox·ane
ble·o·my·cin
    b. sulfate
Bleph
bleph·ar·ad·e·ni·tis
bleph·a·ral
bleph·a·rec·to·my
bleph·a·rel·o·sis
bleph·a·rism
bleph·a·ri·tis
    b. angularis
    b. ciliaris
    b. marginalis
    nonulcerative b.
    seborrheic b.
    b. squamosa
    squamous seborrheic b.
    b. ulcerosa
bleph·a·ro·ad·e·ni·tis

bleph·a·ro·ad·e·no·ma
bleph·a·ro·ath·er·o·ma
bleph·a·ro·chal·a·sis
bleph·a·ro·chro·mi·dro·sis
bleph·a·roc·lo·nus
bleph·a·ro·col·o·bo·ma
bleph·a·ro·con·junc·ti·vi·tis
Bleph·a·ro·co·ryn·thi·na
bleph·a·ro·di·a·sta·sis
bleph·a·ron
bleph·a·ron·cus
bleph·a·ro·pach·yn·sis
bleph·a·ro·phi·mo·sis
bleph·a·ro·plast
bleph·a·ro·plas·ty
bleph·a·ro·ple·gia
bleph·a·rop·to·sis
bleph·a·ro·py·or·rhea
bleph·a·ror·rha·phy
bleph·a·ro·spasm
    essential b.
    symptomatic b.
bleph·a·ro·sphinc·ter·ec·to·my
bleph·a·ro·stat
bleph·a·ro·ste·no·sis
bleph·a·ro·syn·ech·ia
bleph·a·rot·o·my
Bles·sig's cysts
Bles·sig's groove
Bles·sig's lacunae
Bles·sig's spaces
blind
    color b.
blind·gut
blind·ism
blind·ness
    amnesic color b.
    apperceptive b.
    blue b.
    blue-yellow b.
    Bright's b.
    central b.
    color b.
    concussion b.
    cortical b.
    cortical psychic b.
    day b.

blind·ness *(continued)*
    eclipse b.
    electric-light b.
    epidemic b.
    flash b.
    flight b.
    functional b.
    green b.
    hysterical b.
    legal b.
    letter b.
    mind b.
    moon b.
    musical b.
    night b.
    note b.
    object b.
    psychic b.
    pure word b.
    red b.
    red-green b.
    river b.
    sign b.
    snow b.
    solar b.
    soul b.
    syllabic b.
    taste b.
    text b.
    total b.
    twilight b.
    word b.
    yellow b.
blis·ter
    blood b.
    burn b.
    fever b.
    Marochetti's b's
    water b.
bloat
bloat·er
    blue b.
Blo·ca·dren
Bloch, Konrad
Bloch-Sulz·ber·ger syndrome
block
    adrenergic b.
    affect b.

block *(continued)*
air b.
alveolar-capillary b.
anesthetic b.
ankle b.
anode b.
anterograde b.
arborization b.
articular b.
Atkinson-type lid b.
atrioventricular b.
Bier b.
brachial b.
brachial plexus b.
bundle-branch b.
caudal b.
cerebrospinal fluid b.
cervical plexus b.
comparator b.
complete heart b.
cryogenic b.
dynamic b.
ear b.
elbow b.
entrance b.
epidural b.
exit b.
femoral b.
field b.
ganglionic b.
heart b.
hyperpolarization b.
incomplete heart b.
intercostal nerve b.
interventricular b.
intra-atrial b.
intranasal b.
intraspinal b.
intravenous (IV) b.
intraventricular b.
lumbar plexus b.
manometric b.
meningeal b.
mental b.
metabolic b.
methadone b.
nerve b.
neuromuscular b.

block *(continued)*
paracervical b.
paraffin b.
paraneural b.
parasacral b.
paravertebral b.
partial b.
peri-infarction b.
perineural b.
portal b.
presacral b.
protective b.
pudendal b.
regional b.
retrograde b.
sacral b.
saddle b.
segmental b.
shock b.
sinoatrial b.
sinus b.
sphenopalatine b.
spinal b.
spinal subarachnoid b.
splanchnic b.
stellate b.
subarachnoid b.
sympathetic b.
transsacral b.
tubal b.
unidirectional b.
uterosacral b.
vagal b.
vagus nerve b.
ventricular b.
vertebral b.
Wenckebach b.
Wilson's b.
wrist b.
block·ade
adrenergic b.
adrenergic neuron b.
alpha-b.
alpha-adrenergic b.
beta-b.
beta-adrenergic b.
cholinergic b.
lymphatic b.

block·ade *(continued)*
    narcotic b.
    neuromuscular b.
    renal b.
    reticuloendothelial b.
    sympathetic b.
    virus b.
block·age
    tendon b.
Block·ain
block·er
    α-b.
    β-b.
    bronchial b.
    calcium channel b.
    neuromuscular b.
    starch b.
block·ing
    adrenergic b.
    thought b.
block·out
Blocq's disease
Blom-Sin·ger valve
Blond·lot rays
blood
    arterial b.
    banked b.
    cord b.
    defibrinated b.
    laky b.
    occult b.
    oxalated b.
    peripheral b.
    sludged b.
    splanchnic b.
    strawberry-cream b.
    venous b.
    whole b.
blood bank
Blood·good's disease
blood group
    ABO b. g.
    Auberger b. g.
    Bombay b. g.
    Cartwright b. g.
    CDE b. g.
    Diego b. g.
    Dombrock b. g.

blood group *(continued)*
    Duffy b. g.
    high frequency b. g.
    I b. g.
    Kell b. g.
    Kidd b. g.
    Lewis b. g.
    low frequency b. g.
    Lutheran b. g.
    MN b. g.
    MNSs b. g.
    P b. g.
    Rh b. g.
    Sutter b. g.
    Xg b. g.
blood·less
blood·let·ting
blood plas·ma
blood pres·sure
blood·root
blood se·rum
    glycerin b. s.
    Löffler's b. s.
blood stream, blood·stream
blood type
Bloom's syndrome
blotch
Blount's disease
blow·fly
blow·pipe
BLS — basic life support
blue
    alcian b.
    alizarin b.
    alkali b.
    aniline b.
    aniline b., W. S.
    anthracene b.
    azidine b., 3 B.
    benzamine b., 3 B.
    benzo b.
    Berlin b.
    b. bloater
    Borrel's b.
    brilliant b., C.
    brilliant cresyl b.
    bromchlorphenol b.
    bromophenol b.

blue *(continued)*
    bromothymol b.
    china b.
    chlorazol b., 3 B.
    Congo b., 3 B.
    Coomassie b.
    cresyl b.
    cyanol b.
    diamine b.
    dianil b., H. 3 G.
    Evans b.
    Helvetia b.
    indigo b.
    indigo b., soluble
    indophenol b.
    isamine b.
    isosulfan b.
    Kühne's methylene b.
    Löffler's methylene b.
    marine b.
    methylene b.
    methylene b., N. N.
    methylene b., O.
    naphthamine b., 3 B. X.
    new methylene b., N.
    Niagara b., 3 B.
    Nile b., A., Nile b. sulfate
    polychrome methylene b.
    Prussian b.
    pyrrole b.
    quinaldine b.
    spirit b.
    sulfan b.
    Swiss b.
    tetrabromophenol b.
    thymol b.
    toluidine b., toluidine b., O
    trypan b.
    Victoria b.
    b. vitriol
    water b.
blu·en·so·my·cin
Blum·berg, Baruch Samuel
Blum·berg's sign
Blu·men·au's nucleus
Blu·men·thal's disease
Blu·mer shelf
blunt·hook

blur
    spectacle b.
blush
    angiographic b.
    tumor b.
BM — bowel movement
BMA — British Medical Association
BMG — benign monoclonal gammopathy
BMI — body mass index
BMR — basal metabolic rate
BMS — Bachelor of Medical Science
BNA — Basle Nomina Anatomica
BOA — British Orthopaedic Association
board
    alphabet b.
    angle b.
    back b.
    bed b.
    powder exercise b.
    spine b.
    transfer b.
board certified
board eligible
Bo·a·ri's operation
Bo·as' algesimeter
Bo·as' point
Bo·as' test
Bo·as' test meal
Bo·as-Op·pler bacillus
Bo·bath method
Boch·da·lek's duct
Boch·da·lek's foramen
Boch·da·lek's ganglion
Boch·da·lek's gap
Boch·da·lek's hernia
Boch·da·lek's pseudoganglion
Boch·da·lek's sinus
Boch·da·lek's valve
Bock's ganglion
Bock's nerve
Bock·hart's impetigo
Bo·dan·sky unit

Bo·dech·tel-Gutt·mann
  disease
bo·den·plat·te
Bo·di·an method
Bo·do
body
  acetone b's
  accessory b.
  adipose b. of cheek
  adipose b. of ischiorectal
    fossa
  adipose b. of orbit
  adrenal b.
  Alder-Reilly b's
  alkapton b's
  Amato b's
  amygdaloid b.
  amylaceous b's
  amyloid b's
  anococcygeal b.
  anti-immune b.
  aortic b.
  apical b.
  b's of Arantius
  Arnold's b's
  asbestos b's
  Aschoff b's
  asteroid b.
  Auer b's
  Babès-Ernst b.
  bacillary b.
  Balbiani's b.
  Balfour b's
  bamboo b's
  Barr b.
  Bartonia b's
  basal b.
  Behla's b's
  Bence Jones b's
  Bichat's fatty b. of cheek
  Bollinger's b's
  Borrel b's
  Bracht-Wächter b's
  brassy b.
  "bull's eye" b.
  Cabot's ring b's
  Call-Exner b's
  cancer b's

body *(continued)*
  carotid b.
  cavernous b. of clitoris
  cavernous b. of penis
  cell b.
  central b.
  central fibrous b. of heart
  chromaffin b.
  chromatin b's
  chromatinic b.
  chromatoid b.
  chromophilous b's
  ciliary b.
  Civatte b.
  coccoid x b's
  coccygeal b.
  colloid b's
  compressible cavernous b's
  colostrum b's
  Councilman b's
  Cowdry type I inclusion b's
  creola b's
  crystalloid b.
  cytoid b's
  cytomegalic inclusion b.
  cytoplasmic inclusion b.
  Deetjen's b's
  demilune b.
  dense b's
  Döhle's inclusion b's
  Donné's b's
  Donovan's b.
  Dutcher b.
  elementary b.
  Elschnig b's
  Elzholz b's
  b. of epididymis
  epithelial b.
  falciform b.
  fatty b. of acetabular fossa
  fatty b. of orbit
  ferruginous b's
  fibrin b's of pleura
  filling b's
  foreign b.
  fruiting b.
  fuchsin b's
  b. of gallbladder

body *(continued)*

    Gamna-Favre b's
    Gamna-Gandy b's
    gastric b.
    geniculate b.
    Giannuzzi's b's
    glass b.
    glomus b.
    Golgi b.
    Gordon's elementary b.
    Guarnieri's b's
    habenular b.
    Halberstaedter-Prowazek
     b's
    Harting b's
    Hassall's b's
    Hassall-Henle b's
    Heinz b's
    Heinz-Ehrlich b's
    hematoxylin b's
    Hensen's b.
    Herring b's
    b. of Highmore
    Hirano b.
    Hollenhorst b's
    Howell's b's
    Howell-Jolly b's
    hyaline b's
    hyaloid b.
    immune b.
    inclusion b's
    infrapatellar fatty b.
    infundibular b.
    inner b's
    intermediate b. of
     Flemming
    interrenal b.
    intravertebral b.
    Jaworski b's
    Joest's b's
    Jolly's b's
    jugulotympanic b.
    juxtaglomerular b.
    juxtarestiform b.
    ketone b's
    Kurloff's b's
    Lafora's b's
    Lallemand's b's

body *(continued)*

    Lallemand-Trousseau b's
    Laveran b's
    L.C.L. b's
    Leishman-Donovan b.
    Levinthal-Coles-Lillie b's
    Lewy b's
    Lieutaud's b.
    Lindner's initial b's
    Lipschütz b's
    Lostorfer's b's
    Luschka's b.
    Luys' b.
    lyssa b's
    Mallory's b's
    malpighian b's
    mamillary b.
    Marchal b's
    Masson b's
    medullary b.
    melon-seed b.
    metachromatic b's
    Michaelis-Gutmann b's
    mitochondrial b.
    Miyagawa b's
    molluscum b's
    Mooser b's
    Mott b's
    multilamellar b.
    multivesicular b.
    Negri b's
    Neill-Mooser b.
    nemaline b's
    nigroid b.
    Nissl b's
    Nothnagel's b's
    no-threshold b's
    Odland b.
    Oken's b.
    olivary b.
    onion b's
    oryzoid b's
    pacchionian b's
    pampiniform b.
    b. of pancreas
    Pappenheimer b's
    para-aortic b's
    parabasal b.

body *(continued)*
    parabigeminal b.
    paranuclear b.
    paraphyseal b.
    pararenal b.
    paraterminal b.
    parathyroid b.
    parietal b.
    parolivary b's
    Paschen b's
    pearly b's
    penile b.
    perineal b.
    pheochrome b.
    phi b's
    Pick b's
    pineal b.
    pituitary b.
    platelet dense b.
    Plimmer's b's
    polar b's
    postbranchial b's
    presegmenting b's
    primitive perineal b.
    Prowazek's b's
    Prowazek-Greeff b's
    psammoma b.
    pseudolutein b.
    psittacosis inclusion b.
    purine b's
    pyknotic b's
    quadrigeminal b's
    Reilly b's
    Renaut's b's
    residual b.
    residual b. of Regnaud
    restiform b.
    reticulate b.
    b. of Retzius
    rice b's
    Rosenmüller's b.
    Ross's b's
    Russell b's
    sand b's
    Sandström's b's
    Savage's perineal b.
    Schaumann's b's
    Schmorl b.

body *(continued)*
    Seidelin b's
    semilunar b's
    spongy b.
    Stieda b.
    b. of stomach
    striate b.
    supracardial b's
    suprarenal b.
    Symington's b.
    telobranchial b's
    threshold b's
    thyroid b.
    tigroid b's
    tingible b.
    Todd b's
    Torres-Teixeira b's
    touch b.
    trachoma b's
    trapezoid b.
    Trousseau-Lallemand b's
    turbinated b.
    tympanic b.
    ultimobranchial b's
    vagal b.
    vermiform b's
    Verocay b's
    b. of Vicq d'Azyr
    Virchow-Hassall b.
    vitelline b.
    vitreous b.
    Winkler's b.
    wolffian b.
    xanthine b's
    X chromatin b.
    yellow b. of ovary
    zebra b.
    Zuckerkandl's b's
body rock·ing
body snatch·ing
Boeck's disease
Boeck's sarcoid
Boer·haa·ve's syndrome
Bo·go·mo·lets serum
Bo·gros' space
Bo·grov's fiber
Bohr effect
Bo·hun upas

boil
  Aleppo b.
  Bagdad b.
  Biskra b.
  blind b.
  Delhi b.
  gum b.
  Jericho b.
  Madura b.
  Oriental b.
  salt water b.
  sea water b.
  shoe b.
Bol. — L. bolus (pill)
bol·a·ster·one
bol·de·none un·dec·y·len·ate
bol·dine
bol·do
bol·doa
bol·e·nol
Bo·le·tus
  B. satanas
Bolk's retardation theory
Bol·lin·ger's bodies
Bol·lin·ger's granules
bo·lom·e·ter
Bol·ton's plane
Bol·ton's point
Bol·ton's triangle
bo·lus
  b. alba
  alimentary b.
bom·bé
bom·be·sin
bom·bi·ces·ter·ol
bom·by·kol
Bombyx mori
bond
  conjugated double b's
  coordinate covalent b.
  covalent b.
  disulfide b.
  energy-rich b.
  glycosidic b's
  high-energy b.
  high-energy phosphate b.
  high-energy sulfur b.
  hydrogen b.

bond *(continued)*
  hydrophobic b.
  ionic b.
  isopeptide b.
  pair b.
  peptide b.
  phosphodiester b.
  pi b.
  sigma b.
  Van der Waals b.
bond·ing
  direct b.
  tooth b.
Bon·dy mastoidectomy
Bon·dy operation
bone
  accessory b.
  acetabular b.
  acromial b.
  alar b.
  Albers-Schönberg marble
    b's
  Albrecht's b.
  alisphenoid b.
  alveolar b.
  ankle b.
  astragaloid b.
  astragaloscaphoid b.
  basal b.
  basihyal b.
  basilar b.
  basioccipital b.
  basiotic b.
  basisphenoid b.
  Bertin's b.
  blade b.
  breast b.
  bregmatic b.
  Breschet's b.
  brittle b's
  bundle b.
  calcaneal b.
  calf b.
  cancellated b.
  cancellous b.
  capitate b.
  carpal b's
  cartilage b.

bone *(continued)*
    cavalry b.
    central b.
    cheek b.
    coccygeal b.
    collar b.
    compact b.
    cortical b.
    costal b.
    cotyloid b.
    cranial b's, b's of cranium
    cribriform b.
    cuboid b.
    cuckoo b.
    cuneiform b.
    dermal b.
    ectethmoid b's
    ectocuneiform b.
    endochondral b.
    entocuneiform b.
    epactal b's
    epactal b., proper
    epihyal b.
    epipteric b.
    episternal b.
    ethmoid b.
    exercise b.
    exoccipital b.
    exocranial wormian b.
    facial b's
    femoral b.
    fetal b.
    fibular b.
    flank b.
    flat b.
    Flower's b.
    frontal b.
    funny b.
    Goethe's b.
    hamate b.
    heterotopic b.
    hyoid b.
    iliac b.
    inca b.
    incarial b.
    incisive b.
    innominate b.
    intermaxillary b.

bone *(continued)*
    intermediate b.
    interparietal b.
    intrachondrial b.
    irregular b.
    ischial b.
    ivory b's
    jaw b., lower
    jaw b., upper
    jugal b.
    Krause b.
    lacrimal b.
    lamellated b.
    lenticular b. of hand
    lentiform b.
    lingual b.
    long b.
    lunate b.
    malar b.
    marble b's
    mastoid b.
    maxillary b.
    maxillary b., inferior
    maxillary b., superior
    maxilloturbinal b.
    membrane b.
    mesethmoid b.
    mesocuneiform b.
    metacarpal b's
    metatarsal b's
    mosaic b.
    multangular b., accessory
    multangular b., larger
    multangular b., smaller
    nasal b.
    navicular b. of foot
    navicular b. of hand
    nonlamellated b.
    occipital b.
    odontoid b.
    orbital b.
    orbitosphenoidal b.
    palatine b.
    parietal b.
    pelvic b.
    perichondral b.
    periosteal b.
    petrous b.

bone *(continued)*
    phalangeal b's
    Pirie's b.
    pisiform b.
    pneumatic b.
    postsphenoidal b.
    postulnar b.
    prefrontal b.
    preinterparietal b.
    premaxillary b.
    presphenoidal b.
    primary b.
    primitive b.
    pterygoid b.
    pubic b.
    pyramidal b.
    radial b.
    replacement b.
    resurrection b.
    reticulated b.
    rider's b.
    Riolan's b's
    rudimentary b.
    sacral b.
    scaphoid b.
    scapular b.
    scroll b's
    secondary b.
    secondary cuboid b.
    semilunar b.
    septal b.
    sesamoid b's
    shank b.
    shin b.
    short b.
    sieve b.
    solid b.
    sphenoid b.
    sphenoturbinal b.
    splint b's
    spoke b.
    spongy b.
    squamo-occipital b.
    squamous b.
    subperiosteal b.
    substitution b.
    supernumerary b.
    suprainterparietal b.

bone *(continued)*
    supraoccipital b.
    suprapharyngeal b.
    suprasternal b's
    sutural b's
    tabular b.
    tarsal b's
    temporal b.
    tongue b.
    trabecular b.
    trapezoid b.
    trapezoid b. of Henle
    trapezoid b. of Lyser
    turbinate b.
    tympanic b.
    ulnar b.
    ulnar carpal b.
    unciform b.
    uncinate b.
    vesalian b.
    whirl b.
    wormian b's
    woven b.
    xiphoid b.
    zygomatic b.
bone·let
Bon·hoef·fer's symptom
Bo·nine
    gluteal b.
Bon·net's capsule
Bon·net's sign
Bon·ni·er's syndrome
Bon·not's gland
Bon·will crown
Bon·will triangle
Böök's syndrome
boom·slang
Boor·man gastric cancer typing system (I-IV)
boost·er
boot
    air b.
    bunny b.
    gelatin compression b.
    Gibney's b.
    moon b.
    pneumatic b.
    Unna's paste b.

Booth·by's mask
bo·rac·ic acid
bo·rate
bo·rax
bor·bo·ryg·mus *pl.* bor·bo·ryg·mi
bor·deaux B
bor·der
  b. of acetabulum
  alveolar b. of mandible
  alveolar b. of maxilla
  anterior b.
  brush b.
  denture b.
  external b. of tibia
  inferior b. of mandible
  interosseous b.
  lacrimal b.
  lambdoid b.
  lateral b.
  medial b.
  orbital b. of sphenoid bone
  b. of oval fossa
  peripheral b.
  posterior b. of petrous
    portion of temporal bone
  posterointernal b. of fibula
  striated b.
  superior b. of patella
  superior b. of petrous
    portion of temporal bone
  vermilion b.
Bor·det, Jules Jean Baptiste
  Vincent
Bor·det-Gen·gou agar
Bor·det-Gen·gou bacillus
Bor·det-Gen·gou culture
  medium
Bor·det-Gen·gou phenomenon
Bor·det-Gen·gou reaction
Bor·de·tel·la
  B. bronchiseptica
  B. parapertussis
  B. pertussis
Bor·di·er-Fränk·el sign
bo·ric acid
bo·rism
Bor·na disease

Born·holm disease
bor·nyl
  b. salicylate
bo·ro·cain
bo·ron
  b. carbide
bo·ro·sal·i·cyl·ic acid
Bor·re·lia
  B. berbera
  B. buccalis
  B. burgdorferi
  B. carteri
  B. caucasica
  B. crocidurae
  B. dipodilli
  B. duttonii
  B. hermsii
  B. hispanica
  B. kochii
  B. latyschewii
  B. mazzottii
  B. merionesi
  B. microti
  B. neotropicalis
  B. novyi
  B. obermeyeri
  B. parkeri
  B. persica
  B. recurrentis
  B. turicatae
  B. venezuelensis
  B. vincentii
bor·rel·i·o·sis
Bor·si·eri's line
Bor·si·eri's sign
Bor·then's operation
Bose's hook
boss
  frontal b.
  parietal b's
  sanguineous b.
bos·se·lat·ed
bos·se·la·tion
boss·ing
  b. of cranium
Bos·tock's catarrh
Bos·tock's disease
Bos·ton's sign

Bos·worth procedure
Bo·tal·lo's duct
Bo·tal·lo's foramen
Bo·tal·lo's ligament
bo·tan·ic
bot·a·ny
    medical b.
bot·fly
both·rid·i·um
both·rio·ceph·a·li·a·sis
Both·rio·ceph·a·lus
    B. mansoni
    B. mansonoides
both·ri·um
both·rop·ik
Both·rops
    B. atrox
bo·tog·e·nin
bot·ry·oid
Bot·ryo·my·ces
bot·ryo·my·co·ma
bot·ryo·my·co·sis
bot·ryo·my·cot·ic
bo·try·ti·my·co·sis
Bo·try·tis
    B. bassiana
    B. tenella
Bött·cher's cells
Bött·cher's crystals
Bött·cher's ganglion
Bött·cher's space
bot·tle
    Castaneda b.
    Junker b.
    Spritz b.
    wash b.
    Woulfe's b.
bot·tom
    weavers' b.
bot·tro·my·cin
bot·u·li·form
bot·u·lin
bot·u·li·nal
bot·u·lin·o·gen·ic
bot·u·lism
    food-borne b.
    infant b.
    wound b.

bot·u·lis·mo·tox·in
bou·ba
Bou·chard's coefficient
Bou·chard's disease
Bou·chard's nodes
Bou·chard's nodules
Bou·chard's sign
Bou·char·dat's test
Bou·char·dat's treatment
bouche
    b. de tapir
Bou·chut's respiration
Bou·chut's tubes
bouf·fée
    b. délirante
bou·gie
    b. à boule
    acorn-tipped b.
    bulbous b.
    caustic b.
    conic b.
    cylindrical b.
    dilating b.
    elastic b.
    elbowed b.
    filiform b.
    fusiform b.
    Hurst's b's
    Maloney b's
    olive-tipped b.
    rosary b.
    wax-tipped b.
    whip b.
bou·gie·nage
Bouil·laud's disease
Bouil·laud's sign
Bouil·laud's syndrome
bouil·lon
Bou·in's fluid
Bou·in's solution
bou·lim·ia
bou·quet
    b. of Riolan
Bour·gery's ligament
Bourne·ville's disease
Bourne·ville-Bris·saud disease
Bourne·ville-Prin·gle
    syndrome

bou·ton
    b. en passage
    b's terminaux
bou·ton·neuse
bou·ton·niére
Bou·ve·ret's disease
Bou·ve·ret's syndrome
Bou·ve·ret-Du·guet ulcer
Bo·vet, Daniel
bo·vied
Bo·vi·my·ces pleu·ro·pneu·
    mo·niae
bow
    Birnberg b.
    cupid's b.
    hypochordal b.
    labial b.
    Logan b.
Bow·ditch's law
bow·el
bow·en·oid
Bow·en's disease
Bow·en's precancerous
    dermatosis
bowl
    mastoid b.
    mastoidectomy b.
bow·leg
    nonrachitic b.
Bow·man's capsule
Bow·man's lamina
Bow·man's muscle
Bow·man's probe
Bow·man's theory
Bow·man's tube
box
    anatomical snuff-b.
    Bárány's b.
    black b.
    CAT b.
    glove b.
    Hogness b.
    homeo b.
    hot air b.
    obstruction b.
    Pribnow b.
    Skinner b.
    TATA b.

box *(continued)*
    voice b.
    Yerkes discrimination b.
box·car·ring
box·i·dine
box-note
Boyce's sign
Boy·den sphincter
Boy·den test
Boy·er's bursa
Boy·er's cyst
Boyle's law
Boze·man's catheter
Boze·man's operation
Boze·man's position
Boze·man's speculum
Boze·man-Fritsch catheter
Boz·zo·lo's sign
BP — blood pressure
       British Pharmacopoeia
b.p. — boiling point
bp — base pair
BPA — British Paediatric
    Association
B Ph — British
    Pharmacopoeia
BPIG — bacterial
    polysaccharide immune
    globulin
Bq — becquerel
Braasch catheter
brace
    Bledsoe b.
    Blount b.
    Boston b.
    clam-shell b.
    dropfoot b.
    Fisher b.
    Goldthwait b.
    Jewett b.
    Jones b.
    Klenzak b.
    49er knee b.
    Knight-Taylor b.
    Kydex b.
    Lenox Hill b.
    LSU reciprocation-gait
      orthosis b.

brace *(continued)*
    McKee b.
    Milwaukee b.
    Moe b.
    Roylan tibia fracture b.
    Seton hip b.
    SMo (stainless steel and
      molybdenum) b.
    SOMI b.
    Taylor b.
    UBC (University of British
      Columbia) b.
brace·let
    Nageotte's b's
Bra·chet's mesolateral fold
bra·chia
bra·chi·al
bra·chi·al·gia
    b. statica paresthetica
brach·i·form
bra·chio·ce·phal·ic
bra·chio·cru·ral
bra·chio·cu·bi·tal
bra·chio·cyl·lo·sis
bra·chio·cyr·to·sis
bra·chio·fa·cio·lin·gual
bra·chio·gram
bra·chi·um *pl.* bra·chia
    anterior conjunctival b.
    b. colliculi cranialis
    b. colliculi inferioris
    b. colliculi rostralis
    b. colliculi superioris
    b. conjunctivum cerebelli
    b. of cranial colliculus
    b. of inferior colliculus
    b. opticum
    b. pontis
    b. quadrigeminum inferius
    b. quadrigeminum superius
    b. of rostral colliculus
    b. of superior colliculus
Bracht's maneuver
Bracht-Wäch·ter lesion
brachy·ba·sia
brachy·car·dia
brachy·ce·pha·lia
brachy·ce·phal·ic
brachy·ceph·a·lism
brachy·ceph·a·lous
brachy·ceph·a·ly
brachy·chei·lia
brachy·chron·ic
brachy·cne·mic
brachy·cra·ni·al
brachy·cra·nic
brachy·dac·ty·ly
brachy·don·tia
brachy·esoph·a·gus
brachy·fa·cial
brachy·glos·sal
brach·yg·na·thia
brach·yg·na·thous
brachy·ker·kic
brachy·kne·mic
brachy·meta·car·pal·ism
brachy·meta·car·pia
brachy·me·tap·o·dy
brachy·meta·tar·sia
brachy·me·tro·pia
brachy·me·tro·pic
brachy·mor·phic
brachy·pha·lan·gia
brachy·po·dous
brachy·ra·dio·ther·a·py
brachy·rhin·ia
brachy·rhyn·cus
brachy·skel·ous
brachy·staph·y·line
brachy·sta·sis
brachy·ther·a·py
    interstitial b.
    intracavitary application b.
    remote afterloading b.
brachy·typ·i·cal
brachy·uran·ic
Brack·in technique
bract
Brad·ford frame
brady·acu·sia
brady·ar·rhyth·mia
brady·ar·thria
brady·aux·e·sis
Brady·bae·na
brady·car·dia
    Branham's b.

brady·car·dia *(continued)*
   central b.
   essential b.
   fetal b.
   nodal b.
   physiologic b.
   postinfective b.
   sinoatrial b.
   sinus b.
   vagal b.
brady·car·di·ac
brady·crot·ic
brady·di·as·to·le
brady·ecoia
brady·es·the·sia
brady·gen·e·sis
brady·glos·sia
brady·ki·ne·sia
brady·ki·net·ic
brady·ki·nin
brady·la·lia
brady·lex·ia
brady·lo·gia
brady·men·or·rhea
brady·pha·gia
brady·pha·sia
brady·phe·mia
brady·phra·sia
brady·phre·nia
brady·pnea
brady·pra·gia
brady·rhyth·mia
brady·sper·ma·tism
brady·sphyg·mia
brady·stal·sis
brady·tachy·car·dia
brady·tel·eo·ci·ne·sia
brady·tel·eo·ki·ne·sis
brady·to·cia
brady·tro·phia
brady·troph·ic
brady·uria
brady·zo·ite
Bra·gard's sign
braid·ism
Brai·ley's operation
braille

brain
   cyclopean b.
   isolated b.
   respirator b.
Brain's reflex
brain stem
brain·case
brain-dam·aged
brain·wash·ing
brake
   duodenal b.
branch
   b's of bundle of His
   gluteal b. of MacAlister
   left bundle b.
   right bundle b.
   b's of suprascapular artery
   sural communicating b.
   thenar b. of median nerve
   b's of vertebral artery
branched-chain α-ke·to ac·id
  de·hy·dro·gen·ase
branch·er deficiency
branch·er en·zyme
bran·chia
bran·chi·al
branch·ing en·zyme
bran·chi·o·gen·ic
bran·chi·og·e·nous
bran·chi·o·ma
bran·chio·mere
bran·chio·mer·ic
bran·chi·om·er·ism
Bran·chio·sto·ma
Brand bath
Brandt-An·drews maneuver
Bran·ham's bradycardia
Bran·ham's sign
Bran·ha·mel·la
   B. catarrhalis
brash
   water b.
   weaning b.
Bras·si·ca
bras·sid·ic acid
Braun's anastomosis
Braun's canal

Braun's hook
Braun von Fer·wald sign
Brau·ne's canal
Brau·ne's muscle
Brau·ne's ring
Brau·ne's vein
Braun·wald's sign
Bra·vais-jack·so·ni·an
  epilepsy
brawny
Brax·ton Hicks contraction
Brax·ton Hicks sign
Brax·ton Hicks version
breadth
  b. of accommodation
  bizygomatic b.
break
  chromatid b.
  isochromatid b.
  single chain b.
  single strand b.
break·age and re·un·ion
break·off
breast
  broken b.
  caked b.
  chicken b.
  Cooper's irritable b.
  cystic b.
  funnel b.
  gathered b.
  irritable b.
  keeled b.
  pigeon b.
  proemial b.
  shoe-makers' b.
  shotty b.
  supernumerary b.
  thrush b.
breast-feed·ing
breath
  lead b.
  saturnine b.
Breath·a·ly·zer
breath-hold·ing
  blue b.
  white b.

breath·ing
  apneustic b.
  ataxic b.
  autonomous b.
  Biot's b.
  bronchial b.
  Cheyne-Stokes b.
  cogwheel b.
  continuous positive
    pressure b.
  diaphragmatic b.
  frog b.
  glossopharyngeal b.
  intermittent positive
    pressure b.
  Kussmaul b.
  mouth-to-mouth b.
  periodic b.
  shallow b.
  suppressed b.
  vesicular b.
Bre·da's disease
bre·douille·ment
breech
  complete b.
  frank b.
  incomplete b.
  single footling b.
breg·ma
breg·mat·ic
breg·ma·to·dym·ia
Breh·mer's method
Breh·mer's treatment
brei
Brei·sky's disease
brems·strah·lung
Brenne·mann's syndrome
Bren·ner's formula
Bren·ner's test
Bren·ner tumor
breph·ic
brepho·plas·tic
brepho·plas·ty
brepho·troph·ic
Bre·schet's canals
Bre·schet's hiatus
Bre·schet's sinus

Bre·schet's veins
Bre·scia-Ci·mi·no fistula
Breth·ine
Bre·ton·neau's angina
Bre·ton·neau's disease
bre·tyl·i·um to·sy·late
Breus mole
Bre·vi·bac·te·ri·um
    B. linens
brev·i·col·lis
brev·i·flex·or
brevi·lin·e·al
brevi·ra·di·ate
Brev·i·tal
Brew·er's infarcts
Brew·er's point
Bric·a·nyl
Brick·er's operation
Brick·ner's sign
brick·pox
bridge
    anaphase b.
    arteriolovenular b.
    Bellevue b.
    cantilever b.
    cell b's
    chromatid b.
    chromosome b.
    conjugative b.
    cytoplasmic b.
    dentin b.
    disulfide b.
    extension b.
    fixed b.
    fixed-fixed b.
    fixed-movable b.
    Gaskell's b.
    intercellular b.
    b. of the nose
    protoplasmic b.
    removable b.
    salt b.
    stationary b.
    tarsal b.
    ureteric b.
    b. of Varolius
bridge·work
    fixed b.

bridge·work *(continued)*
    removable b.
bri·dle
Brie·ger's cachexia
Brie·ger's reaction
Brie·ger's test
Bright's blindness
Bright's disease
Bright's eye
bright·ic
bright·ism
Brill's disease
Brill-Sym·mers disease
Brill-Zins·ser disease
Bri·nell hardness number
Brin·ker·hoff speculum
bri·no·lase
Brin·ton's disease
Bri·on-Kay·ser disease
Bri·quet's syndrome
brise·ment
    b. forcé
Bris·saud's dwarf
Bris·saud's infantilism
Bris·saud's reflex
Bris·saud's scoliosis
Bris·saud-Ma·rie syndrome
Bris·saud-Si·card syndrome
Bris·ta·cy·cline
Bris·ta·min
Bris·tow procedure
broach
    barbed b.
    pathfinder b.
    root canal b.
    smooth b.
Broad·bent's sign
Broad·bent-Bol·ton plane
Bro·ca's amnesia
Bro·ca's aphasia
Bro·ca's area
Bro·ca's band
Bro·ca's center
Bro·ca's convolution fissure
Bro·ca's formula
Bro·ca's gyrus
Bro·ca's plane
Bro·ca's point

Bro·ca's pouch
Bro·ca's region
Brock's infundibulectomy
Brock's operation
Brock's syndrome
Brock·en·brough's sign
Brocq's lupoid sycosis
Brocq's pseudopelade
Brö·del's white line
Bro·ders' classification
Bro·ders' index
Bro·die's abscess
Bro·die's disease
Bro·die's knee
Bro·die's ligament
Brod·mann's area
Broe·si·ke's fossa
bro·fox·ine
bro·ma·to·ther·a·py
bro·ma·ze·pam
brom·chlor·e·none
bro·me·lain
bro·mel·in
bro·meth·ol
brom·hex·ine hy·dro·chlo·ride
brom·hi·dro·sis
bro·mic
bro·mide
    hydrogen b.
    methyl b.
bro·mi·dism
bro·mi·dro·sis
bro·mi·nat·ed
brom·in·di·one
bro·mine
bro·mism
brom·iso·val·um
bro·mi·za·tion
bro·mized
bro·mo·ben·zene
bro·mo·chlo·ro·tri·flu·o·ro·
    eth·ane
bro·mo·crip·tine
5-bro·mo·de·oxy·uri·dine
bro·mo·der·ma
bro·mo·di·phen·hy·dra·mine
    hy·dro·chlo·ride
bro·mo·io·dism

bro·mo·ma·nia
bro·mo·men·or·rhea
bro·mo·meth·ane
brom·op·nea
5-bro·mo·ura·cil
bro·mox·a·nide
brom·per·i·dol
brom·phen·ir·amine
    b. maleate
brom·phe·nol
    b. blue
Bromp·ton cocktail
Bromp·ton mixture
Bromp·ton solution
Brom·sul·pha·lein
brom·thy·mol
    b. blue
brom·urat·ed
bronch·ad·e·ni·tis
bron·chi
bron·chia
bron·chi·al
bron·chi·arc·tia
bron·chi·ec·ta·sia
bron·chi·ec·tas·ic
bron·chi·ec·ta·sis
    capillary b.
    cystic b.
    dry b.
    follicular b.
bron·chi·ec·tat·ic
bron·chil·o·quy
bron·chio·cele
bron·chio·cri·sis
bron·chio·gen·ic
bron·chi·ole
    alveolar b.
    lobular b.
    respiratory b.
    terminal b.
bron·chio·lec·ta·sis
bron·chi·o·li
bron·chi·o·li·tis
    acute obliterating b.
    b. exudativa
    b. fibrosa obliterans
    vesicular b.

bron·chi·o·lus *pl.* bron·chi·o·
li
    bronchioli respiratorii
bron·chio·spasm
bron·chio·ste·no·sis
bron·chi·sep·ti·cin
bron·chis·mus
bron·chit·ic
bron·chi·tis
    acute b.
    acute laryngotracheal b.
    acute suppurative b.
    arachidic b.
    capillary b.
    Castellani's b.
    catarrhal b.
    cheesy b.
    chronic b.
    croupous b.
    dry b.
    ether b.
    exudative b.
    fibrinous b.
    hemorrhagic b.
    infectious asthmatic b.
    mechanic b.
    membranous b.
    b. obliterans
    parasitic b.
    phthinoid b.
    plastic b.
    productive b.
    pseudomembranous b.
    putrid b.
    suffocative b.
    summer b.
    vesicular b.
bron·chi·um *pl.* bron·chia
bron·cho·ad·e·ni·tis
bron·cho·al·ve·o·lar
bron·cho·al·ve·o·li·tis
bron·cho·as·per·gil·lo·sis
bron·cho·blas·to·my·co·sis
bron·cho·blen·nor·rhea
bron·cho·can·di·di·a·sis
bron·cho·cav·ern·ous
bron·cho·cele
bron·cho·con·stric·tion

bron·cho·con·stric·tor
bron·cho·di·la·ta·tion
bron·cho·di·la·tion
bron·cho·di·la·tor
bron·cho·egoph·o·ny
bron·cho·esoph·a·ge·al
bron·cho·esoph·a·gol·o·gy
bron·cho·esoph·a·gos·co·py
bron·cho·fi·ber·scope
bron·cho·fi·ber·sco·py
bron·cho·fi·bros·co·py
bron·cho·gen·ic
bron·cho·gram
    air b.
    tantalum b.
bron·cho·graph·ic
bron·chog·ra·phy
bron·cho·lith
bron·cho·li·thi·a·sis
bron·cho·log·ic
bron·chol·o·gy
bron·cho·ma·la·cia
bron·cho·mo·ni·li·a·sis
bron·cho·mo·tor
bron·cho·mu·co·trop·ic
bron·cho·my·co·sis
bron·cho·no·car·di·o·sis
bron·cho-oid·io·sis
bron·cho·pan·cre·at·ic
bron·chop·a·thy
bron·choph·o·ny
    pectoriloquous b.
    sniffling b.
    whispered b.
bron·cho·plas·ty
bron·cho·ple·gia
bron·cho·pleu·ral
bron·cho·pleu·ro·pneu·mo·
nia
bron·cho·pneu·mo·nia
    inhalation b.
    postoperative b.
    subacute b.
    virus b.
bron·cho·pneu·mon·ic
bron·cho·pneu·mo·ni·tis
bron·cho·pneu·mop·a·thy
bron·cho·pul·mo·nary

bron·cho·ra·di·og·ra·phy
bron·chor·rha·gia
bron·chor·rha·phy
bron·chor·rhea
bron·cho·scope
    fiberoptic b.
bron·cho·scop·ic
bron·chos·co·py
    fiberoptic b.
bron·cho·si·nus·itis
bron·cho·spasm
bron·cho·spi·ro·che·to·sis
bron·cho·spi·rog·ra·phy
bron·cho·spi·rom·e·ter
bron·cho·spi·rom·e·try
    differential b.
bron·cho·stax·is
bron·cho·ste·no·sis
bron·chos·to·my
bron·cho·tome
bron·chot·o·my
bron·cho·tra·che·al
bron·cho·ve·sic·u·lar
bron·chus *pl.* bron·chi
    apical b.
    cardiac b.
    dorsal b.
    eparterial b.
    extrapulmonary b.
    hyparterial bronchi
    intermediate b.
    intrapulmonary b.
    left superior ventral b.
    lingular b.
    b. lingularis
    lobar bronchi
    bronchi lobares
    primary bronchi
    right ventral b.
    secondary bronchi
    segmental bronchi
    bronchi segmentales
    stem b.
    subapical b.
    tracheal b.
Brøn·sted acid
Brøn·sted base
bron·to·pho·bia

Brooke's disease
Brooke's tumor
Bro·phy's operation
broth
    carbohydrate b.
    dextrose b.
    heart infusion b.
    infusion b.
    laurel sulfate b.
    nitrate b.
    nutrient b.
    selenite b.
    Stuart b.
    sugar b.
brow
Brown, Michael Stuart
brown
    aniline b.
    Bismarck b.
    Bismark b. R
    Bismark b. Y
    Manchester b.
    phenylene b.
Brown Kel·ly sign
Brown-Sé·quard's paralysis
Brown-Sé·quard's treatment
Brown-Sym·mers disease
Browne operation
brown·i·an move·ment
brown·i·an-Zsig·mon·dy
    movement
Brown·ing's vein
Brox·o·lin
BRS — British Roentgen
    Society
Bruce's tract
Bru·cel·la
    B. abortus
    B. bronchiseptica
    B. canis
    B. melitensis
    B. rangiferi tarandi
    B. suis
bru·cel·la
Bru·cel·la·ceae
bru·cel·lar
bru·cel·ler·gen
bru·cel·lin

bru·cel·lo·sis
Bruch's glands
bru·cine
Bruck's disease
Brücke's lines
Brücke's muscle
Brücke's reagent
Brücke's test
Brücke's tunic
Brud·zin·ski's reflex
Brud·zin·ski's sign
Bru·gia
    B. malayi
    B. pahangi
Bru·hat maneuver
bruise
    stone b.
bruisse·ment
bruit
    abdominal b.
    aneurysmal b.
    b. d'airain
    b. de bois
    b. de canon
    carotid b.
    b. de choc
    b. de clapotement
    b. de claquement
    cranial b.
    b. de craquement
    b. de cuir neuf
    b. de diable
    b. de drapeau
    femoral b.
    b. de froissement
    b. de frolement
    b. de frottement
    b. de galop
    b. de grelot
    b. de lime
    b. de moulin
    b. de parchemin
    b. de piaulement
    b. de pot fêlé
    b. de rape
    b. de rappel
    b. de Roger
    b. de scie

bruit *(continued)*
    b. de soufflet
    b. de tabourka
    b. de tambour
    false b.
    b. placentaire
    Roger's b.
    b. skodique
    seagull b.
    spinal b.
    systolic b.
    Verstraeten's b.
bru·nes·cent
Brunn's epithelial nests
Brunn's membrane
Brun·ner's glands
Bruns' sign
Bruns' syndrome
Brun·schwig's operation
Brun·sting's syndrome
brush
    Ayre's b.
    electrical b.
    Haidinger's b.
    b's of Ruffini
    stomach b.
Brushfield's spots
Brush·field-Wy·att disease
Brush·field-Wy·att syndrome
brush·ing
    bronchial b.
Bru·ton's agamma-
  globulinemia
Bru·ton's disease
brux
brux·ism
    centric b.
bruxo·ma·nia
Bry·ant's line
Bry·ant's traction
Bryce-Teach·er ovum
Bry·o·bia
    B. praetiosa
bry·o·nia
BS — Bachelor of Science
    Bachelor of Surgery
    blood sugar
    bowel sounds

BS — Bachelor of Science
(continued)
    breath sounds
BSA — body surface area
BSAER — brain stem
  auditory evoked response
B-scan
BSER — brain stem-evoked
  response
BSP — Bromsulphalein
BSS — balanced salt solution
BTU, BThU — British
  thermal unit
bub·ble ven·tric·u·log·ra·phy
bu·bo
    bullet b.
    chancroidal b.
    climatic b.
    indolent b.
    malignant b.
    nonvenereal b.
    pestilential b.
    strumous b.
    syphilitic b.
    tropical b.
    virulent b.
bu·bon
    b. d'emblée
bu·bon·ad·e·ni·tis
bu·bon·ic
bu·bono·cele
bu·bon·u·lus
bu·cai·nide mal·e·ate
bu·car·dia
buc·ca pl. buc·cae
buc·cal
buc·ci·na·tor
buc·co·ax·i·al
buc·co·ax·io·cer·vi·cal
buc·co·ax·io·gin·gi·val
buc·co·clu·sion
buc·co·cer·vi·cal
buc·co·clu·sal
buc·co·clu·sion
buc·co·dis·tal
buc·co·fa·cial
buc·co·gin·gi·val
buc·co·glos·so·phar·yn·gi·tis

buc·co·glos·so·phar·yn·gi·tis
    b. sicca
buc·co·la·bi·al
buc·co·lin·gual
buc·co·lin·gual·ly
buc·co·max·il·lary
buc·co·me·si·al
buc·co·phar·yn·ge·al
buc·co·place·ment
buc·co·pul·pal
buc·cos·to·my
buc·co·ver·sion
Buch·ner's extract
Buch·ner's tuberculin
Buck's extension
Buck's operation
buck·eye
buck·ling
    scleral b.
Bucky diaphragm
Bucky rays
Bucky-Potter diaphragm
bu·cli·zine hy·dro·chlo·ride
bu·cry·late
bud
    appendage b.
    appendicular b.
    bronchial b.
    dorsal pancreatic b.
    end b.
    epidermal b.
    epithelial b.
    gustatory b.
    hepatic b.
    limb b.
    liver b.
    lung b.
    mammary b.
    metanephric b.
    periosteal b.
    placental syncytial b's
    skin b.
    tail b.
    taste b.
    tooth b.
    ureteric b.
    b. of urethra
    vascular b.

bud *(continued)*
    ventral pancreatic b.
    wing b.
Budd-Chiari disease
Budd-Chiari syndrome
Budge's center
Bu·din's joint
Bu·din's rule
BUDR — 5-bromodeoxy-
    uridine
Buer·ger's disease
Buer·ger's symptom
Buer·gi's theory
Buer·henne stone basket
    technique
bu·fa·di·en·o·lide
bu·fa·ge·nin
bu·fa·gin
bu·fa·no·lide
büf·fel·seu·che
buf·fer
    bicarbonate b.
    cacodylate b.
    phosphate b.
    protein b.
    TRIS b.
    veronal b.
bu·fil·con A
bu·fin
Bu·fo
bu·for·min
bu·fo·tal·in
bu·fo·te·nin
bu·fo·ther·a·py
bu·fo·tox·in
bug
    assassin b.
    barley b.
    blister b.
    blue b.
    cocaine b.
    cone-nose b.
    croton b.
    harvest b.
    hematophagous b.
    kissing b.
    Malay b.
    miana (Mianeh) b.

bug *(continued)*
    red b.
    wheat b.
Buhl's desquamative
    pneumonia
Buhl's disease
Buhl-Dit·trich law
bulb
    b. of aorta
    auditory b.
    b. of corpus cavernosum
    b. of corpus spongiosum
    dental b.
    duodenal b.
    end b.
    end b's of Krause
    b. of eye
    gustatory b.
    b. of hair
    b. of heart
    b. of jugular vein, inferior
    b. of jugular vein, superior
    b's of Krause
    b. of occipital horn of
        lateral ventricle
    olfactory b.
    onion b.
    b. of ovary
    b. of penis
    b. of posterior horn of
        lateral ventricle
    Rouget's b.
    sinovaginal b.
    spinal b.
    taste b.
    terminal b's of Krause
    b. of urethra
    vaginal b.
    vestibulovaginal b.
    b. of vestibule of vulva
bul·bar
bul·bi
bul·bi·form
bul·bi·tis
bul·bo·atri·al
bul·bo·cap·nine
bul·bo·cav·er·no·sus
bul·bo·gas·trone

bul·boid
bul·bo·mem·bra·nous
bul·bo·nu·cle·ar
bul·bo·pon·tine
bul·bo·spi·nal
bul·bo·spon·gi·o·sus
bul·bo·ure·thral
bul·bous
Bul·bu·li·an mask
bul·bus *pl.* bul·bi
    b. aortae
    b. arteriosus
    b. caroticus
    b. cordis
    b. cornus occipitalis
      ventriculi lateralis
    b. cornus posterioris
      ventriculi lateralis
    b. corporis spongiosi
    b. inferior venae jugularis
    b. oculi
    b. olfactorius
    b. penis
    b. pili
    b. superior venae jugularis
    b. urethrae
    b. venae jugularis inferior
    b. venae jugularis superior
    b. vestibuli vaginae
bu·lim·ia
    b. nervosa
bu·lim·ic
Bu·lim·i·nae
bu·lim·o·rex·ia
Bu·li·mus
    B. fuchsianus
    B. leachii
Bu·li·nus
    B. africanus
    B. truncatus
Bull. — L. bulliat (let it boil)
bul·la *pl.* bul·lae
    emphysematous b.
    ethmoid b.
    b. ethmoidalis cavi nasi
    b. ethmoidalis ossis
      ethmoidalis
    b. mastoidea

bul·la *(continued)*
    b. ossea
bul·lae
bul·late
bul·la·tion
bul·lec·to·my
Bul·ler's bandage
Bul·ler's shield
bull·neck
bul·lo·sis
    diabetic b.
    b. diabeticorum
bul·lous
bu·met·a·nide
Bu·mi·nate
Bum·ke's pupil
bumps
    goose b's
    pump b's
BUN — blood urea nitrogen
bu·na·mi·dine hy·dro·chlo·ride
bu·nam·io·dyl
bun·dle
    aberrant b's
    Arnold's b.
    atrioventricular b.
    A-V b.
    axial b. of muscle spindle
    Bachmann's b.
    basis b's
    Bruce's b.
    cornucommissural b.
    central tegmental b.
    circumolivary b. of
      pyramid
    cleidoepitrochlear b.
    crossed olivocochlear b.
    b. of Flechsig
    forebrain b., medial
    Helweg's b.
    b. of His
    Keith's b.
    Kent's b.
    Kent-His b.
    Killian's b.
    lateral pontine b.
    longitudinal medial b.

bun·dle *(continued)*
    Mahaim's b.
    mamillotegmental b.
    marginal b.
    medial forebrain b.
    Meynert's b.
    Monakow's b.
    muscle b.
    olfactory b.
    olivocochlear b. of
      Rasmussen
    b. of Oort
    oval b.
    papillomacular b's
    Pick's b.
    posterior longitudinal b.
    precommissural b.
    b. of Probst
    proprius b's of spinal cord
    b. of Rasmussen
    Schultze's b.
    Schutz's b.
    sinoatrial b.
    solitary b.
    b. of Stanley Kent
    subcallosal b.
    tendon b.
    thalamomamillary b.
    Thorel's b.
    Türck's b.
    uncinate b.
    b. of Vicq d'Azyr
    Weissmann's b.
bun·dle branch
bun·ga·ro·tox·in
Bun·ga·rus
Bun·ge's amputation
Bun·ge's law
Bun·ge sponge
Büng·ner's bands
Büng·ner's cell cordons
bu·ni·o·dyl
bun·ion
    tailor's b.
bun·ion·ec·to·my
bun·ion·ette
Bun·nell splints
Bun·nell tendon transfer

Bun·nell's suture
bu·no·dont
bu·no·lol hy·dro·chlo·ride
Bun·sen burner
Bun·sen coefficient
Bun·ya·vi·ri·dae
bun·ya·vi·rus
buph·thal·mia
buph·thal·mos
bu·pic·o·mide
bu·piv·a·caine hy·dro·chlo·ride
bu·pre·nor·phine hy·dro·chlo·ride
bu·pro·pi·on hy·dro·chlo·ride
bu·quin·o·late
bur
    diamond b.
bu·ra·mate
Bur·chard-Lie·ber·mann reaction
Bur·chard-Lie·ber·mann test
Bur·dach's columns
Bur·dach's fasciculus
Bur·dach's fiber
Bur·dach's fissure
Bur·dach's nucleus
Bur·dach's tract
bu·ret, bu·rette
Bür·ger-Grütz syn·drome
Burg·hart's sign
Burg·hart's symptom
bu·rim·amide
Bur·kitt's lymphoma
burn
    arc b.
    brush b.
    chemical b.
    closed space b.
    coagulation b.
    contact b.
    corneal b.
    electrical b.
    first degree b.
    flash b.
    fourth degree b.
    friction b.
    full thickness b.

burn *(continued)*
    high tension b.
    immersion b.
    partial thickness b.
    powder b.
    radiation b.
    respiratory b.
    second degree b.
    sun b.
    thermal b.
    third degree b.
    x-ray b.
Bur·net, Sir Frank Macfarlane
Bur·nett's disinfecting fluid
Bur·nett's solution
Bur·nett's syndrome
bur·nish·er
bur·nish·ing
Burns' ligament
Burns' space
Bu·row's operation
Bu·row's solution
Bu·row's vein
burr
bur·sa *pl.* bur·sae
    b. of Achilles (tendon)
    acromial b.
    adventitious b.
    anconeal b.
    b. anserina
    bicipital b.
    bicipitofibular b.
    bicipitoradial b.
    b. bicipitoradialis
    Boyer's b.
    Brodie's b.
    calcaneal b.
    Calori's b.
    copulatory b.
    b. copulatrix
    coracobrachial b.
    coracoid b.
    b. cubitalis interossea
    deltoid b.
    epiploic b.
    b.-equivalent
    b. of Fabricius
    fibular b.

bur·sa *(continued)*
    Fleischmann's b.
    gastrocnemiosemimembra-
      nous b.
    genual b.
    gluteal b.
    gluteal intermuscular
      bursae
    gluteofascial bursae
    gluteofemoral bursae
    gluteotuberosal b.
    His b.
    humeral b.
    hyoid b.
    b. iliopectinea
    infracardiac b.
    infracondyloid b., external
    infragenual b.
    infrahyoid b.
    b. infrahyoidea
    infrapatellar b.
    interosseous cubital b.
    intertubercular b.
    b. intratendinea olecrani
    ischiadic b.
    Luschka's b.
    Monro's b.
    b. mucosa
    b. mucosa submuscularis
    mucous b.
    multilocular b.
    b. of olecranon
    omental b.
    b. omentalis
    ovarian b.
    b. ovarica
    patellar b., deep
    patellar b., middle
    patellar b., prespinous
    patellar b., subcutaneous
    peroneal b., common
    b. pharyngea
    popliteal b.
    postcalcaneal b.
    postcalcaneal b., deep
    postgenual b., external
    prepatellar b., middle

bur·sa *(continued)*
    prepatellar b.,
      subcutaneous
    prepatellar b., subfascial
    prepatellar b.,
      subtendinous
    bursae prepatellares
    pretibial b.
    radial b.
    retrocondyloid b.
    retrohyoid b.
    b. retrohyoidea
    retromammary b.
    rider's b.
    sacral b.
    semimembranosogastro-
      cnemial b.
    semimembranous b.
    semitendinous b.
    sternohyoid b.
    b. sternohyoidea
    subachilleal b.
    subacromial b.
    b. subacromialis
    subacromiodeltoid b.
    subcalcaneal b.
    subclavian b.
    subcoracoid b.
    subcrural b.
    b. subcutanea
    subcutaneous synovial b.
    b. subcutanea acromialis
    b. subcutanea calcanea
    b. subcutanea
      infrapatellaris
    b. subcutanea olecrani
    b. subcutanea prepatellaris
    b. subcutanea sacralis
    b. subcutanea
      trochanterica
    subcutaneous acromial b.
    subcutaneous calcaneal b.
    subcutaneous infrapatellar
      b.
    subcutaneous patellar b.
    subcutaneous synovial b.
    subcutaneous trochanteric
      b.

bur·sa *(continued)*
    subdeltoid b.
    b. subdeltoidea
    subfascial b.
    subfascial synovial b.
    b. subfascialis
    b. subfascialis prepatellaris
    subhyoid b.
    subiliac b.
    subligamentous b.
    b. sublingualis
    submuscular b.
    submuscular synovial b.
    b. submuscularis
    subpatellar b.
    b. subtendinea
    b. subtendinea iliaca
    b. subtendinea
      prepatellaris
    subtendinous iliac b.
    subtendinous prepatellar b.
    subtendinous b.
    subtendinous synovial b.
    supragenual b.
    suprapatellar b.
    b. suprapatellaris
    synovial b.
    b. synovialis
    b. synovialis subcutanea
    b. synovialis subfascialis
    b. synovialis submuscularis
    b. synovialis subtendinea
    b. tendinis Achillis
    b. tendinis calcanei
    b. of tendon of Achilles
    b. of testes
    thyrohyoid b.
    thyrohyoid b., anterior
    Tornwaldt's b.
    trochanteric b.,
      subcutaneous
    b. trochanterica
      subcutanea
    trochlear synovial b.
    tuberoischiadic b.
    ulnar b.
    ulnoradial b.
    vesicular b., ileopubic

bur·sa *(continued)*
    vesicular b. of
      sternohyoideus muscle
bur·sae
bur·sal
bur·sal·o·gy
Bur·sa·ta
bur·sate
bur·sec·to·my
bur·si·con
bur·si·tis
    Achilles b.
    adhesive b.
    calcaneal b.
    calcific b.
    ischial b.
    ischiogluteal b.
    olecranon b.
    omental b.
    pharyngeal b.
    popliteal b.
    prepatellar b.
    radiohumeral b.
    retrocalcaneal b.
    scapulohumeral b.
    subacromial b.
    subdeltoid b.
    superficial calcaneal b.
    Thornwaldt's (Tornwaldt's)
      b.
bur·so·lith
bur·sop·a·thy
bur·sot·o·my
burst
    bilaterally synchronous b.
    metabolic b.
    respiratory b.
bur·su·la
Burton's line
Burton's sign
BUS — Bartholin's, urethral,
  Skene's (glands)
Busch·ke's disease
Busch·ke's scleredema
Busch·ke-Lö·wen·stein's
  tumor
Busch·ke-Ol·len·dorff
  syndrome

bush·mas·ter
bu·spi·rone hy·dro·chlo·ride
Bus·quet's disease
Bus·se-Busch·ke disease
bu·sul·fan
But. — L. butyrum (butter)
bu·ta·bar·bi·tal
bu·ta·bar·bi·tal so·di·um
bu·ta·caine sul·fate
bu·tac·e·tin
bu·ta·cla·mol hy·dro·chlo·
  ride
bu·ta·di·az·amide
bu·tal·bi·tal
bu·tal·lyl·o·nal
bu·tam·ben
bu·ta·mi·rate cit·rate
bu·tam·i·sole hy·dro·chlo·
  ride
bu·ta·mox·ane hy·dro·chlo·
  ride
bu·tane
    normal b.
bu·ta·no·ic acid
bu·ta·per·a·zine
    b. maleate
Bu·ta·zol·i·din
Butch·er's saw
bu·te·thal
bu·teth·amine hy·dro·chlo·
  ride
bu·thi·a·zide
Bu·thus
    B. carolinianus
    B. quinquestriatus
bu·tir·o·sin sul·fate
Bu·ti·sol so·di·um
bu·to·nate
bu·to·pro·zine hy·dro·chlo·
  ride
bu·to·py·ro·nox·yl
bu·tor·pha·nol
    b. tartrate
bu·tox·amine hy·dro·chlo·ride
bu·trip·ty·line hy·dro·chlo·
  ride
Bütsch·li's nuclear spindle
But·ti·aux·el·la

but·tock
but·ton
    Aleppo b.
    belly b.
    Biskra b.
    bone b.
    bromide b.
    dog b.
    iodide b.
    Jaboulay b.
    mescal b's
    Murphy's b.
    Oriental b.
    Panje voice b.
    peritoneal b.
    quaker b.
    synaptic b.
    terminal b's
but·ton·hole
    mitral b.
bu·tyl
    b. acetate
    b. aminobenzoate
    b. chloride
    b. formate
    b. hydride
bu·ty·lene
bu·tyl·par·a·ben
Bu·tyn
bu·ty·rate
bu·tyr·ic
bu·tyr·ic acid
bu·ty·rin
bu·ty·rine
bu·ty·roid
bu·ty·ro·phe·none
bu·ty·ro·scope
bu·ty·ryl-CoA dehydrogenase
By·ers flap

by·pass
    aortobifemoral b.
    aortocoronary b.
    aortofemoral b.
    aortoiliac b.
    aortorenal b.
    axillo-axillary b.
    axillobifemoral b.
    axillofemoral b.
    axillopopliteal b.
    cardiopulmonary b.
    carotid-subclavian b.
    coronary b.
    coronary artery b.
    extra-anatomic b.
    extracranial/intracranial
      (EC/IC) b.
    femorofemoral b.
    femorofemoropopliteal b.
    femoropopliteal b.
    gastric b.
    ileojejunal b.
    infrapopliteal b.
    in situ b.
    intestinal b.
    jejunal b.
    jejunoileal b.
    left heart b.
    obturator b.
    partial b.
    partial ileal b.
    percutaneous biliary b.
    right heart b.
    saphenous vein b.
    subclavian-subclavian b.
bys·si·no·sis
bys·si·not·ic
bys·soid
Byth·nia
By·wa·ters' syndrome

C — Calorie
carbon
cervical vertebrae (C1–C7)
closure
complement (C1–C9)
contraction
coulomb
cytidine
cytosine
C. — L. congius (gallon)
C — capacitance
clearance
°C — degree Celsius
c — centi-
contact
small calorie
c. — L. cibus (food)
L. cum (with)
c — molar concentration
specific heat capacity
velocity of light in a
vacuum
c̄ — L. cum (with)
CA — cancer
carcinoma
cardiac arrest
chronologic age
coronary artery
croup-associated (virus)
Ca — calcium
cancer
carcinoma
cathode
ca. — L. circa (about)
CA15-3 RIA — A15-3
radioimmunoassay
CABG — coronary artery
bypass graft
cab·in·et
Sauerbruch's c.
ca·ble
coaxial c.
Cab·ot's ring bodies
cab·u·fo·con A
ca·cao
cac·a·tion

cac·a·to·ry
CaCC — cathodal closure
contraction
cac·es·then·ic
ca·chec·tic
ca·chec·tin
ca·chet
ca·chex·ia
addisonian c.
amyotrophic c.
Brieger's c.
cancerous c.
cardiac c.
c. exophthalmica
fluoric c.
Grawitz c.
hypophyseal c.
c. hypophysiopriva
hypothalamic pituitary c.
malarial c.
c. mercurialis
neurogenic c.
pituitary c.
psychogenic c.
saturnine c.
c. suprarenalis
uremic c.
cach·in·na·tion
caco·de·mono·ma·nia
cac·o·dyl
c. cyanide
c. hydride
cac·o·dyl·ate
cac·o·dyl·ic acid
caco·ethic
caco·gen·e·sis
cac·o·gen·ic
caco·gen·ics
caco·geu·sia
caco·la·lia
caco·me·lia
caco·plas·tic
caco·rhyth·mic
cac·os·mia
caco·then·ic
caco·then·ics

cac·ot·ro·phy
cac·u·men
cac·u·mi·nal
CAD — coronary artery
  disease
ca·dav·er
ca·dav·er·ic
ca·dav·er·ine
ca·dav·er·ous
cad·dis
cad·mi·o·sis
cad·mi·um
    c. anthranilate
    c. bromide
CaDTe — cathodal duration
  tetanus
ca·du·ca
ca·du·ce·us
ca·du·cous
cae·cum
    cupular c. of cochlear duct
    c. cupulare ductus
      cochlearis
    vestibular c. of cochlear
      duct
    c. vestibulare ductus
      cochlearis
cae·cus
    c. minor ventriculi
ca·fard
caf·fein·at·ed
caf·feine
    c. citrate
    citrated c.
    c. and sodium benzoate
caf·fein·ism
Caf·fey's disease
Caf·fey-Sil·ver·man syndrome
cage
    population c.
    thoracic c.
ca·hin·cic acid
Cairns syndrome
Ca·jal's cells
Ca·jal's interstitial nucleus
Ca·jal's stain
Cal — large calorie
  (kilocalorie)

cal — calorie
ca·lage
cal·a·mine
cal·a·mus
    c. scriptorius
Cal·an·druc·cio compression
  apparatus
cal·ca·ne·al
cal·ca·ne·an
cal·ca·ne·itis
cal·ca·neo·apoph·y·si·tis
cal·ca·neo·as·trag·a·loid
cal·ca·neo·ca·vus
cal·ca·neo·cu·boid
cal·ca·ne·odyn·ia
    c. sodium lactate
cal·ca·neo·fib·u·lar
cal·ca·neo·na·vic·u·lar
cal·ca·neo·plan·tar
cal·ca·neo·scaph·oid
cal·ca·neo·tib·i·al
cal·ca·neo·val·go·ca·vus
cal·ca·ne·um *pl.* cal·ca·nea
cal·ca·ne·us *pl.* cal·ca·nei
cal·ca·no·dyn·ia
cal·car
    c. avis
    c. femorale
    c. pedis
cal·car·ea
    c. chlorata
    c. hydrica
    c. phosphorica
    c. usta
cal·car·e·ous
cal·ca·rine
cal·ca·ri·uria
cal·ca·roid
cal·ce·mia
cal·ci·bil·ia
Cal·ci·bind
cal·cic
cal·ci·co·sil·i·co·sis
cal·ci·co·sis
cal·ci·di·ol
cal·cif·a·mes
cal·cif·e·di·ol
cal·cif·er·ol

cal·cif·ic
cal·ci·fi·ca·tion
   aortic c.
   conjunctival metastatic c.
   coronary c.
   dystrophic c.
   eggshell c.
   habenular c.
   intracranial c.
   metastatic c.
   Mönckeberg's c.
   myocardial c.
   periarticular c.
   pericardial c.
   pulmonary c.
   valvular c.
cal·ci·fied
cal·cig·er·ous
Cal·ci·mar
cal·cim·e·ter
cal·ci·na·tion
cal·cine
cal·ci·no·sis
   c. circumscripta
   c. cutis
   c. interstitialis
   c. intervertebralis
   tumoral c.
   c. universalis
cal·cio·ki·ne·sis
cal·cio·ki·net·ic
cal·ci·or·rha·chia
cal·ci·pec·tic
cal·ci·pe·nia
cal·ci·pe·nic
cal·ci·pex·ic
cal·ci·pex·is
cal·ci·pexy
cal·ci·phile
cal·ci·phil·ia
cal·ci·phy·lac·tic
cal·ci·phy·lax·is
   systemic c.
   topical s.
cal·ci·priv·ia
cal·ci·priv·ic
cal·ci·py·eli·tis
cal·cite

cal·ci·to·nin
cal·ci·tri·ol
cal·ci·um
   c. acetylsalicylate carbamide
   c. alginate
   c. aminosalicylate
   c. benzamidosalicylate
   c. benzoylpas
   c. carbaspirin
   c. carbimide
   c. carbonate
   c. caseinate
   c. chloride
   c. cyanamide
   c. cyclamate
   c. disodium edathamil
   c. disodium edetate
   c. disodium ethylenediaminetetra-acetate
   c. Disodium Versenate
   c. EDTA
   c. fluoride
   c. glubionate
   c. gluceptate
   c. gluconate
   c. hydroxide
   c. lactate
   c. levulinate
   c. novobiocin
   c. oxalate
   c. oxide
   c. pantothenate
   c. phosphate
   c. polycarbophil
   c. propionate
   c. pyrophosphate
   radioactive c.
   c. stearate
   c. sulfate
   c. superphosphate
   c. trisodium pentetate
cal·ci·um·ed·e·tate so·di·um
cal·ci·um-mag·ne·si·um aden·o·sine tri·phos·phate
cal·ci·uria
calc·odyn·ia

cal·co·glob·u·lin
cal·co·spher·ite
cal·cu·lary
cal·cu·li
cal·cu·lif·ra·gous
cal·cu·lo·gen·e·sis
cal·cu·lo·sis
cal·cu·lous
cal·cu·lus *pl.* cal·cu·li
  alternating c.
  alvine c.
  articular c.
  biliary calculi
  blood c.
  branched c.
  bronchial c.
  calcareous renal c.
  calcium oxalate c.
  cardiac c.
  cholesterol c.
  combination c.
  cystic c.
  cystine c.
  decubitus c.
  dental c.
  encysted c.
  fibrin c.
  fusible c.
  gastric c.
  gonecystic c.
  hemic c.
  hemp seed c.
  hepatic c.
  indigo c.
  intestinal c.
  joint c.
  lacrimal c.
  lacteal c.
  lung c.
  mammary c.
  matrix c.
  metabolic c.
  mulberry c.
  nasal c.
  nephritic c.
  noncalcareous renal c.
  oxalate c.
  pancreatic c.

cal·cu·lus *(continued)*
  phosphate c.
  pocketed c.
  preputial c.
  prostatic c.
  renal c.
  salivary c.
  serumal c.
  shellac c.
  spermatic c.
  staghorn c.
  stomachic c.
  struvite c.
  subgingival c.
  submorphous c.
  supragingival c.
  tonsillar c.
  urate c.
  ureteral c.
  urethral c.
  uric acid c.
  urinary c.
  urostealith c.
  uterine c.
  vesical c.
  vesicoprostatic c.
  xanthic c.
Cal·da·ni's ligament
Cald·well's protection
Cald·well-Luc operation
Cald·well-Mo·loy classification
Calef. — L. calefac (make
  warm)
    L. calefactus (warmed)
cal·e·fa·cient
calf
cal·i·ber
cal·i·brate
cal·i·bra·tion
    Békésy c.
    pure tone c.
cal·i·bra·tor
    dose c.
cal·i·ce·al
cal·i·cec·ta·sis
cal·i·cec·to·my
ca·li·ces
cal·i·cine

cal·i·ci·vi·rus
ca·lic·u·lus *pl.* ca·lic·u·li
    c. gustatorius
    c. ophthalmicus
ca·li·ec·ta·sis
ca·li·ec·to·my
cal·i·for·ni·um
cal·i·pers
    Jameson c.
    Lange skin-fold c.
    Machemer c.
    Oscher c.
    skinfold c.
    Stahl c.
    ultrasonic c.
    Vernier c.
    walking c.
cal·is·then·ics
ca·lix *pl.* ca·li·ces
    renal calices
    calices renales
    calices renales majores
    calices renales minores
CALLA — common acute
  lymphoblastic leukemia
  antigen
Cal·la·han's method
Cal·lan·der's amputation
Cal·la·way's test
Cal·le·ja's islands
Cal·le·ja's islets
Call-Ex·ner body
Cal·liph·o·ra
    C. vomitoria
Cal·li·phor·i·dae
Cal·li·son's fluid
cal·lo·sal
cal·los·i·tas
cal·los·i·ty
cal·lo·so·mar·gin·al
cal·lo·sum
cal·lous
cal·lus
    bony c.
    central c.
    definitive c.
    ensheathing c.
    external c.

cal·lus *(continued)*
    inner c.
    intermediate c.
    internal c.
    medullary c.
    myelogenous c.
    permanent c.
    provisional c.
    temporary c.
cal·ma·tive
Cal·mette's conjunctival
  reaction
Cal·mette's opthalmic reaction
Cal·mette's test
Cal·mette's vaccine
Cal·mette-Gué·rin bacillus
cal·mod·u·lin
Ca·lo·ba·ta
cal·o·mel
    vegetable c.
ca·lor
    c. febrilis
    c. fervens
    c. innatus
    c. internus
    c. mordax
    c. mordicans
cal·o·ra·di·ance
cal·o·res·cence
Ca·lo·ri's bursa
ca·lo·ric
cal·o·ric·i·ty
Cal·o·rie
cal·o·rie
    15°C c.
    gram c.
    International Table (IT) c.
    large c.
    mean c.
    small c.
    standard c.
    thermochemical c.
ca·lor·i·fa·cient
cal·o·rif·ic
ca·lor·i·gen·ic
cal·o·rim·e·ter
    Atwater-Benedict c.
    bomb c.

cal·o·rim·e·ter *(continued)*
   compensating c.
   respiration c.
ca·lor·i·met·ric
cal·o·rim·e·try
   direct c.
   indirect c.
   partitional c.
cal·o·ri·punc·ture
ca·lor·i·scope
ca·lor·i·trop·ic
Ca·lot's triangle
ca·lotte
cal·pain
cal·pas·ta·tin
cal·se·ques·trin
cal·u·ster·one
cal·var·ia
cal·var·i·al
cal·va·sin
Cal·va·tia gi·gan·tea
Cal·vé's disease
Cal·vé-Per·thes disease
Cal·vin cycle
cal·vi·ti·es
calx
Ca·lym·ma·to·bac·te·ri·um
   C. granulomatis
Cam·ba·roi·des
cam·ben·da·zole
cam·bi·um
cam·era *pl.* cam·eras, cam·
   erae
      Anger c.
      c. anterior bulbi
      electron diffraction c.
      gamma c.
      c. lucida
      c. obscura
      c. oculi
      c. oculi anterior
      c. oculi posterior
      positron c.
      c. posterior bulbi
      powder c.
      c. pulpi
      radionuclide c.
      recording c.

cam·era *(continued)*
   scintillation c.
   c. vitrea bulbi
cam·erae
Cam·er·er's law
Ca·mey ileocystoplasty
cam·i·sole
Cam·mann's stethoscope
CA (cardiac-apnea) monitor
Cam·o·quin
cAMP — cyclic adenosine
   monophosphate
cam·pan·u·la
Camp·bell's ligament
Cam·per's angle
Cam·per's fascia
Cam·per's ligament
cam·pes·ter·ol
cam·phene
cam·phor
cam·pho·ra·ceous
cam·pho·rat·ed
cam·phor·ism
cam·pim·e·ter
cam·pim·e·try
cam·po·spasm
cam·pot·o·my
3′,5′-cAMP syn·the·tase
camp·to·cor·mia
camp·to·cor·my
camp·to·dac·tyl·ia
camp·to·dac·tyl·ism
camp·to·dac·ty·ly
camp·to·me·lia
camp·to·me·lic
camp·to·spasm
camp·to·the·cin
Cam·py·lo·bac·ter
      C. coli
      C. fetus
      C. pylori
cam·py·lo·bac·te·ri·o·sis
   bovine genital c.
   ovine genital c.
cam·py·log·na·thia
cam·sy·late
Cam·u·ra·ti-En·gel·mann
   disease

Can·a·da-Cronk·hite
  syndrome
ca·nal
    abdominal c.
    accessory palatine c's
    adductor c.
    Alcock's c.
    alimentary c.
    alisphenoid c.
    alveolar c's
    alveolodental c's
    anal c.
    c. of Arantius
    archenteric c.
    archinephric c.
    Arnold's c.
    arterial c.
    atrioventricular c.
    auditory c., external
    auditory c., internal
    auricular c.
    basipharyngeal c.
    Bichat's c.
    biliary c's, interlobular
    biliary c's, intralobular
    birth c.
    blastoporic c.
    c. of Bochdalek
    bony c's of ear
    branching c.
    Braun's c.
    Breschet's c's
    calciferous c's
    caroticotympanic c's
    carotid c.
    carpal c.
    c's of cartilage
    caudal c.
    central c. of modiolus
    central c. of spinal cord
    central c. of Stilling
    central c. of vitreous
    cerebrospinal c.
    cervicoaxillary c.
    cervical c. of uterus
    cervicouterine c.
    chordal c.
    c. of chorda tympani

ca·nal *(continued)*
    ciliary c's
    Civinini's c.
    Cloquet's c.
    cochlear c.
    collateral pulp c.
    condylar c.
    condyloid c.
    connecting c.
    corneal c.
    c. of Corti
    c. of Cotunnius
    craniopharyngeal c.
    craniovertebral c.
    crural c.
    crural c. of Henle
    c. of Cuvier
    dental c., inferior
    dental c's, posterior
    dentinal c's
    digestive c.
    diploic c's
    Dorello's c.
    entodermal c.
    c. of epididymis
    ethmoid c., anterior
    ethmoid c., posterior
    eustachian c.
    eustachian c., osseous
    external acoustic c.
    facial c.
    c. for facial nerve
    fallopian c.
    femoral c.
    Ferrein's c.
    flexor c.
    ganglionic c.
    Gartner's c.
    gastric c.
    genital c.
    gubernacular c's
    c. of Guidi
    Guyon's c.
    gynecophoral c.
    gynecophorous c.
    hair c.
    Hannover's c.
    haversian c.

ca·nal *(continued)*
 hemal c.
 Henle's c's
 Hensen's c.
 c's of Hering
 hernial c.
 Hirschfeld's c's
 His c.
 Holmgren-Golgi c's
 c. of Hovius
 Huguier's c.
 Hunter's c.
 Huschke's c.
 hyaloid c.
 hypoglossal c.
 hypophyseal c.
 iliac c.
 incisive c.
 infraorbital c.
 inguinal c.
 intercellular c's
 interdental c's
 interfacial c's.
 interlobular biliary c.
 internal acoustic c.
 intersacral c's
 intestinal c.
 intracytoplasmic c's
 intralobular biliary c.
 Jacobson's c.
 c. for Jacobson's nerve
 Kovalevsky's c.
 lacrimal c.
 Laurer's c.
 Lauth's c.
 Leeuwenhoek's c.
 longitudinal c's of modiolus
 Löwenberg's c.
 lumbrical c's of Kanavel
 mandibular c.
 maxillary c., superior
 medullary c.
 mental c.
 Müller's c.
 musculotubal c.
 nasal c.
 nasolacrimal c.
 nasopalatine c.

ca·nal *(continued)*
 neural c.
 neurenteric c. (of
  Kovalevsky)
 notochordal c.
 c. of Nuck
 nutrient c. of bone
 obstetric c.
 obturator c.
 c. of Oken
 olfactory c.
 omphalomesenteric c.
 optic c.
 orbital c's
 osseous cochlear c.
 osseous eustachian c.
 palatine c's, accessory
 palatine c., anterior
 palatine c's, lesser
 palatine c's, posterior
 palatomaxillary c.
 palatovaginal c.
 paraurethral c's of male
  urethra
 parturient c.
 pelvic c.
 peritoneovaginal c.
 perivascular c.
 persistent common
  atrioventricular c.
 Petit's c.
 pharyngeal c.
 pharyngotracheal c.
 plasmatic c.
 pleural c's
 pleuropericardial c.
 pleuroperitoneal c.
 portal c.
 pterygoid c.
 pterygopalatine c.
 pudendal c.
 pulmoaortic c.
 pulp c.
 pyloric c.
 c's of Recklinghausen
 recurrent c.
 Reichert's c.
 c's of Rivinus

ca·nal *(continued)*
  root c.
  root c., accessory
  sacculocochlear c.
  sacculoutricular c.
  sacral c.
  Santorini's c.
  Scarpa's c.
  Schlemm's c.
  scleral c.,
    scleroticochoroidal c.
  semicircular c's
  seminal c.
  serous c.
  sheathing c.
  Sondermann's c's
  spermatic c.
  sphenopalatine c.
  sphenopharyngeal c.
  spinal c.
  spiral c.
  spiroid c.
  Steno's c.
  Stensen's c.
  c. of Stilling
  c. of stomach
  subsartorial c.
  Sucquet-Hoyer c.
  supraciliary c.
  supraoptic c.
  supraorbital c.
  tarsal c.
  Theile's c.
  thymopharyngeal c.
  Tourtual's c.
  tubal c.
  tubotympanic c.
  tympanic c. of cochlea
  umbilical c.
  urogenital c's
  uterine c.
  uterocervical c.
  uterovaginal c.
  utriculosaccular c.
  vaginal c.
  vaginoperitoneal c.
  Van Hoorne's c.
  Velpeau's c.

ca·nal *(continued)*
  ventricular c.
  Verneuil's c's
  vertebral c.
  vesicourethral c.
  vestibular c.
  vidian c.
  Volkmann's c's
  vomerine c.
  vomerobasilar c., lateral
    inferior
  vomerobasilar c., lateral
    superior
  vomerorostral c.
  vomerovaginal c.
  vulvar c.
  vulvouterine c.
  c's of Walther
  c's of Wearn
  c. of Wirsung
  zygomaticofacial c.
  zygomatico-orbital c.
  zygomaticotemporal c.
ca·na·les
can·a·lic·u·lar
can·a·lic·u·li
can·a·lic·u·li·tis
can·a·lic·u·li·za·tion
can·a·lic·u·lo·rhi·nos·to·my
can·a·lic·u·lus *pl.* can·a·lic·
  u·li
  apical c.
  auricular c.
  bile canaliculi
  biliary canaliculi
  bone canaliculi
  caroticotympanic
    canaliculi
  canaliculi
    caroticotympanici
  c. of chorda tympani
  c. chordae tympani
  c. of cochlea
  c. cochleae
  dental canaliculi
  canaliculi dentales
  haversian c.
  incisor c.

can·a·lic·u·lus *(continued)*
   innominate c.
   c. innominatus
   c. innominatus of Arnold
   intercellular c.
   intracellular canaliculi of
     parietal cells
   c. lacrimalis
   c. laqueiformis
   mastoid c.
   mastoid c. for Arnold's
     nerve
   c. mastoideus
   c. of osteocytes
   c. petrosus
   petrous c.
   pseudobile c.
   secretory c.
   Thiersch's c.
   tympanic c.
   tympanic c. for Jacobson's
     nerve
   c. tympanicus
ca·na·lis *pl.* ca·na·les
   c. adductorius
   c. alimentarius
   canales alveolares
   c. analis
   c. basipharyngeus
   c. caroticus
   canales paraurethrales
   c. carpalis
   c. carpi
   c. centralis medullae
     spinalis
   c. centralis osteoni
   c. cervicis uteri
   c. chordae tympani
   c. communis
   c. condylaris
   c. condyloideus
   canales diploici
   c. facialis
   c. facialis [Fallopii]
   c. femoralis
   c. gastricus
   c. hyaloideus
   c. hypoglossalis

ca·na·lis *(continued)*
   c. incisivus
   c. infraorbitalis
   c. inguinalis
   canales longitudinales
     modioli
   c. mandibulae
   c. musculotubarius
   c. nasolacrimalis
   c. nutricius ossis
   c. nutriens ossis
   c. obturatorius
   c. opticus
   canales palatini
   c. palatovaginalis
   c. pharyngeus
   c. portalis
   c. pterygoideus
   c. pterygopalatinus
   c. pudendalis
   c. pyloricus
   c. radicis dentis
   c. reuniens
   c. sacralis
   c. spinalis
   c. spiralis cochleae
   c. spiralis modioli
   c. subsartorialis
   c. ventricularis
   c. ventriculi
   c. vertebralis
   c. vomerorostralis
   c. vomerovaginalis
can·a·li·za·tion
ca·nalo·plas·ty
ca·na·ry·pox
Can·a·val·ia
can·a·val·in
Can·a·van's disease
Can·a·van's sclerosis
Can·a·van's spongy
   degeneration
Can·a·van-van Bo·gaert-Ber·
   trand disease
can·av·a·nase
can·av·a·nine
can·cel·lat·ed
can·cel·li

can·cel·lous
can·cel·lus *pl.* can·cel·li
can·cer
  acinar c.
  acinous c.
  adenoid c.
  c. à deux
  alveolar c.
  aniline c.
  apinoid c.
  arsenic c.
  asbestos c.
  c. atrophicans
  3,4-benzpyrene c.
  betel c.
  black c.
  boring c.
  branchiogenous c.
  Butter's c.
  buyo cheek c.
  cellular c.
  cerebriform c.
  chimney-sweeps' c.
  chondroid c.
  chromate c.
  chutta c.
  claypipe c.
  colloid c.
  contact c.
  corset c.
  cystic c.
  dendritic c.
  duct c.
  dye workers' c.
  encephaloid c.
  c. en cuirasse
  endothelial c.
  epidermal c.
  epithelial c.
  glandular c.
  green c.
  hard c.
  c. in situ
  jacket c.
  kang c.
  kangri c.
  latent c.
  medullary c.

can·cer *(continued)*
  melanotic c.
  metastatic c.
  mineral oil c.
  mule-spinners' c.
  multicentric c.
  nickel c.
  occult c.
  osteoblastic c.
  osteolytic c.
  paraffin c.
  pitch-workers' c.
  radiologists' c.
  radium c.
  retrograde c.
  rodent c.
  roentgenologist's c.
  Schneeberg's c.
  scirrhous c.
  shale oil c.
  shale-workers' c.
  smokers' c.
  soft c.
  soot c.
  spindle cell c.
  swamp c.
  tar c.
  tubular c.
  ulcer c.
  ulcerated c.
  villous duct c.
  vinyl chloride c.
  x-ray c.
can·cer·emia
can·cer·i·ci·dal
can·cer·i·gen·ic
can·cer·iza·tion
can·cer·ol·o·gist
can·cer·ol·o·gy
can·cer·o·sis
can·cer·ous
can·cer·pho·bia
can·cer-ul·cer
can·cri·form
can·croid
can·crum
  c. nasi
  c. oris

can·crum *(continued)*
    c. pudendi
can·dela
    c. steradian
Can·dep·tin
can·di·ci·din
Can·di·da
    C. albicans
    C. mesenterica
    C. parapsilosis
    C. tropicalis
    C. vini
can·di·dal
can·di·de·mia
can·di·di·a·sis
    acute pseudomembranous
      c.
    atrophic c.
    chronic mucocutaneous c.
    cutaneous c.
    endocardial c.
    oral c.
can·di·did
can·di·din
can·di·do·sis
can·did·u·lin
can·did·uria
can·dle
    Chamberland's c.
    foot c.
    meter c.
    vaginal c.
can·dle-gut·ter·ing
can·dol
cane
    adjustable c.
    broad-based c.
    English c.
    glider c.
    quadripod c.
    tripod c.
ca·nes·cent
ca·nine
ca·ni·ni·form
ca·ni·nus
ca·ni·ti·es
can·ker

can·na
    c. major
    c. minor
can·na·bi·di·ol
can·nab·i·noid
can·nab·i·nol
can·na·bis
can·na·bism
Can·niz·za·ro's reaction
Can·non's point
Can·non's ring
Can·non-Bard theory
can·nu·la
    Bellocq's c.
    Concorde suction c.
    Flexicath c.
    infusion c.
    irrigation c.
    Kanavel brain-exploring c.
    Karman c.
    Lifemed c.
    Mercedes tip c.
    Packo pars plana c.
    Padgett shark-mouth c.
    perfusion c.
    Polystan c.
    Portnoy c.
    Scheie c.
    Tulevech c.
    USCI c.
    Veirs c.
    ventricular c.
    Verres c.
    washout c.
can·nu·late
can·nu·la·tion
can·nu·li·za·tion
can·ren·o·ate po·tas·si·um
can·ren·one
cant
    c. of mandible
can·thal
can·tha·ri·a·sis
can·tha·ric acid
can·thar·i·dal
can·thar·i·date

can·thar·i·des
can·tha·rid·ic acid
can·thar·i·din
can·thar·i·dism
can·thec·to·my
can·thi
can·thi·tis
Can·tho·bac·ter
can·thol·y·sis
can·tho·plas·ty
can·thor·rha·phy
can·thot·o·my
can·thus *pl.* can·thi
    c. inversus
Can·til
Can·tor tube
can·tus gal·li
can·u·la
CAP — catabolite activator
  protein
Cap. — L. capiat (let him take)
cap. — L. capsula (capsule)
cap
    acrosomal c.
    bishop's c.
    5' c.
    chin c.
    cradle c.
    Dumas c.
    duodenal c.
    dutch c.
    enamel c.
    fibrin c.
    fibrinoid c.
    germinal c.
    head c.
    head c., anterior
    knee c.
    metanephric c's
    phrygian c.
    polar c.
    postnuclear c.
    pulp c.
    pyloric c.
    root c.
    skull c.
    c. of Zinn

ca·pac·i·tance
    membrane c.
ca·pac·i·ta·tion
ca·pac·i·tor
ca·pac·i·ty
    antigen-binding c.
    carbon monoxide diffusing
      c.
    cranial c.
    diffusing c.
    diffusion c.
    forced vital c. (FVC)
    functional residual c.
    heat c.
    inspiratory c.
    maximal breathing c.
    maximal tubular excretory
      c.
    maximal tubular
      reabsorptive c.
    maximal tubular secretory
      c.
    maximum lung c.
    mental c.
    molar heat c.
    respiratory c.
    specific heat c.
    testamentary c.
    thermal c.
    timed vital c.
    total iron-binding c. (TIBC)
    total lung c.
    virus neutralizing c.
    vital c.
Cap·a·stat
CAPD — continuous
  ambulatory peritoneal
  dialysis
cap·e·let
cap·e·line
Cap·gras syndrome
cap·il·lar·ec·ta·sia
Cap·il·lar·ia
    C. contorta
    C. hepatica
    C. philippinensis
cap·il·la·ri·a·sis
    intestinal c.

cap·il·lar·io·mo·tor
cap·il·lar·i·os·co·py
cap·il·lar·itis
cap·il·lar·i·ty
cap·il·la·rop·a·thy
cap·il·la·ros·co·py
cap·il·lary
    arterial c's
    arteriolar c.
    bile c's
    continuous c's
    erythrocytic c's
    fenestrated c's
    glomerular c.
    junctional c.
    lymph c.
    lymphatic c.
    Meigs' c's
    peritubular c.
    secretory c's
    sheathed c's
    sinusoidal c.
    venous c's
cap·il·li
cap·il·li·ti·um
cap·il·lo·mo·tor
cap·il·lo·ve·nous
cap·il·lus *pl.* ca·pil·li
cap·i·stra·tion
cap·i·ta
cap·i·tal
cap·i·tate
cap·i·ta·tion
cap·i·ta·tum
cap·i·tel·lum
cap·i·ton·nage
cap·i·to·ped·al
Cap·i·trol
ca·pit·u·la
ca·pit·u·lar
ca·pit·u·lum *pl.* ca·pit·u·la
    c. costae
    c. fibulae
    c. humeri
    c. mallei
    c. radii
    c. stapedis
    c. ulnae

Cap·la
Cap·lan's nodules
Cap·lan's syndrome
cap·ne·ic
Cap·no·cy·toph·a·ga
cap·no·gram
cap·no·graph
cap·nog·ra·phy
cap·no·hep·a·tog·ra·phy
cap·nom·e·ter
cap·nom·e·try
cap·no·phil·ic
cap·o·ben·ate so·di·um
cap·o·ben·ic acid
ca·pote·ment
cap·ping
    pulp c.
cap·rate
cap·reo·lary
cap·reo·late
cap·reo·my·cin
    c. sulfate, sterile
cap·ric acid
ca·pril·lic
ca·pril·o·quism
Cap·ri·pox·vi·rus
cap·ri·zant
cap·ro·ate
ca·pro·ic acid
ca·pro·in
cap·rone
cap·ro·yl
cap·ro·yl·amine
cap·ry·late
ca·pryl·ic acid
cap·ry·lin
CAPS — carbamoyl phosphate
   synthetase
    caffeine, alcohol, pepper,
    spicy foods
CAPS-free diet
cap·sa·i·cin
Cap·se·bon
cap·si·cin
cap·si·cism
Cap·si·cum
cap·si·cum
cap·sid

cap·si·tis
cap·so·mer
cap·sot·o·my
Capsul. — L. capsula (capsule)
cap·su·la *pl.* cap·su·lae
    c. adiposa
    c. adiposa renis
    c. articularis
    c. bulbi
    c. cordis
    c. externa
    c. extrema
    c. fibrosa
    c. ganglii
    c. glandulae thyroideae
    c. glomeruli
    c. interna
    c. lentis
    c. nuclei dentati
    capsulae nuclei lentiformis
    c. pancreatis
    c. prostatica
    capsulae renis
    c. serosa lienis
    c. tonsillaris
cap·su·lae
cap·su·lar
cap·su·la·tion
cap·sule
    acoustic c.
    adherent c.
    adipose c.
    adrenal c.
    adrenal c's, accessory
    anthrax c.
    articular c.
    articular c., fibrous
    articular c. of shoulder
      joint
    atrabiliary c.
    auditory c.
    bacterial c.
    biopsy c.
    Bonnet's c.
    Bowman's c.
    brood c's
    cartilage c.

cap·sule *(continued)*
    cartilaginous ear c.
    central c.
    cricoarytenoid articular c.
    cricothyroid articular c.
    Crosby c.
    Crosby-Kugler c.
    crystalline c.
    decavitamin c.
    dental c.
    enteric c.
    external c.
    extreme c.
    fibrous c.
    formalized c.
    Gerota's c.
    Glisson's c.
    glomerular c.
    glutoid c.
    hepatobiliary c.
    internal c.
    joint c.
    malpighian c.
    Müller's c.
    müllerian c.
    nasal c.
    ocular c.
    olfactory c.
    optic c.
    otic c.
    pelvioprostatic c.
    perinephric c.
    periotic c.
    perivascular fibrous c.
    polar c.
    radiotelemetering c.
    renal c.
    serous c. of spleen
    sodium iodide [131]I c's
    suprarenal c.
    sympathoblastic c.
    synovial c.
    telemetering c.
    Tenon's c.
    c. of thymus
    tonsillar c.
    triasyn B c's
cap·su·lec·to·my

cap·su·li·tis
    adhesive c.
    hepatic c.
cap·su·lo·len·tic·u·lar
cap·su·lo·ma
cap·su·lo·plas·ty
cap·su·lor·rha·phy
cap·su·lo·tome
cap·su·lot·o·my
    renal c.
cap·ta·mine hy·dro·chlo·ride
cap·to·di·ame hy·dro·chlo·ride
cap·to·di·amine hy·dro·chlo·ride
cap·to·pril
cap·ture
    electron c.
    ventricular c.
cap·u·let
cap·ur·ide
cap·ut *pl.* cap·i·ta
    c. coli
    c. costae
    c. deformatum
    c. distortum
    c. epididymidis
    c. femoris
    c. fibulae
    c. galeatum
    c. gallinaginis
    c. humeri
    c. lienis
    c. mallei
    c. mandibulae
    c. medusae
    c. metacarpalis
    c. metatarsalis
    c. musculi
    c. natiforme
    c. nuclei caudati
    c. ossis femoris
    c. ossis metacarpalis
    c. ossis metatarsalis
    c. pancreatis
    c. penis
    c. planum
    c. progeneum

cap·ut *(continued)*
    c. quadratum
    c. radii
    c. stapedis
    c. succedaneum
    c. tali
    c. ulnae
CAR — Canadian Association
  of Radiologists
Ca·ra·bel·li cusp
Ca·ra·bel·li sign
Ca·ra·bel·li tubercle
car·a·mel
ca·ram·i·phen
    c. edisylate
    c. ethanedisulfonate
    c. hydrochloride
car·a·way
car·ba·chol
car·ba·dox
car·ba·mate
car·ba·maz·e·pine
car·bam·ic acid
car·bam·ide
carb·ami·no
car·bam·i·no·he·mo·glo·bin
car·bam·o·yl
car·ba·moyl·as·par·tic acid
car·bam·o·yl·a·tion
car·bam·o·yl-phos·phate syn·thase (ammonia)
car·bam·o·yl phos·phate syn·the·tase (CAPS) deficiency
car·bam·o·yl-phos·phate syn·the·tase (glutamine-hydrolyzing)
car·bam·o·yl·trans·fer·ase
car·ba·myl
car·ba·myl·cho·line chlo·ride
car·ban·tel laur·yl sul·fate
car·ba·ril
car·bar·sone
car·ba·ryl
car·ba·sal·ate cal·ci·um
car·ba·zide
car·baz·o·chrome sal·i·cyl·ate
car·ba·zo·cine
car·baz·o·tate

car·ben·i·cil·lin
  c. disodium
  c. indanyl sodium
  c. phenyl sodium
  c. potassium
  c. sodium
car·ben·ox·o·lone so·di·um
car·be·ta·pen·tane cit·rate
car·beth·yl sal·i·cyl·ate
carb·he·mo·glo·bin
car·bide
  metallic c.
car·bi·do·pa
car·bi·ma·zole
car·bi·nol
  acetylmethyl c.
  dimethyl c.
car·bin·ox·amine mal·e·ate
car·bo·ben·zoxy
Car·bo·caine
car·bo·ca·tion
car·bo·cho·line
car·bo·clo·ral
car·bo·cro·men hy·dro·chlo·ride
car·bo·cy·clic
car·bo·cys·te·ine
car·bo·di·im·ide
car·bo·gas·e·ous
car·bo·gen
car·bo·he·mia
car·bo·he·mo·glo·bin
car·bo·hy·drase
car·bo·hy·drate
  C c.
  reserve c's
car·bo·hy·dra·tu·ria
car·bo·hy·dro·gen·ic
car·bo·late
car·bol·fuch·sin
  Ziehl-Neelsen c.
car·bol·ic acid
car·bol·ism
car·bol·ize
car·bol·uria
car·bol·xy·lene
car·bo·mer
  car·bo·mer 934 P

car·bo·my·cin
car·bon
  ^{13}C
  ^{14}C
  c. dioxide
  c. disulfide
  c. monoxide
  c. oxysulfide
  c. tetrachloride
car·bo·na·ceous
car·bon·ate
car·bon·ate-ap·a·tite
car·bon·ate de·hy·dra·tase
car·bon·emia
car·bon·ic acid
car·bon·ic an·hy·drase
car·bon·ize
car·bon·uria
  dysoxidative c.
car·bon·yl
car·bo·prost
  c. methyl
  c. tromethamine
Car·bo·run·dum
Car·bo·wax
car·boxy·bi·o·tin
car·boxy·dis·mu·tase
γ-car·boxy·glu·ta·mate [gam·ma-]
γ-car·boxy·glu·tam·ic acid [gam·ma-]
car·boxy·he·mo·glo·bin
car·box·y·he·mo·glo·bin·e·mia
car·box·yl
car·box·yl (acid) pro·tein·ase
car·box·y·lase
  amino acid c.
  multiple c. deficiency (MCD)
car·box·y·late
car·box·y·la·tion
  reductive c.
car·box·yl·es·ter·ase
car·box·yl·ic acid
car·box·yl·ic es·ter hy·dro·lase
car·box·yl-ter·mi·nal

car·box·yl·trans·fer·ase
car·box·y-ly·ase
car·boxy·meth·yl
car·boxy·meth·yl·cel·lu·lose
　so·di·um
car·boxy·myo·glo·bin
car·boxy·pep·ti·dase
car·boxy·pep·ti·dase A
car·boxy·pep·ti·dase B
car·boxy·poly·pep·ti·dase
car·bro·mal
car·bun·cle
　malignant c.
　renal c.
car·bun·cu·lar
car·bun·cu·loid
car·bun·cu·lo·sis
car·bu·ta·mide
car·bu·ter·ol hy·dro·chlo·ride
Car·cas·sonne's ligament
Car·cas·sonne's perineal
　ligament
car·ci·nec·to·my
car·cin·emia
car·cin·o·gen
　direct-reacting c.
car·ci·no·gen·e·sis
car·cin·o·gen·ic
car·ci·no·ge·nic·i·ty
car·ci·noid
　bronchial c.
　enterochromaffin c.
　G-cell c.
car·ci·nol·y·sin
car·ci·nol·y·sis
car·ci·no·lyt·ic
car·ci·no·ma *pl.* car·ci·no·
　mas, car·ci·no·ma·ta
　acinar c.
　acinous c.
　adenocystic c.
　adenoid cystic c.
　c. adenomatosum
　adenosquamous c.
　c. of adrenal cortex
　alveolar c.
　alveolar cell c.
　anaplastic c.

car·ci·no·ma *(continued)*
　apocrine c.
　argentaffin c.
　c. asbolicum
　basal cell c.
　basaloid c.
　c. basocellulare
　basosquamous cell c.
　betel-nut c.
　brachiogenic c.
　bronchioalveolar c.
　bronchiolar c.
　bronchogenic c.
　cerebriform c.
　cholangiocellular c.
　chorionic c.
　clear cell c.
　cloacogenic c.
　colloid c.
　comedo c.
　corpus c.
　cribriform c.
　c. en cuirasse
　c. cuniculatum
　c. cutaneum
　cylindrical c.
　cylindrical cell c.
　desmoplastic c.
　duct c.
　ductal papillary c.
　embryonal c.
　endometrioid c.
　epibulbar c.
　epidermoid c.
　c. epitheliale adenoides
　erysipeloid c.
　exophytic c.
　fibrosing basal cell c.
　c. fibrosum
　follicular c.
　fungating c.
　gelatiniform c.
　gelatinous c.
　giant cell c.
　c. gigantocellulare
　glandular c.
　glottic c.
　granular cell c.

car·ci·no·ma *(continued)*
  granulosa cell c.
  hair-matrix c.
  hepatocellular c.
  Hürthle cell c.
  hypernephroid c.
  infantile embryonal c.
  inflammatory c.
  c. in situ
  intermediary c.
  intermediate-cell c.
  intraepidermal c.
  intraepithelial c.
  intrahepatic bile duct c.
  Krompecher's c.
  Kulchitzky-cell c.
  large-cell c.
  c. lenticulare
  lenticular c.
  lobular c.
  lymphoepithelial c.
  c. mastitoides
  c. medullare
  medullary c.
  melanotic c.
  Merkel cell c.
  metatypical c.
  c. molle
  morphea-type basal cell c.
  mucinous c.
  c. muciparum
  c. mucocellulare
  mucoepidermoid c.
  mucoid c.
  c. mucosum
  mucous c.
  c. myxomatodes
  nasopharyngeal c.
  nonencapsulated sclerosing
    c.
  oat cell c.
  occult c.
  oncocytic c.
  c. ossificans
  osteoid c.
  oxyphilic c.
  papillary c.
  parafollicular thyroid c.

car·ci·no·ma *(continued)*
  periportal c.
  polypoid c.
  postcricoid c.
  preinvasive c.
  prickle cell c.
  pseudomucinous c.
  pyriform fossa c.
  renal cell c. of kidney
  reserve cell c.
  schneiderian c.
  scirrhous c.
  c. scroti
  sebaceous c.
  seminal c.
  signet-ring cell c.
  c. simplex
  small-cell c.
  spheroidal cell c.
  spindle cell c.
  spinous cell c.
  c. spongiosum
  squamous c.
  squamous cell c.
  string c.
  c. telangiectaticum
  c. telangiectodes
  teratoid c.
  trabecular c.
  transitional cell c.
  c. tuberosum
  tuberous c.
  undifferentiated c.
  V2 c.
  verrucous c.
  c. villosum
  VX2 c.
car·ci·no·ma·ta
car·ci·nom·a·toid
car·ci·no·ma·toi·des al·veo·
  gen·i·ca mul·ti·cen·tri·ca
car·ci·no·ma·to·pho·bia
car·ci·no·ma·to·sis
  c. of meninges
  c. pleurae
car·ci·nom·a·tous
car·ci·no·phil·ia
car·ci·no·phil·ic

car·ci·no·pho·bia
car·ci·no·sar·co·ma
    embryonal c.
    Flexner-Jobling c.
    Walker c. 256
car·ci·no·sec·to·my
car·ci·no·sis
    miliary c.
    c. pleurae
    pulmonary c.
car·ci·no·stat·ic
car·ci·nous
car·da·mom
Car·da·rel·li's sign
Car·da·rel·li's symptom
car·del·my·cin
Car·den's amputation
car·de·no·lide
car·dia
    c. of stomach
car·di·ac
car·dial
car·di·al·gia
car·di·ant
car·di·asth·ma
car·di·ec·ta·sis
car·di·ec·to·mized
car·di·ec·to·my
Car·di·late
car·di·nal
car·dio·ac·cel·er·a·tor
car·dio·ac·tive
car·dio·an·gi·og·ra·phy
car·dio·an·gi·ol·o·gy
car·dio·aor·tic
car·dio·ar·te·ri·al
Car·di·o·bac·te·ri·um
    C. hominis
car·dio·cai·ro·graph
car·dio·cele
car·dio·cen·te·sis
car·dio·cha·la·sia
car·dio·cir·cu·la·tory
car·dio·cir·rho·sis
car·dio·di·a·phrag·mat·ic
car·dio·di·la·tin
car·dio·di·la·tor
car·dio·na·trin

car·dio·di·o·sis
car·dio·dy·nam·ics
car·di·odyn·ia
car·dio·esoph·a·ge·al
car·dio·gen·e·sis
car·dio·ge·net·ic
car·di·o·gen·ic
Car·dio·gra·fin
car·dio·gram
    apex c.
    esophageal c.
    negative c.
    precordial c.
    vector c.
car·dio·graph
car·dio·graph·ic
car·di·og·ra·phy
    apex c.
    radionuclide c.
    ultrasonic c.
    vector c.
Car·dio-Green
car·dio·he·pat·ic
car·dio·hep·a·to·meg·a·ly
car·di·oid
car·dio·in·hib·i·tor
car·dio·in·hib·i·to·ry
car·dio·ki·net·ic
car·dio·ky·mo·graph·ic
car·dio·ky·mog·ra·phy
car·dio·lip·in
car·dio·lith
car·di·ol·o·gist
car·di·ol·o·gy
car·di·ol·y·sis
car·dio·ma·la·cia
car·dio·meg·a·ly
    glycogenic c.
    idiopathic c.
car·dio·mel·a·no·sis
car·di·om·e·ter
car·di·om·e·try
car·dio·mo·til·i·ty
car·dio·myo·li·po·sis
car·dio·my·op·a·thy
    alcoholic c.
    Becker's c.
    beer-drinker's c.

car·dio·my·op·a·thy
  (continued)
    congestive c.
    familial c.
    fatty c.
    hypertrophic c.
    infiltrative c.
    nephropathic c.
    nonobstructive
      hypertrophic c.
    obstructive hypertrophic c.
    peripartum c.
    postpartum c.
    restrictive c.
    thyrotoxic c.
    toxic c.
car·dio·myo·pexy
car·dio·my·ot·o·my
car·dio·ne·cro·sis
car·dio·nec·tor
car·dio·neph·ric
car·dio·neu·ral
car·dio-omen·to·pexy
car·dio·pal·u·dism
car·dio·path
car·dio·path·ic
car·di·op·a·thy
    infarctoid c.
car·dio·peri·car·dio·pexy
car·dio·peri·car·di·tis
car·dio·pho·bia
car·dio·phre·nia
car·dio·plas·ty
car·dio·ple·gia
car·dio·ple·gic
car·dio·pneu·mat·ic
car·dio·pneu·mo·graph
car·dio·pneu·mono·pexy
car·di·op·to·sis
car·dio·pul·mo·nary
car·dio·pul·mon·ic
car·dio·punc·ture
car·dio·py·lo·ric
Car·dio·quin
car·dio·re·nal
car·di·or·rha·phy
car·di·or·rhex·is
car·dio·scle·ro·sis

car·dio·scope
car·dio·se·lec·tive
car·dio·spasm
car·dio·sphyg·mo·gram
car·dio·sphyg·mo·graph
car·dio·spleno·pexy
car·dio·ta·chom·e·ter
car·dio·ta·chom·e·try
car·dio·ther·a·py
car·dio·thy·ro·tox·i·co·sis
car·dio·to·co·graph
car·dio·to·cog·ra·phy
car·di·ot·o·my
car·dio·ton·ic
car·dio·to·pog·ra·phy
car·dio·to·pom·e·try
car·dio·tox·ic
car·dio·val·vu·lar
car·dio·val·vu·li·tis
car·dio·val·vu·lo·tome
car·di·o·val·vu·lot·o·my
car·dio·vas·cu·lar
car·dio·vas·cu·lar-re·nal
car·dio·vas·ol·o·gy
car·dio·vec·tor·gra·phy
car·dio·ver·sion
car·dio·vert
car·dio·ver·ter
car·dio·vi·rus
car·di·tis
    rheumatic c.
    streptococcal c.
    verrucous c.
care
    acute c.
    ambulatory c.
    continuity of c.
    custodial c.
    extended c.
    follow-up c.
    home health c.
    primary c.
    respiratory c.
    secondary c.
    skilled nursing c.
    tertiary c.
Carey Coombs murmur
car·fe·cil·lin so·di·um

car·fen·ta·nil cit·rate
car·i·cous
car·ies
    arrested c.
    backward c.
    cemental c.
    central c.
    dental c.
    dentinal c.
    dry c.
    enamel c.
    c. fungosa
    internal c.
    lateral c.
    necrotic c.
    pit c.
    rampant c.
    senile dental c.
    c. sicca
    spinal c.
    c. tuberculosa
ca·ri·na *pl.* ca·ri·nae
    c. fornicis
    c. of trachea
    c. tracheae
    urethral c. of vagina
    c. urethralis vaginae
ca·ri·nae
car·i·nate
car·i·na·tion
car·in·da·cil·lin so·di·um
car·io·gen·e·sis
car·i·o·gen·ic
car·io·ge·nic·i·ty
car·i·ol·o·gy
car·i·os·i·ty
car·io·stat·ic
ca·ri·ous
car·iso·pro·dol
Car·lens tube
Carle·ton's spots
car·mal·um
Carman's sign
car·man·ta·dine
car·min·a·tive
car·mine
    alizarin c.
    indigo c.

car·mine *(continued)*
    lithium c.
    Schneider's c.
car·min·ic acid
car·min·o·phil
car·mus·tine
car·ne·ous
car·nid·a·zole
car·ni·fi·ca·tion
car·ni·tine
car·ni·tine pal·mi·to·yl trans·
    fer·ase
Car·noch·an's operation
car·no·sin·ase
car·no·sine
car·no·si·ne·mia
car·no·sin·uria
car·nos·i·ty
Car·not's test
car·nu·tine
Ca·ro·li's disease
car·o·tene
    beta c.
β-car·o·tene 15,15-di·oxy·gen·
    ase
car·o·ten·emia
car·ot·eno·der·ma
car·ot·eno·der·mia
ca·rot·e·noid
car·o·te·no·sis
ca·rot·ic
ca·rot·i·co·cli·noid
ca·rot·i·co·tym·pan·ic
ca·rot·id
car·o·tin·emia
ca·rot·i·no·der·ma
car·o·ti·no·sis
ca·rot·odyn·ia
ca·rox·a·zone
car·pal
car·pa·le
car·pec·to·my
car·pel
Car·pen·ter syndrome
Car·pen·tier-Ed·wards valve
car·phen·a·zine mal·e·ate
car·phol·o·gy
car·pi·tis

car·po·car·pal
Car·po·gly·phus
   C. passularum
car·po·go·ni·um
car·po·meta·car·pal
car·po·pe·dal
car·po·pha·lan·ge·al
car·pop·to·sis
car·pro·fen
Car·pue's operation
Car·pue's rhinoplasty
Car·pule
car·pus
   c. curvus
Carr-Price test
Carr-Pur·cell-Mei·boom-Gill
  sequence
car·ra·geen
car·ra·gee·nan
Car·rel
Car·rel's method
Car·rel's treatment
Car·rel's tube
Car·rel-Da·kin fluid
Car·rel-Da·kin treatment
Car·rel-Lind·berg pump
car·ri·er
   active c.
   amalgam c.
   chronic c.
   closed c.
   contact c.
   convalescent c.
   electron c.
   enteric c.
   foil c.
   gallbladder c.
   gametocyte c.
   healthy c.
   hemophilia c.
   incubation c.
   intermittent c.
   intestinal c.
   isotopic c.
   lentulo paste c.
   ligature c.
   oxygen c.
   paste c.

car·ri·er *(continued)*
   urinary c.
car·ri·er-free
Car·rión's disease
Car·roll bone-holding forceps
car·rot
Cars·well's grapes
cart
   crash c.
   dressing c.
   resuscitation c.
car·taz·o·late
car·te·o·lol hy·dro·chlo·ride
Car·ter's mycetoma
car·ti·lage
   alar c., greater
   alar c's, lesser
   annular c.
   aortic c.
   arthrodial c.
   articular c.
   arytenoid c.
   c. of auditory tube
   auricular c.
   basal c.
   branchial c.
   calcified c.
   cariniform c.
   cellular c.
   ciliary c's
   circumferential c.
   conchal c.
   condylar c.
   connecting c.
   corniculate c.
   costal c.
   cricoid c.
   cuneiform c.
   dentinal c.
   diarthrodial c.
   ectethmoid c.
   elastic c.
   embryonic c.
   ensiform c.
   epactal c's
   epiglottic c.
   epiphyseal c.
   episternal c.

car·ti·lage *(continued)*
    eustachian c.
    falciform c's
    fetal c.
    floating c.
    gingival c.
    growth c.
    guttural c.
    innominate c.
    interarticular c.
    interarytenoid c.
    intermediary c.
    interosseous c.
    intervertebral c's
    intrathyroid c.
    investing c.
    Jacobson's c.
    laryngeal c's
    laryngeal c. of Luschka
    lateral c's
    lateral c. of nose
    Luschka's c.
    mandibular c.
    meatal c.
    Meckel's c.
    mesethemoid c.
    minor c's
    c. of Morgagni
    nasal c's
    obducent c.
    ossifying c.
    palpebral c's
    parachordal c's
    paranasal c.
    paraseptal c.
    parenchymatous c.
    periotic c.
    permanent c.
    posterior cricoarytenoid c.
    precricoid c.
    precursory c.
    pulmonary c.
    pyramidal c.
    Reichert's c's
    reticular c.
    Santorini's c.
    scutiform c.
    semilunar c.

car·ti·lage *(continued)*
    septal c. of nose
    sesamoid c. of larynx
    sesamoid c's of nose
    sesamoid c. of vocal
      ligament
    sigmoid c's
    slipping rib c.
    sphenobasilar c.
    spheno-occipital c.
    sternal c.
    stratified c.
    subvomerine c's
    supra-arytenoid c.
    suprascapular c.
    synarthrodial c.
    tarsal c's
    temporary c.
    tendon c.
    thyroid c.
    tracheal c's
    triangular c. of nose
    triquetral c.
    triradiate c.
    triticeal c.
    tubal c.
    tympanomandibular c.
    uniting c.
    vomerian c. of Hirschfeld
    vomerian c. of Huschke
    vomerine c.
    vomeronasal c.
    Weitbrecht's c.
    Wrisberg's c.
    xiphoid c.
    Y c.
    yellow c.
car·ti·lag·in
car·ti·lag·i·nes
car·ti·la·gin·i·fi·ca·tion
car·ti·la·gin·i·form
car·ti·lag·i·noid
car·ti·lag·i·nous
car·ti·la·go *pl.* car·ti·lag·i·nes
    c. articularis
    c. arytenoidea
    c. auriculae
    c. corniculata

car·ti·la·go *(continued)*
   c. corniculata [Santorini]
   c. costalis
   c. cricoidea
   c. cuneiformis
   c. cuneiformis [Wrisbergi]
   c. ensiformis
   c. epiglottica
   c. epiphysialis
   cartilagines falcatae
   c. jacobsoni
   cartilagines laryngis
   cartilagines nasales
     accessoriae
   cartilagines nasi
   c. santorini
   c. sesamoidea laryngis
     Luschka
   c. sesamoidea ligamenti
     vocalis
   cartilagines sesamoideae
     nasi
   c. thyroidea
   cartilagines tracheales
   c. triquetra
   c. triticea
   c. vomeronasalis
   c. vomeronasalis
     [Jacobsoni]
   c. wrisbergi
car·ti·la·go·trop·ic
car·un·cle
   amniotic c's
   hymenal c's
   lacrimal c.
   major c. of Santorini
   Morgagni's c.
   morgagnian c.
   myrtiform c's
   salivary c.
   sublingual c.
   urethral c.
ca·run·cu·la *pl.* ca·run·cu·lae
   carunculae hymenales
   c. lacrimalis
   c. sublingualis
ca·run·cu·lae
ca·run·cu·lar

Ca·rus' circle
Ca·rus' curve
Car·val·lo sign
car·ver
car·vone
caryo·phil
car·ze·nide
Ca·sal's necklace
Cas·ami·no acids
ca·san·thra·nol
cas·cade
   electron c.
   extrinsic coagulation c.
   intrinsic coagulation c.
cas·cara
   c. amarga
   c. sagrada
case
   borderline c.
   coroner's c.
   index c.
   primary c.
   secondary c.
   trial c.
ca·se·a·tion
case·book
case-con·trol
case his·to·ry
ca·sein
   c.-calcium
   gluten c.
   c. hydrolysate
   c.-sodium
   vegetable c.
ca·sei·nate
ca·sein·o·gen
ca·sein·og·e·nate
ca·se·og·e·nous
ca·se·ous
ca·se·um
case·worm
Ca·so·ni's intradermal test
Ca·so·ni's reaction
C-as·par·a·gin·ase
Cas·sel·ber·ry's position
Cas·ser's (Casserio's, Casserius)
   fontanelle

Cas·ser's (Casserio's, Casserius)
   ligament
Cas·ser's (Casserio's, Casserius)
   muscle
cas·se·ri·an
cas·sette
Cas·sia
Cas·si·dy syndrome
Cas·si·dy-Schol·te syndrome
cast
   bacterial c.
   blood c.
   broad c.
   coma c.
   decidual c.
   dental c.
   diagnostic c.
   epithelial c.
   false c.
   fatty c.
   fibrinous c.
   gnathostatic c.
   granular c.
   hair c.
   hanging c.
   hemoglobin c.
   Hexcelite c.
   hyaline c.
   investment c.
   Külz's c.
   leukocyte c.
   master c.
   mucous c.
   pigmented c's
   plaster of Paris c.
   preextraction c.
   preoperative c.
   pus c.
   quarter c.
   red cell c.
   refractory c.
   renal c.
   Risser localizer c.
   Sarmiento c.
   spica c.
   spiral c.
   spurious c.
   spurious tube c.

cast *(continued)*
   study c.
   tube c.
   urate c.
   urinary c.
   waxy c.
Cas·ta·ne·da bottle
Cas·ta·ne·da forceps
Cas·tel·la·ni's bronchitis
Cas·tel·la·ni's disease
Cas·tel·la·ni's paint
Cas·tel·la·ni's test
Cas·tel·la·ni-Low symptom
cast·ing
   vacuum c.
Cas·tle's factors
cas·trate
cas·tra·tion
   parasitic c.
   radiologic c.
cas·u·al·ty
cas·u·is·tics
CAT — computerized axial
   tomography
ca·ta·ba·si·al
ca·tab·a·sis
ca·ta·bat·ic
ca·ta·bi·o·sis
ca·ta·bi·ot·ic
ca·ta·bol·ic
ca·tab·o·lism
   antibody c.
ca·tab·o·lite
ca·tab·o·lize
cata·chro·no·bi·ol·o·gy
ca·ta·crot·ic
ca·tac·ro·tism
ca·ta·di·crot·ic
cata·di·cro·tism
cata·di·op·tric
cat·a·gen
cata·gen·e·sis
cata·ge·net·ic
cat·ag·mat·ic
cat·a·lase
cat·a·lep·sy
cat·a·lep·tic
cat·a·lep·ti·form

cat·a·lep·toid
cat·a·lo·gia
ca·tal·y·sis
    contact c.
    heterogeneous c.
    superacid c.
    surface c.
cat·a·lyst
    negative c.
cat·a·lyt·ic
cat·a·lyze
cat·a·me·nia
cat·a·me·ni·al
cat·a·men·o·gen·ic
cat·am·ne·sis
cat·am·nes·tic
cat·a·pasm
cata·pha·sia
ca·taph·o·ra
cata·pho·re·sis
cata·pho·ret·ic
cata·pho·ria
cata·phor·ic
cat·a·phre·nia
cata·phy·lax·is
cat·a·pla·sia
cat·a·plasm
    kaolin c.
cat·a·plec·tic
cat·a·plexie du ré·veil
cat·a·plexy
cat·a·poph·y·sis
Cat·a·pres
cat·a·ract
    after-c.
    aminoaciduria c.
    arborescent c.
    atopic c.
    axial fusiform c.
    axillary c.
    black c.
    blue c.
    blue dot c.
    bottlemakers' c.
    brown c.
    brunescent c.
    calcareous c.
    capsular c.

cat·a·ract *(continued)*
    capsulolenticular c.
    cerulean c.
    complete c.
    complicated c.
    concussion c.
    congenital c.
    contusion c.
    coralliform c.
    coronary c.
    cortical c.
    cuneiform c.
    cupuliform c.
    cystic c.
    dermatogenic c.
    developmental c.
    diabetic c.
    dry-shelled c.
    duplication c.
    electric c.
    embryonal nuclear c.
    embryopathic c.
    evolutionary c.
    fibroid c.
    floriform c.
    fluid c.
    fusiform c.
    galactosemic c.
    glassblowers' c.
    glaucomatous c.
    gray c.
    hard c.
    heat c.
    heat-ray c.
    heterochromic c.
    hypermature c.
    hypocalcemic c.
    immature c.
    incipient c.
    infantile c.
    intumescent c.
    irradiation c.
    juvenile c.
    lamellar c.
    lenticular c.
    mature c.
    membranous c.
    metabolic c.

cat·a·ract *(continued)*
    milky c.
    morgagnian c.
    nuclear c.
    nutritional deficiency c.
    occupational c.
    overripe c.
    perinuclear c.
    peripheral c.
    polar c.
    postinflammatory c.
    c's of prematurity
    presenile c.
    primary c.
    puddlers' c.
    punctate c.
    pyramidal c.
    radiation c.
    reduplication c.
    ringform congenital c.
    ripe c.
    rubella c.
    secondary c.
    sedimentary c.
    senile c.
    senile nuclear sclerotic c.
    siliculose c.
    snowflake c.
    snowstorm c.
    Soemmering's ring c.
    spindle c.
    stationary c.
    stellate c.
    subcapsular c.
    sunflower c.
    supranuclear c.
    sutural c.
    syndermatotic c.
    thermal c.
    total c.
    toxic c.
    traumatic c.
    zonular c.
cat·a·rac·to·gen·ic
cat·a·rac·tous
cat·a·ria
ca·tarrh
    atrophic c.

ca·tarrh *(continued)*
    autumnal c.
    Bostock's c.
    epidemic c.
    hypertrophic c.
    Laënnec's c.
    malignant c. of cattle
    postnasal c.
    sinus c.
    spring c.
    suffocative c.
    summer c.
    vernal c.
ca·tar·rhal
cat·ar·rhine
cat·a·stal·tic
cat·a·stat·ic
cat·a·stroph·ic
cat·a·ta·sis
cata·ther·mom·e·ter
cata·thy·mia
cata·thy·mic
cata·to·nia
cata·ton·ic
cat·a·to·noid
cata·tri·crot·ic
cata·tri·cro·tism
cat·a·tro·pia
cat·e·chin
cat·e·chol
    c. methyl ester
cat·e·chol·amine
cat·e·chol·am·in·er·gic
cat·e·chol ox·i·dase
cat·e·chu
    pale c.
cat·e·chu·ic acid
cat·elec·trot·o·nus
Cat·e·na·bac·te·ri·um
cat·e·nat·ing
cat·e·noid
ca·ten·u·late
cat·gut
    carbolized c.
    chromic c.
    I.K.I. c.
    iodine c.
    iodochromic c.

cat·gut *(continued)*
   silverized c.
Cath. — L. catharticus
   (cathartic)
Catha
   C. edulis
cath·a·rom·e·ter
ca·thar·sis
ca·thar·tic
   bulk c.
   lubricant c.
   saline c.
   stimulant c.
ca·thar·tic acid
ca·thec·tic
Cath·e·lin's method
Cath·e·lin's segregator
cath·emo·glo·bin
ca·thep·sin
ca·ther·e·sis
cath·e·ret·ic
cath·e·ter
   Abramson c.
   acorn-tipped c.
   Amplatz cardiac c.
   angiographic c.
   balloon c.
   bicoudate c.
   c. bicoudé
   Bozeman's c.
   Bozeman-Fritsch c.
   Braasch bulb c.
   Broviac c.
   cardiac c.
   central venous c.
   conical c.
   c. coudé
   DeLee c.
   c. à demeure
   de Pezzer c.
   double-current c.
   double-lumen c.
   Double-J stent c.
   Drew-Smythe c.
   elbowed c.
   eustachian c.
   female c.
   filiform-tipped c.

cath·e·ter *(continued)*
   flexible c.
   Fogarty c.
   Foley c.
   Fritsch's c.
   Garceau c.
   Gouley's c.
   Groshong c.
   Gruntzig c.
   indwelling c.
   intracardiac c.
   Intracath c.
   Jackson-Pratt c.
   Karman c.
   Malecot c.
   Mixtner c.
   Nélaton's c.
   Nutricath c.
   olive-tip c.
   opaque c.
   oropharyngeal c.
   Pezzer's c.
   Phillips' c.
   pigtail c.
   prostatic c.
   Robinson c.
   self-retaining c.
   spiral-tip c.
   split sheath c.
   Swan-Ganz c.
   Tenckhoff peritoneal c.
   Texas c.
   toposcopic c.
   tracheal c.
   two-way c.
   ventricular c.
   vertebrated c.
   whip c.
   whistle-tip c.
   winged c.
cath·e·ter·iza·tion
   cardiac c.
   eustachian c.
   hepatic vein c.
   laryngeal c.
   retrourethral c.
   suprapubic c.
   transseptal c.

cath·e·ter·ize
cath·e·tero·stat
cath·e·tom·e·ter
ca·thex·is
cath·iso·pho·bia
cath·o·dal
cath·ode
ca·thod·ic
ca·thol·i·con
cath·o·lyte
Cath·o·my·cin
cat·ion
cat·ion·ic
cat·i·on·o·gen
cat·lin
ca·top·tric
ca·top·trics
ca·top·tro·scope
Cat·tani se·rum
Cat·tel Infant Intelligence
   Scale
cau·da *pl.* cau·dae
   c. corporis striati
   c. epididymidis
   c. equina
   c. helicis
   c. nuclei caudati
   c. pancreatis
cau·dad
cau·dae
cau·dal
cau·da·lis
cau·dal·ward
Cau·da·moe·ba si·nen·sis
cau·date
cau·da·to·len·tic·u·lar
cau·da·tum
cau·dec·to·my
cau·dex
cau·do·ceph·a·lad
caul
Cau·lo·bac·ter
cau·mes·the·sia
cau·sal·gia
cau·sa·tion
   legal c.
cause
   constitutional c.

cause *(continued)*
   contributory c. of death
   c. of death
   exciting c.
   immediate c.
   local c.
   precipitating c.
   predisposing c.
   primary c.
   proximate c.
   remote c.
   secondary c.
   specific c.
   ultimate c.
   underlying c. of death
caus·tic
   Churchill's iodine c.
   Filhos's c.
   Landolfi's c.
   Lugol's c.
   lunar c.
   mitigated c.
   Plunket's c.
   Rousselot's c.
   Vienna c.
   zinc c.
caus·ti·cize
cau·ter·ant
cau·ter·iza·tion
   cold c.
   c. by points
   punctuate c.
cau·tery
   actual c.
   bicap c.
   bipolar c.
   chemical c.
   cold c.
   Corrigan's c.
   electric c.
   galvanic c.
   gas c.
   potential c.
   virtual c.
   wet field c.
   Ziegler c.
ca·va
ca·val

cav·a·scope
ca·ve·o·la *pl.* ca·ve·o·lae
cav·er·na *pl.* ca·ver·nae
 cavernae corporis spongiosi
 cavernae corporum
  cavernosorum penis
cav·er·nil·o·quy
cav·er·ni·tis
 fibrous c.
cav·er·no·ma
 c. lymphaticum
cav·er·no·scope
cav·er·nos·co·py
cav·er·no·si·tis
cav·er·nos·to·my
cav·er·nous
Ca·via
 C. cobaya
cav·i·ta·ry
cav·i·tas *pl.* cav·i·ta·tes
 c. abdominalis
 c. articularis
 c. conchae
 c. coronalis
 c. cranii
 c. dentis
 c. epiduralis
 c. glenoidalis
 c. infraglottica
 c. laryngis
 c. medullaris
 c. medullaris ossium
 c. nasi
 c. oris
 c. oris externa
 c. oris propria
 c. pelvis
 c. pericardialis
 c. peritonealis
 c. pharyngis
 c. pleuralis
 c. pulparis
 c. septi pellucidi
 c. subarachnoidealis
 c. thoracis
 c. tympanica
 c. uteri

cav·i·ta·tes
cav·i·ta·tion
 c. of septum pellucidum
ca·vi·tis
Cav·i·tron aspiration unit
Cav·i·tron dissector
cav·i·ty
 abdominal c.
 absorption c's
 allantoic c.
 alveolar c's
 amniotic c.
 articular c.
 Baer's c.
 body c.
 buccal c.
 cleavage c.
 coelomic c.
 complex c.
 compound c.
 cotyloid c.
 cranial c.
 dental c.
 distal c.
 ectoplacental c.
 epidural c.
 epiploic c.
 faucial c.
 fibrotic c's
 fissure c.
 gastrovascular c.
 gastrulation c.
 glandular c.
 glenoid c.
 hemal c.
 incisal c.
 infraglottic c.
 ischiorectal c.
 joint c.
 labial c.
 laryngeal c.
 laryngopharyngeal c.
 lingual c.
 lymph c's
 marrow c.
 mastoid c.
 Meckel's c.

cav·i·ty *(continued)*
    mediastinal c.
    medullary c.
    mesial c.
    nasal c.
    occlusal c.
    oral c.
    orbital c.
    pectoral c.
    pelvic c.
    pericardial c.
    pericardiopleuroperitoneal
      c.
    peritoneal c.
    pharyngeal c.
    pharyngolaryngeal c.
    pharyngonasal c.
    pharyngo-oral c.
    pit c.
    pleural c.
    pleuroperitoneal c.
    popliteal c.
    prepared c.
    proximal c.
    pulp c.
    rectoischiadic c.
    Retzius's c.
    Rosenmüller's c.
    segmentation c.
    serous c.
    sigmoid c.
    simple c.
    smooth surface c.
    somatic c.
    somite c.
    splanchnic c.
    Stafne's c.
    subarachnoid c.
    subdural c.
    tension c's
    thoracic c.
    trigeminal c.
    tympanic c.
    uterine c.
    visceral c.
    yolk c.
ca·vog·ra·phy
ca·vo·sur·face

ca·vo·val·gus
ca·vum *pl.* ca·va
    c. trigeminale
ca·vus
Cay·tine
Ca·ze·nave's disease
Ca·ze·nave's vitiligo
CB — L. Chirurgiae
    Baccalaureus (Bachelor of
    Surgery)
CBC — complete blood count
cbc — complete blood count
CBF — cerebral blood flow
CBG — corticosteroid-binding
    globulin
CBS — chronic brain
    syndrome
CC — chief complaint
cc — cubic centimeter
CCA — chimpanzee coryza
    agent (respiratory syncytial
    virus)
    congenital contractural
    arachnodactyly
CCAT — conglutinating
    complement absorption test
CCC — cathodal closure
    contraction
CCF — crystal-induced
    chemotactic factor
CCCl — cathodal closure
    clonus
CCK — cholecystokinin
c cm — cubic centimeter
CCU — coronary care unit
CD — cluster designation
    L. conjugata diagonalis
    (diagonal conjugate
    diameter)
    curative dose
cd — candela
CDC — Centers for Disease
    Control
CDC/AIDS — Centers for
    Disease Control definition of
    acquired immune deficiency
    syndrome

cdf — cumulative distribution
   function
cDNA — complementary
   DNA
      copy DNA
CDP — cytidine diphosphate
CEA — carcinoembryonic
   antigen
ce·as·mic
ce·bo·ceph·a·lus
ce·bo·ceph·a·ly
ce·ca
ce·cal
ce·cec·to·my
Ce·cil's operation
Ce·cil-Culp repair
ce·ci·tis
ce·co·cele
ce·co·cen·tral
ce·co·col·ic
ce·co·co·lon
ce·co·co·lo·pexy
ce·co·co·los·to·my
ce·co·cys·to·plas·ty
ce·co·fix·a·tion
ce·co·il·e·ost·o·my
Ce·con
ce·co·pexy
ce·co·pli·ca·tion
ce·cor·rha·phy
ce·co·sig·moid·os·to·my
ce·cos·to·my
ce·cot·o·my
ce·cum
      cupular c. of cochlear duct
      gastric ceca
      high c.
      c. mobile
      mobile c.
      vestibular c. of cochlear
         duct
Ce·de·cea
Ce·di·lan·id
Ce·di·lan·id-D
Ce·dio·psyl·la
CeeNU
cef·a·clor
cef·a·drox·il

Cef·a·dyl
cef·a·man·dole
      c. nafate
cef·a·pa·role
cef·a·tri·zine
ce·faz·a·flur so·di·um
ce·faz·o·lin
      c. sodium
cef·met·a·zole
cef·on·i·cid
cef·o·per·a·zone
ce·for·a·nide
cef·o·tax·ime
cef·o·tax·ime so·di·um
cef·o·ti·am
ce·fox·i·tin
cef·su·lo·din
cef·ta·zi·dime
cef·ti·zox·ime so·di·um
cef·tri·a·xone so·di·um
ce·fu·rox·ime
Cel — Celsius
ce·la·ri·um
Cel·be·nin
ce·len·ter·on
Cel·es·tin's tube
Ce·les·tone
ce·li·ac
ce·li·ec·to·my
ce·lio·cen·te·sis
ce·lio·col·pot·o·my
ce·lio·ely·trot·o·my
ce·lio·en·ter·ot·o·my
ce·lio·gas·trot·o·my
ce·lio·hys·ter·ec·to·my
ce·li·o·ma
ce·lio·myo·mec·to·my
ce·lio·myo·mot·o·my
ce·lio·myo·si·tis
ce·lio·para·cen·te·sis
ce·li·op·a·thy
ce·lio·py·o·sis
ce·li·or·rha·phy
ce·lio·sal·pin·gec·to·my
ce·lio·sal·pin·got·o·my
ce·lio·scope
ce·li·os·co·py

ce·li·ot·o·my
    vaginal c.
    ventral c.
ce·li·tis
cell
    A c.
    Abbé-Zeiss counting c.
    absorptive c., intestinal
    accessory c's
    acidophilic c.
    acinar c.
    acinous c.
    acoustic hair c.
    activated reticular c.
    adipose c.
    adventitial c's
    agger nasi c's
    agranular c.
    air c.
    albuminous c.
    algoid c's
    alpha c's
    alveolar c.
    alveolar c's, type I
    alveolar c's, type II
    Alzheimer's c's
    amacrine c's
    ameboid c.
    amine precursor uptake and decarboxylation c's
    amphophilic c.
    anaplastic c.
    Anichkov's (Anitschkow's) c.
    anterior ethmoidal air c's
    anterior horn c.
    antigen-presenting c's
    antigen-reactive c's
    antigen-sensitive c's
    antipodal c's
    apocrine c's
    apolar c.
    apotrophic c's
    APUD [amine precursor uptake and decarboxylation system] c's
    argentaffin c's

cell *(continued)*
    argyrophilic c's
    Arias-Stella c's
    arkyochrome c.
    Armanni-Ebstein c's
    Aschoff's c's
    Askanazy c.
    auditory c's
    autologous lymphokine activated killer c.
    B c's
    balloon c's
    band c.
    basal c.
    basal granular c's
    basilar c.
    basket c.
    basophilic c.
    beaker c.
    Beale's ganglion c's
    Bergmann's c's
    berry c.
    beta c's
    Betz's c's
    Bevan-Lewis c's
    biochemical fuel c.
    bipolar c.
    bipolar retinal c's
    bite c.
    Bizzozero c's
    bladder c's
    blast c.
    bloated c.
    blood c's
    border c's
    Böttcher's c's
    breviradiate c's
    bristle c's
    bronchic c.
    brood c.
    brush bipolar c.
    buffy coat c's
    bulliform c.
    burr c.
    C c's
    Cajal c.
    caliciform c.
    cameloid c.

cell *(continued)*
- capsule c.
- cardiac failure c's
- cartilage c's
- caryochrome c's
- Caspersson type B c's
- castration c's
- caudate c's
- caveolated c's
- cement c.
- central c.
- centrifugal bipolar c.
- centroacinar c's
- chalice c.
- chief c's
- Chinese hamster ovary (CHO) c's
- CHO c's
- chromaffin c's
- chromophobe c's
- chromophobic c's
- ciliated c.
- Clara c's
- Clarke's c's
- Claudius' c's
- clear c's
- cleavage c.
- clue c.
- clump c's
- collenchyma c's
- columnar c.
- cometal c's
- commissural c's
- committed c.
- companion c.
- compound granule c.
- cone c.
- cone bipolar c.
- conjunctival c.
- connective tissue c's
- contractile fiber c's
- contrasuppressor c's
- corneal c.
- c's of Corti
- corticotroph c.
- corticotroph-lipotroph c.
- counting c.
- cover c.

cell *(continued)*
- crescent c's
- cribrate c.
- Crooke's c's
- cuboid c.
- Custer c's
- cylindric c.
- cytomegalic c.
- cytotoxic T c's
- D c's
- daughter c.
- Davidoff's c's
- decidual c's
- deep c.
- Deiters' c's
- delta c's
- demilune c's
- dendritic c's
- dentin c.
- diffuse ganglion c.
- diploid c.
- displaced ganglion c.
- dome c's
- Dorothy Reed c's
- Downey c's
- dust c's
- EAC rosette-forming c.
- ectoblastic c.
- ectodermal c.
- effector c.
- electrochemical c.
- electrolytic c.
- electromotive force c.
- elementary c's
- embryonic c's
- emigrated c.
- enamel c.
- encasing c.
- end c.
- endocrine c's of gut
- endothelioid c's
- enterochromaffin c's
- ependymal c's
- epidermic c's
- epithelial c's
- epithelioid c's
- E rosette-forming c.
- erythroid c's

cell *(continued)*
eta c.
ethmoidal c's, bony
eukaryotic c.
F c.
faggot c.
c. of Fañanás
fat c.
fat-storing c's of liver
fatty granule c.
Ferrata's c.
fiber c.
fixed c.
flagellate c.
flat bipolar c.
floor c's
foam c's
follicle c's
follicular c's
follicular epithelial c's
foot c's
foreign body giant c's
formative c.
Foulis' c's
free c.
fuchsinophil c.
fusiform c.
G c's
galvanic c.
gametoid c's
gamma c's of hypophysis
ganglion c.
Gaucher's c.
Gegenbaur's c.
gemistocytic c.
generative c.
germ c's
germinal c.
ghost c.
c's of Giannuzzi
giant c.
giant pyramidal c's
Gierke's c's
gitter c.
glandular c.
Gley's c's
glia c.
glitter c's

cell *(continued)*
glomerular c.
glomus c.
goblet c.
Golgi's c's
gonadotroph c.
Goormaghtigh c's
granular c.
granule c's
granulosa c's
granulosa-lutein c's
grape c.
guard c.
gustatory c's
gyrochrome c.
H c.
hair c's
hairy c.
Hammar's myoid c's
haploid c.
heart-disease c's
heart-failure c's
heart-lesion c's
hecatomeral c's
heckle c.
Heidenhain's c's
HEK (human embryo
   kidney) c.
HEL (human embryo lung)
   c.
HeLa c's
helmet c.
helper c's
hemopoietic c.
Hensen's c's
hepatic c's
heteromeral c's
hilus c's
Hodgkin's c's
Hofbauer c's
homozygous typing c's
   (HTC)
horizontal c.
horizontal c. of Cajal
horn c's
Hortega c.
hot c.
Hürthle c's

cell *(continued)*
- hyperchromatic c.
- I-c.
- immunocompetent c.
- immunologically competent c.
- incasing c's
- indifferent c.
- inducer c.
- inflammatory c.
- initial c's
- inner hair c.
- inner phalangeal c.
- integrator c.
- intercalary c's
- intercapillary c's
- interdental c's
- interdigitating c's
- interfollicular c's
- internuncial c.
- interstitial c's
- islet c's
- juvenile c.
- juxtaglomerular c's
- K c's
- karyochrome c's
- killer c's
- killer T c's
- koilocytotic c.
- Kulchitsky's c's
- Kupffer's c's
- Kurloff c.
- L c's
- lacis c.
- lacrimoethmoid c's
- lactotroph c.
- lacunar c.
- Langerhans c's
- Langhans' c's
- Langhans' giant c's
- large cleaved follicular center c.
- large granule c's
- large noncleaved follicular center c.
- LE c.
- Leclanché c.
- Leishman's chrome c's

cell *(continued)*
- lepra c.
- Leydig's c's
- light c's
- littoral c's
- liver c's
- locomotive c.
- longiradiate c's
- lupus erythematosus c.
- luteal c's
- lutein c's
- lymph c.
- lymphadenoma c's
- lymphoblastic plasma c.
- lymphoid c.
- macroglial c.
- malpighian c.
- Marchand's c.
- marginal c's
- marrow c.
- Martinotti's c's
- mast c.
- mastoid c's
- matrix c's
- Mauthner's c.
- medullary interstitial c.
- medulloepithelial c.
- megaspore mother c.
- melanotropic c.
- memory c's
- Merkel's c's
- Merkel-Ranvier c's
- Merkel tactile c.
- mesangial c's
- mesenchymal c's
- mesothelial c's
- metallophil c's
- Mexican hat c.
- Meynert's c's
- microglial c.
- microspore mother c.
- midget bipolar c.
- migratory c's
- Mikulicz's c's
- mitral c's
- monocytoid c.
- monosynaptic bipolar c.
- Mooser c.

cell *(continued)*
  mop bipolar c.
  morular c.
  mossy c.
  mother c.
  motile c.
  motor c.
  Mott c.
  mouth c's
  mucoalbuminous c's
  mucoserous c's
  mucous c's
  mucous neck c's
  mulberry c.
  c's of Müller
  multipolar c.
  mural c.
  muscle c.
  mycosis c.
  myeloid c.
  myeloma c.
  myoepithelial c's
  myoepithelioid c's
  myogenic c.
  myoid c's
  myointimal c.
  Nageotte's c's
  natural killer c.
  nerve c.
  neuroepithelial c's
  neuroglia c's
  neuroglial c's
  neuromuscular c.
  neurosecretory c.
  neutrophilic c.
  nevus c.
  niche c.
  Niemann-Pick c's
  NK c's
  noble c's
  normal c.
  nucleated c.
  nucleated red blood c.
  null c's
  nurse c's
  oat c's
  olfactory c's
  osseous c.

cell *(continued)*
  osteochondrogenic c.
  osteoprogenitor c's
  outer hair c.
  outer phalangeal c.
  owl's eye c's
  oxyntic c's
  oxyphil c's
  oxyphilic c's
  packed human blood c's
  Paget's c.
  pagetoid c.
  palatine c's
  palisade c's
  Paneth's c's
  oligodendroglial c.
  Opalski c.
  parafollicular c's
  osteogenic c.
  paraluteal c's
  paralutein c's
  parenchymal hepatic c's
  parenchymal liver c's
  parent c.
  parietal c's
  pathologic c.
  pavement c's
  pediculated c's
  peg c's
  Pelger-Huët c.
  peptic c's
  pericapillary c's
  pericellular c's
  perineurial c.
  perithelial c.
  peritoneal exudate c.
  peritubular contractile c's
  perivascular c's
  pessary c.
  petrosal c's
  phagocytic c.
  phalangeal c's
  phantom c.
  pheochrome c's
  photoautotrophic c's
  photoreceptor c's
  physaliferous c's
  Pick's c's

cell *(continued)*
    pigment c.
    pillar c's
    pineal c.
    plaque-forming c's
    plasma c's
    pluripotent c.
    pneumatic c's
    PNH c's
    polar c's
    Polyak's i-type c.
    polychromatic c's
    polychromatophil c's
    polyhedral c's
    polyplastic c.
    postmitotic c.
    PP c.
    pre-B c's
    prefollicle c's
    pregnancy c.
    pregranulosa c.
    pre-T c.
    prickle c.
    primary c.
    primitive granulosa c's
    primitive wandering c.
    primordial germ c's
    principal c's
    prokaryotic c.
    prolactin c.
    prop c's
    psychic c's
    pulmonary epithelial c's
    pulpar c's
    Purkinje's c's
    pyknotic c.
    pyramidal c.
    pyroninophilic blast c.
    RA c.
    radial c's of Müller
    Raji c's
    red c.
    red blood c.
    Reed c's
    Reed-Sternberg c's
    regeneration c.
    renal tubular c.
    Renshaw c's

cell *(continued)*
    reproductive c.
    reserve c's
    residential c.
    responder c.
    resting c.
    resting wandering c.
    reticular c's
    reticuloendothelial c.
    reticulum c.
    rhagiocrine c.
    Rieder's c.
    rod c's
    Rohon-Beard c's
    Rolando's c's
    root c's
    Rouget c's
    round c.
    S c's
    Sala's c's
    sarcogenic c's
    satellite c's
    scavenger c.
    Schultze's c's
    Schwann c.
    sclerenchyma c's
    segmented c.
    seminal c's
    seminoma c.
    sensitized c.
    sensory c.
    sentinel c's
    septal c.
    serous c.
    Sertoli's c's
    sexual c's
    Sézary c.
    shadow c.
    sickle c.
    signet-ring c.
    silver c's
    skein c.
    skeletogenous c.
    small cleaved follicular
      center c.
    small granule c's
    small noncleaved follicular
      center c.

cell *(continued)*
  smooth muscle c.
  smudge c's
  somatic c's
  somatostatin c's
  somatotropic c.
  sperm c.
  spermatogenic c's
  spermatogonial c.
  sphenoid c's
  spider c.
  spindle c.
  splenic c.
  spur c.
  squamous c.
  stab c.
  staff c.
  star c's
  static balance receptor c.
  stave c's.
  stellate c's
  stem c.
  Sternberg's giant c's
  Sternberg-Reed c's
  stimulator c.
  stipple c.
  strap c.
  stroma c.
  supporting c's
  suppressor c's
  sustentacular c's
  sympathetic formative c.
  sympathicotrophic c's
  sympathochromaffin c's
  sympathotropic c.
  syncytial c.
  synovial c's
  T c's
  tactile c.
  tadpole c's
  tanned red c's
  tapetal c.
  target c.
  tart c.
  taste c's
  tautomeral c's
  T_{DTH} c's
  teardrop c.

cell *(continued)*
  tegmental c's
  tendon c's
  $T\gamma$ c's
  theca c's
  theca-lutein c's
  Thoma-Zeiss counting c.
  thymus-dependent c.
  thymus-derived c.
  thyroidectomy c's
  thyrotroph c.
  Tiselius electrophoresis c.
  $T\mu$ c's
  totipotential c.
  Touton giant c.
  transitional c.
  trophochrome c's
  tubal air c's
  tube c.
  Türk's c.
  tympanic c's
  Tzanck c.
  ultimobranchial c's
  umbrella c.
  undifferentiated c.
  unipolar c.
  unit c.
  vacuolated c.
  c's of van Gehuchten
  van Hansemann c's
  vasofactive c's
  vasoformative c's
  vegetative c.
  veil c's
  ventricular c.
  Vero c's
  vestibular hair c's
  veto c's
  Vignal's c's
  Virchow c's
  visual c's
  voltaic c.
  von Kupffer's c's
  wandering c's
  Warthin-Finkeldey c's
  wasserhelle c's
  water-clear c.
  Wedl c's

cell *(continued)*
    white c.
    white blood c.
    wing c's
    xanthoma c.
    Zander's c's
    zymogenic c's
cel·la *pl.* cel·lae
cel·la·bur·ate
cel·lae
Cel·lase 1000
Cell·fal·cic·u·la
cel·lic·o·lous
cel·lif·er·ous
cel·li·form
cel·lif·u·gal
cel·lip·e·tal
cel·lo·bi·ose
cel·lo·bi·uron·ic acid
cel·lo·hex·ose
cel·loi·din
cel·lo·phane
cel·lo·tet·rose
cel·lo·tri·ose
Cell Sa·ver Hae·mo·lite
cell·tri·fuge
cel·lu·la *pl.* cel·lu·lae
    cellulae ethmoidales
    cellulae lentis
    cellulae mastoideae
    cellulae pneumaticae tubae
      auditivae
    c. sensoria pilosa
    cellulae tympanicae
cel·lu·lae
cel·lu·lar
cel·lu·lar·i·ty
cel·lu·lase
cel·lule
    c. claire
cel·lu·lic·i·dal
cel·lu·lif·er·ous
cel·lu·lif·u·gal
cel·lu·lip·e·tal
cel·lu·li·tis
    anaerobic c.
    clostridial anaerobic c.
    dissecting c. of scalp

cel·lu·li·tis *(continued)*
    facial c.
    finger c.
    gangrenous c.
    gaseous c.
    indurated c.
    necrotizing c.
    nonclostridial anaerobic c.
    orbital c.
    pelvic c.
    periurethral c.
    phlegmonous c.
    streptococcus c.
    ulcerative c.
cel·lu·lo·fi·brous
cel·lu·lo·neu·ri·tis
    acute anterior c.
cel·lu·lo·ra·dic·u·lo·neu·ri·tis
cel·lu·lo·sa
cel·lu·lose
    absorbable c.
    c. acetate phthalate
    acid c.
    microcrystalline c.
    oxidized c.
    starch c.
    tetranitrate c.
cel·lu·los·ic acid
cel·lu·los·i·ty
cel·lu·lo·tox·ic
cel·lu·lous
Ce·lon·tin
ce·lo·phle·bi·tis
ce·los·chi·sis
celo·scope
ce·los·co·py
ce·lo·so·mia
ce·lo·so·mus
ce·lo·thel
ce·lo·the·li·o·ma
ce·lo·the·li·um
ce·lot·o·my
celo·vi·rus
ce·lo·zo·ic
Cel·si·us scale
Cel·sus, Aulus Cornelius

ce·ment
    black copper c.
    calcium hydroxide c.
    dental c.
    glass ionomer c.
    intercellular c.
    methylmethacrylate c.
    oxyphosphate c.
    polycarboxylate c.
    resin c.
    root canal c.
    silicate c.
    silicophosphate c.
    zinc oxide–eugenol c.
    zinc phosphate c.
ce·men·ta·tion
ce·men·ti·cle
    adherent c.
    attached c.
    free c.
    interstitial c.
ce·men·ti·fi·ca·tion
ce·men·tin
ce·men·ti·tis
ce·men·to·blast
ce·men·to·blas·to·ma
ce·men·to·cla·sia
ce·men·to·clast
ce·men·to·cyte
ce·men·to·gen·e·sis
ce·men·toid
ce·men·to·ma
    gigantiform c.
ce·men·to·path·ia
ce·men·to·peri·os·ti·tis
ce·men·to·phyte
ce·men·to·sis
ce·men·tum
    acellular c.
    afibrillar c.
    cellular c.
    uncalcified c.
cen·a·del·phus
ce·nen·ceph·a·lo·cele
ce·nes·the·sia
ce·nes·the·sic
ce·nes·the·si·op·a·thy
ce·nes·thet·ic

ce·nes·thop·a·thy
ce·no·bi·um
ce·no·cyte
ce·no·gen·e·sis
Cen·o·late
Ce·no·phe·les bal·a·ba·cen·sis
ce·no·psych·ic
ce·no·sis
ce·not·ic
ce·no·type
cen·sor
cen·ter
    accelerating c.
    acoustic c.
    active c.
    anospinal c's
    apneustic c.
    appetite c.
    association c.
    auditopsychic c.
    auditory c.
    basioccipital c.
    basiotic c.
    basisphenoid c.
    Béclard's ossification c.
    birthing c.
    brain c.
    Broca's c.
    Budge's c.
    bulbar respiratory c.
    burn c.
    cardioaccelerating c.
    cardioinhibitory c.
    cardiomotor c.
    cardiovascular c.
    cell c.
    cheirokinesthetic c.
    chiral c.
    c's of chondrification
    ciliospinal c.
    community mental health
      c. (CMHC)
    convergence c.
    coordination c.
    correlation c.
    cortical c.
    costal c.
    coughing c.

cen·ter *(continued)*
  defecation c.
  deglutition c.
  dentary c.
  C's for Disease Control
    (CDC)
  dominating c.
  ejaculation c.
  epiotic c.
  erection c.
  eupraxic c.
  exoccipital c.
  facial c.
  feeding c.
  Flemming c.
  foot clonus c.
  ganglionic c.
  genital c.
  genitospinal c.
  germinal c.
  glossokinesthetic c.
  glycogenic c.
  gustatory c.
  health c.
  heat-regulating c's
  hunger c.
  hypothalamic c's
  ideomotor c.
  inactivation c.
  inhibitory c.
  interim accommodation c.
  interparietal c.
  Kerckring's c.
  kinesthetic c.
  kinetic c.
  Kronecker's c.
  Kupressoff's c.
  Lumsden's c.
  mastication c.
  medullary c. of cerebellum
  medullary respiratory c.
  micturition c.
  motor c.
  negative reward c.
  nerve c.
  olfactory c.
  optic c.
  orbitosphenoid c.

cen·ter *(continued)*
  ossification c.
  pacemaker c.
  panting c.
  parenchymatous c.
  parturition c.
  phrenic c.
  plantar reflex c.
  pneumotaxic c.
  poison control c.
  polypneic c.
  pontine c. for lateral gaze
  pteriotic c.
  punishment c.
  reaction c.
  rectovesical c.
  reflex c.
  respiratory c's
  reward c.
  rotation c.
  salivary c.
  satiety c.
  semioval c.
  sensory c.
  Setchenow's (Sechenoff's)
    c's
  sex-behavior c.
  somatosensory c's
  speech c.
  sphenotic c.
  spinal cardioaccelerator c.
  spinogenital c.
  splenial c.
  suboccipital c.
  sudorific c's
  sweat c's
  swallowing c.
  taste c.
  tendinous c.
  thermoregulatory c's
  thirst c.
  trophic c.
  vascular c.
  vasoconstrictor c.
  vasodilator c.
  vasomotor c's
  vasotonic c.
  vesical c.

cen·ter *(continued)*
    vesicospinal c.
    visuopsychic c.
    vital c's
    vomiting c.
    Wernicke's c.
    winking c.
    word c., auditory
    word c., visual
cen·tes·i·mal
cen·te·sis
cen·ti·grade
cen·ti·gray
cen·ti·li·ter
cen·ti·me·ter
    cubic c.
cen·ti·mor·gan
cen·ti·nem
cen·ti·pede
cen·ti·poise
cen·ti·stoke
cen·ti·u·nit
cen·tra
cen·trad
cen·trage
cen·tral
cen·tra·lis
cen·tra·phose
cen·tra·tion
cen·trax·o·ni·al
cen·tren·ce·phal·ic
cen·tric
    power c.
    true c.
cen·tric·i·put
cen·trif·u·gal
cen·trif·u·ga·li·za·tion
cen·trif·u·gate
cen·trif·u·ga·tion
    cesium chloride gradient c.
    density gradient c.
    differential c.
    isopyknic c.
    zonal c.
cen·tri·fuge
    microscope c.
cen·tri·lob·u·lar

cen·tri·ole
    anterior c.
    distal c.
    posterior c.
    proximal c.
    ring c.
cen·trip·e·tal
cen·tro·ac·i·nar
cen·tro·blast
cen·tro·ce·cal
cen·tro·cyte
cen·tro·des·mose
cen·tro·des·mus
cen·tro·ki·ne·sia
cen·tro·ki·net·ic
cen·tro·lec·i·thal
cen·tro·lob·u·lar
cen·tro·mere
cen·tro·mer·ic
cen·tro·nu·cle·us
cen·tro-os·teo·scle·ro·sis
cen·tro·phen·ox·ine
cen·tro·phose
cen·tro·plasm
cen·tro·scle·ro·sis
cen·tro·some
cen·tro·sphere
cen·tro·stal·tic
cen·tro·ther·a·py
cen·trum *pl.* cen·tra
    c. medianum of Luys
    c. medullare
    c. ossificationis
    c. semiovale
    c. tendineum
    c. vertebrae
Cen·tru·roi·des
ceph·a·ce·trile so·di·um
Ceph·a·e·lis
ceph·a·lad
ceph·a·lal·gia
    histamine c.
    pharyngotympanic c.
    quadrantal c.
ceph·al·ede·ma
ceph·a·lex·in

ceph·al·he·mat·o·cele
    Stromeyer's c.
ceph·al·he·ma·to·ma
    c. deformans
ceph·al·hy·dro·cele
    c. traumatica
ce·phal·ic
ceph·a·lin
ceph·a·li·za·tion
ceph·a·lo·ca·thar·tic
ceph·a·lo·cau·dad
ceph·a·lo·cau·dal
ceph·a·lo·cele
    orbital c.
ceph·a·lo·cen·te·sis
ceph·a·lo·cyst
ceph·a·lo·dac·ty·ly
    Vogt's c.
ceph·a·lo·did·y·mus
ceph·a·lo·di·pros·o·pus
ceph·a·lo·dym·ia
ceph·a·lod·y·mus
ceph·al·odyn·ia
ceph·a·lo·gen·e·sis
ceph·a·lo·ge·net·ic
ceph·a·lo·gly·cin
ceph·a·lo·gram
ceph·a·lo·gy·ric
ceph·a·lo·hem·a·to·cele
ceph·a·lo·he·ma·to·ma
ceph·a·lo·meg·a·ly
ceph·a·lom·e·lus
ceph·a·lo·me·nia
ceph·a·lo·men·in·gi·tis
ceph·a·lom·e·ter
ceph·a·lo·met·ric
ceph·a·lom·e·try
    fetal c.
    radiographic c.
    ultrasonic c.
ceph·a·lo·mo·tor
ceph·a·lo·nia
ceph·a·lop·a·gus
ceph·a·lo·pa·thia splanch·no·cys·ti·ca
ceph·a·lop·a·thy
ceph·a·lo·pel·vic
ceph·a·lo·pel·vim·e·try

ceph·a·lo·pha·ryn·ge·us
ceph·a·lo·ple·gia
ceph·a·lo·ra·chid·i·an
ceph·a·lo·rha·chid·i·an
ceph·a·lor·i·dine
ceph·a·lo·spo·rin
    c. C
    c. N
    c. P
ceph·a·lo·spor·in·ase
ceph·a·lo·spo·ri·o·sis
Ceph·a·lo·spo·ri·um
    C. falciforme
    C. granulomatis
ceph·a·lo·stat
ceph·a·lo·tet·a·nus
ceph·a·lo·thin
    c. sodium
ceph·a·lo·tho·rac·ic
ceph·a·lo·tho·ra·co·ili·op·a·gus
ceph·a·lo·tho·ra·cop·a·gus
    c. dibrachius
    c. disymmetros
    c. monosymmetros
ceph·a·lo·tho·rax
ceph·a·lo·tome
ceph·a·lot·o·my
ceph·a·lo·trop·ic
ceph·a·lox·ia
ceph·a·my·cin
ceph·a·pi·rin
    c. sodium
ceph·ra·dine
cep·tor
    chemical c.
    contact c.
    distance c.
    nerve c.
CERA — cortical-evoked response audiometry
ce·ra·ceous
ce·ra·ce·ra·ti·tis
ce·ram·ic
    glass c.
ce·ram·ics
    dental c.
cer·am·i·dase

cer·a·mide
    galactosyl c.
    c. glucoside
    c. trihexoside
cer·a·mide tri·hex·o·si·dase
ce·ram·odon·tics
cer·a·sin
cer·a·sine
cer·a·sus
ce·rate
    blistering c.
    lead subacetate c.
    simple c.
    Turner's c.
cer·a·tec·to·my
cer·a·tin
Ce·ra·ti·um
cer·a·to·cri·coid
cer·a·to·cri·coi·de·us
cer·a·to·hy·al
cer·a·to·pha·ryn·ge·us
Cer·a·to·phyl·lus
    C. gallinae
    C. punjabensis
    C. tesquorum
Cer·a·to·po·gon·i·dae
ce·ra·tum
cer·car·ia *pl.* cer·car·iae
cer·car·i·ci·dal
cer·car·i·en·hul·len·re·ak·
  tion
cerci
cer·clage
cer·co·cyst
cer·co·cys·tis
cer·coid
cer·co·mer
Cer·co·mo·nas hom·in·is
cer·co·pith·e·coid
Cer·co·pith·e·coi·dea
Cer·cos·pora apii
Cer·cos·po·ral·la vex·ans
cer·co·spo·ra·my·co·sis
cer·cus *pl.* cer·ci
ce·rea flex·i·bil·i·tas
cer·e·bel·la
cer·e·bel·lar
cer·e·bel·lif·u·gal

cer·e·bel·lip·e·tal
cer·e·bel·li·tis
cer·e·bel·lo-ol·i·vary
cer·e·bel·lo·pon·tile
cer·e·bel·lo·pon·tine
cer·e·bel·lo·ret·i·nal
cer·e·bel·lo·ru·bral
cer·e·bel·lo·ru·bro·spi·nal
cer·e·bel·lo·spi·nal
cer·e·bel·lo·tha·lam·ic
cer·e·bel·lo·ves·tib·u·lar
cer·e·bel·lum
cer·e·bra
cer·e·bral
cer·e·bra·tion
cer·e·bri·form
cer·e·brif·u·gal
cer·e·brip·e·tal
cer·e·bri·tis
    saturnine c.
cer·e·bro·car·di·ac
cer·e·bro·cer·e·bel·lar
cer·e·bro·cu·pre·in
cer·e·bro·ga·lac·tose
cer·e·bro·ga·lac·to·side
cer·e·bro·hy·phoid
cer·e·broid
cer·e·brol·o·gy
cer·e·bro·ma
cer·e·bro·mac·u·lar
cer·e·bro·ma·la·cia
cer·e·bro·med·ul·lary
cer·e·bro·me·nin·ge·al
cer·e·bro·men·in·gi·tis
cer·e·bron·ic acid
cer·e·bro-oc·u·lar
cer·e·bro·path·ia
    c. psychica toxemica
cer·e·brop·a·thy
cer·e·bro·phys·i·ol·o·gy
cer·e·bro·pon·tile
cer·e·bro·pon·tine
cer·e·bro·psy·cho·sis
cer·e·bro·ra·chid·i·an
cer·e·bro·ret·i·nal
cer·e·bro·scle·ro·sis
cer·e·brose
cer·e·bro·side

cer·e·bro·side sul·fa·tase
cer·e·bro·si·do·sis
cer·e·bro·sis
cer·e·bro·spi·nal
cer·e·bro·spi·nant
cer·e·bros·to·my
cer·e·bro·ten·di·nous
cer·e·brot·o·my
cer·e·bro·to·nia
cer·e·bro·vas·cu·lar
cer·e·brum
cere·cloth
Cer·en·kov radiation
cer·e·o·li
cer·e·o·lus *pl.* cer·e·o·li
cer·e·vi·sia *pl.* cer·e·vi·siae
   cerevisiae fermentum
   cerevisiae fermentum
   compressum
Cer·i·thid·ia
   C. cingulata
ce·ri·um
ce·roid
ce·roid lip·o·fus·cin
ce·roid-lip·o·fus·ci·no·sis
   Finnish-type c.
   Hagberg-Santavuori
     variant of c.
   Jansky-Bielschowsky type
     c.
   Kufs-type c.
ce·ro·li·poid
ce·ro·ma
ce·ro·plas·ty
cer·ti·fi·a·ble
Ce·ru·bi·dine
ce·ru·le·an
ce·ru·le·in
ce·ru·le·us
ce·ru·lo·plas·min
ce·ru·men
   impacted c.
   inspissated c.
ce·ru·mi·nal
ce·ru·min·ol·y·sis
ce·ru·mino·ly·tic
ce·ru·mi·no·ma
ce·ru·mi·no·sis

ce·ru·mi·nous
ce·ruse
cer·vi·cal
cer·vi·cal·gia
cer·vi·ca·lis
cer·vi·cec·to·my
cer·vi·ces
cer·vi·ci·spi·nal
cer·vi·ci·tis
   granulomatous c.
   traumatic c.
cer·vi·co·ax·il·lary
cer·vi·co·bra·chi·al
cer·vi·co·bra·chi·al·gia
cer·vi·co·buc·cal
cer·vi·co·col·pi·tis
   c. emphysematosa
cer·vi·co·dor·sal
cer·vi·co·dyn·ia
cer·vi·co·fa·cial
cer·vi·co·hu·mer·al
cer·vi·co·la·bi·al
cer·vi·co·lin·gual
cer·vi·co·mus·cu·lar
cer·vi·co-oc·cip·i·tal
cer·vi·co·plas·ty
cer·vi·co·scap·u·lar
cer·vi·co·tho·rac·ic
cer·vi·co·vag·i·ni·tis
cer·vi·co·ves·i·cal
Cer·vi·lax·in
cer·vim·e·ter
cer·vix *pl.* cer·vi·ces
   c. of axon
   c. dentis
   double c.
   c. glandis
   incompetent c.
   c. mallei
   tapiroid c.
   c. uteri
   c. vesicae
ce·ryl
ces — central excitatory state
ce·sar·e·an
CESD — cholesteryl ester
  storage disease
ce·si·um

Ces·tan sign
Ces·tan syndrome
Ces·tan-Che·nais syndrome
Ces·tan-Ray·mond syndrome
ces·ti·ci·dal
Ces·to·da
Ces·to·dar·ia
ces·tode
ces·to·di·a·sis
ces·to·dol·o·gy
ces·toid
Ces·toi·dea
ce·ta·ben so·di·um
cet·al·ko·ni·um chlo·ride
ce·ta·nol
ce·ti·e·dil cit·rate
ce·to·cy·cline hy·dro·chlo·ride
ce·tri·mide
cet·ri·mo·ni·um bro·mide
ce·tyl
ce·tyl·pyr·i·din·i·um chlo·ride
ce·tyl·tri·meth·yl·am·mo·ni·um bro·mide
Ce·va·lin
Ce·vex
Ce-Vi-Sol
ce·vi·tam·ic acid
ceys·sa·tite
CF — calibration factor
  carbolfuchsin
  cardiac failure
  Christmas factor
  citrovorum factor
  complement fixation
  cystic fibrosis
cf — L. confer (bring together, compare)
CFA — complement-fixation antibody
  complete Freund's adjuvant
cff — critical fusion frequency
CFT — complement-fixation test
CFU — colony-forming unit

CGD — chronic granulomatous disease
CGL — chronic granulocytic leukemia
cGMP — cyclic guanosine monophosphate
cGy — centigray
CH — crown-heel (length of fetus)
Chad·dock's reflex
Chad·dock's sign
Chad·wick sign
Cha·gas' disease
Cha·gas-Cruz disease
Cha·gas·ia
cha·gas·ic
cha·go·ma
Chain, Ernst Boris
chain
    A c.
    α c.
    amino-acid side c.
    β c.
    branched c.
    closed c.
    δ c.
    ϵ c.
    electron transport c.
    food c.
    γ c.
    H c.
    heavy c.
    hemolytic c.
    immunoglobulin c.
    J c.
    kappa c.
    L c.
    lambda c.
    lateral c.
    light c.
    μ c.
    nascent polypeptide c.
    nuclear c.
    open c.
    ossicular c.
    respiratory c.
    side c.
    sympathetic c.

chain *(continued)*
    transport polypeptide c.
chair
    birthing c.
    Gardner c.
    pendular c.
cha·la·sia
cha·la·za
cha·la·zi·on *pl.* cha·la·zia,
    cha·la·zi·ons
cha·la·zo·der·mia
chal·co·my·cin
chal·cone
chal·co·sis
    c. corneae
    c. oculi
chal·i·co·sis
chalk
    precipitated c.
    prepared c.
chalk·i·tis
chal·lenge
    fluid c.
chal·one
cha·lon·ic
cha·lu·ni
cha·lyb·e·ate
cham·ae·ce·phal·ic
cham·ae·ceph·a·ly
cham·ae·pro·so·pic
cham·ae·pros·o·py
cham·ber
    Abbé-Zeiss counting c.
    acoustic c.
    air-equivalent ionization c.
    altitude c.
    anterior c. of eye
    aqueous c.
    Atwater's c.
    Atwater-Benedict c.
    Boyden c.
    counting c.
    decompression c.
    diffusion c.
    c's of eye
    free-air ionization c.
    Haldane c.
    hyperbaric c.

cham·ber *(continued)*
    ionization c.
    lethal c.
    multiwire proportional c.
    Petroff-Hauser counting c.
    pocket c.
    posterior c. of eye
    pronephrotic c.
    pulp c.
    rabbit-ear c.
    relief c.
    Sandison-Clark c.
    Storm Van Leeuwen c.
    thimble c.
    Thoma-Zeiss counting c.
    tissue-equivalent
      ionization c.
    vitreous c.
    Zappert's c.
Cham·ber·lain's line
Cham·ber·land's candle
Cham·ber·land's filter
Cham·ber·len forceps
Cham·pe·tier de Ribes' bag
chan·cre
    hard c.
    hunterian c.
    mixed c.
    monorecidive c.
    c. redux
    erosive c.
    fungating c.
    soft c.
    sporotrichotic c.
    sulcus c.
    tuberculous c.
    tularemic c.
chan·cri·form
chan·croid
    phagedenic c.
    serpiginous c.
chan·croi·dal
chan·crous
Chand·ler's disease
change
    Alzheimer's neurofibrillary
      c.
    Armanni-Ebstein c.

change *(continued)*
    Crooke's c's
    Crooke-Russell c's
    E to A c's
    fatty c.
    free energy c.
    harlequin color c.
    tubular hydropic c.
Ch'ang Shan
chan·nel
    acetylcholine c.
    blood c's
    calcium c.
    calcium-sodium c.
    central c.
    fast c.
    gated c.
    c. of Haller
    ligand-gated c.
    lymph c's
    perineural c.
    perivascular c.
    potassium c.
    protein c.
    slow c.
    sodium c.
    thoroughfare c.
    voltage-gated c.
Chante·messe' reaction
Chao·bor·us
    C. lacustris
Cha·oul therapy
Cha·oul tube
chapped
Cha·put's operation
char·ac·ter
    acquired c.
    anal c.
    compound c.
    dominant c.
    epileptic c.
    imvic c's
    mendelian c.
    monogenic c.
    polygenic c.
    primary sex c's
    quantitative c.
    recessive c.

char·ac·ter *(continued)*
    secondary sex c's
    sex-influenced c.
    sex-limited c.
    sex-linked c.
    unit c.
char·ac·ter·ist·ic
    demand c's
char·coal
    activated c.
    animal c.
    dextran-coated c.
    purified animal c.
Char·cot's arthropathy
Char·cot's bath
Char·cot's cirrhosis
Char·cot's disease
Char·cot's fever
Char·cot's foot
Char·cot's gait
Char·cot's joint
Char·cot's syndrome
Char·cot's triad
Char·cot-Bött·cher crystalloid
Char·cot-Bou·chard aneurysm
Char·cot-Ley·den crystals
Char·cot-Ma·rie atrophy
Char·cot-Ma·rie type
Char·cot-Ma·rie-Tooth atrophy
Char·cot-Ma·rie-Tooth disease
Char·cot-Ma·rie-Tooth type
Char·cot-Ma·rie-Tooth-Hoff·man disease
Char·cot-Neu·mann crystals
Char·cot-Weiss-Ba·ker syndrome
char·la·tan
char·la·tan·ism
char·la·tan·ry
Charles' law
Charles' operation
char·ley horse
Char·lin syndrome
Char·lou·is' disease
Charn·ley's hip arthroplasty
Charn·ley's prosthesis
Charn·ley-Muel·ler hip prosthesis

Char·rière scale
Chart. — L. charta (paper)
chart
  alignment c.
  Amsler's c's
  E-type c.
  exposure c.
  flow c.
  Guibor's c.
  Landolt ring c.
  reading c.
  Reuss' color c's
  Snellen's c.
char·tu·la pl. char·tu·lae
chas·ma
chas·ma·to·plas·son
Chas·sai·gnac's tubercle
chaude-pisse
Chauf·fard's syndrome
Chauf·fard-Still syndrome
Chau·li·ac, Guy de
chaul·moo·gric acid
Chaus·sier's areola
Chaus·sier's line
Chau·veau's bacillus
Chau·veau's bacterium
ChB — L. Chirurgiae
  Baccalaureus (Bachelor of
  Surgery)
CHD — congenital heart
  disease
    congestive heart disease
    coronary heart disease
ChD — L. Chirurgiae Doctor
  (Doctor of Surgery)
ChE — cholinesterase
Chea·dle's disease
Chea·tle slit
Chea·tle-Hen·ry hernia
check-bite
Ché·di·ak-Hi·ga·shi syndrome
Ché·di·ak-Stein·brinck-Hi·ga·
  shi anomaly
cheek
  cleft c.
cheek·bone
chei·lec·to·my

chei·lec·tro·pi·on
chei·li·tis
  actinic c.
  allergic c.
  angular c.
  apostematous c.
  commissural c.
  c. exfoliativa
  c. glandularis
  c. glandularis
    apostematosa
  c. granulomatosa
  impetiginous c.
  migrating c.
  mycotic c.
  solar c.
  c. venenata
chei·lo·al·ve·o·los·chi·sis
chei·lo·an·gi·os·co·py
chei·lo·car·ci·no·ma
chei·lo·gnatho·glos·sos·chi·sis
chei·lo·gnatho·pal·a·tos·chi·
  sis
chei·lo·gnatho·pros·o·pos·
  chi·sis
chei·lo·gnath·os·chi·sis
chei·lo·gnatho·ura·nos·chi·sis
chei·lo·pha·gia
chei·lo·plas·ty
chei·lor·rha·phy
chei·los·chi·sis
chei·lo·sis
  angular c.
chei·lo·sto·ma·to·plas·ty
chei·lot·o·my
chei·ra·gra
chei·ral·gia
  c. paresthetica
cheir·ar·thri·tis
chei·ro·bra·chi·al·gia
  c. paresthetica
chei·ro·cin·es·the·sia
chei·rog·no·my
chei·rog·nos·tic
chei·ro·kin·es·the·sia
chei·ro·kin·es·thet·ic
chei·rol·o·gy

chei·ro·meg·a·ly
chei·ro·plas·ty
chei·ro·po·dal·gia
chei·ro·pom·pho·lyx
chei·ro·scope
chei·ro·spasm
che·late
che·la·tion
che·lic·era *pl.* che·lic·erae
chel·i·don
Chel-Iron
chem·abra·sion
chem·a·ne·sia
chem·as·the·nia
chem·ex·fo·li·a·tion
chem·i·cal
    radiomimetic c.
chem·i·co·gen·e·sis
chem·i·co·phys·i·cal
chem·i·co·phys·i·o·log·ic
chemi·lu·mi·nes·cence
chem·ism
chemi·sorp·tion
chem·ist
chem·is·try
    analytical c.
    applied c.
    biological c.
    blood c.
    clinical c.
    colloid c.
    ecological c.
    forensic c.
    histologic c.
    industrial c.
    inorganic c.
    medical c.
    metabolic c.
    mineral c.
    organic c.
    pharmaceutical c.
    physical c.
    physiological c.
    radiation c.
    structural c.
    surface c.
    synthetic c.
che·mo·at·trac·tant

che·mo·au·to·troph
che·mo·au·to·troph·ic
che·mo·bi·ot·ic
che·mo·cau·tery
che·mo·cep·tor
che·mo·co·ag·u·la·tion
che·mo·dec·to·ma
che·mo·dif·fer·en·ti·a·tion
che·mo·dy·ne·sis
che·mo·het·ero·troph
che·mo·het·ero·troph·ic
che·mo·hor·mo·nal
che·mo·im·mu·nol·o·gy
che·mo·ki·ne·sis
che·mo·ki·net·ic
che·mo·litho·troph
che·mo·litho·troph·ic
che·mo·lu·mi·nes·cence
che·mol·y·sis
che·mo·mor·pho·sis
che·mo·nu·cle·ol·y·sis
che·mo-or·gano·troph
che·mo--or·gano·troph·ic
che·mo·pal·li·dec·tomy
che·mo·pal·li·do·thal·a·mec·
    to·my
che·mo·pal·li·dot·o·my
che·mo·phar·ma·co·dy·nam·
    ic
che·mo·phys·i·ol·o·gy
che·mo·pre·ven·tion
che·mo·pro·phy·lax·is
    primary c.
    secondary c.
che·mo·psy·chi·a·try
che·mo·re·cep·tion
che·mo·re·cep·tor
che·mo·re·sis·tance
che·mo·re·sis·tant
che·mo·sen·si·tive
che·mo·sen·sory
che·mo·se·ro·ther·a·py
che·mo·sis
chem·os·mo·sis
chem·os·mot·ic
che·mo·sorp·tion
che·mo·sphere
che·mo·stat

che·mo·ster·il·ant
che·mo·ster·il·iza·tion
che·mo·sup·pres·sion
che·mo·sur·gery
    Mohs'c.
che·mo·syn·the·sis
che·mo·syn·thet·ic
che·mo·tac·tic
che·mo·tax·in
che·mo·tax·is
che·mo·thal·a·mec·to·my
che·mo·thal·a·mot·o·my
che·mo·ther·a·peu·tic
che·mo·ther·a·peu·tics
che·mo·ther·a·py
    adjuvant c.
che·mot·ic
che·mo·trans·mit·ter
che·mo·troph
che·mo·troph·ic
che·mo·trop·ic
che·mo·trop·ism
che·nic acid
che·no·de·oxy·cho·late
che·no·de·oxy·cho·lic acid
che·no·de·oxy·cho·lyl·tau·
  rine
che·no·di·ol
Che·no·po·di·um
che·no·ther·a·py
Cher·chev·ski's (Cher·chew·
  ski's) disease
Che·ron serum
cher·ub·ism
Cher·vin's method
chest
    alar c.
    barrel c.
    blast c.
    cobbler's c.
    emphysematous c.
    fissured c.
    flail c.
    flat c.
    foveated c.
    funnel c.
    hourglass c.
    keeled c.

chest *(continued)*
    paralytic c.
    pendelluft c.
    phthinoid c.
    pigeon c.
    pterygoid c.
    rachitic c.
    stove-in c.
    tetrahedron c.
Chey·le·ti·el·la
    C. blakei
    C. parasitovorax
    C. yasguri
Cheyne's nystagmus
Cheyne-Stokes asthma
Cheyne-Stokes nystagmus
Cheyne-Stokes psychosis
Cheyne-Stokes respiration
CHF — congestive heart
  failure
Chi·a·ri's disease
Chi·a·ri's network
Chi·a·ri's reticulum
Chi·a·ri's syndrome
Chi·a·ri-Ar·nold syndrome
Chi·a·ri-From·mel disease
Chi·a·ri-From·mel syndrome
chi·asm
    campers' c.
    optic c.
    tendinous c. of flexor
      digitorum sublimis
      muscle
chi·as·ma *pl.* chi·as·ma·ta
    c. opticum
chi·as·mal
chi·as·ma·ta
chi·as·mat·ic
chi·as·ma·ty·py
chi·as·mic
chi·as·mom·e·ter
chi·as·tom·e·ter
Chi·ba needle
chick·en·pox
Chie·vitz's layer
Chie·vitz's organ
chig·ger
chig·oe

chik·un·gun·ya
Chi·lai·di·ti's sign
Chi·lai·di·ti's syndrome
chil·blain
Child's hepatic risk
  classification
child·bed
child·birth
child·proof
chi·li·tis
chill
    brass c.
    brazier's c.
    creeping c.
    shaking c.
    spelter c's
    urethral c.
    zinc c.
Chi·log·na·tha
chi·lo·mas·ti·gi·a·sis
Chi·lo·mas·tix
    C. mesnili
chi·lo·mas·to·sis
chi·lo·pa
Chi·lop·o·da
chi·me·ra
    heterologous c.
    homologous c.
    isologous c.
    radiation c.
    tetraparental c.
chi·mer·ism
    blood group c.
chin
    galoche c.
chin·cap
chi·on·ablep·sia
chip
    bone c's
Chi·ra·can·thi·um
chi·ral
chi·ral·i·ty
chi·ro·bra·chi·al·gia
chi·rog·nos·tic
chi·ro·meg·a·ly
Chi·ro·nom·i·dae
Chi·ron·o·mus
chi·ro·plas·ty

chi·ro·po·dal·gia
chi·ro·pod·i·cal
chi·rop·o·dist
chi·rop·o·dy
chi·ro·prac·tic
chi·ro·prac·tor
chi·ro·scope
chi·ro·spasm
chis·el
    binangled c.
    periodontal c.
chi-squared
chi·tin
chi·tin·ase
chi·tin·ous
chi·to·bi·ose
chi·to·san
chi·tose
chi·to·tri·ose
chi·u·fa
chla·my·de·mia
Chla·myd·ia
    C. psittaci
    C. trachomatis
chla·myd·ia *pl.* chla·myd·iae
Chla·myd·i·a·ceae
chla·myd·i·ae
chla·myd·i·al
Chla·myd·i·al·es
chla·myd·i·o·sis
chlam·y·do·spore
chlo·as·ma
    c. gravidarum
chlo·phe·di·a·nol hy·dro·
  chlo·ride
chlor·ac·e·tate es·ter·ase
chlor·a·ce·tic acid
chlor·ac·e·ti·za·tion
chlor·ac·ne
chlo·ral
    c. betaine
    c. hydrate
chlo·ral·ism
chlo·ra·li·za·tion
chlo·ral·ize
chlo·ra·lose
chlor·am·bu·cil
chlo·ra·mine-T

chlor·am·phen·i·col
    c. palmitate
    c. sodium succinate
chlo·rate
chlor·a·zan·il hy·dro·chlo·ride
chlor·bu·tol
chlor·cy·cli·zine hy·dro·chlo·ride
chlor·dan
chlor·dane
chlor·dan·to·in
chlor·de·cone
chlor·di·az·ep·ox·ide
    c. hydrochloride
chlor·dim·or·ine hy·dro·chlo·ride
chlo·rel·lin
chlor·emia
chlor·en·chy·ma
chlor·et·ic
Chlo·re·tone
chlor·gua·nide
chlor·hex·i·dine
    c. acetate
    c. gluconate
    c. hydrochloride
chlor·his·tech·ia
chlor·hy·dria
chlo·ric
chlo·ric acid
chlo·ride
    acid c.
    ferric c.
    mercuric c.
    mercurous c.
    stannous c.
    thallous c. Tl 201
chlo·ri·de·mia
chlo·ri·dim·e·ter
chlo·ri·dim·e·try
chlo·rid·i·on
chlo·ri·dom·e·ter
chlor·id·or·rhea
    familial c.
chlo·ri·du·ria
chlo·ri·nat·ed

chlo·rine
    c. dioxide
chlor·io·dized
chlor·i·son·da·mine chlo·ride
chlo·rite
chlor·mad·i·none ac·e·tate
chlor·mer·o·drin
    c. Hg 197
    c. Hg 203
chlor·meth·az·a·none
chlor·meth·yl
chlor·mez·a·none
chlo·ro·ace·tic acid
chlo·ro·az·o·din
chlo·ro·bright·ism
chlo·ro·bu·ta·nol
chlo·ro·cru·o·rin
chlo·ro·di·ni·tro·ben·zene
chlo·ro·eryth·ro·blas·to·ma
chlo·ro·eth·ane
chlo·ro·form
    acetone c.
    liniment of c.
chlo·ro·form·ism
chlo·ro·form·iza·tion
chlo·ro·gen·ic acid
chlo·ro·gua·nide hy·dro·chlo·ride
chlo·ro·labe
chlo·ro·leu·ke·mia
chlo·ro·lym·pho·sar·co·ma
chlo·ro·ma
p-chlo·ro·mer·cu·ri·ben·zo·ate
chlo·ro·meth·ane
chlo·ro·meth·a·py·ri·line cit·rate
chlo·rom·e·try
Chlo·ro·my·ce·tin
chlo·ro·my·elo·ma
chlo·ro·naph·tha·lene
chlo·ro·pe·nia
chlo·ro·pex·ia
chlo·ro·phane
chlo·ro·phyll
chlo·ro·phyl·lin
chlo·ro·pia
Chlo·rop·i·dae

chlo·ro·plast
chlo·ro·plas·tid
chlo·ro·priv·ic
chlo·ro·pro·caine hy·dro·chlo·
ride
chlo·ro·pro·caine pen·i·cil·lin
chlo·rop·sia
Chlor·op·tic
chlo·ro·pyr·i·lene cit·rate
chlo·ro·quine
    c. hydrochloride
    c. phosphate
chlo·ro·sis
    Egyptian c.
    tropical c.
Chlo·ro·stig·ma
chlo·ro·stig·mine
chlo·ro·sul·fon·ic acid
chlo·ro·then cit·rate
chlo·ro·then·i·um cit·rate
chlo·ro·thi·a·zide
chlo·ro·thy·mol
chlo·rot·ic
chlo·ro·tri·an·i·sene
chlo·rous
chlo·rous acid
chlo·ro·vi·nyl·di·chlo·ro·ar·
sine
chlo·rox·ine
chlo·ro·xy·le·nol
chlor·phen·e·sin
    c. carbamate
chlor·phen·ir·amine
    c. maleate
chlor·phen·ox·amine hy·dro·
chlo·ride
chlor·phen·ter·mine hy·dro·
chlo·ride
chlor·prom·a·zine
    c. hydrochloride
chlor·pro·pa·mide
chlor·pro·phen·py·rid·amine
chlor·pro·thix·ene
chlor·quin·al·dol
chlor·tet·ra·cy·cline
    c. hydrochloride
chlor·thal·i·done
Chlor-Tri·me·ton

chlor·ure·sis
chlor·uret·ic
chlor·uria
chlor·zox·a·zone
ChM — L. Chirurgiae
    Magister (Master of Surgery)
CHO — Chinese hamster
    ovary
cho·a·na *pl.* cho·a·nae
    c. ossae
cho·a·nae
cho·a·nal
cho·a·nate
cho·a·no·cyte
cho·a·no·flag·el·late
cho·a·noid
cho·a·no·mas·ti·gote
choke
    ophthalmovascular c.
    thoracic c.
    water c.
chol·a·gog·ic
chol·a·gogue
cho·la·ic acid
Cho·lan-DH
cho·lane
cho·lan·e·re·sis
cho·lan·ge·itis
cho·lan·gi·ec·ta·sis
cho·lan·gio·ad·e·no·ma
cho·lan·gio·car·ci·no·ma
cho·lan·gio·cho·le·cys·to·cho·
le·doch·ec·tomy
cho·lan·gio·en·ter·os·to·my
cho·lan·gio·gas·tros·to·my
cho·lan·gio·gram
cho·lan·gi·og·ra·phy
    cystic duct c.
    fine needle transhepatic c.
        (FNTC)
    intravenous c.
    operative c.
    transhepatic c.
    transjugular c.
    T-tube c.
cho·lan·gio·hep·a·ti·tis
cho·lan·gio·hep·a·to·ma

cho·lan·gio·je·ju·nos·to·my
  intrahepatic c.
cho·lan·gi·o·lar
cho·lan·gi·ole
cho·lan·gi·o·li·tis
cho·lan·gi·o·ma
cho·lan·gio·pan·cre·a·tog·ra·
  phy
    endoscopic retrograde c.
    (ERCP)
cho·lan·gi·os·to·my
cho·lan·gi·ot·o·my
cho·lan·gi·tis
    chronic nonsuppurative
      destructive c.
    c. lenta
    primary sclerosing c.
    progressive
      nonsuppurative c.
cho·lan·ic acid
cho·lano·poi·e·sis
cho·lano·poi·et·ic
cho·lan·threne
cho·late
cho·le·bil·i·ru·bin
Cho·le·brine
cho·le·cal·ci·fer·ol
cho·le·chro·mo·poi·e·sis
cho·le·cy·a·nin
cho·le·cyst
cho·le·cyst·a·gog·ic
cho·le·cyst·a·gogue
cho·le·cys·tal·gia
cho·le·cys·tat·o·ny
cho·le·cys·tec·ta·sia
cho·le·cys·tec·to·my
cho·le·cys·ten·ter·ic
cho·le·cyst·en·tero·anas·to·
  mo·sis
cho·le·cyst·en·ter·or·rha·phy
cho·le·cyst·en·ter·os·to·my
cho·le·cyst·gas·tros·to·my
cho·le·cys·tic
cho·le·cys·tis
cho·le·cys·ti·tis
    acute c.
    chronic c.
    c. cystica

cho·le·cys·ti·tis *(continued)*
    c. emphysematosa
    emphysematous c.
    follicular c.
    gaseous c.
    c. glandularis proliferans
cho·le·cyst·ne·phros·to·my
cho·le·cys·to·cele
cho·le·cys·to·cho·lan·gio·
  gram
cho·le·cys·to·co·lon·ic
cho·le·cys·to·co·los·to·my
cho·le·cys·to·co·lot·o·my
cho·le·cys·to·du·o·de·nos·to·
  my
cho·le·cys·to-en·dy·sis
cho·le·cys·to·en·ter·os·to·my
cho·le·cys·to·en·ter·ot·o·my
cho·le·cys·to·gas·tric
cho·le·cys·to·gas·tros·to·my
cho·le·cys·to·gog·ic
cho·le·cys·to·gram
cho·le·cys·tog·ra·phy
    post fatty meal c.
cho·le·cys·to·il·e·os·to·my
cho·le·cys·to·in·tes·ti·nal
cho·le·cys·to·je·ju·nos·to·my
cho·le·cys·to·ki·net·ic
cho·le·cys·to·ki·nin
cho·le·cys·to·li·thi·a·sis
cho·le·cys·to·li·thot·o·my
cho·le·cys·to·litho·trip·sy
cho·le·cys·to·ne·phros·to·my
cho·le·cys·top·a·thy
cho·le·cys·to·pexy
cho·le·cys·top·to·sis
cho·le·cys·to·py·elos·to·my
cho·le·cys·tor·rha·phy
cho·le·cys·to·sis
    hyperplastic c.
cho·le·cys·tos·to·my
cho·le·cys·tot·o·my
cho·le·doch·al
cho·le·do·chec·to·my
cho·le·do·chen·dy·sis
cho·le·do·chi·tis
cho·led·o·cho·cele

cho·led·o·cho·chol·e·do·chos·
  to·my
cho·led·o·cho·cys·tos·to·my
cho·led·o·cho·do·chor·rha·
  phy
cho·led·o·cho·du·o·de·nos·to·
  my
cho·led·o·cho·en·ter·os·to·
  my
cho·led·o·cho·gas·tros·to·my
cho·led·o·cho·gram
cho·led·o·chog·ra·phy
cho·led·o·cho·hep·a·tos·to·
  my
cho·led·o·cho·il·e·os·to·my
cho·led·o·cho·je·ju·nos·to·my
cho·led·o·cho·lith
cho·led·o·cho·li·thi·a·sis
cho·led·o·cho·li·thot·o·my
cho·led·o·cho·litho·trip·sy
cho·led·o·cho·neph·ro·scope
cho·led·o·cho·plas·ty
cho·led·o·chor·rha·phy
cho·led·o·cho·scope
cho·led·o·chos·co·py
cho·led·o·chos·to·my
cho·led·o·chot·o·my
cho·led·o·chus
Cho·led·yl
cho·le·glo·bin
cho·le·hem·a·tin
cho·le·ic
cho·le·lith
cho·le·li·thi·a·sis
cho·le·lith·ic
cho·le·li·thot·o·my
cho·le·litho·trip·sy
cho·le·li·thot·ri·ty
cho·lem·e·sis
cho·le·mia
  familial c.
  Gilbert c.
cho·le·mic
cho·le·mim·e·try
cho·le·peri·to·ne·um
cho·le·peri·to·ni·tis
cho·le·poi·e·sis
cho·le·poi·et·ic

cho·le·pra·sin
chol·era
  Asiatic c.
  bilious c.
  dry c.
  European c.
  c. fulminans
  c. infantum
  c. morbus
  pancreatic c.
  c. sicca
  summer c.
chol·er·a·gen
chol·e·ra·ic
chol·er·a·phage
cho·ler·e·sis
cho·ler·et·ic
cho·ler·ia
chol·er·ic
cho·ler·i·form
chol·er·i·gen·ic
chol·er·ig·e·nous
chol·er·oid
chol·er·rha·gia
chol·er·rha·gic
cho·le·scin·ti·gram
cho·le·scin·tig·ra·phy
cho·les·tane
cho·les·ta·nol
  beta-c.
cho·le·sta·sia
  familial intraheptic c.
cho·le·stat·ic
cho·le·ste·a·to·ma
  congenital c.
  intracranial c.
  paranasal sinus c.
  c. tympani
cho·le·ste·a·to·ma·tous
cho·le·ste·a·to·sis
cho·les·tene
cho·les·tero·gen·e·sis
cho·les·tero·his·tech·ia
cho·les·tero·hy·dro·tho·rax
cho·les·ter·ol
  radioiodinated c.
cho·les·ter·ol acyl·trans·fer·
  ase

cho·les·ter·ol des·mol·ase
cho·les·ter·ol·emia
cho·les·ter·ol·er·e·sis
cho·les·ter·ol es·ter·ase
cho·les·ter·ol·es·ter·sturz
cho·les·ter·ol mono·oxy·gen·
ase (side-chain cleaving)
cho·les·ter·olo·poi·e·sis
cho·les·ter·ol sul·fa·tase
cho·les·ter·ol·uria
cho·les·ter·o·sis
    c. cutis
    extracellular c.
cho·les·ty·ra·mine res·in
cho·let·e·lin
cho·le·ther·a·py
cho·le·ver·din
cho·lic
cho·lic acid
cho·line
    acetyl glyceryl ether
      phosphoryl c.
    c. chloride carbamate
    c. magnesium trisalicylate
    phosphatidyl c.
    c. salicylate
    c. theophyllinate
cho·line acet·y·lase
cho·line ac·e·tyl·trans·fer·ase
cho·line·phos·pho·trans·fer·
  ase
cho·lin·er·gic
cho·lin·es·ter·ase
cho·li·no·cep·tive
cho·li·no·cep·tor
cho·li·no·gen·ic
cho·li·no·lyt·ic
cho·li·no·mi·met·ic
cho·li·no·re·ac·tive
cho·li·no·re·cep·tors
cholo·chrome
cholo·cy·a·nin
cholo·ge·net·ic
Cho·lo·gra·fin
cholo·hem·a·tin
cho·lo·he·mo·tho·rax
cholo·tho·rax
Cho·lox·in

chol·uria
chol·uric
cho·lyl·gly·cine
cho·lyl·tau·rine
Chon·do·den·dron
    C. tomentosum
chon·dral
chon·dral·gia
chon·dral·lo·pla·sia
chon·drec·to·my
chon·dric
chon·dri·fi·ca·tion
chon·dri·gen
chon·drin
Chon·dri·na
chon·dri·ome
chon·drio·some
chon·dri·tis
    costal c.
    ear c.
    c. intervertebralis calcanea
chon·dro·ad·e·no·ma
chon·dro·an·gi·o·ma
chon·dro·blast
chon·dro·blas·to·ma
    benign c.
chon·dro·cal·ci·no·sis
chon·dro·car·ci·no·ma
chon·dro·cla·sis
chon·dro·clast
chon·dro·cos·tal
chon·dro·cra·ni·um
chon·dro·cyte
    isogenous c's
chon·dro·der·ma·ti·tis
    c. nodularis chronica
      helicis
chon·dro·dyn·ia
chon·dro·dys·pla·sia
    genotypic c.
    hereditary deforming c.
    hyperplastic c.
    McKusick-type
      metaphyseal c.
    metaphyseal c.
    c. punctata
    rhizomelic type c.

chon·dro·dys·tro·phia
    c. calcificans congenita
    c. congenita punctata
    c. fetalis calcificans
chon·dro·dys·tro·phy
    familial c.
    hereditary deforming c.
    hyperplastic c.
    hypoplastic c.
    hypoplastic fetal c.
    c. malacia
chon·dro·en·do·the·li·o·ma
chon·dro·epi·phys·e·al
chon·dro·epi·phys·itis
chon·dro·fi·bro·ma
chon·dro·gen
chon·dro·gen·e·sis
chon·dro·gen·ic
chon·dro·glos·sus
chon·dro·glu·cose
chon·drog·ra·phy
chon·droid
chon·dro·it·ic
chon·dro·i·tin sul·fate
chon·dro·i·tin·sul·fa·tase
chon·dro·i·tin·uria
chon·dro·li·po·ma
chon·drol·o·gy
chon·drol·y·sis
chon·dro·ma
    joint c.
    c. of lung
    medullary c.
    c. sarcomatosum
    synovial c.
    true c.
chon·dro·ma·la·cia
    c. fetalis
    c. of larynx
    c. patellae
chon·dro·ma·to·sis
    synovial c.
chon·dro·ma·tous
chon·dro·mere
chon·dro·meta·pla·sia
    synovial c.
    tenosynovial c.
chon·dro·mu·cin

chon·dro·mu·coid
chon·dro·mu·co·pro·tein
chon·dro·my·o·ma
chon·dro·myxo·fi·bro·ma
chon·dro·myx·o·ma
chon·dro·myxo·sar·co·ma
chon·dro·ne·cro·sis
chon·dro·os·se·ous
chon·dro·os·teo·dys·tro·phy
chon·dro·path·ia
    c. tuberosa
chon·dro·pa·thol·o·gy
chon·drop·a·thy
chon·dro·phyte
chon·dro·pla·sia
    c. punctata
chon·dro·plast
chon·dro·plas·tic
chon·dro·plas·ty
chon·dro·po·ro·sis
chon·dro·pro·tein
chon·dro·sa·mine
chon·dro·sar·co·ma
    central c.
    juxtacortical c.
    mesenchymal c.
chon·dro·sar·co·ma·to·sis
chon·dro·sar·co·ma·tous
chon·dro·sep·tum
chon·dro·sin
chon·dro·sis
chon·dro·skel·e·ton
chon·dros·te·o·ma
chon·dro·ster·nal
chon·dro·ster·no·plas·ty
chon·dro·tome
chon·drot·o·my
chon·dro·troph·ic
chon·dro·xi·phoid
chon·drus
cho·ne·chon·dro·ster·non
Cho·part's amputation
Cho·part's articulation
Cho·part's joint
Cho·part's operation
Cho·pra's antimony test
cho·ran·gi·o·ma

chord
  condyle c.
chor·da *pl.* chor·dae
  c. dorsalis
  c. gubernaculum
  c. magna
  c. spermatica
  c. spinalis
  c. tendineae cordis
  c. tympani
  c. umbilicalis
  c. vertebralis
  c. vocalis
  chordae Willisii
chor·dae
chor·dal
chor·da-meso·derm
chor·dec·to·my
chor·dee
chor·di·tis
  c. cantorum
  c. fibrinosa
  c. nodosa
  c. tuberosa
  c. vocalis
  c. vocalis inferior
chor·do·blas·to·ma
chor·do·car·ci·no·ma
chor·do·epi·the·li·o·ma
chor·doid
chor·do·ma
chor·do·pexy
chor·do·sar·co·ma
chor·do·skel·e·ton
chor·dot·o·my
chord·ure·thri·tis
cho·rea
  acute c.
  atonic c.
  Bergeron's c.
  chronic progressive
    nonhereditary c.
  c. cordis
  c. cruciata
  dancing c.
  degenerative c.
  diaphragmatic c.
  c. dimidiata

cho·rea *(continued)*
  Dubini c.
  electric c.
  epidemic c.
  c. festinans
  fibrillary c.
  c. gravidarum
  c. gravis
  habit c.
  hemilateral c.
  hemiplegic c.
  Henoch's c.
  hereditary c.
  Huntington's c.
  hyoscine c.
  hysterical c.
  infective c.
  jumping c.
  juvenile c.
  laryngeal c.
  limp c.
  malleatory c.
  methodic c.
  mimetic c.
  c. minor
  c. mollis
  c. nocturna
  c. nutans
  one-sided c.
  paralytic c.
  polymorphous c.
  posthemiplegic c.
  prehemiplegic c.
  rheumatic c.
  saltatory c.
  Schrötter's c.
  senile c.
  simple c.
  Sydenham's c.
  tetanoid c.
cho·re·al
cho·re·at·ic
cho·re·ic
cho·re·i·form
cho·reo·ath·e·toid
cho·reo·ath·e·to·sis
  paroxysmal familial c.
  paroxysmal kinesogenic c.

cho·re·oid
cho·reo·ma·nia
cho·ri·al
cho·rio·ad·e·no·ma
   c. destruens
cho·rio·al·lan·to·ic
cho·rio·al·lan·to·is
cho·rio·am·ni·on·ic
cho·rio·am·ni·o·ni·tis
cho·rio·an·gio·fi·bro·ma
cho·rio·an·gi·o·ma
cho·rio·an·gi·op·a·gus par·a·
  si·ti·cus
cho·rio·blas·to·ma
cho·rio·blas·to·sis
cho·rio·cap·il·la·ris
cho·rio·car·ci·no·ma
cho·rio·cele
cho·rio·epi·the·li·o·ma
   c. malignum
cho·rio·gen·e·sis
cho·ri·oid
cho·ri·oi·dea
cho·ri·o·ma
cho·rio·mam·mo·tro·pin
cho·rio·men·in·gi·tis
   lymphocytic c.
cho·ri·on
   c. avillosum
   c. frondosum
   c. laeve
   primitive c.
   shaggy c.
   c. villosum
cho·ri·on·epi·the·li·o·ma
cho·ri·on·ic
cho·rio·pla·cen·tal
cho·rio·plaque
Cho·ri·op·tes
cho·rio·ret·i·nal
cho·rio·ret·i·ni·tis
   c. sclopetaria
   toxoplasmic c.
cho·rio·ret·i·nop·a·thy
chor·is·mate
cho·ris·mic acid
cho·ris·ta
cho·ris·to·blas·to·ma

cho·ris·to·ma
cho·roid
cho·roi·dal
cho·roi·dea
cho·roi·dec·to·my
cho·roi·der·e·mia
cho·roi·di·tis
   anterior c.
   areolar c.
   central c.
   diffuse c.
   disseminated c.
   Doyne's familial
    honeycombed c.
   exudative c.
   focal c.
   Förster's c.
   c. guttata senilis
   Jensen's c.
   juxtapapillary c.
   macular c.
   metastatic c.
   senile macular exudative c.
   c. serosa
   suppurative c.
   Tay's c.
cho·roi·do·cyc·li·tis
cho·roi·do·iri·tis
cho·roi·dop·a·thy
   areolar c.
   guttate c.
cho·roi·do·ret·i·ni·tis
cho·rol·o·gy
chor·tos·ter·ol
Chot·zen syndrome
Chris·ten·sen-Krab·be disease
Chris·ten·sen-Krab·be
  poliodystrophy
Chris·tian's disease
Chris·tian's syndrome
Chris·tian-Web·er disease
Christ·i·son's formula
Christ·mas disease
Christ·mas factor
Christ·mas tree pattern
Christ-Sie·mens-Tou·raine
  syndrome
Chro·bak's test

chro·maf·fin
chro·maf·fin·i·ty
chro·maf·fi·no·ma
    medullary c.
chro·maf·fi·nop·a·thy
chro·man
chro·ma·phil
chro·mar·gen·taf·fin
chro·mate
chro·mat·ic
chro·ma·tid
    nonsister c's
    sister c's
chro·ma·tin
    nucleolar-associated c.
    nucleolus-associated c.
    sex c.
chro·ma·tin·ic
chro·ma·tin-neg·a·tive
chro·ma·tin-pos·i·tive
chro·ma·tism
chro·ma·tize
chro·ma·to·blast
chro·ma·to·cyte
chro·ma·to·ge·nous
chro·ma·to·gram
chro·ma·to·graph
chro·ma·to·graph·ic
chro·ma·tog·ra·phy
    adsorption c.
    affinity c.
    antibody affinity c.
    column c.
    electric c.
    filter paper c.
    gas c. (GC)
    gas-liquid c. (GLC)
    gas-solid c. (GSC)
    gel-filtration c.
    gel-permeation c.
    high-performance liquid c.
    high-pressure liquid c.
      (HPLC)
    ion-exchange c.
    liquid-liquid c.
    molecular sieve c.
    paper c.
    partition c.

chro·ma·tog·ra·phy
    (continued)
    thin-layer c. (TLC)
    two-dimensional c.
chro·ma·toid
chro·ma·to·ki·ne·sis
chro·ma·tol·o·gy
chro·ma·tol·y·sis
chro·ma·tom·e·ter
chro·ma·to·pec·tic
chro·ma·to·pex·is
chro·ma·toph·a·gus
chro·ma·to·phil
chro·ma·to·phil·ia
chro·ma·to·phil·ic
chro·ma·toph·i·lous
chro·ma·to·phore
chro·ma·to·pho·ro·trop·ic
chro·ma·to·plasm
chro·ma·to·plast
chro·ma·top·sia
chro·ma·top·tom·e·ter
chro·ma·top·tom·e·try
chro·ma·to·scope
chro·ma·tos·co·py
    gastric c.
chro·ma·to·sis
chro·ma·to·ski·am·e·ter
chro·ma·to·tax·is
chro·ma·to·trop·ism
chro·ma·tu·ria
chrome he·ma·toxy·lin
1,2-chro·mene
chro·mes·the·sia
chrom·hi·dro·sis
chro·mic acid
chro·mi·cize
chro·mid·i·um
chro·mi·um
    c. trioxide
Chro·mo·bac·te·ri·um
    C. violaceum
chro·mo·blast
chro·mo·blas·to·my·co·sis
chro·mo·cen·ter
chro·mo·cho·los·co·py
chro·mo·clas·to·gen·ic
chro·mo·cys·tos·co·py

chro·mo·cyte
chro·mo·dac·ry·or·rhea
chro·mo·di·ag·no·sis
chro·mo·fla·vine
chro·mo·gen
    Porter-Silber c's
chro·mo·gene
chro·mo·gen·e·sis
chro·mo·gen·ic
chro·mo·gran·in
chro·mo·hy·dro·tu·ba·tion
chro·mo·isom·er·ism
chro·mo·lip·oid
chro·mol·y·sis
chro·mo·mere
chro·mom·e·ter
chro·mo·my·co·sis
chro·mo·nar hy·dro·chlo·ride
chro·mone
chro·mo·ne·ma *pl.* chro·mo·
  ne·ma·ta
chro·mo·ne·mal
chro·mo·ne·ma·ta
chro·mo·nu·cle·ic acid
chro·mo·par·ic
chro·mo·pec·tic
chro·mo·per·tu·ba·tion
chro·mo·pex·ic
chro·mo·pexy
chro·mo·phage
chro·mo·phane
chro·mo·phil
chro·mo·phil·ic
chro·moph·i·lous
chro·mo·phobe
chro·mo·pho·bia
chro·mo·phore
chro·mo·phor·ic
chro·moph·o·rous
chro·mo·phose
chro·mo·pho·to·ther·a·py
chro·mo·plasm
chro·mo·plast
chro·mo·plas·tid
chro·mo·pro·tein
chro·mop·sia
chro·mop·tom·e·ter
chro·mo·ret·i·nog·ra·phy

chro·mo·rhi·nor·rhea
chro·mo·san·to·nin
chro·mo·scope
chro·mos·co·py
chro·mo·so·mal
chro·mo·some
  accessory c's
  acentric c.
  acrocentric c.
  B c.
  bivalent c.
  daughter c's
  dicentric c.
  fragile X c.
  gametic c.
  giant c's
  heteromorphic c.
  heterotypical c's
  homologous c's
  lampbrush c's
  late replicating X c.
  m-c.
  metacentric c.
  mitochondrial c.
  mitotic c.
  monocentric c.
  nonhomologous c's
  nucleolar c's
  odd c's
  Ph^1 c.
  Philadelphia c.
  polytene c's
  ring c.
  sex c's
  small c.
  somatic c.
  submetacentric c.
  subtelocentric c.
  supernumerary c.
  telocentric c.
  W c's
  X c.
  Y c.
  Z c's
chro·mo·sperm·ism
chro·mo·ther·a·py
chro·mo·tox·ic
chro·mo·trich·ia

chro·mo·trich·i·al
chro·mo·trop·ic
chro·mo·ure·ter·os·co·py
chro·mo·uri·nog·ra·phy
chro·naxy
chron·ic
chro·nic·i·ty
chro·nio·sep·sis
chrono·bio·log·ic
chron·o·bi·ol·o·gist
chron·o·bi·ol·o·gy
chron·og·no·sis
chron·o·graph
chro·nom·e·try
    mental c.
chron·o·pho·bia
chron·o·pho·to·graph
chron·o·scope
chron·o·sphyg·mo·graph
chro·no·tar·ax·is
chron·o·trop·ic
chron·o·trop·ism
chro·to·plast
chrys·a·lis
chrys·a·ro·bin
chrys·a·zin
chry·si·a·sis
chryso·der·ma
chryso·mo·nad
Chryso·mo·nad·i·da
Chryso·my·ia
    C. albiceps
    C. bezziana
    C. macellaria
chryso·pho·re·sis
Chrys·ops
    C. cecutiens
    C. dimidiata
    C. discalis
    C. silacea
Chryso·spo·ri·um
    C. pruinosum
chryso·ther·a·py
chryso·tile
Chryso·zo·na
Churg-Strauss syndrome
chur·gan·ja
Chvos·tek's sign

Chvos·tek's symptom
Chvos·tek's test
Chvos·tek-Weiss sign
chy·lan·gi·o·ma
chyl·aque·ous
chyle
chyl·ec·ta·sia
chy·le·mia
chy·li·fa·cient
chy·li·fac·tion
chy·li·fac·tive
chy·lif·er·ous
chy·li·fi·ca·tion
chy·li·form
chy·lo·cele
    parasitic c.
chy·lo·cyst
chy·lo·der·ma
chy·loid
chy·lol·o·gy
chy·lo·me·di·as·ti·num
chy·lo·mi·cro·graph
chy·lo·mi·cron *pl.* chyl·lo·mi·
    crons, chy·lo·mi·cra
chy·lo·mi·cro·ne·mia
chy·lo·peri·car·di·tis
chy·lo·peri·car·di·um
chy·lo·peri·to·ne·um
chy·lo·phor·ic
chy·lo·pleu·ra
chy·lo·pneu·mo·tho·rax
chy·lo·poi·e·sis
chy·lo·poi·et·ic
chy·lor·rhea
chy·lo·sis
chy·lo·tho·rax
chy·lous
chy·lu·ria
chy·lus
Chy·mar
chy·mase
chyme
Chy·mex
chy·mi·fi·ca·tion
chy·mo·nu·cle·ol·y·sis
chy·mo·pa·pa·in
chy·mor·rhea
chy·mo·sin

chy·mo·tryp·sin
   c. alpha
   sterile c.
chy·mo·tryp·sin·o·gen
chy·mo·tryp·tic
chy·mous
chy·mus
Chy·trid·i·a·les
Chy·trid·io·my·ce·tes
Chy·trid·i·um
CI — color index
   Colour Index
   coronary insufficiency
Ci — curie
Ciac·cio's glands
Ciac·cio's method
Ciac·cio's stain
Cib. — L. cibus (food)
cic·a·trec·to·my
ci·ca·tri·ces
ci·ca·tri·cial
cic·a·tri·cot·o·my
cic·a·trix *pl.* cic·a·tri·ces
   filtering c.
   hypertrophic c.
   manometric c.
   meningocerebral c.
   vicious c.
cic·at·ri·zant
cic·a·tri·za·tion
cic·a·trize
cic·la·frine hy·dro·chlo·ride
cic·lo·pir·ox ol·amine
ci·clo·pro·fen
Cic·u·ta
   C. maculata
   C. virosa
cic·u·tism
cic·u·tox·in
CID — cytomegalic inclusion
   disease
Ci·dex
CIE — counterimmunoelectro-
   phoresis
CIF — clonal inhibitory factor
ci·gua·te·ra
CIH — Certificate in
   Industrial Health

Ci-hr — curie-hour
cil·ia
cil·i·a·ris
cil·i·ar·i·scope
cil·i·ar·ot·o·my
cil·i·ary
cil·ia·static
Cil·i·a·ta
cil·i·ate
cil·i·at·ed
cil·i·a·tion
cil·i·ec·to·my
cil·io·cy·to·phor·ia
cil·io·gen·e·sis
Cil·i·oph·o·ra
cil·i·oph·o·ran
cil·io·ret·i·nal
cil·io·scle·ral
cil·io·spi·nal
cil·i·ot·o·my
cil·io·tox·ic·i·ty
cil·i·um *pl.* cil·ia
   olfactory cilia
cil·lo
Cil·lo·bac·te·ri·um
cil·lo·sis
cim·bia
ci·met·i·dine
Ci·mex
   C. boueti
   C. hemipterus
   C. lectularius
   C. pilosellus
   C. pipistrella
   C. rotundatus
ci·mex *pl.* ci·mi·ces
ci·mi·cid
Ci·mic·i·dae
Cim·i·cif·u·ga
cim·i·co·sis
CIN — cervical intraepithelial
   neoplasia
cin·an·es·the·sia
cinch·ing
Cin·cho·na
cin·cho·na
cin·chon·ic

cin·chon·ic ac·id hy·dro·chlo·ride
cin·cho·ni·dine
cin·cho·nine
cin·cho·nin·ic acid
cin·cho·nism
cin·cli·sis
cinc·tured
cine-esoph·a·go·gram
cine·an·gio·car·diog·ra·phy
cine·an·gio·gram
cine·an·gio·graph
cine·an·gi·og·ra·phy
    radionuclide c.
cine·den·sig·ra·phy
cine·flu·o·rog·ra·phy
cine·flu·o·ros·co·py
cine·mi·crog·ra·phy
    time-lapse c.
cin·e·ol
cin·e·paz·et mal·e·ate
cine·phle·bog·ra·phy
cine·ra·di·og·ra·phy
ci·ne·rea
ci·ne·re·al
cin·er·i·tious
cine·roent·geno·flu·o·rog·ra·phy
cine·roent·gen·og·ra·phy
cin·es·al·gia
cine·urog·ra·phy
cin·ges·tol
cin·gu·la
cin·gule
cin·gu·lec·to·my
cin·gu·lot·o·my
cin·gu·lum *pl.* cin·gu·la
    c. athleticum
    c. dentis
    c. extremitatis inferioris
    c. extremitatis superioris
    c. hemispherii
    c. membri inferioris
    c. pelvicum
    c. membri superioris
    c. pectorale
cin·gu·lum·ot·o·my
cin·na·bar

cin·na·mal·de·hyde
cin·na·mene
cin·nam·ic
cin·nam·ic acid
cin·na·mol
Cin·na·mo·mum
cin·na·mon
cin·nar·i·zine
cin·no·pen·ta·zone
cin·ox·a·cin
cin·ox·ate
cin·ro·mide
cin·ta·zone
ci·o·nec·to·my
Ci·o·nel·la
Ci·o·nel·li·dae
ci·o·ni·tis
ci·on·op·to·sis
ci·o·nor·rha·phy
ci·on·o·tome
ci·o·not·o·my
cip·ro·ci·no·nide
ci·pro·fi·brate
cir·ca·di·an
cir·can·nu·al
cir·cel·lus
cir·ci·nate
cir·cle
    arterial c.
    arterial c. of Willis
    Berry's c's
    c. of Carus
    c. of confusion
    defensive c.
    c. of dispersion
    c. of dissipation
    c. of Haller
    c. of Hovius
    Huguier's c.
    Latham's c.
    Minsky's c's
    Robinson's c.
    sensory c.
    vascular c.
    venous c. of mammary
      gland
    Vieth-Müller c.
    c's of Weber

cir·cle *(continued)*
    c. of Willis
    c. of Zinn
cir·clet
Circ·O·lec·tric bed
cir·cuit
    analog c.
    Bain c.
    breathing c.
    coincidence c.
    constant potential c.
    full-wave c.
    gate c.
    Magill-Mapleson c.
    open c.
    Papez c.
    quenching c.
    reflex c.
    reverberating c.
    scaling c.
    short c.
cir·cu·lar
cir·cu·la·tion
    allantoic c.
    assisted c.
    chorionic c.
    collateral c.
    compensatory c.
    coronary c.
    cross c.
    derivative c.
    embryonic c.
    enterohepatic c.
    extracorporeal c.
    fetal c.
    first c.
    fourth c.
    greater c.
    hypophyseoportal c.
    intervillous c.
    lesser c.
    lymph c.
    omphalomesenteric c.
    persistent fetal c.
    placental c.
    plasmatic c.
    portal c.
    portoumbilical c.

cir·cu·la·tion *(continued)*
    primitive c.
    pulmonary c.
    sinusoidal c.
    systemic c.
    thebesian c.
    umbilical c.
    vertebral-basilar c.
    vitelline c.
cir·cu·la·to·ry
cir·cu·lus *pl.* cir·cu·li
    c. arteriosus
    c. arteriosus halleri
    c. arteriosus [Willisi]
    c. umbilicalis
    c. vasculosus
    c. venosus halleri
    c. venosus hovii
    c. venosus ridleyi
    c. willisii
    c. zinnii
cir·cum·anal
cir·cum·ar·tic·u·lar
cir·cum·ax·il·lary
cir·cum·buc·cal
cir·cum·bul·bar
cir·cum·cal·lo·sal
cir·cum·cise
cir·cum·ci·sion
    female c.
    pharaonic c.
    Sunna c.
cir·cum·clu·sion
cir·cum·cor·ne·al
cir·cum·cres·cent
cir·cum·duc·tion
cir·cum·fer·ence
    articular c.
    occipitofrontal c. (OFC)
cir·cum·fer·en·tia
    c. articularis
    c. articularis capitis ulnae
    c. articularis capituli ulnae
    c. articularis radii
cir·cum·fer·en·tial
cir·cum·flex
cir·cum·flex·us
cir·cum·gem·mal

cir·cum·in·su·lar
cir·cum·in·tes·ti·nal
cir·cum·len·tal
cir·cum·nu·cle·ar
cir·cum·oc·u·lar
cir·cum·ol·i·vary
cir·cum·oral
cir·cum·or·bi·tal
cir·cum·pen·nate
cir·cum·po·la·ri·za·tion
cir·cum·re·nal
cir·cum·scribed
cir·cum·scrip·tus
cir·cum·stan·ti·al·i·ty
Cir·cum·straint
cir·cum·val·late
cir·cum·vas·cu·lar
cir·cum·vo·lute
cir·cus se·nil·is
cir·rhog·e·nous
cir·rhon·o·sus
cir·rho·sis
    acholangic biliary c.
    acute juvenile c.
    alcoholic c.
    atrophic c.
    bacterial c.
    biliary c.
    calculus c.
    cardiac c.
    Charcot's c.
    congenital hepatic c.
    congestive c.
    Cruveilhier-Baumgarten c.
    cryptogenic c.
    decompensated c.
    fatty c.
    Glisson c.
    Hanot's c.
    hypertrophic c.
    Indian childhood c.
    Laënnec's c.
    macronodular c.
    malarial c.
    c. mammae
    metabolic c.
    micronodular c.
    multilobular c.

cir·rho·sis *(continued)*
    obstructive c.
    pericholangiolitic c.
    periportal c.
    pigment c.
    pigmentary c.
    pipe stem c.
    portal c.
    posthepatitic c.
    postnecrotic c.
    primary biliary c.
    pulmonary c.
    secondary biliary c.
    stasis c.
    syphilitic c.
    Todd's c.
    toxic c.
    unilobular c.
    vascular c.
cir·rhot·ic
cir·rus *pl.* cir·ri
cir·sec·to·my
cir·sen·chy·sis
cir·so·cele
cir·sod·e·sis
cir·soid
cir·som·pha·los
cir·soph·thal·mia
cir·so·tome
cir·sot·o·my
CIS — carcinoma in situ
cis·clo·mi·phene
cis·pla·tin
cis-plat·i·num
11-*cis* ret·i·nal
cis·sa
Cis·sam·pe·los
cis·tern
    anterolateral cerebellar c.
    basal c.
    cerebellomedullary c.
    chiasmatic c.
    chyle c.
    great c.
    interpeduncular c.
    lumbar c.
    c. of Pecquet
    pontine c.

cis·tern *(continued)*
    posterior c.
    subarachnoidal c's
    supracallosal c.
    c. of Sylvius
    terminal c's
cis·ter·na *pl.* cis·ter·nae
    c. ambiens
    c. basalis
    c. caryothecae
    c. cerebellomedullaris
    c. chiasmatis
    c. chyli
    c. corporis callosi
    c. fossae lateralis cerebri
    c. fossae Sylvii
    c. intercruralis profunda
    c. interpeduncularis
    c. laminae terminalis
    c. lateralis pontis
    c. lumbalis
    c. magna
    perinuclear c.
    cisternae
      subarachnoideales
    c. sulci lateralis
    c. Sylvii
    c. valleculae lateralis
      cerebri
    c. venae magnae cerebri
cis·ter·nae
cis·ter·nal
cis·ter·no·gram
cis·ter·no·graph·ic
cis·ter·nog·ra·phy
    oxygen c.
    radionuclide c.
cis·tron
Ci·ta·nest
Ci·tel·li-Melt·zer atticus
  punch
Ci·tel·li's syndrome
cit·rate
    cupric c.
    ferric c.
    c. phosphate dextrose
    (CPD)

cit·rate *(continued)*
    c. phosphate dextrose
    adenine (CPDA-1)
cit·rate lyase
cit·rat·ed
cit·rate syn·thase
cit·rate (si)-syn·thase
ci·treo·vir·i·din
cit·ric acid
Cit·ro·bac·ter
    C. amalonaticus
    C. diversus
    C. freundii
    C. intermedius
cit·ron·el·la
cit·ro·phos·phate
cit·rul·line
cit·rul·lin·emia
cit·rul·lin·uria
ci·tru·ria
Cit·rus
cit·ta
cit·to·sis
Civ·atte's poikiloderma
Civ·i·a·le's operation
Ci·vi·ni·ni's ligament
Ci·vi·ni·ni's process
Ci·vi·ni·ni's spine
CK — creatine kinase
clad·i·o·sis
Cla·do's anastomosis
Cla·do's band
Cla·dor·chis wat·so·ni
clad·o·spo·ri·o·sis
Clado·spo·ri·um
cla·moxy·quin hy·dro·chlo·
  ride
clamp
    anastomosis c.
    Berens muscle c.
    bone c.
    cervical punch biopsy c.
    Cope's c.
    cotton roll rubber dam c.
    Crile's c.
    crushing c.
    Crutchfield c.
    Doyen's c.

clamp *(continued)*
    fenestrated c.
    Gant's c.
    gingival c.
    Goldblatt's c.
    hemostatic c.
    Joseph's c.
    lever-compression c.
    Liddle aorta c.
    Martel's c.
    microvascular c.
    Mikulicz's c.
    Noon AV fistula c.
    occlusion c.
    Payr c.
    pedicle c.
    Potts' c.
    Rankin c.
    rubber dam c.
    Sehrt's c.
    Selverstone c.
    towel c.
    vascular c.
    voltage c.
    Willett c.
    Yellen c.
clamping
    euglycemic c.
clang
clang·ing
clap·o·tage
cla·pote·ment
claque·ment
    c. d'ouverture
Clara cells
clar·if·i·cant
clar·i·fi·ca·tion
clar·i·fy
Clark-Col·lip method
Clarke's cells
Clarke's column
Clarke's nucleus
Clarke-Mon·a·kow nucleus
clas·mato·cyte
clas·mato·cy·to·sis
clas·mato·den·dro·sis
clas·ma·to·sis

clas·mo·cy·to·ma
clasp
    Adams c.
    arrow c.
    arrowhead c.
    bar c.
    circumferential c.
    continuous c.
    continuous lingual c.
    Crozat c.
    wrought c.
class-in·ter·val
clas·si·fi·ca·tion
    adansonian c.
    Angle's c.
    Arneth's c.
    Astler-Coller c.
    Bergey's c.
    Berman c. of pelves
    Black's c.
    Broders' c.
    Caldwell-Moloy c.
    Chicago c.
    Child's hepatic risk c.
    Clark c.
    Denver c.
    Duane's c.
    Dukes' c.
    FIGO c.
    French-American-British
      (FAB) c.
    Gell and Coombs c.
    Goldstein's c.
    Griffith's c.
    Head's c.
    Henry's c.
    Hunt and Hess
      neurological c.
    Jansky's c.
    Jewett's c.
    Karnofsky status c.
    Kauffman-White c.
    Keith-Wagener (K-W) c.
    Keith-Wagener-Barker c.
    Kennedy c.
    Kiel c.
    Kleist's c.

clas·si·fi·ca·tion *(continued)*
 Kraepelin's c.
 Lancefield c.
 Landsteiner c.
 Lukes-Butler c.
 Lukes-Collins c.
 Luria's c.
 McNeer c.
 Migula's c.
 Moss'c.
 Neer c.
 New York Heart
  Association (NYHA) c.
 numerical c.
 Papanicolaou c.
 Paris c.
 Rappaport c.
 Reese-Ellsworth c.
 Runyon c.
 Rye c.
 Schilling c.
 Skinner c.
 TNM (tumor, node,
  metastasis) c.
 van Heuven's c.
 White's c.
 Wiberg c.
 Wullstein c.
clas·tic
clas·to·gen·ic
clas·to·thrix
clath·rate
clath·rin
Clau·berg's test
Claude, Albert
Claude's hyperkinesis sign
Claude's syndrome
Claude and Lher·mitte
 syndrome
clau·di·cant
clau·di·ca·tion
 intermittent c.
 jaw c.
 venous c.
clau·di·ca·tory
Clau·di·us' cell
claus·tra
claus·tral

claus·tro·phil·ia
claus·tro·pho·bia
claus·trum *pl.* claus·tra
 c. gutturis
 c. oris
 c. virginale
cla·va
cla·va·cin
cla·val
cla·vate
cla·va·tion
Clavi·ceps
Clav·i·cip·i·ta·ceae
Clav·i·cip·i·ta·les
clav·i·cle
clav·i·cot·o·my
cla·vic·u·la
cla·vic·u·lar
cla·vic·u·lec·to·my
cla·vic·u·lus *pl.* cla·vic·u·li
clav·i·for·min
clav·i·pec·to·ral
cla·vus *pl.* cla·vi
 c. hystericus
claw·foot
claw·hand
cla·zo·lam
cla·zo·li·mine
clear·ance
 p-aminohippurate c.
 blood-urea c.
 creatinine c.
 fractional c. of dextran
 free water c.
 immune c.
 interocclusal c.
 inulin c.
 occlusal c.
 osmolal c.
 plasma iron c.
 sodium *p*-aminohippuric
  (PAH) acid c.
 urea c.
cleav·age
 accessory c.
 adequal c.
 complete c.
 determinate c.

cleav·age *(continued)*
    discoidal c.
    equal c.
    equatorial c.
    holoblastic c.
    incomplete c.
    indeterminate c.
    latitudinal c.
    meridional c.
    meroblastic c.
    partial c.
    radial c.
    spiral c.
    superficial c.
    total c.
    unequal c.
cleft
    anal c.
    branchial c.
    cervical c's
    cholesterol c.
    clunial c.
    coelomic c.
    corneal c.
    facial c.
    fetal c.
    genal c.
    genital c.
    gill c.
    gingival c.
    gluteal c.
    hyobranchial c.
    hyoid c.
    hyomandibular c.
    interdental c.
    intergluteal c.
    Lanterman's c's
    Larrey's c.
    Maurer's c's
    middle ear c.
    natal c.
    orbitonasal c.
    pharyngeal c.
    posthyoidean c.
    pudendal c.
    Santorini's c.
    Schmidt-Lanterman c's
    Sondergaard's c.

cleft *(continued)*
    Stillman's c.
    submucous c.
    synaptic c.
    tubotympanic c.
    visceral c's
    vulval c.
clegs
clei·dag·ra
clei·dal
clei·dar·thri·tis
clei·do·cos·tal
clei·do·cra·ni·al
clei·do·mas·toid
clei·do-oc·cip·i·tal
clei·dor·rhex·is
clei·do·scap·u·lar
clei·do·ster·nal
clei·do·hu·mer·al
clei·sag·ra
cleis·to·the·ci·um
Cle·land's ligament
clem·as·tine
    c. fumarate
Clem·a·tis
clem·i·zole
    c. hydrochloride
    c. penicillin
clench·ing
Cle·o·cin
cle·oid
Clé·ram·bault-Kan·din·sky
    complex
Clé·ram·bault-Kan·din·sky
    syndrome
Cleth·ri·ono·mys
    C. glariolus
Clev·en·ger's fissure
click
    ejection c's
    mitral c.
    Ortolani's c.
    systolic c's
cli·din·i·um bro·mide
cli·mac·ter·ic
cli·ma·to·ther·a·peu·tics
cli·ma·to·ther·a·py
clin·ar·thro·sis

clin·da·my·cin
    c. hydrochloride
    c. palmitate hydrochloride
    c. phosphate
cline
clin·ic
    ambulant c.
    dry c.
clin·i·cal
cli·ni·cian
    nurse c.
clin·i·co·ge·net·ic
clin·i·co·patho·log·ic
clin·i·co·pa·thol·o·gy
Clin·i·stix
Clin·i·test
Cli·ni·tron bed
cli·no·ceph·a·lism
cli·no·ceph·a·ly
cli·no·dac·tyl·ism
cli·no·dac·ty·ly
cli·nog·ra·phy
cli·noid
cli·nol·o·gy
cli·nom·e·ter
cli·no·scope
cli·no·stat·ic
cli·no·stat·ism
cli·no·ther·a·py
cli·o·quin·ol
cli·ox·a·nide
CLIP — corticotropin-like
  intermediate lobe peptide
clip
    Acland c.
    catheter c.
    dura c.
    Hulka c.
    skin c.
    towel c.
cli·pro·fen
clis·e·om·e·ter
Clis·tin
cli·tel·lum
clit·i·on
Cli·to·cy·be
clit·o·cy·bine
clit·o·ral

clit·o·ral·gia
clit·o·rec·to·my
clit·o·rid·auxe
clit·o·rid·e·an
clit·o·ri·dec·to·my
clit·o·ri·di·tis
clit·o·ri·dot·o·my
clit·o·ri·meg·a·ly
clit·o·ris
clit·o·rism
clit·o·ri·tis
clit·o·ro·plas·ty
clit·o·rot·o·my
clit·or·rha·gia
cli·val
cli·vog·ra·phy
cli·vus
    basilar c.
    c. basilaris
    Blumenbach's c.
    c. monticuli
    c. ossis occipitalis
    c. ossis sphenoidalis
CLL — chronic lymphocytic
  leukemia
clo
clo·a·ca *pl.* clo·a·cae
    congenital c.
    ectodermal c.
    entodermal c.
    persistent c.
    ventral c.
clo·a·cal
clo·a·ci·tis
clo·a·co·gen·ic
clo·ba·zam
clock
    aging c.
    biological c.
clo·cor·to·lone
clo·dan·o·lene
clo·da·zon hy·dro·chlo·ride
clo·dron·ic acid
clo·fa·zi·mine
clo·fen·am·ic acid
clo·fi·brate
clo·ges·tone ac·e·tate
clo·ma·cran phos·phate

Clo·mid
clo·mi·phene cit·rate
clo·mip·ra·mine hy·dro·chlo·
    ride
clon·al
clo·nal·i·ty
clo·naz·e·pam
clone
    forbidden c.
clon·ic
clo·nic·i·ty
clon·i·co·ton·ic
clo·ni·dine hy·dro·chlo·ride
clon·ing
    DNA c.
clon·ism
clo·nis·mus
clo·nix·er·il
clo·nix·in
clo·no·gen·ic
clono·graph
Clon·o·pin
clo·nor·chi·a·sis
clo·nor·chi·o·sis
Clo·nor·chis si·nen·sis
clono·spasm
clo·no·type
clo·nus
    ankle c.
    anodal closure c. (ACCl)
    anodal opening c. (AOCl)
    cathodal closure c. (CCCl)
    cathodal opening c. (COCl)
    drawn ankle c.
    foot c.
    patellar c.
    toe c.
    wrist c.
C-loop of duodenum
clo·pa·mide
Clo·pane
clo·pen·thix·ol
clo·pi·dol
clo·pim·o·zide
clo·pi·rac
clo·pred·nol
clo·pros·te·nol
Clo·quet's canal

Clo·quet's fascia
Clo·quet's ganglion
Clo·quet's hernia
Clo·quet's ligament
Clo·quet's pseudoganglion
clor·az·e·pate
    c. dipotassium
    c. monopotassium
clor·a·zep·ic acid
clor·ex·o·lone
clo·ro·per·one hy·dro·chlo·
    ride
clor·o·phene
Clor·pac·tin XCB
clor·pren·a·line hy·dro·chlo·
    ride
clor·ter·mine hy·dro·chlo·ride
clo·san·tel
clo·sir·amine ac·e·tur·ate
clos·trid·ia
clos·trid·i·al
clos·trid·io·pep·ti·dase
Clos·trid·i·um
    C. bifermentans
    C. botulinum
    C. butyricum
    C. cadaveris
    C. clostridiiforme
    C. difficile
    C. haem-olyticum
    C. histolyticum
    C. innocuum
    C. kluyveri
    C. limosum
    C. novyi
    C. perfringens
    C. ramosum
    C. septicum
    C. sordellii
    C. sphenoides
    C. sporogenes
    C. subterminale
    C. tertium
    C. tetani
    C. welchii
clos·trid·i·um *pl.* clos·trid·ia
clo·sure
    delayed primary c.

clo·sure *(continued)*
    flask c.
    Tom Jones c.
    velopharyngeal c.
clo·sy·late
clot
    agonal c.
    antemortem c.
    autologous c.
    blood c.
    chicken fat c.
    currant jelly c.
    distal c.
    external c.
    heart c.
    internal c.
    laminated c.
    marantic c.
    muscle c.
    passive c.
    plasma c.
    plastic c.
    postmortem c.
    proximal c.
    Schede's c.
    spider-web c.
    stratified c.
    washed c.
    white c.
clo·thi·a·pine
clo·trim·a·zole
cloud·ing
    c. of consciousness
CMR — cerebral metabolic
    rate
Cloud·man's melanoma S91
Clou·ston's syndrome
clove
Clow·ard back fusion
clox·a·cil·lin so·di·um
clox·y·quin
clo·za·pine
club·bing
    c. of calix
    c. of fingers
club·foot
club·hand
    radial c.

club·hand *(continued)*
    ulnar c.
clump·ing
clu·ne·al
clu·nis *pl.* clu·nes
clu·pan·o·don·ic acid
clu·pe·ine
clut·ter·ing
Clut·ton's joint
cly·sis
    subeschar c.
clys·ma *pl.* clys·ma·ta
Cly·so·drast
clys·ter
cly·to·cy·bine
CM — L. Chirurgiae Magister
    (Master of Surgery)
cM — centimorgan
cm — centimeter
cm^2 — square centimeter
cm^3 — cubic centimeter
CMA — Canadian Medical
    Association
    Certified Medical Assistant
CMAP — compound muscle
    action potential
CMD — cerebromacular
    degeneration
CMHC — community mental
    health center
CMI — cell-mediated
    immunity
CML — cell-mediated
    lympholysis
c mm — cubic millimeter
CMP — cytidine
    monophosphate
c.m.s. — L. cras mane
    sumendus (to be taken
    tomorrow morning)
CMT — Certified Medical
    Transcriptionist
CMV — cytomegalovirus
CN — L. cras nocte (tomorrow
    night)
CNA — Canadian Nurses'
    Association
CN-Cbl — cyanocobalamin

cne·mi·al
cne·mis
cne·mi·tis
cne·mo·sco·li·o·sis
Cni·dar·ia
cni·dar·i·an
cni·do·blast
cni·do·cil
CNM — Certified
  Nurse-Midwife
CNS — central nervous
  system
c.n.s. — L. cras nocte
  sumendus (to be taken
  tomorrow night)
COA — Canadian Orthopaedic
  Association
CoA — coenzyme A
co·ac·er·vate
co·ac·er·va·tion
Co·ac·tin
co·ad·ap·ta·tion
co·ad·u·na·tion
co·ad·u·ni·tion
co·ag·glu·ti·na·tion
co·ag·u·la
co·ag·u·la·bil·i·ty
co·ag·u·la·ble
co·ag·u·lant
co·ag·u·lase
co·ag·u·late
co·ag·u·la·tion
    blood c.
    disseminated intravascular
      c. (DIC)
    electric c.
    infrared c.
    massive c.
co·ag·u·la·tive
co·ag·u·la·tor
co·ag·u·lo·gram
co·ag·u·lop·a·thy
    consumption c.
co·ag·u·lo·vis·co·sim·e·ter
co·ag·u·lum *pl.* co·ag·u·la
    closing c.
co·a·les·cence
co·apt

co·ap·ta·tion
co·arc·tate
co·arc·ta·tion
    c. of aorta
    c. of aorta, adult type
    c. of aorta, infantile type
    reversed c.
co·ar·tic·u·la·tion
CoA-SH — coenzyme A
coat
    adventitial c.
    adventitious c. of uterine
      tube
    albugineous c.
    buffy c.
    cremasteric c. of testis
    dartos c.
    extraneous c.
    fibrous c.
    fuzzy c.
    mucous c.
    mucous c. of tympanic
      cavity
    muscular c.
    pharyngobasilar c.
    proper c.
    sclerotic c.
    serous c.
    spore c.
    subendothelial c.
    submucous c.
    subserous c.
    uveal c.
    vaginal c. of testis
    vascular c.
    villous c. of small intestine
    white c.
coat·ing
    enteric c.
CoA-trans·fer·ase
Coats' disease
Coats' retinitis
co·ax·i·al
co·bal·a·min
    c. concentrate
co·b(1)al·a·min ad·e·no·syl·
    trans·fer·ase
co·bal·oph·i·lin

co·balt
    c. 57
    c. 58
    c. 60
    radioactive c.
    c. salipyrine
co·bal·to·sis
co·bal·tous
co·ba·mide
co·ban
cob·ble·ston·ing
co·bra
    black-necked c.
    Indian c.
    king c.
    spitting c.
co·bra·ism
co·bra·ly·sin
COC — calcifying odontogenic cyst
co·ca
co·caine
    c. hydrochloride
co·cain·ism
co·cain·iza·tion
co·cain·ize
co·car·box·y·lase
co·car·cin·o·gen
co·car·cino·gen·e·sis
coc·cal
coc·ce·rin
coc·ci
Coc·cid·ia
coc·cid·ia
coc·cid·i·al
coc·cid·i·an
coc·cid·i·oi·dal
Coc·cid·i·oi·des
    C. immitis
coc·cid·i·oi·din
coc·cid·i·oi·do·ma
coc·cid·i·oi·do·me·nin·gi·tis
coc·cid·i·oi·do·my·co·sis
    disseminated c.
    latent c.
    primmary extrapulmonary c.
coc·cid·i·oi·do·sis

coc·cid·i·o·sis
coc·cid·io·stat
coc·cid·io·stat·ic
coc·ci·gen·ic
coc·ci·nel·lin
coc·co·bac·il·lary
coc·co·bac·il·li
coc·co·ba·cil·lus pl. coc·co·ba·cil·li
coc·co·bac·te·ria
coc·code
coc·co·gen·ic
coc·co·gen·ous
coc·coid
coc·cu·lin
Coc·cus
coc·cus pl. coc·ci
    pyogenic c.
coc·cy·ceph·a·lus
coc·cy·gal·gia
coc·cyg·e·al
coc·cy·gec·to·my
coc·cy·ge·rec·tor
coc·cyg·e·us
coc·cy·go·dyn·ia
coc·cy·got·o·my
coc·cy·odyn·ia
coc·cyx
Coch·i·cel·la
coch·i·neal
cochl. — L. cochleare (a spoonful)
cochl. cochl. amp. — L. cochleare amplum (a heaping spoonful)
cochl. cochl. mag. — L. cochleare magnum (a tablespoonful)
cochl. cochl. med. — L. cochleare medium (a dessertspoonful)
cochl. cochl. parv. — L. cochleare parvum (a teaspoonful)
coch·lea
    membranous c.
    Mondini's c.
coch·le·ar

Coch·le·ar·ia
coch·le·ar·i·form
coch·le·itis
coch·le·og·ra·phy
    acoustic c.
coch·le·os·to·my
coch·leo·top·ic
coch·leo·ves·tib·u·lar
Coch·lio·my·ia
    C. *americana*
    C. *bezziana*
    C.*hominivorax*
    C. *macellaria*
coch·li·tis
co·cil·la·na
Cock·ayne's syndrome
cock·tail
    GI c.
    lytic c.
    McConckey c.
    Philadelphia c.
    Rivers' c.
COCl — cathodal opening
  clonus
co·coa
co·con·scious
co·con·trac·tion
Coct. — L. coctio (boiling)
coc·tion
coc·to·an·ti·gen
coc·to-im·mu·no·gen
coc·to·la·bile
coc·to·pre·cip·i·tin
coc·to·pro·tein
coc·to·sta·bile
coc·to·sta·ble
coc·u·line
co·cul·ti·va·tion
COD — cause of death
code
    degeneracy of c.
    degenerate c.
    genetic c.
    triplet c.
co·deine
    c. phosphate
    c. sulfate
    c. valerianate

co·dex *pl.* co·di·ces
Co·di·vil·la's operation
Cod·man's sign
Cod·man's triangle
co·dom·i·nance
co·dom·i·nant
co·don
    amber c.
    chain-initiation c's
    chain-termination c's
    initiator c.
    nonsense c's
    ochre c.
    stop c.
    umber c.
co·ef·fi·cient
    absorption c.
    activity c.
    atomic attenuation c.
    Baumann's c.
    binomial c.
    biological c.
    Bouchard's c.
    Bunsen c.
    Chick-Martin c.
    confidence c.
    c. of consanguinity
    correlation c.
    creatinine c.
    cryoscopic c.
    c. of demineralization
    diffusion c.
    dilution c.
    distribution c.
    extinction c.
    Falta's c.
    c. of friction
    Haines' c.
    Häser's c.
    Hill c.
    homogeneity c.
    hygienic laboratory c.
    c. of inbreeding
    intensity transmission c.
    isometric c. of lactic acid
    isotonic c.
    Kendall's rank correlation
      c.

co·ef·fi·cient *(continued)*
    c. of kinship
    Lancet c.
    lethal c.
    linear absorption c.
    linear attenuation c.
    Loebisch's c.
    Long's c.
    Maillard's c.
    mass absorption c.
    mass attenuation c.
    osmotic c.
    Ostwald's c.
    c. of partage
    partition c.
    Pearson's correlation c.
    phenol c.
    product-moment c.
    reflection c.
    c. of relationship
    Rideal-Walker c.
    sedimentation c.
    selection c.
    solubility c.
    Spearman's rank
     correlation c.
    Svedberg c.
    temperature c.
    c. of thermal conductivity
    c. of thermal expansion
    Trapp's c.
    urohemolytic c.
    urotoxic c.
    c. of utilization of oxygen
    c. of variation (CV)
    velocity c.
    c. of viscosity
    volume c.
coe·la·ri·um
Coe·len·ter·a·ta
coe·len·ter·ate
coe·len·ter·on
coe·li·ac
coe·lio·cy·e·sis
coe·lo·blas·tu·la
coe·lom
    extraembryonic c.
coe·lo·ma

coe·lo·mate
coe·lom·ic
coe·los·o·my
coe·nu·ri·a·sis
coe·nu·ro·sis
Coe·nu·rus
    C. cerebralis
coe·nu·rus
co·en·zyme
    c. I
    c. II
    c. A
    nucleotide c.
    c. Q
    c. R
coe·ru·le·us
coeur
    c. en sabot
co·ex·ci·ta·tion
co·fac·tor
    platelet c. I
    platelet c. II
    c. V
    ristocetin c.
Cof·fey suspension
Cof·fey technique
Cof·fey-Hum·ber treatment
Co·gan's disease
Co·gan's syndrome
co·ge·ner
Co·gen·tin
cog·ni·tion
cog·ni·tive
cog·wheel
cog·wheel·ing
co·he·sion
co·he·sive
Cohn's solution
Cohn·heim's areas
Cohn·heim's theory
co·ho·ba·tion
co·hort
coil
    choke c.
    chromosome c.
    crossed c.
    Gianturco wool-tufted wire
     c.

coil *(continued)*
    Golay c.
    Helmholtz c.
    induction c.
    paranemic c.
    plectonemic c.
    random c.
    relational c.
    resistance c.
    spark c.
co·in·di·ca·tion
co·in·fec·tion
coin·o·site
co·iso·ge·ne·ic
co·i·so·gen·ic
co·i·tal
Coi·ter's muscle
co·i·tion
co·i·to·pho·bia
co·i·tus
    c. incompletus
    c. interruptus
    c. reservatus
Col. — L. cola (strain)
col
Co·lace
co·la·mine
Colat. — L. colatus (strained)
col·a·ture
ColBENEMID
col·ce·mide
col·chi·cine
Col·chi·cum
cold
    allergic c.
    common c.
    June c.
    rose c.
cold·sore
Cole's sign
co·lec·to·my
Cole·man-Shaf·fer diet
co·leo·cys·ti·tis
Col·e·op·tera
co·les·ti·pol
    c. hydrochloride
Colet. — L. coletur (let it be
    strained)

co·li·bac·il·le·mia
co·li·bac·il·lo·sis
    c. gravidarum
co·li·bac·il·lu·ria
co·li·bac·il·lus
col·ic
    appendicular c.
    biliary c.
    bilious c.
    copper c.
    cystic c.
    Devonshire c.
    endemic c.
    flatulent c.
    gallstone c.
    gastric c.
    hepatic c.
    infantile c.
    intestinal c.
    kidney c.
    lead c.
    menstrual c.
    milk c.
    nephric c.
    ovarian c.
    painters' c.
    pancreatic c.
    Poitou c.
    renal c.
    salivary c.
    sand c.
    saturnine c.
    stercoral c.
    tubal c.
    ureteral c.
    uterine c.
    vermicular c.
    verminous c.
    wind c.
    worm c.
    zinc c.
col·i·cin
col·i·cin·o·gen
col·i·cin·o·gen·ic
col·i·ci·nog·e·ny
col·icky
col·i·co·ple·gia
co·li·cys·ti·tis

co·li·cys·to·py·eli·tis
col·i·form
co·lin·e·ar·i·ty
co·li·ne·phri·tis
col·i·phage
co·li·pli·ca·tion
co·li·punc·ture
co·li·sep·sis
co·lis·ti·meth·ate so·di·um
co·lis·tin
    c. sulfate
    c. sulfomethate sodium
co·li·tis *pl.* co·lit·i·des
    amebic c.
    antibiotic-associated c.
    balantidial c.
    cathartic c.
    collagenous c.
    c. cystica profunda
    c. cystica superficialis
    diversion c.
    granulomatous c.
    c. gravis
    irradiation c.
    ischemic c.
    mucous c.
    c. polyposa
    pseudomembranous c.
    radiation c.
    regional c.
    segmental c.
    transmural c.
    c. ulcerativa
    ulcerative c.
    uremic c.
col·i·tose
co·li·tox·emia
co·li·tox·i·co·sis
co·li·tox·in
co·li·uria
col·la
col·la·cin
col·la·gen
    fibrous long-spacing (FLS) c.
    segment long-spacing (SLS) c.

col·la·gen·ase
    Clostridium histolyticum c.
    vertebrate c.
col·la·ge·na·tion
col·la·gen·ic
col·lag·e·ni·tis
col·lag·e·no·blast
col·lag·e·no·cyte
col·la·gen·o·gen·ic
col·la·gen·ol·y·sis
col·lag·e·no·ly·tic
col·la·ge·no·ma
    familial cutaneous c.
col·la·gen·o·sis
    reactive perforating c.
col·lag·e·nous
col·lapse
    alveolar c.
    cardiovascular c.
    circulatory c.
    heat c.
    massive c.
col·lar
    abrasion c.
    Biett's c.
    Casal's c.
    four-poster c.
    c. of pearls
    perichondral bony c.
    periosteal bone c.
    renal c.
    Spanish c.
    c. of Stokes
    venereal c.
    c. of Venus
col·lar·bone, col·lar bone
col·lar·ette
    iris c.
col·las·tin
col·lat·er·al
    Schaffer c's
Col·les' fascia
Col·les' fracture
Col·les' ligament
Col·les' space
Col·let's syndrome

Col·let-Si·card syndrome
col·lic·u·lec·to·my
col·lic·u·li
col·lic·u·li·tis
col·lic·u·lus *pl.* col·lic·u·li
    c. abducentis
    c. of arytenoid cartilage
    c. of Barkow
    bulbar c.
    c. cartilaginis arytenoideae
    caudal c.
    c. caudalis
    c. caudatus
    cervical c. of female
      urethra
    facial c.
    c. facialis
    c. inferior
    inferior c.
    rostral c.
    c. rostralis
    seminal c.
    c. seminalis
    c. superior
    superior c.
    c. superior laminae
      quadrigeminae
Col·lier's tract
col·lig·a·tive
col·li·ma·tion
col·li·ma·tor
Col·lin's osteoclast
col·lin·e·ar
Col·lin·so·nia
col·li·ot·o·my
Col·lip unit
col·li·qua·tion
    ballooning c.
    reticulating c.
col·liq·ua·tive
col·li·sion
    elastic c.
    scattering c.
col·lo·chem·is·try
col·lo·di·a·phys·e·al
col·lo·di·on
    c. elastique
    flexible c.

col·lo·di·on *(continued)*
    hemostatic c.
    salicylic acid c.
    simple c.
    styptic c.
col·loid
    antimony trisulfide c.
    association c.
    bovine c.
    dispersion c.
    emulsion c.
    hydrophilic c.
    hydrophobic c.
    irreversible c.
    lyophilic c.
    lyophobic c.
    lyotropic c.
    protective c.
    reversible c.
    stable c.
    stannous sulfur c.
    suspension c.
    technetium-sulfur c.
    thyroid c.
col·loi·dal
col·loi·din
col·loi·do·pexy
col·loid·oph·a·gy
col·lox·y·lin
col·lum *pl.* col·la
    c. anatomicum humeri
    c. chirurgicum humeri
    c. costae
    c. dentis
    c. distortum
    c. fibulae
    c. folliculi pili
    c. glandis penis
    c. mallei
    c. mandibulae
    c. ossis femoris
    c. radii
    c. scapulae
    c. tali
    c. vesicae biliaris
Collut. — L. collutorium
  (mouth wash)
col·lu·to·ry

Collyr. — L. collyrium (eye wash)

col·lyr·i·um *pl.* col·lyr·ia

col·o·bo·ma *pl.* col·o·bo·mas, col·o·bo·ma·ta

  atypical c's
  c. auriculae
  bridge c.
  c. of choroid
  c. of ciliary body
  complete c.
  facial c.
  Fuchs's c.
  c. of fundus
  c. iridis
  c. of iris
  c. of lens
  c. lentis
  c. lobuli
  c. of optic disk
  c. of optic nerve
  c. at optic nerve entrance
  c. palpebrale
  peripapillary c.
  c. of retina
  c. retinae
  retinochoroidal c.
  typical c.
  c. of vitreous

co·lo·ce·cos·to·my

co·lo·cen·te·sis

co·lo·cho·le·cys·tos·to·my

co·lo·cly·sis

co·lo·clys·ter

co·lo·col·ic

co·lo·co·los·to·my

co·lo·cu·ta·ne·ous

colo·cynth

colo·cyn·thi·dism

colo·cyn·thin

co·lo·dys·pep·sia

co·lo·en·ter·itis

co·lo·fix·a·tion

Col·o·gel

co·lo·hep·a·to·pexy

co·lo·il·e·al

co·lol·y·sis

co·lo·me·trom·e·ter

co·lon
  c. ascendens
  ascending c.
  c. descendens
  descending c.
  giant c.
  iliac c.
  irritable c.
  lead-pipe c.
  left c.
  pelvic c.
  redundant c.
  right c.
  sigmoid c.
  c. sigmoideum
  spastic c.
  transverse c.
  c. transversum

co·lon·al·gia

co·lon·ic

col·o·ni·za·tion

Co·lon·na's operation

co·lo·nop·a·thy

co·lon·or·rha·gia

co·lono·scope

co·lo·nos·co·py
  fiberoptic c.

col·o·ny
  checker c.
  D. c.
  daisy-head c.
  daughter c.
  dwarf c.
  fried-egg c.
  G c.
  Gheel c.
  glossy c.
  gonidial c.
  gregaloid c.
  H c.
  M. c.
  matte c.
  mother c.
  motile c.
  mucoid c.
  O c.

col·o·ny *(continued)*
    R c.
    rough c.
    S c.
    smooth c.
    satellite c.
    secondary c.
co·lop·a·thy
co·lo·pex·os·to·my
co·lo·pex·ot·o·my
co·lo·pexy
co·lo·pli·ca·tion
co·lo·proc·tec·to·my
co·lo·proc·ti·tis
co·lo·proc·tos·to·my
co·lop·to·sis
co·lo·punc·ture
Color. — L. coloretur (let it be
  colored)
col·or
    complementary c's
    confusion c's
    contrast c.
    incidental c.
    metameric c's
    Munsell's c's
    primary c's
    pseudoisochromatic c's
    pure c.
    saturation c.
co·lo·rec·tal
co·lo·rec·ti·tis
co·lo·rec·tos·to·my
co·lo·rec·tum
col·or·im·e·ter
    Duboscq's c.
    photoelectric c.
    titration c.
col·or·im·e·try
co·lor·rha·phy
co·lor·rhea
co·lo·scope
co·los·co·py
co·lo·sig·moid·os·to·my
co·los·to·my
    dry c.
    end c.
    Hartmann's c.

co·los·to·my *(continued)*
    ileotransverse c.
    Mikulicz c.
    wet c.
co·los·tric
co·los·tror·rhea
co·los·trous
co·los·trum
    c. gravidarum
    c. puerperarum
co·lot·o·my
co·lo·vag·i·nal
co·lo·ves·i·cal
col·pal·gia
col·pa·tre·sia
col·pec·ta·sia
col·pec·to·my
col·pe·de·ma
col·peu·ryn·ter
col·peu·ry·sis
col·pis·mus
col·pi·tis
    c. emphysematosa
    emphysematous c.
    c. granulosa
    c. mycotica
col·po·cele
col·po·cel·io·cen·te·sis
col·po·ce·li·ot·o·my
col·po·clei·sis
col·po·cys·ti·tis
col·po·cys·to·cele
col·po·cys·to·plas·ty
col·po·cys·tot·o·my
col·po·cys·to·ure·tero·cys·
  tot·o·my
col·po·cys·to·ure·thro·pexy
col·po·cy·to·gram
col·po·cy·tol·o·gy
Col·po·di·da
col·po·dyn·ia
col·po·epis·i·or·rha·phy
col·po·hy·per·pla·sia
    c. cystica
    c. emphysematosa
col·po·mi·cro·scope
col·po·mi·cro·scop·ic
col·po·mi·cros·co·py

col·po·myo·mec·to·my
col·po·my·o·mot·o·my
col·po·par·ovar·io·cys·tec·to·my
col·po·per·i·neo·plas·ty
col·po·per·i·ne·or·rha·phy
col·po·pexy
col·po·plas·ty
col·po·poi·e·sis
col·po·poly·pus
col·pop·to·sis
col·po·rec·to·pexy
col·por·rha·gia
col·por·rha·phy
col·por·rhex·is
col·po·scope
col·po·scop·ic
col·pos·co·py
col·po·spasm
col·po·stat
col·po·ste·no·sis
col·po·ste·not·o·my
col·po·therm
col·pot·o·my
    posterior c.
col·po·ure·tero·cys·tot·o·my
col·po·ure·ter·ot·o·my
col·po·xe·ro·sis
col·te·rol mes·y·late
Col·u·ber
col·u·brid
Col·u·bri·dae
col·u·mel·la *pl.* col·u·mel·lae
    c. cochleae
    c. nasi
col·u·mel·lae
col·umn
    c's of abdominal ring
    anal c's
    anterolateral c.
    c's of Bertin
    branchial efferent c.
    c. of Burdach
    Clarke's c.
    c's of Cotunnius
    dorsal c.
    enamel c's
    fat c's

col·umn *(continued)*
    fleshy c's of heart
    c. of fornix
    fractionating c.
    fundamental c.
    general somatic afferent c.
    general somatic efferent c.
    c. of Goll
    Gowers' c.
    gray c's
    ion exchange c.
    c. of Kölliker
    c. of Lissauer
    c's of Morgagni
    muscle c.
    c. of nose
    positive c.
    posteroexternal c.
    Rathke's c's
    rectal c's
    renal c's of Bertin
    c. of Rolando
    c. of Sertoli
    somatic motor c.
    somatic sensory c.
    spinal c.
    c. of Spitzka-Lissauer
    Stilling's c.
    striomotor c.
    thoracic c.
    Türck's c.
    ventral c. of spinal cord
    vertebral c.
    visceral motor c.
    visceral sensory c.
co·lum·na *pl.* co·lum·nae
    columnae adiposae
    columnae anales
    columnae bertini
    columnae carneae cordis
    c. fornicis
    columnae griseae
    c. nasi
    c. posterolateralis
    c. posteromediana
    columnae rectales
    [Morgagnii]
    columnae renales

co·lum·na *(continued)*
  columnae renales [Bertini]
  c. thoracica
  c. vertebralis
co·lum·nae
co·lum·ni·za·tion
Coly-My·cin M
Coly-My·cin S
co·ma
  agrypnodal c.
  alcoholic c.
  alpha c.
  apoplectic c.
  deanimate c.
  diabetic c.
  epileptic c.
  hepatic c.
  c. hepaticum
  hyperosmolar nonketotic c.
  hypoglycemic c.
  hypopituitary c.
  hypothermic c.
  irreversible c.
  Kussmaul's c.
  metabolic c.
  myxedema c.
  c. somnolentium
  thyrotoxic c.
  uremic c.
  c. vigil
com·a·tose
Com·bi·pres
Com·by sign
com·e·do *pl.* com·e·do·nes
  closed c.
  open c.
  polyporous c.
  solar c.
com·e·do·car·ci·no·ma
com·e·do·gen·ic
com·e·do·mas·ti·tis
co·mes *pl.* com·i·tes
co·mi·tance
com·i·tes
co·mi·tial
com·men·sal
com·men·sal·ism
  epizoic c.

com·mi·nut·ed
com·mi·nu·tion
Com·miph·o·ra
com·mis·su·ra *pl.* com·mis·su·rae
  c. anterior cerebri
  c. bulborum
  c. of bulbs of vestibule of vagina
  c. cerebelli
  c. colliculorum anteriorum
  c. colliculorum caudalium
  c. colliculorum cranialium
  c. colliculorum inferiorum
  c. colliculorum rostralium
  c. colliculorum superiorum
  c. epithalamica
  c. fornicis
  c. grisea medullae spinalis
  c. habenularis
  c. habenularum
  c. hippocampi
  c. inferior guddeni
  c. labiorum oris
  c. labiorum pudendi
  c. magna cerebri
  c. media cerebri
  c. mollis
  c. olivarum
  c. optica
  c. palpebrarum lateralis
  c. palpebrarum medialis
  c. palpebrarum nasalis
  c. palpebrarum temporalis
  c. posterior cerebri
  c. rostralis cerebri
  c. superior meynerti
  c. supraoptica dorsalis
  c. supraoptica ventralis
com·mis·su·rae
com·mis·su·ral
com·mis·sure
  c. of bulb
  c. of caudal colliculi
  c. of cerebrum, anterior
  c. of cerebrum, middle
  c. of cerebrum, posterior
  c. of cerebrum, rostral

com·mis·sure *(continued)*
    chiasmatic posterior c.
    c. of cranial colliculi
    dorsal c. of cerebellum
    c. of epithalamus
    c. of eyelids, lateral
    c. of eyelids, medial
    Forel's c.
    c. of fornix
    Ganser's c.
    gray c.
    great c.
    Gudden's c.
    c. of habenulae
    habenular c.
    hippocampal c.
    c. of inferior colliculi
    interthalamic c.
    intrachiasmatic c.
    c. of labia, posterior
    laryngeal c.
    lateral c. of cerebellum
    lateral c. of eyelids
    lateral palpebral c.
    c. of lips of mouth
    medial c. of eyelids
    medial palpebral c.
    Meynert's c.
    c. of rostral colliculi
    c. of superior colliculi
    supraoptic c's
    supraoptic c., dorsal
    supraoptic c., ventral
    c. of vestibule
    c's of vulva
com·mis·su·ror·rha·phy
com·mis·sur·ot·o·my
    mitral c.
com·mit·ment
com·mo·tio
    c. cerebri
    c. retinae
    c. spinalis
com·mu·ni·ca·ble
com·mu·ni·cans
com·mu·nis
com·mu·ni·ty
    therapeutic c.

Com·ol·li's sign
Comp. — L. *compositus*
   (compound)
com·pac·tion
com·pa·ges
    c. thoracis
com·par·a·scope
com·par·a·tor
com·part·ment
    extracellular c.
    intracellular c.
    muscular c.
    vascular c.
com·part·men·ta·li·za·tion
Com·pa·zine
com·pen·di·um *pl.* com·pen·
dia
    drug c.
com·pen·sat·ed
com·pen·sa·tion
    attenuation c.
    Bekhterev c.
    broken c.
    dosage c.
    electronic distance c.
    time gain c.
    Workers' C.
com·pen·sa·tor
com·pen·sa·to·ry
com·pe·tence
    embryonic c.
    immunologic c.
com·pe·ti·tion
    antigenic c.
com·pim·e·ter
com·plaint
    chief c.
    summer c.
com·ple·ment
    chromosome c.
com·ple·men·tal
com·ple·men·tar·i·ty
    dominant c.
    recessive c.
com·ple·men·ta·ry
com·ple·men·ta·tion
    in vitro c.
    interallelic c.

com·ple·men·ta·tion
　(continued)
　　intercistronic c.
　　intergenic c.
　　intracistronic c.
　　intragenic c.
com·plex
　　abortive c.
　　adrenochrome
　　　monosemicarbazone
　　　sodium salicylate c.
　　AIDS-related c. (ARC)
　　amniotic band disruption c.
　　amygdaloid c.
　　amyotrophic lateral
　　　sclerosis–parkinsonism–de-
　　　mentia c.
　　anomalous c.
　　antigen-antibody c.
　　apical c.
　　atrial c.
　　avian leukosis c.
　　basal c. of choroid
　　Behçet triple symptom c.
　　calcarine c.
　　castration c.
　　Clérambault-Kandinsky c.
　　diphasic c.
　　EAHF c.
　　Eisenmenger c.
　　Electra c.
　　equiphasic c.
　　factor IX c.
　　father c.
　　flocculonodular c.
　　Friedmann's c.
　　Ghon c.
　　Golgi c.
　　H-2 c.
　　hapten-carrier c.
　　hemoglobin-haptoglobin c.
　　HLA c.
　　hydrocodone resin c.
　　immune c.
　　inclusion c's
　　inferior olivary c.
　　inferiority c.
　　iron-dextran c.

com·plex *(continued)*
　　jumped process c.
　　junctional c.
　　K c.
　　α-ketoglutarate
　　　dehydrogenase c.
　　α-ketoisovalerate
　　　dehydrogenase c.
　　Lutembacher's c.
　　major histocompatibility c.
　　　(MHC)
　　membrane attack c. (MAC)
　　Meyenburg's c's
　　oculomotor nuclear c.
　　Oedipus c.
　　Parkinson dementia c.
　　perihypoglossal c.
　　pore c.
　　primary inoculation c.
　　primary tuberculous c.
　　QRS c.
　　QRST c.
　　Ranke c.
　　sicca c.
　　ribosome-lamella c.
　　rSr c.
　　Steidele's c.
　　symptom c.
　　synaptonemal c.
　　ureterotrigonal c.
　　urobilin c.
　　ventricular c's
　　ventricular depolarization
　　　c.
　　Wilks symptom c.
com·plex·us
　　c. basalis choroideae
com·pli·ance
　　dynamic
　　motor c.
　　patient c.
　　pulmonary c.
　　somatic c.
　　static c.
com·pli·cat·ed
com·pli·ca·tion
Com·po·cil·lin-VK

com·po·nent
    anterior c.
    complement c's
    G c.
    group-specific c.
    M c.
    plasma thromboplastin c.
      (PTC)
    secretory c. (SC)
    somatic motor c.
    somatic sensory c.
    splanchnic motor c.
    splanchnic sensory c.
    Woodbridge's c's of
      anesthesia
com·pos men·tis
com·po·si·tion
com·pound
    acyclic c.
    addition c.
    aliphatic c.
    APC c.
    aromatic c.
    benzene c's
    binary c.
    clathrate c's
    closed-chain c.
    coal-tar c.
    condensation c.
    cyclic c.
    diazo c.
    endothermic c.
    energy-rich c's
    exothermic c.
    fatty c.
    c. G-11
    genetic c.
    Grignard c.
    heterocyclic c.
    high-energy c's
    Hurler-Scheie c.
    impression c.
    inorganic c.
    isocyclic c.
    isopropyl alcohol rubbing c.
    low-energy c's
    methonium c's
    nonpolar c's

com·pound (continued)
    occlusion c's
    open-chain c.
    organic c.
    organometallic c.
    paraffin c.
    polar c's
    quaternary c.
    quaternary ammonium c.
    ring c.
    saturated c.
    substitution c.
    sulfonylurea c's
    ternary c.
    tertiary c.
    unsaturated c.
com·press
    cribriform c.
    fenestrated c.
com·pres·si·bil·i·ty
com·pres·sion
    cardiac c.
    cerebral c.
    digital c.
    instrumental c.
    jugular c.
    renal artery c.
    spinal c.
    sponge stick c.
com·pres·sor
    aortic c.
    Deschamps' c.
    c. naris
    Sehrt's c.
    shot c.
    c. urethrae
    c. vaginae
    c. venae dorsalis
com·pro·mise
Comp·ton effect
Comp·ton scattering
com·pul·sion
    repetition c.
com·pul·sive
ConA — concanavalin A
con·al·bu·min
co·na·ri·um
co·na·tion

con·a·tive
con·a·van·ine
con·cam·er·a·tion
con·ca·nav·a·lin A
con·cas·sa·tion
con·cat·e·mer
con·cat·e·nate
con·cat·e·na·tion
Con·ca·to's disease
con·cave
con·cav·i·ty
con·ca·vo·con·cave
con·ca·vo·con·vex
con·ceive
con·cen·trate
    liver c.
    plant protease c.
    vitamin c.
con·cen·tra·tion
    bicarbonate ion c.
    hydrogen ion c.
    ionic c.
    limiting isorrheic c. (LIC)
    mass c.
    maximum cell (MC) c.
    maximum allowable c.
      (MAC)
    maximum urinary c.
      (MUC)
    mean corpuscular
      hemoglobin c.
    minimal alveolar c. (MAC)
    minimal bactericidal c.
      (MBC)
    minimal inhibitory c. (MIC)
    minimal isorrheic c. (MIC)
    minimal lethal c. (MLC)
    minimum alveolar c.
      (MAC)
    molar c.
    selective c.
    substance c.
con·cen·tric
con·cept
    no-threshold c.
con·cep·tion
con·cep·tive

con·cep·tus
con·cha *pl.* con·chae
    c. of auricle
    c. auriculae
    c. bullosa
    c. of cranium
    ethmoidal c., inferior
    ethmoidal c., superior
    ethmoidal c., supreme
    inferior nasal c.
    inferior turbinate c.
    middle nasal c.
    c. nasalis inferior
    c. nasalis media
    c. nasalis superior
    c. nasalis suprema
    nasoturbinal c.
    Santorini's c.
    sphenoidal c.
    c. sphenoidalis
    superior nasal c.
con·chae
con·chi·form
con·chio·lin·os·teo·my·eli·tis
con·chi·tis
con·choi·dal
con·cho·scope
con·cho·tome
con·chot·o·my
Concis. — L. concisus (cut)
con·cli·na·tion
con·com·i·tant
con·cor·dance
con·cor·dant
con·cre·ment
con·cres·cence
con·cre·tio
    c. cordis
    c. pericardii
con·cre·tion
    alvine c.
    calculous c.
    preputial c.
    prostatic c's
    tophic c.
con·cre·tism
con·cre·ti·za·tion

con·cus·sion
 abdominal c., hydraulic
 acceleration c.
 c. of the brain
 compression c.
 c. of the labyrinth
 pulmonary c.
 c. of the retina
 c. of the spinal cord
con·den·sa·tion
 aldol c.
con·den·ser
 Abbe's c.
 automatic c.
 back-action c.
 cardioid c.
 darkfield c.
 foil c.
 foot c.
 gold c.
 mechanical c.
 paraboloid c.
 reverse c.
con·di·tion·ing
 aversive c.
 classical c.
 higher-order c.
 instrumental c.
 operant c.
 pavlovian c.
 reinforcement c.
 respondent c.
con·dom
Con·do·rel·li syndrome
con·duct
con·duc·tance
 airway c.
con·duc·tion
 aberrant c.
 accelerated c.
 aerial c.
 aerotympanal c.
 air c.
 anomalous c.
 anterograde c.
 antidromic c.
 atrial c.
 atrioventricular c.

con·duc·tion *(continued)*
 avalanche c.
 bone c.
 cardiac c.
 concealed c.
 cranial c.
 decremental c.
 delayed c.
 ephaptic c.
 forward c.
 His-Purkinje c.
 intra-atrial c.
 intraventricular c.
 nerve c.
 osteotympanic c.
 retrograde c.
 saltatory c.
 synaptic c.
 tissue c.
 ventricular c.
 ventriculoatrial c.
con·duc·tiv·i·ty
con·duc·tor
con·du·it
 ileal c.
con·du·pli·cate
con·du·pli·ca·tio
 c. corporis
con·du·pli·ca·to cor·po·re
con·dy·lar
con·dy·lar·thro·sis
con·dyle
 extensor c. of humerus
 external c. of femur
 external c. of humerus
 external c. of tibia
 fibular c. of femur
 flexor c. of humerus
 c. of humerus
 internal c. of femur
 internal c. of humerus
 internal c. of tibia
 lateral c. of femur
 lateral c. of humerus
 lateral c. of tibia
 c. of mandible
 medial c. of femur
 medial c. of humerus

con·dyle *(continued)*
    medial c. of tibia
    occipital c.
    radial c. of humerus
    c. of scapula
    tibial c. of femur
    ulnar c. of humerus
con·dy·lec·to·my
con·dy·li
con·dyl·i·cus
con·dyl·i·on
con·dy·loid
con·dy·lo·ma *pl.* con·dy·lo·ma·ta
    c. acuminatum
    flat c.
    c. latum
    pointed c.
    c. subcutaneum
con·dy·lo·ma·ta
con·dy·lo·ma·toid
con·dy·lo·ma·to·sis
con·dy·lom·a·tous
con·dy·lot·o·my
con·dy·lus *pl.* con·dy·li
cone
    acrosomal c.
    adjusting c's
    antipodal c.
    arterial c.
    attraction c.
    bifurcation c.
    cerebellar pressure c.
    Dunham's c's
    ectoplacental c.
    elastic c. of larynx
    fertilization c.
    graduated c.
    growth c.
    gutta-percha c.
    Haller's c's
    implantation c.
    c. of light
    long c.
    medullary c.
    ocular c.
    pilar c.
    Politzer's c.

cone *(continued)*
    pressure c.
    primitive c.
    pulmonary c.
    retinal c.
    sarcoplasmic c.
    short c.
    silver c.
    tentorial pressure c.
    terminal c. of spinal cord
    theca interna c.
    treatment c.
    twin c's
    Tyndall c.
    ureteral c.
    vascular c's
    visual c.
cone-mono·chro·mat
cone-nose
Con·es·tron
con·fab·u·la·tion
con·fer·tus
con·fig·u·ra·tion
    cis c.
    trans c.
con·fine·ment
con·flict
    approach-approach c.
    approach-avoidance c.
    avoidance-avoidance c.
    extrapsychic c.
    intrapersonal c.
    intrapsychic c.
con·flu·ence
    c. of sinuses
con·flu·ens
    c. sinuum
con·flu·ent
con·fo·cal
con·for·ma·tion
con·form·er
    neck c.
con·fri·ca·tion
con·fron·ta·tion
cong. — L. congius (gallon)
con·ge·la·tion
con·gen·ic
con·ge·ner

con·ge·ner·ic
con·gen·er·ous
con·gen·i·tal
con·gest·ed
con·gest·in
con·ges·tion
    active c.
    cerebral c.
    circulatory c.
    functional c.
    hypostatic c.
    neuroparalytic c.
    neurotonic c.
    passive c.
    physiologic c.
    pulmonary c.
    rebound c.
    renal c.
    venous c.
con·ges·tive
con·glo·bate
con·glo·ba·tion
con·glom·er·ate
con·glu·tin
con·glu·ti·nant
con·glu·ti·na·tio
    c. orificii externi
    c. of cervix
con·glu·ti·na·tion
con·glu·ti·nin
    immune c.
con·glu·ti·no·gen
co·ni
co·nid·ia
co·nid·i·al
co·nid·io·phore
Co·nid·io·spo·ra·les
co·nid·io·spore
co·nid·i·um *pl.* co·nid·ia
co·ni·ine
co·ni·ism
co·nio·fi·bro·sis
co·ni·ol·o·gy
co·nio·lymph·sta·sis
co·ni·om·e·ter
co·nio·phage
co·ni·o·sis
Co·nio·spor·i·um

co·nio·spo·ro·sis
co·ni·ot·o·my
co·nio·tox·i·co·sis
Co·ni·um
    C. maculatum
con·iza·tion
    cold c.
con·ju·gal
con·ju·gant
con·ju·ga·ta
    c. anatomica
    c. diagonalis
    c. vera
    c. vera obstetrica
con·ju·gate
    anatomic c.
    available c.
    diagonal c.
    effective c.
    external c.
    false c.
    c. of inlet
    internal c.
    obstetric c.
    c. of outlet
    true c.
con·ju·ga·tion
con·junc·ti·va *pl.* con·junc·ti·vae
    bulbar c.
    corneal c.
    ocular c.
    palpebral c.
    scleral c.
con·junc·ti·val
con·junc·ti·vi·plas·ty
con·junc·ti·vi·tis
    actinic c.
    acute contagious c.
    acute epidemic c.
    acute hemorrhagic c.
    allergic c.
    anaphylactic c.
    angular c.
    arc-flash c.
    atopic c.
    atropine c.
    blennorrheal c.

con·junc·ti·vi·tis *(continued)*
   calcareous c.
   catarrhal c.
   caterpillar c.
   chemical c.
   chronic catarrhal c.
   croupous c.
   diphtheritic c.
   diplobacillary c.
   eczematous c.
   Egyptian c.
   epidemic c.
   follicular c.
   glare c.
   gonococcal c.
   gonorrheal c.
   granular c.
   hypertrophic c.
   inclusion c.
   infantile purulent c.
   infectious c.
   klieg c.
   Koch-Weeks c.
   larval c.
   lithiasis c.
   c. medicamentosa
   membranous c.
   meningococcus c.
   molluscum c.
   Morax-Axenfeld c.
   mucopurulent c.
   necrotic infectious c.
   c. nodosa
   nodular c.
   Parinaud's c.
   Pascheff's c.
   c. petrificans
   phlyctenular c.
   prairie c.
   pseudomembranous c.
   purulent c.
   scrofular c.
   shipyard c.
   simple c.
   spring c.
   squirrel plague c.
   swimming pool c.
   trachomatous c.

con·junc·ti·vi·tis *(continued)*
   tularemic c.
   uratic c.
   vaccinial c.
   vernal c.
   welder's c.
   Widmark's c.
con·junc·ti·vo·dac·ryo·cys·tos·to·my
con·junc·ti·vo·ma
con·junc·ti·vo·plas·ty
con·junc·ti·vo·rhi·nos·to·my
Conn's syndrome
con·na·tal
con·nate
con·nec·tion
   clamp c.
   intertendinous c.
   thalamostriate c.
con·nec·tor
   major c.
   minor c.
   saddle c.
Con·nell's suture
con·nex·us *pl.* con·nex·us
   c. intertendineus
co·noid
   Sturm's c.
co·no·my·oi·din
con·oph·thal·mus
Co·no·po·di·na
con·qui·nine
Con·radi's disease
Con·radi's line
Con·radi's syndrome
Con·ray
Cons. — L. conserva (keep)
con·san·guin·e·ous
con·san·guin·i·ty
con·scious
con·scious·ness
   colon c.
   double c.
con·scious-se·da·tion
con·sent
   informed c.
con·ser·va·tion
con·ser·va·tive

con·serve
con·sis·ten·cy
con·sol·i·dant
con·sol·i·da·tion
con·sol·i·da·tive
con·so·lute
con·so·na·tion
con·spe·ci·fic
con·sper·gent
con·sper·sus
con·stan·cy
    cell c.
    object c.
con·stant
    absorption c.
    affinity c.
    association c.
    Avogadro's c.
    binding c.
    Boltzmann's c.
    catalytic c.
    decay c.
    dielectric c.
    diffusion c.
    disintegration c.
    dissociation c.
    equilibrium c.
    Faraday's c.
    flotation c.
    gas c.
    gravitational c.
    growth rate c.
    Lapicque's c.
    Michaelis c.
    Newtonian c. of gravitation
    Planck's c.
    quantum c.
    radioactive c.
    sedimentation c.
    specific gamma-ray c.
    specificity c.
    velocity c.
con·sti·pat·ed
con·sti·pa·tion
    atonic c.
    gastrojejunal c.
    proctogenous c.
    spastic c.

con·sti·tu·ent
con·sti·tu·tion
    lymphatic c.
    vasoneurotic c.
con·sti·tu·tion·al
con·strict
con·stric·tion
    congenital ring c's
    duodenopyloric c.
    primary c.
    pyloric c.
    Ranvier's c's
    secondary c.
con·stric·tive
con·stric·tor
    c. isthmi faucium
    c. naris
    c. urethrae
    c. vaginae
con·strin·gent
con·struc·tive
con·sult
con·sul·tant
con·sul·ta·tion
con·sump·tion
    galloping c.
    luxus c.
con·sump·tive
Cont. — L. contusus (bruised)
con·tact
    balancing c.
    centric c.
    complete c.
    deflective c.
    direct c.
    immediate c.
    indirect c.
    initial c.
    mediate c.
    occlusal c.
    premature c.
    proximal c., proximate c.
    weak c.
    working c.
con·tac·tant
con·tac·tol·o·gist
con·tac·tol·o·gy
con·ta·gia

con·ta·gion
  psychic c.
con·ta·gi·os·i·ty
con·ta·gious
con·ta·gi·um *pl.* con·ta·gia
con·tam·i·nant
con·tam·i·na·tion
con·tent
  catalytic c.
  effective radium c.
  equivalent radium c.
  latent c.
  manifest c.
  polymorphism information
    c. (PIC)
  substance c.
  volume c.
con·ti·gu·i·ty
con·tig·u·ous
Contin. — L. continuetur (let
  it be continued)
con·ti·nence
  fecal c.
  urinary c.
con·ti·nent
con·tor·tion
con·tour
  equal loudness c.
  height of c.
con·toured
con·tour·ing
  occlusal c.
con·tra-an·gle
con·tra-ap·er·ture
con·tra·cep·tion
  intrauterine c.
  rhythm c.
con·tra·cep·tive
  barrier c.
  chemical c.
  intrauterine c.
  oral c.
con·tract
con·trac·tile
con·trac·til·i·ty
  cardiac c.
  galvanic c.
  idiomuscular c.

con·trac·til·i·ty *(continued)*
  neuromuscular c.
con·trac·tion
  aerobic c.
  anaerobic c.
  anisometric c.
  anodal closure c.
  anodal opening c.
  atrial c.
  automatic ventricular c.
  bladder neck c.
  blocked arterial c.
  Braxton Hicks c's
  cardiac c.
  carpopedal c.
  cathodal closure c.
  cathodal opening c.
  cicatricial c.
  clonic c.
  closing c.
  concentric c.
  Dupuytren's c.
  escaped ventricular c.
  false uterine c.
  faradic c.
  fibrillary c's
  galvanotonic c.
  Hicks c's
  hourglass c.
  hunger c.
  idiomuscular c.
  isokinetic c.
  isometric c.
  isotonic c.
  isovolumetric c.
  lengthening c.
  myoclonic c.
  myotatic c.
  opening c.
  palmar c.
  paradoxical c.
  postural c.
  premature c.
  segmentation c.
  shortening c.
  tetanic c.
  tone c.
  tonic c.

con·trac·tion *(continued)*
    tumultuous c's
    twitch c.
    uterine c.
    wound c.
con·trac·ture
    burn scar c.
    Dupuytren's c.
    extrapyramidal c.
    flexion c.
    functional c.
    hypertonic c.
    hysterical c.
    ischemic c.
    muscle c.
    organic c.
    postpoliomyelitic c.
    Volkmann's c.
con·tra·fis·sure
con·tra·in·ci·sion
con·tra·in·di·cant
con·tra·in·di·cate
con·tra·in·di·ca·tion
con·tra·in·su·lar
con·tra·lat·er·al
con·tra·pa·ret·ic
con·tra·sex·u·al
con·trast
    film c.
    high c.
    long-scale c.
    low c.
    object c.
    radiographic c.
    short-scale c.
    subject c.
con·tra·stim·u·lant
con·tra·stim·u·lism
con·tra·stim·u·lus
con·tre·coup
con·trec·ta·tion
Cont. rem. — L. continuetur
  remedium (let the medicine
  be continued)
con·trol
    associative automatic c.
    astigmatism c.
    automatic gain c.

con·trol *(continued)*
    aversive c.
    biologic c.
    birth c.
    Diack c.
    feedback c.
    fine c.
    idiodynamic c.
    multivalent c.
    reflex c.
    relaxed c.
    Schick test c.
    sex c.
    stimulus c.
    stringent c.
    synergic c.
    tonic c.
    vestibuloequilibratory c.
    volitional c.
    voluntary c.
Con·trolled Sub·stan·ces Act
con·tund
con·tuse
con·tu·sion
    brain c.
    cerebral c.
    contrecoup c.
con·tu·sive
con·u·lar
Co·nus
co·nus *pl.* co·ni
    c. arteriosus
    distraction c.
    c. elasticus
    coni epididymidis
    c. medullaris
    myopic c.
    supertraction c.
    c. terminalis
    coni vasculosi
con·va·lesce
con·va·les·cence
con·va·les·cent
con·vec·tion
con·ver·gence
    accommodative c.
    amplitude of c.
    conjugate c.

con·ver·gence *(continued)*
    far point of c.
    fusional c.
    near point of c.
    negative c.
    positive c.
    proximal c.
    tonic c.
con·ver·gent
con·ver·gi·om·e·ter
Con·verse method
con·ver·sion
con·ver·tase
    C3 c.
    C3 proactivator c.
      (C3PAase)
    C5 c.
con·vert·er
    analog-to-digital (A/D) c.
    digital-to-analog (D/A) c.
    scan c.
con·ver·tin
con·vex
con·vex·i·ty
con·vexo·ba·sia
con·vexo·con·cave
con·vexo·con·vex
con·vo·lut·ed
con·vo·lu·tio
con·vo·lu·tion
    Broca's c.
    callosal c.
    c's of cerebrum
    first temporal c.
    c's of Gratiolet
    Heschl's c.
    occipitotemporal c.
    second temporal c.
    transitional c.
    Zuckerkandl's c.
con·vo·lu·tion·al
con·vo·lu·tion·ary
con·vul·sant
con·vul·si·bil·i·ty
con·vul·sion
    audiogenic c.
    central c.
    choreic c.

con·vul·sion *(continued)*
    clonic c.
    coordinate c.
    crowing c.
    epileptiform c.
    essential c.
    febrile c's
    hypoglycemic c.
    hysterical c.
    hysteroid c.
    infantile c.
    jackknife c.
    lightning major c.
    local c.
    mimetic c.
    mimic c.
    puerperal c.
    salaam c.
    spontaneous c.
    static c.
    tetanic c.
    tonic c.
    toxic c.
    traumatic c.
    uremic c.
con·vul·sive
Coo·ley's anemia
Coo·ley's disease
Coo·lidge tube
Coombs' test
Coo·per's disease
Coo·per's fascia
Coo·per's hernia
Coo·per's irritable breast
Coo·per's irritable testis
Coo·per's ligament
Coo·per·nail's sign
co·or·di·na·tion
co·os·si·fi·ca·tion
co·os·si·fy
co·pal
co·par·af·fin·ate
COPD — chronic obstructive
    pulmonary disease
Cope's sign
co·pe·pod
Co·pep·o·da
Co·per·ni·cia

cop·ing
　　transfer c.
co·pi·opia
Cop·lin's jar
copo·dys·ki·ne·sia
co·poly·mer
cop·per
　　c. abietinate
　　c. citrate
　　c. sulfate
　　c.-wiring
cop·per·as
cop·per·head
cop·ra·cra·sia
cop·ra·gogue
co·pre·cip·i·tin
cop·rem·e·sis
cop·ro·an·ti·body
Cop·ro·coc·cus
cop·ro·lag·nia
cop·ro·la·lia
cop·ro·lith
cop·rol·o·gy
cop·ro·ma
Cop·ro·mas·tix
　　C. prowazeki
Cop·ro·mo·nas
cop·ro·pha·gia
cop·roph·a·gous
cop·roph·a·gy
cop·ro·phil
cop·ro·phil·ia
cop·ro·phil·ic
cop·roph·i·lous
cop·ro·pho·bia
cop·ro·phra·sia
cop·ro·por·phy·ria
　　erythropoietic c.
　　hereditary c.
cop·ro·por·phy·rin
cop·ro·por·phy·rin·o·gen
cop·ro·por·phy·rin·o·gen ox·
　　i·dase
cop·ro·por·phy·rin·uria
co·pros·ta·nol
cop·ro·sta·sis
cop·ro·ste·rin
co·pros·ter·ol

cop·ro·zoa
cop·ro·zo·ic
cop·u·la
　　c. linguae
cop·u·la·tion
Coq. — L. coque (boil)
Coq. in s. a. — L. coque in
　　sufficiente aqua (boil in
　　sufficient water)
Coq. s. a. — L. coque
　　secundum artem (boil
　　properly)
co·quille
cor
　　c. adiposum
　　c. arteriosum
　　c. biloculare
　　c. bovinum
　　c. dextrum
　　c. hirsutum
　　c. pendulum
　　c. pseudotriloculare
　　　biatriatum
　　c. pulmonale
　　c. sinistrum
　　c. taurinum
　　c. triatriatum
　　c. triloculare
　　c. triloculare biatriatum
　　c. triloculare
　　　biventriculare
　　c. venosum
　　c. villosum
cor·a·cid·ia
cor·a·cid·i·um *pl.* cor·a·cid·ia
cor·a·co·acro·mi·al
cor·a·co·bra·chi·al·is
cor·a·co·cla·vic·u·lar
cor·a·co·hu·mer·al
cor·a·coid
cor·a·coi·di·tis
cor·a·co·ra·di·a·lis
cor·a·co·ul·nar·is
cor·al·li·form
cor·al·lin
　　yellow c.
cor·al·loid
Co·ra·mine

cor·asth·ma
Cor·bus' disease
cord
    Bergmann's c's
    Billroth's c's
    c. of Hippocrates
    condyle c.
    dental c.
    enamel c.
    Ferrein's c's
    ganglionated c.
    genital c.
    germinal c.
    gubernacular c.
    hepatic c's
    lateral c.
    lateral c. of brachial plexus
    lumbosacral c.
    lymph c's
    medial c.
    medullary c's
    mesonephrogenic c.
    metanephrogenic c.
    nasolacrimal c.
    nephrogenic c.
    nerve c.
    oblique c. of elbow joint
    ovigerous c's
    Pflüger's c's
    posterior c.
    pronephrogenic c.
    psalterial c.
    red pulp c's
    rete c's
    scirrhous c.
    sex c's
    sexual c's
    spermatic c.
    spinal c.
    splenic c's
    tendinous c.
    testis c's
    umbilical c.
    urogenital c.
    vocal c., false
    vocal c., true
    Weitbrecht's c.
    Willis' c's

cord·al
cor·date
cor·dec·to·my
cor·di·form
cor·di·tis
cor·do·meso·blast
cor·do·pexy
cor·dot·o·my
Cor·dran
Cor·dy·ceps
    C. sinensis
Cor·dy·lo·bia
core
    cast c.
    spore c.
core·cli·sis
cor·ec·ta·sis
cor·ec·tome
co·rec·to·me·di·al·y·sis
co·rec·to·my
cor·ec·to·pia
core·di·al·y·sis
core·di·as·ta·sis
co·reg·o·nin
co·rel·y·sis
cor·e·mor·pho·sis
cor·en·cli·sis
cor·e·om·e·ter
cor·e·om·e·try
cor·eo·plas·ty
cor·e·pexy
co·re·pres·sor
cor·e·ste·no·ma
    c. congenitum
co·re·to·me·di·al·y·sis
co·ret·o·my
Co·ri, Carl Ferdinand
Co·ri, Gerty Theresa Radnitz
Co·ri cycle
Co·ri ester
co·ri·a·ceous
cori·a·myr·tin
cor·i·an·der
Co·ri·a·ria
co·ri·in
co·ri·um
    lingual c.
Cor·mack, Allan MacCleod

cor·meth·a·sone ac·e·tate
corn
    hard c.
    soft c.
cor·nea
    conical c.
    c. farinata
    flat c.
    c. globata
    c. globosa
    c. guttata
    c. opaca
    c. plana
    c. verticillata
cor·ne·al
cor·ne·itis
cor·neo·bleph·a·ron
cor·neo·iri·tis
cor·neo·scle·ra
cor·neo·scle·ral
cor·ne·ous
Cor·ner-Al·len test
Cor·ner-Al·len unit
Cor·ner's tampon
Cor·net's forceps
cor·ne·um
cor·nic·u·late
cor·nic·u·lum
cor·ni·fi·ca·tion
cor·ni·fied
Cor·ning's anesthesia
Cor·ning's method
cor·noid
cor·nu *pl.* cor·nua
    c. Ammonis
    c. coccygeale
    c. coccygeum
    c. cutaneum
    c. descendens
    ethmoid c.
    sacral c.
    c. sacrale
    cornua of spinal cord
    c. uteri
cor·nua
cor·nu·al
cor·nu·ate
cor·nu·com·mis·sur·al

cor·nu·co·pia
co·ro·di·as·ta·sis
co·rol·la
co·rom·e·ter
co·ro·na *pl.* co·ro·nas, co·ro·nae
    c. capitis
    c. ciliaris
    c. clinica
    dental c.
    c. dentis
    c. glandis penis
    c. of glans penis
    c. radiata
    c. seborrheica
    c. veneris
    Zinn's c.
co·ro·nad
co·ro·nae
co·ro·nal
cor·o·na·le
cor·o·na·lis
cor·o·na·ri·tis
cor·o·nary
    café c.
co·ro·na·vi·rus
co·ro·ne
cor·o·ner
co·ro·ni·on
co·ro·ni·tis
cor·o·noid
cor·o·noi·dec·to·my
co·ro·par·el·cy·sis
co·ro·plas·ty
co·ros·co·py
co·rot·o·my
cor·po·ra
cor·por·ic
corps
    medical c.
    c. ronds
corpse
cor·pu·len·cy
cor·pus *pl.* cor·po·ra
    c. adiposum
    c. albicans
    corpora allata
    c. amygdaloideum

cor·pus *(continued)*
  corpora amylacea
  corpora arantii
  corpora atretica
  corpora bigemina
  c. calcanei
  c. callosum
  c. cavernosum
  c. cerebelli
  c. ciliare
  c. claviculae
  c. clitoridis
  c. coccygeum
  c. costae
  c. delicti
  c. dentatum
  c. epididymidis
  c. femoris
  c. fibrosum
  c. fibulae
  c. fimbriatum
  corpora flava
  c. fornicis
  c. gastricum
  c. geniculatum
  c. glandulae
    bulbourethralis
  c. glandulae sudoriferae
  c. glandulare prostatae
  c. hemorrhagicum
  c. Highmori
  c. highmorianum
  c. humeri
  c. hypothalamicum
  c. incudis
  c. interpedunculare
  c. linguae
  corpora lutea atretica
  c. luteum
  c. Luysii
  c. mamillare
  c. mammae
  c. mandibulae
  c. maxillae
  c. medullare cerebelli
  c. medullare vermis
  c. metacarpalis
  c. metatarsalis

cor·pus *(continued)*
  c. nuclei caudati
  c. of Oken
  corpora oryzoidea
  c. ossis femoris
  c. ossis hyoidei
  c. ossis ilii
  c. ossis ischii
  c. ossis metacarpalis
  c. ossis metatarsalis
  c. ossis pubis
  c. ossis sphenoidalis
  c. pampiniforme
  c. pancreatis
  corpora para-aortica
  c. paraterminalis
  c. penis
  c. pineale
  c. pontobulbare
  c. pyramidale medullae
  corpora quadrigemina
  c. radii
  corpora restiformia
  c. rhomboidale
  corpora santoriana
  c. sphenoidale
  c. spongiosum
  c. sterni
  c. striatum
  c. subthalamicum
  c. tali
  c. tibiae
  c. trapezoideum
  c. triticeum
  c. ulnae
  c. unguis
  c. uteri
  c. ventriculare
  c. ventriculi
  c. vertebrae
  c. vertebralis
  c. vesicae biliaris
  c. vesicae felleae
  c. vesicae urinariae
  c. vitreum
  c. Wolffi
cor·pus·cal·los·to·my

cor·pus·cle
- Alzheimer's c's
- amylaceous c's
- amyloid c's
- articular c's
- Babès-Ernst c.
- basal c.
- Bennet's large c's
- Bennet's small c's
- Bizzozero's c.
- blood c's
- bridge c.
- bulboid c's
- cartilage c.
- cement c.
- chorea c's
- chromophil c.
- chyle c.
- colloid c's
- colostrum c's
- concentric c's
- corneal c's
- Dogiel's c.
- Donné's c's
- Drysdale's c's
- dust c's
- genital c's
- Gierke's c's
- Gluge's c's
- Golgi's c's
- Golgi-Mazzoni c's
- Grandry's c's
- Grandry-Merkel c's
- Guarnieri's c's
- Hassall's c's
- Hayem's elementary c.
- Herbst's c's
- Jaworski's c's
- Krause's c's
- lamellar c's
- lamellated c's
- Laveran's c's
- Leber's c's
- lingual c.
- Lostorfer's c's
- lymph c's
- lymphoid c's

cor·pus·cle *(continued)*
- malpighian c's
- Mazzoni's c's
- meconium c's
- Meissner's c's
- Merkel's c's
- milk c's
- mucous c's
- Norris' c's
- Nunn's gorged c's
- oval c.
- Pacini's c's
- pacinian c's
- Paschen's c's
- pessary c.
- phantom c.
- Purkinje's c's
- pus c.
- Rainey's c.
- red c.
- renal c's
- reticulated c's
- Röhl's marginal c's
- Ruffini's c's
- Russell c's
- salivary c.
- Schwalbe's c.
- splenic c's
- tactile c's
- taste c's
- tendon c's
- terminal nerve c's
- thymus c's
- Timofeew's c's
- touch c's
- Toynbee's c's
- Tröltsch's c's
- typhic c's
- Valentin's c's
- Vater's c's
- Vater-Pacini c's
- Virchow's c's
- Wagner's c's
- Weber's c.
- white c.

cor·pus·cu·la
cor·pus·cu·lar

cor·pus·cu·lum *pl.* cor·pus·cu·
la
    corpuscula articularia
    corpuscula bulboidea
    corpuscula genitalia
    corpuscula lamellosa
    corpuscula nervosa
      terminalia
    c. nervosum acapsulatum
    corpuscula renis
    corpuscula tactus
cor·rec·tion
    Yates c.
cor·rec·tor
    function c.
cor·re·la·tion
    zero c.
cor·re·spon·dence
    anomalous retinal c.
    harmonious retinal c.
    normal retinal c.
    retinal c.
Cor·ri·gan's disease
Cor·ri·gan's line
Cor·ri·gan's pulse
Cor·ri·gan's respiration
Cor·ri·gan's sign
cor·ri·gent
cor·rin
cor·ri·noid
cor·ro·dens
    Bacteroides c.
    Eikenella c.
cor·roid
cor·ro·sion
cor·ro·sive
cor·ru·ga·tion
cor·ru·ga·tor
cor·set
    Milwaukee c.
Cort. — L. cortex (bark)
Cor·tate
Cort-Dome
Cor·tef
Cor·ten·e·ma
cor·tex *pl.* cor·ti·ces
    aberrant suprarenal c.
    adrenal c.

cor·tex *(continued)*
    agranular c.
    auditory c.
    calcarine c.
    cerebellar c.
    c. cerebelli
    cerebral c.
    c. cerebri
    cingulate c.
    driftwood c.
    entorhinal c.
    eulaminate c.
    fetal c.
    frontal premotor c.
    c. glandulae suprarenalis
    c. of hair shaft
    heterotypical c.
    homogenetic c.
    homotypical c.
    interpyramidal c.
    c. lentis
    limbic c.
    motor c.
    c. nodi lymphatici
    nonolfactory c.
    olfactory c.
    c. ovarii
    periamygdaloid c.
    piriform c.
    precentral motor c.
    premotor c.
    provisional c.
    renal c.
    c. renis
    retrosplenial c.
    sensorimotor c.
    somatosensory c.
    somesthetic c.
    striate c.
    supplementary motor c.
    tertiary c.
    c. thymi
    visual c.
Cor·ti's arch
Cor·ti's canal
Cor·ti's cell
Cor·ti's fiber
Cor·ti's ganglion

Cor·ti's membrane
Cor·ti's organ
Cor·ti's rod
Cor·ti's tunnel
cor·ti·cal
cor·ti·cal·iza·tion
cor·ti·cal·os·te·ot·o·my
cor·ti·cate
cor·ti·cec·to·my
cor·ti·ces
cor·ti·cif·u·gal
cor·ti·cip·e·tal
cor·ti·co·ad·re·nal
cor·ti·co·af·fer·ent
cor·ti·co·au·to·nom·ic
cor·ti·co·bul·bar
cor·ti·co·can·cel·lous
cor·ti·co·cer·e·bral
cor·ti·co·di·en·ce·phal·ic
cor·ti·co·ef·fer·ent
cor·ti·co·gram
cor·ti·coid
cor·ti·co·lib·er·in
cor·ti·co·med·ul·lary
cor·ti·co·mes·en·ce·phal·ic
cor·ti·co·pe·dun·cu·lar
cor·ti·cop·e·tal
cor·ti·co·pleu·ri·tis
cor·ti·co·pon·tine
cor·ti·co·pon·to·cer·e·bel·lar
cor·ti·co·ru·bral
cor·ti·co·spi·nal
cor·ti·co·ster·oid
cor·ti·cos·ter·one
cor·ti·co·stri·ate
cor·ti·co·ten·sin
cor·ti·co·tha·lam·ic
cor·ti·co·troph
cor·ti·co·troph·ic
cor·ti·co·troph-li·po·troph
cor·ti·co·trop·ic
cor·ti·co·tro·pin
cor·ti·lymph
cor·ti·sol
cor·ti·sone
    c. acetate
cor·tiv·a·zol
Cor·tone

Cor·tril
Cor·tro·phin
Cor·tro·syn
co·run·dum
cor·us·ca·tion
Cor·vi·sart's disease
cor·y·ban·ti·asm
cor·y·ban·tism
co·ryd·a·line
co·ryd·a·lis
co·rym·bi·form
co·rym·bose
cor·y·ne·bac·te·ria
Cor·y·ne·bac·te·ri·a·ceae
cor·y·ne·bac·te·rio·phage
Cor·y·ne·bac·te·ri·um
    C. diphtheriae
    C. genitalium
    C. haemolyticum
    C. minutissimum
    C. parvum
    C. pseudodiphtheriticum
    C. pseudotuberculosis
    C. pyogenes
    C. tenuis
    C. ulcerans
    C. xerosis
cor·y·ne·bac·te·ri·um *pl.* cor·
    y·ne·bac·te·ria
    group JK c.
    group 3 c.
Cor·y·ne·form
cor·y·ne·form
cor·y·tu·ber·ine
co·ry·za
    allergic c.
    c. foetida
    infectious avian c.
    c. oedematosa
co·ry·za·vi·rus
COS — Canadian
    Ophthalmological Society
co·sen·si·tize
Cos·me·gen
cos·mid
cos·mo·pol·i·tan
cos·ta *pl.* cos·tae
    c. cervicalis

cos·ta *(continued)*
    c. fluctuans
    c. fluctuans decima
    costae fluitantes
    c. prima
    costae spuriae
    costae verae
cos·tae
cos·tal
cos·tal·gia
cos·ta·lis
cos·tate
cos·ta·tec·to·my
cos·tec·to·my
Cos·ten's syndrome
cos·ti·car·ti·lage
cos·ti·cer·vi·cal
cos·tif·er·ous
cos·ti·form
cos·ti·spi·nal
cos·tive
cos·to·ab·dom·i·nal
cos·to·cen·tral
cos·to·cer·vi·ca·lis
cos·to·chon·dral
cos·to·chon·dri·tis
cos·to·cla·vic·u·lar
cos·to·cor·a·coid
cos·to·di·a·phrag·mat·ic
cos·to·gen·ic
cos·to·in·fe·ri·or
cos·to·lum·bar
cos·to·phren·ic
cos·to·plas·ty
cos·to·pleu·ral
cos·to·pneu·mo·pexy
cos·to·scap·u·lar
cos·to·scap·u·lar·is
cos·to·ster·nal
cos·to·ster·no·plas·ty
cos·to·su·pe·ri·or
cos·to·tome
cos·tot·o·my
cos·to·trans·verse
cos·to·trans·ver·sec·to·my
cos·to·ver·te·bral
cos·to·xiph·oid
co·syn·tro·pin

Co·tard's syndrome
Cot·a·zym
COTe — cathodal opening tetanus
co·throm·bo·plas·tin
co·ti·nine
    c. fumarate
co·trans·duc·tion
Co·trel-Du·bous·set spinal instrumentation
co-tri·mox·a·zole
Cotte's operation
Cot·ting's operation
Cot·ton's effect
cot·ton
    absorbent c.
    capsicum c.
    collodion c.
    gun c.
    gun c., soluble
    purified c.
    salicylated c.
    styptic c.
cot·ton·mouth
cot·ton·pox
cot·ton-wool
Co·tu·gno's disease
Co·tun·ni·us' canal
Co·tun·ni·us' nerve
Co·tun·ni·us' space
co·tur·nism
co-twin
cot·y·le
cot·y·le·don
    placental c.
cot·y·le·don·tox·in
cot·y·loid
cot·y·lo·pu·bic
cot·y·lo·sa·cral
co·type
cough
    aneurysmal c.
    Balme's c.
    barking c.
    bovine c.
    brassy c.
    compression c.
    dog c.

cough *(continued)*
  dry c.
  ear c.
  extrapulmonary c.
  hacking c.
  mechanical c.
  Morton's c.
  nonproductive c.
  paroxysmal c.
  privet c.
  productive c.
  reflex c.
  smoker's c.
  stomach c.
  Sydenham's c.
  tea taster's c.
  trigeminal c.
  weavers' c.
  wet c.
  whooping c.
  winter c.
cou·lomb
Cou·ma·din
cou·ma·my·cin
cou·mar·ic acid
cou·ma·rin
cou·mer·my·cin
cou·mes·trol
Coun·cil·man's bodies
Coun·cil·man's lesions
coun·sel·ing
  genetic c.
  nondirective c.
count
  Addis c.
  Arneth c.
  bleeding point c.
  blood c.
  complete blood c.
  differential c.
  direct platelet c.
  dust c.
  filament-nonfilament c.
  indirect platelet c.
  kick c's
  leukocyte c.
  neutrophil lobe c.
  pollen c.

count *(continued)*
  red cell c.
  reticulocyte c.
  ridge c.
  total white c.
coun·ter
  automated differential leukocyte c.
  colony c.
  Coulter c.
  crystal c.
  electronic cell c.
  end-window c.
  gamma scintillation c.
  gamma well c.
  gas-flow c.
  Geiger c.
  Geiger-Müller c.
  immersion c.
  liquid-flow c.
  proportional c.
  scintillation c.
  whole-body c.
coun·ter·ac·tion
coun·ter·bal·ance
  renal c.
coun·ter·cur·rent
coun·ter·de·pres·sant
coun·ter·die
coun·ter·elec·tro·pho·re·sis
coun·ter·ex·ten·sion
coun·ter·fis·sure
coun·ter·im·mu·no·elec·tro·pho·re·sis
coun·ter·in·ci·sion
coun·ter·in·vest·ment
coun·ter·ir·ri·tant
coun·ter·ir·ri·ta·tion
coun·ter·open·ing
coun·ter·pho·bia
coun·ter·pho·bic
coun·ter·poi·son
  intra-aortic balloon c.
coun·ter·punc·ture
coun·ter-roll·ing
coun·ter·stain
coun·ter·stroke
coun·ter·trac·tion

coun·ter·trans·fer·ence
coup
    c. de fouet
    c. de sabre
    en c. de sabre
    c. de sang
    c. Highmori
    c. sur coup
coup·ler
    acoustic c.
coup·ling
    contact c.
    electrochemical c.
    excitation-contraction c.
    fixed c.
    immersion c.
    liquid c.
cour·ba·ture
Cour·nand, André Frédéric
Cour·tois sign
Cour·voi·si·er's law
Cour·voi·si·er's sign
Cour·voi·si·er-Ter·rier
    syndrome
Cou·tard's method
cou·vade
Cou·ve·laire uterus
cou·ver·cle
co·va·lence
co·va·lent
co·var·i·ance
co·var·i·ate
cov·er·glass
cov·er·slip
cow·age
Cow·den disease
Cow·den syndrome
Cow·dry's type A inclusion
    bodies
Cow·dry's type B inclusion
    bodies
Cow·per's gland
Cow·per's ligament
cow·pe·ri·an
cow·per·itis
cow·pox
coxa
    c. adducta

coxa *(continued)*
    c. flexa
    c. magna
    c. plana
    c. valga
    c. vara
    c. vara luxans
cox·al·gia
    Mediterranean c.
cox·an·ky·lom·e·ter
cox·ar·thria
cox·ar·thri·tis
cox·ar·throc·a·ce
cox·ar·throp·a·thy
cox·ar·thro·plas·ty
cox·ar·thro·sis
Cox·i·el·la
    C. burnetii
cox·itis
    c. fugax
    senile c.
    transient c.
cox·odyn·ia
coxo·fem·o·ral
coxo·tu·ber·cu·lo·sis
cox·sack·ie·vi·rus
co·zy·mase
CP — candle power
    chemically pure
cp — centipoise
CPAP — continuous positive
    airway pressure
CPC — clinicopathological
    conference
CPD — citrate phosphate
    dextrose
CPDA-1 — citrate phosphate
    dextrose adenine
CPDD — calcium
    pyrophosphate deposition
    disease
C Ped — Certified Pedorthist
CPH — Certificate in Public
    Health
CPK — creatine
    phosphokinase
CPM — continuous passive
    motion

CPR — cardiopulmonary resuscitation
CPS — carbamoyl phosphate synthetase
    carbamoyl phosphate synthetase II
cps — cycles per second
CR — complement receptor
    conditioned response
    crown-rump
Crab·tree effect
crack·le
    pleural c's
cra·dle
    electric c.
    heat c.
    ice c.
Crafts' test
Crai·gia
Cra·mer's splint
cramp
    accessory c.
    heat c.
    menstrual c's
    muscle c.
    nocturnal c's
    occupational c.
    recumbency c's
    seamstresses' c.
    stoker's c.
    tailors' c.
    watchmakers' c.
    writers'c.
Cramp·ton's muscle
Cramp·ton's test
cra·ni·ad
cra·ni·al
cra·ni·a·lis
cra·ni·am·phit·o·my
cra·ni·ec·to·my
cra·nio·acro·mi·al
cra·nio·au·ral
cra·nio·buc·cal
cra·nio·cau·dal
cra·nio·cele
cra·nio·cer·e·bral
cra·nio·cer·vi·cal
cra·nio·cla·sis

cra·nio·clast
cra·nio·clas·ty
cra·nio·did·y·mus
cra·nio·fa·cial
cra·nio·fe·nes·tria
cra·ni·og·no·my
cra·nio·graph
cra·ni·og·ra·phy
cra·nio·la·cu·nia
cra·ni·ol·o·gy
cra·nio·ma·la·cia
cra·nio·man·dib·u·lar
cra·nio·me·nin·go·cele
cra·ni·om·e·ter
cra·nio·met·ric
cra·ni·om·e·try
cra·ni·op·a·gus
    c. frontalis
    c. occipitalis
    c. parasiticus
    c. parietalis
cra·ni·op·a·thy
    metabolic c.
cra·nio·pha·ryn·ge·al
cra·nio·pha·ryn·gi·o·ma
cra·nio·phore
cra·nio·plas·ty
cra·nio·punc·ture
cra·nio·ra·chis·chi·sis
    c. totalis
cra·nio·sa·cral
cra·ni·os·chi·sis
cra·nio·scle·ro·sis
cra·nio·spi·nal
cra·nio·ste·no·sis
cra·ni·os·to·sis
cra·nio·syn·os·to·sis
cra·nio·ta·bes
cra·nio·tome
cra·ni·ot·o·my
cra·nio·to·nos·co·py
cra·nio·to·pog·ra·phy
cra·nio·try·pe·sis
cra·nio·tym·pan·ic
cra·nio·ver·te·bral
cra·ni·tis
cra·ni·um *pl.* cra·nia
    c. bifidum

cra·ni·um *(continued)*
    c. bifidum occultum
    cerebral c.
    c. cerebrale
    visceral c.
    c. viscerale
crap·u·lent
crap·u·lous
Crast. — L. crastinus (for tomorrow)
cra·ter·i·form
cra·ter·iza·tion
crau·nol·o·gy
crau·no·ther·a·py
craw-craw
Craw·ford-Ad·ams acetabular cup
Craw·ford-Ad·ams cup arthroplasty
craz·ing
CRD — chronic respiratory disease
cream
    barrier c.
    cold c.
    c. of tartar
Cream·a·lin
crease
    ear lobe c.
    gluteofemoral c.
    flexion c.
    palmar c.
    Sidney c.
    simian c.
cre·a·sote
cre·a·tine
    c. phosphate
cre·a·tine ki·nase
cre·a·tin·emia
cre·a·tine phos·pho·ki·nase
cre·a·tine phos·pho·trans·fer·ase
cre·at·i·nine
cre·a·tin·uria
cre·a·tor·rhea
cre·a·to·tox·ism
cre·a·tox·i·con
cre·a·tox·in

crèche
Cre·dé's ointment
CREG — cross-reactive group (of HLA antigens)
cre·mas·ter
    internal c. of Henle
crem·as·ter·ic
cre·ma·tion
cre·ma·to·ri·um
crem·no·cele
cre·na *pl.* cre·nae
    c. ani
    c. clunium
    c. cordis
cre·nae
cre·na·tion
cre·no·cyte
cre·no·cy·to·sis
creno·ther·a·py
cren·u·la·tion
cre·o·lin
cre·o·sol
cre·o·sote
    c. carbonate
crep·i·tant
crep·i·ta·tion
crep·i·tus
    articular c.
    bony c.
    false c.
    c. indux
    joint c.
    c. redux
    silken c.
    c. uteri
cre·pus·cu·lar
cre·scen·do-de·cres·cen·do murmur
cres·cent
    articular c.
    blastoporal c.
    cellular c.
    congenital c. of choroid
    epithelial c.
    fibrous c.
    c's of Giannuzzi
    gray c.
    malarial c's

cres·cent *(continued)*
  myopic c.
  sublingual c.
cres·cen·tic
cre·sol
cre·sol·phtha·lein
cre·sor·cin
cre·sor·cin·ol
cres·oxy·di·ol
cres·oxy·pro·pane·di·ol
crest
  acoustic c.
  acusticofacial c.
  alveolar c.
  anterior c. of fibula
  anterior c. of tibia
  arcuate c. of arytenoid
    cartilage
  basilar c.
  buccinator c.
  cerebral c's of cranial bone
  c. of cochlear window
  conchal c. of maxilla
  conchal c. of palatine bone
  deltoid c.
  dental c.
  dermal c's
  ethmoid c. of maxilla
  ethmoid c. of palatine bone
  falciform c.
  femoral c.
  fimbriated c.
  frontal c.
  ganglionic c.
  gingival c.
  glandular c. of larynx
  gluteal c.
  iliac c.
  iliopectineal c. of iliac bone
  iliopectineal c. of pelvis
  iliopectineal c. of pubis
  infratemporal c.
  infundibuloventricular c.
  inguinal c.
  c. of insertion
  interosseous c.
  intertrochanteric c.

crest *(continued)*
  intertrochanteric c.,
    anterior
  interureteric c.
  jugular c. of great wing of
    sphenoid bone
  lacrimal c., anterior
  lacrimal c., posterior
  c. of larger tubercle
  lateral c. of fibula
  marginal c.
  medial c. of fibula
  mental c., external
  mitochondrial c's
  nasal c. of maxilla
  nasal c. of palatine bone
  nasopalatine c.
  neural c.
  oblique c. of thyroid
    cartilage
  obturator c.
  occipital c., external
  occipital c., internal
  orbital c.
  papillary c.
  pectineal c. of femur
  pharyngeal c. of occipital
    bone
  radial c.
  rough c. of femur
  sacral c.
  seminal c.
  sphenoidal c.
  spinal c. of Rauber
  spiral c.
  spiral c. of cochlea
  supracondylar c.
  supramastoid c.
  supraventricular c.
  temporal c. of frontal bone
  terminal c. of right atrium
  tibial c.
  triangular c.
  trigeminal c.
  turbinal c.
  ulnar c.
  urethral c.

crest *(continued)*
    zygomatic c. of great wing
      of sphenoid bone
cres·to·my·cin sul·fate
cre·syl·ic acid
cre·tin
cre·tin·ism
    athyreotic c.
    endemic c.
    goitrous c.
    nonendemic goitrous c.
    sporadic goitrous c.
    sporadic nongoitrous c.
cre·tin·ist·ic
cre·tin·oid
cre·tin·ous
crev·ice
    gingival c.
cre·vic·u·lar
CRF — corticotropin-releasing
  factor
CRH — corticotropin-releasing hormone
crib
    clinical c.
    Jackson c.
    tongue c.
crib·bing
crib·ra
crib·ral
crib·rate
crib·ra·tion
crib·ri·form
cri·brum *pl.* cri·bra
    cribra orbitalia of Welcker
Cri·ce·tu·lus
Cri·ce·tus
Crich·ton-Browne's sign
Crick, Francis Harvey Compton
cri·co·ar·y·te·noid
cri·coid
cri·coi·dec·to·my
cri·coi·dyn·ia
cri·co·pha·ryn·ge·al
cri·co·pha·ryn·ge·us
cri·co·thy·re·ot·o·my
cri·co·thy·roid
cri·co·thy·roi·dot·o·my

cri·co·thy·rot·o·my
cri·cot·o·my
cri·co·tra·che·ot·o·my
cri du chat
Crig·ler-Naj·jar syndrome
crim·in·al·is·tics
crim·i·nol·o·gy
cri·nes
crin·in
cri·nis *pl.* cri·nes
cri·nol·o·gy
crin·oph·a·gy
Cri·num
cri·sis *pl.* cri·ses
    abdominal c.
    adolescent c.
    adrenal c.
    adrenocortical c.
    anaphylactoid c.
    aplastic c.
    blast c.
    brainstem c.
    bronchial c.
    cardiac c.
    cataleptic c.
    catathymic c.
    celiac c.
    cholinergic c.
    clitoris c.
    decerebrate c.
    deglobulinization c.
    developmental c.
    Dietl's c.
    false c.
    febrile c.
    gastric c.
    genital c. of newborn
    glaucomatocyclitic c.
    hemolytic c.
    hepatic c.
    hypertensive c.
    identity c.
    intestinal c.
    laryngeal c.
    myasthenic c.
    nefast c.
    nephralgic c.
    ocular c.

cri·sis *(continued)*
  oculogyric c.
  parkinsonian c.
  Pel's c's
  pharyngeal c.
  physiologic c.
  posterior c.
  rectal c.
  reflex anoxic c.
  reflex hypoxic c.
  renal c.
  salt-depletion c.
  salt-losing c.
  situational c.
  tabetic c.
  thoracic c.
  utricular c.
  vesical c.
  visceral c.
cris·pa·tion
cris·pa·tu·ra
cris·ta *pl.* cris·tae
  c. acustica
  c. ampullaris
  c. anterior fibulae
  c. anterior tibiae
  c. arcuata
  c. basilaris ductus
    cochlearis
  c. buccinatoria
  c. capitis costae
  c. colli costae
  c. conchalis maxillae
  c. conchalis ossis palatini
  cristae cutis
  c. dividens
  c. ethmoidalis maxillae
  c. ethmoidalis ossis palatini
  c. falciformis
  c. femoris
  c. fenestrae cochleae
  c. frontalis
  c. galli
  c. helicis
  c. iliaca
  c. infratemporalis
  c. interossea fibulae
  c. interossea radii

cris·ta *(continued)*
  c. interossea tibiae
  c. interossea ulnae
  c. intertrochanterica
  c. lacrimalis anterior
  c. lacrimalis posterior
  c. lateralis fibulae
  c. marginalis
  c. matricis unguis
  c. medialis fibulae
  c. musculi supinatoris
  c. nasalis maxillae
  c. nasalis ossis palatini
  c. obturatoria
  c. occipitalis externa
  c. occipitalis interna
  c. palatina
  c. pubica
  c. sacralis intermedia
  c. sacralis lateralis
  c. sphenoidalis
  c. spiralis
  c. spiralis cochleae
  c. supramastoidea
  c. supraventricularis
  c. temporalis
  c. terminalis atrii dextri
  c. transversa
  c. transversalis
  c. triangularis
  c. tuberculi majoris
  c. tuberculi minoris
  c. tympanica
  c. ulnae
  c. urethralis femininae
  c. urethralis masculinae
  c. vestibuli
cris·tae
cris·tal
cris·tate
cris·to·ba·lite
Crit·chett's operation
cri·te·ri·on
  Cooke's c.
  Jones' c.
  Spiegelberg's c.
crith
crit·i·cal

CRM — cross-reacting material
CRNA — Certified Registered Nurse Anesthetist
cro·ce·in
cro·ci·dis·mus
cro·cid·o·lite
cro·fil·con A
Crohn's disease
cro·mo·gly·cate
cro·mo·gly·cic acid
cro·mo·lyn
    c. sodium
Cro·nin method
Cron·khite-Can·a·da syndrome
Crooke's changes
cro·pro·pa·mide
CROS — contralateral routing of signals
Cros·by's capsule
cross
    occipital c.
    phage c.
    Ranvier's c's
    silver c.
    two-factor c.
    yellow c.
cross-ab·sorp·tion
cross·bite
    anterior c.
    buccal c.
    lingual c.
    posterior c.
cross·breed·ing
cross-bridges
cross-dress·ing
cross-eye
cross-feed·ing
cross·foot
cross·ing over
cross-link·ing
cross·match
cross·match·ing
cross·over, cross-over
cross-re·ac·tion
cross-re·ac·ti·va·tion
cross-re·ac·tiv·i·ty
cross-sec·tion
    capture c.
    nuclear c.
    total atomic attenuation c.
cross-sen·si·tiv·i·ty
cross-sen·si·ti·za·tion
cross-stri·a·tions
cross·talk
cross·way
crot·a·lid
Cro·tal·i·dae
crot·a·lin
Cro·tal·i·nae
cro·ta·line
cro·tal·ism
cro·ta·lo·tox·in
Crot·a·lus
cro·ta·mine
cro·ta·mi·ton
cro·taph·i·on
cro·teth·a·mide
cro·tin
Cro·ton
cro·ton·ic acid
cro·ton·ism
cro·tox·in
crou·no·ther·a·py
croup
    catarrhal c.
    diphtheritic c.
    false c.
    spasmodic c.
croup·ous
croupy
Crou·zon's disease
crown
    anatomical c.
    artificial c.
    basket c.
    bell c.
    Bischoff's c.
    Bonwill c.
    cap c.
    celluloid c.
    ciliary c.
    clinical c.

crown *(continued)*
    collar c.
    complete c.
    dental c.
    dowel c.
    extra-alveolar c.
    faced c.
    half-cap c.
    jacket c.
    open-face c.
    overlay c.
    physiological c.
    pinledge c.
    post c.
    radiating c.
    Richmond c.
    shell c.
    steel c.
    tapered c.
    three-quarter c.
    veneered c.
    window c.
crown·ing
CRP — C-reactive protein
CRS — Chinese restaurant syndrome
CRT — cathode ray tube
cru·ces
cru·ci·ate
cru·ci·ble
cru·ci·form
cru·fo·mate
crunch
    mediastinal c.
    xiphisternal c.
cru·or *pl.* cru·o·res
cru·ra
cru·ral
cru·re·us
cru·ri·tis
cru·ro·gen·i·tal
cru·ro·scro·tal
cru·rot·o·my
crus *pl.* cru·ra
    ampullary osseous crura
    anterior c. of stapes
    c. anterius stapedis
    crura anthelicis

crus *(continued)*
    c. breve incudis
    c. cerebelli ad pontem
    c. cerebri
    c. clitoridis
    common osseous c.
    c. dextrum diaphragmatis
    c. of diaphragm, left
    c. of diaphragm, right
    c. fornicis
    c. glandis clitoridis
    c. helicis
    long c. of incus
    c. longum incudis
    crura membranacea
    membranous crura
    crura ossea
    crura ossea ampullaria
    osseous crura
    c. osseum commune
    c. osseum simplex
    c. penis
    posterior c. of stapes
    c. posterius stapedis
    short c. of incus
    simple osseous c.
    c. sinistrum diaphragmatis
    superior c. of cerebellum
crust
    milk c.
crus·ta *pl.* crus·tae
    c. inflammatoria
    c. lactea
    c. petrosa dentis
    c. phlogistica
    c. radicis
Crus·ta·cea
crus·ta·cean
crus·ta·ceo·ru·bin
crus·tae
crus·tal
crus·to·sus
crutch
    Canadian c.
    perineal c.
Crutch·field tongs
crux *pl.* cru·ces
    c. of heart

crux *(continued)*
    cruces pilorum
Cruz's trypanosomiasis
Cruz-Chag·as disease
cry
    cephalic c.
    epileptic c.
    hydrocephalic c.
    joint c.
    night c.
cry·al·ge·sia
cry·an·es·the·sia
Cry·er's elevator
cry·es·the·sia
cry·mo·an·es·the·sia
cry·mo·dyn·ia
cry·mo·phil·ic
cryo·ab·la·tion
cryo·an·al·ge·sia
cryo·an·es·the·sia
cryo·bank
cryo·bi·ol·o·gy
cryo·car·dio·ple·gia
cryo·cau·tery
cryo·crit
cry·ode
cryo·ex·trac·tion
cryo·ex·trac·tor
cry·o·fi·brin·o·gen
cryo·fi·brin·o·gen·emia
cryo·gam·ma·glob·u·lin
cry·o·gen
cry·o·gen·ic
cryo·glob·u·lin
cryo·glob·u·lin·emia
cryo·hy·drate
cryo·hy·po·phys·ec·to·my
cryo·mag·net
cry·om·e·ter
cryo·pal·li·dec·to·my
cry·op·a·thy
cryo·pexy
cryo·phake
cryo·phile
cryo·phil·ic
cryo·phy·lac·tic
cryo·pre·cip·i·ta·bil·i·ty
cryo·pre·cip·i·tate

cryo·pre·cip·i·ta·tion
cryo·pres·er·va·tion
cryo·probe
cryo·pro·tec·tive
cryo·pro·tein
cryo·scope
cryo·scop·i·cal
cry·os·co·py
cryo·spasm
cryo·stat
cryo·sty·let
cryo·sur·gery
cryo·thal·a·mec·to·my
cryo·thal·a·mot·o·my
cryo·ther·a·py
cryo·tol·er·ant
cryo·tome
cryo·ul·tra·mi·crot·o·my
crypt
    anal c's
    bony c.
    dental c.
    enamel c.
    c's of Fuchs
    c's of Haller
    c's of iris
    c's of Lieberkühn
    lingual c's
    c's of Littre
    Luschka's c's
    c. of Morgagni
    mucous c's of duodenum
    multilocular c.
    odoriferous c's of prepuce
    c's of palatine tonsil
    c's of pharyngeal tonsil
    synovial c.
    c's of tongue
    tonsillar c's
    tonsillar c's of palatine
      tonsil
    tonsillar c's of pharyngeal
      tonsil
    tooth c.
    c's of Tyson
cryp·ta *pl.* cryp·tae
    cryptae mucosae
    cryptae tonsillares

crypt·an·am·ne·sia
cryp·tec·to·my
cryp·ten·amine
   c. acetates
   c. tannates
cryp·tes·the·sia
cryp·tic·i·ty
cryp·ti·tis
   anal c.
cryp·to·ceph·a·lus
Cryp·to·coc·ca·ceae
cryp·to·coc·cal
cryp·to·coc·co·ma
cryp·to·coc·co·sis
Cryp·to·coc·cus
   C. neoformans
cryp·to·crys·tal·line
cryp·to·de·ter·min·ant
cryp·to·did·y·mus
cryp·to·em·py·ema
cryp·to·gam
cryp·to·ge·net·ic
cryp·to·gen·ic
cryp·to·gli·o·ma
cryp·to·lith
cryp·to·men·or·rhea
cryp·to·mere
cryp·to·me·ro·ra·chis·chi·sis
cryp·tom·ne·sia
cryp·tom·ne·sic
cryp·to·mo·nad
cryp·to·neu·rous
cryp·toph·thal·mos
cryp·to·plas·mic
cryp·to·po·dia
cryp·to·por·ous
cryp·to·py·ic
cryp·tor·chid
cryp·tor·chi·dec·to·my
cryp·tor·chi·dism
cryp·tor·chi·do·pexy
cryp·tor·chism
cryp·to·scope
   Satvioni's c.
cryp·tos·co·py
cryp·to·spo·rid·i·o·sis
Cryp·to·spo·ri·di·um

cryp·tos·ter·ol
Cryp·to·stro·ma
   C. corticale
cryp·to·stro·mo·sis
cryp·to·tia
cryp·to·tox·ic
cryp·to·xan·thin
cryp·to·zo·ite
cryp·to·zy·gous
Crys. — crystal
crys·tal
   asthma c's
   blood c's
   Böttcher's c's
   calcium pyrophosphate
      dihydrate (CPPD) c's
   Charcot-Leyden c's
   Charcot-Neumann c's
   coffin lid c's
   CPPD c's
   dumbbell c's
   ear c.
   hedgehog c's
   hydroxyapatite c.
   knife rest c's
   liquid c's
   Lubarsch's c's
   Platner's c's
   c's of Reinke
   scintillation c.
   Teichmann's c's
   thorn-apple c's
   Virchow's c's
   whetstone c's
crys·tal·bu·min
crys·tal·lin
crys·tal·line
crys·tal·li·tis
crys·tal·li·za·tion
   fern-leaf c.
crys·tal·log·ra·phy
   x-ray c.
crys·tal·loid
   Charcot-Böttcher
      (Boettcher) c.
   c's of Reinke
crys·tal·lu·ria

Crys·ti·cil·lin
Crys·to·dig·in
CS — cesarean section
    conditioned stimulus
CSAA — Child Study
    Association of America
CSC — coup sur coup
CSF — cerebrospinal fluid
    colony-stimulating factor
CSGBI — Cardiac Society of
    Great Britain and Ireland
CSM — cerebrospinal
    meningitis
CST — contraction stress test
CT — computerized
    tomography
CTA — Canadian
    Tuberculosis Association
CTBA — cetrimonium
    bromide
ctei·no·phyte
Cte·no·ce·phal·i·des
    C. canis
    C. felis
Cten·oph·o·ra
cten·o·phore
Cte·noph·thal·mus
    C. agrytes
Cte·nus
C-ter·mi·nal
Cte·si·as of Cni·dus
CTL — cytotoxic T
    lymphocytes
CTP — cytidine triphosphate
cua·ja·ni
cu·bi·tal
cu·bi·ta·lis
cu·bi·to·car·pal
cu·bi·to·ra·di·al
cu·bi·tus
    c. valgus
    c. varus
cu·boid
cu·boi·dal
cu·boi·deo·na·vic·u·lar
cu·boi·des
cu·bo·na·vic·u·lar
cu cm — cubic centimeter

cu·cur·bo·cit·rin
cu·co·line
cu·cul·la·ris
cud·bear
cuff
    epithelial c.
    musculotendinous c.
    rotator c.
cuff·ing
    peribronchial c.
Cui·gnet's method
cui·rass
    tabetic c.
Cuj. — L. cujus (of which)
cul-de-sac
    conjunctival c.
    Douglas' c.
    dural c.
    Gruber's c.
    inferior c.
    lesser c.
cul·do·cen·te·sis
cul·do·plas·ty
cul·do·scope
cul·dos·co·py
cul·dot·o·my
Cu·lex
    C. nigripalpus
    C. pipiens
    C. quinquefasciatus
    C. tarsalis
    C. tritaeniorhychnus
Cu·lic·i·dae
cu·li·ci·dal
cu·li·cide
cu·lic·i·fuge
Cu·li·ci·nae
cu·li·cine
Cu·li·ci·ni
Cu·li·coi·des
cu·li·co·sis
Cu·li·se·ta
    C. inorata
    C. melanura
Cul·len's sign
cull·ing
cul·men *pl.* cul·mi·na
cul·mi·na

Culp-De Weerd
   ureteropelvioplasty
cul·tur·a·ble
cul·ture
   asynchronous c.
   attenuated c.
   blood c.
   cell c.
   chorioallantoic c.
   continuous flow c.
   direct c.
   embryo c.
   enrichment c.
   hanging-block c.
   hanging-drop c.
   mixed c.
   mixed lymphocyte c. (MLC)
   needle c.
   plate c.
   primary c.
   pure c.
   quantitative c.
   radioisotopic c.
   roll-tube c.
   secondary c.
   selective c.
   sensitized c.
   shake c.
   slant c.
   slope c.
   stab c.
   stock c.
   streak c.
   subculture c.
   surface c.
   suspension c.
   synchronized c.
   tissue c.
   type c.
cul·ture me·di·um
   defined c. m.
   N.N.N. (Novoy, McNeal,
     Nicolle) c. m.
cu mm — cubic millimeter
cu·mu·la·tive
cu·mu·lus *pl.* cu·mu·li
   c. oophorus
cu·ne·ate

cu·nei
cu·ne·i·form
cu·neo·cu·boid
cu·neo·na·vic·u·lar
cu·neo·scaph·oid
cu·ne·us *pl.* cu·nei
cu·nic·u·lar
cu·nic·u·lus *pl.* cu·nic·u·li
   c. internus
cun·ni·lin·gus
cun·nus
cup
   acetabular c.
   Aufranc-Turner c.
   chin c.
   Crawford-Adams
     acetabular c.
   Diogenes c.
   dry c.
   eye c.
   favus c.
   glaucomatous c.
   McKee-Farrar acetabular
     c.
   optic c.
   perilimbal suction c.
   physiologic c.
   wet c.
cu·po·la
cup·ping
   c. of calix
   pathologic c.
cu·pre·mia
cu·pric
Cup·ri·mine
cup·ri·myx·in
cu·pri·uria
cu·pro·phane
cu·pro·pro·teins
cu·prous
cu·pru·re·sis
cu·pru·ret·ic
cu·pu·la *pl.* cu·pu·lae
   c. of ampullary crest
   c. cristae ampullaris
cu·pu·lae
cup·u·lar
cup·u·late

cu·pu·lo·gram
cu·pu·lo·li·thi·a·sis
cu·pu·lom·e·try
cu·ra·re
cu·ra·re·mi·met·ic
cu·ra·ri·form
cu·rar·iza·tion
cur·a·tive
cur·cu·min
    alum c.
    alum c. of Riverius
cure
cu·ret
    adenoid c.
    Beckmann c.
    Delstanche c.
    Gottstein c.
    Hartmann's c.
    St. Clair Thompson c.
cu·ret·tage
    apical c.
    gingival c.
    medical c.
    periapical c.
    root c.
    subgingival c.
    suction c.
    surgical c.
    ultrasonic c.
    vacuum c.
cu·rette
cu·rette·ment
    physiologic c.
Cu·rie, Marie Sklodowska
Cu·rie, Pierre
cu·rie
cu·rie-hour
cu·rie·ther·a·py
cur·ing
    denture c.
cu·ri·os·co·py
cu·ri·um
Curl·ing's ulcer
cur·rent
    abnerval c.
    action c.
    alternating c.
    anelectrotonic c.

cur·rent *(continued)*
    anionic c.
    anodal c.
    ascending c.
    axial c.
    blaze c.
    catelectrotonic c.
    centrifugal c.
    centripetal c.
    coagulating c.
    combined c.
    compensating c.
    d'Arsonval c.
    damped c.
    demarcation c.
    depolarization c.
    descending c.
    diphasic action c.
    direct c.
    eddy c's
    electric c.
    electrotonic c.
    ephaptic c.
    fault c.
    fulguration c.
    galvanic c.
    high-frequency c.
    induced c.
    c. of injury
    interaxonal c.
    inverse c.
    ionization c.
    monophasic action c.
    nerve-action c.
    oscillating c.
    Oudin c.
    resting c.
    rising c.
    saturation c.
    sine-wave c.
    sinusoidal c.
    static-wave c.
    surgical c.
    undamped c.
cur·ric·u·lum *pl.* cur·ric·u·la
Cur·tis and Fitz-Hugh
    syndrome
Cur·ti·us' syndrome

cur·va·ture
   anterior c.
   backward c.
   compensating c.
   c. of field
   greater gastric c.
   greater c. of stomach
   hyperopia of c.
   lateral c.
   lesser gastric c.
   lesser c. of stomach
   occlusal c.
   Petzval's c.
   Pott's c.
   spinal c.
curve
   alignment c.
   anti-Monson c.
   audibility c.
   auditory c.
   Barnes's c.
   bell-shaped c.
   biphasic c.
   Bragg c.
   buccal c.
   camel c.
   c. of Carus
   compensating c.
   cystometric c.
   Damoiseau's c.
   decay c.
   dental c.
   diabetic glucose tolerance c.
   diphasic c.
   dromedary c.
   dye-dilution c.
   c. of Ellis and Garland
   Frank-Starling c.
   Friedman's c.
   Garland's c.
   gaussian c.
   Gompertz c.
   growth c.
   Harrison's c.
   indicator-dilution c.
   intracardiac pressure c.
   inverted-U c. of arousal

curve (continued)
   isodose c's
   isoresponse c.
   isovolume pressure-flow c.
   Kaplan-Meier survival c.
   labial c.
   learning c.
   leutic c.
   logistic c.
   modified exponential c.
   Monson c.
   muscle c.
   c. of occlusion
   paretic c.
   photopic sensitivity c.
   Price-Jones c.
   pulse c.
   regression c.
   reverse c.
   ROC (receiver operating characteristics) c.
   saddleback temperature c.
   Starling's c.
   stress-strain c.
   survival c.
   temperature c.
   tension c's
   titration c.
   visibility c.
   Wunderlich's c.
cur·vi·lin·e·ar
CUSA — Cavitron ultrasonic aspirator
cus·cam·i·dine
cus·cam·ine
Cush·ing's suture
Cush·ing-Ro·ki·tan·sky ulcer
cush·ing·oid
cush·ion
   air c.
   atrioventricular canal c.
   coronary c.
   digital c.
   endocardial c's
   c. of epiglottis
   intimal c's
   levator c.
   Passavant's c.

Stimulite Contour cushion

cush·ion *(continued)*
    plantar c.
    polar c. of glomerulus
    sucking c.
cusp
    aortic c.
    Carabelli c.
    dental c.
    c. of mitral valve
    plunger c.
    semilunar c.
    shearing c.
    stamp c.
    c. of tricuspid valve
cus·pid
cus·pi·date
cus·pi·des
cus·pis *pl.* cus·pi·des
    c. anterior valvae
      atrioventricularis dextrae
    c. anterior valvae
      atrioventricularis
      sinistrae
    c. anterior valvulae
      bicuspidalis
    c. anterior valvulae
      tricuspidalis
    c. coronae
    c. dentalis
    c. dentis
    c. medialis valvulae
      tricuspidalis
    c. posterior valvae
      atrioventricularis dextrae
    c. posterior valvae
      atrioventricularis
      sinistrae
    c. posterior valvulae
      bicuspidalis
    c. posterior valvulae
      tricuspidalis
    c. septalis valvae
      atrioventricularis dextrae
    tangential c.
cu·ta·ne·ous
cut·down
Cu·ter·e·bra

Cu·te·reb·ri·dae
cu·ti·cle
    dental c.
    enamel c.
    Gottlieb's c.
    keratose c.
    primary c.
    prism c.
    c. of root sheath
    secondary c.
cu·tic·u·la *pl.* cu·tic·u·lae
    c. dentis
cu·tic·u·lae
cu·tic·u·lar
cu·tic·u·lin
cu·tic·u·lum
    Flechsig's c.
cu·ti·dure
cu·ti·du·ris
cu·tif·i·ca·tion
cu·tin
cu·ti·re·ac·tion
    von Pirquet c.
cu·tis
    c. anserina
    c. elastica
    c. hyperelastica
    c. laxa
    c. marmorata
    c. rhomboidalis nuchae
    c. vera
    c. verticis gyrata
cu·vette
CV — cardiovascular
    coefficient of variation
C.V. — conjugata vera (true
    conjugate diameter of the
    pelvic inlet)
    L. cras vespere (tomorrow
    evening)
CVA — cardiovascular
accident
    cerebrovascular accident
    costovertebral angle

CVP — central venous
   pressure
      cyclophosphamide,
      vincristine, and
      prednisone
CVS — cardiovascular system
      chorionic villus sampling
CW — continuous wave
Cx — cervix
      convex
Cy — cyanogen
cy·an·amide
cy·a·nate
cy·an·hem·a·tin
cy·an·he·mo·glo·bin
cy·a·nide
cy·an·met·he·mo·glo·bin
cy·an·met·myo·glo·bin
cy·a·no·ac·ryl·ate
cy·a·no·al·co·hol
Cy·a·no·bac·te·ria
cy·a·no·co·bal·a·min
      radioactive c.
cy·a·no·crys·tal·lin
cy·ano·form
cy·an·o·gen
      c. bromide
      c. chloride
cy·a·no·gen·e·sis
cy·a·no·ge·net·ic
cy·a·no·hy·drin
cy·a·no·labe
cy·a·no·phil
cy·a·noph·i·lous
cy·a·no·phor·ic
cy·a·no·phose
Cy·a·no·phy·ceae
cy·a·no·phytes
cy·a·no·pia
cy·a·nop·sia
cy·a·nop·sin
cy·a·nose
      c. tardive
cy·a·nosed
cy·a·no·sis
      autotoxic c.
      c. bulbi
      central c.

cy·a·no·sis (continued)
      compression c.
      enterogenous c.
      false c.
      hereditary
        methemoglobinemic c.
      c. lienis
      peripheral c.
      pulmonary c.
      c. retinae
      shunt c.
      tardive c.
      toxic c.
cy·a·not·ic
Cy·an·tin
cy·an·uria
cy·an·uric acid
cy·an·urin
Cyath. — L. cyathus (a
   glassful)
cy·ber·net·ics
CYC — cyclophosphamide
cy·ca·sin
cy·cla·cil·lin
Cy·claine
cy·cla·mate
Cyc·la·men
cy·clam·ic acid
cyc·la·min
Cy·cla·my·cin
cy·clan·de·late
cyc·lar·thro·di·al
cyc·lar·thro·sis
cy·clase
cy·cla·zo·cine
cy·cle
      aberrant c.
      anovulatory c.
      asexual c.
      biliary c.
      breakage-fusion-bridge c.
      Calvin c.
      carbon c.
      cardiac c.
      cell c.
      chewing c.
      citrate-pyruvate c.
      citric acid c.

cy·cle *(continued)*
    Cori c.
    cytoplasmic c.
    Embden-Meyerhof c.
    endogenous c.
    endometrial c.
    estrous c.
    exogenous c.
    fatty acid oxidation c.
    forced c.
    futile c.
    gastric c.
    genesial c.
    glucose-lactate c.
    glycine succinate c.
    glyoxylate c.
    gonotrophic c.
    hair c.
    Hodgkin c.
    isohydric c.
    Krebs' c.
    Krebs-Henseleit c.
    lactation c.
    life c.
    mammary c.
    menstrual c.
    mitotic c.
    mosquito c.
    nasal c.
    nitrogen c.
    oogenetic c.
    ornithine c.
    ovarian c.
    pentose phosphate c.
    pregnancy c.
    reproductive c.
    restored c.
    returning c.
    Ross c.
    Schiff's biliary c.
    tricarboxylic acid c.
    urea c.
    uterine c.
    vaginal c.
    visual c.
cyc·lec·to·my
cyc·len·ceph·a·lus
cy·clen·ceph·a·ly

cyc·lic
cyc·lic AMP
3′,5′-cyc·lic AMP syn·the·tase
cyc·lic GMP
cyc·li·cot·o·my
cy·clin·dole
cyc·li·tis
    heterochromic c.
    plastic c.
    pure c.
    purulent c.
    serous c.
cy·cli·za·tion
cy·cli·zine
    c. hydrochloride
    c. lactate
cy·clo·ar·te·nol
cy·clo·bar·bi·tal
    c. calcium
cy·clo·ben·da·zole
cy·clo·ben·za·prine hy·dro·chlo·ride
cy·clo·bu·ta·nol
cy·clo·ceph·a·lus
cy·clo·cer·a·ti·tis
cy·clo·cho·roid·itis
cy·clo·cryo·ther·a·py
cy·clo·cu·ma·rol
cy·clo·cyt·i·dine
cy·clo·da·mia
cy·clo·de·vi·a·tion
cy·clo·di·al·y·sis
cy·clo·di·a·ther·my
cy·clo·duc·tion
cy·clo·elec·trol·y·sis
cy·clo·er·gom·e·ter
cy·clog·e·ny
cy·clo·guan·ide em·bo·nate
cy·clo·guan·il pam·o·ate
Cy·clo·gyl
cy·clo·hex·ane·hex·ol
cy·clo·hex·ane·sul·fam·ic acid
cy·clo·hex·a·nol
cy·clo·hex·i·mide
cy·cloid
cy·clo·isom·er·ase
cy·clo·ker·a·ti·tis
cy·clo-li·gase

cy·clo·mas·top·a·thy
cy·clo·meth·y·caine sul·fate
cy·clo·oxy·gen·ase
cy·clo·pe·an
cy·clo·pen·ta·mine hy·dro·
  chlo·ride
cy·clo·pen·tane
cy·clo·pen·te·no·phe·nan·
  threne
cy·clo·pen·thi·a·zide
cy·clo·pen·to·late hy·dro·
  chlo·ride
cy·clo·phen·a·zine hy·dro·
  chlo·ride
cy·clo·pho·ria
    accommodative c.
    minus c.
    plus c.
cy·clo·pho·rom·e·ter
cy·clo·phos·pha·mide
Cy·clo·phyl·lid·ea
cy·clo·pia
cy·clo·pin
cy·clo·ple·gia
cy·clo·ple·gic
cy·clo·pro·pane
Cy·clops
cy·clops
    c. hypognathus
cy·close
cy·clo·ser·ine
cy·clo·sis
cy·clo·spasm
Cy·clo·spas·mol
cy·clo·spor·in A
cy·clo·spor·ine
cy·clo·stat
cy·clo·tate
cy·clo·ther·a·py
cy·clo·thi·a·zide
cy·clo·thyme
cy·clo·thy·mia
cy·clo·thym·i·ac
cy·clo·thy·mic
cy·clo·tia
cy·clo·tol
cy·clo·tome
cy·clot·o·my

cy·clo·tor·sion
cy·clo·tron
cy·clo·tro·pia
cy·clo·zoo·no·sis
cy·cri·mine hy·dro·chlo·ride
cy·e·sis
cy·es·te·in
cy·es·the·in
cyl — cylinder
    cylindrical lens
cyl·i·cot·o·my
cyl·in·der
    Bence Jones c's
    crossed c's
    Külz's c.
    Leydig's c's
    Ruffini's c's
    terminal c's
    urinary c.
cyl·in·drar·thro·sis
cyl·in·drax·ile
cyl·in·dri·cal
cy·lin·dri·form
cyl·in·dro·cel·lu·lar
cyl·in·dro·den·drite
cyl·in·droid
cyl·in·dro·ma
    eccrine dermal c.
cy·lin·drom·a·tous
Cy·lin·dro·tho·rax
    C. melanocephala
cyl·in·dru·ria
cy·lite
cyl·lo·sis
cyl·lo·so·ma
cyl·lo·so·mus
cy·ma·rose
cym·ba *pl.* cym·bae
    c. conchae auriculae
cym·bi·form
cym·bo·ce·pha·lia
cym·bo·ce·phal·ic
cym·bo·ceph·a·lous
cym·bo·ceph·a·ly
cyme
cy·mo·graph
cy·nan·che
    c. maligna

cy·nan·che *(continued)*
   c. tonsillaris
cy·nan·thro·py
cyn·ic
cy·no·ce·phal·ic
cy·no·ceph·a·ly
cy·no·dont
cyn·odon·tism
cyn·o·mol·gus
Cy·no·my·ia
Cy·no·mys
cy·no·pho·bia
cy·o·gen·ic
cy·o·pho·ria
cy·o·phor·ic
cy·o·pin
cy·ot·ro·phy
Cy·pe·rus
cyp·i·o·nate
cy·po·thrin
cy·pra·ze·pam
cyp·ri·nin
cy·pro·hep·ta·dine hy·dro·chlo·ride
cy·pro·quin·ate
cy·pro·ter·one ac·e·tate
cyr·to·graph
cyr·toid
cyr·tom·e·ter
cyr·tos
cyr·to·sis
Cys
Cys — cysteine
Cys-Cys — cystine
cyst
   adventitious c.
   allantoic c.
   alveolar c's
   alveolar hydatid c.
   amnionic c.
   aneurysmal bone c.
   angioblastic c.
   antral c.
   apical c.
   apoplectic c.
   arachnoid c.
   atheromatous c.
   Baker's c.

cyst *(continued)*
   Blessig's c's
   blue dome c.
   bone c.
   Boyer's c.
   bronchial c's
   bronchogenic c.
   bronchopulmonary c.
   bursal c.
   cervical c.
   cervical lymphoepithelial c.
   chocolate c.
   choledochal c.
   choledochus c.
   chyle c.
   colloid c.
   compound c.
   corpus luteum c.
   Cowper c.
   craniobuccal c.
   craniopharyngeal duct c.
   cutaneous c.
   cuticular c.
   daughter c.
   dental c.
   dentigerous c.
   dermoid c.
   dilatation c.
   distention c.
   duplication c.
   echinococcus c.
   endometrial c.
   endothelial c.
   ependymal c.
   epidermal c.
   epidermal inclusion c.
   epidermoid c.
   epithelial c.
   eruption c.
   extra-axial leptomeningeal c.
   extravasation c.
   exudation c.
   false c.
   fissural c.
   follicular c.
   ganglionic c.

cyst *(continued)*

gas c.
germinal inclusion c.
gingival c.
globulomaxillary c.
glomerular c.
granddaughter c.
hemorrhagic c.
heterotopic oral
  gastrointestinal c.
hydatid c.
implantation c.
incisive canal c.
inclusion c.
intracranial parasitic c.
intraepithelial c's
intraluminal c's
intrapituitary c's
involution c.
Iwanoff's c's
lacteal c.
laryngeal c.
lateral periodontal c.
leptomeningeal c.
lutein c.
lymphoepithelial c.
median anterior maxillary
  c.
median mandibular c.
median palatal c.
meibomian c.
mesenteric c.
milk c.
morgagnian c.
mother c.
mucous c.
multilocular c.
myxoid c.
nasopalatine duct c.
necrotic c.
neural c.
neurenteric c.
nevoid c.
odontogenic c.
oil c.
omental c's
oophoritic c.
osseous hydatid c's

cyst *(continued)*

ovarian c.
pancreatic c.
paranephric c.
parapyelitic c's
parasitic c.
paratracheal c.
paratubal c.
parovarian c.
pearl c.
periapical c.
pericardial c.
perineurial c.
periodontal c.
perirenal c.
perisalpingian c.
phaeomycotic c.
pilar c.
placental c.
porencephalic c.
post-traumatic
  leptomeningeal c.
preauricular c., congenital
primordial c.
proligerous c.
pseudomucinous c.
pyelogenic renal c.
radicular c.
Rathke's c's
renal c.
residual c.
retention c.
retroperitoneal c.
root c.
root-end c.
sacral c.
Sampson's c.
sanguineous c.
sarcosporidian c.
sebaceous c.
secretory c.
seminal c.
septal c.
sequestration c.
serous c.
simple bone c.
soapsuds c's
solitary bone c.

cyst *(continued)*
    springwater c.
    steatoid c.
    sterile c.
    subchondral c.
    sublingual c.
    subsynovial c.
    suprasellar c.
    synovial c.
    Tarlov c.
    tarry c.
    tarsal c.
    thecal c.
    theca-lutein c.
    thymic c's
    tissue c.
    Tornwaldt's c.
    traumatic bone c.
    trichilemmal c.
    true c.
    tubo-ovarian c.
    tubular c.
    umbilical c.
    unicameral c.
    unilocular c.
    urachal c.
    urinary c.
    vaginal c.
    vitelline c.
    vitellointestinal c.
    wolffian c.
cys·tad·e·no·car·ci·no·ma
cyst·ad·e·no·fi·bro·ma
cys·tad·e·no·ma
    c. adamantinum
    c. cylindrocellulare
      celloides ovarii
    mucinous c.
    papillary c.
    papillary c.
      lymphomatosum
    c. phyllodes
    pseudomucinous c.
    serous c.
cyst·ad·e·no·sar·co·ma
cys·tal·gia
cys·ta·thi·o·nase
cys·ta·thi·o·nine

cys·ta·thi·o·nine γ-ly·ase
cys·ta·thi·o·nine β-syn·thase
cys·ta·thi·o·nin·uria
cys·ta·tro·phia
cys·tau·che·ni·tis
cys·tau·che·not·o·my
cys·te·amine
cys·tec·to·my
cys·te·ic acid
cys·te·ine
    c. hydrochloride
cys·te·in·yl
cys·tel·co·sis
cys·ten·ceph·a·lus
cyst·er·e·thism
cyst·hy·per·sar·co·sis
cys·tic
cys·ti·cer·ci
cys·ti·cer·coid
cys·ti·cer·co·sis
    spinal c.
Cys·ti·cer·cus
    C. bovis
    C. cellulosae
    C. ovis
    C. tenuicollis
cys·ti·co·li·thec·to·my
cys·ti·co·li·tho·trip·sy
cys·ti·cor·rha·phy
cys·ti·cot·o·my
cys·ti·des
cys·ti·do·ce·li·ot·o·my
cys·ti·do·lap·a·rot·o·my
cys·ti·do·tra·chel·o·to·my
cys·ti·fel·lot·o·my
cys·tif·er·ous
cys·ti·form
cys·tig·er·ous
cys·tine
cys·tin·emia
cys·ti·no·sis
    benign c.
    intermediate c.
    nephrogenic c.
cys·tin·uria
    familial c.
cys·tin·uric
cys·tir·rha·gia

cys·tir·rhea
cys·tis *pl.* cys·ti·des
    c. fellea
cys·ti·stax·is
cys·ti·tis
    allergic c.
    bacterial c.
    catarrhal c., acute
    c. colli
    croupous c.
    diphtheritic c.
    c. emphysematosa
    eosinophilic c.
    exfoliative c.
    c. follicularis
    gangrenous c.
    c. glandularis
    incrusted c.
    interstitial c., chronic
    mechanical c.
    panmural c.
    c. papillomatosa
    postpartum c.
    c. senilis feminarum
    submucous c.
    ulcerative c.
cys·ti·tome
cys·tit·o·my
cys·to·blast
cys·to·blas·te·ma
cys·to·car·ci·no·ma
    pseudomucinous c.
cys·to·cele
cys·to·chrome
cys·to·chro·mos·co·py
cys·to·co·los·to·my
Cys·to-Con·ray
cys·to·di·a·pha·nos·co·py
cys·to·du·od·e·nos·to·my
cys·to·dyn·ia
cys·to·elyt·ro·plas·ty
cys·to·en·tero·cele
cys·to·epip·lo·cele
cys·to·epi·the·li·o·ma
cys·to·fi·bro·ma
    c. papillare
cys·to·gas·tros·to·my
cys·to·gen·e·sis

Cys·to·graf·in
cys·to·gram
cys·tog·ra·phy
    delayed c.
    voiding c.
cys·toid
cys·to·je·ju·nos·to·my
cys·to·lith
cys·to·li·thec·to·my
cys·to·li·thi·a·sis
cys·to·lith·ic
cys·to·li·thot·o·my
cys·to·lu·te·in
cys·to·ma
    c. serosum simplex
    colloid ovarian c.
cys·to·ma·ti·tis
cys·to·ma·tous
cys·tom·e·ter
cys·to·met·ro·gram
cys·to·me·trog·ra·phy
cys·tom·e·try
cys·to·mor·phous
cys·to·ne·phro·sis
cys·to·neu·ral·gia
cys·to·pa·ral·y·sis
cys·to·pexy
cys·toph·o·rous
cys·to·pho·tog·ra·phy
cys·toph·thi·sis
cys·to·plas·ty
    augmentation c.
cys·to·ple·gia
cys·to·proc·tos·to·my
cys·to·pros·ta·tec·to·my
cys·top·to·sis
cys·to·py·eli·tis
cys·to·py·elog·ra·phy
cys·to·py·elo·ne·phri·tis
cys·to·ra·di·og·ra·phy
cys·to·rec·to·cele
cys·to·rec·tos·to·my
cys·tor·rha·gia
cys·tor·rha·phy
cys·tor·rhea
cys·to·sar·co·ma
    c. phyllodes
cys·tos·chi·sis

cys·to·scle·ro·sis
cys·to·scope
cys·to·scop·ic
cys·tos·co·py
cys·tose
cys·to·spasm
Cys·to·spaz
cys·to·sper·mi·tis
cys·to·stax·is
cys·tos·to·my
    tubeless c.
cys·to·tome
cys·tot·o·my
    suprapubic c.
cys·to·tra·chel·ot·o·my
cys·to·ure·ter·itis
cys·to·ure·ter·o·cele
cys·to·ure·tero·gram
cys·to·ure·tero·py·elo·neph·ri·tis
cys·to·ure·ter·o·py·elo·neph·ri·tis
cys·to·ure·thri·tis
cys·to·ure·thro·cele
cys·to·ure·thro·gram
cys·to·ure·throg·ra·phy
    chain c.
    micturating c.
    retrograde c.
    voiding c.
cys·to·ure·thro·scope
cys·tyl
Cy·ta·dren
cyt·a·phe·re·sis
cy·tar·a·bine
cyt·ar·me
Cy·tel·lin
cyth·ero·ma·nia
cy·ti·dine
    c. diphosphate (CDP)
    c. diphosphate choline
    c. diphosphate
      ethanolamine
    c. monophosphate (CMP)
    c. triphosphate (CTP)
cy·ti·dine de·am·i·nase
cy·ti·dyl·ate
cy·ti·dyl·ic acid

cy·ti·dyl·yl
cyt·i·sine
cyt·i·sism
Cyt·i·sus
cy·to·an·a·ly·zer
cy·to·ar·chi·tec·ton·ic
cy·to·ar·chi·tec·tu·ral
cy·to·ar·chi·tec·ture
cy·to·bi·ol·o·gy
cy·to·bio·tax·is
cy·to·blast
cy·to·chal·a·sin
    c. B
cy·to·chem·ism
cy·to·chem·is·try
cy·to·chrome
    c. b
    c. b_5
    c. c
    c. c_1
cy·to·chrome ox·i·dase
cy·to·chrome *c. ox·i·dase*
cy·to·chrome b_5 *re·duc·tase*
cy·to·chrome P-450 re·duc·tase
cy·to·chy·le·ma
cy·to·ci·dal
cy·to·cide
cy·to·cla·sis
cy·to·clas·tic
cy·to·cle·sis
cy·to·clet·ic
cy·to·crit
cy·toc·to·ny
cy·to·cu·prein
cy·tode
cy·to·des·ma
cy·to·di·ag·no·sis
    exfoliative c.
cy·to·di·ag·nos·tic
cy·to·di·er·e·sis
cy·to·dif·fer·en·ti·a·tion
cy·to·dis·tal
cy·to·flav
cy·to·fla·vin
cy·to·gene
cy·to·gen·e·sis
cy·to·ge·net·i·cal

cy·to·ge·net·i·cist
cy·to·ge·net·ics
   clinical c.
cy·to·gen·ic
cy·tog·e·nous
cy·tog·e·ny
cy·to·glom·er·a·tor
cy·to·gly·co·pe·nia
cy·tog·o·ny
cy·to·his·to·gen·e·sis
cy·to·his·to·log·ic
cy·to·his·tol·o·gy
cy·to·hor·mone
cy·to·hy·a·lo·plasm
cy·toid
cy·to·in·hi·bi·tion
cy·to·kal·i·pe·nia
cy·to·ke·ras·tic
cy·to·kine
cy·to·ki·ne·sis
cy·to·ki·nin
cy·to·lem·ma
cy·to·log·ic
cy·tol·o·gist
cy·tol·o·gy
   aspiration biopsy c. (ABC)
   exfoliative c.
   nuclear c.
cy·tol·y·sate
   blood c.
cy·tol·y·sin
cy·tol·y·sis
   immune c.
cy·to·ly·so·some
cy·to·lyt·ic
cy·to·ma
cy·to·me·gal·ic
cy·to·meg·a·lo·vir·u·ria
cy·to·meg·a·lo·vi·rus
cy·to·meg·a·ly
Cy·to·mel
cy·to·mem·brane
cy·to·mere
cy·to·meta·pla·sia
cy·tom·e·ter
   eyepiece c.
   stage c.

cy·tom·e·try
   flow c.
cy·to·mi·cro·some
cy·to·mi·tome
cy·to·mor·phol·o·gy
cy·to·mor·pho·sis
cy·ton
cy·to·ne·cro·sis
cy·to·path·ic
cy·to·patho·gen·e·sis
cy·to·patho·ge·net·ic
cy·to·path·o·gen·ic
cy·to·patho·ge·nic·i·ty
cy·to·pa·thol·o·gist
cy·to·pa·thol·o·gy
cy·to·pe·nia
cy·to·phago·cy·to·sis
cy·toph·a·gous
cy·toph·a·gy
cy·to·phar·ynx
cy·to·phil
cy·to·phil·ic
cy·to·pho·tom·e·ter
cy·to·pho·to·met·ric
cy·to·pho·tom·e·try
cy·to·phy·lac·tic
cy·to·phy·lax·is
cy·to·phy·let·ic
cy·to·phys·ics
cy·to·phys·i·ol·o·gy
cy·to·pig·ment
cy·to·pi·pette
cy·to·plasm
cy·to·plas·mic
cy·to·plast
cy·to·pre·pa·ra·tion
cy·to·proct
cy·to·prox·i·mal
cy·to·pyge
cy·to·re·tic·u·lum
cy·tor·rhyc·tes
Cy·to·sar-U
cy·tos·co·py
cy·to·sid·er·in
cy·to·sine
   c. arabinoside
   5-hydroxymethyl c.
   c. deoxyriboside

cy·to·skel·e·tal
cy·to·skel·e·ton
cy·to·smear
cy·to·sol
cy·to·sol ami·no·pep·ti·dase
cy·to·sol·ic
cy·to·some
cy·to·spon·gi·um
cy·tost
cy·to·sta·sis
cy·to·stat·ic
cy·to·ste·a·to·ne·cro·sis
cy·to·stome
cy·to·stro·mat·ic
cy·to·tac·tic
cy·to·tax·i·gen
cy·to·tax·in
cy·to·tax·is
cy·to·tech·nol·o·gist

cy·to·ther·a·py
cy·toth·e·sis
cy·to·tox·ic
cy·to·tox·ic·i·ty
cy·to·tox·in
cy·to·tropho·blast
cy·to·trop·ic
cy·to·tro·pism
Cy·tox·an
cy·to·zoa
cy·to·zo·ic
cy·to·zo·on
cyt·u·la
cy·tu·lo·plasm
cy·tu·ria
Cza·pek-Dox solution
Czer·ny's suture
Czer·ny-Lem·bert suture
CZI — crystalline zinc insulin

D

D — dalton
  deciduous (teeth)
  decimal reduction time
  density
  deuterium
  died
  diffusing capacity
  diopter
  distal
  dorsal vertebrae (D1–D12)
  dose
  duration
  dwarf (colony)
2,4-D — 2,4-dichlorophenoxy-
  acetic acid
D. — L. da (give)
  L. detur (let it be given)
  L. dexter (right)
  L. dosis (dose)
d — day
  deci-
  deoxyribose

d. — L. da (give)
  L. detur (let it be given)
  L. dexter (right)
  L. dosis (dose)
d — density
  diameter
Δ — increment
δ — the heavy chain of IgD
  the δ chain of hemoglobin
DA — developmental age
  diphenylchlorarsine
Da — dalton
dA — deoxyadenosine
da- — deka-
Daae-Fin·sen disease
Dab·ney's grip
Da·boia
  D. russelli
da·car·ba·zine
Da·Cos·ta's syndrome
d'Acosta's disease

Dacron
dac·ry·ad·e·nal·gia
dac·ry·ad·e·no·scir·rhus
dac·ry·a·gog·atre·sia
dac·ry·a·gog·ic
dac·ry·a·gogue
dac·ry·cys·tal·gia
dac·ry·cys·ti·tis
dac·ry·el·co·sis
dac·ryo·ad·e·nal·gia
dac·ryo·ad·e·nec·to·my
dac·ryo·ad·e·ni·tis
dac·ryo·blen·nor·rhea
dac·ryo·cana·lic·u·li·tis
dac·ryo·cele
dac·ryo·cyst
dac·ryo·cys·tal·gia
dac·ryo·cys·tec·ta·sia
dac·ryo·cys·tec·to·my
dac·ryo·cys·tis
dac·ryo·cys·ti·tis
dac·ryo·cys·ti·tome
dac·ryo·cys·to·blen·nor·rhea
dac·ryo·cys·to·cele
dac·ryo·cys·tog·ra·phy
dac·ryo·cys·top·to·sis
dac·ryo·cys·to·rhi·nos·to·my
dac·ryo·cys·to·rhi·not·o·my
dac·ryo·cys·to·ste·no·sis
dac·ryo·cys·tos·to·my
dac·ryo·cys·to·tome
dac·ryo·cys·tot·o·my
dac·ryo·cyte
dac·ry·o·gen·ic
dac·ryo·hel·co·sis
dac·ryo·hem·or·rhea
dac·ry·oid
dac·ryo·lith
dac·ryo·li·thi·a·sis
dac·ry·o·ma
dac·ry·on
dac·ry·ops
dac·ryo·py·or·rhea
dac·ryo·py·o·sis
dac·ryo·rhi·no·cys·tot·o·my
dac·ry·or·rhea
dac·ryo·scin·tig·ra·phy
dac·ryo·si·nus·itis

dac·ryo·so·le·ni·tis
dac·ryo·ste·no·sis
dac·ryo·syr·inx
Dac·til
dac·ti·no·my·cin
dac·tyl
dac·tyl·al·gia
dac·ty·late
dac·ty·le·de·ma
dac·tyl·ic
dac·tyl·i·on
dac·ty·li·tis
    d. strumosa
    d. tuberculosa
dac·ty·lo·camp·so·dyn·ia
dac·tyl·ody·nia
dac·ty·lo·dys·tro·phy
dac·tylo·gram
dac·ty·log·ra·phy
dac·ty·lo·gry·po·sis
dac·ty·loid
dac·ty·lol·o·gy
dac·ty·lol·y·sis
    d. spontanea
dac·ty·lo·meg·a·ly
dac·ty·lo·pha·sia
dac·ty·los·co·py
dac·ty·lose
dac·ty·lo·spasm
dac·ty·lo·sym·phy·sis
dac·ty·lus
DADDS — diacetyl
    diaminodiphenylsulfone
dADP — deoxyadenosine
    diphosphate
Dag·e·nan
dahl·ia
    d. B.
dahl·in
Da·kin's antiseptic solution
Da·kin's fluid
Da·kin-Car·rel method
dak·ry·on
Dale, Sir Henry Hallett
Dale's phenomenon
Dale's reaction
Dale-Feld·berg law
da·le·da·lin to·sy·late

D'Al·le·san·dro serial suture
　holding forceps
Dal·mane
Dal·rym·ple's disease
Dal·rym·ple's sign
dal·ton
Dal·ton's law
Dal·ton-Hen·ry law
dal·ton·ism
Dam, Carl Peter Henrik
dam
　　rubber d.
da·mi·a·na
dam·mar
Da·moi·seau's curve
Da·moi·seau's sign
dAMP — deoxyadenosine
　monophosphate
damp
　　after-d.
　　black d.
　　choke d.
　　cold d.
　　fire d.
　　white d.
damp·ing
Da·na's operation
da·na·zol
Dan·bolt-Closs syndrome
dance
　　brachial d.
　　hilar d.
　　hilus d.
　　St. Anthony's d.
　　St. Guy's d.
　　St. John's d.
　　St. Vitus' d.
Dan·cel's treatment
D and C — dilation and
　curettage
dan·der
dan·druff
Dan·dy scissors
Dan·dy-Walk·er deformity
Dan·dy-Walk·er syndrome
Dane particle
Dan·forth sign
dan·iell

Dan·iels·sen-Boeck disease
Dan·iels·sen-Boeck sarcoidosis
Dan·i·lone
Dan·los' disease
Dan·los' syndrome
dan·syl chlo·ride
dan·thron
dan·tro·lene so·di·um
Dan·ysz's effect
Dan·ysz's phenomenon
Daph·ne
daph·ne·tin
Daph·nia
daph·nin
daph·nism
dap·sone
Dar·a·nide
Dar·a·prim
Dar·bid
Dar·dik Bio·graft
Dar es Sa·laam bacterium
Dar·i·con
Da·rier's disease
Da·rier's sign
Da·rier-Rous·sy sarcoid
Da·rier-White disease
Dark·she·vich's fibers
Dark·she·vich's nucleus
Dar·ling's disease
Dar·rach procedure
Dar·row solution
d'Ar·son·val current
Dar·tal
dar·to·ic
dar·toid
dar·tos
Dar·von
Dar·win's reflex
dar·win·ism
D'As·sump·ção rhytidoplasty
　marker
das·ym·e·ter
DAT — direct antiglobulin
　test
da·ta
　　censored d.
da·ta·base, data base

dATP — deoxyadenosine
  triphosphate
da·tum *pl.* da·ta
Da·tu·ra
  D. metel
da·tu·rine
da·tu·rism
Dau·ben·ton's angle
Dau·ben·ton's line
Dau·ben·ton's plane
daugh·ter
  DES d.
dau·no·my·cin
dau·no·ru·bi·cin
  d. hydrochloride
dau·no·sa·mine
Daus·set, Jean Baptiste
  Gabriel
Da·vai·nea
  D. madagascariensi
  D. proglottina
Da·vai·ne·i·dae
Dav·en·port stain
Da·vid's disease
Da·vid·off's (Da·vid·ov's) cells
Da·vid·sohn differential
  absorption test
Da·vid·sohn's sign
Da·vi·el's operation
Da·vi·el's spoon
Da·vis graft
Daw·barn's sign
dawn phe·nom·e·non
Daw·son's encephalitis
da·za·drol mal·e·ate
dB — decibel
db — decibel
DBA — dibenzanthracene
DBM — demineralized bone
  matrix
DC — direct current
  Doctor of Chiropractic
D & C — dilation and
  curettage
dC — deoxycytidine
DCA — desoxycorticosterone
  acetate
DCc — double concave

dCDP — deoxycytidine
  diphosphate
DCF — direct centrifugal
  flotation
DCH — Diploma in Child
  Health
DCI — dichloroisoproterenol
dCMP — deoxycytidine
  monophosphate
DCOG — Diploma of the
  College of Obstetricians and
  Gynaecologists (British)
dCTP — deoxycytidine
  triphosphate
DCx — double convex
d.d. — L. detur ad (let it be
  given to)
DDS — Doctor of Dental
  Surgery
DDSc — Doctor of Dental
  Science
DDT — dichlorodiphenyltrichlo-
  roethane
D & E — dilation and
  evacuation
de·ac·e·tyl·la·nat·o·side C
de·acid·i·fi·ca·tion
de·ac·ti·va·tion
de·acyl·ase
dead
deaf
de·af·fer·en·ta·tion
deaf-mute
deaf-mut·ism
  endemic d.
deaf·ness
  acoustic trauma d.
  Alexander's d.
  apoplectiform d.
  bass d.
  Bing-Stibenmann type
    genetic d.
  boilermakers' d.
  central d.
  cerebral d.
  cochlear d.
  conduction d.
  congenital d.

deaf·ness *(continued)*
    cortical d.
    familial perceptive d.
    functional d.
    genetic d.
    heredodegenerative d.
    high-frequency d.
    hysterical d.
    immune complex
      associated d.
    labyrinthine d.
    malarial d.
    Michel's d.
    midbrain d.
    Mondini's d.
    music d.
    nerve d.
    neural d.
    noise-induced d.
    organic d.
    ototoxic d.
    pagetoid d.
    paradoxic d.
    perceptive d.
    postlingual d.
    prelingual d.
    retrocochlear d.
    Scheibe's d.
    sensorineural d.
    syphilitic d.
    tone d.
    toxic d.
    transmission d.
    traumatic d.
    vascular d.
    word d.
de·al·ba·tion
de·al·co·hol·iza·tion
de·al·ler·gi·za·tion
de·am·i·dase
de·am·i·da·tion
de·am·i·di·za·tion
de·am·i·nase
de·am·i·na·tion
de·am·i·ni·za·tion
de·ami·no-oxy·to·cin
Dea·ner

de·a·nol ac·et·am·i·do·ben·zo·ate
de·aqua·tion
de·ar·te·ri·al·iza·tion
de·ar·tic·u·la·tion
death
    apparent d.
    associated d.
    black d.
    brain d.
    cell d.
    cot d.
    crib d.
    direct maternal d.
    fetal d.
    functional d.
    genetic d.
    indirect maternal d.
    instantaneous d.
    intrauterine d.
    liver d.
    local d.
    molecular d.
    neonatal d.
    nonmaternal d.
    perinatal d.
    somatic d.
    thymineless d.
    voodoo d.
death-cap
death-cup
Dea·ver's incision
de·band·ing
De·bar·yo·my·ces
    D. hansenii
    D. hominis
    D. neoformans
de·bil·i·ta·tion
de·bil·i·ty
dé·bouche·ment
Dé·bove's disease
Dé·bove's membrane
Dé·bove's treatment
de·branch·ing en·zyme
De·bré-de To·ni-Fan·co·ni syndrome
De·bré-Se·me·laigne syndrome
dé·bride

dé·bride·ment
   enzymatic d.
   surgical d.
   tangential d.
de·bris
   dermal d.
   d. of Malassez
   word d.
De·bri·san
deb·ris·o·quin sul·fate
Deb. spis. — L. debita
   spissitudine (of the proper
   consistency)
debt
   oxygen d.
de·bulk·ing
de·bye
Dec. — L. decanta (pour off)
Dec·a·derm
Dec·a·dron
Dec·a·dron-LA
Deca-Dur·ab·o·lin
de·cal·ci·fi·ca·tion
de·cal·ci·fy
dec·a·me·tho·ni·um
   d. bromide
   d. iodide
dec·ane
de·can·nu·la·tion
de·can·ta·tion
deca·pep·tide
de·cap·i·tate
de·cap·i·ta·tion
de·cap·i·ta·tor
De·ca·po·da
Dec·a·pryn
de·cap·su·la·tion
de·car·box·y·lase
de·car·box·y·la·tion
   oxidative d.
deca·vi·ta·min
de·cay
   beta d.
   branching d.
   dental d.
   free induction d.
   isomeric level d.
   radioactive d.

de·cay *(continued)*
   tone d.
de·ce·dent
de·cel·er·a·tion
   early d.
   late d.
   variable d's
de·cen·ter
de·cen·tra·tion
de·ce·ra·tion
de·cer·e·bel·la·tion
de·cer·e·brate
de·cer·e·bra·tion
de·cer·e·brize
de·chlo·ri·da·tion
de·chlo·ri·na·tion
de·chlo·ru·rant
de·chlo·ru·ra·tion
de·cho·les·ter·in·iza·tion
de·cho·les·ter·ol·iza·tion
De·cho·lin
dec·i·bel
   d. A
   A-weighted d.
de·cid·ua
   basal d.
   d. basalis
   capsular d.
   d. capsularis
   d. compacta
   ectopic d.
   d. marginalis
   menstrual d.
   d. menstrualis
   parietal d.
   d. parietalis
   d. polyposa
   reflex d.
   d. reflexa
   d. serotina
   d. spongiosa
   d. subchorialis
   true d.
   d. tuberosa papulosa
   d. vera
de·cid·u·al
de·cid·u·ate
de·cid·u·a·tion

de·cid·u·itis
de·cid·u·o·ma
 Loeb's d.
 d. malignum
de·cid·u·o·ma·to·sis
de·cid·u·o·sis
de·cid·u·ous
dec·ile
dec·i·li·ter
de·cip·a·ra
de·ci·sion
 Brawner d.
 Durham d.
deck·platte
dec·li·na·tion
dec·li·na·tor
de·clive
de·cli·vis
Dec·lo·my·cin
de·co·ag·u·lant
Decoct. — L. decoctum (a
 decoction)
de·coc·tion
de·coc·tum
de·col·la·tion
de·col·or·a·tion
de·col·or·ize
de·com·bus·tion
de·com·pen·sa·tion
 Bekhterev d.
 corneal d.
de·com·ple·men·ta·tion
de·com·ple·men·tize
de·com·po·si·tion
 anaerobic d.
 d. of movement
de·com·pres·sion
 abdominal d.
 cardiac d.
 cerebral d.
 explosive d.
 d. of heart
 Heyns' d.
 intestinal d.
 Naffziger orbital d.
 nerve d.
 d. of pericardium

de·com·pres·sion (continued)
 d. of rectum
 d. of spinal cord
 suboccipital d.
 subtemporal d.
 trigeminal d.
de·con·den·sa·tion
de·con·di·tion·ing
de·con·ges·tant
de·con·ges·tive
de·con·tam·i·na·tion
de·co·quin·ate
de·cor·ti·cate
de·cor·ti·ca·tion
 arterial d.
 chemical d.
 enzymatic d.
 d. of lung
 renal d.
dec·re·ment
de·crep·i·tate
de·crep·i·ta·tion
de·cru·des·cence
de·crus·ta·tion
dec·ta·flur
Decub. — L. decubitus (lying
 down)
de·cu·ba·tion
de·cu·bi·tal
de·cu·bi·tus pl. de·cu·bi·tus
 d. acutus
 Andral's d.
 d. chronicus
 dorsal d.
 lateral d.
 sacral d.
 ventral d.
de·cum·bin
de·cur·rent
de·cus·sate
de·cus·sa·tio pl. de·cus·sa·ti·
 o·nes
 d. brachii conjunctivi
 d. lemniscorum medialium
 d. motoria
 d. nervorum trochlearium
 d. pedunculorum
  cerebellarium cranialium

de·cus·sa·tio *(continued)*
  d. pedunculorum
    cerebellarium
    superiorum
  d. pyramidum
  d. sensoria
  d. supraoptica dorsalis
  d. supraoptica ventralis
  decussationes tegmenti
  d. trochlearis
de·cus·sa·tion
  anterior hypothalamic d.
  d. of brachia conjunctiva
  d. of cranial cerebellar
    peduncles
  d. of fillet
  Forel's d.
  fountain d. of Meynert
  Held's d.
  inferior hypothalamic d.
  d. of medial lemnisci
  motor d.
  optic d.
  posterior hypothalamic d.
  d. of pyramids
  pyramidal d.
  rubrospinal d.
  sensory d.
  d. of superior cerebellar
    peduncles
  superior hypothalamic d.
  superior supraoptic d.
  suprachiasmatic d.
  supramammillary d.
  tectospinal d.
  tegmental d's
  trochlear d.
  d. of trochlear nerves
  ventral supraoptic d.
de·cus·sa·ti·o·nes
de·den·ti·tion
de·dif·fer·en·ti·a·tion
de d. in d. — L. de die in diem
  (from day to day)
ded·o·la·tion
de Duve
de-ef·fer·en·ta·tion
de·em·a·nate

de-epi·car·di·al·iza·tion
deet
Deet·jen's bodies
de·fat·i·ga·tion
de·fat·ted
de·faun·ate
def·e·ca·tion
  fragmentary d.
de·fect
  acquired d.
  aortic septal d.
  aorticopulmonary septal d.
  aortopulmonary d.
  atrial septal d's
  atrioseptal d's
  atrioventricular septal d.
  birth d.
  congenital d.
  congenital pericardial d.
  congenital reading d.
  cortical d.
  dehalogenase d.
  developmental d.
  ectodermal d., congenital
  endocardial cushion d's
  fibrous cortical d.
  filling d.
  galactokinase d.
  genetic d.
  3β-hydroxysteroid
    dehydrogenase d.
  interatrial septal d.
  iodine transport d.
  iodotyrosine coupling d.
  iodotyrosine deiodinase d.
  limb reduction d.
  lucent d.
  luteal phase d.
  metaphyseal fibrous d.
  neural-tube d.
  obstructive ventilatory d.
  organification d.
  ostium primum d.
  ostium secundum d.
  polytropic field d.
  restrictive ventilatory d.
  retention d.
  salt-losing d.

de·fect *(continued)*
    septal d.
    serum iodoprotein d.
    subcortical d.
    subperiosteal cortical d.
    ventricular septal d.
de·fec·tive
de·fem·i·ni·za·tion
de·fense
    character d.
    insanity d.
    muscular d.
    Ur-d.
def·er·ens
def·er·ent
def·er·en·tec·to·my
def·er·en·tial
def·er·en·ti·tis
de·fer·ox·amine
    d. hydrochloride
    d. mesylate
def·er·ves·cence
def·er·ves·cent
de·fib·ril·la·tion
de·fib·ril·la·tor
de·fi·bri·nat·ed
de·fi·bri·na·tion
de·fi·bri·no·gen·a·tion
de·fi·cien·cy
    debrancher d.
    IgA d., isolated
    IgA d., selective
    immune d.
    leukocyte G6PD d.
    mental d.
    oxygen d.
    vitamin d.
def·i·cit
    base d.
    oxygen d.
    pulse d.
    reversible ischemic
      neurologic d.
    saturation d.
Def·i·nate
def·i·ni·tion
de·fin·i·tive

de·flec·tion
    atrial d.
    His bundle d.
    intrinsic d.
    QRS d.
def·lo·ra·tion
de·flo·res·cence
de·flu·vi·um
    postpartum d.
    d. unguium
de·flux·io
de·flux·ion
de·form·a·bil·i·ty
de·for·ma·tion
de·form·ing
de·form·i·ty
    Åkerlund d.
    Arnold-Chiari d.
    boutonnière d.
    buttonhole d.
    cloverleaf d.
    coup de sabre b.
    crossbar d.
    Dandy-Walker d.
    dishface d.
    equinus d.
    Erlenmeyer flask d.
    funnel d.
    gun stock d.
    Haglund's d.
    hitchhiker's thumb d.
    Ilfeld-Holder d.
    intrinsic minus d.
    intrinsic plus d.
    lobster-claw d.
    Madelung's d.
    mermaid d.
    Michel d.
    parachute d.
    pinched tip d.
    polly-beak d.
    recurvatum d.
    reduction d.
    riding breeches d.
    rocker-bottom d.
    rolled edge d.
    round back d.

de·form·i·ty *(continued)*
  saddle d. of nose
  seal-fin d.
  silver fork d.
  simian d.
  split-foot d.
  split-hand d.
  Sprengel's d.
  swan-neck d.
  thumb-in-palm d.
  torsional d.
  ulnar drift d.
  Velpeau's d.
  Volkmann's d.
  whistling d.
Deg — degeneration
  degree
de·gan·gli·on·ate
de·gas·sing
de·gen·er·a·cy
  d. of code
de·gen·er·ate
de·gen·er·a·tio
  d. micans
de·gen·er·a·tion
  Abercrombie's d.
  adipose d.
  adiposogenital d.
  albuminoid d.
  albuminous d.
  Alzheimer's neurofibrillary
    d.
  amyloid d.
  angiolithic d.
  Armanni-Ehrlich's d.
  ascending d.
  atheromatous d.
  atrophic pulp d.
  axonal d.
  bacony d.
  ballooning d.
  basic d.
  basophilic d.
  Best's macular d.
  black d. of brain
  blastophthoric d.
  calcareous d.
  Canavan spongy d.

de·gen·er·a·tion *(continued)*
  carneous d.
  caseous d.
  cellulose d.
  central d. of the corpus
    callosum
  cerebellar d. of late onset
  cerebellofugal d.
  cerebromacular d.
  cerebroretinal d.
  cheesy d.
  chitinous d.
  cloudy-swelling d.
  cobblestone d.
  colloid d.
  colloid d. of choroid
  comma d.
  congenital macular d.
  corticostriatal-spinal d.
  corticostriatonigral d.
  Crooke's hyaline d.
  cystic d.
  cystic d. of adventitia
  cystoid d.
  descending d.
  disciform macular d.
  Doyne's familial colloid d.
  Doyne's honeycomb d.
  dystrophic d.
  earthy d.
  elastoid d.
  familial colloid d.
  fascicular d.
  fatty d.
  fibrinous d.
  fibroid d.
  fibrous d.
  floccular d.
  gelatiniform d.
  glassy d.
  glistening d.
  glycogenic d.
  Gombault's d.
  granular d.
  granulovacuolar d.
  granulovascular d.
  gray d.
  hematohyaloid d.

de·gen·er·a·tion *(continued)*
  hepatolenticular d.
  heredomacular d.
  Holmes's d.
  Horn's d.
  hyaline d.
  hyaloid d.
  hydropic d.
  Kuhnt-Junius d.
  lardaceous d.
  lattice d.
  lattice d. of retina
  lenticular d.
  lipoidal d.
  liquefaction d.
  macular d.
  macular disciform d.
  Mönckeberg's d.
  mucinoid d.
  mucinous d.
  mucoid d.
  mucous d.
  multisystem d.
  myelinic d.
  myxomatous d.
  neurosomatic d.
  Nissl d.
  olivopontocerebellar d.
  pallidal d.
  paraneoplastic subacute
    cerebellar d.
  parenchymatous d.
  paving stone d.
  pigmental d.
  pigmentary d.
  pigmentary d. of globus
    pallidus
  polychromatophilic d.
  polypoid d.
  primary progressive
    cerebellar d.
  progressive
    pyramidopallidal d.
  Quain's d.
  red d.
  retrograde d.
  rim d.
  Rosenthal's d.

de·gen·er·a·tion *(continued)*
  sclerotic d.
  secondary d.
  senile d.
  senile disciform d.
  senile exudative macular d.
  spinocerebellar d.
  spongy d. of central
    nervous system
  spongy d. of white matter
  Stock's pigmentary d.
  striatonigral d.
  subacute combined d. of
    spinal cord
  system d.
  tapetoretinal d.
  Terrien's d.
  trabecular d.
  transneuronal d.
  traumatic d.
  Türck's d.
  turbid-swelling d.
  uratic d.
  vacuolar d.
  van Bogaert's familial
    axonal spongy d.
  Virchow's d.
  vitelliform d. of Best
  vitelliform macular d.
  vitelline macular d.
  vitreous d.
  wallerian d.
  waxy d.
  Wilson's d.
  Zenker's d.
de·gen·er·a·tive
de·germ
de·glov·ing
Deglut. — L. deglutiatur (let it
  be swallowed)
de·glu·ti·ble
de·glu·ti·tion
de·glu·ti·tive
de·glu·ti·to·ry
De·gos' disease
De·gos' syndrome
de·gra·da·ble
deg·ra·da·tion

de·gran·u·la·tion
de·gree
    d. absolute
    d. Celsius
    d. Fahrenheit
    d's of freedom
    prism d.
de·growth
de·gus·ta·tion
de·hab
de·he·ma·tized
de·he·mo·glo·bin·ized
de·hep·a·tized
De·hio's test
de·his·cence
    d. of alveolar process
    Killian's d.
    root d.
    d. of uterus
    wound d.
    Zuckerkandl's d's
de·hu·mid·i·fi·er
de·hy·drant
de·hy·drase
de·hy·dra·tase
    serine d.
de·hy·drate
de·hy·dra·tion
    absolute d.
    hypernatremic d.
    relative d.
    voluntary d.
de·hy·dro·an·dros·ter·one
de·hy·dro·as·cor·bic acid
de·hy·dro·bil·i·ru·bin
de·hy·dro·cho·lan·er·e·sis
de·hy·dro·cho·late
de·hy·dro·cho·les·ter·ol
    7-d., activated
de·hy·dro·cho·lic acid
11-de·hy·dro·cor·ti·cos·ter·one
de·hy·dro·co·ryd·a·line
de·hy·dro·em·e·tine res·in·ate
de·hy·dro·epi·an·dros·ter·one
    d. sulfate
de·hy·dro·gen·ase

de·hy·dro·gen·ate
de·hy·dro·gen·a·tion
de·hy·dro·iso·an·dros·ter·one
de·hy·dro·mor·phine
de·hy·dro·pep·ti·dase
de·hy·dro·ret·i·nal
de·hy·dro·ret·i·nol
de·hyp·no·tize
de·io·din·a·tion
de·ion·iza·tion
dei·ter·al
Dei·ters' cells
Dei·ters' frame
Dei·ters' nucleus
Dei·ters' phalanx
Dei·ters' process
Dei·ters' tract
dé·jà en·ten·du
dé·jà éprou·vé
dé·jà fait
dé·jà pen·sé
dé·jà ra·con·té
dé·jà vé·cu
dé·jà vou·lu
dé·jà vu
de·jec·ta
de·jec·tion
De·jer·ine's disease
De·jer·ine's sign
De·jer·ine's syndrome
De·jer·ine's type
De·jer·ine-Klump·ke paralysis
De·jer·ine-Klump·ke syndrome
De·jer·ine-Lan·dou·zy dystrophy
De·jer·ine-Lan·dou·zy type
De·jer·ine-Licht·heim phenomenon
De·jer·ine-Rous·sy syndrome
De·jer·ine-Sot·tas atrophy
De·jer·ine-Sot·tas disease
De·jer·ine-Sot·tas syndrome
De·jer·ine-Thom·as atrophy
de·la·cri·ma·tion
de·lac·ta·tion
Del·a·field's fluid
Del·a·field's hematoxylin

Del·a·lu·tin
de·lam·i·na·tion
Del·a·tes·tryl
de·lay
    pulse d.
    synaptic d.
Del·bet's sign
del Cas·til·lo syndrome
Del·brück
De Lee catheter
De Lee forceps
De Lee-Hil·lis stethoscope
Del·es·tro·gen
del·e·te·ri·ous
de·le·tion
    antigenic d.
    intercalary d.
    terminal d.
de·lim·i·ta·tion
de·lin·quen·cy
de·lin·quent
    juvenile d.
de·lip·i·da·tion
del·i·ques·cence
del·i·ques·cent
dé·lire onei·rique
de·lir·ia
de·lir·i·ant
de·lir·i·fa·cient
de·lir·i·ous
de·lir·i·um *pl.* de·li·ria
    acute d.
    d. alcoholicum
    alcohol withdrawal d.
    Bell's d.
    collapse d.
    d. cordis
    febrile d.
    d. grandiosum
    d. grave
    low d.
    oneiric d.
    organic d.
    senile d.
    toxic d.
    traumatic d.
    d. tremens
del·i·tes·cence

de·liv·er
de·liv·ery
    abdominal d.
    breech d.
    forceps d.
    forceps d., high
    forceps d., low
    forceps d., outlet
    midforceps d.
    normal spontaneous
        vaginal d. (NSVD)
    postmature d.
    postmortem d.
    premature d.
    spontaneous d.
    vaginal d.
dell
del·le
del·len
dell·ing
del·mad·i·none ac·e·tate
de·lo·mor·phic
de·lo·mor·phous
de·lous·ing
Del·phi·an node
del·phine
del·phi·nine
Del·phin·i·um
del·phi·noid·ine
del·phi·sine
del·ta
    Galton's d.
    d. mesoscapulae
del·ta OD$_{450}$
Del·ta-Cor·tef
del·ta·cor·ti·sone
Del·ta·lin
Del·ta·sone
del·toid
del·to·pec·to·ral
Del·tra
de·lu·sion
    autochthonous d.
    d. of being controlled
    d. of control
    bizarre d.
    depressive d.
    encapsulated d.

de·lu·sion *(continued)*
    erotomaniacal d.
    expansive d.
    fragmentary d's
    d. of grandeur
    grandiose d.
    d. of influence
    messianic d.
    d. of misidentification
    mood-congruent d.
    mood-incongruent d.
    d. of negation
    nihilistic d.
    paranoid d's
    d. of persecution
    persecutory d.
    d. of poverty
    primary d.
    d. of reference
    secondary d.
    self-referential d.
    shared d.
    somatic d.
    systematized d's
de·lu·sion·al
Del·vi·nal
De·man·sia
de·mar·ca·tion
    surface d.
De·mar·quay's sign
de·mas·cu·lin·iza·tion
De·mat·i·a·ceae
de·mat·i·a·ceous
De·ma·ti·um
deme
dem·e·car·i·um
dem·e·car·i·um bro·mide
dem·e·clo·cy·cline
    d. hydrochloride
de·ment·ed
de·men·tia
    alcoholic d.
    Alzheimer's d.
    arteriosclerotic d.
    Binswanger d.
    boxers' d.
    catatonic d.
    chronic d.

de·men·tia *(continued)*
    dialysis d.
    epileptic d.
    hebephrenic d.
    d. infantilis
    multi-infarct d.
    d. myoclonica
    myxedematous d.
    paralytic d.
    d. paralytica
    paretic d.
    post-traumatic d.
    d. praecox
    presenile d.
    primary degenerative d.
    d. pugilistica
    senile d.
    subcortical d.
    toxic d.
    vascular d.
    Wernicke's d.
Dem·er·ol
de·meth·yl·a·tion
de·meth·yl·chlor·tet·ra·cy·cline
demi·bain
demi·fac·et
    inferior d. for head of rib
    superior d. for head of rib
demi·gaunt·let
demi·lune
    d's of Adamkiewicz
    d's of Giannuzzi
    d's of Heidenhain
demi·mon·stros·i·ty
de·min·er·al·iza·tion
demi·pen·ni·form
Demi-Reg·ro·ton
De·moc·ri·tus
dem·o·dec·tic
Dem·o·dex
    D. folliculorum
Dem·o·dic·i·dae
dem·o·dic·i·do·sis
dem·o·di·co·sis
de·mod·u·la·tion
de·mo·gram
dem·o·graph·ic

de·mog·ra·phy
  dynamic d.
  static d.
de·mo·ni·ac
de·mono·pho·bia
dem·on·stra·tor
De Mor·gan's spots
de·mor·phin·iza·tion
de Mor·sier syndrome
de Mor·sier-Gau·thier
  syndrome
De·mours' membrane
de·mox·e·pam
de·mu·co·sa·tion
de·mul·cent
de Mus·set
de Mus·sy's point
de Mus·sy's sign
de·mus·tard·iza·tion
de·mu·ti·za·tion
de·my·e·lin·ate
de·my·e·lin·a·tion
de·my·e·lin·iza·tion
de·my·eli·nol·y·sis
de·nar·co·tize
de·na·sal·i·ty
de·na·tal·i·ty
de·na·to·ni·um ben·zo·ate
de·na·tur·ant
de·na·tur·a·tion
  protein d.
de·na·tured
den·drax·on
den·dric
den·dri·cep·tor
Den·drid
den·dri·form
den·drite
  apical d.
  basal d.
den·drit·ic
den·dri·tum
  d. apicale
  d. basale
Den·dro·as·pis
Den·dro·chi·um
den·dro·den·drit·ic
den·dro·do·chio·tox·i·co·sis

den·droid
den·dron
den·dro·phago·cy·to·sis
de·ner·vate
de·ner·va·tion
den·gue
  hemorrhagic d.
de·ni·al
den·i·da·tion
Den·is Browne splint
Den·is' method
Den·i·so·nia
de·ni·tri·fi·ca·tion
de·ni·tri·fi·er
de·ni·tri·fy
de·ni·tro·ge·na·tion
Den·ker's operation
Den·man's method
Den·man's spontaneous
  evolution
Den·man's version
Den·nie's sign
Den·nis-Brown pouch
Den·ny-Brown syndrome
de·no·fun·gin
De·non·vil·liers' aponeurosis
De·non·vil·liers' fascia
De·non·vil·liers' operation
dens *pl.* den·tes
  dentes acustici
  dentes acuti
  dentes angulares
  d. axis
  dentes canini
  dentes de Chiaie
  dentes decidui
  d. epistrophei
  dentes incisivi
  d. in dente
  d. invaginatus
  dentes molares
  dentes permanentes
  dentes premolares
  d. sapientiae
  d. serotinus
den·sim·e·ter
den·si·tom·e·ter
  gas d.

den·si·tom·e·try
   dual-photon d.
   Norland-Cameron photon
     d.
   photon d.
den·si·ty
   absolute d.
   arciform d.
   background d.
   buoyant d.
   count information d.
   flux d.
   inherent d.
   ionization d.
   ocular d.
   optical d. (OD)
   relative d.
   scan information d.
   superhelix d.
den·sog·ra·phy
den·tag·ra
den·tal
den·tal·gia
den·ta·ta
den·tate
den·ta·to·ru·bral
den·ta·to·tha·lam·ic
den·ta·tum
den·tes
den·tia
   d. praecox
   d. tarda
den·ti·buc·cal
den·ti·cle
   adherent d.
   attached d.
   embedded d.
   false d.
   free d.
   interstitial d.
   true d.
den·tic·u·lat·ed
den·ti·fi·ca·tion
den·ti·form
den·ti·frice
den·tig·er·ous
den·ti·la·bi·al
den·ti·lin·gual

den·tim·e·ter
den·tin
   adventitious d.
   calcified d.
   circumpulpar d.
   cover d.
   functional d.
   hereditary opalescent d.
   hypoplastic d.
   interglobular d.
   irregular d.
   mantle d.
   opalescent d.
   peritubular d.
   primary d.
   reparative d.
   sclerotic d.
   secondary d.
   secondary irregular d.
   secondary regular d.
   tertiary d.
   transparent d.
den·ti·nal
den·tine
den·ti·no·blast
den·ti·no·blas·to·ma
den·ti·no·gen·e·sis
   d. imperfecta
den·ti·no·gen·ic
den·ti·noid
den·ti·no·ma
den·ti·nos·te·oid
den·ti·num
den·tip·a·rous
den·tist
den·tis·try
   cosmetic d.
   esthetic d.
   forensic d.
   four-handed d.
   geriatric d.
   legal d.
   operative d.
   pediatric d.
   preventive d.
   prosthetic d.
   psychosomatic d.
   restorative d.

den·ti·tion
 artificial d.
 deciduous d.
 delayed d.
 first d.
 mixed d.
 natural d.
 permanent d.
 precocious d.
 predeciduous d.
 premature d.
 primary d.
 retarded d.
 secondary d.
 temporary d.
 transitional d.
den·to·al·ve·o·lar
den·to·al·ve·o·li·tis
den·to·fa·cial
den·to·form
den·tog·ra·phy
den·toid
den·to·le·gal
den·to·ma
den·to·me·chan·i·cal
den·ton·o·my
den·to·sur·gi·cal
den·to·trop·ic
den·tu·lous
den·ture
 clasp d.
 complete d.
 conditioning d.
 Every d.
 full d.
 immediate d.
 immediate-insertion d.
 implant d.
 interim d.
 overlay d.
 partial d.
 partial d., distal extension
 partial d., fixed
 partial d., removable
 partial d., unilateral
 provisional d.
 skeleton d.

den·ture *(continued)*
 spoon d.
 telescopic d.
 temporary d.
 tooth-borne partial d.
 transitional d.
 trial d.
den·tur·ism
den·tur·ist
De·nu·cé's ligament
de·nu·cle·at·ed
de·nu·da·tion
de·nu·tri·tion
Den·ver De·vel·op·men·tal
 Screen·ing Test
Den·ver shunt
de·odor·ant
de·odor·ize
de·odor·iz·er
de·on·tol·o·gy
de·op·pi·lant
de·op·pi·la·tion
de·or·sum·duc·tion
de·or·sum·ver·gence
de·or·sum·ver·sion
de·os·si·fi·ca·tion
de·ox·i·da·tion
de·ox·i·dize
de·oxy·aden·o·sine
 d. diphosphate (dADP)
 d. monophosphate (dAMP)
 d. triphosphate (dATP)
5′-de·ox·y·a·den·o·syl trans·
 fer·ase
de·oxy·aden·yl·ate
de·oxy·ad·e·nyl·ic acid
de·oxy·ad·e·nyl·yl
de·ox·y·cho·lan·er·e·sis
de·oxy·cho·late
de·oxy·chol·ic acid
de·oxy·chol·yl·gly·cine
de·oxy·chol·yl·taur·ine
 d. acetate
 d. pivalate
 d. trimethylacetate
de·oxy·cor·tone
11-de·oxy·cor·ti·cos·ter·one
 (DOC)

de·oxy·cy·ti·dine
    d. diphosphate (dCDP)
    d. monophosphate (dCMP)
    d. triphosphate (dCTP)
de·oxy·cy·ti·dyl·ate
de·oxy·cy·ti·dyl·ic acid
de·oxy·cy·ti·dyl·yl
de·oxy·gen·ate
de·ox·y·gen·a·tion
2-de·oxy-D-glu·cose
de·oxy·guan·o·sine
    d. diphosphate (dGDP)
    d. monophosphate (dGMP)
    d. triphosphate (dGTP)
de·oxy·guan·yl·ate
de·oxy·guan·yl·ic acid
de·oxy·guan·yl·yl
de·oxy·he·mo·glo·bin
de·oxy·nu·cleo·tid·yl trans·
  fer·ase (terminal)
de·oxy·nu·cleo·side
de·oxy·pen·tose·nu·cle·ic acid
de·oxy·ri·bo·nu·cle·ase
    d. I
    d. II
de·oxy·ri·bo·nu·cle·ic acid
de·oxy·ri·bo·nu·cleo·pro·tein
de·oxy·ri·bo·nu·cleo·side
de·oxy·ri·bo·nu·cleo·tide
de·oxy·ri·bose
de·oxy·thy·mi·dine
    d. diphosphate (dTDP)
    d. monophosphate (dTMP)
    d. triphosphate (dTTP)
de·oxy·thy·mi·dyl·ate
de·oxy·thy·mi·dyl·ic acid
de·oxy·thy·mi·dyl·yl
Dep. — L. depuratus (purified)
De·page position
De·page-Jane·way gastrostomy
Dep·a·kene
de·pat·tern·ing
de·pen·dence
    psychoactive substance d.
    substance d.
de·pen·den·cy
    drug d.
    psychological d.

de·pen·den·cy (continued)
    pyridoxine d.
de·pen·dent
de·pep·sin·ized
de·per·son·al·iza·tion
de Pez·zer catheter
de·phos·phor·y·la·tion
de·pig·men·ta·tion
dep·i·late
dep·i·la·tion
de·pil·a·to·ry
de·plas·mol·y·sis
de·plas·mo·lyze
de·plete
de·ple·tion
    plasma d.
de·po·lar·iza·tion
de·po·lar·ize
de·po·lar·iz·er
de·po·lym·er·iza·tion
de·po·lym·er·ize
De·po-Pro·vera
de·pos·it
    glomerular d's
    hyaline d.
    mesangial d.
    para-amyloid d.
    subendothelial d.
    subepithelial d.
    tooth d.
de·pot
    fat d.
De·po-Tes·tos·ter·one
dep·ra·va·tion
de·pres·sant
    cardiac d.
de·pressed
de·pres·sion
    agitated d.
    anaclitic d.
    congenital chondrosternal
      d.
    endogenous d.
    freezing point d.
    involutional d.
    Leão spreading d.
    major d.
    neurotic d.

de·pres·sion *(continued)*
    otic d.
    pacchionian d's
    precordial d.
    psychotic d.
    pterygoid d.
    radial d.
    reactive d.
    retarded d.
    situational d.
    supratrochlear d.
    tooth d.
    unipolar d.
    ventricular d.
de·pres·sive
de·pres·so·mo·tor
de·pres·sor
    d. anguli oris
    d. epiglottidis
    d.   labii inferioris
    tongue d.
dep·ri·mens oc·u·li
dep·ri·va·tion
    emotional d.
    maternal d.
    psychosocial d.
    sensory d.
    thought d.
de·pros·til
de·pro·tein·iza·tion
dep·side
dep·si·pep·tide
depth
    focal d.
    d. of focus
dep·u·la
dep·u·li·za·tion
dep·u·rant
dep·u·rate
dep·u·ra·tion
dep·u·ra·tive
dep·u·ra·tor
de·pu·ri·na·tion
de Quer·vain's thyroidosis
der·a·del·phus
der·an·en·ce·pha·lia
de·range·ment
    Hey's internal d.

Der·cum's disease
de·re·al·i·za·tion
de·re·ism
de·re·is·tic
der·en·ceph·a·lo·cele
der·en·ceph·a·lus
der·en·ceph·a·ly
de·re·pres·sion
    gene d.
der·i·vant
der·i·va·tion
de·riv·a·tive
    hematoporphyrin d.
    purified protein d.
    tricyclic d.
der·ma
derm·abrad·er
derm·abra·sion
der·ma·car·ri·er
Der·ma·cen·tor
    D. albipictus
    D. andersoni
    D. halli
    D. hunteri
    D. marginatus
    D. nuttallii
    D. occidentalis
    D. parumapertus
    D. reticulatus
    D. sylvarum
    D. variabilis
Der·ma·cen·trox·e·nus
der·ma·cha·la·sis
der·mad
der·mal
der·mal·gia
der·ma·my·ia·sis
Der·ma·nys·si·dae
Der·ma·nys·sus
    D. gallinae
der·ma·skel·e·ton
der·ma·tan sul·fate
der·mat·ic
der·ma·tit·i·des
der·ma·ti·tis *pl.* der·ma·tit·i·
    des
    actinic d.
    allergic d.

der·ma·ti·tis *(continued)*
allergic contact d.
ammonia d.
ancylostome d.
d. artefacta
ashy d.
atopic d.
autosensitization d.
bathers' d.
berlock d., berloque d.
d. blastomycotica
brown-tail moth d.
d. bullosa striata pratensis
d. calorica
carcinomatous d.
caterpillar d.
cercarial d.
chemical d.
d. congelationis
contact d.
contagious pustular d.
cosmetic d.
cumulative insult d.
dhobie mark d.
diaper d.
dried fruit d.
eczematous d.
d. exfoliativa
d. exfoliativa neonatorum
exfoliative d.
exudative discoid and
  lichenoid d.
factitial d.
d. gangrenosa infantum
grass d.
d. herpetiformis
d. hiemalis
industrial d.
infectious eczematous d.
insect d.
irritant d.
Jacquet's d.
livedoid d.
marine d.
meadow d.
meadow-grass d.
d. medicamentosa
moth d.

der·ma·ti·tis *(continued)*
napkin d.
nummular eczematous d.
occupational d.
onion mite d.
d. papillaris capillitii
perfume d.
periocular d.
perioral d.
photoallergic contact d.
photocontact d.
phototoxic d.
phytophototoxic d.
pigmented purpuric
  lichenoid d.
poison ivy d.
poison oak d.
poison sumac d.
precancerous d.
primary irritant d.
radiation d.
rat-mite d.
d. repens
rhus d.
roentgen-ray d.
sabra d.
schistosome d.
seborrheic d.
d. seborrheica
stasis d.
d. striata pratensis bullosa
swimmer's d.
uncinarial d.
d. vegetans
d. venenata
verminous d.
vesicular d.
x-ray d.

der·ma·to·ar·thri·tis
lipid d.
lipoid d.

der·ma·to·au·to·plas·ty
Der·ma·to·bia
  D. hominis

der·ma·to·bi·a·sis
der·ma·to·con·junc·ti·vi·tis
der·ma·to·dys·pla·sia

der·ma·to·fi·bro·ma
    d. protuberans
der·ma·to·fi·bro·sar·co·ma
    progressive recurrent d.
    d. protuberans
der·ma·to·fi·bro·sis
    d. lenticularis disseminata
der·ma·to·glyph·ics
der·ma·to·graph·ic
der·ma·to·graph·ism
    black d.
    white d.
der·ma·to·het·ero·plas·ty
der·ma·to·log·ic
der·ma·to·log·i·cal
der·ma·tol·o·gist
der·ma·tol·o·gy
der·ma·tol·y·sis
    d. palpebrarum
der·ma·tome
    Brown d.
    Castroviejo d.
    drum d.
    Padgett d.
    Reese d.
der·ma·to·meg·a·ly
der·ma·to·mere
der·ma·tom·ic
der·ma·to·my·ces
der·ma·to·my·cid
der·ma·to·my·cin
der·ma·to·my·co·sis
der·ma·to·my·ia·sis
der·ma·to·my·o·ma
der·ma·to·myo·si·tis
der·ma·to·neu·rol·o·gy
der·ma·to·no·sol·o·gy
der·ma·to-oph·thal·mi·tis
der·ma·to·path·ic
der·ma·to·pa·thol·o·gy
der·ma·top·a·thy
Der·ma·toph·a·goi·des
    D. farinae
    D. pteronyssinus
    D. scheremetewskyi
der·ma·to·phar·ma·col·o·gy
Der·ma·to·phi·la·ceae
der·ma·to·phi·li·a·sis

der·ma·to·phi·lo·sis
Der·ma·toph·i·lus
    D. congolensis
    D. penetrans
der·ma·to·phyte
der·ma·to·phy·tid
der·ma·to·phy·ton
der·ma·to·phy·to·sis
    d. interdigitale
der·ma·to·plas·tic
der·ma·to·plas·ty
    Thompson's d.
der·ma·to·poly·neu·ri·tis
der·ma·tor·rha·gia
    d. parasitica
der·ma·tor·rhex·is
der·ma·to·scle·ro·sis
der·ma·to·sis *pl.* der·ma·to·ses
    acute febrile neutrophilic d.
    ashy d. of Ramirez
    Bowen's precancerous d.
    chick nutritional d.
    cholinogenic d.
    chronic bullous d. of childhood
    chronic hemosideric d.
    d. cinecienta
    contact d.
    dermatolytic bullous d.
    industrial d.
    lichenoid d.
    menstrual d.
    occupational d.
    d. papulosa nigra
    precancerous d.
    progressive pigmentary d.
    radiation d.
    Schamberg's d.
    seborrheic d.
    subcorneal pustular d.
    transient acantholytic d.
    d. vegetans
der·ma·to·some
der·ma·to·spa·rax·is
der·ma·to·syph·i·lis
der·ma·to·ther·a·py

der·ma·to·trop·ic
der·ma·to·zoa
der·ma·to·zo·ia·sis
der·ma·to·zo·on
der·ma·to·zoo·no·sis
der·men·chy·sis
der·mic
der·mis
    reticular d.
der·mo·ac·ti·no·my·co·sis
der·mo·blast
der·mo·cy·ma
der·mo·cy·mus
der·mo·gen·e·sis
der·mo·graph·ia
der·mo·graph·ism
der·mo·hy·grom·e·ter
der·moid
    corneal d.
    implantation d.
    inclusion d.
    intracranial d.
    intramedullary d.
    thyroid d.
    tubal d.
der·moid·ec·to·my
der·mo·li·pec·to·my
der·mo·li·po·ma
der·mol·y·sin
der·mom·e·ter
der·mom·e·try
der·mo·my·co·sis
der·mo·myo·tome
der·mo·neu·ro·trop·ic
der·mo·path·ic
der·mop·a·thy
    diabetic d.
    infiltrative d.
der·mo·phy·ma ve·ner·e·um
der·mo·phyte
der·mo·plas·ty
der·mo·re·ac·tion
der·mor·rha·gia
der·mo·skel·e·ton
der·mo·syn·o·vi·tis
der·mo·tox·in
der·mo·trop·ic
der·mo·vas·cu·lar

der·o·did·y·mus
der·ren·ga·de·ra
der·ri·en·gue
der·ris
DES — diethylstilbestrol
de·sal·i·na·tion
de·sal·i·va·tion
De Sanc·tis-Cac·chi·o·ne
    syndrome
de·sat·u·ra·tion
De·sault's apparatus
De·sault's bandage
De·sault's sign
Des·cartes' law
Des·ce·met's membrane
des·ce·me·ti·tis
des·ce·me·to·cele
des·cen·dens
    d. cervicalis
    d. cervicis
des·cend·ing
des·cen·sus *pl.* des·cen·sus
    d. testis
    d. uteri
de·scent
    d. of testis
    x d.
    y d.
Des·champs' compressor
Des·champs' needle
des·ci·clo·vir
des·cin·o·lone acet·o·nide
de·sen·si·ti·za·tion
    anaphylactic d.
    systematic d.
de·sen·si·tize
de·ser·pi·dine
de·sex·u·al·ize
Des·fer·al
des·fer·ri·ox·amine
des·hy·dre·mia
des·ic·cant
des·ic·cate
des·ic·ca·tion
    electric d.
des·ic·ca·tive
des·ic·ca·tor

de·sip·ra·mine hy·dro·chlo·ride
Des·jar·dins' point
des·lan·o·side
des·mal·gia
des·mec·ta·sis
des·mep·i·the·li·um
des·mid
des·min
des·mi·og·nath·us
des·mi·tis
des·mo·cra·ni·um
des·mo·cyte
des·mo·cy·to·ma
des·mo·don·ti·um
des·mo·dyn·ia
des·mog·e·nous
des·mog·ra·phy
des·mo·he·mo·blast
des·moid
des·mo·lase
    17,20-d.
    20,22-d.
des·mol·o·gy
des·mo·ma
des·mo·neo·plasm
des·mop·a·thy
des·mo·pex·ia
des·mo·pla·sia
des·mo·plas·tic
des·mo·pres·sin
des·mor·rhex·is
des·mose
des·mo·sine
des·mo·sis
des·mo·some
    half d.
des·mos·ter·ol
des·mot·o·my
des·mo·trop·ism
deso·leo·lec·i·thin
deso·mor·phine
des·o·nide
de·sorb
de·sorp·tion
De·Sou·za exercises
des·ox·i·met·a·sone

des·oxy·cor·ti·cos·ter·one
    d. acetate
    d. pivalate
    d. trimethylacetate
des·oxy·cor·tone
    d. acetate
des·oxy·ephed·rine
des·oxy·mor·phine
Des·ox·yn
des·oxy·phe·no·bar·bi·tal
des·oxy·ri·bo·nu·cle·ase
des·oxy·ri·bose
des·oxy-su·gar
de·spe·ci·ate
de·spe·ci·a·tion
de·spe·ci·fi·ca·tion
d'Es·pine's sign
des·pu·ma·tion
des·qua·mate
des·qua·ma·tion
    furfuraceous d.
    lamellar d. of the newborn
des·qua·ma·tive
des·qua·ma·to·ry
dest. — L. destilla (distil)
    destillatus (distilled)
des·thio·bio·tin
destil. — L. destilla (distil)
de·sulf·hy·drase
De·sul·fo·mo·nas
de·sul·fur·ase
2-des·vi·nyl-2-for·myl chlo·ro·phyll
de·sy·nap·sis
de·syn·chron·iza·tion
DET — diethyltryptamine
Det. — L. detur (let it be given)
de·tach·ment
    epiphyseal d.
    exudative retinal d.
    d. of retina
    retinal d.
    rhegmatogenous retinal d.
de·tec·tor
    activation d.

de·tec·tor *(continued)*
    alpha wave d.
    Doppler fetal heart d.
    flame ionization d.
    nonparalyzable d.
    photocell d.
    quadrature d.
    radiation d.
    scintillation d.
    self-quenching d.
    sterility d.
    thermoluminescent d.
    threshold d.
de·ter·e·nol hy·dro·chlo·ride
de·ter·gent
    anionic d.
    cationic d.
de·te·ri·or·a·tion
    d. of affect
    emotional d.
    schizophrenic d.
    simple senile d.
de·ter·mi·nant
    antigenic d.
    germ cell d.
    hidden d.
    immunogenic d.
    inaccessible d.
    resistance d.
    sequential d.
de·ter·mi·na·tion
    embryonic d.
    sex d.
de·ter·min·er
de·ter·min·ism
    psychic d.
de·thy·roid·ize
de To·ni-De·bré-Fan·co·ni syndrome
de To·ni-Fan·co·ni syndrome
Det. in dup., Det. in 2 plo. — L. detur in duplo (let twice as much be given)
de·tor·sion
de·tox·i·cate
de·tox·i·ca·tion
de·tox·i·fi·ca·tion
    metabolic d.

de·tox·i·fy
de·tri·tion
de·tri·tiv·o·rous
de·tri·tus
de·trun·ca·tion
de·tru·sor
    d. urinae
    d. vesicae
D. et s. — L. detur et signetur (let it be given and labeled)
de·tu·ba·tion
de·tu·ber·cu·li·za·tion
de·tu·mes·cence
deu·tan
deu·ter·anom·al
deu·ter·anom·a·lous
deu·ter·anom·a·ly
deu·ter·an·ope
deu·ter·an·o·pia
deu·ter·an·op·ic
deu·ter·an·op·sia
deu·ter·ate
deu·ter·a·tion
deu·te·ri·on
deu·ter·ip·a·ra
deu·te·ri·um
    d. oxide
deu·tero·co·ni·di·um
deu·tero·fat
deu·tero·he·min
deu·tero·he·mo·phil·ia
deu·tero·my·cete
Deu·tero·my·ce·tes
deu·ter·on
deu·tero·path·ic
deu·ter·op·a·thy
deu·tero·pine
deu·tero·plasm
deu·tero·por·phy·rin
deu·tero·some
deu·tero·stome
deu·tero·to·cia
deu·ter·ot·o·ky
deu·thy·alo·some
deu·to·me·rite
deu·ton
deu·to·neph·ron
deu·to·plasm

deu·to·plas·mol·y·sis
Deutsch·län·der's disease
DEV — duck embryo rabies
  vaccine
de·vas·a·tion
de·vas·cu·lar·iza·tion
Dev·e·gan
de·vel·op·ment
  arrested d.
  cognitive d.
  mosaic d.
  postnatal d.
  prenatal d.
  psychomotor d.
  psychosexual d.
  psychosocial d.
  regulative d.
de·vel·op·men·tal
De·ven·ter's diameter
De·ver·gie's attitude
de·vi·ance
de·vi·ant
  sexual d.
de·vi·a·tion
  animal d.
  axis d.
  complement d.
  conjugate d.
  Hering-Hellebrand d.
  immune d.
  latent d.
  d. to the left
  manifest d.
  minimum d.
  ocular conjugate d.
  primary d.
  d. to the right
  sample standard d.
  secondary d.
  sexual d.
  skew d.
  squint d.
  standard d.
  strabismic d.
  ulnar d.
  Vulpian's conjugate d.
Dev·ic's disease

de·vice
  central-bearing d.
  central-bearing tracing d.
  contraceptive d.
  emergency infusion d.
    (EID)
  intrauterine d. (IUD)
  left ventricular assist d.
  MediPort vascular access
    d.
  static imaging d.
de·vi·om·e·ter
de·vis·cer·a·tion
de·vi·tal·iza·tion
  pulp d.
de·vi·tal·ize
dev·o·lu·tion
de·vol·u·tive
De Vries' theory
Dew's sign
Dew·ar flask
de·wa·tered
dex·a·meth·a·sone
  d. acetate
  d. sodium phosphate
dex·am·i·sole
dex·brom·phen·ir·a·mine
  d. maleate
dex·chlor·phen·ir·a·mine
  d. maleate
dex·cla·mol hy·dro·chlo·ride
Dex·e·drine
dex·et·i·mide
dex·im·a·fen
dex·io·car·dia
dex·io·trop·ic
dex·iv·a·caine
Dex·on
Dex·o·val
dex·pan·the·nol
dex·pro·pran·o·lol hy·dro·
  chlo·ride
dex·ter
dex·trad
dex·tral
dex·tral·i·ty
dex·tran

dex·tran
    d. sulfate
dex·trano·mer
dex·trates
dex·trau·ral
dex·tri·fer·ron
dex·trin
    limit d.
dex·trin·ase
α-dex·trin·ase
dex·trin·ate
dex·trin·ize
dex·trin-1,6-glu·co·si·dase
dex·trin·ose
dex·tri·no·sis
    limit d.
dex·trin·uria
dex·tro·am·phet·amine
    d. phosphate
    d. sulfate
dex·tro·car·dia
    isolated d.
    mirror-image d.
    secondary d.
dex·tro·car·dio·gram
dex·tro·cer·e·bral
dex·tro·cli·na·tion
dex·tro·com·pound
dex·troc·u·lar
dex·troc·u·lar·i·ty
dex·tro·cy·clo·duc·tion
dex·tro·duc·tion
dex·tro·gas·tria
dex·tro·glu·cose
dex·tro·gram
dex·tro·gy·ral
dex·tro·gy·ra·tion
dex·tro·man·u·al
dex·tro·men·thol
dex·tro·meth·or·phan hy·dro·bro·mide
dex·trop·e·dal
dex·tro·po·si·tion
dex·tro·pro·poxy·phene
dex·tro·ro·ta·ry
dex·tro·ro·ta·to·ry
dex·trose
dex·tro·sin·is·tral

dex·tro·so·zone
Dex·tro·stix
dex·tros·uria
dex·tro·thy·rox·ine so·di·um
dex·tro·tor·sion
dex·tro·trop·ic
dex·tro·ver·sion
dex·tro·vert·ed
dez·o·cine
DFA — direct fluorescent antibody test
DFMO — difluoromethylorni-thine
DFP — diisopropyl flurophosphate
DF-2 bacillus
dG — deoxyguanosine
dg — decigram
dGDP — deoxyguanosine diphosphate
dGMP — deoxyguanosine monophosphate
dGTP — deoxyguanosine triphosphate
DH — delayed hypersensitivity
DHEA — dehydroepiandro-sterone
d'He·relle phenomenon
DHg — Doctor of Hygiene
DHy — Doctor of Hygiene
DHL — diffuse histiocytic lymphoma
DHPG — dihydroxypropoxyme-thylguanine
DHT — dihydrotestosterone
dhur·rin
DI — diabetes insipidus
di·a·be·tes
    adult-onset d.
    alloxan d.
    brittle d.
    bronze d.
    chemical d.
    class A d.
    gestational d.
    glucophosphatemic d.
    growth-onset d.

di·a·be·tes *(continued)*
   d. insipidus
   d. insipidus, nephrogenic
   insulin-dependent d. (IDD)
   juvenile-onset d.
   ketosis-prone d.
   ketosis-resistant d.
   latent d.
   lipoatrophic d.
   maturity-onset d.
   maturity-onset d. of youth
    (MODY)
   d. mellitus (DM)
   metahypophyseal d.
   neurogenic d.
   non–insulin-dependent d.
    (NIDD)
   obesity-associated d.
   overt d.
   pancreatic d.
   phlorhizin d.
   phosphate d.
   piqûre d.
   preclinical d.
   pregnancy d.
   puncture d.
   renal d.
   renal amino acid d.
   secondary d.
   starvation d.
   steroid d.
   steroidogenic d.
   subclinical d.
   thiazide d.
   type I d.
   type II d.
   vasopressin-resistant d.
    insipidus
   Young's d.
di·a·bet·ic
di·a·be·tid
di·a·be·to·gen·ic
di·a·be·tog·e·nous
di·a·be·to·graph
di·a·be·tom·e·ter
Di·ab·i·nese
di·a·bro·sis
di·a·brot·ic

di·ac·e·tate
di·ac·e·te·mia
di·a·ce·tic acid
di·a·ce·tic·acid·uria
di·ac·e·ton·uria
di·ac·et·uria
di·ac·e·tyl
   d. peroxide
di·ac·e·tyl-*N*-al·lyl·nor·mor·
  phine
di·ac·e·tyl·dap·sone
di·ac·e·tyl·mor·phine
   d. hydrochloride
di·ac·e·tyl·tan·nic acid
Di·a·chlo·rus
di·a·cho·re·ma
di·a·cho·re·sis
di·ac·id
di·ac·la·sis
di·a·clast
di·ac·ri·nous
di·ac·ri·sis
di·a·crit·ic
di·ac·tin·ic
di·ac·tin·ism
di·a·cyl·glyc·er·ol
di·a·der·mic
di·ad·o·cho·ci·ne·sia
di·ad·o·cho·ci·net·ic
di·ad·o·cho·ki·ne·sia
di·ad·o·cho·ki·ne·sis
di·ad·o·cho·ki·net·ic
Di·a·dol
Di·a·fen
di·ag·nose
di·ag·no·sis
   biological d.
   clinical d.
   cytohistologic d.
   cytologic d.
   differential d.
   direct d.
   d. by exclusion
   d. ex juvantibus
   laboratory d.
   niveau d.
   pathologic d.
   physical d.

di·ag·no·sis *(continued)*
   provocative d.
   quick-section d.
   roentgen d.
   serum d.
di·ag·nos·tic
di·ag·nos·ti·cate
di·ag·nos·ti·cian
di·ag·nos·tics
di·a·gram
   Berkow d.
   burn d.
   scatter d.
   vector d.
di·a·gram·mat·ic
di·a·graph
di·a·ki·ne·sis
Di·al
di·al
   astigmatic d.
di·al·lyl
di·al·lyl·bis·nor·tox·i·fer·in
  di·chlo·ride
Di·a·log
Di·a·lume
di·al·y·sance
di·al·y·sate
di·al·y·sis
   chronic d.
   continuous ambulatory
     peritoneal d. (CAPD)
   continuous cycling
     peritoneal d.
   cross d.
   Drake-Willock d.
   equilibrium d.
   intermittent d.
   intermittent peritoneal d.
     (IPD)
   kidney d.
   lymph d.
   maintenance d.
   periodic d.
   peritoneal d.
   d. retinae
   single-needle d.
di·a·lyz·able
di·a·lyzed

di·a·lyz·er
   coil d.
   Dow hollow-fiber d.
   parallel flow (plate) d.
   Terumo d.
dia·mag·net·ic
Di·a·ma·nus
   D. montanus
di·am·e·ter
   anterior sagittal d.
   anteroposterior d.
   anterotransverse d.
   Baudelocque's d.
   biischial d.
   biparietal d.
   bisacromial d.
   bisiliac d.
   bispinous d.
   bitemporal d.
   buccolingual d.
   cervicobregmatic d.
   coccygeopubic d.
   d. conjugata pelvis
   conjugate d.
   conjugate d., anatomic
   conjugate d., diagonal
   conjugate d., external
   conjugate d., internal
   conjugate d., obstetric
   conjugate d. of pelvis
   conjugate d., true
   cranial d's
   craniometric d.
   extracanthic d.
   frontomental d.
   fronto-occipital d.
   intercanthic d.
   intercristal d.
   interspinous d.
   intertrochanteric d.
   intertuberal d.
   longitudinal d., inferior
   mean corpuscular d.
   mento-occipital d.
   mentoparietal d.
   d. obliqua pelvis
   oblique d. of pelvis

di·am·e·ter *(continued)*
  occipitofrontal d.
  occipitomental d.
  parietal d.
  pelvic d.
  posterior sagittal d.
  posterotransverse d.
  pubosacral d.
  pubotuberous d.
  sacropubic d.
  sagittal d.
  suboccipitobregmatic d.
  suboccipitofrontal d.
  suprasubparietal d.
  temporal d.
  d. transversa pelvis
  transverse d.
  transverse d. of pelvis
  transverse d. of pelvic
    outlet
  vertebromammary d.
  vertical d.
di·amide
di·am·i·dine
di·amine
di·amine ox·i·dase
di·ami·no·ac·ri·dine
di·ami·no·di·phen·yl·sul·fone
  diacetyl d.
di·ami·no·di·phos·pha·tide
di·ami·no·mono·phos·pha·
  tide
2,6-di·ami·no·pi·mel·ic acid
di·ami·no·py·rim·i·dine
di·amin·uria
di·am·ni·ot·ic
di·a·mo·caine cy·cla·mate
Di·a·mond-Black·fan
  syndrome
di·a·monds
dia·mond-shaped
dia·mor·phine
Di·a·mox
di·am·tha·zole di·hy·dro·
  chlo·ride
di·am·y·lene
Di·an·a·bol

di·an·hy·dro·an·ti·ar·i·gen·
  in
di·an·ion
di·a·no·et·ic
di·an·te·bra·chia
di·ap·amide
Di·ap·a·rene
di·a·pause
  embryonic d.
di·a·pe·de·sis
di·a·pe·det·ic
di·a·phane
di·a·pha·ne·i·ty
di·aph·a·nog·ra·phy
di·aph·a·nom·e·ter
di·aph·a·nom·e·try
di·aph·a·no·scope
di·aph·a·nos·co·py
di·aph·a·nous
di·aph·e·met·ric
di·aph·o·rase
di·aph·o·re·sis
di·a·pho·ret·ic
di·a·phragm
  accessory d.
  Akerlund d.
  Bucky d.
  Bucky-Potter d.
  compression d.
  condensing d.
  contraceptive d.
  epithelial d.
  filtration slit d. of
    glomerulus
  graduating d.
  iris d.
  d. of mouth
  oral d.
  pelvic d.
  polyarcuate d.
  Potter-Bucky d.
  respiratory d.
  secondary d.
  d. of sella turcica
  thoracoabdominal d.
  urogenital d.
  vaginal d.

di·a·phrag·ma *pl.* dia·phrag·
ma·ta
    d. oris
    d. pelvis
    d. sellae
    d. urogenitale
di·a·phrag·mal·gia
di·a·phrag·ma·ta
di·a·phrag·mat·ic
di·a·phrag·ma·ti·tis
di·a·phrag·mat·o·cele
di·a·phrag·mi·tis
di·a·phrag·mo·dyn·ia
di·aph·y·sary
di·aph·y·se·al
di·a·phys·ec·to·my
di·aph·y·ses
di·aph·y·si·al
di·aph·y·sis *pl.* di·aph·y·ses
di·aph·y·si·tis
    tuberculous d.
Di·a·pid
di·a·pi·re·sis
dia·pla·cen·tal
di·a·plex
di·ap·no·ic
di·a·poph·y·sis
Di·ap·to·mus
di·a·py·e·sis
di·a·py·et·ic
di·ar·rhea
    cachectic d.
    choleraic d.
    chronic bacillary d.
    d. chylosa
    climatic d.
    Cochin-China d.
    colliquative d.
    congenital chloride d.
    crapulous d.
    critical d.
    dientameba d.
    dysenteric d.
    enteral d.
    epidemic d. of newborn
    familial chloride d.
    flagellate d.

di·ar·rhea *(continued)*
    gastrogenic d.
    hill d.
    infantile d.
    inflammatory d.
    irritative d.
    lienteric d.
    mechanical d.
    membranous d.
    morning d.
    mucous d.
    neonatal d.
    osmotic d.
    d. pancreatica
    pancreatogenous fatty d.
    paradoxical d.
    parenteral d.
    putrefactive d.
    secretory d.
    serous d.
    stercoral d.
    summer d.
    toxigenic d.
    traveler's d.
    tropical d.
    tubercular d.
    virus d.
    watery d.
di·ar·rhe·al
di·ar·rhe·ic
di·ar·rhe·o·gen·ic
di·ar·thric
di·ar·thro·di·al
di·ar·thro·ses
di·ar·thro·sis *pl.* di·ar·thro·
ses
    planiform d.
    d. rotatoria
di·ar·tic·u·lar
di·as·chi·sis
di·a·scope
di·as·co·py
Di·a·sone
di·a·spi·ro·nec·ro·bi·o·sis
di·a·spi·ro·nec·ro·sis
di·a·stase
di·a·sta·se·mia
di·as·ta·sic

di·as·ta·sis
    d. cordis
    iris d.
    d. recti abdominis
di·a·stas·uria
di·a·stat·ic
di·a·stem
di·a·ste·ma *pl.* di·a·ste·ma·ta
    anterior d.
di·a·stem·a·ta
di·a·stem·a·to·cra·nia
di·a·stem·a·to·my·e·lia
di·a·stem·a·to·py·e·lia
di·as·ter
dia·ster·eo·iso·mer
dia·ster·eo·iso·mer·ic
dia·ster·eo·iso·mer·ism
dia·ster·eo·mer
Di·a·stix
di·as·to·le
    atrial d.
    end d.
    ventricular d.
di·a·stol·ic
di·a·sto·my·e·lia
di·a·stroph·ic
di·atax·ia
    cerebral d.
    d. cerebralis infantilis
di·a·ther·mal
di·a·ther·mic
dia·ther·mo·co·ag·u·la·tion
di·a·ther·my
    conventional d.
    long wave d.
    microwave d.
    pulsed d.
    short wave d.
    surgical d.
    ultrashort wave d.
di·ath·e·sis
    allergic d.
    asthenic d.
    explosive d.
    exudative d.
    fibroplastic d.
    gouty d.
    hemorrhagic d.

di·ath·e·sis *(continued)*
    lipogenic d.
    ossifying d.
    spasmodic d.
    thromboasthenic d.
    traumatophilic d.
    uric acid d.
di·a·thet·ic
di·a·tom
di·a·to·ma·ceous
di·a·tom·ic
di·a·tor·ic
dia·tri·zo·ate
    d. meglumine
    d. sodium
dia·tri·zo·ic acid
di·auch·e·nos
di·aux·ic
di·aux·ie
dia·ver·i·dine
di·ax·on
di·az·e·pam
di·a·zine
di·azo·ben·zene
di·azo·ben·zene·sul·fon·ic
  acid
di·a·zo·ma
di·azo·meth·ane
di·a·zo·nal
di·a·zone
di·azo·sul·fo·ben·zol
di·az·o·ti·za·tion
di·az·o·tize
di·az·ox·ide
di·ba·sic
Di·ben·amine
di·benz·an·thra·cene
di·benz-di·bu·tyl an·thra·
  quin·ol
di·ben·ze·pin hy·dro·chlo·ride
di·ben·zo·thi·a·zine
di·benz·ox·az·e·pine
di·ben·zyl·chlo·reth·amine
N,N'-di·ben·zyl·eth·yl·ene·
  di·amine pen·i·cil·lin
Di·ben·zy·line
di·blas·tu·la
di·both·rio·ceph·a·li·a·sis

Di·both·rio·ceph·a·lus
    D. latus
di·bra·chia
di·bra·chi·us
di·bro·mide
di·bro·mo·cul·ci·tol
di·bro·mo·ke·tone
di·bro·mo·thy·mol·sul·fon·
  phthal·ein
di·brom·sa·lan
di·bu·caine
    d. hydrochloride
Di·bu·line
di·bu·to·line sul·fate
di·bu·tyl
di·bu·ty·ryl cy·clic AMP
DIC — disseminated
  intravascular coagulation
di·cac·o·dyl
di·cal·cic
di·cal·ci·um phos·phate
di·car·bon·ate
di·ce·lous
di·cen·tric
di·ceph·a·lous
di·ceph·a·lus
    d. diauchenos
    d. dipus dibrachius
    d. dipus tetrabrachius
    d. dipus tribrachius
    d. dipygus
    d. monauchenos
    d. parasiticus
    d. tripus tribrachius
di·ceph·a·ly
di·chei·lia
di·chei·ria
di·chei·rus
di·chlo·ral·phen·a·zone
di·chlor·di·oxy·di·am·i·do·
  ar·seno·ben·zol
di·chlor·hy·drin
di·chlo·ride
    carbonic d.
di·chlo·ri·sone
di·chlo·ro·ace·tic acid
di·chlo·ro·di·eth·yl sul·fide

di·chlo·ro·di·flu·o·ro·meth·
  ane
di·chlo·ro·di·phen·yl·tri·
  chlo·ro·eth·ane
1,1-di·chlo·ro·eth·ane
di·chlo·ro·iso·pro·ter·e·nol
di·chlo·ro·ni·tro·ben·zene
  (DCNB)
di·chlo·ro·phen
2,4-di·chlo·ro·phen·oxy·ace·
  tic acid
di·chlo·ro·tet·ra·flu·o·ro·
  eth·ane
di·chlo·ro·xy·le·nol
di·chlor·phen·a·mide
di·chlor·vos
di·chog·a·mous
di·chog·e·ny
di·cho·ri·al
di·cho·ri·on·ic
di·chot·o·mi·za·tion
di·chot·o·my
di·chro·ic
di·chro·ine
di·chro·ism
di·chro·ma·sy
di·chro·mat
di·chro·mate
di·chro·mat·ic
di·chro·ma·tism
di·chro·ma·top·sia
di·chro·mic
di·chro·mo·phil
di·chro·moph·i·lism
Dick reaction
Dick test
Dick toxin
dic·lid·os·to·sis
di·clo·fen·ac so·di·um
di·clor·al·urea
di·clox·a·cil·lin so·di·um
Di·co·did
di·coe·lous
di·co·ria
di·cot·y·le·don
di·cou·ma·rin
dic·ro·ce·li·a·sis
di·crot·ic

di·cro·tism
dic·ty·o·ki·ne·sis
dic·ty·o·ma
dic·tyo·some
dic·tyo·tene
di·cu·ma·rol
Di·cur·in
di·cy·clic
di·cy·clo·hex·yl·car·bo·di·
   im·ide
di·cy·clo·mine hy·dro·chlo·
   ride
di·cys·te·ine
di·dac·tic
di·dac·tyl·ism
di·dac·ty·lous
di·del·phia
di·del·phic
Di·del·phis
di·de·oxy·cy·ti·dine
di·de·oxy·hex·ose
di·der·mal
di·der·mo·ma
Di·drex
Di·dro·nel
did·y·mal·gia
did·y·mi·tis
did·y·mo·dyn·ia
did·y·mous
did·y·mus
die
   amalgam d.
   electroformed d.
   electroplated d.
   plated d.
   stone d.
   waxing d.
Dieb. alt. — L. diebus alternis
   (on alternate days)
Dieb. tert. — L. diebus tertiis
   (every third day)
di·echo·scope
di·e·cious
Dief·fen·bach's operation
Di·e·go blood group
di·el·drin
di·elec·tric
di·elec·trol·y·sis

di·em·bry·ony
di·en·ce·phal·ic
di·en·ceph·a·lo·hy·po·phys·i·
   al
di·en·ceph·a·lon
die·ner
di·en·es·trol
Di·ent·amoe·ba
   D. fragilis
di·er·e·sis
di·esoph·a·gus
di·es·ter·ase
di·et
   absolute d.
   acid-ash d.
   adequate d.
   alkali-ash d.
   antiketogenic d.
   balanced d.
   basal d.
   basic d.
   bland d.
   BRAT (bananas, rice
      cereal, applesauce, toast)
      d.
   Coleman-Shaffer d.
   convalescent d.
   diabetic d.
   elemental d.
   elimination d.
   Feingold d.
   Gerson d.
   Gerson-Herrmannsdorfer
      d.
   Giordano-Giovannetti d.
   gluten-free d.
   gouty d.
   high calorie d.
   high fat d.
   high fiber d.
   high protein d.
   high sodium d.
   Karell d.
   Keith's low ionic d.
   Kempner's d.
   ketogenic d.
   light d.
   low calorie d.

di·et *(continued)*
    low fat d.
    low oxalate d.
    low purine d.
    low residue d.
    low salt d.
    macrobiotic d.
    Meulengracht d.
    Minot-Murphy d.
    Moro-Heisler d.
    optimal d.
    Petrén's d.
    protein-sparing d.
    provocative d.
    purine-free d.
    rachitic d.
    reducing d.
    rice d.
    salt-free d.
    Schemm d.
    Schmidt d.
    Schmidt-Strassburger d.
    Sippy d.
    smooth d.
    subsistence d.
    Taylor's d.
    Wilder's d.
di·e·tary
di·e·tet·ic
di·e·tet·ics
di·eth·a·zine hy·dro·chlo·ride
di·eth·yl·amine
di·eth·yl·ami·no·eth·yl cel·lu·lose
di·eth·yl·car·bam·a·zine
di·eth·yl·ene·di·amine
di·eth·yl ether
di·eth·yl·pro·pi·on hy·dro·chlo·ride
di·eth·yl·stil·bes·trol
    d. diphosphate
    d. dipropionate
di·eth·yl·tol·u·am·ide
di·eth·yl·tryp·ta·mine
di·e·ti·tian
Die·tl's crisis
di·e·to·ther·a·py
di·e·to·tox·ic

di·e·to·tox·i·ci·ty
Dieu·la·foy's theory
Dieu·la·foy's triad
di·fen·ox·amide hy·dro·chlo·ride
di·fen·ox·in
dif·fer·ence
    alveolar-arterial oxygen d.
    arteriovenous oxygen d.
    cation-anion d.
    interaural intensity d.
    interaural time d.
    just-noticeable d.
    linking d.
    d. threshold
dif·fer·en·tial
dif·fer·en·ti·ate
dif·fer·en·ti·a·tion
    correlative d.
    dependent d.
    functional d.
    invisible d.
    regional d.
    response d.
    self d.
    sexual d.
dif·flu·ence
dif·flu·ent
Diff-Quik
dif·frac·tion
    d. grating
    x-ray d.
dif·fu·sate
dif·fuse
dif·fus·ible
dif·fu·si·om·e·ter
dif·fu·sion
    alveolar capillary d.
    double d.
    double d. in one dimension
    double d. in two dimensions
    exchange d.
    facilitated d.
    free d.
    gel d.
    impeded d.
    single d.

dif·fu·sion *(continued)*
   single radial d.
di·flor·a·sone di·ac·e·tate
di·flu·a·nine hy·dro·chlo·ride
di·flu·cor·to·lone
   d. pivalate
di·flu·mi·done so·di·um
di·flu·ni·sal
di·flu·o·ro·meth·yl·or·ni·
   thine (DMFO)
di·flu·pred·nate
dif·ta·lone
Dig. — L digeratur (let it be
   digested)
di·gal·lic acid
di·ga·met·ic
di·gas·tric
di·gen·e·sis
di·ge·net·ic
di·gen·ic
Di·George's syndrome
di·gest
di·ges·tant
di·ges·tion
   artificial d.
   biliary d.
   gastric d.
   gastrointestinal d.
   intercellular d.
   intestinal d.
   intracellular d.
   lipolytic d.
   pancreatic d.
   parenteral d.
   peptic d.
   primary d.
   salivary d.
   secondary d.
   sludge d.
   tryptic d.
di·ges·tive
dig·it
   binary d.
   sausage d.
dig·i·tal
dig·i·tal·gia par·es·thet·i·ca
dig·i·tal·in
Dig·i·tal·ine Na·ti·velle

Dig·i·ta·lis
dig·i·tal·is
   d. leaf
   powdered d.
   prepared d.
dig·i·tal·iza·tion
dig·i·tal·oid
dig·i·tal·ose
dig·i·tate
dig·i·ta·tio *pl.* dig·i·ta·ti·o·
   nes
   digitationes hippocampi
dig·i·ta·tion
dig·i·ta·ti·o·nes
dig·i·ti
dig·i·ti·form
dig·i·ti·grade
dig·i·tize
dig·i·to·fib·u·lar
dig·i·tog·e·nin
dig·i·to·meta·tar·sal
dig·i·to·nide
dig·i·to·nin
dig·i·to·plan·tar
dig·i·to·ra·di·al
dig·i·to·tib·i·al
dig·i·to·ul·nar
dig·i·tox·ic·i·ty
dig·i·tox·i·gen·in
dig·i·tox·in
dig·i·tox·ose
dig·i·tus *pl.* dig·i·ti
   d. annularis
   d. demonstrativus
   d. extensus
   d. hippocraticus
   d. malleus
   digiti manus
   d. medius
   d. minimus manus
   d. minimus pedis
   d. mortuus
   digiti pedis
   d. postminimus
   d. primus (I) manus
   d. primus (I) pedis
   d. quartus (IV) manus
   d. quartus (IV) pedis

dig·i·tus *(continued)*
 d. quintus (V) manus
 d. quintus (V) pedis
 d. secundus (II) manus
 d. secundus (II) pedis
 d. tertius (III) manus
 d. tertius (III) pedis
 d. valgus
 d. varus
di·glos·sia
di·glos·sus
di·glyc·er·ide
dig·na·thus
di·gox·in
Di·gram·ma brau·ni
Di Gu·gliel·mo disease
Di Gu·gliel·mo syndrome
di·het·ero·xe·nic
di·het·ero·zy·gote
di·hex·y·ver·ine hy·dro·chlo·ride
di·ho·mo·cin·cho·nine
di·hy·brid
di·hy·drate
di·hy·drat·ed
di·hy·dric
di·hy·dro·bi·op·ter·in syn·the·tase deficiency
di·hy·dro·cho·les·ter·ol
di·hy·dro·co·deine
di·hy·dro·co·de·i·none bi·tar·trate
di·hy·dro·col·li·dine
di·hy·dro·cor·ti·sol
di·hy·dro·cor·ti·sone
di·hy·dro·di·eth·yl·stil·bes·trol
di·hy·dro·er·go·cor·nine
di·hy·dro·er·go·cris·tine
di·hy·dro·er·go·cryp·tine
di·hy·dro·er·got·amine mes·y·late
di·hy·dro·fo·late re·duc·tase
di·hy·dro·fo·late re·duc·tase (DHFR) deficiency
di·hy·dro·fol·ic acid
di·hy·dro·fol·lic·u·lin
di·hy·dro·in·do·lone

di·hy·drol
di·hy·dro·lipo·am·ide ac·e·tyl·trans·fer·ase
di·hy·dro·lipo·am·ide de·hy·dro·gen·ase
di·hy·dro·lipo·am·ide suc·cin·yl·trans·fer·ase
di·hy·dro·li·po·ic acid
di·hy·dro·lip·o·yl·trans·ac·e·tyl·ase
di·hy·dro·lu·ti·dine
di·hy·dro·mor·phi·none
di·hy·dro·or·o·tase
di·hy·dro·pter·i·dine re·duc·tase
di·hy·dro·pter·i·dine re·duc·tase (DHPR) deficiency
di·hy·dro·strep·to·my·cin
di·hy·dro·tach·ys·te·rol
di·hy·dro·tes·tos·ter·one
di·hy·dro·uri·dine
di·hy·droxy·ac·e·tone
di·hy·drox·y·ac·e·tone phos·phate
di·hy·droxy·alu·mi·num
 d. aminoacetate
 d. sodium carbonate
di·hy·droxy·cho·le·cal·cif·e·rol
di·hy·droxy·es·trin
di·hy·droxy·flu·o·rane
di·hy·droxy·phen·yl·py·ru·vic acid
3,4-di·hy·droxy·phen·yl·al·a·nine
di·hy·droxy·vi·ta·min D$_3$
di·hys·te·ria
di·io·dide
di·io·do·hy·droxy·quin
di·io·do·meth·ane
di·io·do·phen·yl·ami·no·pro·pi·on·ic acid
di·io·do·sal·i·cyl·ic acid
3,5-di·io·do·thy·ro·nine
di·io·do·ty·ro·sine
di·iso·cy·a·nate
di·iso·pro·pyl flu·ro·phos·phate

di·ka·ry·on
di·ka·ry·ote
di·ka·ry·ot·ic
di·ke·tone
di·ke·to·pi·per·a·zine
dik·ty·o·ma
dik·wak·wadi
dil. — L. dilue (dilute or
    dissolve)
di·lac·er·a·tion
Di·lan·tin
di·la·tan·cy
di·la·tant
dil·a·ta·tion
    balloon d.
    d. of cervix
    digital d.
    gastric d.
    d. of the heart
    idiopathic d.
    intraluminal d.
    post-stenotic d.
    prognathic d.
    prognathion d.
    d. of the stomach
    supradiaphragmatic
        esophageal d.
dil·a·ta·tor
di·late
di·la·tion
    digital d.
di·la·tor
    anal d.
    Bakes d.
    Barnes's d.
    Einhorn's d.
    Hegar's d's
    Kollmann's d.
    laryngeal d.
    Mixter d.
    Mosher d.
    d. naris
    Negus d.
    Negus hydrostatic d.
    Plummer's d.
    Starck d.
    tracheal d.
    Tubbs d.

Di·lau·did
di·le·ca·nus
Dil·e·pid·i·dae
dil·ox·an·ide fu·ro·ate
dil·ti·a·zem hy·dro·chlo·ride
Diluc. — L. diluculo (at
    daybreak)
dil·u·ent
dilut. — L. dilutus (diluted)
di·lute
di·lu·tion
    doubling d.
    nitrogen d.
    serial d.
    triple isotope d.
dim. — L. dimidius (one half)
di·mar·gar·in
di·mef·a·dane
di·me·fil·con A
di·mef·line hy·dro·chlo·ride
di·me·fox
di·me·lia
di·me·lus
di·men·hy·dri·nate
di·men·sion
    vertical d.
    vertical d., contact
    vertical d., occlusal
    vertical d., postural
    vertical d., rest
di·men·sion·less
di·mer
    thymine d.
    UV-induced d.
di·mer·cap·rol
di·mer·ic
dim·er·ous
di·me·tal·lic
Di·me·tane
di·meth·i·cone
    d. 350
    activated d.
di·meth·in·dene mal·e·ate
di·meth·i·so·quin hy·dro·
    chlo·ride
di·meth·is·ter·one
di·meth·ox·a·nate hy·dro·
    chlo·ride

2,5-di·me·thoxy-4-meth·yl·
   am·phet·amine
3,4-di·me·thoxy·phen·yl·eth·
   yl·amine
di·meth·oxy·phen·yl pen·i·
   cil·lin sodium
di·meth·yl·amine
p-di·meth·yl·ami·no·az·o·
   ben·zene
Di·meth·y·lane
di·meth·yl·ar·sine
di·meth·yl·ar·sin·ic acid
7,12-di·meth·yl·benz[a]an·
   thra·cene
di·meth·yl·ben·zene
5,6-di·meth·yl·benz·im·id·az·
   ole
di·meth·yl car·bate
di·meth·yl·car·bi·nol
di·meth·yl·eth·yl·pyr·role
di·meth·yl·guan·i·dine
di·meth·yl·ke·tone
di·meth·yl·mor·phine
di·meth·yl·ni·tros·amine
di·meth·yl·phe·nan·threne
di·meth·yl·phen·yl·pip·er·az·
   in·i·um (DMPP)
di·meth·yl phthal·ate
di·meth·yl sul·fate
di·meth·yl sulf·ox·ide
di·meth·yl·tryp·ta·mine
di·meth·yl·tu·bo·cu·ra·rine
   io·dide
di·me·tria
dim·i·nu·tion
Di·mi·tri's disease
Dim·mer's keratitis
Di·mo·cil·lin
di·mor·phic
di·mor·phism
   physical d.
   sexual d.
di·mor·pho·bi·ot·ic
di·mor·phous
di·mox·amine hy·dro·chlo·
   ride
di·mox·y·line phos·phate

dim·ple
   anal d.
   Fuchs's d's
   postanal d.
   sacrococcygeal d.
dim·pling
di·ner·ic
di·neu·ric
di·ni·trate
di·ni·trat·ed
di·ni·tro·ami·no·phe·nol
di·ni·tro·ben·zene
di·ni·tro·cel·lu·lose
di·ni·tro·chlo·ro·ben·zene
di·ni·tro·cre·sol
di·ni·tro-o-cre·sol
di·ni·tro·flu·o·ro·ben·zene
di·ni·tro·gen
   d. monoxide
di·ni·tro·phe·nol
di·ni·tro·re·sor·cin·ol
di·ni·tro·tolu·ene
Di·no·flag·el·la·ta
di·no·flag·el·late
Di·no·fla·gel·li·da
di·no·gun·el·lin
di·no·prost
   d. trometanol
   d. tromethamine
di·no·prost·one
D. in p. aeq. — L. divide in
   partes aequales (divide into
   equal parts)
din·sed
di·nu·cleo·tide
Di·oc·to·phy·ma
   D. renale
Di·oc·to·phy·moi·dea
di·oc·tyl cal·ci·um sul·fo·suc·
   ci·nate
di·oc·tyl so·di·um sul·fo·suc·
   ci·nate
di·ode
   light-emitting d.
Di·o·don
Di·o·do·quin
Di·o·drast

di·oe·cious
Di·og·e·nes syndrome
di·og·en·ism
di·ol·amine
Di·o·lox·ol
Di·on·o·sil
di·op·sim·e·ter
di·op·ter
    prism d.
di·op·tom·e·ter
di·op·tom·e·try
di·op·tos·co·py
di·op·tric
di·op·trics
di·op·trom·e·ter
di·op·trom·e·try
di·op·tros·co·py
Di·os·co·rea
    D. mexicana
di·ose
di·os·gen·in
di·ov·u·la·to·ry
di·ox·ane
di·ox·ide
di·ox·in
di·oxy·ben·zone
di·ox·y·gen
di·ox·y·gen·ase
di·ox·y·line phos·phate
Di·pax·in
di·pen·tene
di·pep·ti·dase
di·pep·tide
di·pep·ti·dyl car·boxy·pep·ti·dase I
di·pep·ti·dyl pep·ti·dase I
di·per·o·don
    d. hydrochloride
Di·pet·a·lo·ne·ma
di·pet·a·lo·ne·mi·a·sis
di·phal·lia
di·phal·lus
di·pha·sic
di·pheb·u·zol
di·phe·ma·nil meth·yl·sul·fate
di·phen·a·di·one

di·phen·hy·dra·mine hy·dro·chlo·ride
di·phen·i·dol
    d. hydrochloride
    d. pamoate
di·phen·ox·y·late hy·dro·chlo·ride
di·phe·nyl
di·phen·yl·amine
di·phen·yl·amine·ar·sine chlo·ride
di·phen·yl·a·mi·no-azo-ben·zene
di·phen·yl·bu·tyl·pi·per·i·dine
di·phen·yl·chlor·ar·sine
di·phen·yl·hy·dan·to·in
di·phen·yl·pyr·a·line hy·dro·chlo·ride
di·pho·nia
di·phos·gene
di·phos·phate
2,3-di·phos·pho·glyc·er·ate
di·phos·pho·glyc·er·ate mu·tase
di·phos·pho·glyc·er·ate phos·pha·tase
di·phos·pho·pyr·i·dine nu·cleo·tide
di·phos·pho·trans·fer·ase
diph·tha·mide
diph·the·ria
    avian d.
    Bretonneau's d.
    calf d.
    cutaneous d.
    faucial d.
    fowl d.
    d. gravis
    laryngeal d.
    laryngeotracheal d.
    malignant d.
    nasal d.
    nasopharyngeal d.
    pharyngeal d.
    scarlatinal d.
    septic d.
    surgical d.

diph·the·ria *(continued)*
    umbilical d.
    wound d.
diph·the·ri·al
diph·the·ric
diph·the·rin
diph·the·rit·ic
diph·the·roid
diph·the·ro·tox·in
diph·thong
diph·thon·gia
Di·phy·lets
di·phyl·lo·both·ri·a·sis
Di·phyl·lo·both·ri·i·dae
Di·phyl·lo·both·ri·um
    D. cordatum
    D. erinacei
    D. latum
    D. mansoni
    D. mansonoides
    D. parvum
    D. taenioides
di·phy·odont
di·pip·a·none hy·dro·chlo·ride
di·piv·e·frin
dip·la·cu·sia
dip·la·cu·sis
    binaural d.
    d. binauralis dysharmonica
    d. binauralis echoica
    disharmonic d.
    echo d.
    monaural d.
    d. monauralis
di·plas·mat·ic
di·plas·tic
di·ple·gia
    atonic-astatic d.
    cerebellar d.
    cerebral d.
    facial d.
    flaccid d.
    Förster's d.
    hypotonic d.
    infantile d.
    infantile cerebrocerebellar d.

di·ple·gia *(continued)*
    masticatory d.
    spastic d.
    tonic d.
di·ple·gic
dip·lo·al·bu·min·uria
dip·lo·ba·cil·li
dip·lo·ba·cil·lus *pl.* dip·lo·ba·cil·li
    Morax-Axenfeld d.
dip·lo·bac·te·ria
dip·lo·bac·te·ri·um *pl.* dip·lo·bac·te·ria
dip·lo·blas·tic
dip·lo·car·dia
dip·lo·ceph·a·lus
dip·lo·ceph·a·ly
dip·lo·chei·ria
dip·lo·coc·cal
dip·lo·coc·ci
dip·lo·coc·coid
Dip·lo·coc·cus
dip·lo·coc·cus *pl.* dip·lo·coc·ci
    d. of Morax-Axenfeld
    d. of Neisser
dip·lo·co·ria
dip·lo·di·a·tox·i·co·sis
dip·lo·ë
dip·lo·et·ic
Dip·lo·gas·ter
dip·lo·gen·e·sis
Dip·lo·go·nop·o·rus
    D. brauni
    D. grandis
dip·lo·ic
dip·loid
    Sappinia d.
dip·loi·dy
dip·lo·kar·y·on
dip·lo·mate
dip·lo·mo·nad
Dip·lo·mo·nad·i·da
Dip·lo·mo·na·di·na
dip·lo·my·e·lia
dip·lon
dip·lop·a·gus
dip·lo·phase
dip·lo·pho·nia

di·plo·pia
  binocular d.
  crossed d.
  direct d.
  facial fracture d.
  heteronymous d.
  homonymous d.
  horizontal d.
  incongruous d.
  intranasal tumor d.
  monocular d.
  paradoxical d.
  physiological d.
  stereoscopic d.
  torsional d.
  uncrossed d.
  vertical d.
di·plo·pi·om·e·ter
Di·plop·o·da
Dip·lo·py·lid·i·um
dip·lo·scope
dip·lo·so·mia
dip·lo·so·ma·tia
dip·lo·some
dip·lo·tene
dip·lo·ter·a·tol·o·gy
Dip·lur·i·dae
di·po·dia
di·po·lar
di·pole
  magnetic d.
di·po·tas·si·um phos·phate
dip·ping
Di·pro·sone
di·pros·o·pus
  d. parasiticus
  d. tetrophthalmus
di·pro·tri·zo·ate
dip·se·sis
dip·set·ic
dip·sia
dip·slides
dip·so·gen
dip·so·gen·ic
dip·so·sis
dip·so·ther·a·py
dip·stick
Dip·tera

dip·ter·ous
di·pus
di·py·gus
  d. parasiticus
dip·y·li·di·a·sis
Dip·y·lid·i·um
  D. caninum
di·py·rid·a·mole
di·pyr·i·thi·one
di·py·rone
di·rect
di·rec·tive
di·rec·tor
  grooved d.
di·rhi·nic
dir·i·go·mo·tor
Di·ro·fi·lar·ia
  D. immitis
  D. magalhaesi
  D. repens
di·ro·fil·a·ri·a·sis
Dir. prop. — L. directione
  propria (with a proper
  direction)
dis·a·bil·i·ty
  developmental d.
  learning d.
  major d.
dis·able
di·sac·cha·ri·dase
  intestinal d. deficiency
  small-intestinal d's
di·sac·cha·ride
  reducing d's
di·sac·cha·rid·uria
di·sac·cha·rose
dis·ac·id·i·fy
Di·sal·cid
dis·ar·tic·u·la·tion
dis·as·sim·i·late
dis·as·sim·i·la·tion
dis·azo
disc
dis·cal
dis·cec·to·my
dis·charge
  brush d.
  conductive d.

dis·charge *(continued)*
  convective d.
  delta d.
  diencephalic autonomic d.
  disruptive d.
  electroencephalographic d.
  epileptic d.
  hypersynchronous
    neuronal d.
  myotonic d.
  nervous d.
  neural d.
  periodic lateralized
    epileptiform d's (PLED)
  polysynaptic reflex d.
  pseudomyotonic d.
  systolic d.
dis·chro·na·tion
dis·ci
dis·ci·form
dis·cis·sion
  d. of cataract
  d. of cervix uteri
  d. of lens
  posterior d.
dis·ci·tis
dis·cli·na·tion
dis·clos·ing
dis·clu·sion
dis·co·blas·tic
dis·co·blas·tu·la
dis·co·gas·tru·la
dis·co·ge·net·ic
dis·co·gen·ic
dis·co·gram
dis·cog·ra·phy
dis·coid
dis·coid·ec·to·my
dis·col·or·a·tion
Dis·co·my·ce·tes
dis·con·ju·gate
dis·con·nec·tion
  portoazygos d.
dis·con·ti·nu·i·ty
  ossicular d.
dis·cop·a·thy
  traumatic d.
dis·coph·o·rous

dis·co·pla·cen·ta
dis·co·plasm
dis·cord
dis·cor·dance
  atrioventricular d.
  ventriculoarterial d.
dis·cor·dant
dis·co·ria
dis·co·stro·ma
dis·cot·o·my
dis·crep·an·cy
  tooth size d.
dis·crete
dis·crim·i·na·tion
  pitch d.
  2-point d.
  speech d.
  tactile d.
  tonal d.
dis·crim·i·na·tor
  pulse-height d.
dis·cus *pl.* dis·ci
  d. articularis
  d. interpubicus
  disci intervertebrales
  d. nervi optici
  d. oophorus
  d. opticus
dis·cus·sive
dis·cu·ti·ent
dis·di·a·clast
dis·di·ad·o·cho·ki·ne·sia
  Acosta's d.
dis·ease (see also under
  syndrome)
  Adams' d.
  Adams-Stokes d.
  d's of adaptation
  Addison's d.
  adenocystic d.
  adult celiac d.
  airsac d.
  akamushi d.
  Ạkureyri d.
  Åland eye d.
  Albers-Schönberg d.
  Albert's d.
  Albright's d.

dis·ease *(continued)*
Aleutian mink d.
Alexander's d.
alkali d.
allogeneic d.
Almeida's d.
Alpers' d.
alpha chain d.
Alström's d.
altitude d.
alveolar hydatid d.
Alzheimer's d.
amyloid d.
Anders' d.
Andersen's d.
Anderson-Fabry d.
Andes d.
Andrews d.
anti–glomerular basement
    membrane (anti-GBM)
    antibody d.
aortoiliac occlusive d.
apatite deposition d.
Apert's d.
Apert-Crouzon d.
Aran-Duchenne d.
arc-welders' d.
Armenian d.
Armstrong's d.
atheroembolic renal d.
atopic d.
attic d.
Aujeszky's d.
Australian X d.
autoimmune d.
aviators' d.
Ayerza's d.
Azorean d.
Baastrup's d.
Baelz's d.
Ballet's d.
Ballingall's d.
Baló's d.
Bamberger's d.
Bamberger-Marie d.
Bang's d.
Bannister's d.
Banti's d.

dis·ease *(continued)*
Barclay-Baron d.
Barcoo d.
Barlow's d.
barometer-maker's d.
Barraquer's d.
Basedow's d.
Bassen-Kornzweig d.
Bateman's d.
Batten d.
bauxite workers' d.
Bayle's d.
Bazin's d.
Beau's d.
Beauvais' d.
Beck's d.
beetle d.
Begbie's d.
Béguez César d.
Behçet's d.
Behr's d.
Beigel's d.
Bekhterev's d.
Bennett's d.
Benson's d.
Berger's d.
Bergeron's d.
Berlin's d.
Bernard-Soulier d.
Bernhardt's d.
Bernhardt-Roth d.
Besnier-Boeck d.
Besnier-Boeck-Schaumann
    d.
Best's d.
Bettlach May d.
Biedl's d.
Bielschowsky-Jansky d.
big spleen d.
Bilderbeck's d.
Billroth's d.
Binswanger's d.
bird-breeders' d.
black d.
bleeders' d.
blinding filarial d.
Blocq's d.
Bloodgood's d.

dis·ease *(continued)*
- Blount d.
- blue d.
- Blumenthal's d.
- Bodechtel-Guttmann d.
- Boeck's d.
- Bornholm d.
- Bostock's d.
- Boston exanthem d.
- Bouchard's d.
- Bouchet-Gsell d.
- Bouillaud's d.
- Bourneville's d.
- Bourneville-Brissaud d.
- Bourneville-Crouzon d.
- Bouveret's d.
- Bowen's d.
- Bradley's d.
- brancher glycogen storage d.
- brass-founders' d.
- braziers' d.
- Breda's d.
- Breisky's d.
- Bretonneau's d.
- Breutsch's d.
- bridegrooms' d.
- Bright's d.
- Brill's d.
- Brill-Symmers d.
- Brill-Zinsser d.
- Brinton's d.
- Brion-Kayser d.
- brisket d.
- broad-beta d.
- Brodie's d.
- bronzed d.
- Brooke's d.
- Brown-Séquard d.
- Brown-Symmers d.
- Bruck's d.
- Brushfield-Wyatt d.
- Bruton's d.
- Budd-Chiari d.
- Buerger's d.
- buffalo d.
- Buhl's d.
- Buschke's d.

dis·ease *(continued)*
- bush d.
- Busquet's d.
- Buss d.
- Busse-Buschke d.
- Byler's d.
- Cacchi-Ricci d.
- Caffey's d.
- caisson d.
- calcium hydroxyapatite deposition d.
- calcium pyrophosphate deposition d. (CPDD)
- California d.
- caloric d.
- Calvé's d.
- Calvé-Perthes d.
- Camurati-Engelmann d.
- Canavan's d.
- Canavan-van Bogaert-Bertrand d.
- candle wax d.
- Cannon's d.
- carcinoid heart d.
- Caroli's d.
- Carrión's d.
- Castellani's d.
- cat-bite d.
- cat-scratch d.
- Cavare's d.
- Cazenave's d.
- celiac d.
- central core d. of muscle
- ceroid storage d.
- Chabert's d.
- Chagas' d.
- Chagas-Cruz d.
- Chandler's d.
- Charcot's d.
- Charcot-Marie-Tooth d.
- Charcot-Marie-Tooth-Hoffman d.
- Charlouis' d.
- Cheadle's d.
- Chédiak-Higashi d.
- Cherchevski's (Cherchewski's) d.
- Chester's d.

dis·ease *(continued)*
  Chiari's d.
  Chiari-Frommel d.
  Chicago d.
  chignon d.
  cholesteryl ester storage d.
    (CESD)
  Christensen-Krabbe d.
  chronic granulomatous d.
    (CGD)
  chronic granulomatouus d.
    of childhood
  Christian-Weber d.
  Christmas d.
  chronic respiratory d. of
    poultry
  climatic d.
  coast d.
  Coats' d.
  Cogan's d.
  cold agglutinin d.
  cold hemolytic antibody d.
  collagen d.
  combined
    immunodeficiency d.
  combined system d.
  communicable d.
  complicating d.
  compressed-air d.
  Concato's d.
  congenital d.
  congenital cystic d. of liver
  congenital heart d. (CHD)
  congestive heart d. (CHD)
  Conor and Bruch's d.
  Conradi's d.
  constitutional d.
  contagious d.
  convulsive tic d.
  Cooley's d.
  copper storage d.
  Corbus' d.
  Cori's d.
  coronary heart d. (CHD)
  corridor d.
  Corrigan's d.
  Corvisart's d.
  Cotugno's d.

dis·ease *(continued)*
  covering d.
  Cowden's d.
  CPPD d.
  creeping d.
  Creutzfeldt-Jakob d.
  Crigler-Najjar d.
  Crohn's d.
  Crouzon's d.
  Cruveilhier's d.
  Cruz-Chagas d.
  Curschmann's d.
  Cushing's d.
  cyanotic heart d.
  cystic d. of breast
  cystic d. of kidney,
    acquired
  cystic d. of lung
  cysticercus d.
  cystine d.
  cystine storage d.
  cytomegalic inclusion d.
  Czerny's d.
  Daae's d.
  Daae-Finsen d.
  Dalrymple's d.
  Danielssen-Boeck d.
  Danlos' d.
  Darier's d.
  Darling's d.
  David's d.
  debrancher glycogen
    storage d.
  decompression d.
  deer-fly d.
  deficiency d.
  degenerative joint d.
  Degos' d.
  Dejerine's d.
  Dejerine-Sottas d.
  demyelinating d.
  dense deposit d.
  deprivation d.
  de Quervain's d.
  Dercum's d.
  dermopathic herpesvirus d.
  Deutschländer's d.
  Devic's d.

dis·ease *(continued)*
  diatomite d.
  Dieulafoy's d.
  Dimitri's d.
  disappearing bone d.
  Di Guglielmo d.
  diverticular d.
  Döhle d.
  Down's d.
  drug d.
  Dubin-Sprinz d.
  Dubini's d.
  Dubois'd.
  Duchenne's d.
  Duchenne-Aran d.
  Duchenne-Griesinger d.
  Duhring's d.
  Dukes'd.
  Duncan's d.
  Dupré's d.
  Dupuytren's d. of foot
  Durand-Nicolas-Favre d.
  Durante's d.
  Duroziez's d.
  Dutton's d.
  dynamic d.
  Eales d.
  Ebola virus d.
  Ebstein's d.
  echinococcus d.
  Economo's d.
  Edsall's d.
  Ehlers-Danlos d.
  Eisenmenger d.
  elevator d.
  endemic d.
  end-stage renal d.
  Engelmann's d.
  Engel-Recklinghausen d.
  English d.
  English sweating d.
  Engman's d.
  enzootic d.
  eosinophilic
    endomyocardial d.
  epidemic d.
  epizootic d.
  Epstein's d.

dis·ease *(continued)*
  Erb's d.
  Erb-Charcot d.
  Erb-Goldflam d.
  Erb-Landouzy d.
  Eulenburg's d.
  extensor process d.
  extrapyramidal d.
  Fabry's d.
  Fahr-Volhard d.
  Fallot's d.
  familial hypophosphatemic
    bone d.
  Fanconi's d.
  Farber d.
  fat-deficiency d.
  Fauchard d.
  Favre-Durand-Nicholas d.
  Fazio-Londe d.
  Fc fragment d.
  Fede's d.
  Feer's d.
  Fenwick's d.
  fibrocystic d.
  fibrocystic d. of breast
  fibrocystic d. of the
    pancreas
  fibromuscular d.
  Fiedler's d.
  fifth d.
  fifth venereal d.
  Filatov's d.
  Filatov-Dukes d.
  file-cutters' d.
  fish-skin d.
  fish-slime d.
  fish-tapeworm d.
  Flajani's d.
  Flatau-Schilder d.
  flax-dresser's d.
  flecked retina d.
  Flegel's d.
  Fleischner's d.
  flint d.
  floating-beta d.
  fluke d.
  focal d.
  Foix-Alajouanine d.

dis·ease *(continued)*

Følling d.
foot-and-mouth d.
foot process d.
Forbes' d.
Fordyce's d.
Forestier d.
Förster's d.
Fothergill's d.
Fournier's d.
fourth d.
fourth venereal d.
Fox-Fordyce d.
fracture d.
Francis' d.
Frankl-Hochwart's d.
Franklin's d.
Frei's d.
Freiberg's d.
Friedländer's d.
Friedmann's d.
Friedreich's d.
fright d.
Frommel's d.
functional d.
functional cardiovascular d.
Fürstner's d.
fusospirochetal d.
Gaisböck's d.
gamma chain d.
Gamna's d.
Gamstorp's d.
Gandy-Gamna d.
Gandy-Nanta d.
gannister d.
garapata d.
Garré's d.
Gastaut's d.
gastroesophageal reflux d.
Gaucher's d.
Gayet's d.
Gee's d.
Gee-Herter d.
Gee-Herter-Heubner d.
Gee-Thaysen d.
genetic d.
Gerhardt's d.

dis·ease *(continued)*

Gerlier's d.
giant platelet d.
Gibert's d.
Gibney's d.
Gierke's d.
Gilbert's d.
Gilchrist's d.
Gilles de la Tourette's d.
Glanzmann's d.
glassblowers' d.
Glasser's d.
Glisson's d.
glomerular epithelial cell d.
glycogen storage d.
Goldflam's d.
Goldflam-Erb d.
Goldstein's d.
Gowers d.
Graefe's d.
graft-versus-host (GVH) d.
Graves' d.
green monkey d.
Greenfield's d.
grinder's d.
Grisel's d.
Gross d.
guinea worm d.
Guinon's d.
Gull's d.
Gumboro d.
Günther's d.
H d.
Habermann's d.
Haff d.
Hageman's d.
Haglund's d.
Hagner's d.
Hailey-Hailey d.
Hallervorden-Spatz d.
Hamman's d.
Hamman-Rich d.
Hammond's d.
Hand's d.
hand-foot-and-mouth d.
Hand-Schüller-Christian d.
Hanot's d.

dis·ease *(continued)*
    Hansen's d.
    d. of the Hapsburgs
    Harada's d.
    hard-metal d.
    Hartnup d.
    Hashimoto's d.
    heart d.
    heartwater d.
    heavy-chain d's
    Heberden's d.
    Hebra's d.
    Heerfordt's d.
    Heine-Medin d.
    Heller's d.
    Heller-Döhle d.
    helminthic d.
    hemoglobin d.
    hemoglobin C–thalassemia
      d.
    hemiglobin E–thalassemia
      d.
    hemoglobin S-O-Arab d.
    hemolytic d. of newborn
    hemorrhagic d. of the
      newborn
    hempworkers' d.
    Henderson-Jones d.
    Henneberg's d.
    Henoch's d.
    hepatic venous web d.
    hepatolenticular d.
    hepatorenal glycogen
      storage d.
    hereditary d.
    heredoconstitutional d.
    heredodegenerative d.
    Herlitz's d.
    Hers' d.
    Herter's d.
    Herter-Heubner d.
    Heubner's d.
    HIB *(Haemophilus
      influenzae* type B) d.
    hidebound d.
    Hildenbrand's d.
    Heubner-Herter d.
    hip-joint d.

dis·ease *(continued)*
    Hippel's d.
    Hippel-Lindau d.
    Hirschsprung's d.
    His d.
    His-Werner d.
    Hodgkin's d.
    Hodgson's d.
    Hoffa's d.
    Hoffa-Kastert d.
    holoendemic d.
    homologous d.
    homozygous hemoglobin S
      d.
    hoof-and-mouth d.
    hookworm d.
    Horton's d.
    Huchard's d.
    Hünermann's d.
    hungry d.
    Hunt's d.
    Huntington's d.
    Hurler's d.
    Hurst's d.
    Hutchinson's d.
    Hutchinson-Boeck d.
    Hutchinson-Gilford d.
    Hutinel's d.
    hyaline membrane d.
    hydatid d.
    hydatid d., alveolar
    hydatid d., unilocular
    hydrocephaloid d.
    hydroxyapatite d.
    hyperendemic d.
    hypertensive heart d.
    hypertensive renal d.
    hypertensive vascular d.
    hypopigmentation-immu-
      nodeficiency d.
    Iceland d.
    I-cell d.
    idiopathic d.
    immune-complex d's
    immunodeficiency d.
    immunoproliferative small
      intestine d.
    inborn lysosomal d's

dis·ease *(continued)*
  inclusion d.
  infantile celiac d.
  infectious d.
  infectious bursal d.
  inflammatory bowel d.
  inherited d.
  intercurrent d.
  interstitial d.
  interstitial lung d.
  iron storage d.
  irritable bowel d.
  Isambert's d.
  ischemic bowel d.
  ischemic heart d.
  island d.
  itai-itai d.
  itch d.
  Itsenko's d.
  Jaffe's d.
  Jaffe-Lichtenstein d.
  Jakob's d.
  Jakob-Creutzfeldt d.
  Janet's d.
  Jansen's d.
  Jansky-Bielschowsky d.
  Jensen's d.
  Jessner-Kanof d.
  Johne's d.
  Johnson-Stevens d.
  Joseph d.
  jumper d. of Maine
  jumping d.
  juvenile Paget d.
  Kahlbaum's d.
  Kahler's d.
  Kaiserstuhl d.
  Kalischer's d.
  Kaposi's d.
  Kashin-Beck d.
  Katayama d.
  Kawasaki d.
  Kayser's d.
  kedani d.
  Keshan d.
  Kienböck's d.
  Kimmelstiel-Wilson (K-W)
    d.

dis·ease *(continued)*
  Kimura's d.
  kinky hair d.
  Kinnier Wilson d.
  Kirkland's d.
  kissing d.
  Klebs' d.
  Klemperer's d.
  Klippel's d.
  knight's d.
  Köhler's bone d.
  Köhler's second d.
  Köhler-Pellegrini-Stieda d.
  König's d.
  Korsakoff's d.
  Koshevnikoff's
    (Koschewnikow's,
    Kozhevnikov's) d.
  Kostmann's d.
  Krabbe's d.
  Krishaber's d.
  Kufs' d.
  Kugelberg-Welander d.
  Kuhnt-Junius d.
  Kümmell's d.
  Kümmell-Verneuil d.
  Kussmaul's d.
  Kussmaul-Maier d.
  Kwok's d.
  Kyasanur Forest d.
  Kyrle's d.
  laboratory d.
  Laënnec's d.
  Lafora's d.
  Lancereaux-Mathieu d.
  Landouzy's d.
  Landry's d.
  Lane's d.
  Larrey-Weil d.
  Larsen's d.
  Larsen-Johansson d.
  Lauber's d.
  laughing d.
  Leber's d.
  Lederer's d.
  Legal's d.
  Legg's d.
  Legg-Calvé d.

dis·ease *(continued)*
- legionnaires' d.
- Leigh d.
- Leiner's d.
- Lemierre's d.
- Lenegre's d.
- Leri's d.
- Leriche's d.
- Letterer-Siwe d.
- Lev's d.
- Lewandowsky-Lutz d.
- Leyden's d.
- Libman-Sacks d.
- Lichtheim's d.
- Lignac's d.
- Lignac-Fanconi d.
- Lindau's d.
- Lindau-von Hippel d.
- lipid storage d.
- Lipschütz's d.
- Little's d.
- Löffler's d.
- Lobo's d.
- Lobstein's d.
- local d.
- loco d.
- Lorain's d.
- Louis-Bar d.
- Lowe's d.
- L-S d.
- Luft's d.
- lung fluke d.
- lunger d.
- Lutembacher's d.
- Lutz-Splendore-Almeida d.
- Lyell's d.
- Lyme d.
- lymphoproliferative d's
- lymphoreticular d's
- lysosomal storage d.
- McArdle's d.
- Machado-Joseph d.
- Mackenzie's d.
- MacLean-Maxwell d.
- Madelung's d.
- Maher's d.
- Majocchi's d.
- malabsorption d.

dis·ease *(continued)*
- Malassez's d.
- Malibu d.
- Manson's d.
- maple bark d.
- maple syrup urine d. (MSUD)
- marble bone d.
- Marburg d.
- March's d.
- Marchiafava-Bignami d.
- Marchiafava-Micheli d.
- Marek's d.
- margarine d.
- Marie's d.
- Marie-Bamberger d.
- Marie-Strümpell d.
- Marie-Tooth d.
- Marion's d.
- Maroteaux-Lamy d.
- Marsh's d.
- Martin's d.
- mast cell d.
- Mathieu's d.
- Medin's d.
- Mediterranean d.
- medullary cystic d.
- Meige's d.
- Meleda d.
- Ménétrier's d.
- Meniere's d.
- Menkes' d.
- mental d.
- Merzbacher-Pelizaeus d.
- mesangial IgA/IgG d.
- metabolic d.
- metazoan d.
- Meyenburg's d.
- Meyer's d.
- Meyer-Betz d.
- Mianeh d.
- microcystic d.
- microdrepanocytic d.
- Mikulicz's d.
- milk alkali d.
- milk-borne d's
- Miller's d.
- Mills' d.

dis·ease *(continued)*
>
> Milroy's d.
> Milton's d.
> Minamata d.
> minimal change d.
> minimal lesion d.
> Minor's d.
> Mitchell's d.
> mixed connective tissue d.
> mixed cryoglobulin d.
> Möbius' d.
> Moeller-Barlow d.
> molecular d.
> Molten's d.
> Mondor's d.
> Monge's d.
> Morgagni's d.
> Morquio's d.
> Mortimer's d.
> Morquio-Ullrich d.
> Morton's d.
> Morvan's d.
> Moschcowitz's d.
> motor neuron d.
> Mouchet's d.
> mountain d.
> moyamoya d.
> Mozer's d.
> mu chain d.
> Mucha's d.
> Mucha-Habermann d.
> mule spinner's d.
> multisystem d.
> Münchmeyer's d.
> Murray Valley d.
> mushroom picker's d.
> mushroom worker's d.
> Nairobi d.
> nanukayami d.
> navicular d.
> neuropathic joint d.
> Newcastle d.
> Nicolas-Favre d.
> Niemann d.
> Niemann-Pick d.
> nil d.
> Nonne-Milroy d.
> Norrie's d.

dis·ease *(continued)*
>
> Norum-Gjone d.
> nosocomial d.
> notifiable d.
> Novy's rat d.
> oasthouse urine d.
> obstructive small airways
>   d.
> occupational d.
> Oguchi's d.
> Ohara's d.
> oid-oid d.
> Ollier's d.
> Ondiri d.
> Opitz's d.
> organic d.
> Oriental lung fluke d.
> Ormond's d.
> Osgood-Schlatter d.
> Osler's d.
> Osler-Vaquez d.
> Osler-Weber-Rendu d.
> Otto's d.
> ouch-ouch d.
> overeating d.
> Owren's d.
> ox-warble d.
> Paas's d.
> Paget d.
> Paget's d., extramammary
> Panner's d.
> parenchymatous d.
> Parkinson's d.
> Parrot's d.
> parrot d.
> Parry's d.
> Patella's d.
> Payr's d.
> pearl d.
> pearl-worker's d.
> Pel-Ebstein d.
> Pelizaeus-Merzbacher d.
> Pellegrini's d.
> Pellegrini-Stieda d.
> pelvic inflammatory d.
> peptic ulcer d. (PUD)
> periodic d.
> periodontal d.

dis·ease *(continued)*

Perrin-Ferraton d.
Perthes' d.
pestilential d.
Peyronie's d.
Pfeiffer's d.
Phocas' d.
phytanic acid storage d.
Pick's d.
Pictou d.
pink d.
plaster-of-Paris d.
Plummer's d.
pneumatic hammer d.
policeman's d.
polycystic d. of kidneys
polycystic ovary d.
polycystic renal d.
polyendocrine autoimmune
  d.
polyhedral d's
Pompe's d.
Poncet's d.
Portuguese-Azorean d.
Posada-Wernicke d.
Pott's d.
pregnancy d.
Preiser's d.
Pringle's d.
Profichet's d.
pseudo-Hurler's d.
pseudo-Pott's d.
psychosomatic d.
pulmonary heart d.
pulpy kidney d.
pulseless d.
Purtscher's d.
Pyle's d.
pyramidal d.
Quervain's d.
Quincke's d.
ragpicker's d.
ragsorter's d.
railroad d.
Ramsay Hunt d.
rat-bite d.
ray-fungus d.
Raynaud's d.

dis·ease *(continued)*

Recklinghausen's d.
Recklinghausen's d. of
  bone
Recklinghausen-Applebaum-
  d.
Reclus' d.
redwater d.
Reed-Hodgkin d.
Refsum d.
Reiter's d.
renal artery d.
Rendu-Osler-Weber d.
reportable d.
rheumatic heart d.
rheumatoid d.
Ribas-Torres d.
Ribbing's d.
rice d.
Riedel's d.
Riga-Fede d.
Riggs' d.
Ritter's d.
Robles' d.
Roger's d.
Romberg's d.
rose d.
Rossbach's d.
Roth's d.
Roth-Bernhardt d.
Rougnon-Heberden d.
round heart d.
Roussy-Lévy's d.
Royal Free d.
Rubarth's d.
Runeberg's d.
Rust's d.
Ruysch's d.
saccharine d.
Sachs' d.
sacroiliac d.
salivary gland d.
salmon d.
Sanders' d.
Sandhoff d.
sandworm d.
Sanfilippo's d.
San Joaquin Valley d.

dis·ease *(continued)*

Saunders' d.
Schamberg's d.
Schanz's d.
Schaumann's d.
Scheuermann's d.
Schilder's d.
Schimmelbusch's d.
Schlatter's d.
Schlatter-Osgood d.
Schmorl's d.
Scholz's d.
Scholz-Greenfield d.
Schönlein's d.
Schönlein-Henoch d.
Schottmüller's d.
Schroeder's d.
Schüller's d.
Schüller-Christian d.
Schultz's d.
Schwediauer's d.
sclerocystic d.
scleroderma heart d.
secondary d.
Seitelberger's d.
self-limited d.
Selter's d.
senecio d.
septic d.
serum d.
Sever's d.
severe combined
   immunodeficiency d.
   (SCID)
sexually transmitted d.
Shaver's d.
shimamushi d.
shuttlemaker's d.
sickle-cell d.
sickle cell–hemoglobin C d.
sickle cell–hemoglobin D d.
sickle cell–thalassemia d.
silk-stocking d.
silo-filler's d.
Simmonds' d.
Simons' d.
Sinding-Larsen-Johansson
   d.

dis·ease *(continued)*

sixth d.
sixth venereal d.
Sjögren's d.
Skevas-Zerfus d.
skinbound d.
sleeping d.
small airways d.
small vessel d.
Smith-Strang d.
Sneddon-Wilkinson d.
sod d.
specific d.
Spencer's d.
Spielmeyer-Vogt d.
sponge-diver's d.
St. Aignon's d.
St. Anthony's d.
St. Modestus' d.
Stanton's d.
Stargardt's d.
Steinert's d.
sterility d.
Sternberg's d.
Stevens-Johnson d.
Sticker's d.
Stieda's d.
Still's d.
Stokes-Adams d.
storage d.
storage pool d.
Strachan's d.
structural d.
Strümpell's d.
Strümpell-Leichtenstern d.
Strümpell-Marie d.
Stühmer's d.
Sturge's d.
Sturge-Weber d.
Sturge-Weber-Dimitri d.
Stuttgart d.
Sudeck's d.
Sutton's d.
Swediaur's (Schwediauer's)
   d.
Swift's d.
Swift-Feer d.
swineherd's d.

dis·ease *(continued)*
   Sylvest's d.
   Symmers' d.
   systemic d.
   Takahara's d.
   Takayasu's d.
   Talfan d.
   Talma's d.
   Tangier d.
   tarabagan d.
   Tarui d.
   Taussig-Bing d.
   Tay's d.
   Tay-Sachs d. (TSD)
   Teschen d.
   thalassemia–sickle cell d.
   Thaysen's d.
   Theiler's d.
   thick leg d.
   Thiemann's d.
   Thomsen's d.
   Thomson's d.
   thyrocardiac d.
   thyrotoxic heart d.
   Tietze's d.
   Tillaux's d.
   Tommaselli's d.
   Tooth d.
   Tornwaldt's (Thorn-
      waldt's) d.
   Tourette's d.
   transplantation d.
   Traum's d.
   Trevor's d.
   Trinidad d.
   trophoblastic d.
   tropical d.
   tsutsugamushi d.
   tubotympanic d.
   tunnel d.
   twin-lamb d.
   twist d.
   Tyzzer's d.
   Tzaneen d.
   Underwood's d.
   unilocular hydatid d.
   Unna-Thost d.
   Unverricht's d.

dis·ease *(continued)*
   Urbach-Oppenheim d.
   Urbach-Wiethe d.
   uremic bone d.
   uremic medullary cystic d.
   vagabonds' d.
   vagrants' d.
   valvular d.
   van Bogaert-Bertrand d.
   van Bogaert-Nyssen-
      Peiffer d.
   van Buchem's d.
   van Buren's d.
   van den Bergh's d.
   Vaquez' d.
   Vaquez-Osler d.
   venereal d.
   veno-occlusive d. of the
      liver
   Verneuil's d.
   Verse's d.
   vibration d.
   Vidal's d.
   Vincent's d.
   vinyl chloride d.
   Virchow's d.
   Vogt's d.
   Vogt-Kayanagi-Harada d.
   Vogt-Spielmeyer d.
   Volkmann's d.
   Voltolini's d.
   von Economo's d.
   von Gierke's d.
   von Hippel's d.
   von Hippel-Lindau d.
   von Recklinghausen's d.
   von Rokitansky's d.
   von Willebrand's d.
   Voorhoeve's d.
   Vrolik's d.
   Wagner's d.
   Waldenström's d.
   Wartenberg's d.
   Wassilieff's d.
   wasting d.
   Weber's d.
   Weber-Christian d.
   Weber-Dimitri d.

dis·ease *(continued)*
> Wegner's d.
> Weil's d.
> Weir Mitchell's d.
> Werdnig-Hoffmann d.
> Werlhof's d.
> Werner-His d.
> Werner-Schultz d.
> Wernicke's d.
> Wesselsbron d.
> Westphal-Strümpell d.
> Wetherbee's d.
> Whipple's d.
> white muscle d.
> white-spot d.
> Whitmore's d.
> Whytt's d.
> Wilson's d.
> Winckel's d.
> Winiwarter-Buerger d.
> Winkelman's d.
> Winkler's d.
> winter vomiting d.
> Winton d.
> Witkop's d.
> Witkop-Von Sallmann d.
> Wolman d.
> woolsorters' d.
> Woringer-Kolopp d.
> x d.
> X-linked
>   lymphoproliferative d.
> Zahorsky's d.
> Ziehen-Oppenheim d.

dis·en·gage·ment
dis·equil·i·bra·tion
dis·fa·cil·i·ta·tion
dis·equi·lib·ri·um
> linkage d.

dis·es·the·sia
dis·ger·mi·no·ma
dish
> culture d.
> dappen d.
> evaporating d.
> Petri d.
> Stender d.

dis·har·mo·ny
> maxillomandibular d.
> occlusal d.

dis·in·fect
dis·in·fec·tant
> coal-tar d.

dis·in·fec·tion
> concomitant d.
> concurrent d.
> terminal d.

dis·in·fes·ta·tion
dis·in·hi·bi·tion
di·si·nom·e·nine
dis·in·sect·ed
dis·in·sec·tion
dis·in·sec·ti·za·tion
dis·in·sec·tor
dis·in·ser·tion
> d. of the retina

dis·in·te·grant
dis·in·te·gra·tion
> radioactive d.
> spontaneous d.

dis·in·te·gra·tor
dis·in·tox·i·ca·tion
Dis·i·pal
dis·joint
dis·ju·gate
dis·junc·tion
> craniofacial d.

dis·junc·tive
disk
> A d.
> abrasive d.
> acromioclavicular d.
> Amici's d.
> anangioid d.
> anisotropic d.
> articular d.
> Bardeen's primitive d.
> bilaminar embryonic d.
> Blake's d.
> blastodermic d.
> blood d.
> Bowman's d's
> Carborundum d.
> choked d.

disk *(continued)*
    ciliary d.
    cloth d.
    cupped d.
    cutting d.
    cuttlefish d.
    dental d.
    diamond d.
    ectodermal d.
    embryonic d.
    emery d.
    Engelmann's d.
    epiphyseal d.
    equatorial d.
    floppy d.
    gelatin d.
    germinal d.
    growth d.
    hair d.
    Hensen's d.
    herniated d.
    I d.
    interarticular d.
    intercalated d.
    intermediate d.
    interpubic d.
    intervertebral d's
    intra-articular d.
    isotropic d.
    J d.
    M d.
    mandibular d.
    Merkel's d's
    micrometer d.
    Miller d.
    Newton's d.
    nuclear d.
    optic d.
    pinhole d.
    Placido's d.
    polishing d.
    proligerous d.
    protruded d.
    Q d.
    Ranvier's tactile d's
    Rekoss d.
    ruptured d.
    sandpaper d.

disk *(continued)*
    sarcous d.
    Schiefferdecker's d's
    slipped d.
    stenopeic d.
    sternoclavicular d.
    stroboscopic d.
    tactile d's
    thin d.
    transverse d.
    triangular d. of wrist
    Z d.
dis·kec·to·my
dis·ki·form
dis·ki·tis
dis·ko·gram
dis·kog·ra·phy
dis·lo·cate
dis·lo·ca·tio
    d. erecta
dis·lo·ca·tion
    anterior d.
    anterior shoulder d.
    d. of articular processes
    Bell-Dally d.
    Bennett's d.
    central d.
    Chopart d.
    closed d.
    complete d.
    complicated d.
    compound d.
    congenital d.
    consecutive d.
    divergent d.
    fracture d.
    frank d.
    gamekeepers' d.
    habitual d.
    incomplete d.
    incudomallear d.
    incudostapedial d.
    intrauterine d.
    Kienböck's d.
    d. of the lens
    Lisfranc's d.
    Monteggia's d.
    Nélaton's d.

dis·lo·ca·tion *(continued)*
   obturator d.
   old d.
   open d.
   paralytic d.
   partial d.
   pathologic d.
   perilunate d.
   posterior d.
   posterior shoulder d.
   primitive d.
   recent d.
   recurrent d.
   sciatic d.
   simple d.
   Smith's d.
   subastragalar d.
   subclavicular d.
   subcoracoid d.
   subglenoid d.
   subspinous d.
   traumatic d.
   unifacet d.
   unreduced d.
   vertebral d.
   voluntary d.
dis·mem·ber·ment
dis·mu·ta·tion
dis·oc·clude
di·so·di·um
   d. cromoglycate
   d. edetate
di·some
Di·so·mer
di·so·mic
di·so·mus
di·so·my
di·so·pyr·amide
   d. phosphate
dis·or·der
   adjustment d.
   affective d's
   aggressive behavior d.
   alcoholic brain d's
   amnestic d.
   anxiety d's
   appetite d.
   arteriosclerotic brain d.

dis·or·der *(continued)*
   attention deficit d. (ADD)
   attention-deficit
     hyperactivity d.
   autistic d.
   autonomic d.
   avoidant d. of childhood or
     adolescence
   behavior d.
   bipolar d.
   body dysmorphic d.
   brain d.
   cerebelloparenchymal d.
   character d.
   character impulse d.
   collagen d.
   conduct d.
   consumptive
     thrombohemorrhagic d.
   conversion d.
   cyclothymic d.
   delusional (paranoid) d.
   depersonalization d.
   dissociative d's
   dysthymic d.
   eating d.
   emotional d.
   epileptoid personality d.
   equilibratory d.
   extrapyramidal d.
   factitious d.
   functional d.
   generalized anxiety d.
   genetic d.
   gnostic d's
   habit d.
   hereditary d.
   hyperkinetic impulse d.
   identity d.
   immunodeficiency d.
   immunoproliferative d.
   impulse d.
   induced psychotic d.
   intermittent explosive d.
   isolated explosive d.
   late luteal phase dysphoric
     d.
   LDL-receptor d.

dis·or·der *(continued)*
   major mood d's
   manic-depressive d.
   mendelian d.
   mental d.
   monogenic d.
   mood d's
   motility d.
   multifactorial d.
   multiple personality d.
   neurotic depressive d.
   organic mental d's
   overanxious d.
   panic d.
   paranoid d's
   personality d.
   panic d. without
     agoraphobia
   pervasive developmental
     d's
   post-traumatic personality
     d.
   post-traumatic stress d.
   psychoactive
     substance-induced
     organic mental d's
   psychoactive substance use
     d's
   psychogenic pain d.
   psychophysiologic d.
   psychosomatic d.
   schizoaffective d.
   schizophreniform d.
   seasonal mood d.
   separation anxiety d.
   shared paranoid d.
   single-gene d.
   sleep terror d.
   sleepwalking d.
   somatization d.
   somatoform d's
   somatoform pain d.
   stress d.
   substance use d's
   thought d.
   Tourette's d.
   transient situational
     personality d.

dis·or·der *(continued)*
   unipolar d's
   vibration d.
   visceral d.
   XXX d.
   XXXX d.
   XXXXY d.
   XXXY d.
   XXYY d.
dis·or·gan·iza·tion
dis·or·i·en·ta·tion
   right-left d.
   spatial d.
dis·ox·i·da·tion
dis·par
dis·par·a·si·tized
dis·pa·rate
dis·par·i·ty
dis·pen·sa·ry
dis·pen·sa·to·ry
   D. of the United States of
     America
dis·pense
di·sper·my
dis·per·sal
   flash d.
dis·per·sate
dis·perse
dis·per·si·ble
dis·per·sion
   chromatic d.
   colloid d.
   d. of light
   molecular d.
   optical rotatory d.
dis·per·si·ty
dis·per·soid
dis·pert
Dis·phol·i·dus
di·spi·ra
di·spi·reme
dis·place·a·bil·i·ty
dis·place·ment
   character d.
   condylar d.
   fetal d.
   fish-hook d.
   gallbladder d.

dis·place·ment *(continued)*
   mesial d.
   Proetz d.
   tissue d.
dis·play
   bistable d.
   leading edge d.
   real-time d.
di·spore
di·spo·rous
dis·po·si·tion
dis·pro·por·tion
   borderline pelvic d.
   cephalopelvic d.
   fiber-type d.
dis·rup·tion
dis·rup·tive
Dis·se's spaces
dis·sec·ans
dis·sect
dis·sec·tion
   aortic d.
   arterial d.
   block d. of neck
   blunt d.
   elective neck d.
   functional neck d.
   partial neck d.
   prophylactic neck d.
   radical neck d.
   sharp d.
   suprahyoid neck d.
dis·sec·tor
   Cavitron d.
dis·sem·i·nat·ed
dis·sep·i·ment
dis·sim·i·late
dis·sim·i·la·tion
dis·so·ci·able
dis·so·ci·at·ed
dis·so·ci·a·tion
   albuminocytologic d.
   atrial d.
   atrioventricular d.
   auriculoventricular d.
   bacterial d.
   electromechanical d.
   interference d.

dis·so·ci·a·tion *(continued)*
   longitudinal d.
   microbic d.
   Mobitz-type
     atrioventricular d.
   peripheral d.
   syringomyelic d.
   tabetic d.
dis·sog·e·ny
dis·so·lu·tion
dis·solve
dis·sol·vent
dis·so·nance
   cognitive d.
Dist. — L. distilla (distil)
dis·tad
dis·tal
dis·ta·lis
dis·tal·ly
dis·tance
   angular d.
   cone-surface d.
   focal d.
   focal skin d.
   infinite d.
   interarch d.
   interocclusal d.
   interocular d.
   interorbital d.
   interpediculate d.
   interpupillary d.
   interridge d.
   map d.
   object-film d.
   source-skin d.
   target-skin d.
   vertex d.
   working d.
dis·tem·per
dis·tend
dis·ten·si·bil·i·ty
dis·ten·tion
dis·tich·ia
dis·ti·chi·a·sis
dis·ti·chous
dis·til, dis·till
dis·til·late

dis·til·la·tion
  cold d.
  destructive d.
  dry d.
  fractional d.
  molecular d.
  vacuum d.
dis·to·ax·io·gin·gi·val
dis·to·ax·io·in·ci·sal
dis·to·ax·io-oc·clu·sal
dis·to·buc·cal
dis·to·buc·co-oc·clu·sal
dis·to·buc·co·pul·pal
dis·to·cep·tor
dis·to·cer·vi·cal
dis·to·cli·na·tion
dis·to·clu·sal
dis·to·clu·sion
dis·to·gin·gi·val
dis·to·la·bi·al
dis·to·la·bio·in·ci·sal
dis·to·lin·gual
dis·to·lin·guo·in·ci·sal
dis·to·lin·guo-oc·clu·sal
dis·to·lin·guo·pul·pal
Dis·to·ma
di·sto·mia
dis·to·mi·a·sis
  pulmonary d.
dis·to·mo·lar
di·sto·mus
dis·to-oc·clu·sal
dis·to-oc·clu·sion
dis·to·place·ment
dis·to·pul·pal
dis·to·pul·po·la·bi·al
dis·to·pul·po·lin·gual
dis·tor·tion
  apperceptive d.
  parataxic d.
dis·tor·tor
  d. oris
dis·to·ver·sion
dis·trac·ti·bil·i·ty
dis·trac·tion
dis·tress
  fetal d.

dis·tress *(continued)*
  idiopathic respiratory d. of
    newborn
dis·tri·bu·tion
  age d.
  Bernouilli d.
  Boltzmann d.
  chi-squared d.
  contagious d.
  continuous d.
  density d.
  discontinuous d.
  discrete d.
  dose d.
  F-d.
  frequency d.
  gaussian d.
  isodose d.
  Laplace-Gauss d.
  marital status d.
  negative binomial d.
  normal d.
  Poisson d.
  probability d.
  saddle d.
  sampling d.
  skew d.
  standard normal d.
  parity d.
  Pascal d.
  t-d.
dis·tri·chi·a·sis
dis·trix
dis·tur·bance
  d.'s of affectivity
  emotional d.
  personality pattern d.
  personality trait d.
  sexual orientation d.
  transient situational d.
di·sub·sti·tut·ed
di·sul·fate
di·sul·fide
di·sul·fi·ram
di·sul·fur di·chlo·ride
di·thi·az·a·nine io·dide
di·thio
di·thi·ol

di·thio·nite
di·thio·thre·i·tol
dith·ra·nol
Di·tro·pan
Dit·tel's operation
Dit·trich's plugs
Dit·y·len·chus
   D. dipsaci
di·type
   nonparental d.
Di·u·car·din
Di·u·lo
Di·u·pres
di·urea
di·ure·ide
di·urese
di·ure·sis *pl.* di·ure·ses
   alcohol d.
   osmotic d.
   tubular d.
   water d.
di·uret·ic
   cardiac d.
   high-ceiling d's
   loop d.
   mercurial d's
   osmotic d.
   potassium-sparing d's
   thiazide d.
di·uria
Di·uril
di·ur·nal
di·ur·nule
Di·u·ten·sin
Div. — L. divide (divide)
di·va·ga·tion
di·va·lent
di·var·i·ca·tion
di·var·i·ca·tor
di·ver·gence
   beam d.
   dissociated vertical d.
      (DVD)
   negative vertical d.
   positive vertical d.
di·ver·gent
di·ver·sine

di·ver·sion
   antigenic d.
   urinary d.
di·ver·si·ty
   combinatorial d.
di·ver·tic·u·la
di·ver·tic·u·lar
di·ver·tic·u·lar·iza·tion
di·ver·tic·u·lec·to·my
di·ver·tic·u·li·tis
di·ver·tic·u·lo·esoph·a·gos·
   to·my
di·ver·tic·u·lo·gram
di·ver·tic·u·lo·ma
di·ver·tic·u·lo·pexy
di·ver·tic·u·lo·sis
di·ver·tic·u·lum *pl.* di·ver·tic·
   u·la
   acquired d.
   allantoic d.
   bladder d.
   caliceal d.
   cervical d.
   colonic diverticula
   congenital d.
   epiphrenic d.
   false d.
   foregut d.
   functional d.
   ganglion d.
   Ganser's d.
   Graser's d.
   Heister's d.
   hepatic d.
   hypopharyngeal d.
   d. ilei verum
   intestinal d.
   Kirchner's d.
   laryngeal d.
   Meckel's d.
   Nuck's d.
   optic d.
   pancreatic diverticula
   Pertik's d.
   pharyngeal d.
   pharyngoesophageal d.
   pineal d.

di·ver·tic·u·lum *(continued)*
  pituitary d.
  pressure d.
  pulsion d.
  Rokitansky's d.
  supracondylar synovial d.
  supradiaphragmatic d.
  synovial d.
  thyroid d.
  tracheal diverticula
  traction d.
  d. unci
  ureteric d.
  d. of utricle
  vesical d.
  Zenker's d.
di·vi·cine
divi-divi
di·vi·nyl
  d. ether
di·vi·sion
  cell d.
  craniosacral d.
  equational d.
  indirect nuclear d.
  maturation d.
  multiplicative d.
  reduction d.
  Remak's d.
  thoracolumbar d.
  d's of trunks of brachial
    plexus
di·vulse
di·vul·sion
di·vul·sor
Dix-Hall·pike test
Dix·on Mann
di·zy·got·ic
di·zy·gous
diz·zi·ness
djen·kol·ic acid
DLE — discoid lupus
  erythematosus
DM — diabetes mellitus
  diphenylamine-arsine
    chloride
DMBA — 7,12-dimethylbenz[a]-
  anthracene

DMD — Doctor of Dental
  Medicine
DMF — decayed, missing,
  filled (teeth)
DMPE — 3,4-dimethoxyphenyl-
  ethylamine
DMRD — Diploma in Medical
  Radio-Diagnosis (British)
DMRT — Diploma in Medical
  Radio-Therapy (British)
DMSO — dimethyl sulfoxide
DMT — dimethyltryptamine
DN — dibucaine number
  dicrotic notch
dn. — decinem
DNA — deoxyribonucleic acid
  complementary DNA
  double-stranded DNA
  DNA library
  linker DNA
  native DNA
  rapidly reannealing DNA
  recombinant DNA
  repetitive DNA
  satellite DNA
  single-copy DNA
  single-stranded DNA
  transferred DNA
  unique DNA
  Z DNA
DNA-di·rect·ed DNA pol·y·
  mer·ase
DNA-di·rect·ed RNA pol·y·
  mer·ase
DNA li·gase
DNA nu·cleo·tid·yl·exo·
  trans·fer·ase
DNA nu·cleo·tid·yl·trans·fer·
  ase
DNA poly·mer·ase
DNase — deoxyribonuclease
DNA topo·isom·er·ase
DNB — dinitrobenzene
DNCB — dinitrochloro-
  benzene
DNFB — dinitrofluorobenzene
DNOC — dinitro-o-cresol
DNR — do not resuscitate

DO — Doctor of Osteopathy
DOA — dead on arrival
Dobb·hoff feeding tube
Do·bie's globule
Do·bie's layer
Do·bie's line
do·bu·ta·mine
    d. hydrochloride
DOC — 11-deoxycortico-
  sterone
Do·ca
Do·ci·bin
do·ci·ma·sia
do·ci·mas·tic
Docke's murmur
do·co·na·zole
doc·tor
doc·trine
    Arrhenius' d.
    Monro-Kellie d.
    neuron d.
doc·u·sate cal·ci·um
doc·u·sate so·di·um
do·deca·dac·ty·li·tis
do·deca·dac·ty·lon
do·de·cyl sul·fate
Dö·der·lein's bacillus
DOE — dyspnea on exertion
Doer·fler-Stew·art test
Do·gi·el's corpuscles
dog·ma
    central d.
Döh·le's disease
Döh·le's inclusion bodies
Döh·le-Hel·ler aortitis
doigt
    d. mort
Doi·sy, Edward Adelbert
dol
do·lab·rate
do·lab·ri·form
Dol·é·ris' operation
dol·i·cho·ce·pha·lia
dol·i·cho·ce·phal·ic
dol·i·cho·ceph·a·lism
dol·i·cho·ceph·a·ly
dol·i·cho·co·lon
dol·i·cho·cra·ni·al

dol·i·cho·der·us
dol·i·cho·fa·cial
dol·i·cho·hi·er·ic
dol·i·cho·ker·kic
dol·i·cho·kne·mic
dol·i·cho-mega-ar·te·ries
dol·i·cho·mor·phic
dol·i·cho·pel·lic, dol·i·cho·
  pel·vic
dol·i·cho·pro·sop·ic
dol·i·cho·steno·me·lia
dol·i·chu·ran·ic
Döl·ling·er's tendinous ring
Do·lo·bid
Do·lo·phine
do·lor pl. do·lo·res
    d. capitis
    d. coxae
    dolores praesagientes
    d. vagus
do·lo·res
do·lor·if·ic
do·lor·im·e·ter
do·lor·im·e·try
do·lor·o·gen·ic
DOM — 2,5-dimethoxy-4-
  methylamphetamine
Do·magk, Gerhard Johannes
  Paul
do·main
    immunoglobulin d's.
do·ma·zo·line fu·mar·ate
Dom·brock blood group
dome
    pleural d.
Dome·boro
dom·i·cil·i·ary
dom·i·nance
    cerebral d.
    conditioned d.
    incomplete d.
    lateral d.
    ocular d.
    one-sided d.
    partial d.
    reversed d. of eyes
dom·i·nance-sub·mis·sion
dom·i·nant

do·mi·phen bro·mide
dom·per·i·done
Do·nath's test
Do·nath-Land·stein·er test
do·nax·ine
Don·ders' glaucoma
Don·ders' law
do·nee
Don Juan·ism
Don·nan's equilibrium
Donné's bodies
Donné's corpuscles
do·nor
    F d.
    general d.
    hydrogen d.
    universal d.
do·nor-spe·cif·ic
Don·o·van bodies
Don·o·va·nia gran·u·lo·ma·
    tis
don·o·va·no·sis
do·pa
    L-d.
    d. quinone
dopa decarboxylase
do·pa·man·tine
do·pa·mine
    d. hydrochloride
do·pa·mine β-hy·drox·y·lase
do·pa·mine β-mono·oxy·gen·
    ase
do·pa·min·er·gic
do·pa-ox·i·dase
do·pa·quin·one
Do·par
do·pase
Doppler
    directional D.
    pulse D.
Dop·pler effect
Dop·pler phenomenon
Dop·pler principle
Do·pram
dor·as·tine hy·dro·chlo·ride
Dor·bane
Do·rel·lo's canal
Dor·en·dorf's sign

Dor·i·den
dor·man·cy
dor·mant
dor·mi·fa·cient
Dor·na·vac
Dor·no's rays
Dorn-Su·gar·man test
Dor·rance operation
dor·sa
Dor·sa·caine
dor·sad
dor·sal
dor·sal·gia
dor·sa·lis
dor·si·cum·bent
dor·si·duct
dor·si·flex·ion
dor·si·flex·or
dor·si·mes·al
dor·si·spi·nal
dor·so·ab·dom·i·nal
dor·so·an·te·ri·or
dor·so·ceph·a·lad
dor·so·dyn·ia
dor·so·epi·troch·le·ar·is
dor·so·in·ter·cos·tal
dor·so·in·ter·os·se·al
dor·so·lat·er·al
dor·so·lum·bar
dor·so·me·di·al
dor·so·me·di·an
dor·so·me·si·al
dor·so·na·sal
dor·so·nu·chal
dor·so·pos·te·ri·or
dor·so·ra·di·al
dor·so·sa·cral
dor·so·scap·u·lar
dor·so·ven·trad
dor·so·ven·tral
dor·sum *pl.* dor·sa
    d. of foot
    d. of hand
    d. ilii
    d. linguae
    d. manus
    d. nasi
    d. pedis

dor·sum *(continued)*
    d. penis
    d. of scapula
    d. scapulae
    d. sellae
    d. of testis
    d. of tongue
do·sage
    gene d.
dose
    absorbed d.
    air d.
    average d.
    booster d.
    central axis depth d.
    cumulative d.
    curative d.
    curative d., median
    daily d.
    depth d.
    divided d.
    doubling d.
    effective d.
    effective d., median
    entrance d.
    epilating d.
    erythema d.
    exit d.
    exposure d.
    fatal d.
    fractional d's
    fractionation d.
    genetically significant d.
    immunizing d.
    infective d.
    infective d., median
    integral absorbed d.
    invariably lethal d.
    L + d.
    L0 d.
    limes nul d.
    limes zero d.
    lethal d.
    lethal d., median
    lethal d., minimum
    Lf d.
    loading d.
    Lr d.

dose *(continued)*
    maintenance d.
    maximum d.
    maximum permissible d.
    median tissue culture
      infective d.
    minimal hemagglutinating
      d.
    minimal hemolytic d.
    minimal reacting d.
    organ tolerance d.
    permissible d.
    preventive d.
    priming d.
    radiation absorbed d.
    reacting d.
    refractive d.
    sensitizing d.
    skin d.
    therapeutic d.
    threshold d.
    threshold erythema d.
    tissue d.
    tolerance d.
    toxic d.
    unit d.
    volume d.
do·sim·e·ter
    film d.
    integrating d.
    noise d.
    pocket d.
do·si·met·ric
do·sim·e·trist
do·sim·e·try
    photographic d.
    thermoluminescent d.
do·sis
    d. curativa
    d. efficax
    d. refracta
    d. tolerata
dos·sier
dot
    Gunn's d's
    Marcus Gunn's d's
    Maurer's d's
    Mittendorf's d.

dot *(continued)*
    Schüffner's d's
    Trantas' d's
do·tage
do·thi·e·pin hy·dro·chlo·ride
dou·ble-armed
dou·ble-blind
dou·ble-masked
dou·ble-strand·ed
doub·let
    Wollaston's d.
douche
    air d.
    alternating d.
    Betadine d.
    fan d.
    jet d.
    Scotch d.
    Tivoli d.
    transition d.
    vinegar d.
Doug·las bag
Doug·las' mechanism
Doug·las' method
Doug·las' septum
Doug·las' cul-de-sac
Doug·las' fold
Doug·las' ligament
Doug·las' line
Doug·las' pouch
Doug·las' space
doug·las·cele
doug·la·si·tis
dou·rine
Do·ver's powder
dow·el
Down syndrome
down
Dow·ney cell
down·gaze
down·go·ing
Downs' analysis
Downs' Y axis
down·stream
dox·a·pram hy·dro·chlo·ride
dox·a·prost
dox·e·pin hy·dro·chlo·ride
Dox·i·nate

doxo·ru·bi·cin
    d. hydrochloride
doxy·cy·cline
    d. calcium
    d. hyclate
    d. hydrochloride
Doxy-II
dox·yl·amine suc·ci·nate
Doy·en's clamp
Do·yère's eminence
Do·yère's hillock
Doyne's familial honeycombed choroiditis
DP — L. *directione propria* (with proper direction)
    Doctor of Pharmacy
    Doctor of Podiatry
DPH — Diploma in Public Health
DPM — Diploma in Psychological Medicine
    Doctor of Podiatric Medicine
DPT — diphtheria-pertussis-tetanus (vaccine)
DR — diabetic retinopathy
    reaction of degeneration
dr — dram
drachm
drac·on·ti·a·sis
dra·cun·cu·lar
dra·cun·cu·li·a·sis
Dra·cun·cu·loi·dea
dra·cun·cu·lo·sis
Dra·cun·cu·lus
    D. medinensis
drag
    solvent d.
dra·gée
drain
    butterfly d.
    cigarette d.
    controlled d.
    Mikulicz's d.
    Penrose d.
    quarantine d.
    stab wound d.

drain *(continued)*
    sump d.
    sump-Penrose d.
drain·age
    anomalous pulmonary
      venous d.
    basal d.
    button d.
    capillary d.
    closed d.
    continuous suction d.
    dependent d.
    open d.
    percutaneous d.
    postural d.
    suction d.
    through d.
    tidal d.
    ventriculoatrial d.
    Wangensteen d.
Drake-Wil·lock dialysis
dram
    fluid d.
Dram·a·mine
drape
dras·tic
draught
dream
    day d.
    wet d.
drench
Drep·a·nido·tae·nia
drep·a·no·cyte
drep·a·no·cyt·e·mia
drep·a·no·cyt·ic
drep·a·no·cy·to·sis
Dres·bach's anemia
Dres·bach's syndrome
dress·er
dress·ing
    adhesive absorbent d.
    antiseptic d.
    biologic d.
    bolus d.
    cement d.
    cocoon d.
    collodion d.
    cross d.

dress·ing *(continued)*
    dry d.
    fixed d.
    iodoform d.
    Lister's d.
    occlusive d.
    pressure d.
    protective d.
    stent d.
    tie-over d.
    wet-to-dry d.
Dress·ler's syndrome
Drey·er's test
Drey·er and Ben·nett
  hypothesis
DRG — diagnosis-related
  group
drift
    antigenic d.
    genetic d.
    mesial d.
    physiologic d.
    radial d.
    random genetic d.
    ulnar d.
drill
    cannulated d.
    mirror d.
drill·ing
Drin·al·fa
dri·ni·dene
drink
    sham d.
Drink·er respirator
drink·ing
    binge d.
    episodic excessive d.
    habitual excessive d.
    periodic d.
    social d.
drip
    heparin d.
    intravenous d.
    Murphy d.
    nasal d.
    postnasal d.
Dris·dol

drive
    acquired d.
    aggressive d.
    exploratory d.
    learned d.
    meiotic d.
    secondary d.
    sexual d.
dRNA — DNA-like RNA
dro·bu·line
dro·car·bil
dro·cin·o·nide
dro·code
Drol·ban
drom·ic
dromo·graph
dro·mo·stan·o·lone pro·pio·nate
drom·o·trop·ic
dro·mot·ro·pism
    negative d.
    positive d.
Dron·cit
drop
    ankle d.
    capsular d.
    ear d's
    enamel d.
    eye d's
    foot d.
    hanging d.
    Hoffmann's d's
    lid d.
    nose d's
    d. phalangette
    steel d's
    wrist d.
drop·a·cism
dro·per·i·dol
drop·let
    Flügge's d.
    hyaline d.
    lipid d.
    protein d.
drop·per
drop·ping
drop·si·cal

drop·sy
    abdominal d.
    d. of amnion
    articular d.
    d. of belly
    d. of brain
    cardiac d.
    d. of chest
    cutaneous d.
    epidemic d.
    famine d.
    d. of head
    hepatic d.
    nutritional d.
    peritoneal d.
    renal d.
    salpingian d.
    tubal d.
    war d.
    wet d.
Dro·soph·i·la
    D. melanogaster
dro·sop·ter·in
drown·ing
    secondary d.
drox·a·cin so·di·um
drox·i·fil·con A
drug
    antagonistic d.
    controlled d.
    crude d.
    designer d.
    ethical d.
    illicit d.
    investigational d.
    licit d.
    over-the-counter d.
    prescription d.
    proprietary d.
drug-fast
drug·gist
drug-re·sis·tant
drum
    Bárány d.
    blue d.
drum·head
Drum·mond's sign

drum·stick
dru·sen
    giant d. of macula
Drys·dale's corpuscles
DSC — Doctor of Surgical
    Chiropody
DSc — Doctor of Science
dsDNA — double-stranded
    DNA
dsRNA — double-stranded
    RNA
Dt — duration tetany
dT — deoxythymidine
D.T.D. — L. datur talis dosis
    (give of such a dose)
dTDP — deoxythymidine
    diphosphate
DTH — delayed type
    hypersensitivity
DTIC — dacarbazine
dTMP — deoxythymidine
    monophosphate
DTPA — pentetic acid
DTR — deep tendon reflex
dTTP — deoxythymidine
    triphosphate
dU — deoxyuridine
du·al·ism
du·al-pho·ton
Du·ane's syndrome
du·azo·my·cin
    d. A
    d. B
    d. C
Du·bin-John·son syndrome
Du·bi·ni's chorea
Du·bi·ni's disease
Du·bois' abscess
Du·bois' disease
Du Bois' sign
Du·Bois-Rey·mond's law
Du·boi·sia
Du·bos crude crystals
Du·bos enzyme
Du·bos lysin
Du·boscq colorimeter
Du·bo·vitz syndrome

Du·bo·witz infant maturity
    scale
Du·breu·ilh's precancerous
    melanosis
Du·chenne's disease
Du·chenne's dystrophy
Du·chenne's paralysis
Du·chenne's type
Du·chenne-Aran disease
Du·chenne-Aran muscular
    atrophy
Du·chenne-Aran type
Du·chenne-Erb paralysis
Du·chenne-Erb syndrome
Du·chenne-Lan·dou·zy
    dystrophy
Du·chenne-Lan·dou·zy type
Duck·worth's phenomenon
Duck·worth's sign
Du·co·bee
Du·crey's bacillus
duct
    aberrant d.
    accessory bile d's
    acoustic d.
    adipose d.
    alimentary d.
    allantoic d.
    alveolar d's
    amnionic d.
    d. of Arantius
    archinephric d.
    arterial d.
    Bartholin's d.
    Bellini's d's
    Bernard's d.
    bile d.
    bile d., common
    bile d's, interlobular
    biliary d.
    Blasius' d.
    Bochdalek's d.
    d. of Botallo
    branchial d's
    canalicular d's
    cervical d.
    choledochous d.
    chyliferous d.

duct *(continued)*
   cloacal d.
   cochlear d.
   collecting d.
   common bile d.
   common
     pharyngobranchial d.
   cowperian d.
   craniopharyngeal d.
   d's of Cuvier
   cystic d.
   deferent d.
   dorsal pancreatic d.
   efferent d.
   efferent d's of testis
   ejaculatory d.
   endolymphatic d.
   d. of epididymis
   epigenital d.
   d. of epoöphoron
   excretory d.
   extrahepatic bile d.
   frontonasal d.
   galactophorous d's
   gasserian d.
   genital d.
   Guérin's d's
   guttural d.
   Haller's aberrant d.
   Hensen's d.
   hepatic d., common
   hepatic d., left
   hepatic d., right
   hepaticopancreatic d.
   hepatocystic d.
   d. of His
   hypophyseal d.
   incisive d.
   incisor d.
   intercalated d.
   interlobular d's
   lacrimal d.
   lacrimonasal d.
   lactiferous d's
   left d. of caudate lobe
   Leydig's d.
   lingual d.

duct *(continued)*
   longitudinal d. of
     epoöphoron
   Luschka's d's
   lymphatic d's
   mammary d's
   mammillary d's
   mesonephric d.
   metanephric d.
   milk d's
   d. of Müller
   müllerian d.
   nasal d.
   nasofrontal d.
   nasolacrimal d.
   nasopharyngeal d.
   nephric d.
   omphalomesenteric d.
   ovarian d.
   pancreatic d.
   pancreatic d., accessory
   pancreatic d., minor
   papillary d's
   paragenital d.'s
   paramesonephric d's of
     female urethra
   paraurethral d's of female
     urethra
   paraurethral d's of male
     urethra
   parotid d.
   d. of Pecquet
   perilymphatic d's
   periotic d.
   persistent
     craniopharyngeal d.
   persistent mesonephric d.
   persistent
     omphalomesenteric d.
   persistent thyroglossal d.
   primordial d.
   pronephric d.
   prostatic d's
   Rathke's d.
   Reichel's cloacal d.
   renal d.
   right d. of caudate lobe
   d's of Rivinus

duct *(continued)*
  Rokitansky-Aschoff d's.
  sacculoutricular d.
  salivary d's
  d. of Santorini
  Schüller's d's
  sebaceous d.
  secretory d.
  segmental d.
  semicircular d's
  seminal d's
  d. of seminal vesicle
  Skene's d's
  spermatic d.
  d. of Steno
  Stensen's d.
  striated d's
  sublingual d's
  sublingual d., major
  sublingual d's, minor
  submandibular d.
  submaxillary d. of
    Wharton
  sudoriferous d.
  sweat d.
  tear d's
  testicular d.
  thoracic d.
  thoracic d., right
  thyrocervical d.
  thyroglossal d.
  thyrolingual d.
  thyropharyngeal d.
  umbilical d.
  urogenital d's
  utriculosaccular d.
  d. of Vater
  ventral pancreatic d.
  vitelline d.
  vitellointestinal d.
  Walther's d's
  Wharton's d.
  d. of Wirsung
  d. of Wolff
  wolffian d.
duc·tal
duc·tile
duc·til·i·ty

duc·tion
  forced d's
  d's and versions
duct·less
duc·tu·lar
duct·ule
  aberrant d's
  alveolar d's
  bile d's
  biliary d's
  cranial aberrant d.
  efferent d's of testis
  excretory d's of lacrimal
    gland
  Haller's aberrant d.
  interlobular d's
  d's of prostate
  transverse d's of
    epoöphoron
duc·tu·lus *pl.* duc·tu·li
  ductuli aberrantes
  ductuli alveolares
  ductuli biliferi
  ductuli efferentes testis
  ductuli interlobulares
  ductuli prostatici
  ductuli transversi
    epoophori
  ductuli transversi
    epoöphorontis
duc·tus *pl.* duc·tus
  d. aberrans
  d. aberrans halleri
  d. Arantii
  d. arteriosus
  d. arteriosus bilateralis
  d. arteriosus, patent
  d. arteriosus, reversed
  d. biliaris
  d. biliferi
  d. choledochus
  d. cochlearis
  d. cuvieri
  d. cysticus
  d. deferens
  d. deferens vestigialis
  double d. arteriosus

duc·tus *(continued)*
    d. ejaculatorius
    d. endolymphaticus
    d. epididymidis
    d. epoöphori longitudinalis
    d. epoöphorontis
      longitudinalis
    d. excretorius vesiculae
      seminalis
    d. glandulae
      bulbourethralis
    d. hepaticus communis
    d. hepaticus dexter
    d. hepaticus sinister
    d. incisivus
    d. interlobulares
    d. interlobulares bilifer
    d. lacrimales
    d. lactiferi
    d. lingualis
    d. lobi caudati dexter
    d. lobi caudati sinister
    d. lymphatici
    d. lymphaticus dexter
    d. mesonephricus
    d. Muelleri
    d. nasolacrimalis
    d. pancreaticus
    d. pancreaticus accessorius
    d. papillaris
    d. paramesonephricus
    d. paraurethrales urethrae
      femininae
    d. paraurethrales urethrae
      masculinae
    d. parotideus
    patent d. arteriosus
    d. perilymphatici
    d. perilymphaticus
    d. prostatici
    d. reuniens
    reversed d. arteriosus
    d. semicirculares
    d. spermaticus
    d. sublingualis major
    d. sublinguales minores
    d. submandibularis
    d. sudoriferus

duc·tus *(continued)*
    d. thoracicus
    d. thoracicus dexter
    d. thyroglossalis
    d. utriculosaccularis
    d. venosus
    d. Wolffi
Dud·dell's membrane
Duffy blood group
Du·gas' sign
Du·gas' test
Du·hot's line
Duh·ring's disease
Dührs·sen's incisions
Dührs·sen's operation
du·ip·a·ra
Duke's method
Duke's test
Dukes' classification
Dukes' disease
Dul·bec·co, Renato
dul·cin
dul·cite
dul·ci·tol
dul·cose
dull·ness
    Gerhardt's d.
    Grocco's triangular d.
    shifting d.
    tympanitic d.
dulse
dumb
dumb·bell
    d's of Schäfer
dumb·ness
    pure word d.
dum·my
dump·ing
dUMP — deoxyuridine
    monophosphate
Dun·can disease
Dun·can syndrome
Dun·can's folds
Dun·can's position
Dun·can's ventricle
Dun·ferm·line scale
Dun·ham's cones
Dun·ham's fans

Dun·ham's triangles
du·o·de·nal
du·o·de·nec·to·my
du·od·e·ni·tis
du·o·de·no·cho·lan·ge·itis
du·o·de·no·cho·le·cys·tos·to·my
du·o·de·no·cho·led·o·chot·o·my
du·o·de·no·col·ic
du·o·de·no·cys·tos·to·my
du·o·de·no·du·o·de·nos·to·my
du·o·de·no·en·ter·os·to·my
du·o·de·no·gram
du·o·de·nog·ra·phy
    hypotonic d.
du·o·de·no·he·pat·ic
du·o·de·no·il·e·os·to·my
du·o·de·no·je·ju·nos·to·my
du·o·de·nol·y·sis
du·o·de·no·pan·cre·a·tec·to·my
du·o·de·no·plas·ty
du·o·de·nor·rha·phy
du·o·de·no·scope
du·o·de·nos·co·py
du·o·de·nos·to·my
du·o·de·not·o·my
du·o·de·num
du·o·par·en·tal
Du·pha·lac
Du·phas·ton
Du·play's bursitis
Du·play's disease
Du·play's operation
Du·play's syndrome
du·pli·ca·tion
    chromosome d.
    incomplete d. of spinal cord
    tandem d.
du·pli·ca·ture
du·pli·ci·tas
    d. anterior
    d. asymmetros
    d. completa
    d. cruciata
    d. incompleta

du·pli·ci·tas *(continued)*
    d. inferior
    d. media
    d. parallela
    d. posterior
    d. superior
    d. symmetros
dupp
Du·pré's disease
Du·pré's syndrome
Du·puy-Du·temps' operation
Du·puy·tren's amputation
Du·puy·tren's contracture
Du·puy·tren's fracture
Du·puy·tren's hydrocele
Du·puy·tren's sign
du·ra
Du·rab·o·lin
Du·ra·cil·lin
du·ral
du·ra ma·ter
Du·ran-Rey·nals' permeability
    factor
Du·rand's disease
Du·rand and Gi·roud vaccine
Du·rand-Ni·co·las-Fa·vre
    disease
Du·ra·nest
dur·ap·a·tite
du·ra·plas·ty
du·ra·tion
    pulse d.
Dürck's granuloma
Dürck's nodes
Dur. dolor. — L. durante
    dolore (while the pain lasts)
Du·ret's lesion
Dur·ham rule
Dur·ham's tube
du·ro·ar·ach·ni·tis
Du·ro·zi·ez' disease
Du·ro·zi·ez' murmur
Du·ro·zi·ez' sign
dusk·i·ness
dusky
dust
    blood d. (of Müller)
    chromatin d.

Dur-Plex

dust *(continued)*
    ear d.
dust-borne
Dutch·er body
dUTP — deoxyuridine triphosphate
Dut·ton's relapsing fever
Dut·ton's spirochete
Dut·to·nel·la
Du·Val procedure
Du·val's nucleus
Duve, Christian René de
Du·ver·ney's foramen
Du·ver·ney's gland
Du·void
Du·Vries hammer toe repair
DV — dependent variable dilute volume
dv — double vibrations
DVD — dissociated vertical divergence
DVM — Doctor of Veterinary Medicine
DVT — deep venous thrombosis
dwarf
    achondroplastic d.
    acromelic d.
    adrenal d.
    Amsterdam d.
    asexual d.
    ateliotic d.
    bird-headed d. of Seckel
    Brissaud's d.
    camptomelic d.
    chondrodystrophic d.
    cretin d.
    diastrophic d.
    geleophysic d.
    hypophysial d.
    hypopituitary d.
    hypoplastic d.
    hyposomatotropic d.
    hypothyroid d.
    idiopathic d.
    infantile d.
    Laron d.
    Levi-Lorain d.

dwarf *(continued)*
    mesomelic d.
    micromelic d.
    nanocephalic d.
    normal d.
    Paltauf's d.
    panhypopituitary d.
    phocomelic d.
    physiologic d.
    pituitary d.
    Pott's d.
    prepubertal d.
    primordial d.
    pure d.
    rachitic d.
    renal d.
    rhizomelic d.
    Russell d.
    Seckel d.
    senile d.
    sexual d.
    sexual ateliotic d.
    Silver d.
    thanatophoric d.
    thyroid d.
    true d.
dwarf·ism
    cardiac d.
    deprivation d.
    diabetic d.
    exostotic d.
    myxedematous d.
    pituitary d.
    polydystrophic d.
    pseudometatropic d.
    psychosocial d.
    Robinow d.
    thanatophoric d.
    Walt Disney d.
Dy — dysprosium
dy·ad
dy·ad·ic
dy·as·ter
Dy·a·zide
Dy·clone
dy·clo·nine hy·dro·chlo·ride
dy·dro·ges·ter·one

dye
- acid d.
- acidic d.
- amphoteric d.
- anionic d.
- azo d.
- basic d.
- cationic d.
- fluorescein d.
- metachromatic d.
- orthochromatic d.
- vital d.

Dy·me·lor
dy·nam·ic
dy·nam·ics
- group d.
- topological d.

dy·na·mo·gen·e·sis
dy·na·mo·gen·ic
dy·na·mog·e·ny
dy·namo·graph
dy·na·mom·e·ter
- squeeze d.

dy·namo·neure
dy·namo·path·ic
dy·namo·phore
dy·namo·pho·ric
dy·namo·scope
dy·na·mos·co·py
Dy·na·pen
dyne
dy·ne·in
dy·phyl·line
Dy·ren·i·um
dys·acou·sia
dys·acous·ma
dys·acu·sis
dys·ad·ap·ta·tion
dys·ad·re·nal·ism
dys·al·li·log·na·thia
dys·an·ag·no·sia
dys·an·ti·gra·phia
dys·aphia
dys·ap·ta·tion
dys·ar·te·ri·ot·o·ny
dys·ar·thria
- ataxic d.
- cerebellar d.

dys·ar·thria *(continued)*
- developmental d.
- d. literalis
- spastic d.
- d. syllabaris spasmodica

dys·ar·thric
dys·ar·thro·sis
- craniofacial d.

dys·au·to·no·mia
- familial d.

dys·bar·ism
- altitude d.

dys·ba·sia
- d. lordotica progressiva

dys·be·ta·lipo·pro·tein·emia
- familial d.

dys·bi·o·sis
dys·bo·lism
dys·cal·cu·lia
dys·ceph·a·ly
- mandibulo-oculofacial d.

dys·che·zia
dys·chi·a·sia
dys·chi·ria
dys·cho·lia
dys·chon·dro·gen·e·sis
dys·chon·dro·pla·sia
dys·chon·dro·ste·o·sis
dys·chro·ma·sia
dys·chro·ma·top·sia
dys·chro·ma·to·sis
dys·chro·mia
dys·chro·nism
dys·chro·no·me·tria
dys·chro·nous
dys·chy·lia
dys·ci·ne·sia
dys·coi·me·sis
dys·con·trol
- episodic d.

dys·co·ria
dys·cor·ti·cism
dys·cra·sia
- blood d.
- plasma cell d's

dys·cra·sic
dys·crat·ic
dys·di·ad·o·cho·ki·ne·sia

dys·di·ad·o·cho·ki·net·ic
dys·dip·sia
dys·eco·ia
dys·em·bry·o·ma
dys·em·bryo·pla·sia
dys·en·ce·pha·lia splanch·no·
cys·ti·ca
dys·en·ter·ic
dys·en·ter·i·form
dys·en·tery
    amebic d.
    asylum d.
    bacillary d.
    balantidial d.
    bilharzial d.
    catarrhal d.
    chronic d. of cattle
    ciliary d.
    ciliate d.
    epidemic d.
    flagellate d.
    Flexner's d.
    fulminant d.
    giardiasis d.
    helminthic d.
    institutional d.
    Japanese d.
    malarial d.
    malignant d.
    protozoal d.
    schistosomal d.
    scorbutic d.
    Shiga's d.
    Sonne d.
    spirillar d.
    sporadic d.
    viral d.
dys·equi·lib·ri·um
dys·er·e·the·sia
dys·er·e·thism
dys·er·gia
dys·eryth·ro·poi·e·sis
dys·eryth·ro·poi·et·ic
dys·es·the·sia
    auditory d.
dys·es·thet·ic
dys·fi·brin·o·gen·emia

dys·func·tion
    central auditory d.
    constitutional hepatic d.
    hypertonic uterine d.
    hypotonic uterine d.
    minimal brain d.
    myofascial pain d.
    orgasmic d.
    papillary muscle d.
    d. of uterus
dys·func·tion·al
dys·ga·lac·tia
dys·gam·ma·glob·u·lin·emia
dys·gram·ma·tax·ia
dys·ge·ne·sia
dys·gen·e·sis
    disseminated nodular d.
    epiphyseal d.
    gonadal d.
    iridocorneal mesodermal d.
    mixed gonadal d.
    pure gonadal d.
    reticular d.
    Rieger's d.
    seminiferous tubule d.
dys·gen·ic
dys·gen·ics
dys·gen·i·tal·ism
dys·ger·mi·no·ma
dys·geu·sia
dys·glob·u·lin·emia
dys·gly·ce·mia
dys·gna·thia
dys·gnath·ic
dys·gno·sia
dys·go·ne·sis
dys·gon·ic
dys·gram·ma·tism
dys·gra·phia
dys·hem·a·to·poi·e·sis
dys·hem·a·to·poi·e·tic
dys·he·mo·poi·e·sis
dys·he·mo·poi·et·ic
dys·he·pa·tia
    lipogenic d.
dys·he·sion
dys·hi·dro·sis

dys·hy·dro·sis
dys·idro·sis
dys·im·mu·no·glob·u·lin·
  emia
dys·junc·tion
dys·kary·o·sis
dys·kary·ot·ic
dys·ker·a·to·ma
  warty d.
dys·ker·a·to·sis
  d. congenita
  congenital d.
  hereditary benign
    intraepithelial d.
  isolated d. follicularis
dys·ker·a·tot·ic
dys·ki·ne·sia
  biliary d.
  BLM (buccal-lingual-
    masticatory) d.
  facial d.
  d. intermittens
  occupational d.
  orofacial d.
  phenothiazine-induced d.
  tardive d.
  tracheobronchial d.
dys·ki·net·ic
dys·koi·me·sis
dys·la·lia
dys·lex·ia
  congenital d.
  developmental d.
dys·lip·i·do·sis *pl.* dys·lip·i·
  do·ses
dys·lipo·pro·tein·emia
dys·lo·chia
dys·lo·gia
dys·ma·ture
dys·ma·tur·i·ty
  pulmonary d.
dys·meg·a·lop·sia
dys·me·lia
dys·men·or·rhea
  acquired d.
  congestive d.
  essential d.
  inflammatory d.

dys·men·or·rhea *(continued)*
  d. intermenstrualis
  mechanical d.
  membranous d.
  obstructive d.
  ovarian d.
  spasmodic d.
  tubal d.
  ureteric d.
  uterine d.
  vaginal d.
dys·men·tia
  tardive d.
dys·me·tab·o·lism
dys·me·tria
  ocular motor d.
dys·met·rop·sia
dys·mim·ia
dys·mne·sia
dys·mne·sic
dys·mor·phia
dys·mor·phic
dys·mor·phism
dys·mor·pho·gen·e·sis
dys·mor·phol·o·gist
dys·mor·phol·o·gy
dys·mor·pho·pho·bia
dys·mor·phop·sia
dys·mor·pho·sis
dys·my·eli·na·tion
dys·my·elo·poi·et·ic
dys·myo·to·nia
dys·no·mia
dys·odon·ti·a·sis
dys·odyn·ia
dys·on·to·gen·e·sis
dys·on·to·ge·net·ic
dys·opia
  d. algera
dys·op·sia
dys·orex·ia
dys·or·gano·pla·sia
dys·or·ia
dys·or·ic
dys·os·mia
dys·os·teo·gen·e·sis
dys·os·to·sis
  acrofacial d.

dys·os·to·sis *(continued)*
    craniofacial d.
    d. enchondralis
      epiphysaria
    mandibulofacial d.
    maxillonasal d.
    metaphyseal d.
    d. multiplex
    Nager's acrofacial d.
    nasomaxillary d.
    orodigitofacial d.
    otomandibular d.
dys·ox·i·da·tive
dys·ox·i·diz·able
dys·pa·reu·nia
dys·pep·sia
    acid d.
    appendicular d.
    catarrhal d.
    chichiko d.
    cholelithic d.
    colon d.
    fermentative d.
    flatulent d.
    gastric d.
    intestinal d.
dys·pep·tic
dys·per·i·stal·sis
dys·pha·gia
    contractile ring d.
    d. globosa
    d. inflammatoria
    d. lusoria
    d. nervosa
    d. paralytica
    sideropenic d.
    d. spastica
    tropical d.
    vallecular d.
    d. valsalviana
dys·phag·ic
dys·pha·sia
dys·phe·mia
dys·pho·nia
    d. clericorum
    dysplastic d.
    d. plicae ventricularis
    d. puberum

dys·pho·nia *(continued)*
    spasmodic d.
    spastic d.
    d. spastica
dys·phon·ic
dys·pho·ret·ic
dys·pho·ria
dys·pho·ri·ant
dys·phor·ic
dys·phra·sia
dys·phy·lax·ia
dys·pig·men·ta·tion
dys·pla·sia
    anhidrotic ectodermal d.
    anteroposterior facial d.
    asphyxiating thoracic d.
    atriodigital d.
    bronchopulmonary d.
    camptomelic d.
    caudal d.
    d. of cervix
    chondroectodermal d.
    cleidocranial d.
    congenital alveolar d.
    congenital d. of hip
    cranio-carpotarsal d.
    craniodiaphyseal d.
    craniometaphyseal d.
    craniometaphyseal d. of
      Pyle
    craniotelencephalic d.
    cretinoid d.
    dental d.
    dentinal d.
    dentoalveolar d.
    diaphyseal d.
    ectodermal d's
    ectodermal d., hidrotic
    ectodermal d., hypohidrotic
    enamel d.
    encephalo-ophthalmic d.
    epiphyseal d.
    d. epiphysealis hemimelica
    d. epiphysealis multiplex
    d. epiphysealis punctata
    extracranial fibromuscular
      d.
    faciogenital d.

dys·pla·sia *(continued)*
   familial white folded
      mucosal d.
   fibromuscular d.
   fibrous d. (of bone)
   fibrous d. of jaw
   florid osseous d.
   hereditary bone d.
   hereditary renal-retinal d.
   d. linguofacialis
   mammary d.
   metaphyseal d.
   Mondini's d.
   monostotic fibrous d.
   multiple epiphyseal d.
   nuclear d.
   oculoauricular d.
   oculoauriculovertebral
      (OAV) d.
   oculodentodigital d.
   oculodentoosseous d.
   olfactory genital d.
   ophthalmomandibulomelic
      d.
   oral familial white folded
      d.
   osseous d.
   osteodental d.
   periapical cemental d.
   polyostotic fibrous d.
   progressive diaphyseal d.
   pseudoachrondroplastic d.
   renal d.
   retinal d.
   skeletal d.
   skeletodental d.
   spondyloepiphyseal d.
   spondylometaepiphyseal d.
   Streeter's d.
   thanatophoric d.
   thymic d.
   ureteral neuromuscular d.
   ventriculoradial d.
dys·plas·tic
dysp·nea
   cardiac d.
   exertional d.
   expiratory d.

dysp·nea *(continued)*
   functional d.
   inspiratory d.
   nocturnal d.
   nonexpansional d.
   orthostatic d.
   paroxysmal nocturnal d.
   renal d.
   sighing d.
   two-flight d.
dysp·ne·ic
dys·poi·e·sis
dys·poi·et·ic
dys·pon·der·al
dys·po·ne·sis
dys·pra·gia
dys·prax·ia
dys·pro·si·um
dys·pros·o·dy
dys·pro·te·in·emia
dys·pro·throm·bin·emia
dys·ra·phia
   prosencephalic d.
   spinal d.
dys·ra·phism
dys·re·flex·ia
   autonomic d.
dys·rhyth·mia
   cerebral d.
   cortical d.
   electroencephalographic d.
   esophageal d.
   paroxysmal cerebral d.
   d. pneumophrasia
   sinus d.
dys·se·ba·cia
dys·so·mat·og·no·sia
dys·som·nia
dys·sper·mia
dys·sta·sia
   hereditary areflexic d.
dys·stat·ic
dys·sym·bo·lia
dys·sym·me·try
dys·syn·er·gia
   biliary d.
   d. cerebellaris myoclonica
   d. cerebellaris progressiva

dys·syn·er·gy
dys·ta·sia
   hereditary ataxic d.
   Roussy-Lévy hereditary
     ataxic d.
dys·tax·ia
dys·tec·tia
dys·te·le·ol·o·gy
dys·thy·mia
dys·thy·mic
dys·thy·re·o·sis
dys·thy·roid
dys·thy·roid·al
dys·thy·roid·ism
dys·tim·bria
dys·tith·ia
dys·to·cia
   cervical d.
   constriction ring d.
   contraction ring d.
   fetal d.
   maternal d.
   placental d.
dys·to·nia
   attitudinal d.
   autonomic d.
   d. deformans progressiva
   hypersympatheticotonic d.
   kinetic d.
   d. lenticularis
   d. musculorum deformans
   periodic d.
   tardive d.
   torsion d.
dys·ton·ic
dys·to·pia
   crossed d. of kidney
   simple renal d.
dys·top·ic
dys·tro·phia
   d. adiposa corneae
   d. adiposogenitalis
   d. brevicollis
   d. endothelialis corneae
   d. epithelialis corneae
   d. mediana canaliformis
   d. mesodermalis congenita
     hyperplastica

dys·tro·phia *(continued)*
   d. myotonica
   d. unguium
dys·troph·ic
dys·troph·in
dys·tropho·neu·ro·sis
dys·tro·phy
   adiposogenital d.
   Albright's d.
   arthritic d.
   asphyxiating thoracic d.
     (ATD)
   Becker's d.
   Best's macular d.
   Biber-Haab-Dimmer d.
   corneal d.
   craniocarpotarsal d.
   crystalline d. of cornea
   Dejerine-Landouzy d.
   distal muscular d.
   Duchenne type muscular d.
   Duchenne-Landouzy d.
   endothelial corneal d.
   Erb's d.
   facioscapulohumeral
     muscular d.
   familial osseous d.
   Fröhlich's adiposogenital d.
   Fuchs' d.
   Gowers type muscular d.
   Groenouw's corneal d.
   gutter d. of cornea
   hereditary vitelliform d.
   hypophysial d.
   infantile neuroaxonal d.
   juvenile progressive
     muscular d.
   Landouzy's d.
   Landouzy-Dejerine d.
   lattice d. (of cornea)
   Leyden-Möbius d.
   limb-girdle muscular d.
   macular corneal d.
   median canaliform d. of
     nail
   muscular d.
   myotonic d.
   neuroaxonal proteid d.

dys·tro·phy *(continued)*
   ocular muscular d.
   oculocerebrorenal d.
   oculopharyngeal muscular
     d.
   progressive muscular d.
   progressive tapetochoroidal
     d.
   pseudohypertrophic
     muscular d.
   reflex sympathetic d.
   Salzmann's nodular
     corneal d.
   Schlichting d.
   Seitelberger's d.
   sex-linked muscular d.
   Simmerlin's d.

dys·tro·phy *(continued)*
   speckled d. of cornea
   tapetochoroidal d.
   thoracic-pelvic-phalangeal
     d.
   thyroneural d.
   vitelliform macular d.
   wound d.
dys·tryp·sia
dys·ure·sia
dys·uria
   spastic d.
dys·uriac
dys·uric
dys·vi·ta·min·o·sis
dys·zoo·sper·mia

E

E — emmetropia
E — elastance
   electromotive force
   energy
   expectancy
   illumination
   redox potential
E_1 — estrone
E_2 — estradiol
E_3 — estriol
E_4 — estetrol
E_h — redox potential
$E°$ — standard reduction
  potential
e — electron
e — elementary unit of
   electric charge
e^+ — positron
e^- — electron
ϵ — molar absorptivity
η — absolute viscosity
   educational age

EA — erythrocyte antibody
EAC — erythrocyte antibody
  complement
EACA — epsilon-amino-
  caproic acid
ead. — L. eadem (the same)
EAE — experimental allergic
  encephalomyelitis
Ea·gle-Bar·rett syndrome
EAHF — eczema, asthma, hay
  fever (complex)
Eales' disease
EAP — epiallopregnanolone
Ea. R. — Ger.
  Entartungs-Reaktion
  (reaction of degeneration)
ear
   acute e.
   artificial e.
   aviator's e.
   Aztec e.
   bat e.

ear *(continued)*
    beach e.
    Blainville e's
    Cagot e.
    cat's e.
    cauliflower e.
    cockleshell e.
    constricted e.
    cup e.
    Darwin's e.
    dead e.
    diabetic e.
    external e.
    glue e.
    hairy e's
    Hong Kong e.
    hot weather e.
    internal e.
    lop e.
    middle e.
    Morel e.
    Mozart e.
    prizefighter e.
    satyr e.
    scroll e.
    shell e.
    Singapore e.
    Stahl e. No. 1
    Stahl e. No. 2
    swimmer's e.
    tank e.
    tropical e.
    Wildermuth's e.
ear·ache
ear·drum
ear·lobe
ear-mind·ed
ear·wax
EAST — external rotation
    abduction stress test
Ea·ton agent pneumonia
Ea·ton-Lam·bert syndrome
EB — elementary body
Eberth's lines
EBL — estimated blood loss
EBNA — Epstein-Barr
    nuclear antigen (test)
Eb·ner's fibrils

Eb·ner's gland
Eb·ner's line
Eb·ner's reticulum
Ebola hemorrhagic fever
Ebola virus
ebo·na·tion
ébranle·ment
Eb·stein's angle
Eb·stein's anomaly
Eb·stein's disease
eb·ul·li·tion
ebur
    e. dentis
ebur·nat·ed
ebur·na·tion
    e. of dentin
ebur·ne·ous
ebur·ni·tis
EBV — Epstein-Barr virus
EC — Enzyme Commission
écar·teur
ecau·date
ec·bol·ic
ec·bol·i·um
ec·bo·vi·rus
ec·cen·tric
ec·cen·tro·chon·dro·pla·sia
ec·cen·tro-os·teo·chon·dro·
    dys·pla·sia
ec·chon·dro·ma
ec·chon·dro·sis
ec·chon·dro·tome
ec·chor·do·sis phys·a·liph·o·
    ra
ec·chy·mo·ma
ec·chy·mosed
ec·chy·mo·sis *pl.* ec·chy·mo·
    ses
    cadaveric e's
    Roederer's e.
ec·chy·mot·ic
Ec·cles, Sir John Carew
ec·crine
ec·cri·sis
ec·crit·ic
ec·cy·e·sis
ec·dem·ic
ec·do·vi·rus

ec·dy·si·asm
ec·dy·sis
    erythrocyte e.
ec·dy·sone
ECF — extended care facility
  extracellular fluid
ECF-A — eosinophil
  chemotactic factor of
  anaphylaxis
ECG — electrocardiogram
ec·go·nine
echid·nase
echid·nin
Ech·id·noph·a·ga
    E. gallinacea
echid·no·tox·in
echid·no·vac·cine
ech·i·nate
echin·e·none
Ech·i·no·chas·mus
    E. perfoliatus
echi·no·chrome
echi·no·coc·ci·a·sis
echi·no·coc·co·sis
echi·no·coc·cot·o·my
Echi·no·coc·cus
    E. alveolaris
    E. granulosus
    E. multilocularis
echi·no·coc·cus *pl.* echi·no·
  coc·ci
echi·no·cyte
echi·no·derm
Echi·no·lae·laps
    E. echidninus
echin·oph·thal·mia
Echi·no·rhyn·chus
    E. gigas
    E. hominis
    E. moniliformis
ech·i·no·sis
Echi·no·ste·li·ida
Ech·i·no·sto·ma
echi·no·sto·mi·a·sis
echin·u·late
Echis
ech·no·thi·o·phate io·dide

ECHO — enteric
  cytopathogenic human
  orphan (virus)
echo
    amphoric e.
    cochlear e.
    metallic e.
    midline e.
echo·acou·sia
echo·car·dio·gram
echo·car·di·og·ra·phy
    cross-sectional e.
    Doppler e.
    M-mode e.
    real-time e.
    two-dimensional e.
echo·en·ceph·a·lo·gram
echo·en·ceph·a·lo·graph
    midline e.
echo·en·ceph·a·log·ra·phy
echo·gen·ic
echo·ge·ni·ci·ty
echo·gram
echo·gra·phia
echog·ra·phy
echo·ing
    thought e.
echo·ki·ne·sis
echo·la·lia
echo·lam·i·nog·ra·phy
echo·lu·cent
echo·ma·tism
echo·mim·ia
echo·mo·tism
echop·a·thy
echo·pho·no·car·di·og·ra·phy
echoph·o·ny
echo·phot·o·ny
echo·phra·sia
echo·prax·ia
echo·prax·is
echo-rang·ing
echo·scope
echo·thi·o·phate
echo·vi·rus
    e. 28
Eck's fistula
Eck·er's fissure

Eck·er's fluid
Eck·hout vertical gastroplasty
ec·la·bi·um
Ec·la·bron
eclamp·sia
    cerebral e.
    puerperal e.
    superimposed e.
    uremic e.
eclamp·sism
eclamp·tic
eclamp·to·gen·ic
eclec·tic
eclec·ti·cism
eclipse
ec·ly·sis
ec·mne·sia
ECMO — extracorporeal
  membrane oxygenation
ec·mo·vi·rus
eco·ge·net·ics
E. coli — *Escherichia coli*
econ·a·zole ni·trate
Econ·o·mo's disease
Econ·o·mo's encephalitis
econ·o·my
    token e.
eco·par·a·site
écor·ché
eco·site
ecos·tate
eco·tax·is
Ec·o·trin
eco·trop·ic
écou·vil·lon
écou·vil·lo·nage
ec·phy·a·di·tis
ECS — electroconvulsive
  shock
ECSO — enteric
  cytopathogenic swine orphan
  (virus)
écrase·ment
écra·seur
ec·so·mat·ics
ec·so·vi·rus
ec·stro·phy

ECT — electroconvulsive
  therapy
ec·ta·co·lia
ec·tad
ec·tal
ec·ta·sia
    alveolar e.
    annuloaortic e.
    corneal e.
    diffuse arterial e.
    hypostatic e.
    mammary duct e.
    papillary e.
    scleral e.
    senile e.
    tubular e.
ec·ta·sis
ec·tat·ic
ec·ten·tal
ec·tero·graph
ec·teth·moid
ec·thy·ma
    contagious e.
    e. gangrenosum
ec·thy·mi·form
ec·to·an·ti·gen
ec·to·bi·ol·o·gy
ec·to·blast
    primary e.
ec·to·car·dia
ec·to·cer·vi·cal
ec·to·cer·vix
ec·to·co·lon
ec·to·com·men·sal
ec·to·con·dyle
ec·to·cor·nea
ec·to·cra·ni·al
ec·to·cu·ne·i·form
ec·to·cyst
ec·to·cy·tic
ec·to·derm
    amniotic e.
    basal e.
    blastodermic e.
    chorionic e.
    epithelial e.
    extraembryonic e.
    neural e.

ec·to·derm *(continued)*
    primitive e.
    superficial e.
ec·to·der·mal
ec·to·der·ma·to·sis
ec·to·der·mic
ec·to·der·moid·al
ec·to·der·mo·sis
    e. erosiva pluriorificialis
ec·to·en·tad
ec·to·en·zyme
ec·to·gen·ic
ec·tog·e·nous
ec·tog·lia
ec·tog·o·ny
ec·to·hor·mone
ec·to·lec·i·thal
ec·tol·y·sis
ec·to·men·inx
ec·to·mere
ec·to·mes·en·chyme
ec·to·meso·blast
ec·to·morph
ec·to·mor·phic
ec·to·mor·phy
ec·to·my
ec·to·nu·cle·ar
ec·to·pa·gia
ec·top·a·gus
ec·to·par·a·site
ec·to·par·a·sit·i·cide
ec·to·par·a·sit·ism
ec·to·pec·to·ra·lis
ec·to·peri·to·ne·al
ec·to·peri·to·ni·tis
ec·to·phyte
ec·to·phyt·ic
ec·to·pia
    e. cloacae
    e. cordis
    crossed renal e.
    e. lentis
    e. pupillae congenita
    renal e.
    e. renis
    e. testis
    e. vesicae
    visceral e.

ec·top·ic
ec·to·pla·cen·ta
ec·to·plasm
ec·to·plas·mat·ic
ec·to·plast
ec·to·plas·tic
ec·to·pter·y·goid
ec·to·py
ec·to·ret·i·na
ec·to·sarc
ec·tos·co·py
ec·to·skel·e·ton
ec·to·sphere
ec·tos·te·al
ec·to·sto·sis
ec·to·sym·bi·ont
ec·to·therm
ec·to·therm·ic
ec·to·ther·my
ec·to·thrix
ec·to·tox·emia
ec·to·zoa
ec·to·zo·al
ec·to·zo·on *pl.* ec·to·zoa
ec·tro·chei·ry, ec·tro·chi·ry
ec·tro·dac·ty·ly
ec·tro·gen·ic
ec·trog·e·ny
ec·tro·me·lia
    infectious e.
ec·tro·mel·ic
ec·trom·e·lus
ec·tro·meta·car·pia
ec·tro·meta·tar·sia
ec·tro·pha·lan·gia
ec·tro·pi·on
    atonic e.
    cervical e.
    e. cicatriceum
    cicatricial e.
    flaccid e.
    e. luxurians
    mechanical e.
    paralytic e.
    e. of pigment layer
    e. sarcomatosum
    senile e.
    spastic e.

ec·tro·pi·on *(continued)*
    e. uveae
ec·tro·pi·o·nize
ec·trop·o·dy
ec·tro·sis
ec·tro·syn·dac·ty·ly
ec·trot·ic
ec·tyl·urea
ec·ty·on·in
ec·type
ec·typ·ia
ec·ze·ma
    allergic e.
    asteatotic e.
    atopic e.
    autoallergic e.
    bakers' e.
    bullous e. of legs
    e. craquelé
    dry e.
    dyshidrotic e.
    dyskeratotic e. of hand
    facial e. of ruminants
    fissured e.
    flexural e.
    e. herpeticum
    e. hypertrophicum
    infantile e.
    infective e.
    intertriginous e.
    e. intertrigo
    lichenoid e.
    e. marginatum
    e. medicamentosa
    nipple e.
    nummular e.
    occupational e.
    e. parasiticum
    phlyctenular e.
    pustular e.
    e. rhagadiforme
    seborrheic e.
    e. siccum
    stasis e.
    e. vaccinatum
    varicose e.
    xerotic e.
ec·zem·a·ti·za·tion

ec·zem·a·to·gen·ic
ec·zem·a·toid
ec·zem·a·tous
ED — erythema dose
ED_{50} [ED50] — median
  effective dose
edath·a·mil
    calcium disodium e.
    e. disodium
EDB — ethylene dibromide
Ed·dowes' disease
Ed·dowes' syndrome
Ed·e·bohls' position
Edec·rin
ede·itis
Edel·man, Gerald Maurice
Edel·mann's anemia
Edel·mann's cell
ede·ma
    alimentary e.
    angioneurotic e.
    Berlin's e.
    brain e.
    brawny e.
    brown e.
    e. bullosum vesicae
    Calabar e.
    e. calidum
    cardiac e.
    cerebral e.
    circumscribed e.
    dependent e.
    famine e.
    fingerprint e.
    e. frigidum
    e. fugax
    gaseous e.
    gestational e.
    giant e.
    e. glottidis
    hepatic e.
    hereditary angioneurotic e.
      (HANE)
    high-altitude pulmonary e.
    Huguenin's e.
    hunger e.
    hydremic e.
    idiopathic e.

ede·ma *(continued)*
 inflammatory e.
 insulin e.
 interstitial e.
 invisible e.
 lymphatic e.
 malignant e.
 menstrual e.
 Milroy's e.
 Milton's e.
 mucous e.
 e. neonatorum
 nephritic e.
 nephrotic e.
 noninflammatory e.
 nonpitting e.
 nutritional e.
 paroxysmal pulmonary e.
 passive e.
 periodic e.
 periretinal e.
 pitting e.
 placental e.
 prehepatic e.
 pulmonary e.
 purulent e.
 Quincke's e.
 Reinke e.
 renal e.
 rheumatismal e.
 salt e.
 solid e.
 solid e. of lungs
 subglottic e.
 terminal e.
 toxic e.
 tubular e.
 turban e.
 vasogenic e.
 venous e.
 vernal e. of lung
 war e.
 wound e.
ede·ma·gen
edem·a·tig·e·nous
edem·a·ti·za·tion
edem·a·to·gen·ic
edem·a·tous

Eden·ta·ta
eden·tate
eden·tia
eden·tu·late
eden·tu·lous
ed·e·tate
 e. calcium disodium
 e. disodium
 ferric sodium e.
 e. sodium
 e. trisodium
edet·ic acid
 e. a. disodium salt
edge
 cutting e.
 denture e.
 incisal e.
edge-strength
EdGr — Edmondson Grading
 (System)
ed·i·ble
Ed·ing·er's law
Ed·ing·er's nucleus
Ed·ing·er-West·phal nucleus
Ed·i·son effect
edis·y·late
Ed·mond·son Grading (EdGr)
 System
EDR — effective direct
 radiation
EDRF — endothelium-derived
 relaxing factor
ed·ro·pho·ni·um
 e. bromide
 e. chloride
Ed·sall's disease
EDTA — ethylenediaminetetraacetic acid
ed·u·ca·ble
ed·u·ca·tion
 compensatory e.
 health e.
educt
educ·tion
Ed·wards syndrome
Ed·ward·si·el·la
 E. hoshinae
 E. ictaluri

Ed·ward·si·el·la (continued)
  E. tarda
Ed·ward·si·el·leae
EEE — eastern equine
  encephalomyelitis
EEG — electroencephalogram
  electroencephalography
eel·worm
EENT — eye-ear-nose-throat
EERP — extended endocardial
  resection procedure
EFA — essential fatty acids
E-Fer·ol
ef·face·ment
ef·fect
  additive e.
  adverse e.
  anachoretic e.
  Anrep e.
  Auger e.
  Bainbridge e.
  Bezold-Jarisch e.
  Blinks e's
  Bohr e.
  Bruce e.
  cis-trans position e.
  clasp-knife e.
  cohort e.
  columella e.
  Compton e.
  contrary e.
  contrast e.
  copper wire e.
  Cotton e.
  Crabtree e.
  crowding e.
  cumulative e.
  cytopathic e.
  Danysz e.
  Deelman e.
  Donnan e.
  Doppler e.
  Edison e.
  electrophonic e.
  electrotonic e.
  Emerson e.
  experimenter e's
  Fahraeus-Lindqvist e.

ef·fect *(continued)*
  field e.
  founder e.
  gene dose e.
  generation e.
  glucose e.
  graded e.
  Haldane e.
  Hallberg e.
  Hallwachs e.
  heel e.
  Hering e.
  hybrid e.
  hyperchromic e.
  hypochromic e.
  inductive e.
  interpolar e.
  isomorphic e.
  isotope e.
  Köbner's e.
  mass e.
  Mierzejewski e.
  muscarinic e.
  Nagler e.
  nicotine e.
  Orbeli e.
  Pasteur e.
  photechic e.
  photoelectrical e.
  piezoelectric e.
  placebo e.
  polar e.
  position e.
  pressure e.
  Purkinje e.
  quantal e.
  Raman e.
  relative biologic e.
  Russell e.
  second gas e.
  side e.
  silver wire e.
  Somogyi e.
  Soret e.
  specific dynamic e.
  Staub-Traugott e.
  Stiles-Crawford e.
  treppe e.

ef·fect *(continued)*
   Tyndall e.
   variegated position e.
   Venturi e.
   Vulpian's e.
   Wever-Bray e.
   Whitten e.
   Wolff-Chaikoff e.
   Zeeman e.
ef·fec·tive·ness
   relative biological e.
ef·fec·tor
   allosteric e.
ef·fem·i·na·tion
ef·fer·ent
   α-e. [alpha-]
   β-e. [beta-]
   dynamic γ-e. [gamma-]
   general visceral e.
   somatic e.
   special visceral e.
   static γ-e. [gamma-]
ef·fer·en·tial
ef·fer·ves·cent
ef·fi·ca·cy
ef·fi·cien·cy
   counting e.
   detection e.
   intrinsic counter e.
   photopeak e.
   production e.
   window e.
ef·fleu·rage
ef·flo·resce
ef·flo·res·cence
ef·flo·res·cent
ef·fluve
ef·flu·vi·um *pl.* ef·flu·via
   anagen e.
   telluric e.
   telogen e.
ef·frac·tion
ef·fu·ma·bil·i·ty
ef·fuse
ef·fu·sion
   chylous e.
   hemorrhagic e.
   middle ear e.

ef·fu·sion *(continued)*
   pericardial e.
   pleural e.
   subdural e.
Ef·u·dex
EGD — esophagogastroduod-
enoscopy
eger·sim·e·ter
egest
eges·ta
eges·tion
Eg·ger's line
Eg·gers' plate
Eg·gle·ston's method
egi·lops
egland·u·lous
ego
   body e.
ego·bron·choph·o·ny
ego·cen·tric
ego-dys·ton·ic
ego-ide·al
ego·ism
ego·ma·nia
egoph·o·ny
ego-strength
ego-syn·ton·ic
ego·tism
ego·trop·ic
EHBF — estimated hepatic
blood flow
   extrahepatic blood flow
EHDP — ethane-1-hydroxy-
1,1-diphosphonate
Eh·lers-Dan·los disease
Eh·lers-Dan·los syndrome
Ehr·en·rit·ter's ganglion
Ehr·lich's body
Ehr·lich's granule
Ehr·lich's reaction
Ehr·lich's stain
Ehr·lich's test
Ehr·lich's theory
Ehr·lich's tumor
Ehr·lich-Ha·ta preparation
Ehr·lich-Ha·ta remedy
Ehr·lich-Ha·ta treatment
Ehr·lich-Heinz granules

Ehr·lich·ia
  E. canis
Ehr·lich·i·eae
ehr·lich·i·osis
EIA — enzyme immunoassay
Eich·horst's atrophy
Eich·horst's corpuscles
Eich·horst's type
Eic·ken's method
ei·co·nom·e·ter
ei·co·sa·no·ate
ei·co·sa·no·ic acid
ei·co·sa·noid
ei·co·sa·pen·ta·eno·ic acid
  (EPA)
EID — emergency infusion
  device
ei·det·ic
ei·do·gen
ei·dop·tom·e·try
EIEC — enteroinvasive
  Escherichia coli
Eijk·man's test
Ei·ken·el·la
  E. corrodens
ei·ko·nom·e·ter
ei·loid
Ei·me·ri·i·na
Ein·horn's saccharimeter
Ein·horn's string test
ein·stei·ni·um
Ein·tho·ven's formula
Ein·tho·ven's galvanometer
Ein·tho·ven's triangle
eis·an·the·ma
Ei·sen·men·ger's complex
ei·sod·ic
EIT — erythrocyte iron
  turnover
Ei·tel·berg's test
ei·weiss·milch
ejac·u·late
ejac·u·la·tio
  e. deficiens
  e. praecos
  e. retardata
ejac·u·la·tion
  premature e.

ejac·u·la·tor
  e. seminis
ejac·u·la·to·ry
ejac·u·lum
ejec·ta
ejec·tion
  milk e.
ejec·tor
  saliva e.
Ejusd. — L. ejusdem (of the
  same)
Ek·bom syndrome
EKG — electrocardiogram
eki·ri
EKY — electrokymogram
elab·o·rate
elab·o·ra·tion
el·a·cin
el·a·id·ic acid
elai·op·a·thy
  pathomimic e.
el·aio·plast
el·an·trine
el·a·pid
Elap·i·dae
Elaps
elas·so·sis
elas·tance
elas·tic
  intermaxillary e.
  intramaxillary e.
  vertical e.
elas·ti·ca
elas·ti·cin
elas·tic·i·ty
elas·tin
elas·tin·ase
elas·to·blast
elas·to·fi·bro·ma
  e. dorsi
  perforating e.
elas·to·gel
elas·toid
elas·toi·do·sis
  nodular e.
elas·tol·y·sis
  generalized e.

elas·tol·y·sis *(continued)*
    perifollicular e.
    postinflammatory e.
elas·to·lyt·ic
elas·to·ma
    juvenile e.
    Miescher's e.
elas·to·mer
elas·tom·e·ter
elas·tom·e·try
elas·to·mu·cin
elas·top·a·thy
Elas·to·plast
elas·tor·rhex·is
elas·tose
elas·to·sis
    actinic e.
    nodular e. of
      Favre-Racouchot
    nodular e. of skin
    e. perforans serpiginosa
    perforating e.
    senile e.
    solar e.
elas·tot·ic
Elaut's triangle
El·a·vil
el·bow
    baseball pitchers' e.
    beat e.
    capped e.
    dropped e.
    golfer's e.
    little leaguer's e.
    miners' e.
    nursemaids' e.
    pulled e.
    students' e.
    tennis e.
El·da·dryl
El·de·cort
El·do·dram
El·do·paque
El·do·quin
el·drin
elec·tive
Elec·tra com·plex
elec·tro·acu·punc·ture

elec·tro·af·fin·i·ty
elec·tro·an·al·ge·sia
elec·tro·anal·y·sis
elec·tro·an·es·the·sia
elec·tro·aug·men·ta·tion
elec·tro·ba·so·graph
elec·tro·bi·ol·o·gy
elec·tro·bi·os·co·py
elec·tro·cap·il·lar·i·ty
elec·tro·car·dio·gram
    bipolar e.
    scalar e.
    twelve-lead e.
    unipolar e.
elec·tro·car·di·og·ra·phy
    intrabronchial e.
    intracardiac e.
    precordial e.
elec·tro·ca·tal·y·sis
elec·tro·cau·ter·iza·tion
elec·tro·cau·tery
elec·tro·cer·e·bel·lo·gram
elec·tro·chem·is·try
elec·tro·chro·ma·tog·ra·phy
elec·tro·ci·sion
elec·tro·co·ag·u·la·tion
elec·tro·coch·le·o·graph
elec·tro·coch·leo·graph·ic
elec·tro·coch·le·og·ra·phy
elec·tro·co·ma
elec·tro·con·trac·til·i·ty
elec·tro·con·vul·sive
elec·tro·cor·ti·co·gram
elec·tro·cor·ti·cog·ra·phy
elec·tro·cu·tion
elec·tro·cys·tog·ra·phy
elec·trode
    active e.
    calomel e.
    carbon dioxide e.
    central terminal e.
    Clark e.
    depolarizing e.
    dispersing e.
    esophageal e.
    exciting e.
    fixed e.
    glass e.

elec·trode *(continued)*
    impregnated e.
    indifferent e.
    ion-selective e.
    localizing e.
    multiple point e.
    periaqueductal gray e.
    point e.
    scalp e.
    return e.
    reversible e.
    silent e.
    therapeutic e.
    transcutaneous oxygen e.
elec·tro·der·mal
elec·tro·der·ma·tome
elec·tro·des·ic·ca·tion
elec·tro·di·ag·no·sis
elec·tro·di·ag·nos·tics
elec·tro·di·al·y·sis
elec·tro·di·a·ly·zer
elec·tro·di·aph·a·ke
elec·tro·di·a·phane
elec·tro·di·aph·a·no·scope
elec·tro·di·aph·a·nos·co·py
elec·tro·en·ceph·a·lo·gram
    flat e.
    isoelectric e.
elec·tro·en·ceph·a·lo·graph
elec·tro·en·ceph·a·log·ra·phy
elec·tro·en·ceph·a·lo·scope
elec·tro·en·dos·mo·sis
elec·tro·ex·ci·sion
elec·tro·fo·cus·ing
elec·tro·gal·van·ic
elec·tro·gas·tro·gram
elec·tro·gas·tro·graph
elec·tro·gas·trog·ra·phy
elec·tro·gen·ic
elec·tro·glot·tog·ra·phy
elec·tro·go·ni·om·e·ter
elec·tro·gram
    His bundle e.
elec·tro·graph
elec·trog·ra·phy
elec·tro·gus·tom·e·ter
elec·tro·gus·tom·e·try
elec·tro·he·mos·ta·sis

elec·tro·hys·tero·gram
elec·tro·hys·ter·og·ra·phy
elec·tro·im·mu·no·as·say
elec·tro·im·mu·no·dif·fu·sion
elec·tro·ki·net·ic
elec·tro·ky·mo·gram
elec·tro·ky·mo·graph
elec·tro·ky·mog·ra·phy
elec·tro·la·ryn·go·gram
elec·tro·la·ryn·go·graph
elec·tro·lar·yn·gog·ra·phy
elec·tro·lep·sy
elec·tro·li·thot·ri·ty
elec·trol·y·sis
elec·tro·lyte
    amphoteric e.
    colloidal e.
elec·tro·lyt·ic
elec·tro·lyz·a·ble
elec·tro·lyz·er
elec·tro·ma·nom·e·ter
elec·tro·ma·nom·e·try
elec·trom·e·ter
elec·tro·met·ro·gram
elec·tro·mi·gra·to·ry
elec·tro·mo·tive
elec·tro·myo·gram
elec·tro·myo·graph
elec·tro·my·og·ra·phy
    ureteral e.
elec·tron
    Auger e.
    Compton e.
    emission e.
    free e.
    secondary e.
    thermionic e.
    valence e.
elec·tro·nar·co·sis
elec·tron-dense
elec·tro·neg·a·tive
elec·tro·neg·a·tiv·i·ty
elec·tro·neu·rog·ra·phy
elec·tro·neu·rol·y·sis
elec·tro·neu·ro·my·og·ra·phy
elec·tron·ic
elec·tron·ics
elec·tron-mi·cro·scop·ic

elec·tron-mi·cro·scop·i·cal
elec·tron·volt, elec·tron volt (eV)
elec·tro·nys·tag·mo·gram
elec·tro·nys·tag·mo·graph
elec·tro·nys·tag·mog·ra·phy
elec·tro-oc·u·lo·gram
elec·tro-oc·u·log·ra·phy
elec·tro-ol·fac·to·gram
elec·tro-os·mo·sis
elec·tro·para·cen·te·sis
elec·tro·pa·thol·o·gy
elec·tro·phero·gram
elec·tro·phile
elec·tro·phil·ic
elec·tro·pho·re·gram
elec·tro·pho·re·sis
    counter e.
    countercurrent e.
    disc e.
    lipoprotein e.
    paper e.
    polyacrylamide gel e.
    protein e.
    pulsed field gradient e.
    rocket e.
    zone e.
elec·tro·pho·ret·ic
elec·tro·pho·reto·gram
elec·troph·o·rus
elec·tro·pho·tom·e·ter
elec·tro·phys·i·o·log·ic
elec·tro·phys·i·ol·o·gy
elec·tro·plat·ing
elec·tro·plexy
elec·tro·pneu·mo·graph
elec·tro·pos·i·tive
elec·tro·pros·the·sis
elec·tro·ra·di·om·e·ter
elec·tro·re·sec·tion
elec·tro·ret·i·no·gram
    E e.
    I e.
elec·tro·ret·i·nog·ra·phy
elec·tro·sa·li·vo·gram
elec·tro·scis·sion
elec·tro·scope
elec·tro·sec·tion
elec·tro·se·le·ni·um
elec·tro·shock
elec·tro·sleep
elec·tro·sol
elec·tro·spec·tro·gram
elec·tro·spec·trog·ra·phy
elec·tro·spi·no·gram
elec·tro·spi·nog·ra·phy
elec·tro·stat·ic
elec·tro·ste·nol·y·sis
elec·tro·stim·u·la·tion
elec·tro·stri·a·to·gram
elec·tro·sur·gery
elec·tro·syn·er·e·sis
elec·tro·syn·the·sis
elec·tro·tax·is
elec·tro·tha·na·sia
elec·tro·ther·a·peu·tics
elec·tro·ther·a·peu·tist
elec·tro·ther·a·pist
elec·tro·ther·a·py
    cerebral e. (CET)
elec·tro·therm
elec·tro·throm·bo·sis
elec·tro·tome
elec·trot·o·my
elec·tro·ton·ic
elec·trot·o·nus
elec·tro·trans·fer
elec·tro·tre·phine
elec·trot·ro·pism
    negative e.
    positive e.
elec·tro·ul·tra·fil·tra·tion
elec·tro·ure·tero·gram
elec·tro·u·re·ter·og·ra·phy
elec·tro·va·go·gram
elec·tro·va·lence
elec·tro·va·lent
elec·tro·ver·sion
elec·tro·vert
elec·tu·a·ry
    e. of senna
el·e·doi·sin
el·e·i·din
el·e·ment
    anatomic e.
    appendicular e's

el·e·ment *(continued)*
   electronegative e.
   electropositive e.
   formed e's (of the blood)
   labile e.
   morphological e.
   radioactive e.
   rare earth e's
   sarcous e.
   stable e.
   tissue e.
   trace e's
   tracer e's
   transcalifornium e's
   transduced e.
   transition e.
   transposable e.
   transuranic e's
   transuranium e's
el·e·men·ta·ry
el·e·mi·cin
el·e·o·ma
el·e·om·e·ter
el·eo·plast
el·e·op·ten
eleo·sac·cha·rum *pl.* eleo·sac·cha·ra
el·eo·ther·a·py
el·e·phan·ti·as·ic
el·e·phan·ti·a·sis
   e. chirurgica
   e. congenita angiomatosa
   congenital e.
   filarial e.
   e. gingivae
   e. italica
   e. leishmaniana
   lymphangiectatic e.
   e. neuromatosa
   nevoid e.
   e. nostras
   e. oculi
   e. scroti
el·e·phan·toid
El·et·ta·ria car·da·mo·mum
el·e·va·tion
   tactile e's
   tubal e.

el·e·va·tor
   angular e.
   apical e.
   Aufricht e.
   cross bar e.
   Cryer e.
   Cushing periosteal e.
   dental e.
   Freer e.
   Lempert e.
   malar e.
   palatal e.
   periosteum e.
   Pierce e.
   root e.
   screw e.
   straight e.
   T-bar e.
   wedge e.
el·faz·e·pam
elim·i·nant
elim·i·na·tion
   immune e.
el·i·nin
Elip·ten
ELISA — enzyme-linked immunosorbent assay
elix·ir
   adjuvant e.
   aromatic e.
   cascara e.
   high-alcoholic e.
   iso-alcoholic e.
   low-alcoholic e.
Elix·o·phyl·lin
El·ko·sin
el·ko·sis
El·li·ot's operation
El·li·ot's position
El·li·ot's sign
el·lip·sin
el·lip·soid
el·lip·to·cy·ta·ry
el·lip·to·cyte
el·lip·to·cyt·ic
el·lip·to·cy·to·sis
   hereditary e.

el·lip·to·cy·tot·ic
El·lis' curve
El·lis' line
El·lis' sign
El·lis-Gar·land line
El·lis-van Crev·eld syndrome
Ells·worth-Ho·ward test
Eloes·ser flap
elon·ga·tion
Els·berg's test
Elsch·nig's bodies
Elsch·nig's pearls
Els·ner's asthma
El·spar
el·u·ate
elu·caine
elu·ent
elute
elu·tion
　　affinity e.
　　gradient e.
　　membrane e.
elu·tri·a·tion
Ely's sign
Ely's test
ely·tro·ce·li·ot·o·my
ely·tro·plas·ty
ely·tro·poly·pus
Elz·holtz bodies
Em — emmetropia
ema·ci·at·ed
ema·ci·a·tion
email·lo·blast
em·a·nat·ing
em·a·na·tion
eman·ci·pa·tion
emas·cu·la·tion
Em·ba·do·mo·nas
em·balm
em·balm·ing
em·bar·rass
Emb·den es·ter
Emb·den-Mey·er·hof pathway
Emb·den-Mey·er·hof-Par·nas
　pathway
em·bed
em·bed·ding
em·boite·ment

em·bo·la·lia
em·bole
em·bo·lec·to·my
em·bo·li
em·bol·ic
em·bol·i·form
em·bo·lism
　air e.
　amniotic fluid e.
　bacillary e.
　bacterial e.
　bland e.
　bone marrow e.
　capillary e.
　cerebral e.
　coronary e.
　crossed e.
　direct e.
　fat e.
　hematogenous e.
　infective e.
　lymph e.
　lymphogenous e.
　miliary e.
　multiple e.
　oil e.
　pantaloon e.
　paradoxical e.
　plasmodium e.
　pulmonary e.
　retinal e.
　saddle e.
　spinal e.
　trichinous e.
　tumor e.
　venous e.
em·bo·li·za·tion
　poppet e.
em·bo·lo·la·lia
em·bo·lo·my·cot·ic
em·bo·lo·phra·sia
em·bo·lo·ther·a·py
em·bo·lus *pl.* em·bo·li
　air e.
　cancer e.
　cellular e.
　cholesterol e.
　fat e.

em·bo·lus *(continued)*
    foam e.
    obturating e.
    pantaloon e.
    platelet e.
    pulmonary e.
    renal cholesterol e.
    riding e.
    saddle e.
    straddling e.
em·bo·ly
em·bouche·ment
em·bra·sure
    buccal e.
    incisal e.
    interdental e.
    labial e.
    lingual e.
    occlusal e.
em·bro·ca·tion
em·bry·at·rics
em·bry·ec·to·my
em·bryo
    hexacanth e.
    Janošík's e.
    presomite e.
    previllous e.
    somite e.
    Spee's e.
em·bryo·blast
em·bryo·car·dia
em·bryo·ci·dal
em·bry·oc·to·ny
em·bryo·gen·e·sis
    accelerated e.
em·bryo·ge·net·ic
em·bry·o·gen·ic
em·bry·og·e·ny
em·bryo·graph
em·bry·og·ra·phy
em·bry·oid
em·bryo·ism
em·bry·o·log·ic
em·bry·ol·o·gist
em·bry·ol·o·gy
    causal e.
    chemical e.
    comparative e.

em·bry·ol·o·gy *(continued)*
    descriptive e.
    experimental e.
em·bry·o·ma
em·bryo·mor·phous
em·bry·o·nal
em·bry·o·nate
em·bry·on·ic
em·bry·o·nif·er·ous
em·bry·on·i·form
em·bry·o·nism
em·bry·o·ni·za·tion
em·bry·o·noid
em·bry·o·ny
em·bryo·path·ia
    e. rubeolaris
em·bryo·pa·thol·o·gy
em·bry·op·a·thy
    rubella e.
em·bryo·phore
em·bryo·plas·tic
em·bryo·scope
em·bryo·tome
em·bry·ot·o·my
em·bryo·tox·ic
em·bryo·tox·ic·i·ty
em·bryo·tox·on
    anterior e.
    posterior e.
em·bryo·troph
em·bryo·troph·ic
em·bry·ot·ro·phy
EMC — encephalomyocarditis
  (virus)
Em·cyt
emed·ul·late
emeio·cy·to·sis
eme·pro·ni·um bro·mide
emer·gen·cy
emer·gent
em·ery
em·e·sis
    fecal e.
    e. gravidarum
em·e·ta·tro·phia
emet·ic
    central e.
    direct e.

emet·ic *(continued)*
  indirect e.
  mechanical e.
  systemic e.
  tartar e.
emet·i·col·o·gy
em·e·tine
  e. and bismuth iodide
  e. hydrochloride
em·e·to·ca·thar·tic
em·e·tol·o·gy
EMF — electromotive force
EMG — electromyogram
EMI — electromagnetic
  interference
emil·i·um to·sy·late
em·i·nence
  alveolar e's
  antithenar e.
  arcuate e.
  articular e. of temporal
    bone
  bicipital e.
  canine e.
  capitate e.
  caudate e. of liver
  coccygeal e.
  cochlear e. of sacral bone
  collateral e. of lateral
    ventricle
  collateral e. of Meckel
  e. of concha
  cruciate e.
  cruciform e. of occipital
    bone
  cuneiform e. of head of rib
  deltoid e.
  Doyère's e.
  facial e. of eminentia teres
  frontal e.
  genital e.
  gluteal e. of femur
  e. of humerus
  hypobranchial e.
  hypoglossal e.
  hypothenar e.
  iliopectineal e.
  iliopubic e.

em·i·nence *(continued)*
  intercondylar e.
  intercondyloid e.
  intermediate e.
  jugular e.
  lateral e's of tuber
    cinereum
  mamillary e.
  e. of maxilla
  medial e. of fourth
    ventricle
  medial e. of rhomboid fossa
  median e.
  median e. of hypothalamus
  median e. of
    neurohypophysis
  median e's of tuber
    cinereum
  nasal e.
  oblique e. of cuboid bone
  occipital e.
  olivary e. of sphenoid bone
  orbital e. of zygomatic bone
  parietal e.
  postchiasmatic e.
  postfundibular e.
  postinfundibular e.
  pyramidal e.
  radial e. of wrist
  e. of scapha
  e. of superior semicircular
    canal
  supracondylar e.
  terete e.
  thenar e.
  thyroid e.
  triangular e.
  e. of triangular fossa of
    auricle
  trigeminal e.
  e. of triquetral fossa
  trochlear e.
  ulnar e. of wrist
  vagal e.
em·i·nen·tia *pl.* em·i·nen·tiae
  e. arcuata
  e. capitata
  e. carpi radialis

em·i·nen·tia *(continued)*
   e. carpi ulnaris
   e. cinerea cuneiformis
   e. conchae
   e. cruciata
   e. cruciformis
   e. facialis
   e. fallopii
   e. frontale
   e. gracilis
   e. hypoglossi
   e. hypothenaris
   e. iliopectinea
   e. iliopubica
   e. intercondylaris
   e. jugularis
   e. maxillae
   e. medialis fossae
     rhomboideae
   e. orbitalis ossis zygomatici
   e. papillaris
   e. pyramidalis
   e. restiformis
   e. scaphae
   e. styloidea
   e. symphysis
   e. teres
   e. thenaris
   e. triangularis
   e. trigemina
   e. vagi
emio·cy·to·sis
em·is·sa·ri·um *pl.* em·is·sa·ria
   e. condyloideum
   e. mastoideum
   e. occipitale
   e. parietale
em·is·sa·ry
emis·sion
   cold e.
   nasal e.
   nocturnal e.
   thermionic e.
emis·siv·i·ty
EMIT — enzyme-multiplied
immunoassay technique
emit·tance

em·men·a·gog·ic
em·men·a·gogue
   direct e.
   indirect e.
em·me·nia
em·men·ic
em·me·ni·op·a·thy
em·me·nol·o·gy
Em·met's operation
Em·met's retractor
Em·met-Stud·di·ford
   perineorrhaphy
em·me·trope
em·me·tro·pia
em·me·trop·ic
Em·mon·sia
Em·mon·si·el·la
em·o·din
emol·li·ent
emo·tio·mo·tor
emo·tion
emo·tion·al
emo·tio·vas·cu·lar
Emp. — L. emplastrum (a
   plaster)
em·pa·cho
em·pas·ma
em·path·ic
em·pa·thize
em·pa·thy
em·peri·po·le·sis
em·phrax·is
em·phy·se·ma
   aging-lung e.
   alveolar e.
   alveolar duct e.
   atrophic e.
   bullous e.
   centriacinar e.
   centrilobular e.
   chronic hypertrophic e.
   compensating e.
   compensatory e.
   cutaneous e.
   cystic e.
   diffuse e.
   ectatic e.
   false e.

em·phy·se·ma *(continued)*
   familial e.
   focal-dust e.
   gangrenous e.
   generalized e.
   glass blower's e.
   hypoplastic e.
   idiopathic unilobar e.
   interlobular e.
   interstitial e.
   intestinal e.
   lobar e.
   lobar e., infantile
   mediastinal e.
   obstructive e.
   panacinar e.
   panlobular e.
   paracicatricial e.
   paraseptal e.
   pulmonary e.
   senile e.
   skeletal e.
   small-lunged e.
   subcutaneous e.
   subgaleal e.
   surgical e.
   traumatic e.
   unilateral e.
   vesicular e.
em·phy·sem·a·tous
em·pir·ic
em·pir·i·cal
em·pir·i·cism
Em·pi·rin
em·plas·tic
em·plas·tra·tion
em·plas·trum
em·po·ri·at·rics
em·pros·thot·o·nos
em·pros·thot·o·nus
emp·ty·sis
em·py·e·ma
   e. articuli
   e. benignum
   extradural e.
   e. of gallbladder
   interlobar e.
   latent e.

em·py·e·ma *(continued)*
   loculated e.
   mastoid e.
   metapneumonic e.
   e. necessitatis
   pneumococcal e.
   pulsating e.
   putrid e.
   streptococcal e.
   subdural e.
   synpneumonic e.
   thoracic e.
   tuberculous e.
em·py·emic
em·py·e·sis
em·pyo·cele
em·py·reu·ma
em·py·reu·mat·ic
EMS — Emergency Medical
  Service (British)
EMT — emergency medical
  technician
emul. — L. emulsum
  (emulsion)
emul·gent
emul·si·fi·ca·tion
emul·si·fi·er
emul·si·fy
emul·sion
   bacillary e.
   benzyl benzoate e.
   hexachlorophene cleansing
    e.
   kerosene e.
   e. of liquid paraffin with
    cascara
   e. of liquid paraffin with
    phenolphthalein
   liquid petrolatum e.
   mineral oil e.
   perlsucht bacillen e. (PBE)
   photographic e.
emul·sive
emul·soid
emul·sum *pl.* emul·sa
emunc·to·ry
E-My·cin
emyl·ca·mate

ENA — extractable nuclear
  antigens
enal·a·pril
en·am·el
    curled e.
    dental e.
    dwarfed e.
    gnarled e.
    hereditary brown e.
    hypoplastic e.
    mottled e.
    nanoid e.
    straight e.
en·am·elo·blast
en·am·elo·blas·to·ma
enam·e·lo·gen·e·sis
en·am·el·o·ma
enam·el·um
en·an·thate
en·an·them
en·an·the·ma pl. en·an·the·
  mas, en·an·them·a·ta
en·an·them·a·tous
enan·thic acid
en·an·tio·bio·sis
en·an·tio·mer
en·an·ti·om·er·ism
en·an·tio·morph
en·an·tio·mor·phic
en·an·tio·mor·phism
en·an·tio·path·ia
en·ar·kyo·chrome
en·ar·thri·tis
en·ar·thro·di·al
en·ar·thro·sis
en bloc
en·cain·ide
en·can·this
en·cap·si·date
en·cap·su·late
en·cap·su·lat·ed
en·cap·su·la·tion
en·car·di·tis
en·ca·tar·rha·phy
en·ce·li·al·gia
en·ce·li·itis
en·ceph·a·lal·gia
en·ceph·a·lat·ro·phy

en·ceph·a·lauxe
en·céphale isolé
en·ceph·a·le·mia
en·ce·phal·ic
en·ceph·a·lit·ic
en·ceph·a·lit·i·des
en·ceph·a·li·tis pl. en·ceph·a·
  lit·i·des
    acute disseminated e.
    acute necrotizing e.
    American e.
    arbovirus e.
    Australian X e.
    Baló's concentric e.
    benign myalgic e.
    Binswanger's e.
    boutonneuse e.
    Calabrian e.
    California e.
    Central European e.
    cerebellar e.
    chronic subcortical e.
    Condorelli's e.
    cortical e.
    e. corticalis
    Coxsackie e.
    Dawson's e.
    diffuse sclerosing e.
    eastern equine e.
    eastern North American e.
    Economo's e.
    epidemic e.
    e. epidemica
    equine e.
    forest-spring e.
    Hayem's e.
    hemorrhagic e.
    hemorrhagic
      arsphenamine e.
    e. hemorrhagica superior
    herpes e.
    herpes simplex e.
    herpetic e.
    e. hyperplastica
    Ilheus e.
    inclusion body e.
    infantile e.
    influenzal e.

en·ceph·a·li·tis *(continued)*
    Japanese B e.
    lead e.
    Leichtenstern's e.
    lethargic e.
    e. lethargica
    limbic e.
    Mengo e.
    mumps e.
    Murray Valley e.
    e. neonatorum
    otic e.
    e. periaxialis concentrica
    e. periaxialis diffusa
    perivenous e.
    postexanthematous e.
    postinfectious e.
    postvaccinal e.
    Powassan e.
    purulent e.
    pyogenic e.
    Russian autumnal e.
    Russian endemic e.
    Russian forest-spring e.
    Russian spring-summer e.
    Russian tick-borne e.
    Russian vernal e.
    St. Louis e.
    Schilder's e.
    Semliki Forest e.
    Sicilian e.
    e. siderans
    Strümpell-Leichtenstern e.
    subacute inclusion body e.
    e. subcorticalis chronica
    summer e.
    suppurative e.
    tick-borne e.
    torula e.
    toxoplasmic e.
    typhoid e.
    van Bogaert e.
    varicella e.
    Venezuelan equine e.
    vernal e.
    vernoestival e.
    Vienna e.
    viral e.

en·ceph·a·li·tis *(continued)*
    von Economo's e.
    western equine e.
    West Nile e.
    woodcutter's e.
en·ceph·a·lit·o·gen
en·ceph·a·lit·o·gen·ic
en·ceph·a·li·za·tion
en·ceph·a·lo-ar·te·ri·og·ra·phy
en·ceph·a·lo·cele
    orbital e.
en·ceph·a·lo·clas·tic
en·ceph·a·lo·coele
en·ceph·a·lo·cys·to·cele
en·ceph·a·lo·cys·to·me·nin·go·cele
en·ceph·a·lo·di·al·y·sis
en·ceph·al·ody·nia
en·ceph·a·lo·dys·pla·sia
en·ceph·a·lo·ede·ma
en·ceph·a·lo·gen
en·ceph·a·lo·gram
en·ceph·a·log·ra·phy
    air e.
    fractional e.
    gamma e.
    positive contrast e.
en·ceph·a·loid
en·ceph·a·lo·lith
en·ceph·a·lol·o·gy
en·ceph·a·lo·ma
en·ceph·a·lo·ma·la·cia
    avian e.
    periventricular e.
en·ceph·a·lo·men·in·gi·tis
en·ceph·a·lo·me·nin·go·cele
en·ceph·a·lo·men·in·gop·a·thy
en·ceph·a·lo·mere
en·ceph·a·lom·e·ter
en·ceph·a·lo·my·eli·tis
    acute disseminated e.
    benign myalgic e.
    equine e.
    equine e., eastern
    equine e., Venezuelan
    equine e., western

en·ceph·a·lo·my·eli·tis
   (continued)
 experimental allergic e.
  (EAE)
 granulomatous e.
 Kelly's e.
 Mengo e.
 postexanthematous e.
 postimmunization e.
 postinfectious e.
 postvaccinal e.
 toxoplasmic e.
 Venezuelan equine e.
  (VEE)
 viral e.
 western equine e. (WEE)
 zoster e.
en·ceph·a·lo·my·elo·cele
en·ceph·a·lo·my·elo·neu·rop·
 a·thy
en·ceph·a·lo·my·elop·a·thy
 epidemic myalgic e.
 Leigh's necrotizing e.
 postinfection e.
 postvaccinal e.
 subacute necrotizing e.
en·ceph·a·lo·my·elo·ra·dic·
 u·li·tis
en·ceph·a·lo·my·elo·ra·dic·
 u·lo·neu·ri·tis
en·ceph·a·lo·my·elo·ra·dic·
 u·lop·a·thy
en·ceph·a·lo·my·elo·sis
en·ceph·a·lo·myo·car·di·tis
en·ceph·a·lo·lon
en·ceph·a·lo·nar·co·sis
en·ceph·a·lo·path·ic
en·ceph·a·lop·a·thy
 acute infantile e.
 alcoholic e.
 anoxic e.
 arsenical e.
 atonic-astasic e.
 biliary e.
 bilirubin e.
 boxer's e.
 callosal demyelinating e.

en·ceph·a·lop·a·thy
   (continued)
 Creutzfeldt-Jakob
  presenile e.
 cystic multilocular e.
 demyelinating e.
 dialysis e.
 hepatic e.
 hypercalcemic e.
 hypernatremic e.
 hypertensive e.
 hypoglycemic e.
 hypoxic e.
 lead e.
 Leigh's e.
 metabolic e.
 myoclonic e. of childhood
 necrotizing e.
 palindromic e.
 para-Wernicke e.
 pertussis e.
 portal-systemic e.
 portasystemic e.
 portocaval e.
 postanoxic e.
 progressive dialysis e.
 progressive multifocal e.
 progressive subcortical e.
 punch-drunk e.
 rheumatic e.
 saturnine e.
 spongiform e.
 subacute necrotizing e.
 subacute spongiform e.
 subcortical arteriosclerotic
  e.
 toxic e.
 traumatic e.
 uremic e.
 Wernicke's e.
en·ceph·a·lo·punc·ture
en·ceph·a·lo·py·o·sis
en·ceph·a·lo·ra·chid·i·an
en·ceph·a·lo·ra·dic·u·li·tis
en·ceph·a·lor·rha·gia
en·ceph·a·los·chi·sis
en·ceph·a·lo·scle·ro·sis
en·ceph·a·lo·scope

en·ceph·a·los·co·py
en·ceph·a·lo·sep·sis
en·ceph·a·lo·sis
    azotemic e.
en·ceph·a·lo·spi·nal
en·ceph·a·lo·thlip·sis
en·ceph·a·lo·tome
en·ceph·a·lot·o·my
en·chon·dral
en·chon·dro·ma
    multiple congenital e.
    e. petrificum
en·chon·dro·ma·to·sis
    multiple e.
    skeletal e.
en·chon·dro·ma·tous
en·chon·dro·sar·co·ma
en·chon·dro·sis
en·chy·ma
en·clave
en·clit·ic
en·clo·mi·phene
en·clo·sure
    Charnley e.
en·col·pism
en·col·pis·mus
en·co·pre·sis
en·coun·ter
en·cra·ni·us
en·cy·e·sis
en·cyo·py·eli·tis
en·cyst·ed
en·cyst·ment
end·a·del·phos
End·amoe·bi·dae
end·an·gi·itis
end·an·gi·um
end·aor·tic
end·aor·ti·tis
    bacterial e.
end·ar·ter·ec·to·mize
end·ar·ter·ec·to·my
    carotid e.
    eversion e.
    gas e.
    transaortic e.
end·ar·te·ri·al

end·ar·ter·itis
    Heubner's specific e.
    e. obliterans
    e. proliferans
    spinal e.
    syphilitic cerebral e.
end·ar·te·ri·um
end·ar·ter·op·a·thy
    digital e.
end-ar·tery
end·au·ral
end-brush
end-bud
end-bulb
    cylindrical e.-b.
    e.-b. of Held
    e.-b's of Krause
end·chon·dral
en·deic·tic
en·de·mia
en·de·mi·al
en·dem·ic
en·de·mi·ci·ty
en·de·mo·ep·i·dem·ic
end-di·as·tol·ic
end·epi·der·mis
end·er·gic
end·er·gon·ic
en·der·on
en·der·on·ic
En·ders, John Franklin
end-feet
    e. of Held
end-flake
end·ing
    annulospiral e's
    ball-of-thread e's
    basket e's
    calyciform e.
    club e. of Bartelmez
    Dogiel e.
    encapsulated nerve e's
    en plaque e.
    epilemmal e's
    flower-spray e's
    free nerve e's
    Golgi-Mazzoni e's

end·ing *(continued)*
    grape e's
    nerve e's
    nonencapsulated e.
    palisade e.
    primary e.
    Ruffini's e's
    secondary e.
    spiral e.
    spray e's
    synaptic e.
    trail e.
    ultraterminal e.
    unencapsulated e.
end-nu·clei
En·do's agar
en·do·ab·dom·i·nal
en·do·am·y·lase
en·do·an·eu·rys·mo·plas·ty
en·do·an·eu·rys·mor·rha·phy
en·do·ap·pen·di·ci·tis
en·do·aus·cul·ta·tion
en·do·bac·il·lary
en·do·bi·ot·ic
en·do·blast
en·do·blas·tic
en·do·bron·chi·tis
en·do·car·di·al
en·do·car·di·og·ra·phy
en·do·car·di·op·a·thy
en·do·car·dit·ic
en·do·car·di·tis
    abacterial thrombotic e.
    atypical verrucous e.
    bacterial e.
    e. benigna
    e. chordalis
    chronic e.
    constrictive e.
    Coxsackie e.
    fungal e.
    gonococcal e.
    infectious e.
    infective e.
    e. lenta
    Libman-Sacks e.
    Löffler's e.
    malignant e.

en·do·car·di·tis *(continued)*
    marantic e.
    mural e.
    mycotic e.
    nonbacterial thrombotic e.
    nonbacterial verrucous e.
    parietal e.
    prosthetic valve e.
    pulmonic e.
    rheumatic e.
    rickettsial e.
    right-side e.
    septic e.
    syphilitic e.
    tuberculous e.
    ulcerative e.
    valvular e.
    vegetative e.
    verrucous e.
    viridans e.
en·do·car·di·um
en·do·ce·li·ac
en·do·cel·lu·lar
en·do·cer·vi·cal
en·do·cer·vi·ci·tis
en·do·cer·vix
en·do·chon·dral
en·do·chon·dro·ma
en·do·cho·ri·on
en·do·chrome
en·do·chy·le·ma
en·do·co·li·tis
en·do·com·men·sal
en·do·co·nid·io·tox·i·co·sis
en·do·cor·pus·cu·lar
en·do·cra·ni·al
en·do·cra·ni·o·sis
en·do·cra·ni·tis
en·do·cra·ni·um
en·do·crine
en·doc·ri·nism
en·do·crin·i·um
en·do·cri·nol·o·gist
en·do·cri·nol·o·gy
en·do·crino·path·ic
en·do·cri·nop·a·thy
en·do·cri·no·sis
en·do·cri·no·ther·a·py

en·do·crino·trop·ic
en·do·cu·ti·cle
en·do·cyc·lic
en·do·cyst
en·do·cys·ti·tis
en·do·cyte
en·do·cy·tize
en·do·cy·tose
en·do·cy·to·sis
en·do·de·oxy·ri·bo·nu·cle·ase
en·do·derm
en·do·der·mal
en·do·der·mo·re·ac·tion
en·do·di·a·scope
en·do·di·as·co·py
en·do·don·tics
en·do·don·tist
en·do·don·ti·um
en·do·don·tol·o·gy
en·do·du·ral
en·do·dy·og·e·ny
en·do·ec·to·thrix
en·do·elec·tron·ther·a·py
en·do·en·ter·itis
en·do·en·zyme
en·do·epi·der·mal
en·do·epi·the·li·al
en·do·er·gic
en·do·esoph·a·gi·tis
en·do·exo·ter·ic
en·do·far·a·dism
en·do·gal·va·nism
en·dog·a·mous
en·dog·a·my
en·do·gas·tric
en·do·gas·tri·tis
en·do·ge·net·ic
en·do·gen·ic
en·do·ge·note
en·dog·e·nous
en·dog·e·ny
en·do·glo·bar
en·do·glob·u·lar
en·do·gna·thi·on
en·do·go·nid·i·um
en·do·her·ni·or·rha·phy
en·do·in·tox·i·ca·tion
en·do·lab·y·rin·thi·tis

en·do·la·ryn·ge·al
en·do·lar·ynx
En·do·li·max
en·do·lymph
en·do·lym·phan·gi·al
en·do·lym·phan·gi·tis
   e. proliferans
en·do·lym·phat·ic
en·dol·y·sin
   leukocytic e.
en·dol·y·sis
en·do·mas·toid·itis
en·do·me·nin·ges
en·do·meso·derm
en·do·me·trec·to·my
en·do·me·tria
en·do·me·tri·al
en·do·me·tri·oid
en·do·me·tri·o·ma
en·do·me·tri·o·sis
   colonic e.
   cutaneous e.
   cystic e.
   e. externa
   e. interna
   interstitial e.
   ovarian e.
   e. ovarii
   stromal e.
   tubal e.
   e. uterina
   e. vesicae
en·do·me·tri·ot·ic
en·do·me·tri·tis
   bacteriotoxic e.
   decidual e.
   exfoliative e.
   glandular e.
   membranous e.
   puerperal e.
   syncytial e.
   tuberculous e.
   e. tuberosa papulosa
en·do·me·tri·um *pl.* en·do·me·tria
   Swiss-cheese e.
en·do·me·tror·rha·gia
en·dom·e·try

en·do·mi·to·sis
en·do·mi·tot·ic
en·do·mix·is
en·do·morph
en·do·morph·ic
en·do·mor·phy
En·do·my·ces
   E. albicans
En·do·my·ce·ta·les
en·do·my·elog·ra·phy
en·do·myo·car·di·al
en·do·myo·car·di·tis
en·do·myo·me·tri·tis
en·do·mys·i·um
en·do·na·sal
en·do·neu·ral
en·do·neu·ri·al
en·do·neu·ri·tis
en·do·neu·ri·um
en·do·neu·rol·y·sis
en·do·nu·cle·ar
en·do·nu·cle·ase
   restriction e.
en·do·nu·cle·o·lus
en·do·par·a·site
en·do·par·a·sit·ic
en·do·par·a·sit·ism
en·do·pel·vic
en·do·pep·ti·dase
en·do·peri·car·di·al
en·do·peri·car·di·tis
en·do·peri·myo·car·di·tis
en·do·peri·neu·ri·tis
en·do·peri·to·ne·al
en·do·peri·to·ni·tis
en·do·per·ox·ide
   e. isomerase
en·do·pha·sia
en·do·phle·bi·tis
   e. hepatica obliterans
   proliferative e.
en·doph·thal·mi·tis
   phacoanaphylactic e.
en·do·phy·lax·i·na·tion
en·do·phyte
en·do·phyt·ic
en·do·plasm
en·do·plas·mic

en·do·po·lyg·e·ny
en·do·poly·ploid
en·do·poly·ploi·dy
en·do·pred·a·tor
en·do·ra·di·og·ra·phy
en·do·ra·dio·sonde
en·do·ra·dio·ther·a·py
en·do·re·du·pli·ca·tion
end-or·gan
en·do·rhi·ni·tis
en·do·ri·bo·nu·cle·ase
en·dor·phin
en·dor·rha·chis
en·do·sal·pin·gi·tis
en·do·sal·pin·go·ma
en·do·sal·pin·go·sis
en·do·sal·pinx
en·do·scope
en·do·scop·ic
en·dos·co·py
   peroral e.
   transcolonic e.
en·do·se·cre·to·ry
en·do·sep·sis
en·do·skel·e·ton
en·dos·mom·e·ter
en·dos·mo·sis
en·dos·mot·ic
en·do·some
en·do·sperm
en·do·spore
en·do·spor·i·um
en·dos·te·al
en·dos·te·itis
en·dos·teo·hy·per·os·to·sis
en·dos·te·o·ma
en·do·stetho·scope
en·dos·te·um
en·do·sym·bi·ont
en·do·sym·bi·o·sis
en·do·ten·din·e·um
en·do·ten·on
en·do·the·lia
en·do·the·li·al
en·do·the·li·al·iza·tion
en·do·the·li·itis
en·do·the·lio·blas·to·ma
en·do·the·lio·cho·ri·al

en·do·the·lio·cyte
en·do·the·li·oid
en·do·the·li·ol·y·sin
en·do·the·lio·lyt·ic
en·do·the·li·o·ma
    e. angiomatosum
    e. capitis
    e. cutis
    diffuse e.
    dural e.
    perithelial e.
en·do·the·li·o·ma·to·sis
en·do·the·lio·sar·co·ma
en·do·the·li·o·sis
    glomerular capillary e.
en·do·the·lio·tox·in
en·do·the·li·um *pl.* en·do·the·lia
    anterior e. of cornea
    e. anterius corneae
    e. camerae anterioris bulbi
    corneal e.
    e. corneale
    extraembryonic e.
    vascular e.
en·do·therm
en·do·ther·mal
en·do·ther·mic
en·do·ther·my
en·do·tho·rac·ic
en·do·thrix
en·do·thy·roi·do·pexy
en·do·tox·ic
en·do·tox·in
en·do·tox·oid
en·do·tra·che·al
en·do·tra·che·itis
en·do·tra·chel·itis
en·do·ure·thral
en·do·uter·ine
en·do·vac·ci·na·tion
en·do·vas·cu·li·tis
en·do·ve·ni·tis
en·do·ve·nous
En·dox·an
en·do·zo·ite
end plate, end-plate
    motor e.p.

end-plea·sure
En·drate
en·drin
en·dry·sone
end-tidal
En·du·ron
En·dur·o·nyl
en·dy·ma
en·e·ma *pl.* en·e·mas, e·nem·a·ta
    air contrast e.
    barium e.
    blind e.
    contrast e.
    double contrast e.
    Fleet e.
    high e.
    hydrocortisone e.
    nutrient e.
    nutritive e.
    pancreatic e.
    sedative e.
    small bowel e.
    soapsuds e.
    starch e.
    theophylline olamine e.
en·e·ma·tor
en·er·get·ics
en·er·gid
en·er·giz·er
    psychic e.
en·er·gom·e·ter
en·er·gy
    activation e.
    atomic e.
    binding e.
    chemical e.
    disintegration e.
    free e.
    Gibbs free e.
    kinetic e.
    latent e.
    nuclear e.
    phosphate bond e.
    e. of position
    potential e.
    radiant e.
    recoil e.

en·er·gy *(continued)*
    specific nerve e.
en·er·gy-rich
en·er·va·tion
en·flag·el·la·tion
en·flu·rane
ENG — electronystagmog-
    raphy
en·gage·ment
en·gas·tri·us
Eng·el's alkalimetry
En·gel-Reck·ling·hau·sen
    disease
Eng·el·mann's disease
Eng·el·mann's disk
Eng·en orthosis
en·gen·dered
en·gine
    dental e.
en·gi·neer·ing
    biomedical e.
    genetic e.
    human e.
en·globe
en·globe·ment
Eng·man's disease
en·gorged
en·gorge·ment
    breast e.
en·gram
en·graph·ia
en grappe
en·hance·ment
    acoustic e.
    contrast e.
en·hanc·er
En·hy·drina
    E. schistosa
en·keph·a·lin
en·keph·a·lin·er·gic
en·large·ment
    cardiac e.
    cervical e.
    gingival e.
    e. of heart
    tympanic e.
en·ni·a·tin
enol

eno·lase
    neuron-specific e.
eno·li·za·tion
en·oph·thal·mos
en·or·gan·ic
en·os·to·sis
En·o·vid
enoyl-ACP re·duc·tase
enoyl-CoA hy·dra·tase
en plaque
en·pro·mate
en·rich·ment
En·roth's sign
en·si·form
en·sis·ter·num
en·som·pha·lus
en·stro·phe
ENT — ear, nose, and throat
en·tad
en·tal
en·ta·la ção
ent·ame·bi·a·sis
Ent·a·moe·ba
    E. buccalis
    E. coli
    E. dispar
    E. dysenteriae
    E. gingivalis
    E. hartmanni
    E. histolytica
    E. invadens
    E. moshkowskii
    E. polecki
en·ta·sia
en·tel·e·chy
ent·epi·con·dyle
en·te·que
en·ter·ad·en
en·ter·ad·e·ni·tis
en·ter·al
en·ter·al·gia
en·ter·am·ine
en·ter·ec·ta·sis
en·ter·ec·to·my
en·ter·epip·lo·cele
en·ter·ic
en·ter·ic·al·ly

en·ter·ic-coat·ed
en·ter·i·coid
en·ter·i·tis
    choleriform e.
    chronic cicatrizing e.
    e. cystica chronica
    diphtheritic e.
    duck virus e.
    feline e.
    Escherichia coli e.
    e. gravis
    infectious feline e.
    mink viral e.
    mucous e.
    e. necroticans
    necrotizing e.
    e. nodularis
    phlegmonous e.
    e. polyposa
    protozoan e.
    pseudomembranous e.
    radiation e.
    regional e.
    segmental e.
    specific feline e.
    streptococcus e.
    terminal e.
    tuberculous e.
en·tero·anas·to·mo·sis
en·tero·ant·he·lone
en·tero·apo·klei·sis
En·tero·bac·ter
    E. aerogenes
    E. agglomerans
    E. alvei
    E. amnigenus
    E. cloacae
    E. gergoviae
    E. hafnia
    E. intermedium
    E. liquefaciens
    E. sakazakii
En·tero·bac·te·ri·a·ceae
en·tero·bac·te·ri·um *pl.* en·
  tero·bac·te·ria
en·tero·bac·tin
en·tero·bi·a·sis
en·tero·bil·i·ary

En·tero·bi·us
    E. vermicularis
en·tero·cele
en·tero·cen·te·sis
en·tero·cep·tor
en·tero·chel·in
en·tero·chi·rur·gia
en·tero·cho·le·cys·tost·o·my
en·tero·ci·ne·sia
en·tero·ci·net·ic
en·tero·clei·sis
    omental e.
en·ter·oc·ly·sis
en·tero·coc·ce·mia
en·tero·coc·ci
en·tero·coc·cus *pl.* en·tero·
  coc·ci
en·tero·coel
en·tero·coele
en·tero·coe·lic
en·tero·coe·lom
en·tero·coel·om·ate
en·tero·co·lec·to·my
en·tero·col·ic
en·tero·co·li·tis
    antibiotic-associated e.
    hemorrhagic e.
    necrotizing e.
    pseudomembranous e.
    regional e.
en·tero·co·los·to·my
en·ter·oc·ri·nin
en·tero·cu·ta·ne·ous
en·tero·cyst
en·tero·cys·to·cele
en·tero·cys·to·ma
en·tero·cyte
en·ter·odyn·ia
en·tero·en·ter·ic
en·tero·en·ter·os·to·my
en·tero·epip·lo·cele
en·tero·gas·tric
en·tero·gas·tri·tis
en·tero·gas·trone
en·ter·og·e·nous
en·tero·glu·ca·gon
en·tero·gram

en·tero·graph
en·ter·og·ra·phy
en·tero·hep·a·ti·tis
en·tero·hep·a·to·cele
en·tero·hep·a·to·pexy
en·tero·hy·dro·cele
en·ter·oi·dea
en·tero·in·tes·ti·nal
en·tero·in·va·sive
en·tero·ki·nase
en·tero·ki·ne·sia
en·tero·ki·net·ic
en·tero·ki·nin
en·tero·lith
en·tero·li·thi·a·sis
en·ter·ol·o·gy
en·ter·ol·y·sis
    excitation e.
en·tero·me·ga·lia
en·tero·meg·a·ly
en·tero·me·nia
en·tero·mere
en·tero·me·ro·cele
en·tero·my·co·der·mi·tis
en·tero·my·co·sis
    e. bacteriacea
en·tero·my·ia·sis
en·tero·myx·or·rhea
en·ter·on
en·tero·neu·ri·tis
en·tero·ni·tis
en·tero-ox·yn·tin
en·tero·pa·ral·y·sis
en·tero·pa·re·sis
en·ter·o·path·o·gen
en·tero·patho·gen·e·sis
en·ter·o·path·o·gen·ic
en·ter·op·a·thy
    gluten e.
    protein-losing e.
en·tero·pep·ti·dase
en·tero·pexy
en·tero·plas·ty
en·tero·ple·gia
en·tero·plex
en·tero·plexy
en·ter·op·to·sis
en·ter·op·tot·ic

en·tero·pty·chia
en·tero·pty·chy
en·tero·re·nal
en·ter·or·rha·gia
en·ter·or·rha·phy
    circular e.
en·ter·or·rhea
en·ter·or·rhex·is
en·tero·scope
en·tero·sep·sis
en·tero·sorp·tion
en·tero·spasm
en·tero·sta·sis
en·tero·stax·is
en·tero·ste·no·sis
en·tero·sto·mal
en·ter·os·to·my
    gun-barrel e.
en·tero·tome
en·ter·ot·o·my
en·ter·o·tox·e·mia
    hemorrhagic e.
    infectious e. of sheep
en·tero·tox·i·ca·tion
en·ter·o·tox·i·gen·ic
en·tero·tox·in
    cholera e.
    perfringens e.
en·tero·tox·ism
en·tero·trop·ic
en·tero·ty·phus
en·tero·vag·i·nal
en·tero·ve·nous
en·tero·ves·i·cal
En·tero-Vi·o·form
en·tero·vi·ral
en·tero·vi·rus
en·tero·zo·ic
en·ter·o·zo·on pl. en·tero·zoa
en·ter·uria
en·thal·py
en·the·sis
en·the·si·tis
en·the·sop·a·thy
en·thet·ic
en·theto·bio·sis
en·thla·sis
en thyrse

en·tire
en·ti·ris
en·ti·ty
en·to·blast
en·to·cele
en·to·chon·dros·to·sis
en·to·cho·roid·ea
en·to·cne·mi·al
en·to·con·dyle
en·to·cor·nea
en·to·cra·ni·al
en·to·cu·ne·i·form
en·to·cyte
en·to·derm
    primitive e.
    yolk-sac e.
en·to·der·mal
en·to·der·mic
En·to·di·nio·mor·phi·da
en·to·ec·tad
en·to·mere
en·to·meso·derm
en·to·mi·on
en·to·mog·e·nous
en·to·mol·o·gist
en·to·mol·o·gy
    medical e.
en·to·moph·a·gous
En·to·moph·thora
    E. coronata
    E. muscae
En·to·moph·tho·ra·ceae
En·to·moph·tho·ra·les
en·to·moph·tho·ro·my·co·sis
En·to·mos·pi·ra
en·to-oc·cip·i·tal
en·toph·thal·mia
en·to·phyte
en·top·ic
en·to·plasm
en·top·tic
en·top·to·scope
en·top·tos·co·py
en·to·ret·i·na
ent·or·gan·ism
en·to·rhi·nal
en·to·sarc
ent·os·to·sis

en·to·tym·pan·ic
en·to·zoa
en·to·zo·al
en·trap·ment
en·trip·sis
en·tro·pi·on
    cicatricial e.
    spastic e.
    e. uveae
en·tro·pi·on·ize
en·tro·pi·um
en·tro·py
ent·wick·lungs·me·cha·nik
en·ty·py
enu·cle·ate
enu·cle·at·ed
enu·cle·a·tion
en·ure·sis
    epileptic e.
    nocturnal e.
en·uret·ic
en·ve·lope
    basilar membrane e.
    cell e.
    egg e.
    nuclear e.
en·ven·om
en·ven·om·a·tion
en·vi·ron·ment
    controlled e.
    external e.
    internal e.
en·vy
    penis e.
En·zac·tin
en·zo·ot·ic
En·zo·pride
en·zy·got·ic
en·zy·mat·ic
en·zyme
    adaptive e.
    allosteric e.
    angiotensin converting e.
    biotinyl e.
    brancher e.
    branching e.
    catheptic e.
    collagenolytic e.

en·zyme *(continued)*
    constitutive e.
    cryptic e.
    debrancher e.
    debranching e.
    débridement e's
    digestant e's
    early e.
    extracellular e.
    fat-splitting e.
    fibrinolytic e's
    glycolytic e.
    hydrolytic e.
    induced e.
    inducible e.
    intracellular e.
    late e.
    Lohmann's e.
    malic e.
    old yellow e.
    proteolytic e.
    Q e.
    receptor-destroying e.
    redox e.
    regulatory e.
    repair e.
    repressible e.
    respiratory e.
    restriction e.
    Schardinger's e.
    serum e.
    terminal addition e.
    transferring e.
    yellow e's
En·zyme Com·mis·sion (EC)
en·zyme-linked
en·zym·ic
en·zy·mol·o·gy
en·zy·mol·y·sis
en·zy·mop·a·thy
    lysosomal e.
EOG — electro-olfactogram
eo·sin
    e. I bluish
    e. B
    ethyl e.
    e. W
    water-soluble e.

eo·sin *(continued)*
    e. W S
    e. Y
    yellowish e.
eo·sino·blast
eo·sin·o·cyte
eo·sin·o·pe·nia
    hormonal e.
eo·sin·o·phil
eo·sin·o·phile
eo·sin·o·phil·ia
    hereditary e.
    Löffler's e.
    pulmonary infiltration e.
    tropical e.
    tropical pulmonary e.
eo·sin·o·phil·ic
eo·sin·o·philo·cyt·ic
eo·sin·o·philo·poi·e·tin
eo·sin·o·phi·lo·sis
eo·sin·o·philo·tac·tic
eo·sin·oph·i·lous
eo·sin·o·phil·uria
eo·sin·o·tac·tic
eo·so·late
EP — evoked potential
EPA — eicosapentaenoic acid
ep·ac·mas·tic
ep·ac·me
epac·tal
ep·al·lo·bi·o·sis
ep·ar·sal·gia
ep·ar·te·ri·al
ep·ax·i·al
ep·en·ceph·al
ep·en·ce·phal·ic
ep·en·ceph·a·lon
ep·en·dop·a·thy
epen·dy·ma
epen·dy·mal
epen·dy·mi·tis
epen·dy·mo·blast
epen·dy·mo·blas·to·ma
epen·dy·mo·cyte
epen·dy·mo·cy·to·ma
epen·dy·mo·ma
    anaplastic e.
    myxopapillary e.

epen·dy·mo·ma *(continued)*
    papillary e.
    water-in-oil e.
ep·eryth·ro·zoo·no·sis
ephapse
ephap·tic
ep·har·mo·ny
ephe·bi·at·rics
epheb·ic
eph·e·bo·gen·e·sis
eph·e·bo·gen·ic
eph·e·bol·o·gy
Ephed·ra
ephed·rine
    e. hydrochloride
    e. sulfate
ephel·i·des
ephe·lis *pl.* ephel·i·des
ephem·era
ephem·er·al
Ephe·mer·i·da
Eph·y·nal
epi·al·lo·preg·nan·o·lone
epi·an·dros·ter·one
epi·blast
epi·blas·tic
epi·bleph·a·ron
epib·o·le
epib·o·ly
epi·bran·chi·al
epi·bul·bar
ep·i·can·thal
ep·i·can·thic
epi·can·thine
epi·can·thus
    e. inversus
ep·i·car·cin·o·gen
epi·car·dia
epi·car·di·al
epi·car·di·ec·to·my
epi·car·di·um
epi·cau·ma
Epi·cau·ta
epi·cen·tral
epi·chi·to·sa·mine
epi·chor·dal
epi·cho·ri·on
epi·cil·lin

epi·coe·lo·ma
epic·o·mus
epi·con·dy·lal·gia
epi·con·dyle
    external e. of femur
    external e. of humerus
    internal e. of femur
    internal e. of humerus
    lateral e. of femur
    lateral e. of humerus
    medial e. of femur
    medial e. of humerus
epi·con·dy·li
epi·con·dy·li·tis
    external humeral e.
    radiohumeral e.
epi·con·dy·lus *pl.* epi·con·dy·li
    e. lateralis femoris
    e. lateralis humeri
    e. medialis femoris
    e. medialis humeri
epi·cor·a·coid
epi·cor·nea·scle·ri·tis
epi·cos·tal
epi·cot·yl
epi·cra·ni·um
epi·cri·sis
epi·crit·ic
epi·cu·ti·cle
epi·cys·ti·tis
epi·cys·tot·o·my
epi·cyte
ep·i·dem·ic
ep·i·de·mic·i·ty
ep·i·de·mi·og·ra·phy
ep·i·de·mi·o·log·ic
ep·i·de·mi·ol·o·gist
ep·i·de·mi·ol·o·gy
epi·derm
epi·der·mal
epi·der·ma·ti·tis
epi·der·ma·to·plas·ty
epi·der·mic
epi·der·mic·u·la
epi·der·mi·dal·iza·tion
epi·der·mi·des
epi·der·mis *pl.* epi·der·mi·des

epi·der·mi·tis
epi·der·mi·za·tion
epi·der·mo·dys·pla·sia
 e. verruciformis
epi·der·moid
 cerebrospinal e.
epi·der·moi·do·ma
epi·der·mol·y·sin
epi·der·mol·y·sis
 e. bullosa
 e. bullosa, acquired
 e. bullosa acquisita
 e. bullosa dystrophica
 e. bullosa dystrophica,
  albopapuloid
 e. bullosa dystrophica,
  dominant
 e. bullosa dystrophica,
  dysplastic
 e. bullosa dystrophica,
  hyperplastic
 e. bullosa dystrophica,
  polydysplastic
 e. bullosa dystrophica,
  recessive
 e. bullosa hereditaria
 e. bullosa, junctional
 e. bullosa letalis
 e. bullosa simplex
 e. bullosa simplex,
  generalized
 e. bullosa simplex, localized
 toxic bullous e.
 Weber-Cockayne e. bullosa
epi·der·mo·lyt·ic
epi·der·mo·my·co·sis
epi·der·moph·y·tid
Ep·i·der·moph·y·ton
 E. floccosum
 E. purpureum
 E. rubrum
epi·der·mo·phy·to·sis
 e. axillaris
epi·der·mo·poi·e·sis
epi·der·mo·sis
 aural e.
epi·did·y·mal
epi·did·y·mec·to·my

epi·did·y·mis *pl.* epi·did·y·
 mi·des
epi·did·y·mi·tis
 spermatogenic e.
epi·did·y·mo·def·er·en·tec·
 to·my
epi·did·y·mo·def·er·en·tial
epi·did·y·mo-or·chi·tis
epi·did·y·mot·o·my
epi·did·y·mo·vas·ec·to·my
epi·did·y·mo·vas·os·to·my
epi·du·ral
epi·du·ri·tis
epi·du·rog·ra·phy
epi·es·tri·ol
epi·fas·cial
epig·a·mous
epi·gas·ter
epi·gas·tral·gia
epi·gas·tric
epi·gas·tri·um
epi·gas·tri·us
 e. parasiticus
epi·gas·tro·cele
epi·gen·e·sis
epi·ge·net·ic
epi·ge·net·ics
epi·glot·tec·to·my
epi·glot·tic
epi·glot·tid·e·an
epi·glot·ti·dec·to·my
epi·glot·ti·di·tis
epi·glot·tis
epi·glot·ti·tis
epig·na·thous
epig·na·thus
 e. parasiticus
epig·o·nal
epi·guan·ine
epi·hi·dro·sis
epi·hy·al
epi·hy·drin·al·de·hyde
epi·hy·oid
epi·ker·a·to·mi·leu·sis
epi·la·mel·lar
ep·i·late
ep·i·la·tion
epil·a·to·ry

ep·i·lem·ma
ep·i·lem·mal
ep·i·lep·sia
   e. arithmetica
   e. cursiva
   e. gravior
   e. major
   e. minor
   e. mitior
   e. mitis
   e. nutans
   e. partialis continua
   e. procursiva
   e. rotatoria
   e. tarda
ep·i·lep·sy
   abdominal e.
   acquired e.
   activated e.
   adversive e.
   affective e.
   alcoholic e.
   alternating e.
   ambulatory e.
   amygdaloid e.
   aphasic e.
   atonic e.
   automatic e.
   autonomic e.
   Bravais-jacksonian e.
   centrencephalic e.
   cingulate e.
   contraversive e.
   cortical e.
   cryptogenic e.
   cyclical e.
   diurnal e.
   dysmnesic e.
   essential e.
   focal e.
   focal e., chronic
   focal e., minor
   gelastic e.
   generalized e.
   generalized flexion e.
   grand mal e.
   haut mal e.
   hysterical e.

ep·i·lep·sy *(continued)*
   hysteriform e.
   ideational e.
   idiopathic e.
   illusional e.
   insular e.
   jacksonian e.
   Koshevnikoff's
     (Koschewnikow's,
     Kozhevnikov's) e.
   larval e.
   laryngeal e.
   latent e.
   localized e.
   major e.
   masticatory e.
   matutinal e.
   menstrual e.
   metabolic e.
   minor e.
   morning e.
   myoclonus e.
   nocturnal e.
   occipital e.
   opercular e.
   opisthotonic e.
   organic e.
   oropharyngeal e.
   Penfield e.
   petit mal e.
   photogenic e.
   physiologic e.
   postcentral e.
   posthemiplegic e.
   postrolandic e.
   post-traumatic e.
   procursive e.
   progressive familial
     myoclonic e.
   psychic e.
   psychomotor e.
   reflex e.
   rolandic e.
   seesaw e.
   self-induced e.
   sensory e.
   serial e.
   somatomotor e.

ep·i·lep·sy *(continued)*
   somnambulistic e.
   sonosensory e.
   spinal e.
   spontaneous e.
   startle e.
   television e.
   temporal lobe e.
   tonic e.
   tornado e.
   traumatic e.
   uncinate e.
   unilateral e.
   versive e.
   vertiginous e.
ep·i·lep·tic
ep·i·lep·ti·form
ep·i·lep·to·gen·ic
ep·i·lep·tog·e·nous
ep·i·lep·toid
ep·i·lep·tol·o·gist
ep·i·lep·tol·o·gy
ep·i·loia
epi·man·dib·u·lar
epi·mas·ti·gote
epi·men·or·rha·gia
epi·men·or·rhea
ep·i·mer
epim·er·ase
ep·i·mere
epim·er·iza·tion
epi·mes·trol
epi·mor·phic
epi·mor·pho·sis
epi·myo·car·di·um
epi·mys·i·ot·omy
epi·mys·i·um
Ep·i·nal
epi·neph·rine
   e. bitartrate
   racemic e.
epi·neph·rin·emia
epi·neph·ros
epi·neph·ryl bo·rate
epi·neu·ral
epi·neu·ri·al
epi·neu·ri·um
epi·no·sic

epi·or·chi·um
epi·ot·ic
ep·i·pas·tic
epi·peri·car·di·al
epi·pha·ryn·ge·al
epi·pha·ryn·gi·tis
epi·phar·ynx
epi·phe·nom·e·non
epiph·o·ra
epi·phys·e·al
epi·phys·ec·to·my
epi·phys·e·od·e·sis
epiph·y·ses
epi·phys·i·al
epi·phys·i·od·e·sis
epi·phys·i·oid
epi·phys·io·lis·the·sis
epi·phys·i·ol·y·sis
   distraction e.
epi·phys·i·om·e·ter
epi·phys·i·op·a·thy
epiph·y·sis *pl.* epiph·y·ses
   capital e.
   e. cerebri
   slipped e.
   stippled epiphyses
epiph·y·si·tis
   e. juvenilis
   vertebral e.
ep·i·phyte
ep·i·phyt·ic
epi·pi·al
epi·pleu·ral
epip·lo·cele
epip·lo·ec·to·my
epip·lo·en·tero·cele
epip·lo·ic
epip·lo·itis
   Sherlock's e.
epip·lo·me·ro·cele
epi·plom·phalo·cele
epip·lo·on
   great e.
   lesser e.
epip·lo·pexy
epip·lo·plas·ty
epip·lor·rha·phy
epip·los·cheo·cele

epi·py·gus
    e. parasiticus
epi·pyr·a·mis
epir·i·zole
epi·ro·tu·li·an
epi·scle·ra
epi·scle·ral
epi·scle·ri·tis
    e. partialis fugax
epi·scle·ro·ti·tis
epis·io·per·i·neo·plas·ty
epis·io·per·i·ne·or·rha·phy
epis·io·plas·ty
epis·i·or·rha·phy
epis·io·ste·no·sis
epis·i·ot·o·my
    Matsner median e. and
      repair
    median e.
    mediolateral e.
ep·i·sode
    acute schizophrenic e.
    hypomanic e.
    major depressive e.
    manic e.
    psycholeptic e.
    psychomotor e.
ep·i·some
epi·spa·dia
epi·spa·di·ac
epi·spa·di·al
epi·spa·di·as
    balanic e.
    balanitic e.
    clitoric e.
    complete e.
    female e.
    glandular e.
    incomplete e.
    penile e.
    penopubic e.
    subsymphyseal e.
epi·spas·tic
epi·spi·nal
epi·sple·ni·tis
epis·ta·sis
epis·ta·sy
epi·stat·ic

ep·i·stax·is
    Gull's renal e.
epis·te·mol·o·gy
epi·ster·nal
epi·ster·num
epis·thot·o·nos
epi·stro·phe·us
epi·syl·vi·an
epi·tar·sus
epi·taxy
epi·te·la
epi·ten·din·e·um
epi·te·non
epi·tha·lam·ic
epi·thal·a·mus
epi·tha·lax·ia
ep·i·the·lia
ep·i·the·li·al
ep·i·the·li·al·iza·tion
ep·i·the·li·a·lize
ep·i·the·li·itis
ep·i·the·lio·cep·tor
ep·i·the·lio·cho·ri·al
ep·i·the·lio·cy·tus
    e. basalis gustatorius
    e. phalangeus externus
    e. phalangeus internus
    e. pilosus columnaris
    e. sensorius gustatorius
    e. sensorius pilosus
      externus
    e. sensorius pilosus
      internus
    e. sensorius pilosus
      piriformis
    e. sustentans gustatorius
ep·i·the·lio·fi·bril
ep·i·the·lio·ge·net·ic
ep·i·the·li·o·gen·ic
ep·i·the·lio·glan·du·lar
ep·i·the·li·oid
ep·i·the·li·ol·y·sin
ep·i·the·li·ol·y·sis
ep·i·the·lio·lyt·ic
ep·i·the·li·o·ma
    e. adamantinum
    e. adenoides cysticum

ep·i·the·li·o·ma *(continued)*
  basal cell e.
  basisquamous e.
  benign calcifying e.
  calcified e.
  calcifying e.
  calcifying e. of Malherbe
  chorionic e.
  columnar e.
  e. contagiosum
  e. cuniculatum
  cylindrical e.
  diffuse e.
  Ferguson-Smith type e.
  glandular e.
  intraepidermal e.
  Malherbe's calcifying e.
  malignant e.
  e. molluscum
  morpheic e.
  multiple self-healing
    squamous e.
  pigmented basal cell e.
  pseudocystic e.
  self-healing squamous e.
  squamous cell e.
ep·i·the·li·o·ma·to·sis
ep·i·the·li·o·ma·tous
ep·i·the·lio·mus·cu·lar
ep·i·the·li·o·sis
ep·i·the·lio·tox·in
ep·i·the·lio·trop·ic
ep·i·the·lite
ep·i·the·li·um *pl.* ep·i·the·lia
  e. anterius corneae
  Barrett's e.
  capsular e.
  ciliated e.
  coelomic e.
  columnar e.
  e. corneae
  corneal e.
  crevicular e.
  cubical e.
  cuboidal e.
  dental e.
  e. ductus semicircularis
  enamel e.

ep·i·the·li·um *(continued)*
  false e.
  follicular e.
  germinal e.
  gingival e.
  glandular e.
  glomerular e.
  junctional e.
  laminated e.
  e. of lens
  e. lentis
  mesenchymal e.
  e. mucosae
  muscle e.
  myxopleomorphic e.
  nerve e.
  olfactory e.
  oral e.
  pavement e.
  pigmentary e.
  pigmented e.
  pigmented e. of iris
  e. pigmentosum iridis
  e. pigmentosum partis
    ciliaris retinae
  e. posterius pigmentosum
    partis iridicae retinae
  posterior e. of cornea
  e. posterius corneae
  protective e.
  pseudostratified e.
  pyramidal e.
  respiratory e.
  retinal pigment e.
  rod e.
  seminiferous e.
  sense e.
  sensory e.
  simple e.
  squamous e.
  stratified e.
  subcapsular e.
  sulcal e.
  sulcular e.
  e. superficiale ovarii
  surface e.
  tabular e.
  tegumentary e.

ep·i·the·li·um *(continued)*
 visceral e.
 tessellated e.
 transitional e.
ep·i·the·li·za·tion
ep·i·the·lize
epith·e·sis
ep·i·thet
epi·thi·a·zide
ep·i·ton·ic
ep·i·tope
Ep·i·trate
ep·i·trich·i·um
epi·tri·que·trum
epi·troch·lea
epi·troch·le·ar
epi·troch·le·itis
epi·tu·ber·cu·lo·sis
epi·tur·bi·nate
epi·tym·pan·ic
epi·tym·pa·num
ep·i·type
epi·typh·li·tis
epi·ty·phlon
epi·vag·i·ni·tis
epi·zoa
epi·zo·ic
epi·zo·i·cide
epi·zo·on *pl.* epi·zoa
epi·zoo·no·sis
epi·zo·ot·ic
epi·zo·ot·i·ol·o·gy
éplu·chage
Epon
epon·tic
ep·o·nych·i·um
ep·o·nym
ep·o·nym·ic, epon·y·mous
ep·o·oph·o·rec·to·my
ep·o·öph·o·ron
ep·o·pro·sten·ol
ep·or·ni·thol·o·gy
ep·or·nit·ic
epox·ide
epoxy
ep·oxy·meth·amine bro·mide
ep·oxy·tro·pine tro·pate
Ep·py

EPR — electrophrenic respiration
Ep·ro·lin
EPS — electrophysiologic study
 exophthalmos-producing substance
 extrapyramidal signs
 extrapyramidal symptoms
ep·si·lon
EPSP — excitatory postsynaptic potential
Ep·stein's disease
Ep·stein's nephrosis
Ep·stein's pearls
Ep·stein's syndrome
Ep·stein-Barr virus
ep·ta·tre·tin
epu·li·des
epu·lis *pl.* epu·li·des
 congenital e.
 e. fibromatosa
 e. fissurata
 giant cell e.
 e. gigantocellularis
 e. granulomatosa
 e. of newborn
 pigmented e.
 e. of pregnancy
ep·u·lo·fi·bro·ma
ep·u·loid
ep·u·lo·sis
ep·u·lot·ic
eq — equivalent
equal·iza·tion
 pressure e.
Equa·nil
equate
equa·tion
 alveolar gas e.
 Arrhenius' e.
 Ayala's e.
 Bloch e.
 Bohr's e.
 chemical e.
 Gompertz e.
 Harden and Young e.
 Henderson-Hasselbalch e.

equa·tion *(continued)*
   Hill e.
   Larmor e.
   Lineweaver-Burk e.
   Michaelis-Menten e.
   Nernst e.
   Poiseuille e. (Hagenbach
     extension)
   Ussing e.
   van't Hoff e.
equa·tor
   e. bulbi oculi
   e. of cell
   e. of crystalline lens
   e. of eyeball
   e. of lens
   e. lentis
equa·to·ri·al
equi·ax·i·al
equi·ca·lor·ic
equi·lat·er·al
equi·li·bra·tion
   mandibular e.
   occlusal e.
equi·li·bra·tor
equi·lib·ra·tory
equi·lib·ri·um
   acid-base e.
   body e.
   calorie e.
   carbon e.
   Donnan's e.
   dynamic e.
   fluid e.
   genetic e.
   Gibbs-Donnan e.
   Hardy-Weinberg e.
   homeostatic e.
   linkage e.
   metabolic e.
   mutational e.
   nitrogen e.
   nitrogenous e.
   nutritive e.
   physiologic e.
   protein e.
   radioactive e.
   secular e.

equi·lib·ri·um *(continued)*
   transient e.
   water e.
equil·in
equi·mo·lar
equi·mo·lec·u·lar
equi·no·ca·vus
equi·no·pho·bia
equi·no·val·gus
equi·no·va·rus
equi·nus
equi·po·ten·tial
equi·po·ten·ti·al·i·ty
equi·se·to·sis
equi·se·tum
equi·tox·ic
equiv·a·lence
equiv·a·lent
   aluminum e.
   caloric e. of oxygen
   calorie e.
   combustion e.
   concrete e.
   dose e.
   endosmotic e.
   epileptic e.
   genetic lethal e.
   gold e.
   gram e.
   isodynamic e.
   lead e.
   lethal e.
   maximum permissible dose
     e.
   neutralization e.
   nitrogen e.
   protein e.
   psychic e.
   starch e.
   toxic e.
   ventilation e.
   water e.
ER — endoplasmic reticulum
   evoked response
   external resistance
ERA — electric response
  audiometry
erab·u·tox·in

era·sion
Er·a·ty·rus
Erb, Wilhelm Heinrich
Erb's point
Erb's sclerosis
Erb's sign
Erb's spastic paraplegia
Erb's syndrome
Erb-Char·cot disease
Erb-Du·chenne paralysis
Erb-Gold·flam disease
Erb-Lan·dou·zy disease
Erb-Op·pen·heim-Gold·flam
  syndrome
Er·ben's phenomenon
Er·ben's reflex
Er·ben's sign
ERBF — effective renal blood
  flow
er·bi·um
er·cal·ci·ol
ERCP — endoscopic
  retrograde
  cholangiopancreatography
Erd·heim cystic medial
  necrosis
Erd·heim cystic syndrome
erec·tile
erec·tion
erec·tor
er·e·ma·cau·sis
er·e·mo·pho·bia
er·e·thic·al
er·e·this·mic
er·e·this·tic
Ereth·ma·pod·i·tes
ERG — electroretinogram
erg
er·ga·sia
er·gas·tic
er·gas·to·plasm
er·go·ba·sine
er·go·cal·cif·er·ol
er·go·car·dio·gram
er·go·car·di·og·ra·phy
er·go·dy·namo·graph
er·go·es·the·sio·graph
er·go·gen·e·sis

er·go·gen·ic
er·go·gram
er·go·graph
  Mosso's e.
er·go·graph·ic
Er·go·mar
er·gom·e·ter
  bicycle e.
er·go·met·rine
er·gom·e·try
er·gon
er·go·nom·ics
er·go·no·vine
  e. maleate
er·go·plasm
er·go·some
er·go·stat
er·gos·te·rol
  activated e.
  activated irradiated e.
er·go·stet·rine
er·got
  hydrogenated e. alkaloids
er·got·amine
  e. tartrate
er·go·tam·i·nine
er·go·ther·a·py
er·go·thi·o·ne·ine
er·go·tin·in
er·got·ism
er·got·ized
er·go·to·cine
er·go·tox·i·co·sis
er·go·tox·ine
Er·go·trate
er·gu·sia
Er·ich·sen's ligature
Er·ich·sen's sign
Er·ich·sen's test
Er·i·o·dic·ty·on
er·i·o·dic·ty·on
er·is·i·phake
Er·is·ta·lis
  E. tenax
Er·ni's sign
erode
erog·e·nous
erose

ero·sio
  e. interdigitalis
    blastomycetica
ero·sion
  cervical e.
  dental e.
ero·sive
erot·ic
erot·i·cism
erot·i·cize
erot·i·co·ma·nia
er·o·tism
  anal e.
  oral e.
er·o·tize
ero·to·gen·e·sis
ero·to·gen·ic
ero·to·ma·nia
ero·to·pho·bia
ERP — endocardial resection
  procedure
ERPF — effective renal
  plasma flow
er·rat·ic
er·rhine
er·ror
  absolute e.
  biased e.
  copy e.
  experimental e.
  inborn e. of metabolism
  random e.
  sampling e.
  standard e.
  standard e. of the mean
  systematic e.
  Type I e.
  Type II e.
Er·tron
eru·cic acid
eruc·ta·tion
  nervous e.
eru·ga·tion
erup·tion
  active e.
  butterfly e.
  clinical e.
  continuous e.

erup·tion (continued)
  creeping e.
  delayed e.
  demodetic e.
  drug e.
  fixed e.
  fixed drug e.
  Kaposi's varicelliform e.
  morbilliform e.
  partial e.
  passive e.
  polymorphous light e.
  sandworm e.
  seabather's e.
  serum e.
  summer e.
  surgical e.
  tooth e.
  total e.
  vaccinal e.
erup·tive
ERV — expiratory reserve
  volume
Er·win·ia
  E. amylovora
  E. carotovora
  E. herbicola
Er·win·i·eae
er·y·sip·e·las
  e. bullosum
  coast e.
  gangrenous e.
  e. grave internum
  hemorrhagic e.
  malignant e.
  e. migrans
  necrotizing e.
  swine e.
  wandering e.
er·y·si·pel·a·tous
er·y·sip·e·loid
  Rosenbach's e.
Er·y·sip·elo·thrix
  E. insidiosa
  E. rhusiopathiae
er·y·sip·e·lo·tox·in
Er·ys·i·pha·ceae
er·ys·i·phake

er·y·the·ma
acrodynic e.
acute infectious e.
e. annulare
e. annulare centrifugum
e. annulare rheumaticum
e. arthriticum epidemicum
e. caloricum
e. chromicum figuratum melanodermicum
e. chronicum migrans
circinate syphilitic e.
e. circinatum
e. circinatum rheumaticum
cold e.
diaper e.
e. dyschromicum perstans
e. elevatum diutinum
e. endemicum
epidemic e.
epidemic arthritic e.
figurate e.
e. figuratum
e. figuratum perstans
e. fugax
gyrate e.
e. gyratum
e. gyratum perstans
e. gyratum repens
e. ab igne
e. induratum
e. infectiosum
e. iris
Jacquet's e.
e. marginatum
e. marginatum rheumaticum
e. migrans
e. multiforme
e. multiforme bullosum
e. multiforme major
e. multiforme minor
necrolytic migratory e.
e. necroticans
e. neonatorum
e. nodosum
e. nodosum leprosum
e. nodosum migrans

er·y·the·ma *(continued)*
e. nodosum syphiliticum
e. nuchae
nummular e.
palmar e.
e. palmare
e. palmare hereditarium
papuloerosive e.
e. papulosum
pellagroid e.
e. pernio
e. a pudore
rheumatic e.
e. streptogenes
e. subitum
toxic e.
e. toxicum
e. toxicum neonatorum
e. urticans
er·y·them·a·tous
er·y·the·mo·gen·ic
er·y·thral·gia
er·y·thras·ma
eryth·re·de·ma pol·y·neu·rop·a·thy
er·y·thre·mia
high-altitude e.
eryth·re·mo·mel·al·gia
Er·y·thri·na
eryth·rism
er·y·thris·tic
eryth·ri·tol
eryth·ri·tyl
e. tetranitrate
eryth·ro·blast
acidophilic e.
basophilic e.
early e.
eosinophilic e.
intermediate e.
definitive e's
late e.
orthochromatic e.
oxyphilic e.
polychromatic e.
polychromatophilic e.
primitive e's
eryth·ro·blas·te·mia

eryth·ro·blas·tic
eryth·ro·blas·to·ma
eryth·ro·blas·to·ma·to·sis
eryth·ro·blas·to·pe·nia
   idiopathic transitory e.
eryth·ro·blas·to·sis
   e. fetalis
   e. neonatorum
eryth·ro·blas·tot·ic
eryth·ro·ca·tal·y·sis
eryth·ro·chro·mia
Eryth·ro·cin
er·y·throc·la·sis
eryth·ro·clast
eryth·ro·clas·tic
eryth·ro·cru·o·rin
eryth·ro·cu·prein
eryth·ro·cy·a·no·sis
   e. frigida
   e. supramalleolaris
eryth·ro·cy·ta·phe·re·sis
eryth·ro·cyte
   achromic e.
   basophilic e.
   burr e.
   crenated e.
   dichromatic e.
   hypochromic e.
   immature e.
   "Mexican hat" e.
   normochromic e.
   nucleated e.
   orthochromatic e.
   polychromatic e.
   reticulated e.
   target e.
   e. transketolase
eryth·ro·cy·the·mia
eryth·ro·cyt·ic
eryth·ro·cy·to·blast
eryth·ro·cy·tol·y·sin
eryth·ro·cy·tol·y·sis
eryth·ro·cy·tom·e·ter
eryth·ro·cy·tom·e·try
eryth·ro·cy·to-op·so·nin
eryth·ro·cy·to·pe·nia
eryth·ro·cy·toph·a·gous
eryth·ro·cy·toph·a·gy

eryth·ro·cy·to·poi·e·sis
eryth·ro·cy·tor·rhex·is
eryth·ro·cy·tos·chi·sis
eryth·ro·cy·to·sis
   anoxemic e.
   e. megalosplenica
   renal e.
   stress e.
eryth·ro·cy·tu·ria
eryth·ro·de·gen·er·a·tive
eryth·ro·der·ma
   congenital ichthyosiform
      e., bullous
   congenital ichthyosiform
      e., nonbullous
   desquamative e.
   e. desquamativum
   exfoliative e.
   e. ichthyosiforme
      congenitum
   leukemic e.
   e. psoriaticum
   resistant maculopapular
      scaly e.
   Sézary e.
eryth·ro·der·mia
eryth·ro·dex·trin
eryth·ro·don·tia
eryth·ro·gen
eryth·ro·gen·e·sis
   e. imperfecta
eryth·ro·gen·ic
eryth·ro·gone
eryth·ro·go·ni·um
eryth·ro·gran·u·lose
er·y·throid
β-eryth·roi·dine
eryth·ro·ka·tal·y·sis
eryth·ro·ker·a·to·der·mia
   progressive symmetrical
      verrucous e.
   e. variabilis
eryth·ro·ki·net·ics
er·yth·rol
   e. tetranitrate
eryth·ro·labe
er·y·thro·le·in
eryth·ro·leu·ke·mia

eryth·ro·leu·ko·blas·to·sis
eryth·ro·leu·ko·sis
eryth·ro·leu·ko·throm·bo·cy·the·mia
eryth·ro·lit·min
er·y·throl·y·sin
er·y·throl·y·sis
eryth·ro·mel·al·gia
    e. of the head
er·y·throm·e·ter
er·y·throm·e·try
eryth·ro·my·cin
    e. B
    e. estolate
    e. ethylcarbonate
    e. ethylsuccinate
    e. gluceptate
    e. lactobionate
    e. propionate
    e. propionate lauryl sulfate
    e. stearate
eryth·ro·my·e·lo·blas·to·sis
er·y·thron
eryth·ro·neo·cy·to·sis
eryth·ro·no·clas·tic
eryth·ro·par·a·site
eryth·ro·pe·nia
eryth·ro·phage
eryth·ro·pha·gia
eryth·ro·phago·cy·to·sis
er·y·throph·a·gous
eryth·ro·phil
er·y·throph·i·lous
Eryth·ro·phloe·um
eryth·ro·pho·bia
eryth·ro·pho·bic
eryth·ro·phore
eryth·ro·phose
eryth·ro·phyll
er·y·thro·pia
eryth·ro·pla·kia
    speckled e.
eryth·ro·pla·sia
    e. of Queyrat
    Zoon's e.
eryth·ro·plas·tid
eryth·ro·poi·e·sis
eryth·ro·poi·et·ic

eryth·ro·poi·e·tin
eryth·ro·pros·o·pal·gia
er·y·throp·sia
er·y·throp·sin
eryth·ro·pyk·no·sis
eryth·ror·rhex·is
eryth·ro·sar·co·ma
er·y·throse
    e. péribuccale pigmentaire
      of Brocq
eryth·ro·sed·i·men·ta·tion
eryth·ro·sin
eryth·ro·sine so·di·um
er·y·thro·sis
    e. of Bechterew
eryth·ro·sta·sis
eryth·ro·thi·o·ne·ine
eryth·ru·lose
er·y·thru·ria
es·cape
    aldosterone e.
    atrioventricular junctional
      e.
    nasal e.
    nodal e.
    vagal e.
    ventricular e.
es·char
es·cha·rot·ic
es·cha·rot·o·my
Esch·er·ich's bacillus
Esch·er·ich's reflex
Esch·er·ich's sign
Esch·e·rich·ia
    E. aurescens
    E. blattae
    E. coli
    E. fergusonii
    E. freundii
    E. hermanii
    E. intermedia
    E. vulneris
Esch·e·rich·i·eae
Esch·scholt·zia
es·cin
es·cor·cin
es·cu·la·pi·an
es·cu·lent

es·cu·lin
es·cutch·eon
esep·tate
es·er·ine
ESF — erythropoietic
   stimulating factor
Es·i·drix
Es·i·mil
Es·ka·barb
Es·ka·di·a·zine
Es·ka·lith
es·march
Es·march's bandage
Es·march's tourniquet
Es·march's tube
eso·cata·pho·ria
eso·cine
eso·de·vi·a·tion
eso·eth·moi·di·tis
eso·gas·tri·tis
esoph·a·gal·gia
esoph·a·ge·al
esoph·a·gec·ta·sia
esoph·a·gec·ta·sis
esoph·a·gec·to·my
esoph·a·gism
   hiatal e.
esoph·a·gis·mus
esoph·a·gi·tis
   acute corrosive e.
   chronic hyperkeratotic e.
   chronic peptic e.
   e. dissecans superficialis
   reflux e.
   thrush e.
esoph·a·go·bron·chi·al
esoph·a·go·car·dio·my·ot·o·
   my
esoph·a·go·cele
esoph·a·go·co·lo·gas·tros·to·
   my
esoph·a·go·co·lo·plas·ty
esoph·a·go·du·o·de·nos·to·
   my
esoph·a·go·dyn·ia
esoph·a·go·ec·ta·sis
esoph·a·go·en·ter·os·to·my
esoph·a·go·esoph·a·gos·to·my

esoph·a·go·fun·do·pexy
esoph·a·go·gas·trec·to·my
esoph·a·go·gas·tric
esoph·a·go·gas·tro·anas·to·
   mo·sis
esoph·a·go·gas·tro·du·od·
   enos·copy
esoph·a·go·gas·tro·my·ot·o·
   my
esoph·a·go·gas·tro·plas·ty
esoph·a·go·gas·tros·co·py
esoph·a·go·gas·tros·to·my
esoph·a·go·gram
esoph·a·gog·ra·phy
esoph·a·go·hi·a·tal
esoph·a·go·je·ju·no·gas·tros·
   to·mo·sis
esoph·a·go·je·ju·no·gas·tros·
   to·my
esoph·a·go·je·ju·no·plas·ty
esoph·a·go·je·ju·nos·to·my
esoph·a·go·lar·yn·gec·to·my
esoph·a·gol·o·gy
esoph·a·go·ma·la·cia
esoph·a·go·my·co·sis
esoph·a·go·my·ot·o·my
   Heller's e.
esoph·a·go·pha·ryn·go·lar·
   yn·gec·to·my
esoph·a·go·phar·ynx
esoph·a·go·plas·ty
esoph·a·go·pli·ca·tion
esoph·a·gop·to·sis
esoph·a·go·res·pi·ra·to·ry
esoph·a·go·scope
   Negus e.
esoph·a·gos·co·py
esoph·a·go·spasm
esoph·a·go·ste·no·sis
esoph·a·gos·to·ma
esoph·a·gos·to·mi·a·sis
esoph·a·gos·to·my
esoph·a·go·tome
esoph·a·got·o·my
esoph·a·go·tra·che·al
esoph·a·gram
esoph·a·gus
   Barrett's e.

esoph·a·gus *(continued)*
    nutcracker e.
eso·pho·ria
eso·phor·ic
eso·sphe·noid·itis
eso·ter·ic
eso·tro·pia
eso·trop·ic
ESP — extrasensory
  perception
esp·no·ic
es·pon·ja
es·pro·quin hy·dro·chlo·ride
es·pun·dia
es·quil·lec·to·my
ESR — erythrocyte
  sedimentation rate
es·sence
    e. of peppermint
es·sen·tia
es·sen·tial
Es·ser's graft
Es·ser's operation
Es·sic cell band
EST — electroshock therapy
es·ter
    Cori e.
    Embden e.
    Harden-Young e.
    Neuberg e.
    Robison e.
es·ter·a·pe·nia
es·ter·ase
    C1 e.
es·ter·i·fi·ca·tion
es·ter·i·fy
es·ter·ize
Es·ter·man visual function
  score
es·ter·ol·y·sis
es·tero·lyt·ic
    hexosephosphoric e.
Es·tes' operation
es·te·trol
es·them·a·tol·o·gy
es·the·sia
es·the·sic
es·the·sio·blast

es·the·si·od·ic
es·the·si·o·gen
es·the·si·o·gen·ic
es·the·si·og·ra·phy
es·the·si·ol·o·gy
es·the·si·om·e·ter
es·the·si·om·e·try
es·the·sio·neure
es·the·sio·neu·ro·blas·to·ma
es·the·sio·neu·ro·cy·to·ma
es·the·sio·neu·ro·epi·the·li·
  o·ma
es·the·sio·phys·i·ol·o·gy
es·the·sod·ic
es·thet·ic
es·the·tics
es·ti·mate
    biased e.
    consistent e.
    interval e.
    point e.
    product-limit e.
    unbiased e.
es·ti·ma·tion
    magnitude e.
    numerical e.
es·ti·ma·tor
Es·ti·nyl
es·ti·val
es·ti·va·tion
es·ti·vo·au·tum·nal
Est·land flap
Est·lan·der's operation
es·to·late
es·ton
Es·trace
es·tra·di·ol
    e. benzoate
    e. cypionate
    e. dipropionate
    e. enanthate
    ethinyl e.
    e. undecylate
    e. valerate
es·tra·di·ol 6β-hydroxy·lase
es·tra·di·ol 6β-mono·oxy·gen·
  ase
es·tra·mus·tine

es·trane
es·tra·pen·ta·ene
es·tra·tet·ra·ene
es·tra·tri·ene
Es·tra·val
es·tra·zi·nol hy·dro·bro·mide
Es·tren-Dam·e·shek syndrome
es·tre·nol
es·tri·a·sis
Es·tri·dae
es·trin
es·trin·iza·tion
es·tri·ol
es·tro·fur·ate
es·tro·gen
    conjugated e's
    esterified e's
    e. glucuronides
es·tro·gen·ic
es·tro·ge·nic·i·ty
es·trog·e·nous
es·trone
    e. sulfate
es·tro·phil·in
es·tro·pi·pate
es·tro·stil·ben
es·trous
es·tru·al
es·tru·a·tion
Es·tru·gen·one
es·trum
es·trus
es·tu·a·ri·um
e.s.u. — electrostatic unit
ESWL — extracorporeal shock
  wave lithotripsy
es·y·late
Et — ethyl group
etaf·e·drine hy·dro·chlo·ride
et·a·fil·con A
Et·a·mon
état
    é. criblé
    é. dysmelinique
    é. lacunaire
    é. mammelonné
    é. marbré
    é. vermoulu

etaz·o·late hy·dro·chlo·ride
ETEC — enterotoxic
    Escherichia coli
Eter·nod's sinus
eter·o·barb
ETF — electron transfer
  flavoprotein
eth·a·cryn·ate
eth·a·cryn·ic acid
eth·al
etham·bu·tol hy·dro·chlo·ride
eth·am·i·van
etham·oxy·tri·phe·tol
etham·sy·late
eth·a·nal
eth·ane
eth·ane·di·al
eth·a·no·ic acid
eth·a·nol
eth·a·nol·amine
eth·a·nol·ism
eth·a·no·yl
eth·a·ver·ine hy·dro·chlo·ride
eth·chlor·vy·nol
eth·ene
eth·ene·sul·fon·ic ac·id ho·
    mo·poly·mer so·di·um salt
eth·e·noid
eth·e·nyl
ether
    anesthetic e.
    methyl tert-butyl e.
    petroleum e.
    thio e.
ethe·re·al
ether·i·fi·ca·tion
ether·iza·tion
ether·ize
ether·om·e·ter
eth·i·cal
eth·ics
    clinical e.
    medical e.
eth·i·dene
    e. chloride
    e. diamine
ethid·i·um
ethin·a·mate

eth·i·nyl
   e. estradiol
Ethi·o·dol
ethi·on·am·ide
ethi·o·nine
ethis·ter·one
eth·mo·car·di·tis
eth·mo·ceph·a·lus
eth·mo·fron·tal
eth·moid
eth·moi·dal
eth·moid·ec·to·my
   transantral e.
eth·moid·itis
eth·moi·do·fron·tal
eth·moi·do·lac·ri·mal
eth·moi·do·max·il·lary
eth·moi·do·na·sal
eth·moi·do·pal·a·tal
eth·moi·do·pal·a·tine
eth·moi·do·sphe·noid
eth·moid·ot·o·my
eth·moi·do·vo·mer·ine
eth·mo·lac·ri·mal
eth·mo·max·il·lary
eth·mo·na·sal
eth·mo·pal·a·tal
eth·mo·sphe·noid
eth·mo·tur·bi·nal
eth·mo·vo·mer·ine
eth·nic
eth·nics
eth·no·bi·ol·o·gy
eth·nog·ra·phy
eth·no·log·ic
eth·nol·o·gy
eth·no·psy·chi·a·try
etho·brom
etho·caine
etho·glu·cid
etho·hep·ta·zine cit·rate
etho·hex·a·di·ol
eth·o·log·i·cal
eth·ol·o·gist
eth·ol·o·gy
etho·mox·ane hy·dro·chlo·ride
eth·o·nam ni·trate

etho·pro·pa·zine hy·dro·chlo·ride
etho·sux·i·mide
etho·to·in
ethox·a·zene hy·dro·chlo·ride
eth·ox·zol·amide
Eth·rane
Eth·ril
eth·y·benz·tro·pine
eth·yl
   e. acetate
   e. aminobenzoate
   e. biscoumacetate
   e. butyrate
   e. chloride
   e. cyanide
   e. dibunate
   e. eosin
   e. ether
   e. hydrocupreine
   e. iodophenylundecylate
   e. linoleate
   e. mercaptan
   e. oleate
   e. orange
eth·yl·al·de·hyde
eth·yl·amine
eth·yl·ate
eth·yl·a·tion
eth·yl·cel·lu·lose
eth·y·lene
   e. dibromide (EDB)
   e. dichloride
   e. glycol
   e. oxide
eth·y·lene·di·a·mine
eth·y·lene·di·a·mine·tet·ra·ac·e·tate
eth·y·lene·di·a·mine·tet·tra·a·ce·tic ac·id
eth·yl·ene·di·ni·trilo·tet·ra·ace·tic acid
eth·yl·en·i·mine
eth·yl·es·tre·nol
ethyl·ic
eth·yl·i·dene
   e. chloride
eth·yl·ism

eth·yl·mal·o·nyl-adip·ic·ac·i·du·ria
eth·yl·mor·phine hy·dro·chlo·ride
eth·yl·nor·a·dren·a·line
eth·yl·nor·epi·neph·rine hy·dro·chlo·ride
eth·yl·nor·su·pra·ren·in
eth·yl·pa·pav·er·ine hy·dro·chlo·ride
eth·yl·par·a·ben
eth·yl·phen·yl·hy·dan·to·in
eth·yl·stib·amine
ethy·no·di·ol di·ac·e·tate
eth·y·nyl
    e. estradiol
    e. testosterone
eti·do·caine hy·dro·chlo·ride
eti·dro·nate
eti·dro·nic acid
etio·cho·lan·o·lone
eti·o·gen·ic
eti·o·la·tion
eti·o·log·ic
eti·o·log·i·cal
eti·ol·o·gy
etio·path·ic
etio·pa·thol·o·gy
etio·por·phyr·in
eti·o·trop·ic
ET-NANB — enterically transmitted non-A, non-B hepatitis
eto·do·lic acid
eto·fen·a·mate
et·o·for·min hy·dro·chlo·ride
etom·i·date
eto·po·side
eto·prine
etox·a·drol hy·dro·chlo·ride
eto·zo·lin
etrot·o·my
eu·adre·no·cor·ti·cism
eu·an·gi·ot·ic
Eu·as·co·my·ce·ti·dae
eu·bac·te·ria
Eu·bac·te·ri·a·les

Eu·bac·te·ri·um
    E. alactolyticum
    E. lentum
    E. limosum
eu·bac·te·ri·um *pl.* eu·bac·te·ria
eu·bi·ot·ics
eu·bo·lism
eu·caine
eu·ca·lyp·tol
Eu·ca·lyp·tus
eu·cap·nia
eu·cary·on
eu·cary·o·sis
Eu·cary·o·tae
eu·cary·ote
eu·cary·ot·ic
eu·cat·ro·pine hy·dro·chlo·ride
Eu·ces·to·da
eu·chlor·hy·dria
eu·cho·lia
eu·chro·mat·ic
eu·chro·ma·tin
eu·chro·ma·top·sy
eu·chyl·ia
Eu·coc·cid·ia
eu·co·deine
eu·coe·lom
Eu·coe·lo·ma·ta
eu·coe·lo·mate
eu·col·loid
eu·cra·sia
eu·die·mor·rhy·sis
eu·di·om·e·ter
eu·dip·sia
eu·er·ga·sia
eu·es·the·sia
Eu·flag·el·la·ta
eu·fla·vine
eu·ga·my
eu·ge·net·ics
Eu·ge·nia
eu·gen·ic acid
eu·gen·i·cist
eu·gen·ics
    negative e.

eu·gen·ics *(continued)*
   positive e.
eu·gen·ism
eu·gen·ist
eu·gen·ol
eu·gle·nid
Eu·gle·ni·da
eu·gle·noid
eu·glob·u·lin
eu·gly·ce·mia
eu·gly·ce·mic
eu·gna·thia
eu·gnath·ic
eu·gno·sia
eu·gnos·tic
eu·gon·ic
eu·hy·dra·tion
eu·kary·on
eu·kary·o·sis
Eu·kary·o·tae
eu·kary·ote
eu·kary·ot·ic
eu·ker·a·tin
eu·ki·ne·sia
eu·ki·ne·sis
eu·ki·net·ic
eu·lam·i·nate
Eu·len·burg's disease
Eu·ler, Ulf Svante von
eu·men·or·rhea
eu·me·tria
eu·mor·phics
eu·mor·phism
Eu·my·ce·tes
eu·my·ce·to·ma
eu·nuch
   fertile e.
eu·nuch·ism
   pituitary e.
eu·nuch·oid
eu·nuch·oid·ism
   female e.
   hypergonadotropic e.
   hypogonadotropic e.
eu·on·y·min
eu·os·mia
eu·pan·cre·a·tism
eu·par·al

eu·pa·theo·scope
eu·pa·to·rin
Eu·pa·to·ri·um
eu·pep·sia
eu·pep·sy
eu·pep·tic
eu·peri·stal·sis
eu·phen·ics
Eu·phor·bia
eu·pho·ret·ic
eu·pho·ria
eu·pho·ri·ant
eu·phor·ic
eu·phor·i·gen·ic
eu·pho·ris·tic
eu·pla·sia
eu·plas·tic
eu·ploid
eu·ploi·dy
eup·nea
eup·ne·ic
eu·prac·tic
eu·prax·ia
eu·prax·ic
eu·pro·cin hy·dro·chlo·ride
Eu·proc·tis
   E. phaeorrhoea
eu·py·rene
eu·py·rex·ia
eu·py·rous
Eu·rax
Eu·re·sol
eu·rhyth·mia
eu·ro·pi·um
Eu·ro·ti·a·ceae
Eu·ro·ti·a·les
Eu·ro·ti·um
   E. malignum
   E. repens
eu·ry·ce·phal·ic
eu·ry·cra·ni·al
eu·ryg·nath·ic
eu·ryg·na·thism
eu·rym·er·ic
eu·ry·on
eu·ry·opia
Eu·ry·pel·ma
   E. hentzii

eu·ry·ther·mal
eu·ry·ther·mic
Eu·scor·pi·us
   E. italicus
Eu·si·mu·li·um
eu·sit·ia
eu·splanch·nia
eu·sple·nia
eu·sta·chi·an
eu·sta·chi·tis
eu·sta·chi·um
eu·sthen·ia
eu·sthen·uria
eu·sys·to·le
eu·sys·tol·ic
eu·tec·tic
eu·telo·lec·i·thal
eu·tha·na·sia
   passive e.
eu·then·ic
eu·then·ics
eu·ther·a·peu·tic
eu·ther·mic
Eu·throid
eu·thy·mic
eu·thy·mism
Eu·thy·neu·ra
eu·thy·roid
eu·thy·roid·ism
eu·thy·scope
eu·to·cia
Eu·to·nyl
eu·top·ic
Eu·tri·at·o·ma
Eu·trom·bic·u·la
   E. alfreddugesi
   E. splendens
Eu·tron
eu·tro·phia
eu·troph·ic
eu·tro·phi·ca·tion
eu·vo·lia
eV — electron volt
ev — electron volt
evac·u·ant
evac·u·ate
evac·u·a·tion
evac·u·a·tor

evag·i·na·tion
   optic e.
ev·a·nes·cent
Ev·ans blue
Ev·ans syndrome
evap·o·ra·tion
eva·sion
even·om·a·tion
event
   ionizing e.
   positron annihilation e.
   scattering e.
even·tra·tion
   diaphragmatic e.
   umbilical e.
Evers·busch's operation
ever·sion
evert
ever·ter
   Berens lid e.
ever·tor
Evex
évide·ment
évi·deur
Ev·i·pal
evi·ra·tion
evis·cer·ate
evis·cer·a·tion
evis·cero·neu·rot·o·my
evo·ca·tion
evo·ca·tor
evoked
evo·lu·tion
   bathmic e.
   convergent e.
   Denman's spontaneous e.
   determinate e.
   Douglas' spontaneous e.
   emergent e.
   organic e.
   orthogenic e.
   parallel e.
   Roederer's spontaneous e.
   saltatory e.
   spontaneous e.
evul·sio
   e. nervi optici

evul·sion
Ew·art's sign
Ew·ing·el·la
Ew·ing's sarcoma
Ew·ing's tumor
ex·ac·er·ba·tion
ex·air·e·sis
ex·al·ta·tion
ex·am·i·na·tion
    air-contrast e.
    double-contrast e.
ex·a·nia
ex·an·i·ma·tion
ex·an·them
    Boston e.
    e. subitum
    vesicular e.
ex·an·the·ma *pl.* ex·an·the·
    mas, ex·an·them·a·ta
    Boston e.
    e. subitum
ex·an·them·a·tous
ex·an·thrope
ex·an·throp·ic
ex·ar·tic·u·la·tion
ex·ca·la·tion
ex·car·na·tion
ex·ca·va·tio *pl.* ex·ca·va·ti·o·
    nes
    e. disci
    e. papillae nervi optici
    e. rectouterina
    e. rectovesicalis
    e. vesicouterina
ex·ca·va·tion
    atrophic e.
    dental e.
    glaucomatous e.
    ischiorectal e.
    e. of optic disk
    physiologic e.
    rectoischiadic e.
    rectouterine e.
    rectovesical e.
    vesicouterine e.
ex·ca·va·ti·o·nes
ex·ca·va·tor
    dental e.

ex·ca·va·tor *(continued)*
    hatchet e.
    spoon e.
ex·ca·va·tum
ex·cer·e·bra·tion
ex·cer·nent
ex·cess
    antibody e.
    antigen e.
    base e.
ex·change
    ion e.
    plasma e.
    sister chromatid e.
ex·change·a·ble
ex·chang·er
    anion e.
    cation e.
    heat e.
    ion e.
ex·cip·i·ent
ex·cise
ex·ci·sion
    fascial e.
    Ferris Smith e.
    narrow e.
    primary e.
    sequential e.
    tangential e.
    wide e.
ex·ci·ta·bil·i·ty
    exteroceptive e.
    proprioceptive e.
    rhythmic e.
    seismogenic e.
    subliminal e.
ex·ci·ta·ble
ex·cit·ant
ex·ci·ta·tion
    anomalous atrioventricular
        e.
    catatonic e.
    direct e.
    ephaptic e.
    indirect e.
ex·ci·ta·to·ry
ex·cite·ment
    anniversary e.

ex·cite·ment *(continued)*
    catatonic e.
    psychomotor e.
ex·ci·to·an·a·bol·ic
ex·ci·to·cat·a·bol·ic
ex·ci·to·glan·du·lar
ex·ci·to·met·a·bol·ic
ex·ci·to·mo·tor
ex·ci·to·mo·to·ry
ex·ci·to·mus·cu·lar
ex·ci·to·nu·tri·ent
ex·ci·tor
ex·ci·to·se·cre·to·ry
ex·ci·to·vas·cu·lar
ex·clave
ex·clu·sion
    allelic e.
    competitive e.
ex·coch·le·a·tion
ex·con·ju·gant
ex·co·ri·a·tion
    neurotic e.
ex·cor·ti·ca·tion
ex·cre·ment
ex·cre·men·ti·tious
ex·cres·cence
    fungating e.
    fungous e.
    Lambl's e's
ex·cres·cent
ex·cre·ta
ex·crete
ex·cre·ter
ex·cre·tin
ex·cre·tion
    fractional e.
    pseudouridine e.
    renal tubular hydrogen e.
ex·cre·to·ry
ex·cur·rent
ex·cur·sion
    lateral e.
    protrusive e.
    respiratory e.
    retrusive e.
ex·cur·sive
ex·cy·clo·de·vi·a·tion
ex·cy·clo·pho·ria

ex·cy·clo·tro·pia
ex·cyst
ex·cys·ta·tion
ex·cyst·ment
ex·el·cy·mo·sis
ex·e·mia
ex·en·ce·pha·lia
ex·en·ceph·a·lo·cele
ex·en·ceph·a·lon
ex·en·ceph·a·lous
ex·en·ceph·a·lus
ex·en·ceph·a·ly
ex·en·ter·a·tion
    pelvic e.
ex·en·ter·a·tive
ex·en·ter·itis
ex·er·cise
    active e.
    active assisted e.
    active resistive e.
    corrective e.
    DeSouza e's
    Fournier's e.
    free e.
    Frenkel's e's
    graduated resistance e.
    isokinetic e.
    isometric e.
    isotonic e.
    Kegel's e's
    muscle-setting e.
    neuromuscular facilitation
     e.
    passive e.
    static e.
    therapeutic e.
    underwater e.
ex·er·e·sis
ex·er·gic
ex·er·gon·ic
ex·e·sion
ex·fe·ta·tion
ex·flag·el·la·tion
ex·fo·li·ate
ex·fo·li·a·tin
ex·fo·li·a·tio
    e. areata linguae
ex·fo·li·a·tion

ex·fo·li·a·tion
  lamellar e. of newborn
ex·fo·li·a·tive
ex·ha·lant
ex·ha·la·tion
ex·hale
ex·haus·tion
  anhidrotic heat e.
  cold e.
  combat e.
  heat e.
Exhib. — L. exhibeatur (let it
  be given)
ex·hi·bi·tion
ex·hi·bi·tion·ism
ex·hi·bi·tion·ist
ex·hu·ma·tion
ex·i·tus *pl.* ex·i·tus
  e. pelvis
Ex·na
Ex·ner's plex·us
exo-am·y·lase
exo·an·ti·gen
exo·bi·ol·o·gy
exo·car·dia
exo·car·di·al
exo·carp
exo·cata·pho·ria
ex·oc·cip·i·tal
exo·cele
exo·cel·lu·lar
exo·cer·vix
exo·cho·ri·on
exo·coe·lom
exo·coe·lo·ma
exo·co·li·tis
exo·cra·ni·al
exo·crine
exo·cri·nol·o·gy
exo·cri·nos·i·ty
exo·cu·ti·cle
exo·cy·clic
exo·cy·to·sis
exo·de·oxy·ri·bo·nu·cle·ase
exo·de·vi·a·tion
ex·odon·tia
ex·odon·tics
ex·odon·tist

exo·en·er·get·ic
exo·en·zyme
exo·er·gic
exo·eryth·ro·cyte
exo·eryth·ro·cyt·ic
ex·og·a·my
exo·gas·tric
exo·gas·tri·tis
exo·gas·tru·la
exo·gas·tru·la·tion
exo·ge·net·ic
ex·o·gen·ic
ex·og·e·note
ex·og·e·nous
ex·og·na·thia
ex·og·na·thi·on
ex·og·no·sis
exo·hor·mone
ex·om·e·ter
ex·om·pha·los
exo·mys·i·um
ex·on
exo·nu·cle·ase
exo·path·ic
ex·op·a·thy
exo·pep·ti·dase
exo·pho·ria
exo·phor·ic
ex·oph·thal·mic
ex·oph·thal·mo·gen·ic
ex·oph·thal·mom·e·ter
ex·oph·thal·mo·met·ric
ex·oph·thal·mom·e·try
ex·oph·thal·mos
  endocrine e.
  malignant e.
  pulsating e.
  thyrotoxic e.
  thyrotropic e.
exo·phyte
exo·phyt·ic
exo·plasm
ex·or·bi·tism
exo·re·sis
exo·ri·bo·nu·cle·ase
exo·sep·sis
exo·se·ro·sis
exo·skel·e·ton

ex·os·mose
ex·os·mo·sis
exo·som·es·the·sia
exo·sple·no·pex·y
exo·spore
exo·spo·ri·um
ex·os·tec·to·my
ex·os·to·sec·to·my
ex·os·to·sis
    e. bursata
    e. cartilaginea
    dental e.
    hereditary multiple
      exostoses
    ivory e.
    multiple cartilaginous
      exostoses
    multiple exostoses
    osteocartilaginous e.
ex·os·tot·ic
exo·ter·ic
exo·the·li·o·ma
exo·ther·mal
exo·ther·mic
exo·thy·mo·pexy
exo·thy·roi·do·pexy
exo·thy·ro·pex·ia
exo·thy·ro·pexy
ex·ot·ic
exo·tox·ic
exo·tox·in
exo·tro·pia
ex·o·trop·ic
ex·pan·der
    plasma volume e.
    subperiosteal tissue e.
      (STE)
    tissue e.
ex·pan·sion
    aliform e.
    e. of the arch
    clonal e.
    cubical e.
    dorsal digital e.
    extensor e.
    fibrous e's of eye muscles
    hygroscopic e.
    maxillary e.

ex·pan·sion *(continued)*
    setting e.
    thermal e.
    wax e.
ex·pan·sive·ness
ex·pec·tan·cy
    life e.
ex·pec·to·rant
    liquefying e.
    stimulant e.
ex·pec·to·rate
ex·pec·to·ra·tion
    rusty e.
ex·pel
ex·pel·lant
ex·per·i·ment
    bulbocapnine e.
    check e.
    control e.
    cross-over e.
    crucial e.
    Cyon's e.
    defect e.
    double-blind e.
    Goltz's e.
    Küss's e.
    Mariotte's e.
    Müller's e.
    Nussbaum's e.
    O'Beirne's e.
    Scheiner's e.
    Stensen's e.
    Toynbee's e.
    Valsalva's e.
ex·pi·rate
ex·pi·ra·tion
ex·pi·ra·to·ry
ex·pire
ex·plant
    cellular e.
ex·plode
ex·plo·ra·tion
ex·plor·a·to·ry
ex·plor·er
ex·plo·sion
ex·plo·sive
ex·po·nent
ex·po·nen·tial

ex·po·sure
  acute e.
  air e.
  chronic e.
  double e.
  pulp e.
ex·press
ex·pres·sate
ex·pres·sion
  Kristeller e.
  manual e. of placenta
ex·pres·sive
ex·pres·siv·i·ty
ex·pres·sor
ex·pul·sion
  spontaneous e. of placenta
ex·pul·sive
ex·qui·site
ex·san·gui·nate
ex·san·gui·na·tion
ex·san·guine
ex·san·gui·no·trans·fu·sion
ex·sect
ex·sec·tion
ex·sec·tor
ex·sic·cant
ex·sic·cate
ex·sic·ca·tion
ex·sic·co·sis
ex·sorp·tion
ex·stro·phy
  e. of the bladder
  e. of cloaca
  cloacal e.
ex·suf·fla·tion
ex·suf·fla·tor
ext. — extract
ex·tend
ex·ten·der
  artificial plasma e.
ex·ten·sion
  Buck's e.
  nail e.
  e. per contiguitatem
  e. per continuitatem
  e. per saltam
  e. for prevention
  ridge e.

ex·ten·sion (continued)
  skeletal e.
  Steinmann's e.
  tectoseptal e.
ex·ten·sor
  e. carpi radialis accessorius
  e. carpi radialis
    intermedius
  long radial e. of wrist
  ulnar e. of wrist
ex·te·ri·or
ex·te·ri·or·ize
ex·tern
ex·ter·nal
ex·ter·na·lia
ex·ter·nal·iza·tion
ex·ter·nal·ize
ex·terne
ex·ter·nus
ex·tero·cep·tive
ex·tero·cep·tor
ex·tero·fec·tion
ex·tero·fec·tive
ex·tero·ges·tate
ex·ti·ma
ex·tinc·tion
ex·tin·guish
ex·tir·pate
ex·tir·pa·tion
  dental pulp e.
ex·tor·sion
ex·tor·tor
ex·tra-adre·nal
ex·tra-am·ni·on·ic
ex·tra-an·a·tom·ic
ex·tra-an·throp·ic
ex·tra-ar·tic·u·lar
ex·tra·bron·chi·al
ex·tra·buc·cal
ex·tra·bul·bar
ex·tra·cap·su·lar
ex·tra·car·di·al
ex·tra·car·pal
ex·tra·car·ti·lag·i·nous
ex·tra·cel·lu·lar
ex·tra·cer·e·bral
ex·tra·chro·mo·so·mal
ex·tra·cor·po·re·al

ex·tra·cor·pus·cu·lar
ex·tra·cor·ti·co·spi·nal
ex·tra·cra·ni·al
ex·tract
  alcoholic e.
  allergenic e.
  belladonna e.
  Buchner's e.
  cascara sagrada e.
  cell-free e.
  chondodendron
   tomentosum e.
  chondrus e.
  compound e.
  dry e.
  equivalent e.
  euphorbia liquid e.
  fluid e.
  glycyrrhiza e.
  henbane e.
  hydroalcoholic e.
  hyoscyamus e.
  Irish moss e.
  licorice root e.
  liver e.
  liver e., liquid
  e. of male fern
  malt e.
  ox bile e.
  oxgall e., powdered
  parathyroid e.
  pilular e.
  placental e.
  poison ivy e.
  poison oak e.
  pollen e.
  powdered e.
  protein e.
  rice polishings e.
  semiliquid e.
  soft e.
  solid e.
  tikitiki e.
  trichinella e.
  yeast e.
ex·trac·tant
ex·trac·tion
  breech e.

ex·trac·tion *(continued)*
  breech e., partial
  breech e., total
  cataract e.
  cataract e., extracapsular
  cataract e., intracapsular
  flap e.
  menstrual e.
  phenol water e.
  progressive e.
  selected e.
  serial e.
  tooth e.
  vacuum e.
ex·trac·tive
ex·trac·tor
  basket e.
  vacuum e.
ex·tra·cys·tic
ex·tra·du·ral
ex·tra·em·bry·on·ic
ex·tra·epi·phys·e·al
ex·tra·fu·sal
ex·tra·gen·i·tal
ex·tra·he·pat·ic
ex·tra·lig·a·men·tous
ex·tra·mal·le·o·lus
ex·tra·mas·toi·di·tis
ex·tra·med·ul·la·ry
ex·tra·me·nin·ge·al
ex·tra·mu·ral
ex·tra·ne·ous
ex·tra·neu·ral
ex·tra·nu·cle·ar
ex·tra·oc·u·lar
ex·tra·os·se·ous
ex·tra·pan·cre·at·ic
ex·tra·par·en·chy·mal
ex·tra·pel·vic
ex·tra·peri·car·di·al
ex·tra·per·i·ne·al
ex·tra·peri·os·te·al
ex·tra·peri·to·ne·al
ex·tra·phys·io·log·ic
ex·tra·pla·cen·tal
ex·tra·plan·tar
ex·tra·pleu·ral
ex·trap·o·la·tion

ex·tra·pros·tat·ic
ex·tra·pros·ta·ti·tis
ex·tra·psy·chic
ex·tra·pul·mo·na·ry
ex·tra·py·ram·i·dal
ex·tra·rec·tus
ex·tra·re·nal
ex·tra·sen·so·ry
ex·tra·se·rous
ex·tra·so·mat·ic
ex·tra·spi·nal
ex·tra·stri·ate
ex·tra·su·pra·re·nal
ex·tra·sys·to·le
    atrial e.
    atrioventricular e.
    auriclar e.
    auriculoventricular e.
    A-V nodal e.
    infranodal e.
    interpolated e.
    junctional e.
    nodal e.
    retrograde e.
    return e.
    supraventricular e.
    ventricular e.
ex·tra·tho·rac·ic
ex·tra·tra·che·al
ex·tra·tu·bal
ex·tra·tym·pan·ic
ex·tra·uter·ine
ex·tra·vag·i·nal
ex·trav·a·sate
ex·trav·a·sa·tion
    punctiform e.
    pyelosinus e.
ex·tra·vas·cu·lar
ex·tra·ven·tric·u·lar
ex·tra·ver·sion
ex·tra·vert
ex·trem·is
ex·trem·i·tal
ex·trem·i·tas *pl.* ex·trem·i·ta·tes
    e. acromialis claviculae
    e. anterior lienis
    e. anterior splenis

ex·trem·i·tas *(continued)*
    e. inferior
    e. inferior lienis
    e. inferior renis
    e. inferior testis
    e. posterior lienis
    e. posterior splenis
    e. sternalis claviculae
    e. superior
    e. superior lienis
    e. superior renis
    e. superior testis
    e. tubale ovarii
    e. tubaria ovarii
    e. uterina ovarii
ex·trem·i·ta·tes
ex·trem·i·ty
    anterior e. of spleen
    cartilaginous e. of rib
    external e. of clavicle
    fimbriated e. of fallopian tube
    inferior e. of kidney
    inferior e. of testis
    internal e. of clavicle
    lower e.
    pelvic e. of ovary
    posterior e. of spleen
    proximal e. of phalanx of finger
    proximal e. of phalanx of toe
    scapular e. of clavicle
    superior e. of kidney
    superior e. of testis
    tubal e. of ovary
    upper e.
    uterine e. of ovary
ex·trin·sic
ex·tro·gas·tru·la·tion
ex·tro·phia
ex·tro·ver·sion
    e. of bladder
ex·tro·vert
ex·trude
ex·tru·sion
    e. of tooth
ex·tu·bate

ex·tu·ba·tion
ex·u·ber·ant
ex·u·date
    catarrhal e.
    cotton-wool e's
    fibrinous e.
    gingival e.
    hemorrhagic e.
    inflammatory e.
    purulent e.
    sanguineous e.
    serofibrinous e.
    serous e.
ex·u·da·tion
ex·u·da·tive
ex·ude
ex·ul·cer·ans
ex·ul·cer·a·tio
    e. simplex
ex·um·bil·i·ca·tion
ex·u·tory
ex·u·vi·a·tion
ex vi·vo
eye
    aphakic e.
    artificial e.
    black e.
    blear e.
    cinema e.
    compound e.
    crab e.
    crossed e's
    cyclopean e.
    cystic e.
    dark-adapted e.
    deviating e.
    doll's e's
    epiphyseal e.
    exciting e.
    fixating e.
    following e.
    hop e.
    Klieg e.
    lazy e.

eye *(continued)*
    light-adapted e.
    median e.
    monochromatic e.
    parietal e.
    pineal e.
    pink e.
    primary e.
    pseudophakic e.
    raccoon e's
    reduced e.
    schematic e.
    secondary e.
    shipyard e.
    Snellen's reform e.
    squinting e.
    sunset e.
    sympathizing e.
    wall e.
eye·ball
eye·brow
eye·cup, eye cup
eye·glass
eye·glass·es
eye·ground
eye·lash
eye·let
eye·lid
    third e.
eye-mind·ed
eye·piece
    comparison e.
    compensating e.
    demonstration e.
    high-eyepoint e.
    huygenian e.
    Huygens (Huyghens) e.
    negative e.
    positive e.
    Ramsden's e.
    widefield e.
eye·point
eye·spot
eye·strain

F

F — farad
  fertility (plasmid)
  fluorine
  formula
  French (scale)
  visual field
F. — L. fiat (let it be done)
F — faraday
  force
  gilbert
F₁ — first filial generation
F₂ — second filial generation
°F — degree Fahrenheit
f — femto-
  focal length
f — frequency
FA — fatty acid
  femoral artery
  fluorescent antibody
Fab — fragment,
  antigen-binding
fa·bel·la *pl.* fa·bel·lae
Fa·ber's anemia
Fa·ber's syndrome
fa·bism
fab·ri·ca·tion
Fabricius' bursa
Fa·bry's disease
fab·u·la·tion
Facb — fragment,
  antigen-and-complement-bind-
  ing
FACD — Fellow of the
  American College of Dentists
face
  adenoid f.
  bony f.
  bovine f.
  cleft f.
  cow f.
  cushingoid f.
  dish f.
  dished f.
  frog f.
  hatchet f.
  hippocratic f.

face *(continued)*
  masklike f.
  moon f.
face-bow
  adjustable axis f.-b.
  kinematic f.-b.
face-lift, face lift
face·om·e·ter
fac·et
  acromial f.
  articular f.
  clavicular f.
  costal f.
  lateral f's of sternum
  Lenoir's f.
  locked f's of spine
  malleolar f. of tibia,
    internal
  squatting f.
  f. for tubercle of rib
  wear f.
fac·e·tec·to·my
fa·cial
fa·ci·es *pl.* fa·ci·es
  f. abdominalis
  acromegalic f.
  adenoid f.
  f. anterior
  f. anterolateralis
  f. anteromedialis
  f. articularis
  f. bovina
  f. buccalis
  f. cerebralis
  f. colica
  f. contactus dentis
  f. convexa cerebri
  f. costalis
  cushingoid f.
  f. diaphragmatica
  f. digitales
  f. digitales dorsales
  f. digitales fibulares pedis
  f. digitales laterales
  f. digitales mediales
  f. digitales palmares

fa·ci·es *(continued)*
    f. digitales plantares
    f. digitales radiales
    f. digitales tibiales
    f. digitales ulnares
    f. distalis
    f. dolorosa
    f. dorsalis
    f. externa
    f. facialis
    f. frontalis
    f. gastrica
    f. glutea ossis ilii
    f. hepatica
    f. hippocratica
    Hutchinson's f.
    f. inferior
    f. inferolateralis
    f. interlobares pulmonis
    f. interna
    f. intestinalis uteri
    f. labialis dentis
    f. lateralis
    leonine f.
    f. leontina
    f. lingualis
    f. lunata
    f. malaris
    f. malleolaris
    Marshall Hall's f.
    f. masticatoria
    f. maxillaris
    f. medialis
    f. mediastinalis pulmonis
    f. mesialis
    mitral f.
    mitrotricuspid f.
    moon f.
    myasthenic f.
    myopathic f.
    myxedematous f.
    f. nasalis
    f. palatina
    paralytic f.
    f. parietalis ossis parietalis
    Parkinson's f.
    parkinsonian f.
    f. patellaris femoris
    f. pelvina

fa·ci·es *(continued)*
    f. poplitea femoris
    f. posterior
    Potter f.
    f. pulmonalis cordis
    f. renalis
    f. sacropelvina
    f. scaphoidea
    f. sphenomaxillaris alae
      magnae
    f. sternocostalis cordis
    f. superior
    f. superolateralis
    f. symphyseos
    f. symphysialis
    tabetic f.
    f. temporalis
    tortua f.
    typhoid f.
    f. urethralis penis
    f. ventralis
    f. vesicalis uteri
    f. vestibularis
    f. visceralis
    f. volaris
fa·cil·i·ta·tion
    associative f.
    f. of reflexes
    Wedensky f.
fa·cil·i·ta·tive
fa·cil·i·ta·to·ry
fa·cil·i·tory
fa·cil·i·ty
    extended care f. (ECF)
    intermediate care f.
    skilled nursing f. (SNF)
fa·cio·bra·chi·al
fa·cio·ceph·a·lal·gia
fa·cio·cer·vi·cal
fa·cio·lin·gual
fa·cio·plas·ty
fa·cio·ple·gia
fa·cio·scap·u·lo·hu·mer·al
fa·cio·ste·no·sis
FACOG — Fellow of the
    American College of
    Obstetricians and
    Gynecologists

FACP — Fellow of the American College of Physicians

FACS — Fellow of the American College of Surgeons
fluorescence-activated cell sorter

FACSM — Fellow of the American College of Sports Medicine

F-act·in
fac·ti·tial
fac·ti·tious
fac·tor
f. A
accelerator f.
activated clotting f's
activation f.
adrenocorticotropic releasing f. (ACTH-RF)
angiogenesis f.
amplification f.
antigen-specific T-cell helper f.
antigen-specific T-cell suppressor f.
antihemophilic f.
antihemophilic f., cryoprecipitated
antihemophilic f., human
antinuclear f. (ANF)
anti-pernicious anemia f.
atrial natriuretic f. (ANF)
f. B
backscatter f.
basophil chemotactic f. (BCF)
B cell differentiation f's (BCDF)
B cell growth f's (BCGF)
Bittner milk f.
blastogenic f. (BF)
B-lymphocyte stimulatory f's (BSF)
bone f.

fac·tor *(continued)*
buildup f.
C f.
C3 nephritic f. (C3 NeF)
calibration f.
CAMP f.
cardiac risk f's
Castle's f.
chemotactic f.
Christmas f.
citrovorum f.
clearing f.
clonal inhibitory f.
clumping f.
coagulation f's (I–XIII)
colony-stimulating f. (CSF)
conglutinogen activating f. (KAF)
contact f.
contact activation f.
cord f.
corticotropin releasing f. (CRF)
coupling f's
crystal-induced chemotactic f. (CCF)
Curling f.
f. D
Day's f.
decapacitation f.
decay-activating f. (DAF)
depolarization f.
diabetogenic f.
diffusion f.
Duran-Reynals f.
duty f.
elongation f.
eluate f.
endothelium-derived relaxing f.
eosinophil chemotactic f. (ECF)
eosinophil chemotactic f. of anaphylaxis (ECF-A)
epidermal growth f.
erythropoietic stimulating f. (ESF)
extrinsic f.

fac·tor *(continued)*
 F (fertility) f.
 fibrin stabilizing f.
 follicle stimulating
  hormone releasing f.
  (FRF, FSH-RF)
 galactopoietic f.
 glass f.
 glucose tolerance f.
 gonadotropin releasing f.
  (GnRF)
 growth f.
 growth hormone releasing
  f. (GRF, GH-RF)
 growth inhibitory f's
 f. H
 Hageman f. (HF)
 hematopoietic growth f's
 high-molecular-weight
  neutrophil chemotactic f.
  (HMW-NCF)
 histamine releasing f.
 hydrazine-sensitive f.
  (HSF)
 hyperglycemic-glycogenolytic f.
 f. I
 immunoglobulin-binding f.
  (IBF)
 inhibiting f's
 initiation f.
 insulin-like growth f's
  (IGF)
 intrinsic f.
 labile f.
 lactogenic f.
 Laki-Lorand f.
 LE f.
 leukocyte inhibitory f.
  (LIF)
 liver filtrate f.
 LLD f.
 luteinizing hormone
  releasing f. (LRF, LH-RF)
 lymph node permeability f.
  (LNPF)
 lymphocyte activating f.

fac·tor *(continued)*
 lymphocyte blastogenic f.
  (BF)
 lymphocyte mitogenic f.
  (LMF)
 lymphocyte transforming f.
  (LTF)
 lysogenic f.
 macrophage-activating f.
  (MAF)
 macrophage chemotactic f.
  (MCF)
 macrophage-derived
  growth f.
 macrophage growth f.
  (MGF)
 macrophage inhibitory f.
  (MIF)
 migration inhibiting f.
  (MIF)
 milk f.
 mitogenic f.
 mouse mammary tumor f.
 müllerian duct inhibitory f.
 müllerian regression f.
 multiple f's
 myocardial depressant f.
  (MDF)
 N f.
 necrotizing f.
 nerve growth f.
 neutrophil chemotactic f.
  (NCF)
 osteoclast activating f.
  (OAF)
 f. P
 pellagra-preventive f.
 platelet f's (1–4)
 platelet activating f. (PAF)
 platelet-derived growth f.
 P.-P. f.
 prolactin inhibiting f. (PIF)
 prolactin releasing f. (PRF)
 proliferation inhibitory f.
  (PIF)
 prothrombokinase f.
 Prower f.
 R f.

fac·tor *(continued)*
    rat acrodynia f.
    recruitment f.
    releasing f.
    resistance-inducing f.
    resistance transfer f.
    Rh f.
    Rhesus f.
    rheumatoid f. (RF)
    risk f.
    f. S
    sex f.
    Simon's septic f.
    skin reactive f. (SRF)
    somatotropin releasing f. (SRF)
    specific macrophage arming f. (SMAF)
    spreading f.
    stable f.
    Stuart f.
    Stuart-Prower f.
    sulfation f.
    T-cell growth f.
    thyrotropin releasing f. (TRF)
    tissue f.
    transfer f. (TF)
    Trapp's f.
    tumor-angiogenesis f.
    tumor necrosis f. (TNF)
    V f.
    von Willebrand's f.
    f. W
    Wills f.
    X f.
    yeast eluate f.
    yeast filtrate f.
fac·to·ri·al
fac·ul·ta·tive
fac·ul·ty
    fusion f.
FAD — flavin adenine dinucleotide
Fa·get's law
Fa·get's sign
fag·op·y·rism
Fah·rae·us-Lind·qvist effect

Fahr·en·heit scale
Fahr·en·heit thermometer
fail·ure
    acute anuric renal f.
    acute oliguric renal f.
    acute polyuric renal f.
    backward heart f.
    biventricular f.
    congestive heart f. (CHF)
    forward heart f.
    heart f.
    high-output heart f.
    high-output renal f.
    kidney f.
    left-sided heart f.
    low-output heart f.
    peripheral circulatory f.
    prerenal f.
    renal f.
    respiratory f.
    template f.
faint
faint·ing
Fa·jer·sztajn sign
Fa·jer·sztajn test
fal·ca·di·na
fal·cate
fal·ces
fal·cial
fal·ci·form
fal·cu·lar
fal·lo·pi·an aqueduct
fal·lo·pi·an arch
fal·lo·pi·an artery
fal·lo·pi·an ligament
fal·lo·pi·an tube
Fal·lot's disease
Fal·lot's syndrome
Fal·lot's tetrad
Fal·lot's tetralogy
Fal·lot's trilogy
false-neg·a·tive
false-pos·i·tive
    biologic f.p. (BFP)
fal·si·fi·ca·tion
    retrospective f.
Fal·ta's coefficient
Fal·ta's triad

falx *pl.* fal·ces
    aponeurotic f.
    f. aponeurotica
    f. cerebelli
    f. cerebri
    inguinal f.
    f. inguinalis
    f. ligamentosa
    ligamentous f.
    f. septi
fa·mil·i·al
fam·i·ly
    extended f.
    form-f.
    Jukes f.
    Kallikak f.
    nuclear f.
    systematic f.
fam·o·tine hy·dro·chlo·ride
fan
    Dunham's f's
    macular f.
    sea f.
Fanconi syndrome
fang
fan·go
fan·go·ther·a·py
Fan·nia
    F. canicularis
    F. scalaris
Fan·si·dar
fan·ta·scope
fan·tri·done hy·dro·chlo·ride
FAPHA — Fellow of the American Public Health Association
Far·a·beuf's amputation
Far·a·beuf's triangle
far·ad
far·a·day
Far·a·day's constant
Far·a·day's dark space
Far·a·day's law
fa·rad·ic
far·a·dim·e·ter
far·a·dism
    surging f.
far·a·di·za·tion

far·a·dize
far·a·do·con·trac·til·i·ty
far·a·do·mus·cu·lar
far·a·do·pal·pa·tion
far·a·do·ther·a·py
Far·ber's disease
Far·ber's test
far·ne·sol
far·ne·syl py·ro·phos·phate
far·no·quin·one
Farr's law
Farre's tubercles
Farre's white line
far·sight·ed
far·sight·ed·ness
fasc. — L. fasciculus (bundle)
fas·cia *pl.* fas·ciae
    abdominal f., internal
    Abernethy's f.
    f. adherens
    alar f. of pharynx
    anal f.
    anoscrotal f.
    antebrachial f.
    f. antebrachii
    aponeurotic f.
    f. axillaris
    bicipital f.
    brachial f.
    f. brachialis
    f. brachii
    buccinator f.
    f. buccopharyngea
    buccopharyngeal f.
    f. buccopharyngealis
    Buck's f.
    bulbar f.
    f. bulbi [Tenoni]
    f. of Camper
    cervical f.
    f. cervicalis
    cervical visceral f.
    clavipectoral f.
    f. clavipectoralis
    f. clitoridis
    Cloquet's f.
    Colles' f.
    f. colli

fas·cia *(continued)*
   Cooper's f.
   coracoclavicular f.
   f. coracoclavicularis
   coracocostal f.
   cremasteric f.
   f. cremasterica
   cribriform f.
   f. cribrosa
   crural f.
   f. cruris
   Cruveilhier's f.
   dartos f. of scrotum
   deep f.
   deltoid f.
   f. deltoidea
   Denonvilliers' f.
   f. dentata hippocampi
   dentate f.
   dorsal f., deep
   dorsal f. of foot
   dorsal f. of hand
   f. dorsalis manus
   f. dorsalis pedis
   Dupuytren's f.
   endoabdominal f.
   endopelvic f.
   f. endopelvina
   endothoracic f.
   f. endothoracica
   external intercostal f.
   extraperitoneal f.
   f. extraperitonealis
   extrapleural f.
   femoral f.
   fibroareolar f.
   f. of forearm
   fusion f.
   f. of Gerota
   gluteal f.
   Godman's f.
   hypogastric f.
   hypothenar f.
   iliac f.
   f. iliaca
   f. iliopectinea
   iliopectineal f.
   infundibuliform f.

fas·cia *(continued)*
   f. of insertion
   intercolumnar f.
   investing f.
   ischiorectal f.
   lacrimal f.
   f. lata femoris
   f. of leg
   longitudinal f., anterior
   longitudinal f., posterior
   lumbar f.
   lumbodorsal f.
   f. lunata
   masseteric f.
   f. masseterica
   muscular fasciae of eye
   fasciae musculares bulbi
   f. nuchae
   nuchal f.
   f. nuchalis
   obturator f.
   f. obturatoria
   orbital fasciae
   fasciae orbitales
   palmar f.
   palpebral f.
   f. palpebralis
   parietal f. of pelvis
   parotid f.
   f. parotidea
   f. pectinea
   pectineal f.
   pectoral f.
   f. pectoralis
   pelvic f.
   pelviprostatic f.
   f. pelvis
   f. pelvis parietalis
   f. pelvis visceralis
   f. penis profunda
   f. penis superficialis
   f. perinei superficialis
   perirenal f.
   peritoneoperineal f.
   f. peritoneoperinealis
   pharyngobasilar f.
   f. pharyngobasilaris
   phrenicopleural f.

fas·cia *(continued)*
  f. phrenicopleuralis
  plantar f.
  popliteal f.
  pretracheal f.
  prevertebral f.
  f. prevertebralis
  f. profunda
  f. propria colli
  f. propria cooperi
  f. prostatae
  psoas f.
  pubic f.
  rectal f.
  rectoabdominal f.
  rectovaginal f.
  rectovesical f.
  renal f.
  f. renalis
  Richet's f.
  scalene f.
  Scarpa's f.
  semilunar f.
  Sibson's f.
  spermatic f., external
  spermatic f., internal
  f. spermatica externa
  f. spermatica interna
  subcutaneous f.
  subperitoneal f.
  f. subperitonealis
  f. subscapularis
  superficial f.
  f. superficialis
  f. superficialis perinei
  f. of Tarin
  f. tarini
  temporal f.
  f. temporalis
  f. of Tenon
  thenar f.
  thoracic f.
  f. thoracica
  f. thoracolumbalis
  thyrolaryngeal f.
  f. of Toldt
  f. transversalis
  f. of Treitz

fas·cia *(continued)*
  triangular f. of Macalister
  triangular f. of Quain
  Tyrrell's f.
  volar f.
fas·ciae
fas·cia·gram
fas·ci·ag·ra·phy
fas·cial
fas·cia·plas·ty
fas·ci·cle
  gracile f.
  longitudinal f's of
    cruciform ligament
fas·cic·u·lar
fas·cic·u·lat·ed
fas·cic·u·la·tion
fas·cic·u·li
fas·cic·u·li·tis
fas·cic·u·lus *pl.* fas·cic·cu·li
  f. aberrans of Monakow
  f. anterior proprius
  f. anterolateralis
    superficialis gowersi
  f. arcuatus
  f. atrioventricularis
  f. of Burdach
  calcarine f.
  central tegmental f.
  cerebellospinal f.
  f. cerebellospinalis anterior
  f. cerebellospinalis lateralis
  f. circumolivaris
    pyramidalis
  crossed pyramidal f.
  cuneate f. of Burdach
  cuneate f. of medulla
    oblongata
  cuneate f. of spinal cord
  f. cuneatus
  f. cuneatus burdachi
  dorsolateral f.
  f. dorsolateralis
  f. exilis
  extrapyramidal motor f.
  fastigiobulbar f.
  f. of Foville
  f. of Goll

fas·cic·u·lus *(continued)*
 Gowers' f.
 f. gracilis
 gyral f.
 inferior longitudinal f. of
  cerebrum
 interfascicular f.
 f. interfascicularis
 intersegmental fasciculi
 lateral cerebrospinal f.
 lenticular f.
 f. lenticularis
 longitudinal f.
 f. longitudinalis
 maculary f.
 mamillotegmental f.
 f. mamillotegmentalis
 mamillothalamic f.
 f. mamillothalamicus
 medial longitudinal f.
 medial prosencephalic f.
 medial telencephalic f.
 median triangular f.
 Meynert's f.
 Monakow's f.
 f. occipitofrontalis
 occipitothalamic f.
 olivocochlear f.
 oval f.
 f. parieto-occipitopontinus
 f. pedunculomamillaris
 perpendicular f.
 f. pontis longitudinales
 f. precommissuralis
 prerubral f.
 fasciculi proprii
 f. prosencephalicus
  medialis
 pyramidal f. of medulla
  oblongata
 f. pyramidalis medullae
  oblongatae
 f. retroflexus
 f. of Rolando
 semilunar f.
 f. semilunaris
 septomarginal f.
 f. septomarginalis

fas·cic·u·lus *(continued)*
 solitary f.
 subcallosal f.
 f. subcallosus
 subthalamic f.
 f. subthalamicus
 sulcomarginal f.
 f. sulcomarginalis
 f. telencephalicus medialis
 thalamamillary f.
 thalamic f.
 f. thalamicus
 f. thalamomamillaris
 f. triangularis
 f. of Türck
 unciform f.
 uncinate f.
 f. uncinatus
 uncrossed pyramidal f.
 f. ventrolateralis
  superficialis
 f. of Vicq d'Azyr
fas·ci·ec·to·my
fas·ci·itis
 eosinophilic f.
 exudative calcifying f.
 necrotizing f.
 nodular f.
 perirenal f.
 proliferative f.
 pseudosarcomatous f.
fas·ci·od·e·sis
Fas·ci·o·la
 F. gigantica
 F. hepatica
fas·ci·o·la *pl.* fas·ci·o·lae
 f. cinerea
fas·ci·o·lar
Fas·ci·o·let·ta
 F. iliocana
fas·cio·li·a·sis
Fas·ci·o·li·dae
Fas·ci·o·loi·des
 F. magna
fas·ci·o·lop·si·a·sis
Fas·ci·o·lop·sis
 F. buski
fas·cio·plas·ty

fas·ci·or·rha·phy
fas·ci·ot·o·my
fas·ci·tis
fast-gly·co·lyt·ic
fas·ti·ga·tum
fas·tig·i·al
fas·tig·io·bul·bar
fas·tig·i·um
fast-ox·i·da·tive-gly·co·lyt·ic
fat
    bound f.
    brown f.
    chyle f.
    corpse f.
    depot f.
    fetal f.
    grave f.
    masked f.
    milk f.
    molecular f.
    moruloid f.
    mulberry f.
    neutral f.
    paranephric f.
    pararenal f.
    perinephric f.
    perirenal f.
    polyunsaturated f.
    saturated f.
    unsaturated f.
    wool f.
    wool f., hydrous
    wool f., refined
    yellow f.
fa·tal
fa·tal·i·ty
fate
    prospective f.
fat·i·ga·bil·i·ty
fa·tigue
    auditory f.
    battle f.
    combat f.
    flying f.
    industrial f.
    pseudocombat f.
    stance f.
    stimulation f.

fat·ty
fat·ty ac·id
    essential f. a.
    free f. a's (FFA)
    monounsaturated f. a's
    nonesterified f. a's (NEFA)
    polyunsaturated f. a's
    saturated f. a's
fat·ty ac·id syn·thase
fau·ces
Fau·chard's disease
fau·cial
fau·ci·tis
Faught's sphygmomanometer
fau·na
faun·tail
Faust's method
fa·va
fa·ve·o·lar
fa·ve·o·late
fa·ve·o·li
fa·ve·o·lus *pl.* fa·ve·o·li
fa·vic
fa·vid
fa·vism
Fav·re-Ra·cou·chot syndrome
fa·vus
fax·en-psy·cho·sis
Fa·zio-Londe atrophy
Fa·zio-Londe disease
Fa·zio-Londe syndrome
FCA — Freund's complete
    adjuvant
fCi — femtocurie
FD — fatal dose
FDA — Food and Drug
    Administration
    fronto-dextra anterior
    (right frontoanterior)
FDP — fibrin degradation
    products
    fronto-dextra posterior
    (right frontoposterior)
FDT — fronto-dextra
    transversa (right
    frontotransverse)
F-duc·tion

F-dUMP — 5-fluorodeoxy-
  uridine monophosphate
FE _{Na} — excreted fraction of
  filtered sodium
Feath·er's analysis
feb·an·tel
Feb. dur. — L. febre durante
  (while the fever lasts)
feb·ri·cant
feb·ri·cide
fe·bric·i·ty
fe·bric·u·la
feb·ri·fa·cient
fe·brif·ic
fe·brif·u·gal
feb·ri·fuge
feb·rif·u·gine
feb·rile
fe·bris
    f. enteriocoides
    f. melitensis
    f. recurrens
    f. rubra
    f. undulans
fe·cal
fe·ca·lith
fe·cal·oid
fe·ca·lo·ma
fe·cal·u·ria
fe·ces
Fech·ner's law
fec·u·la
fec·u·lent
fe·cun·date
fe·cun·da·tio
    f. ab extra
fe·cun·da·tion
    artificial f.
fe·cun·di·ty
Fede's disease
Fe·de·ri·ci's sign
fee·ble·mind·ed·ness
feed·back
    alpha f.
    delayed auditory f. (DAF)
    negative f.
    positive f.
feed-for·ward

feed·ing
    artificial f.
    breast f.
    demand f.
    drip f.
    extrabuccal f.
    Finkelstein's f.
    forced f.
    intravenous f.
    nasal f.
    sham f.
    tube f.
feel·ing
    f's of estrangement
    f's of unreality
Feer's disease
fee-split·ting
Feg·e·ler syndrome
Feh·leis·en's streptococcus
Feh·ling's solution
Feh·ling's test
Feiss line
Fel·dene
Fel·der·struk·tur
Fe·le·ky's instrument
Fe·lix Vi serum
Fe·lix-Weil reaction
fel·la·tio
fel·on
    bone f.
    deep f.
    subcutaneous f.
    subcuticular f.
    subperiosteal f.
    thecal f.
Fel·sules
Fel·ton's phenomenon
felt·work
    Kaes' f.
Fel·ty's syndrome
fe·male
fem·i·nine
fem·i·nin·i·ty
fem·i·nism
    mammary f.
fem·i·ni·za·tion
    testicular f.

fem·i·nize
Fem·i·none
fem·i·no·nu·cle·us
Fem. intern. — L. femoribus
  internus (at the inner side of
  the thighs)
Fem·o·gen
fem·o·ra
fem·o·ral
fem·o·ro·cele
fem·o·ro·fem·o·ral
fem·o·ro·fem·o·ro·pop·lit·e·
  al
fem·o·ro·il·i·ac
fem·o·ro·pop·lit·e·al
fem·o·ro·tib·i·al
fem·to·cu·rie
fe·mur *pl.* fem·o·ra
fen·al·a·mide
fen·a·mate
fen·ben·da·zole
fen·bu·fen
fen·clo·fen·ac
fen·clo·nine
fen·clor·ac
fen·do·sal
fe·nes·tra *pl.* fe·nes·trae
    f. choledocha
    f. of cochlea
    f. cochleae
    f. nov-ovalis
    f. ovalis
    f. rotunda
    f. vestibuli
fe·nes·trae
fen·es·trate
fen·es·trat·ed
fen·es·tra·tion
    alveolar plate f.
    aortopulmonary f.
    apical f.
fen·es·trel
fen·eth·yl·line hy·dro·chlo·
  ride
fen·flur·amine hy·dro·chlo·
  ride
fen·i·so·rex

fen·met·o·zole hy·dro·chlo·
  ride
fen·o·bam
fen·o·pro·fen
    f. calcium
fen·o·ter·ol
fen·pip·a·lone
fen·spir·ide hy·dro·chlo·ride
fen·ta·nyl cit·rate
fen·ti·clor
Fen·wick's disease
Fen·wick-Hun·ner ulcer
Fe·o·sol
fer-de-lance
Féré·ol's nodes
Fer·gon
Fer·gu·son-Smith epithelioma
Fer-In-Sol
fer·ment
fer·men·ta·tion
    heterolactic f.
    homolactic f.
    mixed acid f.
    stormy f.
Fer·mi's vaccine
Fer·mi-Dir·ac statistics
fer·mi·um
fern·ing
Fer·ra·ta's cell
fer·rate
fer·rat·ed
fer·re·dox·in
Fer·rein's canal
Fer·rein's foramen
Fer·rein's ligament
Fer·rein's pyramid
Fer·rein's tube
Fer·rein's tubule
fer·ri-al·bu·min·ic
fer·ric
    f. fructose
    f. oxide, red
    f. oxide, yellow
fer·ri·cy·a·nide
fer·ri·heme
fer·ri·he·mo·chrome
fer·ri·he·mo·glo·bin
fer·ri·por·phy·rin

fer·ri·pro·to·por·phy·rin
Fer·ris Smith technique
fer·ri·tin
fer·ro·che·la·tase
fer·ro·cho·lin·ate
fer·ro·cy·a·nide
fer·ro·elec·tric
fer·ro·floc·cu·la·tion
fer·rog·ra·phy
fer·ro·ki·net·ic
fer·ro·ki·net·ics
Fer·ro·lip
fer·ro·pro·tein
fer·ro·so·fer·ric
fer·ro·ther·a·py
fer·rous
    f. fumarate
    f. gluconate
    f. sulfate
fer·rox·i·dase
fer·ru·gi·nous
fer·rum
Fer·ry-Por·ter law
fer·tile
fer·til·i·ty
fer·ti·li·za·tion
    cross f.
    external f.
    internal f.
    in vitro f.
fer·ti·li·zin
Ferv. — L. fervens (boiling)
fer·ves·cence
FES — functional electrical
  stimulation
Fe·so·tyme
fes·ter
fes·ti·nant
fes·ti·na·tion
fes·toon
    gingival f.
    McCall's f.
fe·tal
fe·tal·ism
fe·tal·iza·tion
fe·ta·tion
fe·ti·cide
fet·id

fet·ish
fet·ish·ism
    transvestic f.
fet·ish·ist
fet·lock
fe·to·am·ni·ot·ic
fe·tog·ra·phy
fe·tol·o·gist
fe·tol·o·gy
fe·to·ma·ter·nal
fe·tom·e·try
    roentgen f.
fe·top·a·thy
fe·to·pla·cen·tal
fe·to·pro·tein
    α-f.
    β-f.
    γ-f.
fe·tor
    f. ex ore
    f. hepaticus
    f. oris
fe·to·scope
fe·to·scop·ic
fe·tos·co·py
fe·to·tox·ic
fe·tox·y·late hy·dro·chlo·ride
fe·tus
    f. acardiacus
    f. amorphus
    calcified f.
    f. compressus
    harlequin f.
    f. in fetu
    mummified f.
    paper-doll f.
    papyraceous f.
    f. papyraceous
    parasitic f.
    retroperitoneal f. in fetu
    f. sanguinolentis
    sireniform f.
Feul·gen-pos·i·tive
Feul·gen reaction
Feul·gen test
fe·ver
    abortus f.
    Aden f.

fe·ver *(continued)*
    adynamic f.
    African coast f.
    African tick f.
    Andaman A f.
    aphthous f.
    apyretic typhoid f.
    Argentine hemorrhagic f.
    artificial f.
    aseptic f.
    Assam f.
    asthenic f.
    auric f.
    Australian Q f.
    Australian tick f.
    autumn f.
    Bangkok hemorrhagic f.
    barbeiro f.
    biduotertian f.
    black f.
    blackwater f.
    blue f.
    Bolivian hemorrhagic f.
    bouquet f.
    boutonneuse f.
    brain f.
    brassfounder's f.
    Brazilian purpuric f.
    Brazilian spotted f.
    breakbone f.
    Brisbane f.
    Bullis f.
    burdwan f.
    Bushy Creek f.
    Bwamba f.
    cachectic f.
    camp f.
    cane-field f.
    canicola f.
    carbuncular f.
    cat f.
    cat-scratch f.
    central f.
    Central Asian hemorrhagic
      f.
    cerebrospinal f.
    Charcot's f.
    chikungunya f.

fe·ver *(continued)*
    childbed f.
    Choix f.
    Colombian tick f.
    Colorado tick f.
    Congolian red f.
    continued f.
    continuous f.
    cotton-mill f.
    Crimean-Congo
      hemorrhagic f.
    cyclic f.
    Cyprus f.
    dandy f.
    deer fly f.
    dehydration f.
    dengue f.
    dengue hemorrhagic f.
    desert f.
    digestive f.
    diphasic milk f.
    drug f.
    Dumdum f.
    Dutton's relapsing f.
    East Coast f.
    Ebola hemorrhagic f.
    elephantoid f.
    endemic relapsing f.
    enteric f.
    entericoid f.
    ephemeral f.
    epidemic hemorrhagic f.
    equine biliary f.
    eruptive f.
    essential f.
    estivoautumnal f.
    etiocholanolone f.
    exanthematous f.
    exsiccation f.
    familial Mediterranean f.
    famine f.
    Far East hemorrhagic f.
    fatigue f.
    field f.
    five-day f.
    Fort Bragg f.
    foundryman's f.
    Gambian f.

fe·ver *(continued)*
    glandular f.
    Guáitara f.
    Hankow f.
    harvest f.
    Hasami f.
    Haverhill f.
    hay f.
    hay f., nonseasonal
    hay f., perennial
    hectic f.
    hematuric bilious f.
    hemoglobinuric f.
    hemorrhagic f's
    hemorrhagic f. with renal
      syndrome
    herpetic f.
    Herxheimer's f.
    hospital f.
    icterohemorrhagic f.
    Ilheus f.
    inanition f.
    induced f.
    intermenstrual f.
    intermittent f.
    intermittent hepatic f.
    inundation f.
    island f.
    Jaccoud's dissociated f.
    jail f.
    Japanese flood f.
    Japanese river f.
    jungle f.
    jungle yellow f.
    Junin f.
    Katayama f.
    Kedani f.
    Kenya f.
    Kew Gardens spotted f.
    Kinkiang f.
    Korean hemorrhagic f.
    Korin f.
    Kyoto f.
    land f.
    Lassa f.
    lemming f.
    leprotic f.
    Lone Star f.

fe·ver *(continued)*
    louse-borne relapsing f.
    lung f.
    macular f.
    malarial f.
    malignant tertian f.
    Malta f.
    Marburg hemorrhagic f.
    Marseilles f.
    marsh f.
    Mediterranean f.
    Mediterranean Coast f.
    Mediterranean tick f.
    melanuric f.
    metabolic f.
    metal fume f.
    Meuse f.
    Mexican spotted f.
    Mianeh f.
    milk f.
    miniature scarlet f.
    mite f.
    monoleptic f.
    Mossman f.
    mountain tick f.
    mud f.
    Murchison-Pel-Ebstein f.
    nanukayami f.
    neurogenic f.
    nine-mile f.
    North Queensland tick f.
    Omsk hemorrhagic f.
    O'nyong-nyong f.
    Oroya f.
    Pahvant Valley f.
    paludal f.
    pappataci f.
    paramalta f.
    paratyphoid f.
    paraundulant f.
    parenteric f.
    parrot f.
    parturient f.
    Pel-Ebstein f.
    periodic f.
    Persian relapsing f.
    petechial f.
    Pfeiffer's glandular f.

fe·ver *(continued)*

pharyngoconjunctival f.
Philippine hemorrhagic f.
phlebotomus f.
pinta f.
pneumonic f.
polyleptic f.
polymer fume f.
Pomona f.
Pontiac f.
pretibial f.
prison f.
protein f.
puerperal f.
pulmonary f.
pythogenic f.
Q f.
quartan f.
Queensland coastal f.
Queensland tick f.
quintan f.
quotidian f.
rabbit f.
rat-bite f.
recurrent f.
red-water f.
relapsing f.
remittent f.
rheumatic f.
rice-field f.
Rift Valley f.
river f. of Japan
Rocky Mountain spotted f.
Russian headache f.
Sakushu f.
salt f.
sandfly f.
San Joaquin f.
São Paulo f.
scarlet f.
Schottmüller's f.
septic f.
seven-day f.
shin bone f.
ship f.
shoddy f.
Sinbis f.
slime f.

fe·ver *(continued)*

snail f.
solar f.
Songo f.
South African tick-bite f.
South American
    hemorrhagic f.
spelter's f.
spiking f.
spirillum f.
splenic f.
spotted f.
sthenic f.
stiff-neck f.
streptobacillary f.
sulfonamide f.
sweat f.
sylvan yellow f.
tertian f.
tetanoid f.
Texas tick f.
Thai hemorrhagic f.
therapeutic f.
thermic f.
thirst f.
three-day f.
threshing f.
tick f.
tick-borne relapsing f.
Tobia f.
trench f.
trypanosome f.
tsutsugamushi f.
typhoid f.
typhomalarial f.
typhus f.
undulant f.
urban yellow f.
urethral f.
urinary f.
urticarial f.
uveoparotid f.
vaccinal f.
valley f.
viral hemorrhagic f's
Volhynia f.
war f.
West African f.

fe·ver *(continued)*
>West Nile f.
>Whitmore's f.
>Wolhynia f.
>Yangtze Valley f.
>yellow f.
>Zika f.
>zinc fume f.

Fèv·re-Langue·pin syndrome

FF — filtration fraction

FFA — free fatty acids

FFT — flicker fusion threshold

F.h. — L. fiat haustus (let a draught be made)

FIA — fluoroimmunoassay

fi·at *pl.* fi·ant (let there be made)

fi·ber
>A f's
>accelerating f's
>accelerator f's
>accessory f's
>adrenergic f's
>afferent nerve f's
>alpha f's
>alveolar f's
>alveolar crest f's
>anastomosing f's
>anastomotic f's
>apical f's
>archiform f's
>arcuate f's
>argentaffin f's
>argentophil f's
>argyrophilic f.
>asbestos f's
>astral f.
>augmentor f's
>auxiliary f's
>axial f.
>B f's
>basilar f's
>Bergmann's f's
>Bernheimer's f's
>beta f's
>Bogrov's f.
>bone f's

fi·ber *(continued)*
>Brücke's f's
>bulbospiral f's
>Burdach's f's
>C f's
>capsular f's
>cardiac accelerator f's
>cardiac depressor f's
>cardiac pressor f's
>cemental f's
>cementoalveolar f's
>centripetal f.
>cerebrospinal f's
>chief f's
>cholinergic f's
>chromatic f.
>chromosomal f.
>cilioequatorial f's
>cilioposterocapsular f's
>circular f's
>climbing f's
>clinging f's
>collagen f's
>collateral f's of Winslow
>commissural nerve f's
>cone f.
>conjunctival f's
>continuous f's
>Corti's f's
>corticobulbar f's
>corticonuclear f's
>corticofugal f.
>corticopetal f.
>corticopontine f's
>corticoreticular f's
>corticorubral f's
>corticospinal f's
>corticostriate f's
>corticothalamic f's
>dark f's
>Darkshevich's f's
>daughter f.
>decussating f's
>dendritic f's
>dentatorubral f's
>dentatothalamic f's
>dentinal f.
>dentinogenic f's

fi·ber *(continued)*
   depressor f's
   dietary f.
   Dieters f's
   Edinger's f's
   efferent nerve f's
   elastic f's
   endogenous f's
   exogenous f's
   extraciliary f's
   extrafusal f's
   fastigioperiventricular f's
   flocculo-oculomotor f's of
    Wallenberg-Klimoff
   forklike f's
   frontopontine f's
   fusimotor f.
   gamma f's
   Gerdy's f's
   giant f.
   gingival f's
   gingivodental f's
   Goll's f's
   Gottstein's f's
   Gratiolet's radiating f's
   gray f's
   hair f.
   half-spindle f's
   Henle's f's
   Herxheimer's f's
   heterodesmotic f's
   homodesmotic f's
   horizontal f's
   Ia f.
   Ib f.
   IF f.
   impulse-conducting f's
   inhibitory f's
   interciliary f's
   intercolumnar f's
   intercrural f's
   internuncial f's
   interzonal f's
   intrafusal f's
   isotropic f.
   James f.
   Korff f's
   Kühne's f.

fi·ber *(continued)*
   lattice f's
   Lenhossek's f's
   f's of lens
   light f's
   longitudinal f's
   Luschka's f's
   Mahaim f's
   main f's
   mantle f.
   Mauthner's f.
   medullated f's
   meridional f's of ciliary
    muscle
   f's of Meynert
   Monakow's f's
   moss f's
   mossy f's
   motor f.
   Müller's f's
   muscle f.
   myelinated nerve f's
   naked f.
   nerve f.
   neuroglial f.
   nonmedullated nerve f's
   nuclear chain muscle f.
   oblique f's
   odontogenic f's
   olfactory f's
   olivocerebellar f's
   orbiculoanterocapsular f's
   orbiculociliary f's
   orbiculoposterocapsular f's
   osteocollagenous f's
   osteogenetic f's
   osteogenic f's
   oxytalan f.
   pallidohypothalamic f's
   pallidothalamic f's
   palliopontine f's
   paraventriculoventricular
    f's
   parent f.
   parietotemporopontine f's
   perforating f's
   periventricular f's
   pilomotor f's

fi·ber *(continued)*
    pontocerebellar f's
    postcommissural f's
    postganglionic nerve f's
    precollagenous f's
    precommissural f's
    preganglionic nerve f's
    pressor f's
    principal f's
    projection nerve f's
    Prussak's f's
    Purkinje f's
    pyramidal f's of medulla
        oblongata
    radial f's of ciliary muscle
    radiating f's
    radicular f's
    ragged red f's
    Rasmussen's nerve f's
    Reissner's f.
    f's of Remak
    reticular f's
    reticuloreticular f's
    Retzius' f's
    ring f's
    Ritter's f.
    rod f.
    Rolando's f.
    Rosenthal's f's
    Sappey's f's
    Schroeder's f's
    secretomotoric f's
    sensory f.
    Sharpey's f's
    short association f's
    sinospiral f's
    skeletofusimotor f.
    somatic nerve f's
    sphincter f's of ciliary
        muscle
    spinal parasympathetic f's
    spindle f's
    Stilling's f's
    f's of stria terminalis
    sudomotor f's
    supraoptic f's
    sustentacular f's
    T f.

fi·ber *(continued)*
    tangential nerve f's
    temporopontine f's
    tendril f's
    thalamocortical f's
    thalamoparietal f's
    thalamostriate f's
    Tomes f.
    traction f's
    transilient f's
    transseptal f's
    transverse f's of pons
    ultraterminal f.
    unmyelinated nerve f's
    varicose f's
    vasoconstrictor f's
    vasodilatory f's
    vasomotor f's
    visceral nerve f's
    von Monakow's f's
    Weissmann's f's
    white f's
    yellow f's
    zonular f's
fi·ber·co·lono·scope
fi·ber·gas·tro·scope
fi·ber-il·lu·mi·nat·ed
fi·ber·op·tic
fi·ber·op·tics
fi·ber·scope
    gastric f.
Fi·bi·ger, Johannes Andreas
    Grib
fi·bra *pl.* fi·brae
    fibrae annulares
    fibrae arcuatae
    fibrae cerebello-olivares
    fibrae circulares musculi
        ciliaris
    fibrae corticonucleares
    fibrae corticopontinae
    fibrae corticoreticulares
    fibrae corticorubrales
    fibrae corticospinales
    fibrae corticothalamicae
    fibrae dentatorubrales
    fibrae frontopontinae
    fibrae intercrurales

fi·bra *(continued)*
fibrae lentis
fibrae longitudinales
fibrae meridionales
fibrae obliquae
fibrae paraventriculares
fibrae parietotemporopontinae
fibrae periventriculares
fibrae pontis longitudinales
fibrae pontis profundae
fibrae pontis superficiales
fibrae pontis transversae
fibrae pontocerebellares
fibrae propriae
fibrae pyramidales
fibrae radiales
fibrae striae terminalis
fibrae supraopticae
fibrae temporopontinae
fibrae thalamoparietales
fibrae zonulares
fi·bra·tion
fi·bre·mia
fi·bril
Alzheimer f.
anchoring f.
axial f's
border f's
collagen f's
cytoplasmic f's
dentinal f's
Dirck's f's
fibroglia f's
muscle f.
nerve f.
side f. of Golgi
Tomes f.
young collagen f's
fi·bril·la *pl.* fi·bril·lae
fi·bril·lar, fi·bril·lary
fi·bril·late
fi·bril·la·tion
atrial f.
auricular f.
ventricular f.
Fi·bril·len·struk·tur
fi·bril·lo·blast

fi·bril·lo·gen·e·sis
fi·bril·lol·y·sis
fi·bril·lo·lyt·ic
fi·brin
stroma f.
fi·brin·ase
fi·brin·emia
fi·bri·no·cel·lu·lar
fi·brin·o·gen
human f.
fi·brin·og·en·ase
fi·brin·o·gen·emia
fi·bri·no·gen·e·sis
fi·bri·no·gen·ic
fi·bri·no·ge·nol·y·sis
fi·bri·no·geno·lyt·ic
fi·brin·o·geno·pe·nia
fi·brin·o·geno·pe·nic
fi·bri·nog·e·nous
fi·brin·oid
canalized f.
placental f.
fi·bri·no·ki·nase
fi·bri·no·li·gase
fi·bri·nol·y·sin
fi·bri·nol·y·sis
fi·bri·no·lyt·ic
fi·bri·no·pe·nia
fi·bri·no·pep·tide
fi·bri·no·plate·let
fi·bri·no·pu·ru·lent
fi·bri·nor·rhea
fi·bri·nos·co·py
fi·brin·ous
fi·brin·uria
fi·bro·ade·nia
fi·bro·ad·e·no·ma
giant f. of the breast
intracanalicular f.
pericanalicular f.
fi·bro·ad·e·no·sis
fi·bro·ad·i·pose
fi·bro·an·gi·o·ma
nasopharyngeal f.
fi·bro·are·o·lar
fi·bro·at·ro·phy
fi·bro·blast
contractile f.

fi·bro·blast *(continued)*
   pericryptal f's
fi·bro·blas·tic
fi·bro·blas·to·ma
   perineural f.
fi·bro·bron·chi·tis
fi·bro·cal·cif·ic
fi·bro·car·ci·no·ma
fi·bro·car·ti·lage
   f. of auricle
   basal f.
   basilar f.
   circumferential f.
   connecting f.
   cotyloid f.
   elastic f.
   glenoid f.
   interarticular f.
   intervertebral f's
   intra-articular f.
   semilunar f's
   spongy f.
   sternoclavicular f.
   stratiform f.
   white f.
   yellow f.
fi·bro·car·ti·lag·i·nous
fi·bro·car·ti·la·go *pl.* fi·bro·
  car·ti·lag·i·nes
   f. basalis
   f. basilaris
   fibrocartilagines
     intervertebrales
   f. navicularis
fi·bro·ca·se·ous
fi·bro·cav·i·tary
fi·bro·cel·lu·lar
fi·bro·ce·men·to·ma
fi·bro·chon·dri·tis
fi·bro·chon·dro·ma
fi·bro·col·lag·e·nous
fi·bro·con·ges·tive
fi·bro·cyst
fi·bro·cys·tic
fi·bro·cys·to·ma
fi·bro·cyte
fi·bro·cy·to·gen·e·sis

fi·bro·dys·pla·sia
   f. ossificans progressiva
   renal artery f.
fi·bro·elas·tic
fi·bro·elas·to·sis
   f. cordis
   endocardial f.
   endomyocardial f.
fi·bro·en·chon·dro·ma
fi·bro·en·do·the·li·o·ma
fi·bro·ep·i·the·li·o·ma
   premalignant f.
fi·bro·fas·ci·tis
fi·bro·fat·ty
fi·bro·fi·brous
fi·bro·gen·e·sis
   f. imperfecta ossium
fi·bro·gen·ic
fi·brog·lia
fi·bro·gli·o·ma
fi·bro·hem·or·rhag·ic
fi·bro·his·tio·cyt·ic
fi·broid
fi·broid·ec·to·my
fi·bro·in
fi·bro·ker·a·to·ma
fi·bro·la·mel·lar
fi·bro·lam·i·nar
fi·bro·leio·my·o·ma
fi·bro·li·po·ma
fi·bro·li·po·ma·tous
fi·bro·ma
   ameloblastic f.
   calcified f.
   f. cavernosum
   cementifying f.
   chondromyxoid f.
   concentric f.
   f. cutis
   cystic f.
   f. durum
   endoneural f.
   hard f.
   intracanalicular f.
   irritation f.
   juvenile nasopharyngeal f.
   f. molle

fi·bro·ma *(continued)*
  f. mucinosum
  myxoid f.
  f. myxomatodes
  nonossifying f.
  nonosteogenic f.
  odontogenic f.
  ossifying f.
  osteogenic f.
  parasitic f.
  f. pendulum
  periapical f.
  periungual f.
  recurrent digital f. of
    childhood
  f. sarcomatosum
  senile f.
  soft f.
  submucous f.
  telangiectatic f.
  f. of testis
  f. thecocellulare
    xanthomatodes
  f. xanthoma
fi·bro·ma·to·gen·ic
fi·bro·ma·toid
fi·bro·ma·to·sis
  aggressive f.
  f. colli
  congenital generalized f.
  f. gingivae
  gingival f.
  infantile digital f.
  palmar f.
  plantar f.
  subcutaneous
    pseudosarcomatous f.
  f. ventriculi
fi·bro·ma·tous
fi·bro·mec·to·my
fi·bro·mem·bra·nous
fi·bro·mus·cu·lar
fi·bro·my·itis
fi·bro·my·o·ma
  f. uteri
fi·bro·myo·mec·to·my
fi·bro·myo·si·tis
  nodular f.

fi·bro·my·ot·o·my
fi·bro·myxo·li·po·ma
fi·bro·myx·o·ma
fi·bro·myx·o·sar·co·ma
fi·bro·nec·tin
fi·bro·neu·ro·ma
fi·bro·neu·ro·sar·co·ma
fi·bro·nu·cle·ar
fi·bro-odon·to·ma
  ameloblastic f.
fi·bro-os·te·o·ma
fi·bro·pap·il·lo·ma
fi·bro·pi·tu·i·cyte
fi·bro·pla·sia
  intimal f.
  medial f.
  myointimal f.
  retrolental f.
  subadventitial f.
fi·bro·plas·tic
fi·bro·plate
fi·bro·poly·pus
fi·bro·pu·ru·lent
fi·bro·re·tic·u·late
fi·bro·sar·co·ma
  ameloblastic f.
  odontogenic f.
  f. phyllodes
  renal f.
fi·bro·scle·ro·sis
  multifocal f.
fi·brose
fi·bro·se·rous
fi·bro·sis
  African endomyocardial f.
  bauxite pulmonary f.
  condensation f.
  congenital hepatic f.
  cystic f.
  diatomite f.
  diffuse interstitial
    pulmonary f.
  endomyocardial f.
  glomerular f.
  graphite f.
  mediastinal f.
  neoplastic f.
  nodular subepidermal f.

fi·bro·sis *(continued)*
    panmural f. of the bladder
    periureteric f.
    pipestem f.
    pleural f.
    postfibrinous f.
    progressive massive f.
    proliferative f.
    pulmonary f.
    renal f.
    replacement f.
    retroperitoneal f.
    root sleeve f.
    Symmers f.
    Symmers pipestem f.
    f. uteri
fi·bro·si·tis
    traumatic f.
fi·bro·sple·no·meg·a·ly
    congestive f.
fi·bro·tho·rax
fi·brot·ic
fi·brous
fi·bro·vas·cu·lar
fi·bro·xan·tho·ma
fib·u·la
fib·u·lar
fib·u·la·ris
fib·u·la·tion
fib·u·lo·cal·ca·ne·al
FICD — Fellow of the International College of Dentists
fi·cin
Fick formula
Fick method
Fick principle
Fick·er's diagnosticum
fi·co·sis
FICS — Fellow of the International College of Surgeons
fi·dic·i·na·les
Fied·ler's disease
Fied·ler's myocarditis
field
    absolute f.
    adversive f.

field *(continued)*
    auditory f.
    binocular f.
    centrocecal area of f.
    Cohnheim's f's
    dark-f.
    developmental f.
    electromagnetic f.
    electrostatic f.
    far f.
    f. of fixation
    Flechsig's f.
    f's of Forel
    frontal eye f.
    gamma f.
    f. H of Forel
    f. H_1 of Forel
    f. H_2 of Forel
    high-power f.
    individuation f.
    low-power f.
    magnetic f.
    morphogenetic f.
    myelinogenetic f.
    near f.
    occipital eye f.
    penumbra f.
    perceptual f.
    prefrontal eye f.
    prerubral f.
    primary nail f.
    receptive f.
    relative f.
    subicular f's
    surplus f.
    tactile f.
    tegmental f.
    f. of vision
    f. of vision, cribriform
    visual f.
    Wernicke's f.
Field·ing's membrane
field-de·pen·dent
Fies·sin·ger-Le·roy-Rei·ter syndrome
Fies·sin·ger-Ren·du syndrome
fièv·re
    f. boutonneuse

FIGLU — formiminoglutamic acid
fig·u·ra·tum
fig·ure
  achromatic f.
  chromatic f.
  fortification f's
  Minkowski's f.
  mitotic f's
  myelin f.
  nuclear f.
  Purkinje's f's
  star f.
  Stifel's f.
  Zöllner's f's
fi·la
fi·la·ceous
fil·a·ment
  acrosomal f.
  actin f.
  axial f.
  desmin f's
  intermediate f's
  keratin f's
  linin f.
  lymphatic anchoring f's
  meningeal f.
  polar injecting f.
  root f's of spinal nerves
  spermatic f.
  spinal f.
  terminal f.
  vimentin f's
fil·a·men·ta·tion
fil·a·men·tous
fil·a·men·tum *pl.* fil·a·men·ta
fi·lar
Fi·la·ria
  F. conjunctivae
  F. diurna
fi·la·ria *pl.* fi·la·riae
  Bancroft's f.
  Brug's f.
fi·la·riae
fi·la·ri·al
fil·a·ri·a·sis
  Bancroft's f.
  f. bancrofti

fil·a·ri·a·sis *(continued)*
  bancroftian f.
  Brug's f.
  Malayan f.
  occult f.
  Ozzard's f.
  periodic f.
fi·lar·i·cid·al
fi·lar·i·cide
fi·lar·i·form
Fi·lar·i·oi·dea
fi·lar·i·ous
Fi·lat·ov's disease
Fi·lat·ov flap
Fi·lat·ov-Dukes disease
Fi·lat·ov-Gilles tubed pedicle
Fil·des enrichment agar
file
  endodontic f.
  root canal f.
fil·i·al
fi·lic·ic acid
fil·i·cin
fil·i·form
fil·io·pa·ren·tal
fi·li·pin
Fi·li·po·vitch's (Fi·li·po·wicz's) sign
fi·lix *pl.* fi·li·ces
  f. mas
fi·lix·ic acid
fil·let
fill·ing
  complex f.
  composite f.
  compound f.
  direct f.
  direct resin f.
  ditched f.
  indirect f.
  permanent f.
  postresection f.
  retrograde f.
  reverse f.
  root canal f.
  root-end f.
  temporary f.
  treatment f.

film
baseline f.
bite-wing f.
fibrin f.
fixed blood f.
gelatin f., absorbable
lateral jaw f.
nonscreen f.
occlusal f.
panoramic x-ray f.
periapical f.
plain f.
port f.
precorneal f.
preliminary f.
scout f.
spot f.
stripping f.
sulfa f.
x-ray f.
film badge
filo·pod
fi·lo·po·di·um *pl.* fi·lo·po·dia
fi·lo·pres·sure
fi·lo·var·i·co·sis
fil·ter
bandpass f.
band-stop f.
barrier f.
Berkefeld f.
Chamberland's f.
collodion f.
excitation f.
Hemming f.
high-pass f.
intermittent sand f.
Kimray-Greenfield f.
low-pass f.
mechanical f.
membrane f.
Millipore f.
Mobin-Uddin f.
notch f.
percolating f.
roughing f.
scrubbing f.
sintered glass f.
slow sand f.

fil·ter *(continued)*
sprinkling f.
Thoraeus f.
trickling f.
ultraviolet f.
umbrella f.
wedge f.
Wood's f.
fil·ter·a·ble
fil·tra·ble
fil·trate
bacterial f.
Folin's protein-free f.
glomerular f.
fil·tra·tion
gel f.
glomerular f.
fil·trum ven·tricu·li
fi·lum *pl.* fi·la
fila anastomotica nervi acustici
f. durae matris spinale
f. meningeale
f. meningeum
fila olfactoria
fila radicularia nervorum spinalium
f. of spinal dura mater
f. spinale
f. terminale
fim·bria *pl.* fim·briae
f. of fallopian tube
f. hippocampi
ovarian f.
f. ovarica
fimbriae of tongue
fimbriae tubae uterinae
fim·bri·al
fim·bri·at·ed
fim·bri·a·tion
fim·bri·a·tum
fim·bri·ec·to·my
fim·brio·cele
fim·brio·den·tate
fim·brio·plas·ty
Finckh's test
fin·ger
baseball f.

fin·ger *(continued)*
 blubber f.
 bolster f's
 clubbed f.
 dead f.
 drop f.
 drumstick f.
 first f.
 giant f.
 hammer f.
 hippocratic f's
 index f.
 lock f.
 Madonna f's
 mallet f.
 ring f.
 seal f.
 snapping f.
 spade f's
 spider f.
 spring f.
 stuck f.
 trigger f.
 tulip f's
 vibration-induced white f's
 washerwoman's f's
 waxy f.
 webbed f's
 white f.
fin·ger·ag·no·sia
fin·ger·drop
fin·ger·nail
fin·ger·print
Fin·kel·stein's albumin milk
Fin·kel·stein's feeding
Fink·ler-Pri·or spirillium
Fin·ney's operation
Fin·ney's pyloroplasty
Fi·no·chi·et·to's stirrup
Fin·sen apparatus
Fin·sen bath
Fin·sen lamp
Fin·sen light
Fin·sen rays
Fin·zi-Har·mer operation
fire
 St. Anthony's f.
fire·damp

Fir·mi·bac·te·ria
Fir·mic·u·tes
fir·pene
first aid
Fisch·er's sign
Fish·berg concentration test
Fish·er's exact test
Fish·er syndrome
Fiske and Sub·ba·row method
fis·sile
fis·sion
 binary f.
 bud f.
 cellular f.
 multiple f.
 nuclear f.
 simple f.
fis·sion·a·ble
fis·sip·a·rous
fis·su·la
 f. ante fenestram
fis·su·ra *pl.* fis·su·rae
 f. in ano
 f. antitragohelicina
 f. auris congenita
 f. calcarina
 fissurae cerebelli
 f. cerebri lateralis sylvii
 f. choroidea
 f. collateralis
 f. dentata
 f. dorsolateralis cerebelli
 f. hippocampi
 f. horizontalis
 f. longitudinalis
 f. obliqua
 f. orbitalis inferior
 f. orbitalis superior
 f. parietooccipitalis
 f. petro-occipitalis
 f. petrosquamosa
 f. petrotympanica
 f. pterygoidea
 f. pterygomaxillaris
 f. sphenooccipitalis
 f. sphenopetrosa
 f. transversa cerebelli
 f. transversa cerebri

fis·su·ra *(continued)*
   f. tympanomastoidea
   f. tympanosquamosa
fis·su·rae
fis·su·ral
fis·su·ra·tion
fis·sure
   abdominal f.
   adoccipital f.
   Allingham's f.
   Ammon's f.
   amygdaline f.
   anal f.
   angular f.
   f. in ano
   antitragohelicine f.
   f. of aqueduct of vestibule
   arciform f.
   f. of auricle, posterior
   auricular f. of temporal bone
   basal f.
   basilar f.
   basisylvian f.
   f. of Bichat
   branchial f's
   Broca's f.
   Burdach's f.
   calcarine f.
   callosal f.
   callosomarginal f.
   central f.
   cerebral f's
   cerebral f., lateral
   cervical f.
   choroid f.
   choroidal f. of eye
   Clevenger's f.
   collateral f.
   corneal f.
   craniofacial f.
   decidual f.
   dentate f.
   dorsolateral f. of cerebellum
   Ecker's f.
   Duverney's f's
   enamel f.

fis·sure *(continued)*
   entorbital f.
   ethmoid f.
   fetal f. of optic cup
   floccular f.
   genitovesical f.
   glaserian f.
   great f. of cerebrum
   great horizontal f.
   Henle's f's
   hippocampal f.
   intercerebral f.
   intercotyledonary f.
   inferofrontal f.
   interparietal f.
   intratonsillar f.
   lacrimal f.
   lateral f. of cerebrum
   linguogingival f.
   longitudinal f.
   mandibular f's
   maxillary f.
   median f.
   f. of Monro
   oblique f. of lung
   occipital f.
   occipitosphenoidal f.
   optic f.
   oral f.
   orbital f., inferior
   orbital f., superior
   palpebral f.
   Pansch's f.
   parafloccular f.
   parietooccipital f.
   parietosphenoid f.
   petrobasilar f.
   petromastoid f.
   petro-occipital f.
   petrosal f., superficial
   petrosphenoidal f.
   petrosquamosal f.
   petrosquamous f.
   petrotympanic f.
   portal f.
   postcentral f.
   posterior median f. of spinal cord

fis·sure *(continued)*
  posterolateral f. of
    cerebellum
  postlingual f.
  postlunate f.
  postpyramidal f.
  precentral f.
  precuneal f.
  prepyramidal f.
  presylvian f.
  primary f.
  pterygoid f.
  pterygomaxillary f.
  pterygopalatine f.
  pterygotympanic f.
  pudendal f.
  retrocuticular f.
  retrotonsillar f.
  rhinal f.
  f. of Rolando
  f. of round ligament
  sagittal f. of liver
  Santorini's f's
  Schwalbe's f.
  sclerotomic f.
  secondary f.
  sphenoidal f.
  sphenomaxillary f.
  sphenooccipital f.
  sphenopetrosal f.
  squamotympanic f.
  subfrontal f.
  subtemporal f.
  superfrontal f.
  superior anterior f.
  supertemporal f.
  sylvian f.
  f. of Sylvius
  transtemporal f.
  transverse f.
  tympanic f.
  tympanomastoid f.
  tympanosquamous f.
  umbilical f.
  urogenital f.
  f. of the venous ligament
  vestibular f. of cochlea
  f. of the vestibule

fis·sure *(continued)*
  zygal f.
  zygomaticosphenoid f.
fis·tu·la *pl.* fis·tu·lae, fis·tu·
  las
  abdominal f.
  alveolar f.
  amphibolic f.
  anal f.
  f. in ano
  aortocaval f.
  aortoduodenal f.
  aortoenteric f.
  arteriovenous f.
  f. auris congenita
  biliary f.
  f. bimucosa
  blind f.
  branchial f.
  Brescia-Cimino f.
  caroticocavernous f.
  bronchoesophageal f.
  bronchopleural f.
  cervical f.
  cervicoaural f.
  f. cervicovaginalis
    laqueatica
  cholecystoduodenal f.
  chylous f.
  f. cibalis
  f. colli congenita
  colonic f.
  complete f.
  congenital urethrorectal f.
  f. corneae
  coronary arteriovenous f.
  coronary artery f.
  craniosinus f.
  dental f.
  Eck's f.
  Eck's f. in reverse
  enterocutaneous f.
  enterovaginal f.
  enterovesical f.
  esophagobronchial f.
  esophagotracheal f.
  external f.
  fecal f.

fis·tu·la *(continued)*
  frontal sinus f.
  gastric f.
  gastrocolic f.
  gastrojejunal f.
  gingival f.
  hepatic f.
  horseshoe f.
  incomplete f.
  internal f.
  intestinal f.
  lacrimal f.
  f. of lip
  lymphatic f.
  f. lymphatica
  Mann-Bollman f.
  mediastinobronchial f.
  mucus f.
  oroantral f.
  oronasal f.
  parietal f.
  perilymph f.
  perirectal f.
  pharyngeal f.
  pilonidal f.
  pleurobronchial f.
  pleurocutaneous f.
  preauricular f., congenital
  pulmonary f.
  pulmonary arteriovenous
    f., congenital
  radiocephalic f.
  rectovaginal f.
  rectovesical f.
  salivary f.
  spermatic f.
  stercoral f.
  submental f.
  Thiry's f.
  Thiry-Vella f.
  thoracic f.
  tracheal f.
  tracheoesophageal f.
  umbilical f.
  urachal f.
  ureterocervical f.
  urinary f.
  uterovesical f.

fis·tu·la *(continued)*
  Vella's f.
  vesical f.
  vesicoabdominal f.
  vesicocolonic f.
  vesicointestinal f.
  vesicorectal f.
  vesicoumbilical f.
  vesicovaginal f.
  vitelline f.
fis·tu·lae
fis·tu·la·tion
fis·tu·la·tome
fis·tu·lec·to·my
fis·tu·li·za·tion
fis·tu·lize
fis·tu·lo·en·ter·os·to·my
fis·tu·log·ra·phy
fis·tu·lot·o·my
fis·tu·lous
fit
    running f.
FITC — fluorescein
  isothiocyanate
fit·ness
    darwinian f.
    genetic f.
    reproductive f.
Fitz law
Fitz syndrome
Fitz Ger·ald method
Fitz Ger·ald treatment
fix·a·tion
    arch bar f.
    autotrophic f.
    bifoveal f.
    binocular f.
    Bovin f.
    carbon dioxide f.
    complement f.
    elastic band f.
    external pin f.
    intermaxillary f.
    internal f.
    intramedullary f.
    intraosseous f.
    Luque rod f.
    maxillomandibular f.

fix·a·tion *(continued)*
  nasomandibular f.
  nitrogen f.
  open reduction and
    internal f. (ORIF)
  postural f.
  reflex ocular f.
  skeletal f.
  Zickel nail f.
fix·a·tive
  Bouin's f.
  denture f.
  glutaraldehyde f.
  Helly's f.
  Kaiserling's f.
  lanthanum permanganate
    f.
  Maximow's f.
  Palade's f.
  paraformaldehyde f.
  potassium permanganate f.
  Rhodin's f.
  Schaudinn's f.
  Zenker's f.
  Zenker-formol f.
fix·a·tor
  Ace-Fischer f.
Fl. — fluid
FLA — fronto-laeva anterior
  (left frontoanterior)
F.l.a. — L. fiat lege artis (let it
  be done according to rule)
flac·cid
flac·cid·i·ty
flach·e·rie
Flack's node
Flack's test
fla·gel·la
flag·el·lan·tism
fla·gel·lar
flag·el·late
    animal-like f.
    plantlike f.
flag·el·lat·ed
flag·el·la·tion
fla·gel·li·form
flag·el·lin
flag·el·lo·sis

fla·gel·lo·spore
fla·gel·lu·la
fla·gel·lum *pl.* fla·gel·la
Flag·yl
Fla·jani's disease
flame
    capillary f.
flange
  buccal f.
  denture f.
  labial f.
  lingual f.
flank
flap
  Abbe f.
  advancement f.
  axial f.
  axilloabdominal f.
  bilobed f.
  bipedicle f.
  Björk f.
  bone f.
  bridge f.
  buccal f.
  Byers f.
  cellulocutaneous f.
  cervical f.
  cheek f.
  composite f.
  coronal f.
  cross-arm f.
  cross-finger f.
  cross-leg f.
  cross-lip f.
  delayed transfer f.
  deltopectoral f.
  direct transfer f.
  distant f.
  dorsalis pedis f.
  double pedicle f.
  eave f.
  Eloesser f.
  envelope f.
  Estlander f.
  fan f.
  Filatov f.
  forehead f.
  free f.

flap *(continued)*
    free bone f.
    French f.
    gauntlet f.
    Gillies' f.
    groin f.
    hinge f.
    immediate transfer f.
    Indian f.
    intercalated f.
    interpolated f.
    island f.
    Italian f.
    jump f.
    Langenbeck's pedicle
      mucoperiosteal f.
    latissimus dorsi muscle f.
    Limberg f.
    lingual tongue f.
    liver f.
    local f.
    Millard island f.
    mucomuscular f.
    mucoperiosteal f.
    muscle f.
    musculocutaneous f.
    myocutaneous f.
    nasolabial f.
    neurovascular f.
    osteoplastic f.
    pectoral muscle f.
    pedicle f.
    pericoronal f.
    pharyngeal f.
    random f.
    rope f.
    rotation f.
    sandwich f.
    scalping f.
    skin f.
    sliding f.
    split-thickness f.
    subcutaneous pedicle f.
    surgical f.
    Tagliacozzi f.
    temporal f.
    tensor fasciae latae muscle
      f.

flap *(continued)*
    thoracoabdominal f.
    thoracoepigastric f.
    tongue f.
    transposition f.
    trapdoor f.
    tube f.
    tubed pedicle f.
    tunnel f.
    turnover f.
    von Langenbeck's bipedicle
      mucoperiosteal f.
    V-Y f.
    Widman f., modified
    Z-f.
    Zimany's bilobed f.
flaps
flare
    aqueous f.
    nasal f.
flash
flash·blind·ed·ness
flask
    Carrel f.
    casting f.
    crown f.
    denture f.
    Dewar f.
    Erlenmeyer f.
    refractory f.
    vacuum f.
    volumetric f.
flask·ing
flat
    optical f.
Fla·tau's law
Fla·tau-Schid·ler disease
flat·foot
    rocker-bottom f.
    spastic f.
    static f.
flat·ness
flat·u·lence
flat·u·lent
fla·tus
    f. vaginalis
flat·worm
fla·vac·i·din

fla·va·noid
fla·va·none
fla·va·non·ol
fla·vec·to·my
fla·ves·cent
fla·vi·an·ic acid
fla·vi·cin
fla·vin
    f.-adenine dinucleotide
      (FAD)
    f. mononucleotide (FMN)
    f. monooxygenase
fla·vi·vi·rus
Fla·vo·bac·te·ri·um
    F. breve
    F. meningosepticum
    F. odoratum
fla·vo·en·zyme
fla·vone
fla·vo·noid
fla·vo·nol
fla·vo·pro·tein
fla·vo·xan·thin
fla·vox·ate hy·dro·chlo·ride
Flax·e·dil
flax·seed
fla·za·lone
fld — fluid
fl dr — fluid dram
flea
    Asiatic rat f.
    burrowing f.
    cat f.
    cavy f.
    chigger f.
    chigoe f.
    common f.
    common rat f.
    dog f.
    European mouse f.
    European rat f.
    human f.
    Indian rat f.
    jigger f.
    mouse f.
    oriental rat f.
    sand f.
    squirrel f.

flea *(continued)*
    sticktight f.
    suslik f.
    tropical rat f.
    water f.
fle·cai·nide
Flech·sig's area
Flech·sig's cuticulum
Flech·sig's fasciculus
Flech·sig's field
Flech·sig's law
fleck
    tobacco f's
fleck·fie·ber
fleck·milz
flec·tion
fleece
    f. of Stilling
Flei·scher-Strüm·pell ring
Fleisch·man's bursa
Fleisch·ner's disease
Fleisch·ner's line
Flem·ing, Sir Alexander
fle·min·gen
Flem·ming's center
Flem·ming's fixing fluid
Flem·ming's solution
flesh
    goose f.
    live f.
    proud f.
fle·taz·e·pam
flet·cher·ism
flex
flex·i·bil·i·tas
    f. cerea
flex·i·bil·i·ty
    waxy f.
flex·i·ble
flex·ile
flex·im·e·ter
flex·ion
    lateral f.
    mass f.
    plantar f.
    universal f.
Flex·ner's bacillus
Flex·ner's dysentery

Flex·ner-Job·ling
  carcinosarcoma
flex·or
    f. retinaculum
flex·or·plas·ty
flex·u·ose
flex·u·ra *pl.* flex·u·rae
    f. coli dextra
    f. coli sinistra
    f. duodeni inferior
    f. duodeni superior
    f. duodenojejunalis
    f. hepatica coli
    f. lienalis coli
    f. perinealis recti
    f. sacralis recti
flex·u·rae
flex·ur·al
flex·ure
    basicranial f.
    caudal f.
    cephalic f.
    cerebral f.
    cervical f.
    cranial f.
    dorsal f.
    duodenojejunal f.
    encephalic f.
    hepatic f. of colon
    inferior f. of duodenum
    left f. of colon
    lumbar f.
    mesencephalic f.
    nuchal f.
    perineal f. of rectum
    pontine f.
    right f. of colon
    sacral f.
    sacral f. of rectum
    sigmoid f.
    splenic f. of colon
    superior f. of duodenum
flick·er
Fliess therapy
Fliess treatment
flight
    f. into disease
    f. of ideas

Flint's arcade
Flint's law
Flint's murmur
float·ers
float·ing
floc·ci·le·gi·um
floc·cil·la·tion
floc·cose
floc·cu·lar
floc·cu·la·tion
floc·cule
    toxoid-antitoxin f.
floc·cu·lent
floc·cu·li
floc·cu·lus *pl.* floc·cu·li
    accessory f.
floc·ta·fen·ine
Flood's ligament
floor
    jugular f. of tympanic
      cavity
    f. of orbit
Flor. — L. flores (flowers)
flo·ra
    intestinal f.
flor·an·ty·rone
Flor·a·quin
Flo·rence reaction
Flo·rey, Sir Howard Walter
Flo·rey unit
flor·id
Flor·i·din
Flor·i·nef
Flor·o·pryl
Flor·schütz formula
flow
    axoplasmic f.
    cerebral blood f.
    effective pulmonary blood
      f.
    effective renal blood f.
    effective renal plasma f.
      (ERPF)
    gene f.
    laminar f.
    maximum midexpiratory f.
    peak expiratory f.
    renal blood f. (RBF)

flow *(continued)*
    renal plasma f.
Flow·er's index
flow·ers
    f. of arsenic
    f. of benzoin
    f. of camphor
    pyrethrum f's
    f. of sulfur
flow·me·ter
    blood f.
    Doppler f.
    dry f.
    electromagnetic f.
    pulsed Doppler f.
flow tract
flox·a·cil·lin
flox·uri·dine
fl oz — fluid ounce
FLP — fronto-laeva posterior
(left frontoposterior)
FLT — fronto-laeva
transversa (left
frontotransverse)
flu
    intestinal f.
flu·az·a·cort
flu·ben·da·zole
flu·cin·dole
flu·clor·o·nide
flu·clox·a·cil·lin
Flu·cort
flu·cry·late
fluc·tu·ant
fluc·tu·a·tion
flu·cy·to·sine
flu·dal·a·nine
flu·da·zo·ni·um chlo·ride
flu·do·rex
flu·dro·cor·ti·sone
flu·ence
    energy f.
flu·fen·am·ic acid
flu·fen·i·sal
flügel·platte
flu·id
    allantoic f.
    Altmann's f.

flu·id *(continued)*
    amniotic f.
    ascitic f.
    bleaching f.
    Bouin's f.
    Callison's f.
    Carrel-Dakin f.
    cerebrospinal f. (CSF)
    chlorpalladium f.
    crevicular f.
    Dakin's f.
    decalcifying f.
    Delafield's f.
    Ecker's f.
    extracellular f.
    extravascular f.
    Flemming's fixing f.
    follicular f.
    formol-Müller f.
    Gendre's f.
    gingival f.
    Helly's f.
    interstitial f.
    intracellular f.
    intraocular f.
    Kaiserling's f.
    labyrinthine f.
    Lang's f.
    Locke's f.
    Müller's f.
    non-newtonian f.
    Parker's f.
    pericardial f.
    Piazza's f.
    Rees and Ecker diluting f.
    saline f.
    Scarpa's f.
    Schaudinn's f.
    seminal f.
    serous f.
    synovial f.
    Tellyesniczky's f.
    Thoma's f.
    tissue f.
    Toison's f.
    transcellular f.
    ventricular f.
    Waldeyer's f.

flu·id *(continued)*
    Wickersheimer's f.
    Zenker's f.
flu·id dram
flu·id·ex·tract
flu·id·ex·trac·tum *pl.* flu·id·
  ex·trac·ta
flu·id·glyc·er·ates
flu·id ounce
flu·i·drachm
fluke
    blood f.
    bronchial f.
    Chinese liver f.
    digenetic f.
    intestinal f's
    liver f's
    lung f.
    oriental f.
fluk·i·cide
flu·men *pl.* flu·mi·na
    flumina pilorum
flu·me·quine
flu·meth·a·sone piv·a·late
flu·me·thi·a·zide
flu·mi·na
flu·mi·zole
flu·mox·o·nide
flu·nar·i·zine hy·dro·chlo·
  ride
flu·nid·a·zole
flu·nis·o·lide
    f. acetate
flu·ni·traz·e·pam
flu·nix·in
    f. meglumine
flu·o·cin·o·lone acet·o·nide
flu·o·cin·o·nide
flu·o·cor·tin bu·tyl
Flu·o·gen
flu·o·hy·dri·sone
flu·o·hy·dro·cor·ti·sone
Flu·o·nid
flu·or
    f. albus
    plastic f.
flu·or·ane
flu·or·ap·a·tite

flu·o·res·ce·in
    f. isothiocyanate (FITC)
    sodium f.
flu·o·res·ce·in·uria
flu·o·res·cence
    natural f.
    nonspecific f.
    secondary f.
    x-ray f.
flu·o·res·cent
flu·o·res·cin
flu·o·ri·da·tion
flu·o·ride
    stannous f.
    topical f.
flu·o·ri·di·za·tion
flu·o·rim·e·ter
flu·o·rim·e·try
flu·o·rine
flu·o·ro·ac·e·tate
flu·o·ro·ace·tic acid
flu·o·ro·car·bon
flu·o·ro·chrome
flu·o·ro·chrom·ing
flu·o·ro·cit·ric acid
α-flu·o·ro·cor·ti·sol [alpha-]
flu·o·ro·cyte
flu·o·rog·ra·phy
    digital f.
p-flu·o·ro·phen·yl·al·a·nine
flu·o·ro·im·mu·no·as·say
flu·o·rom·e·ter
flu·o·ro·meth·o·lone
flu·o·rom·e·try
flu·o·ro·neph·e·lom·e·ter
flu·o·ro·phos·phate
    diisopropyl f.
flu·o·ro·pho·tom·e·try
    vitreous f.
Flu·or·o·plex
flu·o·ro·roent·ge·nog·ra·phy
flu·o·ro·scope
    biplane f.
flu·o·ro·scop·ic
flu·o·ro·scop·i·cal
flu·o·ros·co·py
flu·o·ro·sil·i·cate

flu·o·ro·sis
    dental f.
    endemic f., chronic
5-flu·o·ro·ura·cil
Flu·o·sol
Flu·o·thane
flu·o·tra·cen hy·dro·chlo·ride
flu·ox·e·tine
flu·ox·y·mes·ter·one
flu·per·a·mide
flu·phen·a·zine
    f. dihydrochloride
    f. enanthate
    f. hydrochloride
flu·pred·nis·o·lone
    f. valerate
flu·pros·te·nol so·di·um
flu·qua·zone
flur·an·dren·o·lide
flur·an·dren·o·lone
flu·raz·e·pam hy·dro·chlo·ride
flur·bip·ro·fen
Flur·o·bate
flu·ro·ci·ta·bine
flu·ro·ges·tone ac·e·tate
flu·ro·thyl
flush
    atropine f.
    breast f.
    carcinoid f.
    flamingo f.
    harlequin f.
    hectic f.
    histamine f.
    limbal f.
    mahogany f.
    malar f.
    menopausal f.
    niacin f.
flu·spip·er·one
flu·spir·i·lene
flu·ta·mide
flu·ti·a·zin
flut·ter
    atrial f.
    auricular f.
    diaphragmatic f.

flut·ter *(continued)*
    impure f.
    mediastinal f.
    pure f.
    ventricular f.
flut·ter-fi·bril·la·tion
flux
    celiac f.
    integral neutron f.
    ionic f.
    luminous f.
    menstrual f.
    neutral f.
    neutron f.
    oxidizing f.
    reducing f.
flux·ion
fly
    black f.
    blackbottle f.
    bloodsucking f's
    blow f.
    bluebottle f.
    bot f.
    caddis f.
    cheese f.
    deer f.
    drone f.
    dung f.
    eye f.
    face f.
    filth f.
    flesh f.
    fruit f.
    gad f.
    green-bottle f.
    heel f.
    horn f.
    horse f.
    house f.
    hover f's
    lake f.
    latrine f.
    louse f.
    mango f.
    mangrove f.
    moth f.
    nose f.

fly *(continued)*
    nostril f.
    owl f.
    ox-warble f.
    phlebotomus f.
    pomace f.
    Russian f.
    sand f.
    screw-worm f.
    Seroot f.
    snipe f.
    soldier f.
    Spanish f.
    stable f.
    tick f.
    tsetse f.
    tumbu f.
    warble f.
F.M. — L. fiat mistura (make a mixture)
FMN — flavin mononucleotide (riboflavin 5-phosphate)
FNH — focal nodular hyperplasia
FNTC — fine needle transhepatic cholangiography
fo·cal
fo·ci
fo·cil, fo·cile
fo·cim·e·ter
fo·cus *pl.* fo·ci
    aplanatic f.
    Assmann f.
    conjugate f.
    epileptogenic f.
    Ghon f.
    negative f.
    principal foci
    real f.
    Simon's foci
    spike f.
    virtual f.
fo·cus·ing
    dynamic f.
    electronic f.
    isoelectric f.

Fo·gar·ty catheter
fog·ging
fo·go
    f. selvagem
foil
    activation f.
    gold f.
    mat f.
    platinum f.
    tin f.
Foix paramedian syndrome
Foix-Ala·jou·a·nine disease
Foix-Ala·jou·a·nine syndrome
Fol. — L. folia (leaves)
fo·la·cin
fo·late
fold
    alar f's
    amniotic f.
    aryepiglottic f.
    aryepiglottic f. of Collier
    arytenoepiglottidean f.
    axillary f.
    Brachet's mesolateral f.
    bulboventricular f.
    caudal genital f.
    caval f.
    cecal f's
    cholecystoduodenocolic f.
    ciliary f's
    circular f's of Kerckring
    conjunctival f.
    costocolic f.
    cranial genital f.
    cutaneous f's of anus
    Douglas' f.
    Duncan's f's
    duodenojejunal f.
    duodenomesocolic f.
    epicanthal f.
    epigastric f.
    falciform f. of fascia lata
    fimbriated f.
    gastric f's
    gastropancreatic f.
    gastropancreatic f's of Huschke
    genital f.

fold *(continued)*
  glossoepiglottic f's
  gluteal f.
  Guérin's f.
  Hasner's f.
  head f.
  Heister's f.
  Hensing's f.
  hepatopancreatic f.
  horizontal f's of rectum
  ileocecal f.
  ileocolic f.
  iliopubic f. of Thompson
  incudal f.
  inferior duodenal f.
  interarticular f. of hip
  inter-arytenoid f.
  interdigital f.
  interureteric f.
  iridial f's
  Jonnesco's f.
  Juvara's f.
  junctional f.
  Kerckring's f's (of small
    intestine)
  Kohlrausch's f's
  lacrimal f.
  f. of laryngeal nerve
  lateral f.
  lateral nasal f.
  longitudinal f. of
    duodenum
  mallear f.
  mammary f.
  Marshall's f.
  medial nasal f.
  medullary f.
  mesolateral f.
  mesonephric f.
  mesouterine f.
  mucobuccal f.
  mucolabial f.
  mucosal f.
  mucosobuccal f.
  mucous f.
  nail f.
  nasolabial f.
  nasopharyngeal f.

fold *(continued)*
  Nélaton's f.
  neural f.
  opercular f.
  palantine f's
  palantine f's, transverse
  palmate f's
  palpebral f.
  palpebronasal f.
  pancreaticogastric f., left
  paraduodenal f.
  parietocolic f.
  parietoperitoneal f.
  Pawlik's f's
  pharyngoepiglottic f.
  pleuroperitoneal f.
  primitive f.
  Rathke's f's
  rectal f's
  rectouterine f.
  rectovaginal f.
  rectovesical f.
  retrotarsal f.
  Rindfleisch's f's
  sacrogenital f.
  salpingopalatine f.
  salpingopharyngeal f.
  Schultze's f.
  f's of scrotum
  semilunar f.
  serosal f.
  serous f.
  sigmoid f's of colon
  spiral f.
  spiral f. of cystic duct
  stapedial f.
  sublingual f.
  superior duodenal f.
  synovial f.
  tail f.
  transverse f's of rectum
  Treves' f.
  triangular f.
  triangular f. of His
  tubal f's of uterine tube
  umbilical f.
  f. of urachus
  urethral f.

fold *(continued)*
    urogenital f.
    uterosacral f.
    vaginal f's
    vascular cecal f.
    Vater's f.
    ventricular f.
    vesical f., transverse
    vestibular f.
    vestigial f. of Marshall
    villous f's of stomach
    vocal f.
    vocal f., false
Fo·ley catheter
fo·lia
fo·li·a·ceous
fo·li·an
fol·ic acid
fo·lie
    f. communiquée
    f. à deux
    f. du doute
    f. gémellaire
    f. des grandeurs
    f. imitative
    f. imposée
    f. induite
    f. du pourquoi
    f. raisonnante
Fo·lin's filtrate
Folin's method
Fo·lin and Sved·berg method
Fo·lin and Wu test
fo·lin·ic acid
fo·li·um *pl.* fo·lia
    folia cerebelli
    folia of cerebellum
    lingual f.
    f. vermis
Fo·li·us' muscle
Fo·li·us' process
fol·li·cle
    aggregated f's
    agminated f's
    anovulvar ovarian f.
    antral f's
    atretic f.
    closed f.

fol·li·cle *(continued)*
    dental f.
    Fleischmann's f.
    gastric f's
    germinal f.
    graafian f's
    hair f.
    intestinal f's
    laryngeal lymphatic f's
    lenticular f's
    Lieberkühn's f's
    lingual f's
    lymph f.
    Montgomery's f's
    mucous f's, nasal
    Naboth's f's
    nabothian f's
    ovarian f.
    pilosebaceous f.
    polyovular ovarian f.
    primordial f.
    sebaceous f.
    secondary f's
    solitary f's
    splenic lymph f's
    f. of Stannius
    tertiary f.
    thyroid f's
    f's of tongue
    tooth f.
    unilaminar f.
fol·li·clis
fol·lic·u·lar
fol·lic·u·li
fol·lic·u·li·tis
    f. abscedens et suffodiens
    agminate f.
    f. barbae
    f. cruris atrophicans
    f. decalvans
    f. decalvans cryptococcia
    eosinophilic pustular f.
    f. gonorrhoeica
    gram-negative f.
    industrial f.
    keloidal f.
    f. keloidalis
    f. nares perforans

fol·lic·u·li·tis *(continued)*
  oil f.
  f. ulerythematosa
    reticulata
  f. varioliformis
fol·lic·u·lo·ma
  f. lipidique
fol·lic·u·lo·sis
fol·lic·u·lo·stat·in
fol·lic·u·lus *pl.* fol·lic·u·li
  folliculi glandulae
    thyroideae
  folliculi linguales
  f. lymphaticus
  f. pili
Foøl·ling's disease
Foøl·ling's phenylketonuria
fol·low·up
Fol·lu·te·in
Foltz's valve
Fol·vite
fo·men·ta·tion
fo·mes *pl.* fo·mi·tes
fo·mite
fom·i·tes
fo·na·zine mes·y·late
Fon·se·caea
fons pul·sa·til·is
fon·tac·to·scope
Fon·tan's operation
Fon·tana's markings
Fon·tana's spaces
Fon·tana stain
fon·ta·nel
fon·ta·nelle
  anterior f.
  anterolateral f.
  bregmatic f.
  Casser's f.
  casserian f.
  Casserio's f.
  cranial f's
  frontal f.
  Gerdy's f.
  lateral f's
  mastoid f.
  occipital f.
  posterior f.

fon·ta·nelle *(continued)*
  posterolateral f.
  posterotemporal f.
  quadrangular f.
  sagittal f.
  sphenoidal f.
  supraoccipital f.
  triangular f.
fon·tic·u·li
fon·tic·u·lus *pl.* fon·tic·u·li
  f. anterior
  f. anterolateralis
  fonticuli cranii
  f. frontalis [major]
  f. gutturis
  f. major
  f. mastoideus
  f. minor
  f. occipitalis
  f. posterior
  f. posterolateralis
  f. quadrangularis
  f. sphenoidalis
  f. triangularis
food
  isodynamic f's
foot
  athlete's f.
  bifid f.
  broad f.
  burning feet
  buttress f.
  cavus f.
  Charcot's f.
  claw f.
  cleft f.
  club f.
  contracted f.
  crooked f.
  dancers' f.
  dangle f.
  drop f.
  end f.
  end f. of Held
  fescue f.
  flat f.
  forced f.
  Friedreich's f.

foot *(continued)*
  fungus f.
  Held's f.
  hollow f.
  Hong Kong f.
  hot f.
  immersion f.
  immersion f., tropical
  Madura f.
  march f.
  Morand's f.
  Morton's f.
  mossy f.
  perivascular feet
  pricked f.
  red f.
  reel f.
  rocker-bottom f.
  root f.
  SACH (single axis cushion
    heel) f.
  sag f.
  septic f.
  spatula f.
  splay f.
  split f.
  spread f.
  strawberry rot f.
  stump f.
  sucker f.
  tabetic f.
  taut f.
  tip f.
  trench f.
  weak f.
foot-can·dle
foot·drop
foot-en·gine
foot lam·bert
foot·plate
  vascular f.
foot-pound
foot·print
for·age
fo·ra·men *pl.* fo·ra·mi·na
  accessory f.
  alveolar foramina of
    maxilla

fo·ra·men *(continued)*
  foramina alveolaria
    maxillae
  aortic f.
  apical f. of tooth
  f. apicis dentis
  arachnoid f.
  auditory f., external
  auditory f., internal
  Bichat's f.
  f. of Bochdalek
  Botallo's f.
  f. bursae omentalis majoris
  f. caecum
  caroticoclinoid f.
  caroticotympanic foramina
  carotid f.
  cecal f.
  condyloid f., anterior
  conjugate f.
  f. costotransversarium
  costotransverse f.
  cotyloid f.
  cribroethmoid f.
  foramina cribrosa ossis
    ethmoidalis
  dental foramina
  f. diaphragmatis [sellae]
  Duverney's f.
  emissary f.
  epiploic f.
  f. epiploicum
  esophageal f.
  ethmoidal foramina
  f. ethmoidale anterius
  f. ethmoidale posterius
  foramina ethmoidalia
  f. of Fallopio
  Ferrein's f.
  frontal f.
  f. frontale
  frontoethmoidal f.
  Galen's f.
  glandular foramina of
    Littre
  glandular f. of Morgagni
  great f.
  Hartigan's f.

fo·ra·men *(continued)*
  hemal f.
  Huschke's f.
  Hyrtl's f.
  incisive f.
  f. incisivum
  incisor f., median
  infraorbital f.
  f. infraorbitale
  infrapiriform f.
  innominate f.
  interatrial f. secundum
  intersacral foramina
  interventricular f.
  f. interventriculare
  intervertebral f.
  f. intervertebrale
  intervertebral foramina of
    sacrum
  ischiadic f., greater
  ischiadic f., lesser
  f. ischiadicum majus
  f. ischiadicum minus
  ischiopubic f.
  jugular f.
  f. of Key and Retzius
  lacerate f.
  f. lacerum
  f. lacerum anterius
  f. lacerum medium
  f. lacerum posterius
  f. of Lannelongue
  lateral f.
  f. of Luschka
  f. of Magendie
  f. magnum
  malar f.
  f. mandibulae
  mastoid f.
  f. mastoideum
  maxillary f.
  medullary f.
  meibomian f.
  mental f.
  f. mentale
  f. of Monro
  Morand's f.
  Morgagni's f.

fo·ra·men *(continued)*
  morgagnian f.
  nasal foramina
  foramina nasalia
  neural f.
  f. nutricium
  nutrient f.
  obturator f.
  f. obturatorium
  f. obturatum
  occipital f., great
  occipital f., inferior
  f. occipitale magnum
  olfactory f.
  omental f.
  f. omentale
  optic f.
  f. opticum ossis
    sphenoidalis
  orbitomalar f.
  oval f.
  f. ovale
  f. of Pacchioni
  pacchionian f.
  foramina palatina minora
  palatine foramina,
    accessory
  palatine f., anterior
  palatine f., greater
  palatine foramina, lesser
  palatine f., posterior
  foramina of palatine tonsil
  f. palatinum majus
  foramina papillaria renis
  parietal f.
  f. parietale
  patent f. ovale
  f. petrosum
  pleuroperitoneal f.
  f. primum
  f. processus transversi
  pterygoalar f.
  pterygopalatine f.
  pulpal f.
  quadrate f.
  f. radicis dentis
  Retzius' f.
  right f.

fo·ra·men *(continued)*
  rivinian f.
  Rivinus' f.
  root f.
  f. rotundum ossis
    sphenoidalis
  sacral foramina, anterior
  f. of sacral canal
  foramina sacralia
    anteriora
  foramina sacralia dorsalia
  foramina sacralia pelvina
  foramina sacralia
    posteriora
  foramina sacralia ventralia
  sacrosciatic f., great
  sacrosciatic f., small
  f. of saphenous vein
  Scarpa's f.
  Schwalbe's f.
  sciatic f., greater
  sciatic f., lesser
  f. sciaticum majus
  f. sciaticum minus
  f. secundum
  f. singulare
  foramina of smallest veins
    of heart
  sphenopalatine f.
  f. sphenopalatinum
  sphenotic f.
  spinal f.
  f. spinosum
  Spöndel's f.
  f. of Stensen
  stylomastoid f.
  f. stylomastoideum
  suborbital f.
  supraorbital f.
  suprapiriform f.
  Tarin's f.
  temporomalar f.
  thebesian foramina
  foramina thebesii
  thyroid f.
  f. thyroideum
  tonsillar foramina
  f. transversarium

fo·ra·men *(continued)*
  transverse accessory f.
  f. venae cavae
  vena caval f.
  foramina venarum
    minimarum cordis
  f. venosum
  venous f.
  vertebral f.
  f. vertebrale
  vertebroarterial f.
  f. vertebroarteriale
  f. Vesalii
  f. of Vesalius
  f. of Vicq d'Azyr
  visceral f.
  Vieussen's foramina
  Weitbrecht's f.
  f. of Winslow
  zygomatic f.
  zygomaticofacial f.
  f. zygomaticofaciale
  zygomatico-orbital f.
  f. zygomatico-orbitale
  zygomaticotemporal f.
  f. zygomaticotemporale
fo·ram·i·na
fo·ram·i·nal
for·am·i·nif·er·an
Fo·ram·i·ni·fer·i·da
for·am·i·nif·er·ous
fo·ram·i·not·o·my
for·a·min·u·late
fo·ra·min·u·lum *pl.* fo·ra·
  min·u·la
For·ane
fo·ra·tion
Forbes disease
Forbes-Al·bright syndrome
force
  bite f.
  catabiotic f.
  catabolic f.
  chewing f.
  electromotive f.
  extraoral f.
  field f's
  masticatory f.

force *(continued)*
    occlusal f.
    radiation f.
    reciprocal f.
    f. of recoil of lung
    reserve f.
    rest f.
    shearing f.
    Van der Waals f's
    vital f.

for·ceps
    ACMI Martin endoscopy f.
    Acufex f.
    Adams f.
    adenoid f.
    alligator f.
    Allis f.
    f. anterior
    artery f.
    Asch f.
    axis-traction f.
    Bailey-Williamson f.
    Ballantine f.
    Ballenger's f.
    Barton f.
    bayonet f.
    bone f.
    bone-cutting f.
    bone-nibbling f.
    Brenner f.
    bulldog f.
    bullet f.
    capsule f.
    Carroll bone-holding f.
    cartilage f.
    Castaneda f.
    chalazion f.
    Chamberlen f.
    clamp f.
    clip f.
    Cornet's f.
    f. of corpus callosum
    D'Allesandro serial suture
      holding f.
    DeLee f.
    dental f.
    depilatory f.
    disk f.

for·ceps *(continued)*
    dissecting f.
    double-action f.
    dressing f.
    dural f.
    ear f.
    Elliot f.
    epilating f.
    extracting f.
    failed f.
    fixation f.
    Foster-Ballenger f.
    f. frontalis
    galea f.
    Garrison's f.
    Good f.
    gouge f.
    Haig Ferguson f.
    Hawks-Dennen f.
    hemostatic f.
    high f.
    Hodge's f.
    inlet f.
    insertion f.
    Jansen f.
    Kazanjian f.
    Kerrison f.
    Kielland's (Kjelland's) f.
    Kocher f.
    Koeberlé's f.
    Levret's f.
    lion-jawed f.
    lithotomy f.
    lock f.
    low f.
    Löwenberg's f.
    Luc f.
    Luikart f.
    f. McKenzie f.
    f. major
    mid f.
    f. minor
    mosquito f.
    mouse-tooth f.
    Negus ligature f.
    nonfenestrated f.
    obstetrical f.
    f. occipitalis

for·ceps *(continued)*
    Ostrom f.
    outlet f.
    ovum f.
    Péan's f.
    Piper f.
    placenta f.
    point f.
    f. posterior
    punch f.
    rat-tooth f.
    rib-cutting f.
    rongeur f.
    root-splitting f.
    rubber dam f.
    Sanders f.
    sequestrum f.
    Simpson's f.
    sinus f.
    speculum f.
    sponge-holding f.
    spring f.
    suture f.
    Tarnier's f.
    tenaculum f.
    thumb f.
    tissue f.
    torsion f.
    towel f.
    tubular f.
    Tucker-McLean f.
    uterine f.
    volsella f.
    vulsellum f.
    Walsham f's
    Willett f.
Forch·heim·er spots
for·ci·pate
for·ci·pres·sure
For·dyce's disease
For·dyce's granule
For·dyce's spot
fore·arm
fore·brain
fore·con·scious
fore·fin·ger
fore·foot
fore·gild·ing

fore·gut
fore·head
Fo·rel's areas
Fo·rel's commissure
Fo·rel's decussation
Fo·rel's fields
fore·milk
fo·ren·sic
fore·play
fore-pleas·ure
fore·see·abil·i·ty of harm
fore·skin
    hooded f.
fore·spore
For·es·tier's disease
fore·wa·ters
For·his·tal
fork
    replication f.
    tuning f.
form
    accolé f.
    appliqué f.
    arch f.
    band f's
    involution f's
    juvenile f.
    L-f.
    racemic f.
    replicative f.
    resistance f.
    retention f.
    ring f.
    spherical f. of occlusion
    tooth f.
    wax f.
    young f.
    Z f.
For·mad's kidney
for·mal·de·hyde
for·mal·de·hyde de·hy·dro·gen·ase
for·mal·de·hyd·o·gen·ic
for·ma·lin
for·ma·lin·ize
for·mam·i·dase
form·ant
for·mate

for·mate de·hy·dro·gen·ase
for·mate hy·dro·gen·ly·ase
for·ma·tio *pl.* for·ma·ti·o·nes
 f. hippocampalis
 f. reticularis
for·ma·tion
 Ammon's f.
 chiasma f.
 coffin f.
 compromise f.
 endochondral bone f.
 Gothic arch f.
 hippocampal f.
 intracartilaginous bone f.
 intramembranous bone f.
 medullary reticular f.
 palisade f.
 reaction f.
 reticular f.
 rouleaux f.
for·ma·ti·o·nes
for·ma·tive
form·board
form-class
forme *pl.* formes
 f. fruste
 f. tardive
form-fam·i·ly
form-ge·nus
for·mic acid
for·mi·cant
for·mi·ca·tion
for·mi·ci·a·sis
For·mi·coi·dea
for·mim·i·no
for·mim·i·no·glu·ta·mate
for·mim·i·no·glu·ta·mic acid
for·mim·i·no·glu·ta·mic·ac·
 id·uria
for·mim·i·no·gly·cine
for·mim·i·no·tet·ra·hy·dro·
 fo·late
for·mim·i·no·trans·fer·ase
For·min
for·mi·ni·tra·zole
for·mo·cor·tal
for·mol
 f. saline

for·mol *(continued)*
 f. sublimate
form-ord·er
for·mu·la *pl.* for·mu·lae, for·
 mu·las
 Arneth's f.
 Arrhenius' f.
 Bazett's f.
 Beckmann's f.
 Bernhardt's f.
 Bird's f.
 Black's f.
 Brenner's f.
 Broca's f.
 Casper's f.
 chemical f.
 Christison's f.
 configurational f.
 constitutional f.
 Demoivre's f.
 dental f.
 digital f.
 Dreser's f.
 Du Bois f.
 Einthoven's f.
 empirical f.
 extemporaneous f.
 Fick f.
 Florschütz's f.
 Gale's f.
 Gompertz f.
 Gorlin's f.
 graphic f.
 Guthrie's f.
 Haines'f.
 Hamilton-Stewart f.
 Häser's f.
 Loebisch's f.
 Long's f.
 Mall's f.
 molecular f.
 official f.
 paretic f.
 Pignet's f.
 Poisson-Pearson f.
 projection f.
 Ranke's f.
 rational f.

for·mu·la *(continued)*
    Read's f.
    Reuss' f.
    Rollier's f.
    Runeberg's f.
    spatial f.
    stereochemical f.
    structural f.
    Trapp's f.
    Van Slyke's f.
    vertebral f.
    Vierdordt-Meeh f.
for·mu·lary
    National F.
for·mu·late
for·mu·la·tion
    American Law Institute f.
for·myl
for·myl·a·tion
for·myl·ky·nu·re·nine hy·
   dro·lase
N-for·myl·me·thi·o·nine
for·myl·tet·ra·hy·dro·fo·late
for·myl·trans·fer·ase
for·ni·cal
for·ni·cate
for·nix *pl.* for·ni·ces
    anterior f.
    f. cerebri
    f. conjunctivae inferior
    f. conjunctivae superior
    gastric f.
    f. gastricus
    f. of lacrimal sac
    lateral f.
    f. longus
    f. pharyngis
    posterior f.
    f. sacci lacrimalis
    f. of stomach
    f. vaginae
    f. ventricularis
    f. ventriculi
For·o·blique
Fors·sell's sinus
Forss·mann, Werner Theodor
   Otto
Forss·man's antigen

För·ster's choroiditis
För·ster's disease
För·ster's photometer
For·taz
For·thane
for·ti·fi·ca·tion
for·tu·i·tous
fos·az·e·pam
fos·fo·my·cin
fos·fo·net so·di·um
Fo·shay's test
fos·pi·rate
fos·sa *pl.* fos·sae
    acetabular f.
    f. acetabuli
    adipose fossae
    anconeal f.
    antecubital f.
    f. anthelicis
    articular f.
    f. axillaris
    axillary f.
    Biesiadecki's f.
    Broesike's f.
    f. caecalis
    f. canina
    f. capitelli
    f. capitis femoris
    cerebellar f.
    cerebral f.
    f. cerebri lateralis [Sylvii]
    f. chordae ductus venosi
    cochleariform f.
    condylar f., condyloid f.
    f. condylaris
    coronoid f. of humerus
    f. coronoidea humeri
    f. of coronoid process
    costal f., inferior
    costal f., superior
    costal f. of transverse
      process
    cranial f., anterior
    cranial f., middle
    cranial f., posterior
    f. cranii anterior
    f. cranii media
    f. cranii posterior

fos·sa *(continued)*
crural f.
Cruveilhier's f.
cubital f.
f. cubitalis
f. cystidis felleae
digastric f.
f. digastrica
digital f.
f. ductus venosi
duodenal f., inferior
duodenal f., superior
duodenojejunal f.
epigastric f.
f. epigastrica
ethmoid f.
f. of eustachian tube
femoral f.
floccular f.
frontal f.
f. of gallbladder
f. of gasserian ganglion
Gerdy's hyoid f.
f. glandulae lacrimalis
glandular f. of frontal bone
glenoid f.
glossoepiglottic f.
greater f. of Scarpa
Gruber's f.
Gruber-Landzert f.
harderian f.
Hartmann's f.
f. of head of femur
f. helicis
f. hemielliptica
f. hemispherica
hyaloid f.
f. hyaloidea
hypogastric f.
hypophyseal f.
f. hypophyseos
f. hypophysialis
ileocecal f., inferior
ileocecal f., superior
ileocolic f.
iliac f.
f. iliaca
iliacosubfascial f.

fos·sa *(continued)*
f. iliacosubfascialis
f. iliopectinea
iliopectineal f.
implantation f.
incisive f. of maxilla
incudal f.
f. incudis
infraclavicular f.
f. infraclavicularis
infraduodenal f.
f. infraspinata
infratemporal f.
f. infratemporalis
inguinal f.
f. inguinalis lateralis
f. inguinalis medialis
innominate f. of auricle
intercondylar f.
f. intercondylaris femoris
f. intercondylica
intercondyloid f.
f. intercondyloidea anterior
  tibiae
f. intercondyloidea femoris
f. intercondyloidea
  posterior tibiae
f. intercruralis
f. intermesocolica
  transversa
interpeduncular f.
f. interpeduncularis
intersigmoid f.
intrabulbar f.
f. ischioanalis
ischiorectal f.
f. ischiorectalis
Jobert's f.
f. of Jonnesco
jugular f.
f. jugularis
lacrimal f.
Landzert's f.
lateral f. of brain
lateral f. of cerebrum
f. lateralis cerebri
f. of lateral malleolus
lateral pharyngeal f.

fos·sa *(continued)*

- lateral f. of preputial space
- lenticular f.
- lesser f. of Scarpa
- f. for ligamentum teres
- f. of little head of radius
- longitudinal fossae of liver, right
- f. longitudinalis hepatis
- Luschka's f.
- Malgaigne's f.
- f. malleoli lateralis
- mandibular f.
- f. mandibularis
- mastoid f.
- maxillary f.
- Merkel's f.
- mesentericoparietal f.
- mesogastric f.
- middle cranial f.
- Mohrenheim's f.
- f. of Morgagni
- f. musculi biventeris
- mylohyoid f. of mandible
- myrtiform f.
- nasal f.
- navicular f.
- navicular f. of Cruveilhier
- f. navicularis urethrae
- occlusal f.
- f. olecrani
- olfactory f.
- oral f.
- orbital f.
- f. ovalis cordis
- f. ovalis femoris
- ovarian f.
- f. ovarica
- f. of Pacchioni
- paraduodenal f.
- parajejunal f.
- pararectal f.
- paravesical f.
- f. paravesicalis
- parietal f.
- patellar f.
- perineal f.
- petrosal f.

fos·sa *(continued)*

- piriform f.
- pituitary f.
- f. poplitea
- popliteal f.
- postauditory f.
- postcondyloid f.
- posterior f. of humerus
- f. praenasalis
- prenasal f.
- prescapular f.
- prespinous f.
- pterygoid f.
- f. pterygoidea
- pterygomaxillary f.
- f. pterygopalatina
- radial f. of humerus
- f. radialis humeri
- retrocecal f.
- retrocolic f.
- retroduodenal f.
- retromandibular f.
- f. retromandibularis
- rhomboid f.
- f. rhomboidea
- Rosenmüller's f.
- f. sacci lacrimalis
- fossae sagittales dextrae hepatis
- fossae sagittales hepatis
- f. sagittalis sinistra hepatis
- scaphoid f.
- f. scaphoidea
- f. scarpae major
- sellar f.
- semilunar f. of ulna
- sigmoid f.
- sphenomaxillary f.
- splenic f. of omental sac
- subcecal f.
- f. subinguinalis
- sublingual f.
- submandibular f.
- submaxillary f.
- suborbital f.
- subpyramidal f.
- subscapular f.
- f. subscapularis

fos·sa *(continued)*
    subsigmoid f.
    supinator f.
    supraclavicular f., greater
    supraclavicular f., lesser
    f. supraclavicularis major
    f. supraclavicularis minor
    supracondyloid f.
    supramastoid f.
    suprasphenoidal f.
    f. supraspinata
    supraspinous f.
    suprasternal f.
    supratonsillar f.
    f. supratonsillaris
    supratrochlear f., posterior
    supravesical f.
    f. supravesicalis
    sylvian f.
    f. of Sylvius
    Tarin's f.
    temporal f.
    f. temporalis
    terminal f.
    tibiofemoral f.
    tonsillar f.
    f. tonsillaris
    f. transversalis hepatis
    f. of Treitz
    triangular f. of auricle
    f. triangularis auriculae
    trochanteric f.
    f. trochanterica
    trochlear f.
    f. trochlearis
    ulnar f.
    umbilical f., medial
    f. umbilicalis hepatis
    urachal f.
    f. venae cavae
    f. venae umbilicalis
    f. vesicae biliaris
    f. vesicae felleae
    vestibular f.
    f. vestibuli vaginae
    Waldeyer's f.
    zygomatic f.
fos·sae

fos·sette
fos·su·la *pl.* fos·su·lae
    f. of cochlear window
    costal f., inferior
    costal f., superior
    f. fenestrae cochleae
    f. fenestrae vestibuli
    f. of oval window
    f. petrosa
    f. post fenestram
    f. of round window
    tonsillar fossulae of
      palatine tonsil
    tonsillar fossulae of
      pharyngeal tonsil
    fossulae tonsillares
      tonsillae palatinae
    fossulae tonsillares
      tonsillae pharyngeae
    f. of vestibular window
fos·su·lae
fos·su·late
Fos·ter Ken·ne·dy syndrome
Foth·er·gill's disease
Foth·er·gill's sore throat
Foth·er·gill's neuralgia
Foth·er·gill's operation
Foth·er·gill-Don·ald operation
Fou·chet's test
fou·lage
foun·da·tion
    denture f.
    medical f.
four·chette
Fou·ri·er analysis
Four·nier's gangrene
Four·nier's disease
Four·nier's sign
Four·nier's test
fo·vea *pl.* fo·veae
    articular f.
    f. articularis
    calcaneal f.
    f. capitis femoris
    f. capituli radii
    f. cardiaca
    caudal f.
    f. caudalis

fo·vea *(continued)*
   central f. of retina
   f. centralis retinae
   f. of condyloid process
   f. of coronoid process
   costal f., inferior
   costal f., superior
   costal f., transverse
   costal foveae of sternum
   f. costalis inferior
   f. costalis superior
   f. costalis processus
     transversus
   cranial f.
   f. cranialis
   crural f.
   dental f. of atlas
   f. dentis atlantis
   digastric f.
   femoral f.
   f. of fourth ventricle
   glandular foveae of
     Luschka
   greater anterior f. of
     humerus
   f. hemielliptica
   f. hemispherica
   inferior f.
   f. inferior
   inguinal f.
   f. limbica
   f. of Morgagni
   f. nuchae
   oblong f. of arytenoid
     cartilage
   f. oblonga cartilaginis
     arytenoideae
   pterygoid f.
   f. pterygoidea mandibulae
   sublingual f.
   f. sublingualis
   submandibular f.
   f. submandibularis
   f. superior
   superior f.
   f. supravesicalis peritonaei
   f. trigemini
   trochlear f.

fo·vea *(continued)*
   f. trochlearis
fo·ve·ate
fo·ve·a·tion
fo·ve·o·la *pl.* fo·ve·o·lae
   f. coccygea
   coccygeal f.
   foveolae gastricae
   granular foveolae
   foveolae granulares
   foveolae papillae
   f. retinae
   f. suprameatalis
   f. suprameatica
   triangular f.
fo·ve·o·lae
fo·ve·o·lar
fo·ve·o·late
Fo·ville's syndrome
Fow·ler's position
Fow·ler's solution
Fow·ler-Mur·phy treatment
fowl·pox
Fox's disease
Fox-For·dyce disease
fox·glove
   Austrian f.
   purple f.
   woolly f.
F.p. — L. fiat potio (let a
  potion be made)
   freezing point
fp — foot-pound
   freezing point
F.pil. — L. fiant pilulae (let
  pills be made)
Fra·cas·to·ri·us
Fract. dos. — L. fracta dosi (in
  divided doses)
frac·tion
   absorbed f.
   blood plasma f.
   dried human plasma
     protein f.
   ejection f.
   Fechner f.
   filtration f.
   human plasma protein f.

frac·tion *(continued)*
   microsome f.
   mol f.
   mole f.
   plasma f's
   plasma protein f.
   recombination f.
   sampling f.
   soluble f.
   substance f.
   Teicholz ejection f.
   volume f.
frac·tion·al
frac·tion·ate
frac·tion·a·tion
   cell f.
   Cohn f.
   dose f.
frac·tog·ra·phy
frac·ture
   abduction f.
   adduction f.
   agenetic f.
   apophyseal f.
   articular f.
   atrophic f.
   avulsion f.
   Barton's f.
   basal neck f.
   basal skull f.
   basocervical f.
   bending f.
   Bennett's f.
   birth f.
   blow-out f.
   boxer's f.
   bucket-handle f.
   bumper f.
   bursting f.
   butterfly f.
   buttonhole f.
   capillary f.
   cemental f.
   cementum f.
   chance f.
   chip f.
   chisel f.
   cleavage f.

frac·ture *(continued)*
   closed f.
   Colles' f.
   comminuted f.
   complete f.
   complicated f.
   compound f.
   compound skull f.
   compression f.
   condylar f.
   congenital f.
   f. by contrecoup
   cortical f.
   cough f.
   craniofacial dysjunction f.
   crush f.
   deferred f.
   dentate f.
   depressed f.
   de Quervain's f.
   diacondylar f.
   diastatic skull f.
   direct f.
   dislocation f.
   displaced f.
   double f.
   Dupuytren's f.
   Duverney's f.
   dyscrasic f.
   f. en coin
   endocrine f.
   f. en rave
   epiphyseal f.
   extracapsular f.
   fatigue f.
   fender f.
   fissure f.
   fissured f.
   freeze f.
   Galeazzi's f.
   Gosselin's f.
   greenstick f.
   grenade-thrower's f.
   Guérin's f.
   gutter f.
   hairline f.
   hangman's f.
   heat f's

frac·ture *(continued)*

hickory-stick f.
horizontal maxillary f.
idiopathic f.
impacted f.
incomplete f.
indirect f.
inflammatory f.
interperiosteal f.
intertrochanteric f.
intra-articular f.
intracapsular f.
intraperiosteal f.
intrauterine f.
Jefferson f.
joint f.
Jones f.
lead pipe f.
Le Fort's f.
linear f.
Lisfranc's f.
longitudinal f.
loose f.
malar f.
mallet f.
march f.
midfacial f.
Monteggia's f.
Moore's f.
multiple f.
nasal f.
neoplastic f.
neurogenic f.
oblique f.
occult f.
open f.
panfacial f.
paratrooper f.
parry f.
pathologic f.
perforating f.
periarticular f.
pertrochanteric f.
pillion f.
ping-pong f.
pond f.
posterior element f.
Pott's f.

frac·ture *(continued)*

pressure f.
puncture f.
pyramidal f. (of maxilla)
Quervain's f.
resecting f.
reverse Colles' f.
ring f.
Salter f. (I–VI)
secondary f.
segmental f.
shaft f.
Shepherd's f.
silver-fork f.
simple f.
simple f., complex
Skillern's f.
Smith's f.
spiral f.
splintered f.
spontaneous f.
sprain f.
sprinter's f.
stellate f.
Stieda's f.
strain f.
stress f.
subcapital f.
subcutaneous f.
subperiosteal f.
subtrochanteric f.
supracondylar f.
surgical neck f.
temporal bone f.
tibial plateau f.
torsion f.
torus f.
transcervical f.
transcondylar f.
transverse f.
transverse facial f.
transverse maxillary f.
trimalleolar f.
trophic f.
tuft f.
ununited f.
vertebra plana f.
Wagstaffe's f.

frac·ture *(continued)*
 willow f.
frac·ture-dis·lo·ca·tion
 Monteggia f.
 posterior f.
frad·i·cin
frag·i·form
fra·gil·i·tas
 f. crinium
 f. ossium
 f. unguium
fra·gil·i·ty
 f. of blood
 capillary f.
 erythrocyte f.
 hereditary f. of bone
 mechanical f.
 osmotic f.
fra·gilo·cyte
fra·gilo·cy·to·sis
frag·ment
 f. A
 Fab f.
 F(ab')$_2$ f.
 f. B
 Fc f.
 Fd f.
 fission f.
 one-carbon f.
 papain f.
 restriction f.
 Spengler's f's
frag·men·ta·tion
 f. of myocardium
frag·men·tog·ra·phy
fraise
 diamond f.
fram·be·sia
 f. tropica
fram·be·si·o·ma
fram·boe·sia
fram·boe·si·o·ma
frame
 Balkan f.
 Bradford f.
 Deiters' terminal f.
 Foster f.
 freeze f.

frame *(continued)*
 occluding f.
 quadriplegic standing f.
 reading f.
 rotating f. of reference
 rubber dam f.
 Stryker f.
 suture f.
 trial f.
 unidentified reading f.
  (URF)
 Whitman's f.
frame·work
 implant f.
 scleral f.
 uveal f.
Fran·ce·schet·ti's syndrome
Fran·ce·schet·ti-Jad·as·sohn
  syndrome
Fran·cis' disease
Fran·ci·sel·la
 F. tularensis
fran·ci·um
Fran·co's operation
frange
fran·gul·ic acid
Frank's operation
Frank-Starling curve
Franke's operation
Frän·kel's sign
Frän·kel's speculum
Frän·kel's test
Frän·kel's treatment
Frank·en·häu·ser's ganglion
Frankl-Hoch·wart's disease
Frank·lin's disease
Frank·lin glasses
Fra·ser syndrome
Fraun·ho·fer zone
Fra·zier-Spil·ler operation
FRC — functional residual
  capacity
FRCP — Fellow of the Royal
  College of Physicians
FRCP(C) — Fellow of the
  Royal College of Physicians
  of Canada

FRCPE — Fellow of the Royal College of Physicians of Edinburgh

FRCP(Glasg) — Fellow of the Royal College of Physicians and Surgeons of Glasgow qua Physician

FRCPI — Fellow of the Royal College of Physicians in Ireland

FRCS — Fellow of the Royal College of Surgeons

FRCS(C) — Fellow of the Royal College of Surgeons of Canada

FRCSE — Fellow of the Royal College of Surgeons of Edinburgh

FRCS(Glasg) — Fellow of the Royal College of Physicians and Surgeons of Glasgow qua Surgeon

FRCSI — Fellow of the Royal College of Surgeons in Ireland

FRCVS — Fellow of the Royal College of Veterinary Surgeons

Fre·Am·ine II

freck·le

    melanotic f. of Hutchinson

Fre·det-Ram·stedt operation

free-liv·ing

Free·man-Shel·don syndrome

free·mar·tin

Freer elevator

freeze-cleav·ing

freeze-dry·ing

freeze-etch·ing

freeze-frac·tur·ing

freeze-sub·sti·tu·tion

Frei's antigen

Frei's disease

Frei's test

Frei·berg's infraction

Frejka pillow

Frejka pillow splint

frem·i·tus

    bronchial f.

    friction f.

    hydatid f.

    pectoral f.

    pericardial f.

    pleural f.

    rhonchal f.

    subjective f.

    tactile f.

    tussive f.

    vocal f.

fre·na

fre·nal

French (scale)

fre·nec·to·my

Fren·kel's movements

Fren·kel's treatment

fre·no·plas·ty

fre·not·o·my

    lingual f.

fren·u·la

fren·u·lum *pl.* fren·u·la

    f. of anterior medullary velum

    f. cerebelli

    f. clitoridis

    f. of duodenal papilla

    f. of Giacomini

    f. of ileocecal valve

    f. of ileocolic valve

    f. of inferior lip

    f. labii inferioris

    f. labii superioris

    f. labiorum pudendi

    f. linguae

    f. linguae cerebelli

    f. of Macdowel

    f. of Morgagni

    f. of prepuce of penis

    f. preputii penis

    f. of pudendal labia

    f. pudendi

    f. of rostral medullary velum

    f. of superior lip

fren·u·lum *(continued)*
 f. of superior medullary
  velum
 f. synoviale
 f. of tongue
 f. valvae ilealis
 f. valvae ileocaecalis
 f. veli medullaris cranialis
 f. veli medullaris rostralis
 f. veli medullaris superius
fre·num *pl.* fre·na
 buccal f.
 f. of labia
 lingual f.
 Macdowel's f.
 f. of Morgagni
 f. of tongue
 f. of valve of colon
fre·quen·cy
 audio f.
 audio Doppler f.
 center f.
 f's of class
 critical flicker fusion f.
 cutoff f.
 dominant f.
 fusion f.
 gene f.
 high f.
 infrasonic f.
 Larmor f.
 low f.
 mutant f.
 nearest neighbor f.
 projection f.
 recombination f.
 relative f.
 respiratory f.
 subsonic f.
 supersonic f.
 ultrasonic f.
 urinary f.
 ventilatory f.
Fre·richs' theory
Fres·nel lens
Fres·nel zone
fress·re·flex
fre·tum *pl.* fre·ta

fre·tum
 f. halleri
Freud, Sigmund
freud·i·an
Freund adjuvant
Freund's anomaly
Freund's operation
Frey's gastric pits
Frey's hairs
Frey's syndrome
Frey-Bail·lar·ger syndrome
Frey·er's operation
FRF — follicle-stimulating
 hormone releasing factor
FRFPSG — Fellow of the
 Royal Faculty of Physicians
 and Surgeons of Glasgow
fri·a·ble
fric·a·tive
Fricke's bandage
Frid·er·ich·sen-Wa·ter·house
 syndrome
Frid·er·i·cia's method
Fried·län·der's bacillus
Fried·län·der's disease
Fried·län·der's pneumobacillus
Fried·län·der's pneumonia
Fried·man curve
Fried·man's test
Fried·man-Lap·ham test
Fried·mann's complex
Fried·mann's vasomotor
 syndrome
Fried·reich's ataxia
Fried·reich's disease
Fried·reich's foot
Fried·reich's sign
Fried·reich's tabes
Friend's vi·rus
fri·gid·i·ty
frigo·la·bile
frigo·rif·ic
frigo·sta·bile
frigo·sta·ble
frig·o·ther·a·py
Frisch, Karl Ritter von
frit
Fritsch's catheter

Fröh·lich's syndrome
Frohn's reagent
Frohn's test
Froin's syndrome
frole·ment
Fro·ment's paper sign
From·mann's lines
From·mel's disease
From·mel-Chi·a·ri syndrome
fron·dose
frons
    f. cranii
    wave f.
fron·tad
fron·tal
fron·ta·lis
fron·tip·e·tal
fron·to·cer·e·bel·lar
fron·to·eth·moid·ec·to·my
    external f.
fron·to·ma·lar
fron·to·max·il·lary
fron·to·men·tal
fron·to·na·sal
fron·to-oc·cip·i·tal
fron·to-or·bi·tal
fron·to·pa·ri·e·tal
fron·to·pon·tine
fron·to·pon·to·cer·e·bel·lar
fron·to·tem·por·al
fron·to·zy·go·mat·ic
Fro·riep's ganglion
Fro·riep's induration
Frost suture
frost
    synovial f.
    urea f.
    uremic f.
frost·bite
    deep f.
    superficial f.
    third degree f.
frot·tage
frot·teur
FRS — Fellow of the Royal Society
fruc·ti·fi·ca·tion

fruc·tiv·o·rous
fruc·to·fu·ra·nose
fruc·to·ki·nase
fruc·to·py·ra·nose
fruc·to·sa·mine
fruc·to·san
fruc·to·sa·zone
fruc·tose
    f. 1,6-bisphosphate
    f. 1,6-diphosphate
    f. 6-phosphate
fruc·tose-1,6-bis·phos·pha·tase
fruc·tose-2,6-bis·phos·pha·tase
fruc·tose 2,6-bis·phos·phate
fruc·tose bis·phos·phate al·do·lase
fruc·tose-1,6-di·phos·pha·tase
fruc·tos·emia
fruc·tose-1-phos·phate al·do·lase
fruc·to·si·dase
fruc·to·side
fruc·tos·uria
    benign f.
    essential f.
fruc·to·syl
fruc·to·syl·trans·fer·ase
fruc·to·veg·e·ta·tive
fru·giv·o·rous
fruit·ar·i·an
fruit·ar·i·an·ism
frus·e·mide
Frust. — L. frustillatim (in small pieces)
F.s.a. — L. fiat secundum artem (let it be made skillfully)
FSH — follicle-stimulating hormone
FSH/LH-RH — follicle-stimulating hormone and luteinizing hormone releasing hormone
FSH-RF — follicle-stimulating hormone releasing factor
FSH-RH — follicle stimulating hormone releasing hormone

ft. — L. fiat or fiant (let there
    be made)
    foot
    feet
Ft. mas. div. in pil. — L. fiat
    massa dividenda in pilulae
    (let a mass be made and
    divided into pills)
Ftor·a·fur
Ft. pulv. — L. fiat pulvis (let a
    powder be made)
5-FU — 5-fluorouracil
Fu·a·din
Fuchs' coloboma
Fuchs' dimple
Fuchs' dystrophy
Fuchs' syndrome
fuch·sin
    acid f.
    aldehyde f.
    aniline f.
    basic f.
    diamond f.
    new f.
fuch·sin·o·phil
fuch·sin·o·phil·ia
fuch·sin·o·phil·ic
fuch·sin·oph·i·lous
fu·co·san
fu·cose
α-L-fu·co·si·dase
fu·co·side
fu·co·si·do·sis
fu·co·xan·thin
FUDR — 5-fluorouracil
    deoxyribonucleoside
fu·gac·i·ty
fu·gi·tive
Fu·gu
fugue
    epileptic f.
    psychogenic f.
fu·gu·ism
fu·gu·is·mus
fu·gu·tox·in
Fu·ka·la's operation
ful·gu·rant
ful·gu·rate

ful·gu·rat·ing
ful·gu·ra·tion
ful·gu·rize
fu·lig·i·nous
Fül·le·born's method
Ful·ler's operation
füll·kör·per
ful·mi·nant
ful·mi·nate
ful·mi·nat·ing
Ful·vi·cin
fu·ma·gil·lin
fu·ma·rase
fu·ma·rate
fu·ma·rate hy·dra·tase
fu·mar·ic acid
fu·mar·o·yl·ace·to·ac·e·tate
    hy·dro·lase
fu·mar·yl·ace·to·ac·e·tase
fu·mi·gant
fu·mi·ga·tion
Fum·i·ron
func·tio
    f. laesa
func·tion
    arousal f.
    Carnot's f.
    carnotic f.
    cumulative distribution f.
      (cdf)
    discriminant f.
    distribution f.
    ego f.
    frequency f.
    group f.
    isometric f.
    life table f.
    linear f.
    line-spread f.
    multiple logistic f.
    probability density f.
func·tion·al
func·ti·o·na·lis
func·tion·at·ing
fun·da
fun·dal
fun·da·ment
fun·da·men·tal

fun·dec·to·my
fun·di
fun·dic
fun·di·form
fun·do·plas·ty
fun·do·pli·ca·tion
Fun·du·lus
fun·dus *pl.* fun·di
   albinotic f.
   f. albipunctatus
   f. of bladder
   f. diabeticus
   f. of eye
   f. flavimaculatus
   f. of gallbladder
   gastric f.
   f. gastricus
   f. of internal acoustic
     meatus
   f. meatus acustici interni
   leopard f.
   f. oculi
   salt and pepper f.
   f. of stomach
   tessellated f.
   t. tigré
   tigroid f.
   f. tympani
   f. of urinary bladder
   f. uteri
   f. of vagina
   f. vaginae
   f. ventricularis
   f. ventriculi
   f. vesicae biliaris
   f. vesicae felleae
   f. vesicae urinariae
fun·du·scope
fun·dus·co·py
fun·du·sec·to·my
fun·gal
fun·gate
fun·gat·ing
fun·ge·mia
fun·gi
Fun·gi Im·per·fec·ti
fun·gi·ci·dal
fun·gi·cide

fun·gi·ci·din
fun·gi·form
fun·gi·my·cin
fun·gi·sta·sis
fun·gi·stat
fun·gi·stat·ic
fun·gi·ster·ol
fun·gi·tox·ic
fun·gi·tox·ic·i·ty
Fun·gi·zone
fun·goid
fun·gos·i·ty
fun·gous
fun·gu·ria
fun·gus *pl.* fun·gi
   beefsteak f.
   biphasic f.
   cerebral f.
   f. cerebri
   club f.
   cutaneous f.
   dimorphic f.
   foot f.
   imperfect f.
   mosaic f.
   mycelial f.
   perfect f.
   proper f.
   ray f.
   sac f.
   slime f.
   f. testis
   thread f.
   thrush f.
   true f.
   umbilical f.
fu·nic
fu·ni·cle
fu·nic·u·lar
fu·nic·u·late
fu·nic·u·li
fu·nic·u·li·tis
   endemic f.
   filarial f.
fu·nic·u·lo·ep·i·did·y·mi·tis
fu·nic·u·lo·pexy
fu·nic·u·lus *pl.* fu·nic·u·li
   f. amnii

fu·nic·u·lus *(continued)*
  f. anterior medullae spinalis
  anterior f. of spinal cord
  cuneate f.
  f. cuneatus [Burdachi]
  f. cuneatus lateralis
  dorsal f. of spinal cord
  f. dorsalis medullae spinalis
  hepatic f.
  hepatic f. of Rauber
  lateral f. of medulla oblongata
  f. lateralis medullae oblongatae
  f. lateralis medullae spinalis
  ligamentous f.
  funiculi medullae spinalis
  f. posterior medullae spinalis
  posterior f. of spinal cord
  f. of Rolando
  ventral f. of spinal cord
  f. separans
  f. spermaticus
  funiculi of spinal cord
  f. of spinal cord, anterior
  f. of spinal cord, lateral
  f. of spinal cord, posterior
  f. umbilicalis
  f. ventralis medullae spinalis
fu·ni·form
fu·nis
  f. brachii
  f. hippocratis
fun·nel
  accessory müllerian f.
  mitral f.
  muscular f.
  pial f.
  vascular f.
FUO — fever of undetermined origin
Fu·ra·cin
Fur·a·dan·tin

fu·ran, fu·rane
fu·ra·nose
fu·ra·no·side
fu·ra·zol·i·done
fur·a·zo·li·um
  f. chloride
  f. tartrate
fur·az·o·sin
Für·bring·er's sign
Für·bring·er's test
fur·ca *pl.* fur·cae
fur·cal
fur·ca·tion
fur·co·cer·cous
fur·cu·la
fur·fu·ra·ceous
fur·fu·ran
fur·fu·rol
fur·o·bu·fen
fu·ro·cou·ma·rin
fur·o·da·zole
fu·ror
  f. epilepticus
fu·ro·sem·ide
Fur·ox·one
fur·row
  atrioventricular f.
  digital f.
  division f.
  genital f.
  gluteal f.
  Jadelot's f's
  Liebermeister's f's
  mentolabial f.
  nympholabial f.
  primitive f.
  Schmorl's f.
  scleral f.
  Sibson's f.
  skin f's
fur·sa·lan
Fürst·ner's disease
Furth's tumor
fu·run·cle
fu·run·cu·lar
fu·run·cu·loid
fu·run·cu·lo·sis
  f. blastomycetica

fu·run·cu·lo·sis *(continued)*
   f. cryptococcica
fu·run·cu·lous
fu·run·cu·lus *pl.* fu·run·cu·li
fu·sa·rid·i·o·sis
fu·sar·io·tox·i·co·sis
Fu·sar·i·um
   F. oxysporum
   F. solanae
   F. sporotrichiella
fus·cin
fu·seau *pl.* fu·seaux
fu·si
fu·si·ble
fu·si·cel·lu·lar
fu·si·date
fu·si·dic acid
fu·si·form
fu·si·mo·tor
fu·sion
   binocular f.
   cell f.
   centric f.
   Cloward back f.
   diaphyseal-epiphyseal f.
   flicker f.
   f. of joint
   renal f.

fu·sion *(continued)*
   spinal f.
fu·sion·al
Fu·so·bac·te·ri·um
   F. fusiformis
   F. gonidiaformans
   F. mortiferum
   F. naviforme
   F. necrophorum
   F. nucleatum
   F. plauti-vincenti
   F. russii
   F. varium
fu·so·bac·te·ri·um *pl.* fu·so·bac·te·ria
fu·so·cel·lu·lar
fu·so·spi·ril·lary
fu·so·spi·ril·lo·sis
fu·so·spi·ro·che·tal
fu·so·spi·ro·che·to·sis
fus·ti·ga·tion
fu·sus *pl.* fu·si
   cortical fusi
   fracture fusi
   f. neuromuscularis
   f. neurotendineus
FVC — forced vital capacity

G

G — gauss
   giga-
   gravida
   guanine
   guanosine
G — conductance
   G force
   Gibbs free energy
   gravitational constant
g — gram

g — standard gravity
γ — the heavy chain of IgG
   the γ chains of fetal hemoglobin
   former symbol for microgram (now μg)
GABA — γ-aminobutyric acid
G-ac·tin
gad·fly
gad·o·le·ic acid

gad·o·lin·i·um
Ga·dus
    G. *morrhua*
Gaens·len's sign
Gaens·len's test
Gaff·ky scale
Gaff·ky table
GAG — glycosaminoglycan
gag
    Davis g.
    Davis-Crowe mouth g.
    Doyen g.
    incisor g.
    Mason g.
    McIvor g.
    molar g.
    mouth g.
Gail·lard-Arlt suture
gain
    antigen g.
    end g.
    epinosic g.
    near g.
    paranosic g.
    primary g.
    secondary g.
    swept g.
Gaird·ner's test
Gais·böck's disease
Gais·böck's syndrome
gait
    antalgic g.
    ataxic g.
    calcaneous g.
    cerebellar g.
    Charcot's g.
    cogwheel g.
    double step g.
    drag-to g.
    drop-foot g.
    drunken g.
    duck g.
    dystrophic g.
    equine g.
    festinating g.
    footdrop g.
    four-point g.

gait *(continued)*
    glue-footed g.
    gluteal g.
    gluteus maximus g.
    gluteus medius g.
    heel-toe g.
    helicopod g.
    hemiplegic g.
    hysterical g.
    intermittent double-step g.
    listing g.
    myopathic g.
    Oppenheim's g.
    paraparetic g.
    Petren g.
    reeling g.
    scissor g.
    skaters'g.
    spastic g.
    spastic equinus g.
    staggering g.
    stamping g.
    star g.
    steppage g.
    swaying g.
    swing-through g.
    swing-to g.
    tabetic g.
    tandem g.
    three-point g.
    Todd's g.
    Trendelenburg g.
    two-point g.
    waddling g.
gait and sta·tion
Gaj·du·sek, Daniel Carleton
ga·lac·ta·cra·sia
ga·lac·ta·gog·in
ga·lac·ta·gogue
ga·lac·tan
gal·ac·te·mia
ga·lac·tic
gal·ac·tis·chia
ga·lac·ti·tol
ga·lac·to·blast
ga·lac·to·bol·ic
ga·lac·to·cele
ga·lac·to·cer·e·bro·side

ga·lac·to·cer·e·bro·side β-ga·
  lac·to·si·dase
ga·lac·to·chlo·ral
ga·lac·to·cra·sia
ga·lac·to·gen
ga·lac·tog·e·nous
ga·lac·to·gogue
gal·ac·tog·ra·phy
ga·lac·to·ki·nase
ga·lac·to·lip·id
ga·lac·to·lip·in
gal·ac·to·ma
ga·lac·to·met·a·sta·sis
gal·ac·tom·e·ter
ga·lac·to·pex·ic
ga·lac·to·pexy
gal·ac·toph·a·gous
ga·lac·to·phle·bi·tis
gal·ac·toph·ly·sis
ga·lac·to·phore
ga·lac·to·pho·ri·tis
gal·ac·toph·o·rous
gal·ac·toph·y·gous
ga·lac·to·pla·nia
ga·lac·to·poi·e·sis
ga·lac·to·poi·et·ic
ga·lac·to·py·ra
ga·lac·to·py·ra·nose
ga·lac·tor·rhea
ga·lac·to·sa·mine
ga·lac·to·sa·mine-6-sul·fate
  sul·fa·tase
ga·lac·to·san
ga·lac·to·sa·zone
gal·ac·tos·che·sis
ga·lac·to·scope
ga·lac·tose
ga·lac·tose epim·er·ase
ga·lac·tos·emia
ga·lac·tose-1-phos·phate u·ri·
  dyl·trans·fer·ase
α-D-ga·lac·to·si·dase
    α-D-g. A
    α-D-g. B
β-ga·lac·to·si·dase
ga·lac·to·side
  g. acetylase
  g. permease

gal·ac·to·sis
ga·lac·to·sta·sia
gal·ac·tos·ta·sis
ga·lac·tos·uria
ga·lac·to·syl
ga·lac·to·syl·cer·am·i·dase
ga·lac·to·tox·in
ga·lac·to·tox·ism
gal·ac·tot·ro·phy
gal·ac·tox·ism
ga·lac·tox·is·mus
gal·ac·tu·ria
ga·lac·tu·ron·ic acid
Gal·ant's reflex
ga·lan·tha·mine hy·dro·bro·
  mide
ga·lea
    g. aponeurotica
Gal·e·a·ti's glands
gal·e·a·tus
Gal·e·az·zi's fracture
Gal·e·az·zi's sign
Ga·len
Ga·len's anastomosis
Ga·len's foramen
Ga·len's veins
Ga·len's ventricle
ga·len·ic
ga·len·i·ca
ga·len·i·cals
ga·len·ics
Gal·e·o·des ara·ne·oi·des
gal·er·o·pia
gal·er·op·sia
gall
    Aleppo g.
    ox g.
    Smyrna g.
Gall's craniology
gal·lac·e·to·phe·none
gal·la·mine tri·eth·io·dide
gal·late
gall·blad·der
    Courvoisier's g.
    fish-scale g.
    floating g.
    folded fundus g.
    hourglass g.

gall·blad·der *(continued)*
    mobile g.
    phrygian cap g.
    sandpaper g.
    stasis g.
    strawberry g.
    wandering g.
gal·le·in
gal·lic ac·id
Gal·lie transplant
Gal·li Mai·ni·ni test
gall·ing
gal·li·sin
gal·li·um
    g. 67
    g. 68
    g. Ga 67 citrate
gall·nut
gal·lo·cy·a·nin
gal·lop
    atrial g.
    S₃ g.
    summation g.
    systolic g.
    ventricular g.
gal·lo·tan·nic acid
gall·sick·ness
gall·stone
    silent g.
GalNAc — *N*-acetylgalactosam-
    ine
GALT — gut-associated
    lymphoid tissue
Gal·ton's law of regression
Galv. — galvanic
gal·van·ic
gal·va·nism
    dental g.
gal·va·ni·za·tion
gal·va·no·cau·tery
gal·va·no·chem·i·cal
gal·va·no·con·trac·til·i·ty
gal·va·no·gus·tom·e·ter
gal·va·nol·y·sis
gal·va·nom·e·ter
    Einthoven's g.
    string g.
    thread g.

gal·va·no·ner·vous
gal·va·no·pal·pa·tion
gal·va·no·sur·gery
gal·va·no·tax·is
gal·va·no·ther·a·peu·tics
gal·va·no·ther·a·py
gal·va·not·o·nus
gal·va·not·rop·ism
gal·ziek·te
gam·a·sid
Ga·mas·i·des
gam·a·soi·do·sis
Gam·a·stan
gam·bir
gam·ble·gram
gam·boge
Gam·bu·sia
    G. affinis
ga·me·far
gam·e·tan·gia
gam·e·tan·gi·um *pl.* gam·e·
    tan·gia
gam·ete
ga·met·ic
ga·me·to·ci·dal
ga·me·to·cide
ga·me·to·cyst
ga·me·to·cyte
ga·me·to·cy·te·mia
gam·e·to·gen·e·sis
gam·e·to·gen·ic
gam·e·tog·o·ny
gam·e·toid
gam·e·to·ki·net·ic
gam·e·to·pha·gia
gam·e·to·phyte
ga·me·to·trop·ic
Gam·gee tissue
gam·ic
gam·ma
gam·ma-ami·no·bu·tyr·ic acid
gam·ma ben·zene hex·a·chlo·
    ride
gam·ma·cism
Gam·ma·cor·tin
gam·ma-emit·ter
gam·ma glob·u·lin
gam·ma·glob·u·li·nop·a·thy

gam·ma glu·ta·myl trans·fer·
ase (GGT)
gam·ma·gram
gam·ma·graph·ic
gam·ma-lac·tone
gam·ma-pip·ra·dol
gam·mex·ane
gam·mog·ra·phy
　　cerebral g.
gam·mop·a·thy
　　benign monoclonal g.
　　biclonal g.
　　monoclonal g.
Gam·na's disease
Gam·na's nodules
Gam·na-Fav·re bodies
gamo·gen·e·sis
gamo·ge·net·ic
gam·og·o·ny
gam·one
gam·ont
gamo·pha·gia
Gam·per's reflex
gamp·so·dac·ty·ly
Gam·storp's disease
Gam·u·lin Rh
gan·ci·clo·vir
Gan·dy-Gam·na disease
Gan·dy-Gam·na nodules
Gan·dy-Gam·na spleen
Gan·dy-Nan·ta disease
gan·glia
gan·gli·al
gan·gli·at·ed
gan·gli·ec·to·my
gan·gli·form
gan·gli·itis
gan·glio·blast
gan·glio·cyte
gan·glio·cy·to·ma
gan·glio·form
gan·glio·gli·o·ma
gan·glio·glio·neu·ro·ma
gan·glio·lyt·ic
gan·gli·o·ma
gan·gli·on *pl.* gan·glia, gan·
　gli·ons
　　accessory ganglia

gan·gli·on *(continued)*
　acoustic g.
　acousticofacial g.
　Acrel's g.
　Andersch's g.
　aorticorenal g.
　ganglia aorticorenalia
　Arnold's g.
　auditory g.
　Auerbach's g.
　auricular g.
　autonomic ganglia
　ganglia autonomica
　ganglia of autonomic
　　plexuses
　azygous g.
　basal ganglia
　Bezold's g.
　Bidder's ganglia
　Blandin's g.
　Bochdalek's g.
　g. Bochdalekii
　Bock's g.
　Böttcher's (Boettcher's) g.
　cardiac ganglia
　ganglia cardiaca
　carotid g.
　celiac ganglia
　ganglia celiaca
　cephalic g.
　cerebrospinal ganglia
　cervical g., inferior
　cervical g., middle
　cervical g., superior
　cervical g. of uterus
　g. cervicale inferius
　g. cervicale medium
　g. cervicale superius
　cervicothoracic g.
　g. cervicothoracicum
　cervicouterine g.
　g. ciliare
　Cloquet's g.
　coccygeal g.
　cochlear g.
　g. cochleare
　g. coeliaca
　collateral ganglia

gan·gli·on *(continued)*
  compound g.
  Corti's g.
  craniospinal ganglia
  ganglia craniospinalia
  diaphragmatic g.
  diffuse g.
  dorsal root g.
  g. of duct of Botallo
  Ehrenritter's g.
  encephalospinal ganglia
  ganglia encephalospinalia
  g. extracraniale
  g. of facial nerve
  false g.
  Frankenhäuser's g.
  Froriep's g.
  ganglia of autonomic
    plexuses
  Ganser's g.
  Gasser's g.
  gasserian g.
  geniculate g.
  g. geniculatum nervi
    facialis
  g. of glossopharyngeal
    nerve
  g. of habenulae
  hepatic g.
  Huber's g.
  hypogastric g.
  hypoglossal g.
  g. impar
  inferior g. of
    glossopharyngeal nerve
  inferior thyroid g.
  g. inferius nervi
    glossopharyngei
  g. inferius nervi vagi
  inhibitory g.
  intercrural g.
  ganglia intermedia
  g. intermédiaire
  interpeduncular g.
  g. intervertebrale
  intracranial g.
  jugular g. of
    glossopharyngeal nerve

gan·gli·on *(continued)*
  jugular g. of vagus nerve
  g. jugulare nervi vagi
  Küttner's g.
  Langley's g.
  Laumonier's g.
  Lee's g.
  lesser g. of Meckel
  Lobstein's g.
  Loetwig's g.
  lower g. of
    glossopharyngeal nerve
  lower g. of vagus nerve
  Ludwig's g.
  ganglia lumbalia
  ganglia lumbaria
  Luschka's g.
  ganglia lymphatica
  Meckel's g.
  Meissner's g.
  mesenteric g., inferior
  mesenteric g., superior
  g. mesentericum inferius
  g. mesentericum superius
  g. of Müller
  nasal g.
  nerve g.
  g. nervi splanchnici
  neural g.
  nodose g.
  g. nodosum
  nonpermanent g.
  olfactory g.
  ophthalmic g.
  optic g.
  orbital g.
  otic g.
  g. oticum
  parasympathetic g.
  g. parasympatheticum
  g. parasympathicum
  paravertebral g.
  pelvic ganglia
  ganglia pelvina
  periosteal g.
  permanent g.
  petrosal g.
  petrous g.

gan·gli·on *(continued)*
  phrenic g.
  ganglia phrenica
  ganglia plexuum
    autonomicorum
  ganglia plexuum
    visceralium
  posterior root g.
  prevertebral ganglia
  primary g.
  prostatic g.
  pterygopalatine g.
  g. pterygopalatinum
  Remak's g.
  renal ganglia
  ganglia renalia
  g. retinae
  Ribes' g.
  g. rostralis nervi
    glossopharyngei
  g. rostralis nervi vagi
  sacral ganglia
  ganglia sacralia
  Scarpa's g.
  Schacher's g.
  Schmiedel's g.
  semilunar g.
  g. semilunare [Gasseri]
  g. sensoriale
  sensory g.
  simple g.
  sinoatrial g.
  sinus g.
  sphenomaxillary g.
  sphenopalatine g.
  g. sphenopalatinum
  spinal g.
  g. spinale
  spiral g.
  g. spirale cochleae
  splanchnic g.
  splanchnic g. of Arnold
  splanchnic thoracic g.
  g. splanchnicum
  stellate g.
  g. stellatum
  sublingual g.
  g. sublinguale

gan·gli·on *(continued)*
  submandibular g.
  g. submandibulare
  superior g. of
    glossopharyngeal nerve
  g. superius nervi
    glossopharyngei
  g. superius nervi vagi
  suprarenal g.
  sympathetic ganglia
  g. sympatheticum
  g. sympathicum
  synovial g.
  terminal g.
  g. terminale
  ganglia thoracalia
  thoracic ganglia
  ganglia thoracica
  trigeminal g.
  g. trigeminale
  g. of trigeminal nerve
  Troisier's g.
  ganglia trunci sympathici
  tympanic g.
  tympanic g. of Valentin
  g. tympanicum
  upper g.
  vagal g., inferior
  vagal g., superior
  g. of vagus nerve
  Valentin's g.
  ventricular g.
  vertebral g.
  g. vertebrale
  vestibular g.
  g. vestibulare
  vestibulocochlear g.
  ganglia visceralia
  Walther's g.
  Wrisberg's g.
  g. Wrisbergi
  wrist g.
gan·gli·on·ated
gan·gli·on·ec·to·my
gan·glio·neure
gan·glio·neu·ro·blas·to·ma
gan·glio·neu·ro·fi·bro·ma
  melanotic g.

gan·glio·neu·ro·ma
    dumbbell g.
    hourglass g.
gan·glio·neu·ro·ma·to·sis
gan·gli·on·ic
gan·gli·on·itis
    acute posterior g.
    gasserian g.
gan·gli·ono·pleg·ic
gan·gli·on·os·to·my
gan·glio·pleg·ic
gan·glio·side
    g. GM_1
    g. GM_2
gan·gli·o·si·do·sis *pl.* gan·gli·
  o·si·do·ses
    generalized g.
    GM_1 g.
    GM_1 g., adult
    GM_1 g., infantile
    GM_1 g., juvenile
    GM_2 g.
    GM_2 g., adult
    GM_2 g., juvenile
gan·glio·spore
gan·glio·sym·pa·thec·to·my
gan·glio·sym·pa·thet·i·co·
  blas·to·ma
Gan·glophe sign
gan·go·sa
gan·grene
    angiosclerotic g.
    chemical g.
    circumscribed g.
    cold g.
    cutaneous g.
    decubital g.
    diabetic g.
    disseminated cutaneous g.
    dry g.
    embolic g.
    emphysematous g.
    epidemic g.
    Fournier's g.
    gas g.
    glycemic g.
    hospital g.
    hot g.

gan·grene *(continued)*
    humid g.
    inflammatory g.
    ischemic g.
    Meleney's g.
    mephitic g.
    moist g.
    oral g.
    presenile spontaneous g.
    pressure g.
    primary g.
    progressive g.
    progressive bacterial
      synergistic g.
    progressive postoperative
      g.
    progressive synergistic g.
    pulp g.
    Raynaud's g.
    secondary g.
    senile g.
    static g.
    symmetric g.
    sympathetic g.
    thrombotic g.
    traumatic g.
    trophic g.
    venous g.
    wet g.
gan·gre·no·sis
gan·gre·nous
gan·ja
gan·o·blast
Gan·ser's commissure
Gan·ser's ganglion
Gan·ser's symptom
Gan·ser's syndrome
Gant's clamp
Gant's line
Gan·ta·nol
Gan·tri·sin
gan·try
gap
    air g.
    air-bone g.
    anion g.
    auscultatory g.
    Bochdalek's g.

gap *(continued)*
  chromatid g.
  interocclusal g.
  isochromatid g.
  silent g.
GAPD — glyceraldehyde-3-pho-
  sphate dehydrogenase
gapes
Ga·ra·my·cin
Gar·din·er-Brown's test
Gard·ner chair
Gard·ner's syndrome
Gard·ner·el·la
Ga·rel's sign
Garg. — L. gargarismus
  (gargle)
gar·gal·an·es·the·sia
gar·gal·es·the·sia
gar·gal·es·thet·ic
gar·gle
gar·goyl·ism
  X-linked recessive g.
Gar·land's curve
Gar·land's triangle
gar·ment
  elastic g.
  pneumatic antishock g.
gar·net
Gar·ré's disease
Gar·ré's osteitis
Gar·ré's osteomyelitis
gar·rot
Gärt·ner's bacillus
Gart·ner's canal
Gart·ner's cyst
Gart·ner's duct
Gärt·ner's phenomenon
Gärt·ner's tonometer
Gar·y·mi·cin
gas
  alveolar g.
  arterial blood g's (ABG)
  blood g.
  carrier g.
  choking g.
  coal g.
  ethyl g.
  expired g.

gas *(continued)*
  hemolytic g.
  inert g.
  lacrimator g.
  laughing g.
  marsh g.
  mustard g.
  nerve g.
  noble g.
  sewer g.
  sneezing g.
  suffocating g.
  sweet g.
  tear g.
  vesicating g.
  war g.
gas·e·ous
gas·i·form
Gas·kell's bridge
gas·o·gen·ic
gas·om·e·ter
gas·o·met·ric
gas·om·e·try
Gass scleral punch
Gas·ser, Herbert Spencer
Gas·ser's ganglion
Gas·ser's syndrome
gas·ser·ec·to·my
gas·se·ri·an
Gas·taut's disease
gas·ter
Gas·tero·my·ce·tes
Gas·ter·oph·i·lus
  G. intestinalis
gas·trad·e·ni·tis
gas·tral·gia
gas·tral·go·ke·no·sis
gas·tra·mine hy·dro·chlo·ride
gas·tra·tro·phia
gas·trec·to·my
  antecolic g.
  phsyiologic g.
gas·tric
gas·tric·sin
gas·trin
gas·tri·no·ma
gas·trit·ic

gas·tri·tis
  antral g.
  atrophic g.
  atrophic-hyperplastic g.
  catarrhal g.
  chemical g.
  chronic cystic g.
  chronic follicular g.
  cirrhotic g.
  corrosive g.
  eosinophilic g.
  erosive g.
  exfoliative g.
  follicular g.
  giant hypertrophic g.
  granulomatous g.
  hemorrhagic g.
  hypertrophic g.
  phlegmonous g.
  polypous g.
  pseudomembranous g.
  radiation g.
  superficial g.
  suppurative g.
  toxic g.
  uremic g.
  zonal g.
gas·tro·aceph·a·lus
gas·tro·ad·e·ni·tis
gas·tro·ady·nam·ic
gas·tro·amor·phus
gas·tro·anas·to·mo·sis
gas·tro·cam·era
gas·tro·car·di·ac
gas·tro·cele
gas·troc·ne·mi·us
gas·tro·coele
gas·tro·col·ic
gas·tro·co·li·tis
gas·tro·co·los·to·my
gas·tro·co·lot·o·my
gas·tro·cu·ta·ne·ous
gas·tro·di·a·phane
gas·tro·di·aph·a·nos·co·py
gas·tro·di·aph·a·ny
gas·tro·did·y·mus
gas·tro·dis·ci·a·sis
Gas·tro·dis·coi·des

Gas·tro·dis·coi·des
  G. hominis
gas·tro·disk
gas·tro·du·o·de·nal
gas·tro·du·o·de·nec·to·my
gas·tro·du·o·de·ni·tis
gas·tro·du·o·de·no·en·ter·os·
  to·my
gas·tro·du·o·de·nos·co·py
gas·tro·du·o·de·nos·to·my
gas·tro·dyn·ia
gas·tro·en·ter·al·gia
gas·tro·en·ter·ic
gas·tro·en·ter·i·tis
  acute infectious g.
  eosinophilic g.
  infantile g.
  Norwalk g.
gas·tro·en·tero·anas·to·mo·
  sis
gas·tro·en·tero·co·li·tis
gas·tro·en·tero·co·los·to·my
gas·tro·en·tero·log·ic
gas·tro·ent·er·ol·o·gist
gas·tro·en·ter·ol·o·gy
gas·tro·en·ter·op·a·thy
  allergic g.
gas·tro·en·tero·plas·ty
gas·tro·en·ter·op·to·sis
gas·tro·en·ter·os·to·my
  Billroth g.
  Hofmeister g.
  Roux's g.
  Roux-en-Y g.
gas·tro·en·ter·ot·o·my
gas·tro·ep·i·plo·ic
gas·tro·esoph·a·ge·al
gas·tro·esoph·a·gi·tis
gas·tro·esoph·a·go·plas·ty
gas·tro·esoph·a·gos·to·my
gas·tro·fi·ber·scope
gas·tro·gas·tros·to·my
gas·tro·ga·vage
gas·tro·gen·ic
Gas·tro·graf·in
gas·tro·graph
gas·tro·he·pat·ic
gas·tro·hep·a·ti·tis

gas·tro·hy·dror·rhea
gas·tro·hy·per·ton·ic
gas·tro·il·e·ac
gas·tro·il·e·itis
gas·tro·il·e·os·to·my
gas·tro·in·tes·ti·nal
gas·tro·je·ju·no·col·ic
gas·tro·je·ju·no·esoph·a·gos·
   to·my
gas·tro·je·ju·nos·to·my
   Roux-en-Y g.
gas·tro·ki·neso·graph
gas·tro·la·vage
gas·tro·li·e·nal
gas·tro·lith
gas·tro·li·thi·a·sis
gas·trol·o·gist
gas·trol·o·gy
gas·trol·y·sis
gas·tro·ma·la·cia
gas·tro·meg·a·ly
gas·trom·e·lus
gas·tro·me·nia
gas·tro·my·co·sis
gas·tro·my·ot·o·my
gas·tro·myx·or·rhea
gas·trone
gas·tro·nes·te·os·to·my
gas·tro-omen·tal
gas·trop·a·gus
   g. parasiticus
gas·tro·pan·cre·a·ti·tis
gas·tro·pa·ral·y·sis
gas·tro·pa·re·sis
gas·tro·pa·ri·e·tal
gas·tro·path·ic
gas·trop·a·thy
gas·tro·peri·odyn·ia
gas·tro·peri·to·ni·tis
gas·tro·pexy
   Hill posterior g.
gas·tro·phore
gas·tro·pho·tog·ra·phy
gas·tro·phren·ic
gas·tro·phthis·is
gas·tro·plas·ty
   Eckhout vertical g.
   Mason g.

gas·tro·plas·ty *(continued)*
   vertical banded g.
gas·tro·ple·gia
gas·tro·pli·ca·tion
gas·tro·pneu·mon·ic
gas·tro·pod
Gas·trop·o·da
gas·trop·to·sis
gas·trop·tyx·is
gas·tro·pul·mo·nary
gas·tro·py·lo·rec·to·my
gas·tro·py·lor·ic
gas·tro·ra·dic·u·li·tis
gas·tror·rha·gia
gas·tror·rha·phy
gas·tror·rhea
gas·tror·rhex·is
gas·tros·chi·sis
gas·tro·scope
   fiberoptic g.
gas·tro·scop·ic
gas·tros·co·py
gas·tro·se·lec·tive
gas·tro·sia
   g. fungosa
gas·tro·sis
gas·tro·spasm
gas·tro·splen·ic
gas·tro·stax·is
gas·tro·ste·no·sis
gas·tros·to·ga·vage
gas·tros·to·la·vage
gas·tros·to·ma
gas·tros·to·my
   Beck g.
   Depage-Janeway g.
   Glassman g.
   Stamm g.
   Witzel g.
gas·tro·suc·cor·rhea
   digestive g.
gas·tro·tho·ra·cop·a·gus
   g. dipygus
gas·tro·tome
gas·trot·o·my
gas·tro·to·nom·e·ter
gas·tro·to·nom·e·try
gas·tro·tox·in

Gas·tro·tricha
gas·tro·trop·ic
gas·tro·tym·pa·ni·tes
gas·tru·la
gas·tru·la·tion
Gatch bed
gate
gat·ing
gat·ism
gat·tine
Gau·cher's cells
Gau·cher's disease
Gau·cher's splenomegaly
gauge
    beta ray g.
    bite g.
    Boley g.
    catheter g.
    strain g.
    x-ray thickness g.
Gaul·the·ria
gaunt·let
gauss
gauss·i·an curve
Gau·vain's fluid
gauze
    absorbable g.
    absorbent g.
    antiseptic g.
    Iodoform g.
    petrolatum g.
    ribbon g.
    tullegras g.
    Xeroform g.
    zinc gelatin impregnated
ga·vage
Ga·vard's muscle
Gay's glands
Gay-Lus·sac's law
gaze
    conjugate g.
    disconjugate g.
GBG — glycine-rich β glycoprotein
GBGase — glycine-rich β glycoproteinase
GBM — glomerular basement membrane

GBq — gigabecquerel
GC — gas chromatography
g-cal. — gram calorie
GCS — Glasgow Coma Scale
GDP — guanosine diphosphate
gear
    cervical g.
    head g.
Ge·ast·er
Gee's disease
Gee-Her·ter disease
Gee-Her·ter-Heub·ner disease
Gee-Her·ter-Heub·ner syndrome
Gee-Thay·sen disease
Ge·gen·baur's cell
ge·gen·hal·ten
Gei·gel's reflex
Gei·ger counter
Gei·ger-Mül·ler counter
Gei·ger-Nut·tall law
Geiss·ler's tube
gel
    aluminum hydroxide g.
    aluminum hydroxide g., dried
    aluminum carbonate g., basic
    aluminum phosphate g.
    betamethasone benzoate g.
    corticotropin g.
    fluocinonide g.
    polyacrylamide g.
    silica g.
    sodium fluoride and orthophosphoric acid g.
    sodium fluoride and phosphoric acid g.
    tolnaftate g.
    tretinoin g.
Gel. quav. — L. gelatina quavis (in any kind of jelly)
ge·las·mus
ge·las·tic
gel·ate
ge·lat·i·fi·ca·tion
gel·a·tig·e·nous

gel·a·tin
  formalin g.
  glycerinated g.
  medicated g.
  silk g.
  g. of Wharton
  zinc g.
ge·lat·i·nase
gel·a·ti·nif·er·ous
ge·lat·i·nize
ge·lat·i·noid
gel·a·ti·no·lyt·ic
ge·lat·i·no·sa
ge·lat·i·nous
ge·la·tion
Gel·film
Gel·foam
gel·i·du·si
Gé·li·neau's syndrome
Gel·lé's test
gel·om·e·ter
gel·ose
ge·lo·sis *pl.* ge·lo·ses
gelo·trip·sy
gel·se·mine
gel·sem·ism
Gel·tabs
Gé·ly's suture
ge·mäs·te·te
gem·ca·di·ol
Ge·mel·la
  G. haemolysans
gem·el·lary
gem·el·lip·a·ra
gem·el·lol·o·gy
gem·fib·ro·zil
gem·i·nate
gem·i·na·tion
  false g.
gem·i·ni
gem·i·nous
gem·i·nus *pl.* gem·i·ni
  gemini aequales
ge·mis·to·cyte
ge·mis·to·cyt·ic
ge·mis·to·cy·to·ma
gem·ma
gem·man·gi·o·ma

gem·ma·tion
Gem·min·ges
gem·mule
Gem·o·nil
ge·na
ge·nal
gen·der
gene
  allelic g's
  amorphic g.
  antimutator g.
  autosomal g.
  cell interaction (CI) g's
  CI g's
  codominant g's
  complementary g's
  g. complex
  cumulative g's
  cytoplasmic g.
  derepressed g.
  dominant g.
  H g.
  histocompatibility g.
  hemizygous g.
  holandric g's
  hologynic g's
  homeotic g.
  immune response (Ir) g's
  immune suppressor (Is) g's
  immunoglobulin g's
  Ir g's
  Is g's
  leaky g.
  lethal g.
  major g.
  marker g.
  mimic g.
  modifying g.
  mutant g.
  mutator g.
  nonstructural g's
  operator g.
  pleiotropic g.
  recessive g.
  reciprocal g's
  regulator g.
  regulatory g.
  repressed g.

gene *(continued)*
  repressor g.
  resistance g.
  sex-conditioned g.
  sex-influenced g.
  sex-limited g.
  sex-linked g.
  silent g.
  split g.
  structural g.
  sublethal g.
  supplementary g's
  suppressor g.
  switch g.
  syntenic g's
  transposable g.
  uninducible g.
  wild-type g.
  X-linked g.
  Y-linked g.
gen·e·og·e·nous
gen·era
gen·er·al
gen·er·al·iza·tion
  stimulus g.
gen·er·al·ize
gen·er·a·tion
  alternate g.
  asexual g.
  direct g.
  filial g., first
  filial g., second
  nonsexual g.
  parental g.
  sexual g.
  spontaneous g.
gen·er·a·tive
gen·er·a·tor
  asynchronous pulse g.
  atrial synchronous pulse g.
  demand pulse g.
  fixed-rate pulse g.
  pattern g.
  pulse g.
  radionuclide g.
  standby pulse g.
  supervoltage g.

gen·er·a·tor *(continued)*
  ventricular inhibited pulse
    g.
  ventricular triggered pulse
    g.
ge·ner·ic
ge·ne·si·al
ge·nes·ic
ge·ne·si·ol·o·gy
gen·e·sis
gen·e·sis·ta·sis
gene-splic·ing
gen·e·sta·tic
ge·net·ic
ge·net·i·cist
ge·net·ics
  bacterial g.
  behavioral g.
  biochemical g.
  clinical g.
  developmental g.
  human g.
  mathematical g.
  medical g.
  microbial g.
  molecular g.
  population g.
  reverse g.
  statistical g.
ge·neto·troph·ic
gen·e·tous
Ge·ne·va Con·ven·tion
Gen·gou phenomenon
ge·ni·al
ge·ni·an
gen·ic
ge·nic·u·la
ge·nic·u·lar
ge·nic·u·late
ge·nic·u·lo·cal·ca·rine
ge·nic·u·lo·tem·po·ral
ge·nic·u·lum *pl.* ge·nic·u·la
  g. canalis facialis
  g. of facial nerve
  g. nervi facialis
gen·in
ge·nio·chei·lo·plas·ty
ge·nio·glos·sus

ge·nio·hyo·glos·sus
ge·nio·hy·oid
ge·nio·hy·oi·de·us
ge·nio·plas·ty
gen·i·tal
gen·i·ta·lia
    external g.
    indifferent g.
    internal g.
gen·i·tal·oid
gen·i·to·cru·ral
gen·i·to·fem·o·ral
gen·i·tog·ra·phy
gen·i·to·in·fec·tious
gen·i·to·plas·ty
gen·i·to·uri·nary
ge·nius
Gen·na·ri's band
Gen·na·ri's line
Gen·na·ri's stria
Gen·na·ri's stripe
geno·blast
geno·copy
geno·der·ma·tol·o·gy
geno·der·ma·to·sis
ge·nome
ge·nom·ic
geno·tox·ic
geno·type
geno·typ·ic
gen·ta·mi·cin
    g. sulfate
gen·ta·my·cin
gen·tian
    g. violet
gen·tian·o·phil
gen·tian·o·phil·ic
gen·tian·oph·i·lous
gen·tian·o·pho·bic
gen·tian·oph·o·bous
gen·tian·ose
gen·tia·vern
gen·tio·pic·rin
gen·ti·sate
gen·tis·ic acid
Gen·tran
gen·tro·gen·in

genitorectal

ge·nu *pl.* ge·nua
    g. capsulae internae
    g. corporis callosi
    g. extrorsum
    g. of facial canal
    g. of facial nerve
    g. impressum
    g. of internal capsule
    g. [internum] radicis nervi
      facialis
    g. introrsum
    g. nervi facialis
    g. recurvatum
    g. valgum
    g. varum
gen·ua
gen·u·al
genu·cu·bi·tal
genu·fa·cial
genu·pec·to·ral
ge·nus *pl.* gen·era
geo·bi·ol·o·gy
geo·chem·is·try
geo·cil·lin
ge·ode
ge·o·gen
geo·med·i·cine
geo·pa·thol·o·gy
Ge·o·pen
geo·pha·gia
ge·oph·a·gism
ge·oph·a·gy
geo·phil·ic
geo·tac·tic
geo·tax·is
geo·tri·cho·sis
Ge·ot·ri·chum
ge·o·trop·ic
ge·ot·ro·pism
ge·ra·ni·ol
ge·ra·nyl py·ro·phos·phate
ge·rat·ic
ger·a·tol·o·gy
ger·bil
Ger·dy's fibers
Ger·dy's fontanelle
Ger·dy's fossa

Ger·dy's ligament
Ger·dy's loop
ger·e·ol·o·gy
Ger·hardt's disease
Ger·hardt's phenomenon
Ger·hardt's reaction
Ger·hardt's sign
Ger·hardt's test
Ger·hardt-Se·mon law
ger·i·at·ric
ger·i·atri·cian
ger·i·at·rics
    dental g.
geri·odon·tics
geri·odon·tist
ger·io·psy·cho·sis
Ger·lach's network
Ger·lach's valve
Ger·lier's disease
germ
    dental g.
    enamel g.
    hair g.
    tooth g.
    wheat g.
ger·ma·nin
ger·ma·ni·um
ger·mer·ine
germ-free
ger·mi·ci·dal
ger·mi·cide
ger·mi·nal
ger·mi·na·tion
ger·mi·na·tive
ger·mi·no·blast
ger·mi·no·cyte
ger·mi·no·ma
    pineal g.
ger·mi·trine
germ·line, germ line
ger·o·der·ma
    g. osteodysplastica
ger·odon·tia
ger·odon·tic
ger·odon·tics
ger·odon·tist
ger·odon·tol·o·gy
gero·ma·ras·mus

gero·mor·phism
    cutaneous g.
ger·on·tal
ge·ron·tin
ger·on·tol·o·gist
ger·on·tol·o·gy
ger·on·to·phil·ia
ger·on·to·pia
ger·on·to·ther·a·peu·tics
ger·on·to·ther·a·py
ger·on·to·tox·on, ger·on·tox·on
    g. lentis
gero·psy·chi·a·try
Ge·ro·ta's capsule
Ge·ro·ta's method
Ger·son diet
Ger·son-Herr·manns·dorf·er diet
Gerst·mann's syndrome
ge·rüst·mark
Ge·sell developmental schedule
ges·ta·clone
ges·ta·gen
ge·stalt
    Bender g. test
ge·stal·tism
ges·ta·tion
    abdominal g.
    exterior g.
    interior g.
ges·ta·tion·al
ges·to·dene
ges·to·sis *pl.* ges·to·ses
ges·tri·none
GeV — giga electron volt
Gev — giga electron volt
GFAP — glial fibrillary acidic protein
GFR — glomerular filtration rate
GGT — γ-glutamyltransferase
GH — growth hormone
GH-IH — growth hormone inhibiting hormone
Ghi·lar·duc·ci's reaction
Ghon's complex

Ghon's focus
Ghon's primary lesion
Ghon's tubercle
Ghon-Sachs bacillus
ghost
      erythrocyte g.
      red cell g.
GH-RH — growth hormone
   releasing hormone
GH-RIH — growth hormone
   release inhibiting hormone
GHz — gigahertz
GI — gastrointestinal
Gia·co·mi·ni's band
Gia·nel·li's sign
Gian·nuz·zi's bodies
Gian·nuz·zi's cells
Gian·nuz·zi's crescents
Gian·nuz·zi's demilune
Gia·not·ti-Cros·ti syndrome
gi·ant
gi·ant·ism
Gi·ar·dia
      G. lamblia
gi·ar·di·a·sis
Gib·bon-Lan·dis test
gib·bos·i·ty
gib·bous
Gibbs' free energy theory
Gibbs-Don·nan equilibrium
gib·bus
Gib·ert's disease
Gib·ert's pityriasis
Gib·ney's bandage
Gib·ney's disease
Gib·ney's perispondylitis
Gib·ney's strapping
Gib·son's murmur
Gib·son's rule
gid·di·ness
Giem·sa stain
Giem·sa-Wright stain
Gier·ke's corpuscles
Gier·ke's disease
Gif·ford's operation
Gif·ford's reflex
Gif·ford's sign
Gif·ford-Ga·las·si reflex

giga·bec·que·rel (GBq)
giga·hertz (GHz)
gi·gan·tism
      acromegalic g.
      cerebral g.
      constitutional g.
      digital g.
      eunuchoid g.
      fetal g.
      hyperpituitary g.
      hypothalamic g.
      normal g.
      pituitary g.
Gi·gan·to·bil·har·zia
gi·gan·to·mas·tia
gi·gan·to·so·ma
Gi·gli's operation
Gi·gli's wire saw
gi·ki·yami
gil·bert
Gil·bert's cholemia
Gil·bert's disease
Gil·bert's sign
Gil·bert's syndrome
Gil·bert-Behçet syndrome
Gil·christ's disease
Gil·christ's mycosis
gil·da·ble
Gill's operation
Gilles de la Tou·rette's disease
Gilles de la Tou·rette's
   syndrome
Gil·li·am's operation
Gil·lies' flap
Gil·lies' operation
Gil·mer's splint
Gim·ber·nat's ligament
Gim·ber·nat's reflex ligament
gin·ger
gin·gi·va *pl.* gin·gi·vae
      alveolar g.
      areolar g.
      attached g.
      buccal g.
      cemental g.
      cleft g.
      free g.
      interdental g.

gin·gi·va *(continued)*
  interproximal g.
  labial g.
  lingual g.
  marginal g.
  papillary g.
  septal g.
  unattached g.
gin·gi·vae
gin·gi·val
gin·gi·val·gia
gin·gi·val·ly
gin·gi·vec·to·my
gin·gi·vi·tis
  acute necrotizing
    ulcerative g. (ANUG)
  acute ulcerative g.
  acute ulceromembranous g.
  atrophic senile g.
  bismuth g.
  catarrhal g.
  cotton-roll g.
  desquamative g.
  Dilantin g.
  diphenylhydantoin g.
  eruptive g.
  fusospirochetal g.
  g. gravidarum
  hemorrhagic g.
  herpetic g.
  hormonal g.
  hyperplastic g.
  marginal g.
  marginal g., generalized
  marginal g., simple
  g. marginalis suppurativa
  necrotizing ulcerative g.
  papillary g.
  phagedenic g.
  pregnancy g.
  puberty g.
  scorbutic g.
  streptococcal g.
  suppurative marginal g.
  tuberculous g.
  ulceromembranous g.
  Vincent's g.
gin·gi·vo·buc·co·ax·i·al

gin·gi·vo·glos·si·tis
gin·gi·vo·la·bi·al
gin·gi·vo·lin·guo·ax·i·al
gin·gi·vo·peri·odon·ti·tis
  necrotizing ulcerative g.
gin·gi·vo·plas·ty
gin·gi·vo·sis
gin·gi·vo·sto·ma·ti·tis
  herpetic g.
  necrotizing ulcerative g.
  white folded g.
gin·gi·vo·sto·ma·to·sis
  white folded g.
gin·gly·form
gin·gly·mo·ar·thro·di·al
gin·gly·moid
gin·gly·mus
  helicoid g.
  lateral g.
gin·seng
Gior·da·no's sphincter
GIP — gastric inhibitory
  polypeptide
Gi·ral·dés' organ
Gir·ard's method
Gir·ard's treatment
gir·dle
  hip g.
  Hitzig's g.
  limbus g.
  Neptune's g.
  pectoral g.
  pelvic g.
  shoulder g.
  thoracic g.
  upper limb g.
  white limbal g. of Vogt
Gir·dle·stone operation
Gir·dle·stone resection
Gird·ner's electric probe
gi·tal·i·gen·in
Gi·tal·i·gin
git·a·lin
git·a·lox·in
gith·a·gism
git·og·e·nin
git·o·nin
gi·tox·i·gen·in

gi·tox·in
Git·ter·fas·ern
Giuf·fri·da-Rug·gi·eri stigma
Giv·ens' method
Gjess·ing syndrome
GL — greatest length (an axis
   of measurement or
   dimension used for small
   flexed embryos)
gl. — L. glandula (gland)
gla·bel·la
gla·bel·lad
gla·bel·lum
gla·brous
gla·cial
gla·di·ate
glad·i·o·lic acid
gla·di·o·lus
gla·dio·ma·nu·bri·al
glair·in
glairy
gland
      absorbent g.
      accessory g.
      acid g's
      acinar g.
      acinotubular g.
      acinous g.
      admaxillary g.
      adrenal g.
      adrenal g's, accessory
      aggregate g's
      agminated g's
      Albarrán's g.
      albuminous g.
      alveolar g.
      anal g's
      anteprostatic g.
      apical g's of tongue
      apocrine g.
      aporic g.
      areolar g's
      arterial g.
      arteriococcygeal g.
      arytenoid g's
      Aselli's g's
      axillary g's
      Bartholin's g.

gland (continued)
      Bauhin's g's
      Baumgarten's g's
      g's of biliary mucosa
      Blandin's g's
      Blandin and Nuhn's g's
      blood g's
      blood vessel g's
      Boerhaave's g's
      Bonnot's g.
      Bowman's g's
      brachial g's
      bronchial g's
      Bruch's g's
      Brunner's g's
      buccal g's
      bulbocavernous g.
      bulbourethral g.
      BUS (Bartholin's, urethral,
         and Skene's) g's
      cardiac g's
      carotid g.
      g's of the caruncle
      celiac g's
      ceruminous g's
      cervical g's of uterus
      cheek g's
      Ciaccio's g's
      ciliary g's
      circumanal g's
      Cloquet's g.
      closed g's
      Cobelli's g's
      coccygeal g.
      coil g.
      compound g.
      conglobate g.
      conjunctival g's
      convoluted g.
      Cowper's g.
      cutaneous g's
      cytogenic g.
      ductless g.
      duodenal g's
      Duverney's g.
      Ebner's g's
      eccrine g.
      Eglis' g's

gland (continued)

endocrine g's
endoepithelial g.
endometrial g's
epithelial g.
esophageal g's
excretory g.
exocrine g.
follicular g's of tongue
Fraenkel's g's
fundic g's
fundus g's
Galeati's g's
gastric g's
gastroepiploic g's
Gay's g's
genal g's
genital g.
gingival g's
Gley's g's
globate g.
glomerate g's
glomiform g.
glossopalatine g's
Guérin's g's
gustatory g's
guttural g.
g's of Haller
Harder's g's
harderian g's
haversian g's
hedonic g's
hemal g's
hemal lymph g's
hemolymph g's
Henle's g's
hepatic g's
heterocrine g's
hibernating g.
holocrine g.
Home's g.
incretory g's
inguinal g.
intercarotid g.
intermediate g's
interscapular g.
interstitial g.
intestinal g's

gland (continued)

intraepithelial g.
intramuscular g's of tongue
jugular g.
Kölliker's g.
Krause's g's
labial g's of mouth
lacrimal g.
lacrimal g's, accessory
lactiferous g.
g's of large intestine
large sweat g.
laryngeal g's
lateral nasal g. of Stensen
lenticular g's of stomach
lenticular g's of tongue
g's of Lieberkühn
lingual g's
Littre's g's
Luschka's g.
lymph g.
lymphatic g.
lymph g's, extraparotid
malar g's
malpighian g's
mammary g.
mammary g's, accessory
mandibular g.
master g.
Mehlis' g.
meibomian g's
merocrine g.
mesenteric g's
mesocolic g's
metrial g.
mixed g's
molar g's
Moll's g's
monoptychic g.
Montgomery's g's
Morgagni's g's
g's of mouth
mucilaginous g's
muciparous g.
mucous g.
multicellular g.
myometrial g.
Naboth's g's

gland *(continued)*

nabothian g's
nasal g's
g. of neck
Nuhn's g's
odoriferous g's of prepuce
oil g's
olfactory g's
oxyntic g's
palatine g's
palpebral g's
pancreaticosplenic g's
parafrenal g's
parathyroid g's
paraurethral g's
parotid g.
parotid g., accessory
pectoral g's
peptic g's
Peyer's g's
pharyngeal g's
Philip's g's
pineal g.
pituitary g.
Poirier's g's
polyptychic g.
pregnancy g's
prehyoid g's
preputial g's
prostate g.
pyloric g's
racemose g's
retrolingual g.
retromolar g's
Rivinus g.
Rosenmüller's g.
saccular g.
salivary g's
Sandström's g's
Schüller's g's
sebaceous g's
seminal g.
sentinel g.
seromucous g.
serous g.
Serres' g's
sexual g.
g's of Shambaugh

gland *(continued)*

Sigmund's g's
simple g.
Skene's g's
solitary g's
splenoid g.
splenolymph g.
Stahr's g.
staphyline g's
subauricular g's
sublingual g.
submandibular g.
submaxillary g.
subtrigonal g.
sudoriferous g's
sudoriparous g's
suprahyoid accessory
    thyroid g.
suprarenal g.
Suzanne's g.
sweat g's
synovial g's
target g.
tarsal g's
tarsoconjunctival g's
Theile's g's
thymus g.
thyroid g.
thyroid g's, accessory
Tiedemann's g.
g's of tongue
tracheal g's
trachoma g's
tubular g.
tubuloacinar g.
tympanic g's
g's of Tyson
ultimobranchial g's
unicellular g.
urethral g's
uropygial g.
uterine g's
utricular g's
vaginal g.
vascular g.
vesical g's
vestibular g., greater
vestibular g's, lesser

gland *(continued)*
    Virchow's g.
    vitelline g.
    vulvovaginal g.
    Waldeyer's g's
    Wasmann's g.
    Weber's g's
    Wepfer's g's
    Willis g.
    g's of Wolfring
    g's of Zeis
    Zuckerkandl's g.
glan·der·ous
glan·ders
glan·des
glan·di·lem·ma
glan·du·la *pl.* glan·du·lae
    g. adrenalis
    glandulae areolares
    g. arytenoidea
    g. atrabiliaris
    g. basilaris
    glandulae bronchiales
    glandulae buccales
    g. bulbourethralis
    g. cardiaca esophagi
    g. cardiaca gastrica
    glandulae ceruminosae
    glandulae cervicales uteri
    glandulae ciliares
    glandulae circumanales
    glandulae conjunctivales
    glandulae cutis
    glandulae duodenales
    glandulae endocrinae
    g. epiglottica
    glandulae esophageae
    glandulae gastricae
      [propriae]
    g. glomiformis
    g. gustatoria
    glandulae hepaticae
    g. incisiva
    g. intercarotica
    glandulae intestinales
    glandulae labiales oris
    g. lacrimalis
    glandulae laryngeae

glan·du·la *(continued)*
    glandulae linguales
    g. mammaria
    glandulae molares
    g. mucosa
    glandulae nasales
    glandulae oesophageae
    glandulae olfactoriae
    glandulae oris
    glandulae palatinae
    glandulae parathyroideae
    g. parotidea
    glandulae pharyngeae
    glandulae pharyngeales
    g. pinealis
    g. pituitaria
    glandulae preputiales
    g. prostata
    g. prostatica
    glandulae pyloricae
    g. sacculi laryngis
    glandulae salivariae
      majores
    glandulae salivariae
      minores
    glandulae sebaceae
    g. seminalis
    g. seromucosa
    g. serosa
    glandulae sine ductibus
    g. sublingualis
    g. submandibularis
    glandulae sudoriferae
    g. suprarenalis
    glandulae tarsales
    g. thyroidea
    glandulae tracheales
    g. trigoni vesicae
    glandulae tubariae
    g. tympanicae
    glandulae urethrales
      [Littrei]
    g. uropygialis
    glandulae uterinae
    g. ventriculi laryngis
    g. vestibularis major
    glandulae vestibulares
      minores

glan·du·lae
glan·du·lar
glan·dule
glan·du·lous
glans *pl.* glan·des
 g. clitoridis
 g. penis
glan·u·lar
Glanz·mann's disease
Glanz·mann's thrombasthenia
glare
 direct g.
 indirect g.
glar·om·e·ter
gla·se·ri·an fissure
Glas·gow Coma Scale
Glas·gow's sign
glass
 cover g.
 crown g.
 cupping g.
 flint g.
 lithium g.
 object g.
 optical g.
 quartz g.
 test g.
 Wood's g.
glass·es
 bifocal g.
 contact g.
 crutch g.
 Frenzel g.
 Hallauer's g.
 hyperbolic g.
 safety g.
 trifocal g.
glassy
Glau·ber's salt
glau·co·ma
 absolute g.
 acute congestive g.
 air-block g.
 angle-closure g.
 angle-recession g.
 aphakic g.
 apoplectic g.
 auricular g.

glau·co·ma *(continued)*
 capsular g.
 g. capsulare
 chronic narrow-angle g.
 chymotrypsin-induced g.
 closed-angle g.
 congenital g.
 congestive g.
 g. consummatum
 contusion g.
 Donders'g.
 enzyme g.
 ghost cell g.
 hemolytic g.
 hemorrhagic g.
 incompensated g.
 infantile g.
 inflammatory g.
 inverse g.
 juvenile g.
 lenticular g.
 low-tension g.
 malignant g.
 melanomalytic g.
 narrow-angle g.
 neovascular g.
 noncongestive g.
 obstructive g.
 open-angle g.
 phacogenic g.
 phacolytic g.
 pigmentary g.
 postinflammatory g.
 primary g.
 prodromal g.
 pseudoexfoliative capsular
  g.
 pupillary block g.
 secondary g.
 simple g.
 steroid g.
 traumatic g.
 vitreous-block g.
 wide-angle g.
glau·co·ma·tous
glau·com·fleck·en
glau·co·sis
glau·co·sur·ia

glau·kom·fleck·en
glaze
GLC — gas-liquid
  chromatography
GlcNAc — N-acetylglucos-
  amine
Glea·son score
Glé·nard's disease
Glenn operation
Glenn procedure
Glenn shunt
gle·no·hu·mer·al
gle·noid
Gley's cells
Gley's glands
GLI — glucagon-like
  immunoreactivity
glia
    ameboid g.
    cytoplasmic g.
    g. of Fañana
    fibrillary g.
glia·cyte
gli·a·din
gli·al
gli·am·i·lide
gli·a·rase
gli·ben·cla·mide
gli·born·ur·ide
gli·cen·tin
gli·cet·a·nile so·di·um
glide
    mandibular g.
    occlusal g.
gli·flu·mide
glio·bac·te·ria
glio·blast
glio·blas·to·ma
    giant cell g.
    magnocellular g.
    g. multiforme
glio·coc·cus
glio·cyte
    retinal g's
glio·cy·to·ma
glio·fi·bril·lary
glio·fi·bro·sar·co·ma
gli·og·e·nous

gli·o·ma
    astrocytic g.
    g. endophytum
    ependymal g.
    g. exophytum
    extramedullary g.
    ganglionic g.
    heterotopic g.
    malignant peripheral g.
    mixed g.
    nasal g.
    optic g.
    peripheral g.
    g. retinae
    g. sarcomatosum
    telangiectatic g.
gli·o·ma·to·sis
    g. cerebri
gli·o·ma·tous
glio·neu·ro·ma
glio·pha·gia
glio·pil
glio·sar·co·ma
    g. retinae
gli·o·sis
    basilar g.
    cerebellar g.
    diffuse g.
    g. endometrii
    hemispheric g.
    hypertrophic nodular g.
    isomorphic g.
    lobar g.
    perivascular g.
    progressive subcortical g.
    spinal g.
    unilateral g.
    g. uteri
glio·some
glio·tox·in
glip·i·zide
glis·chrin
glis·chru·ria
glis·sade
glis·sad·ic
Glis·son's capsule
Glis·son's disease

Glis·son's sling
glis·so·ni·tis
glo·bal
globe·fish
glo·bi
glo·bid·i·o·sis
glo·bin
glo·bi·nom·e·ter
glo·boid
glo·bose
glob·o·side
glob·u·lar
Glob·u·lar·ia
glob·u·lar·i·a·cit·rin
glob·ule
    dentin g's
    Dobie's g.
    Marchi's g's
    milk g's
    Morgagni's g's
    myelin g's
    polar g's
glob·u·li
glob·u·lin
    AC g.
    accelerator g.
    alpha g's
    antihemophilic g. (AHG)
    anti–human g. serum
    antilymphocyte g. (ALG)
    antithymocyte g. (ATG)
    Bence Jones g.
    beta g's
    corticosteroid-binding g.
    cortisol-binding g.
    D antigen immune g.
    gamma g's
    hepatitis B immune g.
    human gamma g.
    immune g.
    immune human serum g.
    measles immune g.
    pertussis immune g.
    rabies immune g.
    $Rh_0(D)$ immune g.
    testosterone-estradiol–binding g. (TEBG)
    tetanus immune g.

glob·u·lin *(continued)*
    thyroxine-binding g.
    vaccinia immune g. (VIG)
    varicella-zoster immune g. (VZIG)
    vitamin D-binding g.
    g. X
    zoster immune g. (ZIG)
glob·u·lin·uria
glob·u·lose
glob·u·lus *pl.* glob·u·li
    globuli ossei
glo·bus *pl.* glo·bi
    g. abdominalis
    g. of the heel
    g. hystericus
    g. major epididymidis
    g. minor epididymidis
    g. pallidus
glo·man·gi·o·ma
glo·man·gi·o·sis
    pulmonary g.
glo·mec·to·my
glom·era
glom·er·ate
glo·mer·u·lar
glo·mer·u·li
glo·mer·u·li·tis
    focal g.
    segmental g.
glo·mer·u·lo·ne·phri·tis
    acute g.
    chronic hypocomplementemic g.
    crescentic g.
    diffuse g.
    diffuse lupus g.
    diffuse proliferative g.
    extracapillary g.
    focal g.
    focal embolic g.
    focal necrotizing g.
    focal proliferative g.
    focal sclerosing g.
    IgA g.
    immune complex g.
    lobular g.
    lobulonodular g.

glo·mer·u·lo·ne·phri·tis
  (*continued*)
    lupus g.
    malignant g.
    membranoproliferative g.
    membranous g.
    mesangial IgA/IgG g.
    mesangiocapillary g.
    nodular g.
    rapidly progressive g.
    segmental g.
    subacute g.
glo·mer·u·lo·ne·phrop·a·thy
glo·mer·u·lop·a·thy
    diabetic g.
    membranous g.
    minimum change g.
glo·mer·u·lo·scle·ro·sis
    congenital g.
    diabetic g.
    diffuse g.
    focal segmental g.
    intercapillary g.
    nodular g.
glo·mer·u·lose
glo·mer·u·lo·tro·pin
glo·mer·u·lus *pl.* glo·mer·u·li
    glomeruli arteriosi
      cochleae
    caudal arterial g.
    glomeruli of kidney
    malpighian glomeruli
    g. of mesonephros
    nonencapsulated nerve g.
    olfactory g.
    g. of pronephros
    renal glomeruli
    glomeruli renis
    Ruysch's glomeruli
glo·mic
glo·moid
glo·mus *pl.* glo·me·ra
    glomera aortica
    g. caroticum
    carotid g.
    choroid g.
    g. choroideum
    coccygeal g.

glo·mus (*continued*)
    g. coccygeum
    digital g.
    g. intravagale
    jugular g.
    g. jugulare
    neuromyoarterial g.
glos·sa
glos·sa·gra
glos·sal
glos·sal·gia
glos·san·thrax
glos·sec·to·my
Glos·si·na
    G. fuscipes
    G. morsitans
    G. pallidipes
    G. palpalis
    G. swynnertoni
    G. tachinoides
glos·si·tis
    g. areata exfoliativa
    atrophic g.
    benign migratory g.
    chronic superficial g.
    Clarke-Fournier g.
    cortical superficial sclerotic
      g.
    exfoliative g.
    Fournier's g.
    gummatous g.
    Hunter's g.
    idiopathic g.
    interstitial sclerous g.
    median rhomboid g.
    g. migrans
    Moeller's g.
    monilial g.
    g. rhomboidea mediana
    syphilitic g.
    ulceromembranous g.
glos·so·cele
glos·so·cin·es·thet·ic
glos·soc·o·ma
glos·so·des·mus
glos·so·dy·na·mom·e·ter
glos·so·dyn·ia
    g. exfoliativa

glos·so·dyn·ia *(continued)*
    psychogenic g.
glos·so·epi·glot·tic
glos·so·epi·glot·tid·e·an
glos·so·graph
glos·so·hy·al
glos·so·hy·oid·al
glos·so·kin·es·thet·ic
glos·so·la·lia
glos·sol·o·gy
glos·sol·y·sis
glos·so·man·tia
glos·son·cus
glos·so·pal·a·ti·nus
glos·sop·a·thy
glos·so·pexy
glos·so·pha·ryn·ge·al
glos·so·pha·ryn·ge·um
glos·so·pha·ryn·ge·us
glos·so·pho·bia
glos·so·phyt·ia
glos·so·plas·ty
glos·so·ple·gia
glos·sop·to·sis
glos·so·py·ro·sis
glos·sor·rha·phy
glos·sos·co·py
glos·so·spasm
glos·so·ster·e·sis
glos·so·tilt
glos·sot·o·my
glos·so·trich·ia
glot·tal
glot·tic
glot·tis *pl.* glot·ti·des
    false g.
    intercartilaginous g.
    respiratory g.
    true g.
glot·to·gram
glot·to·graph
glot·tog·ra·phy
glot·tol·o·gy
glou-glou
glove
    Biobrane g.
glox·a·zone
Glu — glutamic acid

glu·ca·gon
    gut g.
    g. hydrochloride
glu·ca·gon·o·ma
glu·cal
glu·can
$1,4$-α-glu·can branch·ing en·zyme
α–glu·can–branch·ing gly·co·syl·trans·fer·ase
α-$1,4$-glu·can: α-$1,4$-glu·can 6-glu·co·syl-trans·fer·ase deficiency
glu·can-$1,4$-α-glu·co·si·dase
α-glu·can gly·co·syl 4:6-trans·fer·ase
glu·car·ic acid
glu·ca·to·nia
glu·cep·tate
Gluck's incision
glu·co·ascor·bic acid
glu·co·cer·e·bro·si·dase
glu·co·cer·e·bro·side
glu·co·cer·e·bro·si·do·sis
glu·co·cin·in
glu·co·cor·ti·coid
Glu·co-Fer·rum
glu·co·fu·ra·nose
glu·co·gen·e·sis
glu·co·gen·ic
glu·co·he·mia
glu·co·ki·nase
glu·co·ki·net·ic
glu·co·kin·in
glu·co·lac·tone
glu·col·y·sis
glu·co·lyt·ic
glu·co·nate
glu·co·neo·gen·e·sis
glu·co·neo·ge·net·ic
glu·con·ic acid
glu·co·no·lac·tone
glu·co·pe·nia
glu·co·phe·net·i·din
glu·co·phore
glu·co·phyl·line
glu·co·pro·tein

glu·co·py·ra·nose
glu·co·reg·u·la·tion
glu·co·sa·mine
   acetyl g.
glu·co·sa·mine·phos·phate
   isom·er·ase
α-glu·cos·am·i·nide-*N*-ac·e·
   tyl·trans·fer·ase
glu·co·san
glu·co·sa·zone
glu·cose
   Brun's g.
   gamma g.
   liquid g.
   g. 1-phosphate
   g. 6-phosphate
glu·cose ox·i·dase
glu·cose-6-phos·pha·tase
glu·cose-6-phos·phate de·hy·
   dro·gen·ase (G6PD)
glu·cose-6-phos·phate isom·er·
   ase
glu·cose-1-phos·phate phos·
   pho·dis·mu·tase
glu·cose-1-phos·phate uri·dyl·
   yl·trans·fer·ase
α-glu·co·si·dase
   lysosomal α-g.
α-1,4-glu·co·si·dase
glu·co·side
glu·co·si·do·lyt·ic
glu·co·sin
glu·co·si·no·late pro·goi·trin
glu·cos·te·roid
glu·co·sul·fone so·di·um
glu·co·sum
glu·cos·uria
glu·co·syl
glu·co·syl·cer·am·i·dase
glu·co·syl·trans·fer·ase
glu·co·xy·lose
glu·cu·ro·nate
glu·cu·ron·ic acid
β-glu·cu·ron·i·dase
glu·cu·ron·ide
glu·cu·ron·ide trans·fer·ase
glu·cu·ron·o·side
glu·cu·ron·o·syl·trans·fer·ase

glu·cu·ron·yl trans·fer·ase
Gluge's corpuscles
glu·ta·mate
glu·ta·mate de·car·box·y·lase
glu·ta·mate de·hy·dro·gen·
   ase
glu·ta·mate for·mim·i·no·
   trans·fer·ase
glu·ta·mate ox·a·lo·ace·tate
   trans·am·i·nase
glu·ta·mate py·ru·vate trans·
   am·i·nase
glu·tam·ic acid
   g.a. hydrochloride
glu·tam·ic-ox·alo·ace·tic
   trans·am·i·nase (GOT)
glu·tam·ic-py·ru·vic trans·
   am·i·nase (GPT)
glu·tam·ic semi·al·de·hyde
glu·tam·i·nase
glu·ta·mine
   g. synthase
glu·tam·i·nyl
glu·tam·i·nyl-pep·tide-γ-glu·
   ta·myl·trans·fer·ase
glu·ta·myl
γ-glu·ta·myl·cy·clo·trans·fer·
   ase
γ-glu·ta·myl·cys·te·ine syn·
   the·tase deficiency
γ-glu·ta·myl·trans·fer·ase
   (GGT)
glu·ta·myl trans·pep·ti·dase
glu·ta·ral
   g. concentrate
glu·ta·ral·de·hyde
glu·tar·e·dox·in
glu·tar·gin
glu·tar·ic acid
glu·ta·ryl-CoA syn·the·tase
glu·ta·thi·one
glu·ta·thi·one per·ox·i·dase
glu·ta·thi·one re·duc·tase
   (NAD(P)H)
glu·ta·thi·one syn·the·tase
glu·ta·thi·on·emia
glu·ta·thi·on·uria
glu·te·al

glu·ten
glu·te·nin
glu·teo·fem·o·ral
glu·teo·in·gui·nal
glu·teth·i·mide
glu·te·us max·i·mus
glu·te·us me·di·us
glu·te·us min·i·mus
glu·ti·nous
glu·ti·tis
glu·tose
Glu·zin·ski's test
Gly — glycine
gly·bur·ide
gly·cal
gly·can
gly·ce·mia
gly·ce·min
gly·cen·tin
glyc·er·al·de·hyde
    g. phosphate
glyc·er·al·de·hyde-3-phos·
    phate de·hy·dro·gen·ase
    (GAPD)
glyc·er·ate
gly·cer·ic acid
glyc·er·i·dase
glyc·er·ide
glyc·er·in
glyc·er·in·at·ed
glyc·er·ite
    starch g.
    tannic acid g.
glyc·ero·gel
glyc·ero·gel·a·tin
glyc·er·ol
    iodinated g.
    g. phosphate
glyc·er·ol·ize
glyc·er·ol ki·nase
glyc·er·ol-3-phos·phate de·hy·
    dro·gen·ase
glyc·er·one phos·phate
glyc·ero·phil·ic
glyc·ero·phos·pha·tase
glyc·ero·phos·phate
    ferric g.
glyc·er·ose

glyc·er·yl
    g. guaiacolate
    g. monostearate
    g. triacetate
    g. trinitrate
gly·cin·amide ri·bo·nu·cleo·
    tide
gly·cin·ate
gly·cine
    g. amidinotransferase
gly·cin·emia
glyc·i·nin
gly·ci·nol
gly·cin·uria
    de Vries-type renal g.
    hereditary g.
gly·co·bi·ar·sol
gly·co·cal·ix
gly·co·che·no·de·oxy·cho·late
gly·co·che·no·de·oxy·cho·lic
    acid
gly·co·cho·late
gly·co·cho·lic acid
gly·co·clas·tic
gly·co·cy·amine
gly·co·gel·a·tin
gly·co·gen
    hepatic g.
    tissue g.
gly·co·gen·ase
gly·co·gen·e·sis
gly·co·ge·net·ic
gly·co·gen·ic
gly·co·ge·nol·y·sis
gly·co·geno·lyt·ic
gly·co·ge·no·sis
    brancher deficiency g.
    generalized g.
    hepatophosphorylase
        deficiency g.
    hepatorenal g.
    myophosphorylase
        deficiency g.
gly·cog·e·nous
gly·co·gen phos·phor·y·lase
gly·co·gen phos·phor·y·lase
    ki·nase

gly·co·gen syn·thase
gly·co·gen syn·the·tase
gly·co·geu·sia
gly·co·he·mia
gly·co·he·mo·glo·bin
gly·col
 g. methacrylate
 polyethylene g.
gly·co·late
gly·col·ic acid
gly·co·lip·id
gly·col·ur·ic acid
gly·co·lyl
gly·col·y·sis
gly·co·lyt·ic
gly·co·met·a·bol·ic
gly·co·me·tab·o·lism
gly·cone
gly·co·nu·cleo·pro·tein
gly·co·pe·nia
gly·co·pep·tide
gly·co·pex·ia
gly·co·pex·ic
gly·co·pex·is
gly·co·phil·ia
gly·co·phor·in
gly·co·poly·uria
gly·co·pri·val
gly·co·pro·tein
 glycine-rich β g. (GBG)
 variable surface g. (VSG)
gly·co·pty·al·ism
gly·co·pyr·ro·late
gly·co·pyr·ro·ni·um bro·mide
gly·co·reg·u·la·tion
gly·co·reg·u·la·to·ry
gly·cor·rha·chia
gly·cor·rhea
gly·co·sam·ine
gly·cos·ami·no·gly·can
gly·cos·ami·no·lip·id
gly·co·se·cre·to·ry
gly·co·se·mia
gly·co·sene
gly·co·si·a·lia
gly·co·si·a·lor·rhea
gly·co·si·dase

gly·co·side
 cardiac g.
 cyanophoric g.
 sterol g.
gly·co·som·e·ter
gly·co·sphingo·lip·id
gly·co·sphing·o·lip·i·do·sis
gly·co·sta·sis
gly·co·stat·ic
gly·cos·uria
 alimentary g.
 artificial g.
 benign g.
 diabetic g.
 digestive g.
 emotional g.
 epinephrine g.
 factitious g.
 hyperglycemic g.
 magnesium g.
 nervous g.
 nondiabetic g.
 nonhyperglycemic g.
 normoglycemic g.
 orthoglycemic g.
 pathologic g.
 phlorhizin g.
 pituitary g.
 renal g.
 toxic g.
gly·cos·uric acid
gly·co·syl
gly·co·syl·at·ed
gly·co·syl·a·tion
gly·co·syl·trans·fer·ase
gly·co·tax·is
gly·co·trop·ic
gly·cu·re·sis
gly·cu·ron·ic acid
gly·cu·ro·nide
gly·cu·ron·uria
glyc·yl
glyc·yl·glyc·ine
glyc·yl·tryp·to·phan
Gly·cyph·a·gus
 G. domesticus
Glyc·yr·rhi·za

glyc·yr·rhi·za
glyc·yr·rhi·zic acid
glyc·yr·rhi·zin
gly·da·nile so·di·um
gly·mi·dine so·di·um
gly·ox·al
gly·ox·a·lin
gly·ox·i·some
gly·ox·o·some
gly·ox·y·late
gly·ox·yl·ic acid
gly·oxy·some
gly·phyl·line
Gly·the·o·nate
gm — gram
GMC — General Medical Council (British)
Gme·lin's test
GMP — guanosine monophosphate
3'5'-GMP — cyclic guanosine monophosphate
gnat
    buffalo g.
    eye g.
    turkey g.
gnath·al·gia
gnath·ic
gnath·i·on
gnath·itis
Gnath·ob·del·li·dae
gnatho·ceph·a·lus
gnatho·dy·nam·ics
gnatho·dy·na·mom·e·ter
    bimeter g.
gnath·odyn·ia
gnath·og·ra·phy
gnatho·log·ic
gnath·ol·o·gy
gna·tho·pal·a·tos·chi·sis
gnatho·plas·ty
gna·tho·ple·gia
gnath·os·chi·sis
gnatho·so·ma
gnatho·stat
gnatho·stat·ics
Gnath·os·to·ma
    G. spinigerum

gnatho·sto·mi·a·sis
gno·sia
gno·sis
gno·to·bi·ol·o·gy
gno·to·bio·ta
gno·to·bi·ote
gno·to·bi·ot·ic
gno·to·bi·ot·ics
gno·to·phor·e·sis
gno·to·phor·ic
Gn-RH — gonadotropin-releasing hormone
Goa powder
Go·dé·lier's law
God·man's fascia
Goeck·er·man treatment
Goe·the's bone
Gof·man's test
Gog·gia's sign
goi·ter
    aberrant g.
    adenomatous g.
    Basedow's g.
    cabbage g.
    colloid g.
    congenital g.
    cystic g.
    diffuse g.
    diving g.
    endemic g.
    exophthalmic g.
    familial g.
    fibrous g.
    follicular g.
    intrathoracic g.
    iodide g.
    lingual g.
    lymphadenoid g.
    multinodular g.
    myxedematous g.
    nontoxic g.
    parenchymatous g.
    perivascular g.
    plunging g.
    retrovascular g.
    simple g.
    substernal g.
    suffocative g.

goi·ter *(continued)*
    thoracic g.
    toxic multinodular g.
    vascular g.
    wandering g.
goi·trin
goi·tro·gen
goi·tro·gen·ic
goi·tro·ge·nic·i·ty
goi·trog·e·nous
goi·trous
gold
    g. 198
    g. aurothiosulfate
    cohesive g.
    colloidal g.
    fibrous g.
    inlay g.
    mat g.
    radioactive g.
    g. sodium thiomalate
    g. sodium thiosulfate
    g. thioglucose
Gold·blatt's clamp
Gold·blatt's hypertension
Gold·blatt's kidney
Gol·den sign
Gol·den·har syndrome
Gold·flam's disease
Gold·flam-Erb disease
Gold·schei·der's percussion
Gold·schei·der's test
Gold·stein, Joseph Leonard
Gold·stein's classification
Gold·stein's disease
Gold·stein's hematemesis
Gold·stein's hemoptysis
Gold·stein rays
Gold·stein's sign
Gold·stein's syndrome
Gold·stein-Reich·mann
  syndrome
Gold·thwait's brace
Gold·thwait's sign
Gold·thwait's symptom
Gol·gi, Camillo
Gol·gi's complex
Gol·gi's corpuscle

Gol·gi's neuron
Gol·gi's organ
Gol·gi's stain
Gol·gi's theory
gol·gio·some
Goll's column
Goll's fasciculus
Goll's fibers
Goll's nucleus
Goll's tract
Goltz's experiment
Goltz syndrome
Goltz's theory
Gom·bault's degeneration
Gom·bault's neuritis
Gom·bault-Phi·lippe triangle
go·mit·o·li
Gom·ori methods
Gom·ori stains
Gom·pertz formula
Gom·pertz law
gom·pho·sis
gon·a·cra·tia
go·nad
    indifferent g.
    primitive g.
    streak g's
go·nad·al
go·na·dec·to·mize
go·na·dec·to·my
go·nad·i·al
gon·a·do·blas·to·ma
go·nado·cen·tric
gon·a·do·gen·e·sis
gon·a·do·in·hib·i·to·ry
gon·a·do·ki·net·ic
go·na·do·ma
    dysgenetic g.
gon·a·dop·a·thy
gon·a·do·pause
go·nado·rel·in
go·nado·trope
go·nado·troph
gon·a·do·troph·ic
gon·a·do·tro·phin
gon·a·do·trop·ic
gon·a·do·tro·pin
    chorionic g.

gon·a·do·tro·pin *(continued)*
    equine g.
    human chorionic g. (hCG)
    human menopausal g.
     (hMG)
    pituitary g.
    pregnant mare serum g.
    g.-releasing hormone
     (Gn-RH)
gon·a·duct
gon·ag·ra
go·nal·gia
gon·an·gi·ec·to·my
gon·ar·thri·tis
gon·ar·throc·a·ce
gon·ar·thro·men·in·gi·tis
gon·ar·thro·sis
gon·ar·throt·o·my
go·nato·cele
Gon·da sign
gon·e·cyst
gon·e·cys·tis
gon·e·cys·ti·tis
gon·e·cys·to·lith
gon·e·cys·to·py·o·sis
gon·e·itis
gon·e·poi·e·sis
gon·e·poi·et·ic
Gon·gy·lo·ne·ma
    G. pulchrum
gon·gy·lo·ne·mi·a·sis
go·nia
go·ni·al
gon·id·an·gi·um
go·nid·ia
go·nid·io·spore
go·nid·i·um *pl.* go·nid·ia
Go·nin's operation
Go·nio·ba·sis
    G. silicula
go·nio·lens
go·ni·om·e·ter
    finger g.
go·ni·on *pl.* go·nia
go·nio·pho·tog·ra·phy
go·nio·prism
    Allen g.
Gon·i·ops

go·nio·punc·ture
go·nio·scope
go·ni·os·co·py
go·nio·syn·ech·ia
go·ni·ot·o·my
go·ni·tis
    fungous g.
    g. tuberculosa
gono·blen·nor·rhea
gono·camp·sis
gono·cele
gon·och·o·rism
gono·coc·cal
gono·coc·ce·mia
gono·coc·ci
gono·coc·cic
gono·coc·cide
gono·coc·co·cide
gono·coc·cus *pl.* gono·coc·ci
gono·cyte
gon·om·ery
gono·neph·ro·tome
gono·phage
gono·phore
gon·or·rhea
gon·or·rhe·al
gon·os·che·o·cele
gono·to·kont
gono·tome
gono·tox·emia
gony·al·gia
    g. paresthetica
Gony·au·lax
gony·camp·sis
gony·cro·te·sis
gony·ec·ty·po·sis
gonyo·cele
gony·on·cus
Gon·za·les blood group
Good's syndrome
Goo·dell's law
Goo·dell's sign
Good·e·nough test
Good·pas·ture's stain
Good·pas·ture's syndrome
Good·sall's rule
Goor·magh·tigh's apparatus
Goor·magh·tigh cells

goose·flesh, goose flesh
Gop·a·lan syndrome
Gor·di·a·cea
Gor·di·us
    G. *aquaticus*
    G. *robustus*
Gor·don's bodies
Gor·don's reflex
Gor·don's sign
Gor·don's test
gor·get
Gor·lin's formula
Gor·lin's syndrome
Gor·lin-Chau·dhry-Moss
  syndrome
Gor·lin-Goltz syndrome
Gor·lin-Psaume syndrome
Gos·lee tooth
Gosse·lin's fracture
Gos·syp·i·um
gos·sy·pol
GOT — glutamine-oxaloacetic
  transaminase (aspartate
  aminotransferase)
Göth·lin's index
Göth·lin's test
Gott·lieb's epithelial
  attachment
Gott·ron's papules
Gott·ron's sign
Gott·stein's fibers
Gott·stein's process
gouge
    Kelley g.
Gou·ger·ot's triad
Gou·ger·ot-Blum syndrome
Gou·ger·ot-Car·teaud
  syndrome
Gou·lard's extract
Gou·lard's lotion
Gou·lard's water
gono·cy·to·ma
gono·ducts
Gou·ley's catheter
goun·dou
gou·siek·te
gout
    abarticular g.

gout *(continued)*
    articular g.
    calcium g.
    chalky g.
    idiopathic g.
    irregular g.
    latent g.
    lead g.
    masked g.
    misplaced g.
    oxalic g.
    polyarticular g.
    primary g.
    regular g.
    rheumatic g.
    saturnine g.
    secondary g.
    tophaceous g.
    visceral g.
gou·ty
Gow·ers' column
Gow·ers' fasciculus
Gow·ers' sign
Gow·ers' solution
Gow·ers' syndrome
Gow·ers' tract
GP — general paresis
  general practitioner
G6PD — glucose-6-phosphate
  dehydrogenase
GPI — general paralysis of the
  insane
GPT — glutamic-pyruvic
  transaminase
GR — gastric resection
gr — grain
graaf·i·an follicle
graaf·i·an vesicle
grac·ile
Grac·i·lic·u·tes
grac·i·lo·tha·lam·ic
Grad. — L. gradatim (by
  degrees)
gra·da·tim
Gra·de·ni·go's syndrome
Gra·de·ni·go-Lan·nois
  syndrome

gra·di·ent
    g. of approach
    atrioventricular g.
    g. of avoidance
    axial g.
    concentration g.
    density g.
    magnetic g.
    mitral g.
    proton g.
    systolic g.
    ventricular g.
grad·ing
    Karnofsky tumor g.
grad·u·ate
grad·u·at·ed
Grae·fe's knife
Grae·fe's operation
Grae·fe's sign
Gräf·en·berg's ring
graft
    accordion g.
    activated g.
    allogeneic g.
    alloplast g.
    anorganic bone g.
    aortofemoral bypass g.
    aortorenal bypass g.
    autochthonous g.
    autodermic g.
    autoepidermic g.
    autogenous g.
    autologous g.
    autologous fat g.
    autoplastic g.
    avascular g.
    axillofemoral bypass g.
    bifurcated vascular g.
    Blair-Brown g.
    bone g.
    brephoplastic g.
    bridge g.
    cable g.
    cantilever g.
    chondrocutaneous g.
    chorioallantoic g.
    composite g.

graft *(continued)*
    coronary artery bypass g.
     (CABG)
    crossover bypass g.
    cutis g.
    Dardik Biograft
    Davis g.
    delayed g.
    derma-fat-fascia g.
    dermal g.
    dermic g.
    dermis-fat g.
    diced cartilage g's
    epidermic g.
    Esser g.
    extracranial-intracranial
     bypass g.
    fascia g.
    fascicular g.
    fat g.
    femoral-femoral g.
    femoral-tibial bypass g.
    filler g.
    free g.
    free gingival g.
    full-thickness g.
    glutaraldehyde-tanned
     bovine carotid artery g.
    Gore-Tex g.
    heterodermic g.
    heterologous g.
    heteroplastic g.
    heterotopic g.
    homogenous g.
    homologous g.
    homoplastic g.
    hyperplastic g.
    ileal g.
    iliac g.
    inlay g.
    interposition g.
    island g.
    isogeneic g.
    isologous g.
    isoplastic g.
    jump g.
    Kiel bone g.
    Krause-Wolfe g.

graft *(continued)*
    lamellar g.
    mesh g.
    mesocaval H g.
    microvascular free g.
    mucosal g.
    nerve g.
    Nicoll bone g.
    Ollier-Thiersch g.
    omental g's
    onlay g.
    onlay bone g.
    orthotopic g.
    osseous g.
    outlay g.
    panel g.
    parathyroid g.
    patch g.
    pedicle g.
    pedicled bone g.
    penetrating g.
    periosteal g.
    Phemister g.
    pigskin g.
    pinch g.
    polytetrafluoroethylene (PTFE) g.
    preserved bone g.
    prosthetic vascular g.
    razor g.
    Reverdin g.
    seed g.
    sequential g.
    sheet g.
    sieve g.
    skin g.
    sleeve g.
    snake g.
    splenorenal bypass g.
    split-rib g.
    split-skin g.
    split-thickness g.
    Stent g.
    syngeneic g.
    thick-split g.
    Thiersch's g.
    thin-split g.
    tube g.

graft *(continued)*
    tunnel g.
    vascular g.
    vein g.
    white g.
    Wolfe's g.
    Wolfe-Krause g.
    xenogeneic g.
graft·ing
    interfascicular nerve g.
    mesh g.
    skin g.
Gra·ham's law
Gra·ham's test
Gra·ham Lit·tle syndrome
Gra·ham Steell murmur
grain
grain·age
gram
Gram's method
Gram's solution
Gram's stain
gram-atom
gram-cal·o·rie
gram-equiv·a·lent
gram·i·ci·din
gram·ine
gram·i·nin
gram·i·niv·o·rous
gram-ion
gram·me·ter
gram·mole
gram-mol·e·cule
gram-neg·a·tive
gram-pos·i·tive
gram-rad (g-rad)
gram-roent·gen
Gran·cher's system
gran·di·ose
gran·di·os·i·ty
grand mal
Gran·dry's corpuscles
Gran·ger line
Gran·ger sign
Gran·it, Ragnar Arthur
grano·plasm
gran·u·la *pl.* gran·u·lae
    g. iridica

gran·u·lar
gran·u·la·ris
gran·u·late
gran·u·la·tio *pl.* gran·u·la·ti·o·nes
   granulationes arachnoideales
   granulationes cerebrales
   granulationes pacchioni
gran·u·la·tion
   arachnoidal g's
   Bayle's g's
   Bright's g's
   cell g's
   exuberant g's
   hypertrophic g.
   pacchionian g's
   pyroninophilic g's
   Reilly g's
   Virchow's g's
gran·u·la·ti·o·nes
gran·ule
   acidophil g's
   acrosomal g.
   albuminous g's
   aleuronoid g's
   alpha g's
   amphophil g's
   argentaffine g's
   atrial g's
   azurophil g.
   Babès-Ernst g.
   basal g.
   basophil g's
   Bensley specific g's
   beta g's
   Birbeck g's
   Bollinger's g's
   "bull's eye" g.
   Bütschli's g's
   carbohydrate g's
   chromatic g's
   chromophilic g's
   chromophobe g's
   cone g's
   cortical g's
   cytoplasmic g's
   delta g's

gran·ule *(continued)*
   dense g.
   dense core g.
   Ehrlich's g's
   Ehrlich-Heinz g's
   elementary g's
   eosinophil g's
   fuchsinophil g's
   Fordyce's g's
   gamma g's
   glycogen g's
   Heinz g's
   hyperchromatin g.
   interstitial g.
   iodophil g's
   Isaac's g's
   juxtaglomerular g's
   kappa g.
   keratohyalin g's
   Kölliker's interstitial g's
   Kretz's g's
   Langerhans' g's
   Langley's g's
   lipofuscin g.
   mast-cell g.
   melanin g.
   membrane-coating g.
   meningeal g's
   metachromatic g.
   Much's g's
   mucinogen g's
   mucous g.
   neurosecretory g.
   neutrophil g's
   Nissl's g's
   oxyphil g's
   Palade g.
   Paschen's g's
   perichromatin g's
   pigment g's
   polar g's
   proacrosomal g.
   protein g's
   rod g's
   Schrön's g.
   Schrön-Much g's
   Schüffner's g's
   secondary g.

gran·ule *(continued)*
    secretory g's
    seminal g's
    specific atrial g's
    sphere g.
    sulfur g's
    tannophil g's
    thread g's
    toxic g's
    trichohyalin g's
    vermiform g's
    volutin g's
    yolk g's
    zymogen g's
gran·u·li·form
gran·u·lo·ad·i·pose
gran·u·lo·blast
gran·u·lo·blas·to·sis
gran·u·lo·cor·pus·cle
gran·u·lo·cy·ta·phe·re·sis
gran·u·lo·cyte
    band-form g.
    heterophil g.
    neutrophil g.
    polymorphonuclear g.
    segmented g.
gran·u·lo·cyt·ic
gran·u·lo·cy·top·a·thy
gran·u·lo·cy·to·pe·nia
gran·u·lo·cy·to·poi·e·sis
gran·u·lo·cy·to·poi·et·ic
gran·u·lo·cy·to·sis
gran·u·lo·fat·ty
gran·u·lo·ma *pl.* gran·u·lo·
  mas, gran·u·lo·ma·ta
    adjuvant g.
    alum g.
    amebic g.
    g. annulare
    apical g.
    aquarium g.
    beryllium g.
    candida g.
    candidal g.
    cholesterol g.
    chronic g.
    coccidioidal g.
    g. contagiosum

gran·u·lo·ma *(continued)*
    dental g.
    eosinophilic g.
    favic g.
    fish tank g.
    g. fissuratum
    foreign-body g.
    g. fungoides
    g. gangraenescens
    g. gluteale infantum
    Hodgkin's g.
    infectious g.
    g. inguinale
    intubation g.
    iodide g.
    laryngeal g.
    lethal midline g.
    lipoid g.
    lipophagic g.
    Majocchi's g.
    malarial g.
    midline g.
    Mignon's eosinophilic g.
    monilial g.
    g. multiforme
    paracoccidioidal g.
    periapical g.
    plasma cell g.
    g. of prostate
    pseudopyogenic g.
    g. pudendi
    g. pudens tropicum
    pyogenic g.
    g. pyogenicum
    reticulohistiocytic g.
    rheumatic g's
    septic g.
    silicotic g.
    swimming pool g.
    g. telangiectaticum
    trichophytic g.
    g. trichophyticum
    umbilical g.
    g. venereum
    Wegener's g.
    xanthomatous g.
    zirconium g.

gran·u·lo·ma·to·sis
   allergic g.
   beryllium g.
   chronic familial g.
   chronic X-linked g.
   g. disciformis progressiva
     et chronica
   Langerhans cell g.
   lipid g.
   lipophagic intestinal g.
   lymphomatoid g.
   malignant g.
   necrotizing respiratory g.
   reticuloendothelial g.
   g. siderotica
   Wegener's g.
gran·u·lom·a·tous
gran·u·lo·mere
gran·u·lo·pe·nia
gran·u·lo·pexy
gran·u·lo·plasm
gran·u·lo·plas·tic
gran·u·lo·poi·e·sis
gran·u·lo·poi·et·ic
gran·u·lo·poi·e·tin
gran·u·lo·po·tent
Gran·u·lo·re·tic·u·lo·sea
gran·u·lo·sa
gran·u·lose
gran·u·lo·sis
   g. rubra nasi
gran·u·los·i·ty
gran·u·lo·vac·u·o·lar
gra·num *pl.* gra·na
graph·es·the·sia
graph·ic
graph·ite
graph·i·to·sis
Graph·i·um
grapho·anal·y·sis
grapho·kin·es·thet·ic
gra·phol·o·gy
grapho·mo·tor
graph·or·rhea
grapho·spasm
GRAS — generally regarded
  as safe
Grash·ey's aphasia

grasp·ing
   forced g.
grass
   scurvy g.
Gras·set's law
Gras·set's phenomenon
Gras·set's sign
Gras·set-Bychowski sign
Gras·set-Gaus·sel phenomenon
Gras·set-Gaus·sel-Hoo·ver
  sign
gra·ti·cule
   eyepiece g.
grat·ing
   diffraction g.
Gra·ti·o·la
   G. officinalis
Gra·ti·o·let's optic radiati
Gra·ti·o·let's radiating fibers
grat·tage
gra·ve·do
grav·el
Graves' disease
grave-wax
grav·id
grav·i·da
gra·vid·ic
grav·id·ism
gra·vid·i·tas
   g. examnialis
   g. exochorialis
gra·vid·i·ty
grav·i·do·car·di·ac
grav·i·do·pu·er·per·al
gra·vim·e·ter
grav·i·met·ric
grav·i·stat·ic
grav·i·ta·tion
grav·i·tom·e·ter
grav·i·ty
   specific g.
   standard g.
Gra·witz's tumor
gray
   central g.
   periaqueductal g.
   perihypoglossal g.

gray-out
Gray·son's ligament
green
    acid g.
    brilliant g.
    bromocresol g.
    diamond g.
    diazin g. S
    ethyl g.
    fast g. FCF
    fast acid g. N
    Hoffman g.
    indocyanine g.
    iodine g.
    Janus g. B
    light g. 2 G
    light g. 2 GN
    light g. N
    light g. S F yellowish
    malachite g.
    malachite g. G
    methyl g.
    methylene g.
    new solid g.
    Paris g.
    Schweinfurt g.
    solid g.
    Victoria g.
Greene's sign
Green·field's disease
Green·field's syndrome
Green·wood-Yule method
greg·a·loid
Greg·o·ry's mixture
Greig syndrome
Grei·ther syndrome
Greu·lich and Pyle bone age
  staging
Grey Tur·ner sign
GRF — growth hormone
  releasing factor
GRH — growth hormone
  releasing hormone
grid
    Amsler g.
    baby g.
    Bucky's g.
    crossed g.

grid *(continued)*
    fixed g.
    focused g.
    moving g.
    parallel g.
    Potter-Bucky g.
    stationary g.
    Thoms g.
    Wetzel g.
Grid·ley stain
grief
Grie·sin·ger's disease
Grie·sin·ger's sign
Grie·sin·ger's symptom
Grif·fith's classification
Grig·nard's reagent
  (compound)
Gri·ful·vin
Grin·de·lia
grind·ing
    night g.
    selective g.
    spot g.
grind·ing-in
grip
    Dabney's g.
    devil's g.
    hook g.
    power g.
    precision g.
grip·pal
grippe
    g. aurique
Gris·ac·tin
gris·ein
Gris·el's disease
gris·eo·ful·vin
gris·eo·my·cin
Gri·solle's sign
Gris-PEG
Grit·ti's amputation
Grit·ti's operation
Grit·ti-Stokes amputation
Groc·co's sign
Groc·co's triangle
Groc·co's triangular dullness
Groe·nouw's corneal dystrophy
groin

grom·met
Grön·blad-Strand·berg
  syndrome
groove
    alveolingual g.
    alveolobuccal g.
    alveololabial g.
    alveololingual g.
    anal intersphincteric g.
    anterior auricular g.
    anterolateral g.
    anteromedian g.
    arterial g's
    atrioventricular g.
    auriculoventricular g.
    basilar g.
    bicipital g.
    Blessig's g.
    branchial g.
    buccal g.
    buccal developmental g.
    carotid g. of sphenoid bone
    cavernous g. of sphenoid
      bone
    central g.
    central developmental g.
    cerebral g.
    chiasmatic g.
    costal g.
    deltopectoral g.
    dental g., primitive
    developmental g's
    digastric g.
    distobuccal g.
    distobuccal developmental
      g.
    distolingual g.
    distolingual developmental
      g.
    duodenopyloric g.
    enamel g's
    ethmoidal g.
    g. for eustachian tube
    free gingival g.
    genital g.
    hamular g.
    Harrison's g.
    infraorbital g. of maxilla

groove *(continued)*
    g. of helix
    inferior dental g.
    interatrial g.
    interdental g.
    interosseous g. of calcaneus
    intertubercular g. of
      humerus
    interventricular g.,
      anterior
    interventricular g. of heart
    interventricular g., inferior
    interventricular g.,
      posterior
    labial g.
    lacrimal g.
    laryngotracheal g.
    lateral phallic g.
    Liebermeister's g's
    lingual g.
    lingual developmental g.
    g. of Lucas
    mastoid g.
    medullary g.
    mesiobuccal g.
    mesiobuccal developmental
      g.
    meningeal g's
    mesiolingual g.
    mesiolingual
      developmental g.
    musculospiral g.
    mylohyoid g.
    nail g.
    nasal g.
    nasolabial g.
    nasolacrimal g.
    nasomaxillary g.
    naso-optic g.
    nasopalatine g.
    nasopharyngeal g.
    neural g.
    nuchal g.
    nutrient artery g.
    obturator g.
    occipital g.
    occlusal g.
    olfactory g.

groove *(continued)*
  optic g.
  palatine g.
  palatomaxillary g.
  palatovaginal g.
  paracolic g.
  paraglenoid g's of hip bone
  pharyngeal g.
  pharyngotympanic g.
  popliteal g.
  posterior auricular g.
  preauricular g's
  preputiolabial g.
  primitive g.
  pterygopalatine g.
  radial g.
  rhombic g.
  sagittal g.
  secondary branchial g.
  Sibson's g.
  sigmoid g. of temporal bone
  sphenobasilar g.
  spiral g.
  subclavian g.
  g. of subclavius muscle
  subcostal g.
  supplemental g's
  supra-acetabular g.
  tracheobronchial g.
  trigeminal g.
  tympanic g.
  ulnar g.
  urethral g.
  urogenital g.
  venous g's
  Verga's lacrimal g.
  vertebral g.
  visceral g.
  vomeral g.
gross
Gross's disease
Gross's leukemia
Gross's test
Gross·man's sign
ground-glass
group
  alcohol g.
  alkalescens-dispar g.

group *(continued)*
  Arizona g.
  azo g.
  Bethesda-Ballerup g.
  blood g.
  California g.
  closed g.
  CMN g.
  coli-aerogenes g.
  colon-typhoid-dysentery g.
  compatibility g.
  continuous g.
  control g.
  coryneform g.
  diagnosis-related g's
  encounter g.
  experimental g.
  functional g.
  glucophore g.
  Gonzales blood g.
  hemorrhagic-septicemia g.
  incompatibility g.
  leukocyte g.
  linkage g.
  marathon g.
  methyl g.
  open g.
  osmophore g.
  paratyphoid-enteritidis g.
  peptide g.
  PLT g.
  prosthetic g.
  reporter g.
  Runyon g.
  saccharide g.
  sapophore g.
  sensitivity g.
  sulfonic g.
  T g., T-g.
  training g.
  ventral thalamic g.
group·ing
  blood g.
  haptenic g.
group-spe·cif·ic
group-trans·fer
growth
  absolute g.

growth *(continued)*
  accretionary g.
  allometric g.
  appositional g.
  auxetic g.
  balanced g.
  condylar g.
  confluent g.
  differential g.
  heterogonous g.
  histiotypic g.
  interstitial g.
  intrauterine g. retardation
    (IUGR)
  intussusceptive g.
  isometric g.
  multiplicative g.
  organotypic g.
  relative g.
grü·bel·sucht
Gru·ber's bougies
Gru·ber's fossa
Gru·ber's hernia
Gru·ber's reaction test
Gru·ber's speculum
Gru·ber's suture
Gru·ber's test
Gru·ber-Land·zert fossa
Gru·ber-Wi·dal reaction
Gru·ber-Wi·dal test
gru·mose, gru·mous
Grün·baum-Wi·dal test
grund·platte
Gryn·feltt's hernia
Gryn·feltt's triangle
Gryn·feltt-Les·gaft triangle
gryo·chrome
gry·pho·sis
gry·po·sis
  g. penis
  g. unguium
GSC — gas-solid
  chromatography
GSH — reduced glutathione
GSR — galvanic skin response
GSSG — oxidized glutathione
gt. — L. gutta (drop)
GTH — gonadotropic hormone

GTP — guanosine
  triphosphate
GTP cy·clo·hy·dro·lase
gtt. — L. guttae (drops)
GU — genitourinary
gua·co
guai·ac
guai·a·col
  g. carbonate
guai·fen·e·sin
guai·phen·e·sin
guai·thyl·line
guan·a·benz
guan·a·cline sul·fate
γ-gua·ni·di·no·bu·tyr·amide
  [gamma-]
guan·a·drel sul·fate
guan·ase
guan·az·o·lo
guan·cy·dine
guan·eth·i·dine
  g. monosulfate
  g. sulfate
guan·i·dase
guan·i·dine
  g. hydrochloride
  g. phosphate
guan·i·dine-acet·ic acid
guan·i·din·emia
gua·ni·di·no
guan·i·di·no·a·ce·tic acid
gua·ni·di·no·suc·cin·ic acid
guan·i·do-ace·tic acid
guan·i·dyl·ate
guan·ine
  g. deoxyriboside
  g. nucleotide
guan·ine de·am·i·nase
guan·o·chlor sul·fate
guan·o·phore
guan·o·sine
  cyclic g. monophosphate
  g. diphosphate (GDP)
  g. monophosphate (GMP)
  g. triphosphate (GTP)
guan·ox·a·benz
guan·ox·an sul·fate
gua·nyl·ate cy·clase

gua·nyl·ic acid
gua·nyl·o·ri·bo·nu·cle·ase
gua·nyl·yl
    g. methylene
      diphosphonate
gua·ra·na
gua·ra·nine
guard
    bite g.
    mouth g.
    night g.
    occlusal g.
guard·ing
Guar·ni·eri's bodies
Guar·ni·eri's corpuscles
guay·u·le
gu·ber·nac·u·la
gu·ber·nac·u·lar
gu·ber·nac·u·lum *pl.* gu·ber·
  nac·u·la
    chorda g.
    g. dentis
    Hunter's g.
    g. testis
Gub·ler's hemiplegia
Gub·ler's line
Gub·ler's paralysis
Gub·ler's sign
Gub·ler's tumor
Gub·ler-Mil·lard paralysis
Gub·ler-Ro·bin typhus
Gud·den's commissure
Gud·den's law
Gue·del stage
Guel·pa treatment
Gué·neau de Mus·sy's point
Guen·ther stain
Gué·rin's fold
Gué·rin's fracture
Gué·rin's gland
Gué·rin's sinus
Gué·rin's valve
guid·ance
    child g.
    condylar g.
    contact g.
    incisal g.

guide
    adjustable anterior g.
    anterior g.
    condylar g.
    incisal g.
    light g.
    mold g.
guide·line
    clasp g.
Gui·di's canal
Guil·lain-Bar·ré syndrome
Guil·le·min, Roger Charles
  Louis
guil·lo·tine
    tonsil g.
Gui·nard's method
Gui·nard's treatment
guin·ea pig
Gui·non's disease
gulf
    Lecat's g.
Gull's disease
Gull·strand, Allvar
Gull·strand's law
Gull·strand's slit lamp
gu·lon·ic acid
L-gu·lo·no·lac·tone
gu·lose
gum
    acacia g.
    animal g.
    g. arabic
    Australian g.
    g. benjamin
    g. benzoin
    blue g.
    British g.
    g. camphor
    cape g.
    g. dragon
    eucalyptus g.
    free g.
    ghatti g.
    g. guaiac
    guar g.
    Indian g.
    g. juniper

gum *(continued)*
    karaya g.
    Kordofan g.
    mesquite g.
    g. opium
    red g.
    g. senegal
    sterculia g.
    g. thus
    g. tragacanth
    wattle g.
    xanthan g.
gum·boil
Gum·boro disease
gum·ma *pl.* gum·mas, gum·
  ma·ta
    tuberculous g.
gum·ma·ta
gum·mate
gum·ma·tous
gum·mi
gum·my
gum-res·in
gun·cot·ton
Gunn's dots
Gunn's law
Gunn's phenomenon
Gunn's pupillary phenomenon
Gunn's sign
Gunn's syndrome
Gun·ning's splint
Günz's ligament
Günz·berg's test
gur·gu·lio
gur·ney
gus·ta·tion
    colored g.
gus·ta·tism
gus·ta·to·ry
gus·tin
gus·tom·e·ter
gus·tom·e·try
gut
    blind g.
    postanal g.
    preoral g.
    primitive g.
    ribbon g.

gut *(continued)*
    silkworm g.
    surgical g.
    tail g.
Guth·rie's formula
Guth·rie's muscle
Guth·rie test
gut·ta *pl.* gut·tae
    g. ophthalmicae
gut·tae
gut·ta-per·cha
Guttat. — L. guttatim (drop by
    drop)
gut·ta·ta
gut·tate
gut·ta·tim
gut·ta·tion
gut·ter
    paracolic g's
    pleuroperitoneal g's
    synaptic g.
gut·ter·ing
gut-tie
Gutt. quibusd. — L. guttis
  quibusdam (with a few drops)
gut·tur
gut·tur·al
gut·tur·oph·o·ny
gut·turo·tet·a·ny
Gut·zeit's test
Guy de Chau·li·ac
Guye sign
Gu·yon's amputation
Gu·yon's operation
Gu·yon's sign
GVH — graft-versus-host
  (disease, reaction)
Gwath·mey's oil-ether
  anesthesia
Gy — gray
Gym·na·moe·bia
gym·nas·tics
    ocular g.
    Swedish g.
    vocal g.
Gym·ne·ma
Gym·no·as·ca·ceae
Gym·no·as·cus

gym·no·car·pous
gym·no·cyte
Gym·no·din·i·um
gym·no·plast
gym·no·sperm
gym·no·spore
gym·no·the·ci·um
gy·nan·der
gy·nan·dria
gy·nan·drism
gy·nan·dro·blas·to·ma
gy·nan·droid
gy·nan·dro·morph
gy·nan·dro·mor·phism
   bilateral g.
gy·nan·dro·mor·phous
gy·nan·dry
gyn·atre·sia
gy·nec·ic
gy·ne·ci·um
gyne·co·gen
gyne·co·gen·ic
gyne·cog·ra·phy
gyn·e·coid
gy·ne·co·log·ic
gy·ne·co·log·i·cal
gy·ne·col·o·gist
gy·ne·col·o·gy
gyne·co·ma·nia
gyne·co·mas·tia
   nutritional g.
   refeeding g.
   rehabilitation g.
gyne·cop·a·thy
gyne·coph·o·ral
gy·ne·co·phor·ic
gyne·duct
gy·ne·phil·ia
gyne·pho·bia
gyne·plas·ty
Gyn·er·gen
gyn·e·sin
gy·no·gam·on
gyno·gen·e·sis
gyno·mer·o·gon
gyno·mer·o·gone
gyno·me·rog·o·ny
gyno·path·ic

gyn·op·a·thy
gy·no·pho·bia
gy·no·plas·tic
gy·no·plas·tics
gy·no·plas·ty
Gy·no·rest
gyp·sum
gy·ral
gy·rase
gy·rate
gy·ra·tion
gy·rec·to·my
   frontal g.
Gy·ren·ceph·a·la
gy·ren·ce·phal·ic
gy·ri
gy·ro·chrome
gy·ro·mele
gy·rom·e·ter
gy·rose
gy·ro·spasm
gy·ro·trope
gy·rous
gy·rus *pl.* gy·ri
   angular g.
   g. angularis
   annectant gyri
   gyri annectentes
   gyri breves insulae
   Broca's g.
   callosal g.
   g. callosus
   central g., anterior
   central g., posterior
   g. centralis anterior
   g. centralis posterior
   g. cerebelli
   gyri cerebri, gyri of
     cerebrum
   cingulate g.
   g. cingulatus
   g. cinguli
   g. cunei
   cuneolingual g.
   deep transitional g.
   dentate g.
   g. dentatus
   g. descendens

gy·rus *(continued)*
g. epicallosus
external orbital g.
g. fasciolaris
g. fornicatus
frontal g., ascending
frontal g., inferior
frontal g., middle
frontal g., superior
g. frontalis inferior
g. frontalis medialis
g. frontalis medius
g. frontalis superior
fusiform g.
g. fusiformis
g. geniculi
Heschl's gyri
hippocampal g.
g. hippocampi
infracalcarine g.
g. infracalcarinus
gyri insulae
internal orbital g.
g. intralimbicus
g. limbicus
lingual g.
g. lingualis
long g. of insula
g. longus insulae
marginal g.
marginal g. of Turner
g. marginalis
occipital gyri, lateral
occipital g., inferior
occipital g., superior
occipitotemporal g., lateral
occipitotemporal g., medial
g. occipitotemporalis
   lateralis
g. occipitotemporalis
   medialis
gyri olfactorii medialis et
   lateralis
g. olfactorius medialis
olfactory g., lateral
olfactory g., medial
orbital gyri

gy·rus *(continued)*
gyri orbitales
g. orbitalis lateralis
g. orbitalis medialis
paracentral g.
g. paracentralis
parahippocampal g.
g. parahippocampalis
parahippocaudal g.
parasplenial g.
paraterminal g.
g. paraterminalis
parietal g.
parietal g., ascending
g. postcentralis
postrolandic g.
precentral g.
g. precentralis
preinsular gyri
prerolandic g.
gyri profundi cerebri
g. rectus
retrosplenal g.
g. of Retzius
g. rolandicus
short gyri of insula
splenial g.
straight g.
subcalcarine g.
subcallosal g.
g. subcallosus
supracallosal g.
g. supracallosus
supramarginal g.
g. supramarginalis
temporal g.
temporal g., inferior
temporal g., middle
temporal g., superior
temporal gyri, transverse
g. temporalis inferior
g. temporalis medius
g. temporalis superior
gyri temporales transversi
gyri transitivi cerebri
uncinate g.
g. uncinatus

H — Hauch
henry
Holzknecht unit
horizontal
Hounsfield unit
hydrogen
hypermetropia
hyperopia
H — enthalpy
magnetic field strength
H. — L. haustus (a draft)
L. hora (hour)
[H⁺] — hydrogen ion
concentration
h — hecto-
hour
h. — L. hora (hour)
h — Planck's constant
height
H_0 — null hypothesis
H_1 — alternate hypothesis
H & E — hematoxylin and
eosin (stain)
HA — hemadsorbent
HAA — hepatitis-associated
antigen
Haab's magnet
Haab's reflex
Haa·gen·sen's test
haar·scheibe
Ha·bel's method
ha·be·na *pl.* ha·be·nae
ha·be·nal
ha·be·nar
ha·ben·u·la *pl.* ha·ben·u·lae
h. arcuata
h. conarii
Haller's h.
h. pectinata
habenulae perforatae
h. urethralis
ha·ben·u·lae
ha·ben·u·lar
Ha·ber syndrome
Ha·ber·mann's disease
ha·bil·i·ta·tion

hab·it
clamping h.
clenching h.
endothelioid h.
glaucomatous h.
leukocytoid h.
oral h.
position h.
tongue h.
hab·i·tat
ha·bit·u·a·tion
hab·i·tus
Buddha-like h.
h. phthisicus
hab·ro·ne·mi·a·sis
cutaneous h.
ha·bu
hache·ment
HACS — hyperactive child
syndrome
Had·field-Clarke syndrome
Ha·dru·rus
Haeck·el's law
H-Ae in·ter·val
hae·ma
Hae·ma·dip·sa
H. ceylonica
H. chiliani
H. japonica
H. zeylandica
Hae·ma·gog·us
Hae·ma·phys·a·lis
H. cinnabarina
H. concinna
H. humerosa
H. leachi
H. leporispalustris
H. punctata
H. spinigera
Haem·a·to·bia
H. irritans
Haem·a·to·si·phon
H. indorus
Hae·ma·tox·y·lon

Haem·en·te·ria
   H. officinalis
Haemo·dip·sus
   H. ventricosus
Haemo·greg·a·ri·na
Hae·mon·chus
   H. contortus
Hae·moph·i·lus
   H. aegyptius
   H. aphrophilus
   H. bronchisepticus
   H. ducreyi
   H. duplex
   H. haemolyticus
   H. influenzae
   H. parainfluenzae
   H. paraphrophilus
   H. parasuis
   H. suis
Haemo·pho·ruc·tus
Hae·mo·pis
Hae·mo·pro·te·us
haem·or·rha·gia
hae·mo·spo·rid·i·an
Hae·mo·spo·ri·na
hae·mo·zo·in
Hae·nel's symptom
Haff disease
Haff·kine's vaccine
Haf·nia
   H. alvei
haf·ni·um
Hag·e·dorn needle
Hage·man coagulation factor
Hag·lund's disease
Hag·ner bag
Hahn's sign
hah·ne·man·ni·an
hah·ne·man·nism
hah·ni·um
HAI — hemagglutination
  inhibition
Hai·ding·er's brushes
Haig Fer·gu·son forceps
Hai·ley-Hai·ley disease
Haines' coefficient
Haines' formula
Haines' reagent

Haines' test
hair
   auditory h's
   bamboo h.
   bayonet h.
   beaded h.
   burrowing h.
   club h.
   exclamation point h.
   Frey's h's
   gustatory h's
   ingrown h.
   knotted h.
   lanugo h.
   moniliform h.
   h's of nose
   olfactory h's
   pubic h.
   resting h.
   ringed h.
   sensory h's
   stellate h.
   stinging h's
   tactile h's
   taste h's
   terminal h.
   twisted h.
   vellus h.
hair·cap
hair·cast
hair·worm
Ha·jek's operation
hal·a·tion
hal·az·e·pam
hal·a·zone
Hal·ban sign
Hal·brecht's syndrome
hal·cin·o·nide
Hal·dane apparatus
Hal·dane chamber
Hal·dane's law
Hal·dane-Priest·ley samp·ling
Hal·dol
Hal·drone
Hales' piesimeter
half-cy·cle
half-lay·er

half-life
    antibody h.
    biological h.
    effective h.
    physical h.
    radioactive h.
half-moon
    red h.
half-thick·ness
half-time
    plasma iron clearance h.
half-val·ue
half·way house
hal·ide
ha·lis·te·re·sis
    h. cerea
ha·lis·te·ret·ic
hal·i·to·sis
ha·lit·u·ous
hal·i·tus
    h. saturninus
Hall band
Hall's method
Hall's sign
hall·a·chrome
Hal·lau·er's glasses
Hall·berg effect
Hallé's point
Hal·ler's ansa
Hal·ler's arch
Hal·ler's circle
Hal·ler's cone
Hal·ler's crypt
Hal·ler's duct
Hal·ler's fretum
Hal·ler's habenula
Hal·ler's layer
Hal·ler's line
Hal·ler's membrane
Hal·ler's plexus
Hal·ler's rete
Hal·ler's tripod
Hal·ler·vor·den-Spatz
    syndrome
Hall·gren syndrome
Hal·lion's test
Hal·lo·peau's acrodermatitis

Hal·lo·peau-Sie·mens
    syndrome
hal·lu·cal
hal·lu·ces
hal·lu·ci·na·tion
    auditory h.
    autoscopic h.
    blank h.
    epileptic h.
    gustatory h.
    haptic h.
    hypnagogic h.
    hypnopompic h.
    kinesthetic h.
    lilliputian h.
    microptic h.
    olfactory h.
    h. of perception
    psychomotor h.
    somatic h.
    stump h.
    tactile h.
    visual h.
hal·lu·ci·na·tive
hal·lu·ci·na·to·ry
hal·lu·ci·no·gen
hal·lu·ci·no·gen·e·sis
hal·lu·ci·no·ge·net·ic
hal·lu·ci·no·gen·ic
hal·lu·ci·no·sis
    acute alcoholic h.
    drug-induced h.
    ethanolic h.
    organic h.
hal·lu·ci·not·ic
hal·lux *pl.* hal·lu·ces
    h. dolorosa
    h. flexus
    h. malleus
    h. rigidus
    h. valgus
    h. varus
Hall·wachs effect
hal·ma·to·gen·e·sis
ha·lo
    anemic h.
    Fick's h.
    h. glaucomatosus

ha·lo *(continued)*
   glaucomatous h.
   peripapillary senile h.
   h. saturninus
   senile h.
halo·bac·te·ria
Halo·bac·te·ri·a·ceae
Halo·bac·te·ri·um
halo·bac·te·ri·um *pl.* halo·
  bac·te·ria
Halo·coc·cus
halo·der·mia
halo·du·ric
ha·lo·fen·ate
Hal·og
hal·o·gen
halo·gen·a·tion
hal·o·ge·ton
hal·oid
ha·lom·e·ter
ha·lom·e·try
hal·o·pem·ide
hal·o·peri·dol
hal·o·phil
hal·o·phile
hal·o·phil·ic
hal·o·pre·done ac·e·tate
hal·o·pro·gin
ha·los·te·re·sis
Hal·o·tes·tin
Hal·o·tex
hal·o·thane
ha·lox·on
hal·quin·ol
hal·quin·ols
Hal·sted's operation
Hal·sted's suture
hal·zoun
Ham's test
Ham·a·me·lis
ham·a·me·lis
ham·ar·thri·tis
ham·ar·tia
ham·ar·ti·al
ham·ar·to·blas·to·ma
ha·mar·to·chon·dro·ma·to·sis
ham·ar·to·ma
   chondromatous h.

ham·ar·to·ma *(continued)*
   fetal h.
   leiomyomatous h.
   neuromuscular h.
   renal h.
   temporal h.
ham·ar·to·ma·to·sis
ham·ar·to·ma·tous
ham·ate
ha·ma·tum
Ham·ber·ger phenomenon
Ham·ber·ger's schema
Ham·ber·ger test
Ham·bur·ger interchange
Ham·il·ton's bandage
Ham·il·ton method
Ham·il·ton's test
Ham·man's disease
Ham·man's sign
Ham·man's syndrome
Ham·man-Rich syndrome
Ham·mar·sten's test
ham·mer
Ham·mer·schlag's method
Ham·mer·schlag's test
ham·mock
   pelvic h.
Ham·mond's disease
Hamp·ton's maneuver
ham·ster
   Syrian cardiomyopathic h.
ham·string
   inner h.
   lateral h.
   medial h's
   outer h.
ham·u·lar
ham·u·late
ham·u·lus *pl.* ham·u·li
   h. cochleae
   h. ethmoid bone
   frontal h.
   h. frontalis
   h. of hamate bone
   lacrimal h.
   h. lacrimalis
   h. laminae spiralis
   h. ossis hamati

ham·u·lus *(continued)*
  pterygoid h.
  h. pterygoideus
  trochlear h.
ha·my·cin
Han·cock's amputation
hand
  accoucheur's h.
  ape h.
  apostolic h.
  beat h.
  benediction h.
  Charcot's h.
  claw h.
  cleft h.
  club h.
  dead h.
  drop h.
  fakir's h.
  flat h.
  flipper h.
  frozen h.
  ghoul h.
  griffin-claw h.
  Krukenberg's h.
  lobster-claw h.
  Marinesco's succulent h.
  mirror h's
  mitten h.
  monkey h.
  obstetrician's h.
  opera-glass h.
  phantom h.
  preacher's h.
  skeleton h.
  spade h.
  split h.
  succulent h.
  trench h.
  trident h.
  writing h.
Hand's disease
Hand's syndrome
Hand-Schül·ler-Chris·tian disease
Hand-Schül·ler-Chris·tian syndrome

hand·ed·ness
  left h.
  right h.
han·di·cap
hand·i·capped
  perceptually h.
Hand·ley's method
hand·piece
hand·print
HANE — hereditary angioneurotic edema
Hánf·mann-Ka·sa·nin test
Hang·er's test
hang·nail
Han·hart syndrome
Han·no·ver's canal
Han·ot's cirrhosis
Han·ot's disease
Han·ot's syndrome
Ha·not-Chauf·fard syndrome
Han·sen's bacillus
Han·sen's disease
han·sen·ia·sis
Han·sen·u·la
  H. anomala
haph·al·ge·sia
haphe·pho·bia
Hap·lo·chi·lus
  H. panchax
hap·lo·dip·loi·dy
hap·lo·dont
hap·loid
hap·lo·iden·ti·cal
hap·lo·iden·ti·ty
hap·loi·dy
ha·plo·my·co·sis
hap·lont
hap·lop·a·thy
hap·lo·phase
hap·lo·pia
Hap·lor·chis
  H. taichui
hap·lo·scope
  mirror h.
hap·lo·scop·ic
hap·lo·spo·ran·gin
hap·lo·type

Haps·burg jaw
Haps·burg lip
hap·ten
hap·tene
hap·ten·ic
hap·te·pho·bia
hap·tic
hap·tics
hap·to·glo·bin
hap·tom·e·ter
Ha·ra·da's disease
Ha·ra·da's syndrome
ha·rara
hard·en·ing
Har·den-Young ester
Har·der's glands
hard·er·i·an
hard·ness
    diamond pyramid h.
    permanent h.
    temporary h.
Har·dy-Wein·berg equilibrium
Har·dy-Wein·berg law
Hare's syndrome
hare·lip
har·le·quin
Har·ley's disease
har·ma·line
har·mine
har·mo·nia
har·mon·ic
har·mo·ny
    occlusal h.
    occlusal h., functional
Har·mo·nyl
har·ness
    Pavlik h.
    shoulder h.
har·poon
Har·ring·ton instrumentation
Har·ring·ton's solution
Har·ris hematoxylin
Har·ris line
Har·ris' segregator
Har·ris' separator
Har·ris' staining method
Har·ris' syndrome
Har·ris tube

Har·ris and Ben·e·dict
  standard
Har·ri·son's curve
Har·ri·son's groove
Har·ri·son's sulcus
Har·row·er's hypothesis
Har·tel's treatment
Hart·ley-Krause operation
Hart·line
Hart·man solution
Hart·mann's curet
Hart·mann's fossa
Hart·mann's point
Hart·mann's pouch
Hart·mann's procedure
Hart·mann's speculum
Hart·man·nel·la
hart·man·nel·li·a·sis
Hart·nup syndrome
harts·horn
har·vei·an
har·vest
Har·vey, William
Hä·ser's coefficient
Hä·ser's formula
Hash·i·mo·to's disease
Hash·i·mo·to's struma
Hash·i·mo·to's thyroiditis
hash·ish
Has·ner's fold
Has·ner's valve
Has·sall's bodies
Has·sall's corpuscles
Has·sall-Hen·le warts
HAT — hypoxanthine-aminopt-
  erin-thymidine (medium)
Ha·ta's phenomenon
Ha·ta's preparation
hatch·et
  enamel h.
Hau·dek's niche
Hau·dek's sign
haunch
haupt·gan·gli·on of Kütt·ner
Haust. — L. haustus (a draft)
haus·tel·lum *pl.* haus·tel·la
haus·to·ri·um *pl.* haus·to·ria
haus·tra

haus·tral
haus·tra·tion
haus·trum *pl.* haus·tra
   cecal h.
   haustra coli
haut-mal
HAV — hepatitis A virus
Ha·ven syn·drome
Ha·ver·hill fever
Ha·ver·hil·lia mul·ti·for·mis
ha·ver·sian canal
ha·ver·sian glands
ha·ver·sian lamella
ha·ver·sian space
ha·ver·sian system
Hawes-Pal·lis·ter-Lan·dor
   syndrome
haw·kin·sin
haw·kin·sin·u·ria
Haw·ley appliance
Haw·ley retainer
Hay's test
Ha·yem's corpuscles
Ha·yem's encephalitis
Ha·yem's icterus
Ha·yem's jaundice
Ha·yem-Wi·dal syndrome
hay fe·ver
Hay·flick's phenomenon
Hay·garth's nodes
Hay·garth's nodosities
Ha·zen's theorem
HB — hepatitis B
HB_c — hepatitis B core
   (antigen)
HB_e — hepatitis B e (antigen)
HB_s — hepatitis B surface
   (antigen)
Hb — hemoglobin
HB_cAg — hepatitis B core
   antigen
HB_eAg — hepatitis B e
   antigen
HB_sAg — hepatitis B surface
   antigen
HbCV — *Haemophilus
   influenzae* b conjugate
   vaccine

HbO_2 — oxyhemoglobin
HbPV — *Haemophilus
   influenzae* b. polysaccharide
   vaccine
HBV — hepatitis B virus
HC — hospital corps
HCG — human chorionic
   gonadotropin
hCG — human chorionic
   gonadotropin
HCT — hematocrit
H.d. — L. hora decubitus (at
   bedtime)
HDCV — human diploid cell
   rabies vaccine
HDL — high-density
   lipoprotein
HDL_1 — Lp(a) lipoprotein
HDN — hemolytic disease of
   the newborn
H and E — hematoxylin and
   eosin (stain)
head
   articular h.
   h. of astragalus
   box h.
   h. of caudate nucleus
   drum h.
   engaged h.
   h. of epididymis
   h. of femur
   h. of fibula
   floating h.
   hot cross bun h.
   hourglass h.
   h. of humerus
   little h. of humerus
   little h. of mandible
   h. of malleus
   h. of mandible
   medusa h.
   h. of metacarpal
   h. of metatarsal
   h. of muscle
   h. of optic nerve
   overriding h.
   h. of pancreas
   h. of penis

head *(continued)*
   h. of phalanx of fingers
   h. of phalanx of toes
   radial h. of humerus
   h. of radius
   h. of rib
   saddle h.
   h. of spermatozoon
   h. of spleen
   h. of stapes
   steeple h.
   swelled h.
   h. of talus
   h. of thigh bone
   tower h.
   h. of ulna
   white h.
Head's zones
Head-Holmes syndrome
head·ache
   anemic h.
   bilious h.
   blind h.
   cluster h.
   congestive h.
   cough h.
   drainage h.
   dynamite h.
   fibrositic h.
   functional h.
   helmet h.
   histamine h.
   Horton's h.
   hyperemic h.
   jolt h.
   lumbar puncture h.
   meningeal h.
   migraine h.
   miners' h.
   Monday morning h.
   muscle contraction h.
   neuralgic h.
   nitroglycerin h.
   organic h.
   paraplegic h.
   postconcussional h.
   postspinal h.
   pressor h.

head·ache *(continued)*
   puncture h.
   pyrexial h.
   reflex h.
   rhinogenous h.
   sick h.
   spinal h.
   spinal-fluid loss h.
   symptomatic h.
   tension h.
   thunderclap h.
   toxic h.
   traction h.
   traumatic h.
   vacuum h.
   vascular h.
   vasomotor h.
head·cap
head·gear
head·grit
head·gut
head·light
head-nod·ding
Heaf test
heal
heal·ing
   h. by first intention
   h. by granulation
   h. by second intention
health
   holistic h.
   occupational h.
   public h.
health main·te·nance or·ga·
ni·za·tion (HMO)
healthy
hear·ing
   color h.
   double disharmonic h.
   monaural h.
   residual h.
   visual h.
hear·ing loss
   Alexander's h.l.
   conductive h.l.
   pagetoid h.l.
   paradoxic h.l.
   sensorineural h.l.

hear·ing loss *(continued)*
   transmission h.l.
heart
   abdominal h.
   addisonian h.
   amyloid h.
   armored h.
   artificial h.
   athlete's h.
   athletic h.
   atrophic h.
   beer h.
   beriberi h.
   boat-shaped h.
   bony h.
   booster h.
   bovine h.
   cervical h.
   chaotic h.
   crisscross h.
   drop h.
   dynamite h.
   encased h.
   extracorporeal h.
   fat h.
   fatty h.
   fibroid h.
   flask-shaped h.
   frosted h.
   goiter h.
   hairy h.
   hanging h.
   horizontal h.
   hypertensive h.
   hyperthyroid h.
   hypoplastic h.
   icing h.
   intermediate h.
   intracorporeal h.
   irritable h.
   Jarvik h.
   kyphoscoliotic h.
   left h.
   lymph h.
   mechanical h.
   myxedema h.
   ox h.
   paracorporeal h.

heart *(continued)*
   parchment h.
   pear-shaped h.
   pectoral h.
   pendulous h.
   pulmonary h.
   Quain's fatty h.
   rheumatic h.
   right h.
   round h.
   sabot h.
   scleroderma h.
   semihorizontal h.
   semivertical h.
   soldier's h.
   stony h.
   suspended h.
   systemic h.
   tabby cat h.
   three-chambered h.
   thrush breast h.
   tiger h.
   tiger lily h.
   thyroid h.
   thyrotoxic h.
   tobacco h.
   Traube's h.
   triatrial h.
   trilocular h.
   vertical h.
   wandering h.
   wooden-shoe h.
heart·beat
heart block
   atrioventricular h.b.
   bundle-branch h.b.
   complete h.b.
   congenital h.b.
   incomplete h.b.
   interventricular h.b.
   intraventricular h.b.
   Mobitz h.b.
   partial h.b.
   sinoatrial h.b.
   Wenckebach h.b.
heart·burn
heart fail·ure
   acute congestive h.f.

heart fail·ure *(continued)*
    backward h.f.
    congestive h.f.
    forward h.f.
    high output h.f.
    left-sided h.f.
    left ventricular h.f.
    right-sided h.f.
    right ventricular h.f.
heart·wa·ter
heart·worm
heat
    atomic h.
    h. of compression
    conductive h.
    convective h.
    conversive h.
    dry h.
    h. of fusion
    latent h.
    latent h. of fusion
    latent h. of sublimation
    latent h. of vaporization
    molecular h.
    prickly h.
    radiant h.
    specific h.
    h. of sublimation
    h. of vaporization
heat-la·bile
Heath's operation
heat·ing
    reflex h.
    ultrasonic h.
heat·stroke
    parasternal h.
heaves
    dry h.
Hebdom. — L. hebdomada (a week)
heb·dom·a·dal
he·be·phre·nia
he·be·phren·ic
He·ber·den's asthma
He·ber·den's disease
He·ber·den's nodes
He·ber·den's rheumatism
He·ber·den's signs

he·bet·ic
heb·e·tude
he·bi·at·rics
He·bra's disease
He·bra's prurigo
hec·a·tom·er·al
hec·a·to·mer·ic
Hecht's phenomenon
Hecht's pneumonia
Heck·er's law
hec·to·gram
hec·to·li·ter
hec·tom·e·ter
Hed·in·ger syndrome
he·don·ic
he·do·nism
hed·ro·cele
Hed·u·lin
heel
    anterior h.
    basketball h.
    black h.
    contracted h.
    cracked h's
    gonorrheal h.
    painful h.
    policeman's h.
    prominent h.
    Thomas h.
HEENT — head, eyes, ears, nose, and throat
Heer·fordt's disease
Heer·fordt's syndrome
he·fil·con A
Hef·ke-Tur·ner sign
He·gar's dilator
He·gar's sign
Hegg·lin's anomaly
Hei·berg-Es·march maneuver
Hei·den·hain's cells
Hei·den·hain's law
Hei·den·hain's rods
Hei·den·hain's stain
height
    apex h.
    h. of contour
    h. of contour, surveyed
    cusp h.

height *(continued)*
    facial h.
    midparental h.
    sitting h.
    sitting suprasternal h.
    sitting vertex h.
    standing h.
Heil·bron·ner's sign
Heil·bron·ner's thigh
Heim-Krey·sig sign
Heim·lich maneuver
Heine's operation
Hei·ne-Med·in disease
Hei·ne·ke's operation
Hei·ne·ke-Mik·u·licz operation
Hei·ne·ke-Mik·u·licz pyloroplasty
Heinz bodies
Heinz granules
Heinz-Ehr·lich bodies
Heis·rath's operation
Heis·ter's diverticulum
Heis·ter's fold
Heis·ter's valve
HEK — human embryo kidney (cell culture)
Hek·toen phenomenon
HEL — human embryo lung (cell culture)
HeLa cells
Hel·bing's sign
hel·coid
hel·col·o·gy
hel·co·ma
hel·co·sis
Held's end-bulb
Held's foot
Held's striae
He·le·i·dae
hel·e·nine
he·li·an·thin
he·li·a·tion
hel·i·cal
hel·i·case
He·li·cel·la
He·li·cel·li·dae
hel·i·cin

hel·i·cine
He·li·co·bac·ter
    H. pylori
hel·i·coid
hel·i·co·pod
hel·i·co·po·dia
hel·i·co·tre·ma
he·lio·aero·ther·a·py
he·lio·path·ia
he·lio·sin
he·li·o·sis
he·lio·tax·is
he·lio·ther·a·py
He·li·o·ti·a·les
he·lio·trope B
he·li·ot·ro·pism
he·li·um
he·lix
    α-h.
    alpha h.
    double h.
    Pauling-Corey h.
    Watson-Crick h.
Hel·lat's sign
hel·le·bore
    American h.
    black h.
    green h.
    white h.
Hel·len·dall's sign
Hel·ler's disease
Hel·ler's operation
Hel·ler's plexus
Hel·ler's test
Hel·ler-Döh·le disease
Hel·lin's law
Hel·ly's fixative
Hel·ly's fluid
Helm·holtz's ligament
Helm·holtz's theory
hel·minth
hel·min·tha·gogue
hel·min·them·e·sis
hel·min·thi·a·sis
    cutaneous h.
    h. elastica
hel·min·thic
hel·min·thi·cide

hel·min·thism
hel·min·thoid
hel·min·thol·o·gy
hel·min·tho·ma
hel·min·thous
He·lo·der·ma
he·lo·ma
    h. durum
    h. molle
He·loph·i·lus
he·lo·sis
he·lot·o·my
help·less·ness
    learned h.
Hel·vel·la
Hel·vel·la·ceae
hel·vel·lic acid
Hel·ve·ti·us' ligaments
hel·vol·ic acid
Hel·weg's bundle
Hel·weg's tract
he·ma
hema·chro·ma·to·sis
hema·chrome
he·ma·chro·sis
hema·cyte
hema·cy·tom·e·ter
hema·cy·tom·e·try
hem·ado·ste·no·sis
hem·ad·sor·bent
hem·ad·sorp·tion
    mixed h.
hema·dy·na·mom·e·try
hema·fa·cient
hema·fe·cia
hem·ag·glu·ti·na·tion
    indirect h.
    passive h.
    viral h.
hem·ag·glu·ti·na·tive
hem·ag·glu·ti·nin
    cold h.
    warm h.
he·ma·gog·ic
he·ma·go·ni·um
he·mal
hem·al·um
    Mayer's h.

hem·a·nal·y·sis
hem·an·gi·ec·ta·sia
hem·an·gi·ec·ta·sis
hem·an·gio·amelo·blas·to·ma
hem·an·gio·blast
hem·an·gio·blas·to·ma
    h. retinae
hem·an·gio·blas·to·ma·to·sis
hem·an·gio·en·do·the·lio·blas·to·ma
hem·an·gio·en·do·the·li·o·ma
    benign h.
    infantile h.
    malignant h.
    h. tuberosum multiplex
hem·an·gio·en·do·the·lio·sar·co·ma
hem·an·gio·fi·bro·ma
he·man·gio·glio·ma·to·sis ret·i·nae
he·man·gio·lym·phan·gi·o·ma
hem·an·gi·o·ma
    ameloblastic h.
    capillary h.
    h. cavernosum
    cavernous h.
    cirsoid h.
    h. congenitale
    h. hypertrophicum cutis
    multiple hemorrhagic h. of Kaposi
    h. planum extensum
    racemose h.
    renal h.
    sclerosing h.
    h. simplex
    strawberry h.
    venous h.
    verrucous keratotic h.
hem·an·gio·ma·to·sis
    h. retinae
    systemic h.
he·man·gio·myo·li·po·ma
hem·an·gio·peri·cyte
hem·an·gio·peri·cy·to·ma
    renal h.

hem·an·gio·sar·co·ma
hema·phe·ic
hema·phe·in
hema·phe·ism
hema·phe·re·sis
hema·poi·e·sis
hema·poi·et·ic
hem·a·poph·y·sis
hem·ar·thros
hem·ar·thro·sis
hema·stron·ti·um
hem·a·tal
hem·at·a·pos·te·ma
hem·a·te·in
hem·a·tem·e·sis
   Goldstein's h.
hem·at·en·ceph·a·lon
hema·ther·a·py
hema·ther·mal
hema·ther·mous
hema·tho·rax
he·mat·ic
hem·a·tid
hem·at·idro·sis
hem·a·tim·e·ter
hem·a·tim·e·try
hem·a·tin
   acid h.
hem·a·tin·emia
hem·a·tin·ic
hem·a·tin·om·e·ter
hem·a·tin·uria
hem·a·to·bil·ia
hem·a·to·bi·um *pl.* hem·a·to·bia
hem·a·to·blast
   Hayem's h.
hem·a·to·cele
   pudendal h.
   rectouterine h.
   retrouterine h.
   scrotal h.
   vaginal h.
hem·a·to·ce·lia
hem·a·to·ceph·a·lus
hem·a·to·che·zia
hem·a·to·chlo·rin
hem·a·to·chro·ma·to·sis

hem·a·to·chy·lo·cele
hem·a·to·chy·lu·ria
hem·a·to·coe·lia
hem·a·to·col·po·me·tra
hem·a·to·col·pos
he·ma·to·crit
   heelstick h.
   large vessel h.
   total body h.
   whole body h.
   Wintrobe h.
hem·a·toc·ry·al
hem·a·to·cy·a·nin
hem·a·to·cyst
hem·a·to·cys·tis
hem·a·to·cyte
hem·a·to·cy·to·blast
hem·a·to·cy·tol·y·sis
hem·a·to·cy·tom·e·ter
hem·a·to·cy·to·pe·nia
hem·a·to·cy·to·sis
hem·a·to·cy·tu·ria
hem·a·to·di·al·y·sis
hem·a·to·dys·cra·sia
hem·a·to·dys·tro·phy
hem·a·to·en·ce·phal·ic
hem·a·to·gen·e·sis
hem·a·to·gen·ic
hem·a·tog·e·nous
hem·a·to·glo·bin
hem·a·to·glo·bin·uria
hem·a·to·gone
hem·a·to·hid·ro·sis
he·ma·to·his·tio·blast
hem·a·to·hy·a·loid
hem·a·toid
hem·a·toid·in
hem·a·to·kol·pos
hem·a·tol·o·gist
hem·a·tol·o·gy
hem·a·to·lymph·an·gi·o·ma
hem·a·tol·y·sis
hem·a·to·lyt·ic
hem·a·to·ma *pl.* hem·a·tomas
   aneurysmal h.
   h. auris
   cystic h.
   dissecting h.

hem·a·to·ma *(continued)*
    epidural h.
    intracerebral h.
    intramural h.
    nasal septum h.
    pelvic h.
    perianal h.
    perinephric h.
    puerperal h.
    retroperitoneal h.
    retrouterine h.
    subchorionic tuberous h.
    subdural h.
    subungual h.
    tuberous subchorial h.
hem·a·to·ma·nom·e·ter
hem·a·to·me·di·as·ti·num
hem·a·to·meta·ki·ne·sis
hem·a·tom·e·ter
hem·a·tom·e·tra
hem·a·tom·e·try
he·ma·to·mole
hem·at·om·pha·lo·cele
hem·at·om·pha·lus
he·ma·to·my·e·lia
he·ma·to·my·eli·tis
he·ma·to·my·elo·pore
hem·a·to·ne·phro·sis
he·ma·ton·ic
hem·a·to·pa·thol·o·gy
hem·a·to·pe·nia
he·ma·to·peri·car·di·um
he·ma·to·peri·to·ne·um
hem·a·to·phage
hem·a·to·pha·gia
he·ma·to·phago·cyte
hem·a·toph·a·gous
hem·a·toph·a·gy
hem·a·to·phil·ia
hem·a·to·pho·bia
hem·a·to·phyte
hem·a·to·phyt·ic
hem·a·to·pi·e·sis
hem·a·to·plast
hem·a·to·plas·tic
hem·a·to·poi·e·sis
    extramedullary h.
hem·a·to·poi·et·ic

hem·a·to·poi·e·tin
hem·a·to·por·phy·ria
hem·a·to·por·phy·rin
hem·a·to·por·phy·rin·emia
hem·a·to·por·phy·rin·ism
hem·a·to·por·phy·rin·uria
hem·a·tor·rha·chis
    h. externa
    h. interna
hem·a·tor·rhea
hem·a·to·sal·pinx
hem·a·to·sar·co·ma
he·ma·tos·cheo·cele
hem·a·to·sep·sis
hem·a·to·spec·tro·pho·tom·e·ter
hem·a·to·spec·tro·scope
hem·a·to·spec·tros·co·py
he·ma·to·sper·mato·cele
hem·a·to·sper·mia
hem·a·to·spher·in·emia
hem·a·to·stat·ic
hem·a·tos·te·on
hem·a·to·ther·a·py
hem·a·to·ther·mal
hem·a·to·tho·rax
hem·a·to·tox·ic
hem·a·to·tox·i·co·sis
hem·a·to·tox·in
hem·a·to·tra·che·los
hem·a·to·trop·ic
hem·a·to·tym·pa·num
hem·a·tox·ic
he·ma·tox·y·lin
    alum h.
    Delafield's h.
    Ehrlich's h.
    Harris h.
    Heidenhain's iron h.
    iron h.
    Weigert's iron h.
hem·a·to·ze·mia
hem·a·to·zoa
he·ma·to·zo·al
hem·a·to·zo·an
hem·a·to·zo·ic
hem·a·to·zo·on *pl.* hem·a·to·zoa

hem·a·tu·re·sis
hem·a·tu·ria
   benign recurrent h.
   Egyptian h.
   endemic h.
   essential h.
   false h.
   hereditary h.
   initial h.
   microscopic h.
   primary h.
   recurrent h.
   renal h.
   terminal h.
   total h.
   urethral h.
   vesical h.
heme
hem·en·do·the·li·o·ma
hem·er·al·ope
hem·er·a·lo·pia
Hem·ero·cam·pa
   H. leukostigma
hem·eryth·rin
heme syn·the·tase
hemi·acar·di·us
hemi·aceph·a·lus
hemi·ac·e·tal
hemi·achro·ma·top·sia
hemi·ac·i·drin
hemi·agen·e·sis
hemi·ageu·sia
hemi·ageus·tia
hemi·ag·no·sia
   h. for pain
hemi·al·bu·min
hemi·al·bu·mose
hemi·al·bu·mos·uria
hemi·al·gia
hemi·am·bly·o·pia
hemi·amy·os·the·nia
hemi·an·acu·sia
hemi·an·al·ge·sia
hemi·an·en·ceph·a·ly
hemi·an·es·the·sia
   alternate h.
   bulbar h.
   cerebral h.

hemi·an·es·the·sia *(continued)*
   crossed h.
   h. cruciata
   mesocephalic h.
   pontile h.
   peduncular h.
   spinal h.
hemi·an·o·pia
   absolute h.
   altitudinal h.
   bilateral h.
   binasal h.
   binocular h.
   bitemporal h.
   color h.
   complete h.
   congruous h.
   crossed h.
   heteronymous h.
   homonymous h.
   horizontal h.
   incomplete h.
   incongruous h.
   lateral h.
   nasal h.
   quadrant h.
   quadrantic h.
   relative h.
   temporal h.
   true h.
   unilateral h.
hemi·an·op·ic
hemi·an·op·sia
hemi·an·op·tic
hemi·an·os·mia
hemi·aprax·ia
hemi·ar·thro·sis
hemi·as·co·my·ce·ti·dae
hemi·aso·ma·tog·no·sia
hemi·asyn·er·gia
hemi·atax·ia
hemi·ath·e·to·sis
hemi·ato·nia
hemi·at·ro·phy
   facial h.
   progressive lingual h.
   Romberg's progressive
      facial h.

hemi·ax·i·al
hemi·bal·lism
hemi·bal·lis·mus
hemi·blad·der
hemi·block
he·mic
hemi·ca·nit·i·es
hemi·car·dia
   h. dextra
   h. sinistra
hemi·car·di·us
hemi·cel·lu·lose
hemi·cen·trum
hemi·ceph·a·lal·gia
hemi·ce·pha·lia
hemi·ceph·a·lus
hemi·ceph·a·ly
hemi·cer·e·brum
hemi·cho·rea
   paralytic h.
   posthemiplegic h.
   preparalytic h.
hemi·chro·ma·top·sia
hemi·chrome
hemi·co·lec·to·my
   left h.
   right h.
hemi·cor·por·ec·to·my
hemi·cor·ti·cec·to·my
hemi·cra·nia
hemi·cra·ni·ec·to·my
hemi·cra·ni·o·sis
hemi·cra·ni·ot·o·my
hemi·de·cor·ti·ca·tion
hemi·des·mo·some
Hemi·des·mus
hemi·dia·pho·re·sis
hemi·dia·phragm
hem·idro·sis
hemi·dys·er·gia
hemi·dys·es·the·sia
hemi·dys·tro·phy
hemi·ec·tro·me·lia
hemi·elas·tin
hemi·en·ceph·a·lon
hemi·en·ceph·a·lus
hemi·epi·lep·sy
hemi·fa·cial

hemi·gas·trec·to·my
hemi·geu·sia
hemi·gi·gan·tism
hemi·glos·sal
hemi·glos·sec·to·my
hemi·glos·si·tis
hemi·glos·so·ple·gia
hemi·gna·thia
hemi·hep·a·tec·to·my
hemi·hi·dro·sis
hemi·hy·dran·en·ceph·a·ly
hemi·hy·pal·ge·sia
hemi·hy·per·es·the·sia
hemi·hy·per·hi·dro·sis
hemi·hy·per·idro·sis
hemi·hy·per·me·tria
hemi·hy·per·pla·sia
hemi·hy·per·to·nia
hemi·hy·per·tro·phy
   facial h.
hemi·hy·pes·the·sia
hemi·hy·po·es·the·sia
hemi·hy·po·geu·sia
hemi·hy·po·me·tria
hemi·hy·po·pla·sia
hemi·hy·po·ther·mia
hemi·hy·po·to·nia
hemi·kary·on
hemi·ke·tal
hemi·lam·i·nec·to·my
hemi·lar·yn·gec·to·my
   horizontal h.
   vertical h.
hemi·lar·ynx
hemi·lat·er·al
hemi·le·sion
hemi·lin·gual
hemi·mac·ro·ceph·a·ly
hemi·ma·cro·glos·sia
hemi·man·di·ble
hemi·man·dib·u·lec·to·my
hemi·man·dib·u·lo·glos·sec·
   to·my
hemi·max·il·lec·to·my
hemi·me·lia
   axial h.
   fibular h.
   radial h.

hemi·me·lia *(continued)*
    tibial h.
    transverse h.
    ulnar h.
hem·im·e·lus
hemi·me·tab·o·lous
he·min
hemi·ne·phrec·to·my
hemi·neph·ro·ure·ter·ec·to·my
hemi·obe·si·ty
hemi·op·al·gia
hemi·opia
hemi·op·ic
hem·ip·a·gus
hemi·pa·ral·y·sis
hemi·par·an·es·the·sia
hemi·par·a·ple·gia
hemi·pa·re·sis
hemi·par·es·the·sia
hemi·pa·ret·ic
hemi·par·kin·son·ism
hemi·pel·vec·to·my
hemi·pel·vis
hemi·pel·vi·sec·to·my
hemi·pep·tone
hemi·phal·an·gec·to·my
hemi·pla·cen·ta
hemi·ple·gia
    h. alternans hypoglossica
    alternate h.
    alternating oculomotor h.
    ascending h.
    Avellis h.
    bulbar h.
    capsular h.
    cerebellar h.
    cerebral h.
    collateral h.
    congenital h.
    contralateral h.
    crossed h.
    h. cruciata
    facial h.
    faciobrachial h.
    faciolingual h.
    flaccid h.
    functional h.

hemi·ple·gia *(continued)*
    Gubler's h.
    hysterical h.
    infantile h.
    organic h.
    peduncular h.
    pontine h.
    puerperal h.
    spastic h.
    spinal h.
    superior alternate h.
    Wernicke-Mann h.
hemi·ple·gic
hemi·pros·o·ple·gia
hemi·pros·ta·tec·to·my
He·mip·tera
he·mip·ter·ous
hemi·py·lor·ec·to·my
hemi·pyo·cy·a·nin
hemi·pyo·ne·phro·sis
hemi·ra·chis·chi·sis
hemi·sa·cral·iza·tion
hemi·sco·to·sis
hemi·sec·tion
    h. of spinal cord
hemi·sec·to·my
hemi·sep·tum
    h. cerebri
hemi·so·mus
hem·iso·ton·ic
hemi·spasm
    facial h.
    glossolabial h.
hemi·sphere
    cerebellar h.
    cerebral h.
    dominant h.
    nondominant h.
    talking h.
hemi·spher·ec·to·my
hemi·sphe·ri·um *pl.* hemi·sphe·ria
    h. bulbi urethrae
    h. cerebelli
    h. cerebralis
    h. cerebri
hemi·sphyg·mia
Hem·is·po·ra stel·la·ta

hemi·spore
hemi·syn·drome
hemi·ter·a·ta
hemi·ter·at·ic
hemi·ter·pene
hemi·tet·a·ny
hemi·ther·mo·an·es·the·sia
hemi·tho·rax
hemi·thy·roi·dec·to·my
hemi·to·mi·as
hemi·to·nia
hemi·tox·in
hemi·tre·mor
hemi·va·got·o·ny
hemi·ver·te·bra
hemi·zy·gos·i·ty
hemi·zy·gote
hemi·zy·gous
hem·lock
    poison h.
    water h.
he·mo·ac·cess
he·mo·ag·glu·ti·na·tion
he·mo·ag·glu·ti·nin
he·mo·bil·ia
he·mo·bi·lin·uria
he·mo·blast
    lymphoid h. of Pappenheim
he·mo·ca·ther·e·sis
he·mo·cath·er·et·ic
He·moc·cult
he·mo·cho·le·cyst
he·mo·cho·le·cys·ti·tis
he·mo·cho·ri·al
he·mo·chro·ma·to·sis
    exogenous h.
he·mo·chro·ma·tot·ic
he·mo·chrome
he·mo·chro·mo·gen
    hemoglobin h.
he·mo·chro·mom·e·ter
he·mo·chro·mom·e·try
he·mo·cla·sia
he·mo·cla·sis
he·mo·clas·tic
he·mo·clip
he·mo·co·ag·u·lin
he·mo·coel

he·mo·coe·lom
he·mo·coe·lo·ma
he·mo·con·cen·tra·tion
he·mo·co·nia
he·mo·co·ni·o·sis
he·mo·crine
he·mo·cry·os·co·py
he·mo·cul·ture
he·mo·cu·pre·in
he·mo·cy·a·nin
    keyhole-limpet h. (KLH)
he·mo·cyte
he·mo·cy·to·blast
he·mo·cy·to·blas·to·ma
he·mo·cy·to·ca·ther·e·sis
he·mo·cy·to·gen·e·sis
he·mo·cy·to·lyt·ic
he·mo·cy·to·ma
he·mo·cy·tom·e·ter
he·mo·cy·tom·e·try
he·mo·cy·to·pha·gia
he·mo·cy·to·phag·ic
he·mo·cy·to·poi·e·sis
he·mo·cy·to·trip·sis
he·mo·dia·fil·tra·tion
he·mo·di·ag·no·sis
he·mo·di·al·y·sis
    sequential ultrafiltration h.
    simultaneous h. and hemofiltration
he·mo·di·a·lyz·er
    ultrafiltration h.
he·mo·di·a·pe·de·sis
he·mo·di·lu·tion
he·mo·dro·mog·ra·phy
he·mo·dy·nam·ic
he·mo·dy·nam·ics
he·mo·dy·na·mom·e·try
he·mo·dys·cra·sia
he·mo·dys·tro·phy
he·mo·en·do·the·li·al
He·mo·fil
he·mo·fil·ter
he·mo·fil·tra·tion
    continuous arteriovenous h.

he·mo·fil·tra·tion *(continued)*
    simultaneous hemodialysis
      and h.
he·mo·flag·el·late
he·mo·fus·cin
he·mo·gen·e·sis
he·mo·gen·ic
he·mo·glo·bin
    h. A
    h. A_{1c}
    h. A_2
    Bart's h.
    h. C
    h. carbamate
    h. Chesapeake
    h. Constant Spring
    h. D
    deoxygenated h.
    h. E
    h. F
    "fast" h's
    fetal h.
    glycosylated h.
    Gower h.
    h. Gun Hill
    h. H
    homozygous h. (C, D, or E)
    h. I
    h. J
    h. K
    h. Köln
    h. Lepore
    h. M
    mean corpuscular h.
    muscle h.
    h. N
    h. O
    oxidized h.
    oxygenated h.
    pyridoxilated stroma-free
      h.
    h. Rainier
    reduced h.
    h. S
    h. Seattle
    sickle h.
    "slow" h's
    unstable h.

he·mo·glo·bin *(continued)*
    h. Yakima
    h. Zürich
he·mo·glo·bin·at·ed
he·mo·glo·bin·emia
he·mo·glo·bino·cho·lia
he·mo·glo·bin·ol·y·sis
he·mo·glo·bin·om·e·ter
he·mo·glo·bin·om·e·try
he·mo·glo·bin·op·a·thy
he·mo·glo·bi·nous
he·mo·glo·bin·uria
    bacillary h.
    bovine h.
    intermittent h.
    malarial h.
    march h.
    paroxysmal cold h.
    paroxysmal nocturnal h.
      (PNH)
    toxic h.
he·mo·glo·bin·uric
he·mo·gram
he·mo·his·tio·blast
he·mo·ki·ne·sis
he·mo·ki·net·ic
he·mol·o·gy
he·mo·lymph
he·mo·lymph·ad·e·no·sis
he·mo·lymph·an·gi·o·ma
he·mo·lym·pho·cy·to·tox·in
he·mol·y·sate
he·mol·y·sin
    acid h.
    alpha h.
    bacterial h.
    beta h.
    cold h.
    heterophile h.
    hot-cold h.
    immune h.
    natural h.
    specific h.
he·mol·y·sis
    alpha h.
    beta h.
    contact h.
    gamma h.

he·mol·y·sis *(continued)*
   immune h.
   osmotic h.
   passive h.
   siderogenous h.
   venom h.
   viridans h.
he·mo·lyt·ic
he·mo·lyz·a·ble
he·mo·ly·za·tion
he·mo·lyze
he·mo·ma·nom·e·ter
he·mo·ma·nom·e·try
he·mo·me·di·as·ti·num
he·mom·e·ter
he·mo·me·tra
he·mom·e·try
he·mo·my·elo·sis
he·mo·ne·phro·sis
he·mo·nor·mo·blast
he·mo·path·ic
he·mo·pa·thol·o·gy
he·mop·a·thy
he·mo·per·fu·sion
   charcoal h.
   resin h.
he·mo·peri·car·di·um
he·mo·peri·to·ne·um
he·mo·pex·in
he·mo·phage
he·mo·phago·cyte
he·mo·phago·cy·to·sis
he·mo·phil
he·mo·phil·ia
   h. A
   h. B
   h. B, Leyden
   h. C
   classical h.
   h. neonatorum
   vascular h.
he·mo·phil·i·ac
he·mo·phil·ic
he·mo·phil·i·oid
he·moph·i·lus
he·mo·pho·bia
he·mo·pho·re·sis
he·moph·thal·mia

he·moph·thal·mos
he·mo·phthi·sis
he·mo·pi·ezom·e·ter
he·mo·plas·mop·a·thy
he·mo·plas·tic
he·mo·pleu·ra
he·mo·pneu·mo·peri·car·di·um
he·mo·pneu·mo·tho·rax
he·mo·poi·e·sic
he·mo·poi·e·sis
he·mo·poi·et·ic
he·mo·poi·e·tin
he·mo·po·sia
he·mo·pre·cip·i·tin
he·mo·proc·tia
he·mo·pro·tein
he·mo·pro·to·zoa
he·mop·so·nin
he·mop·tic
he·mop·to·ic
he·mop·ty·sic
he·mop·ty·sis
   cardiac h.
   endemic h.
   Goldstein's h.
   Manson's h.
   oriental h.
   parasitic h.
   vicarious h.
he·mo·py·elec·ta·sis
he·mo·re·pel·lant
he·mo·rhe·ol·o·gy
he·mor·rha·chis
he·mor·rhage
   accidental antepartum h.
   alveolar h.
   arterial h.
   brain h.
   capillary h.
   capsular h.
   capsuloganglionic h.
   cerebellar h.
   cerebral h.
   concealed h.
   critical h.
   epidural h.
   essential h.

he·mor·rhage *(continued)*
  expulsive h.
  external h.
  extradural h.
  fetomaternal h.
  fibrinolytic h.
  flame-shaped h's
  glomerular h.
  gravitating h.
  internal h.
  intracerebral h.
  intracranial h.
  intradural h.
  intramedullary h.
  intrapartum h.
  intraventricular h.
  massive h.
  meningeal h.
  nasal h.
  neonatal subdural h.
  parenchymatous h.
  h. per rhexin
  petechial h.
  pontine h.
  postpartum h.
  primary h.
  pulmonary h.
  punctate h.
  recurring h.
  renal h.
  salmon-patch h.
  secondary h.
  slit h.
  splinter h's
  spontaneous h.
  subarachnoid h.
  subconjunctival h.
  subdural h.
  subgaleal h.
  subhyaloid h.
  unavoidable h.
  uterine h., essential
  venous h.
he·mor·rha·gen·ic
he·mor·rha·gic
he·mor·rha·gin
he·mor·rhag·ip·a·rous
he·mor·rhea

he·mor·rhe·ol·o·gy
he·mor·rhoid
  combined h.
  external h.
  internal h.
  mixed h.
  mucocutaneous h.
  prolapsed h.
  strangulated h.
  thrombosed h.
he·mor·rhoi·dal
he·mor·rhoid·ec·to·my
he·mor·rhoi·dol·y·sis
he·mo·sal·pinx
he·mo·sid·er·in
he·mo·sid·er·in·uria
he·mo·sid·er·o·sis
  hepatic h.
  nutritional h.
  pulmonary h.
  transfusional h.
he·mo·sper·mia
he·mo·spo·ri·an
he·mo·spo·rid·i·an
he·mo·spo·rine
he·mo·sta·sia
he·mo·sta·sis
he·mo·stat
he·mo·stat·ic
  capillary h.
he·mo·styp·tic
he·mo·ther·a·peu·tics
he·mo·ther·a·py
he·mo·tho·rax
he·mo·tox·ic
he·mo·tox·ic·i·ty
he·mo·tox·in
  cobra h.
he·mo·troph
he·mo·trophe
he·mo·troph·ic
he·mo·trop·ic
he·mo·tym·pa·num
he·mo·zo·ic
he·mo·zo·in
he·mo·zo·on
  American h.
  Indian h.

hem·ure·sis
hen·bane
Hench, Philip Showalter
Hench-Al·drich index
Hench-Al·drich test
Hen·der·son-Has·sel·balch
  equation
Hen·der·son-Jones disease
Hen·der·so·nu·la
hen·der·so·nu·lo·sis
Hen·ke's space
Hen·ke's triangle
Hen·ke's trigone
Hen·le's ampulla
Hen·le's ansa
Hen·le's canal
Hen·le's cell
Hen·le's fiber
Hen·le's fissure
Hen·le's gland
Hen·le's layer
Hen·le's ligament
Hen·le's loop
Hen·le's membrane
Hen·le's reaction
Hen·le's sheath
Hen·le's sphincter
Hen·le's spine
Hen·le's tubule
Hen·le-Coe·nen sign
Hen·le-Coe·nen test
hen·na
Henne·berg's disease
Henne·bert's sign
Henne·bert's test
Hen·ning's sign
He·noch's chorea
He·noch's disease
He·noch's purpura
He·noch-Schön·lein purpura
He·noch-Schön·lein syndrome
heno·gen·e·sis
hen·pu·ye
hen·ry
Hen·ry's classification
Hen·ry's law
Hen·ry's melanin test
Hen·ry's system

Hen·sen's body
Hen·sen's canal
Hen·sen's cell
Hen·sen's disk
Hen·sen's duct
Hen·sen's knot
Hen·sen's line
Hen·sen's node
Hen·shaw test
Hen·sing's fold
Hen·sing's ligament
he·par
  h. adiposum
  h. lobatum
  h. siccatum
hep·a·ran-α-glu·co·sam·i·
  nide ac·e·tyl·trans·fer·ase
hep·a·ran *N*-sul·fa·tase
hep·a·ran sul·fate
hep·a·ran sul·fate sul·fam·i·
  dase
hep·a·ran sul·fate sul·fa·tase
hep·a·rin
  h. sodium
hep·a·rin·ate
hep·a·rin·emia
hep·ar·i·nize
hep·a·ri·tin sul·fate
hep·a·ri·ti·nur·ia
hep·a·tal·gia
hep·a·ta·tro·phia
hep·a·tat·ro·phy
hep·a·tec·to·mize
hep·a·tec·to·my
he·pat·ic
he·pat·i·co·cho·lan·gio·je·ju·
  nos·to·my
he·pat·i·co·cho·led·o·chos·
  to·my
he·pat·i·co·do·chot·o·my
he·pat·i·co·du·o·de·nos·to·
  my
he·pat·i·co·en·ter·os·to·my
he·pat·i·co·gas·tros·to·my
he·pat·i·co·je·ju·nos·to·my
he·pat·i·co·li·a·sis
he·pat·i·co·li·thot·o·my
he·pat·i·co·litho·trip·sy

he·pat·i·co·pul·mo·nary
he·pat·i·cos·to·my
he·pat·i·cot·o·my
hep·a·tism
he·pa·tit·ic
hep·a·ti·tis *pl.* hep·a·ti·ti·des
  h. A.
  acute parenchymatous h.
  alcoholic h.
  amebic h.
  anicteric h.
  autoimmune h.
  h. B.
  h. C
  cholangiolitic h.
  cholangitic h.
  cholestatic h.
  chronic active h.
  chronic aggressive h.
  chronic interstitial h.
  chronic persisting h.
  h. contagiosa canis
  delta h.
  drug-induced h.
  h. E
  enterically transmitted
    non-A, non-B h.
    (ET-NANB)
  epidemic h.
  h. externa
  familial h.
  fulminant h.
  giant cell h.
  halothane h.
  homologous serum h.
  infectious h.
  inoculation h.
  ischemic h.
  long-incubation h.
  lupoid h.
  neonatal h.
  neonatal giant cell h.
  non-A, non-B h.
  plasma cell h.
  post-transfusion h.
  serum h.
  short-incubation h.
  subacute h.

hep·a·ti·tis *(continued)*
  toxic h.
  toxipathic h.
  transfusion h.
  viral h.
hep·a·ti·za·tion
  gray h.
  red h.
  yellow h.
hep·a·tized
hep·a·to·bil·i·ary
hep·a·to·blast
hep·a·to·blas·to·ma
hep·a·to·bron·chi·al
hep·a·to·car·ci·no·gen·e·sis
hep·a·to·car·cin·o·gen·ic
hep·a·to·car·ci·no·ma
hep·a·to·cele
hep·a·to·cel·lu·lar
hep·a·to·cer·e·bral
hep·a·to·cho·lan·ge·itis
hep·a·to·cho·lan·gio·car·ci·
  no·ma
hep·a·to·cho·lan·gio·du·o·
  de·nos·to·my
hep·a·to·cho·lan·gio·ent·er·
  os·to·my
hep·a·to·cho·lan·gio·gas·
  tros·to·my
hep·a·to·cho·lan·gio·je·ju·
  nos·to·my
hep·a·to·cho·lan·gi·os·to·my
hep·a·to·cho·lan·gi·tis
hep·a·to·cir·rho·sis
hep·a·to·col·ic
hep·a·to·cu·prein
hep·a·to·cys·tic
hep·a·to·cyte
hep·a·to·du·o·de·nal
hep·a·to·du·o·de·nos·to·my
hep·a·to·dyn·ia
hep·a·to·dys·tro·phy
hep·a·to·en·ter·ic
hep·a·to·en·ter·os·to·my
hep·a·to·fla·vin
hep·a·tof·u·gal
hep·a·to·gas·tric
hep·a·to·gen·ic

hep·a·tog·e·nous
hep·a·to·gram
    emission h.
    radionuclide h.
hep·a·tog·ra·phy
hep·a·to·he·mia
hep·a·toid
hep·a·to·jug·u·lar
hep·a·to·len·tic·u·lar
hep·a·to·li·e·nal
hep·a·to·li·e·nog·ra·phy
hep·a·to·li·e·no·meg·a·ly
hep·a·to·lith
hep·a·to·li·thec·to·my
hep·a·to·li·thi·a·sis
hep·a·tol·o·gist
hep·a·tol·o·gy
hep·a·tol·y·sin
hep·a·tol·y·sis
hep·a·to·lyt·ic
hep·a·to·ma
    malignant h.
hep·a·to·ma·la·cia
hep·a·to·me·ga·lia
    h. glycogenica
hep·a·to·meg·a·ly
    glycogenic h.
hep·a·to·mel·a·no·sis
hep·a·tom·e·try
hep·a·tom·pha·lo·cele
hep·a·tom·pha·los
hep·a·to·neph·ric
hep·a·to·ne·phrit·ic
hep·a·to·ne·phri·tis
hep·a·to·neph·ro·meg·a·ly
hep·a·to·pan·cre·as
hep·a·to·path
hep·a·to·path·ic
hep·a·top·a·thy
hep·a·to·peri·to·ni·tis
hep·a·top·e·tal
hep·a·to·pexy
hep·a·to·phage
hep·a·to·phle·bi·tis
hep·a·to·phle·bog·ra·phy
hep·a·to·pleu·ral
hep·a·to·pneu·mon·ic
hep·a·to·por·tal

hep·a·top·to·sis
hep·a·to·pul·mo·nary
hep·a·to·re·nal
hep·a·tor·rha·gia
hep·a·tor·rha·phy
hep·a·tor·rhea
hep·a·tor·rhex·ia
hep·a·tor·rhex·is
hep·a·to·scan
hep·a·tos·co·py
hep·a·to·sis
    serous h.
hep·a·to·so·le·no·trop·ic
hep·a·to·splen·ic
hep·a·to·sple·ni·tis
hep·a·to·sple·nog·ra·phy
hep·a·to·sple·no·meg·a·ly
hep·a·to·sple·nom·e·try
hep·a·to·sple·nop·a·thy
hep·a·tos·to·my
hep·a·to·ther·a·py
hep·a·tot·o·my
    transthoracic h.
hep·a·to·tox·emia
hep·a·to·tox·ic
hep·a·to·tox·i·ci·ty
hep·a·to·tox·in
hep·a·to·trop·ic
hep·a·to·ve·sic·u·lar
hep·a·tox·ic
hep·a·to·zoo·no·sis
Hep·i·ce·brin
hep·ta·bar·bi·tal
hep·ta·chro·mic
hep·tad
hep·ta·dac·ty·ly
hep·ta·ene
hep·ta·nal
hep·ta·pep·tide
hep·ta·tom·ic
hep·ta·va·lent
Hep·ta·vax-B
hep·to·glo·bin
hep·to·glo·bin·emia
hep·tose
hep·tos·uria
hep·tyl·pen·i·cil·lin

herb
    death's h.
    vulnerary h.
her·ba·ceous
her·bal
her·bal·ist
Her·bert's operation
Her·bert's pits
Herb. recent. — L. herbarium
  recentium (of fresh herbs)
Herbst's corpuscles
he·red·i·tary
he·red·i·ty
    autosomal h.
    dominant h.
    sex-linked h.
    X-linked
her·e·do·atax·ia
her·e·do·de·gen·er·a·tion
    spinocerebellar h.
her·e·do·di·ath·e·sis
her·e·do·fa·mil·i·al
her·e·do·in·fec·tion
her·e·do·lu·es
her·e·do·lu·et·ic
her·e·do·path·ia
    h. atactica
      polyneuritiformis
her·e·do·ret·i·no·path·ia
  con·gen·i·ta
her·e·do·syph·i·lis
her·e·do·syph·i·lit·ic
her·e·do·syph·i·lol·o·gy
Her·ing's law
Her·ing's nerve
Her·ing's phenomenon
Her·ing's test
Her·ing's theory
Her·ing-Breu·er reflex
her·i·ta·bil·i·ty
her·i·ta·ble
Her·litz's disease
Her·mann-Pe·rutz reaction
Her·mann-Pe·rutz test
Her·man·sky-Pud·lak
  syndrome
her·maph·ro·dism

her·maph·ro·dite
    pseudo-h.
    true h.
her·ma·phro·dit·ic
her·maph·ro·di·tism
    bilateral h.
    h. with excess
    false h.
    lateral h.
    ovotesticular h.
    protandrous h.
    protogynous h.
    spurious h.
    synchronous h.
    transverse h.
    true h.
    unilateral h.
her·maph·ro·di·tis·mus
    h. verus
    h. verus bilateralis
    h. verus lateralis
    h. verus unilateralis
Her·me·tia il·lu·cens
her·met·ic
her·met·i·cal·ly
her·nia
    abdominal h.
    acquired h.
    h. adiposa
    annular h.
    axial hiatal h.
    Barth's h.
    Béclard's h.
    Birkett's h.
    Bochdalek's h.
    h. of broad ligament of
      uterus
    cecal h.
    h. cerebri
    Cheatle-Henry h.
    Cloquet's h.
    complete h.
    concealed h.
    congenital h.
    congenital diaphragmatic
      h.
    Cooper's h.

her·nia *(continued)*
  crural h.
  diaphragmatic h.
  direct h.
  diverticular h.
  dry h.
  duodenojejunal h.
  encysted h.
  epigastric h.
  exomphalos h.
  external h.
  extrasaccular h.
  fat h.
  femoral h.
  foraminal h.
  funicular h.
  gastroesophageal h.
  Grynfeltt h.
  Hesselbach's h.
  Hey's h.
  hiatal h.
  hiatus h.
  Holthouse's h.
  incarcerated h.
  incisional h.
  incomplete h.
  indirect h.
  infantile h.
  inguinal h.
  inguinocrural h.
  inguinofemoral h.
  inguinoproperitoneal h.
  inguinosuperficial h.
  intermuscular h.
  internal h.
  interparietal h.
  intersigmoid h.
  interstitial h.
  internal hernia
  intra-abdominal h.
  intraperitoneal h.
  irreducible h.
  ischiatic h.
  ischiorectal h.
  Krönlein's h.
  labial h.
  Laugier's h.
  levator h.

her·nia *(continued)*
  Littre's h.
  lumbar h.
  mesenteric h.
  mesocolic h.
  Morgagni's h.
  oblique h.
  obturator h.
  omental h.
  ovarian h.
  paraduodenal h.
  paraesophageal h.
  parahiatal h.
  paraperitoneal h.
  parasaccular h.
  paraumbilical h.
  parietal h.
  pectineal h.
  perineal h.
  Petit's h.
  posterior vaginal h.
  prevascular h.
  properitoneal h.
  pudendal h.
  pulsion h.
  rectal h.
  rectovaginal h.
  reducible h.
  retrocecal h.
  retrograde h.
  retroperitoneal h.
  retrovascular h.
  Richter's h.
  Rieux's h.
  Rokitansky's h.
  rolling h.
  sciatic h.
  scrotal h.
  Serafini's h.
  sliding h.
  sliding hiatal h.
  slip h.
  slipped h.
  spigelian h.
  strangulated h.
  synovial h.
  tentorial h.
  tonsillar h.

her·nia *(continued)*
    transmesenteric h.
    Treitz's h.
    umbilical h.
    h. uteri inguinale
    uterine h.
    vaginal h.
    vaginolabial h.
    Velpeau's h.
    ventral h.
    vesical h.
    W h.
her·ni·al
her·ni·at·ed
her·ni·a·tion
    caudal transtentorial h.
    cingulate h.
    foraminal h.
    painful fat h.
    rostral transtentorial h.
    subfalcial h.
    tentorial h.
    tonsillar h.
    transtentorial h.
    uncal h.
her·nio·ap·pen·dec·to·my
her·nio·en·ter·ot·o·my
her·ni·oid
her·nio·lap·a·rot·o·my
her·ni·ol·o·gy
her·nio·plas·ty
    Cooper's ligament h.
her·nio·punc·ture
her·ni·or·rha·phy
    Shouldice h.
her·ni·ot·o·my
her·o·in
He·roph·i·lus
herp·an·gi·na
her·pes
    buccal h.
    h. corneae
    h. digitalis
    h. disseminatus
    h. facialis
    h. febrilis
    h. generalisatus
    genital h.

her·pes *(continued)*
    h. genitalis
    h. gestationis
    h. gladiatorum
    h. labialis
    lingual h.
    menstrual h.
    h. mentalis
    nasal h.
    neuralgic h.
    ocular h.
    h. ophthalmicus
    orofacial h. simplex
    h. praeputialis
    h. progenitalis
    recurrent h.
    h. simplex
    h. simplex recurrens
    traumatic h.
    wrestler's h.
    h. zoster
    h. zoster auricularis
    h. zoster ophthalmicus
    h. zoster oticus
    h. zoster varicellosus
her·pes·en·ceph·a·li·tis
Her·pes·vi·ri·dae
Her·pes·vi·rus hom·i·nis
her·pes·vi·rus
    h. B
her·pet·ic
her·pet·i·form
her·pe·tol·o·gist
her·pe·tol·o·gy
her·peto·pho·bia
Her·pe·to·so·ma
Her·plex
Her·rick's anemia
Her·ring bodies
Herr·manns·dor·fer diet
her·sage
Her·shey, Alfred Day
Her·ter's disease
Her·ter's infantilism
Her·ter's test
Her·ter-Heub·ner disease
Her·tig-Rock ova
Hert·wig's sheath

Hert·wig-Ma·gen·die phenomenon
Hert·wig-Ma·gen·die sign
hertz
hertz·i·an rays
hertz·i·an waves
Herx·heim·er's fibers
Herx·heim·er's reaction
Herx·heim·er's spirals
Her·yng's sign
Heschl's convolution
Heschl's gyrus
hes·per·i·din
Hess, Walter Rudolf
Hess capillary test
Hes·sel·bach's hernia
Hes·sel·bach's ligament
Hes·sel·bach's triangle
het·a·cil·lin
    h. potassium
het·a·flur
het·a·starch
HETE — hydroxyeicosatetarae-
noic acid
het·er·adel·phia
het·er·a·del·phus
het·er·a·de·nia
het·er·a·den·ic
Het·er·a·kis
het·er·a·li·us
het·er·aux·e·sis
het·er·ax·i·al
het·er·e·cious
het·er·e·cism
het·er·er·gic
het·er·es·the·sia
het·er·in·oc·u·la·tion
het·ero·ag·glu·ti·na·tion
het·ero·ag·glu·ti·nin
het·ero·al·bu·mose
het·ero·al·bu·mos·uria
het·ero·al·lele
het·ero·al·le·lic
het·ero·an·ti·body
het·er·o·an·ti·gen
het·ero·at·om
het·ero·aux·in

Het·ero·ba·sid·io·my·ce·ti·dae
Het·ero·bil·har·zia
    H. americana
het·ero·blas·tic
het·ero·cel·lu·lar
het·ero·cen·tric
het·ero·ceph·a·lus
het·ero·chi·ral
het·ero·chro·ma·tin
    constitutive h.
    facultative h.
    paracentric h.
het·ero·chro·ma·tin·iza·tion
het·ero·chro·ma·ti·za·tion
het·ero·chro·ma·to·sis
het·ero·chro·mia
    binocular h.
    h. iridis
    monocular h.
het·ero·chro·mo·some
het·ero·chro·mous
het·ero·chron
het·ero·chro·nia
het·ero·chron·ic
het·er·och·ro·nous
het·er·och·tho·nous
het·ero·chy·lia
het·ero·clad·ic
het·ero·crine
het·er·oc·ri·sis
het·ero·cy·cle
het·ero·cyc·lic
het·er·o·cy·to·trop·ic
Het·er·od·era rad·i·cic·o·la
het·ero·der·mic
het·ero·des·mot·ic
het·ero·did·y·mus
het·ero·di·mer
het·ero·dont
Het·ero·dox·us
het·er·od·ro·mous
het·ero·du·plex
het·er·od·y·mus
het·er·oe·cious
het·ero·erot·i·cism
het·ero·er·o·tism
het·ero·fer·men·ta·tion

het·ero·fer·men·ta·tive
het·ero·fer·ment·er
het·ero·gam·ete
het·ero·ga·met·ic
het·ero·gam·e·ty
het·er·og·a·mous
het·er·og·a·my
het·ero·gan·gli·on·ic
het·ero·ge·ne·i·ty
   genetic h.
het·ero·ge·ne·ous
het·ero·gen·e·sis
het·ero·ge·net·ic
het·er·o·gen·ic
het·ero·ge·nic·i·ty
het·ero·ge·note
het·er·og·e·nous
het·ero·geu·sia
het·ero·glob·u·lose
het·ero·gon·ic
het·er·og·o·ny
het·ero·graft
   bovine
   porcine h.
het·er·og·ra·phy
het·ero·hem·ag·glu·ti·na·tion
het·ero·hem·ag·glu·ti·nin
het·ero·he·mol·y·sin
het·ero·hex·o·san
het·ero·im·mune
het·ero·im·mu·ni·ty
het·ero·in·tox·i·ca·tion
het·ero·kary·on
het·ero·kary·o·sis
het·ero·ker·a·to·plas·ty
het·ero·ki·ne·sia
het·ero·ki·ne·sis
het·ero·lac·tic
het·ero·la·lia
het·ero·lat·er·al
het·ero·lec·i·thal
het·ero·lit·er·al
het·ero·lith
het·er·ol·o·gous
het·er·ol·o·gy
het·er·ol·y·sin
het·er·ol·y·sis
het·ero·ly·so·some

het·ero·lyt·ic
het·ero·mas·ti·gote
het·er·om·er·al
het·ero·mer·ic
het·er·om·er·ous
het·ero·meta·pla·sia
het·ero·met·ric
het·ero·me·tro·pia
het·ero·mor·phic
het·ero·mor·pho·sis
het·ero·mor·phous
het·er·on·o·mous
het·er·on·y·mous
het·ero-os·teo·plas·ty
het·ero-ov·u·lar
het·er·op·a·gus
het·ero·pan·cre·a·tism
het·er·op·a·thy
het·ero·pen·to·san
het·ero·phago·some
het·er·oph·a·gy
het·er·oph·a·ny
het·ero·pha·sia
het·ero·pha·sis
het·ero·phe·mia
het·ero·phil
het·ero·phile
het·ero·phil·ic
het·ero·pho·nia
het·ero·pho·ral·gia
het·ero·pho·ria
het·ero·phor·ic
het·er·oph·thal·mia
het·er·oph·thal·mos
het·ero·phy·di·a·sis
Het·er·oph·y·es
   H. brevicaeca
   H. heterophyes
   H. katsuradai
het·ero·phy·i·a·sis
Het·ero·phy·i·dae
het·ero·pla·sia
het·ero·plasm
het·ero·plas·tic
het·ero·plas·tid
het·ero·plas·ty
het·ero·ploid
het·ero·ploi·dy

Het·er·op·o·da
   H. venatoria
het·er·op·o·dal
het·ero·poly·mer·ic
het·ero·poly·sac·cha·ride
het·ero·pro·so·pus
het·ero·pro·te·ose
het·er·op·sia
het·ero·psy·chol·o·gy
Het·er·op·tera
het·er·op·tics
het·ero·pyk·no·sis
   negative h.
   positive h.
het·ero·pyk·not·ic
   negatively h.
   positively h.
het·ero·sac·cha·ride
het·ero·sce·das·tic·i·ty
het·ero·scope
het·er·os·co·py
het·ero·sex·u·al
het·ero·sex·u·al·i·ty
het·er·o·sis
het·er·os·mia
het·ero·some
het·ero·spe·cif·ic
het·ero·spore
het·er·os·po·rous
het·ero·sug·ges·tion
het·ero·tax·ia
het·ero·tax·ic
het·ero·tax·is
het·ero·taxy
het·ero·thal·lic
het·ero·thal·lism
het·ero·ther·a·py
het·ero·therm
het·ero·ther·mic
het·ero·ther·my
het·ero·to·nia
het·ero·ton·ic
het·ero·to·pia
   nasal glial h.
   neuronal h.
het·ero·top·ic
het·er·ot·o·py
het·ero·tox·ic

het·ero·tox·in
het·ero·tox·is
het·ero·trans·plant
het·ero·trans·plan·ta·tion
het·ero·tri·cho·sis
   h. superciliorum
het·ero·troph
het·ero·tro·phia
het·ero·troph·ic
het·er·ot·ro·phy
het·ero·tro·pia
het·er·ot·ro·py
het·ero·type
het·ero·typ·ic
het·ero·typ·i·cal
het·ero·vac·cine
het·er·ox·e·nous
het·er·ox·e·ny
het·ero·zo·ic
het·ero·zy·go·sis
het·ero·zy·gos·i·ty
het·ero·zy·gote
   compound h.
   double h.
   inversion h.
   manifesting h.
het·ero·zy·gous
Het·ra·zan
Heub·lein method
Heub·ner's disease
Heub·ner's endarteritis
Heub·ner-Her·ter disease
heu·ris·tic
Heu·ser's membrane
HEW — Department of
   Health, Education, and
   Welfare (now Department of
   Health and Human Services,
   HHS)
hexa·ba·sic
Hexa-Be·ta·lin
hexa·bi·ose
hexa·canth
hexa·chlo·rane
hexa·chlo·ro·ben·zene
hexa·chlo·ro·cy·clo·hex·ane
hexa·chlo·ro·eth·ane
hexa·chlo·ro·phene

hexa·chro·mic
hex·ac·o·sane
hex·ad
hexa·dac·ty·ly
hexa·dec·a·no·ate
hexa·di·meth·rine bro·mide
Hex·a·drol
hex·a·ene
hex·a·flu·o·ren·i·um bro·mide
Hex·a·ge·nia bi·lin·e·a·ta
hexa·hy·dric
hex·a·mer
hexa·me·tho·ni·um
    h. bromide
    h. chloride
hex·a·meth·y·lat·ed
hexa·meth·yl·en·amine
hexa·meth·yl·en·amine·sal·i·cyl·sul·fon·ic acid
hexa·meth·yl·en·di·amine
hex·a·mine
hex·am·i·ti·a·sis
hex·am·y·lose
hex·ane
Hex·a·nic·o·tol
hex·a·no·ic acid
Hex·ap·o·da
hex·atom·ic
hexa·vac·cine
hexa·va·lent
Hexa·vi·bex
hexa·vi·ta·min
hex·ax·i·al
hex·e·dine
hex·en·milch
hex·es·trol
hex·e·thal so·di·um
hex·et·i·dine
hex·hy·dric
hexo·bar·bi·tal
    h. sodium
hexo·bar·bi·tone
hexo·ben·dine
hexo·cy·cli·um meth·yl·sul·fate
hexo·ki·nase
hex·o·nate

hex·one
hex·on·ic acid
hex·os·amine
hex·os·amin·i·dase
    h. A
    h. B
hex·o·san
hexo·sa·zone
hex·ose
    h. diphosphate
    h. monophosphate
hex·ose·di·phos·phor·ic acid
hex·ose·phos·pha·tase
hex·ose·phos·phate
hex·ose·phos·phate isom·er·ase
hex·ose-1-phos·phate uri·dyl·yl·trans·fer·ase
hex·o·syl·trans·fer·ase
hex·uron·ic acid
hex·yl
n-hex·yl·amine
hex·yl·caine hy·dro·chlo·ride
hex·yl·re·sor·ci·nol
Hey's amputation
Hey's derangement
Hey's hernia
Hey's ligament
Hey's operation
Hey's saw
Hey·er valve
Hey·man's technique
Hey·mans, Corneille
Hey·mans' law
Heyn·si·us' test
HF — Hageman factor (coagulation Factor XII)
Hgb — hemoglobin
HGF — hyperglycemic-glycogenolytic factor (glucagon)
HGG — human gamma globulin
HGH — human (pituitary) growth hormone
hGH — human (pituitary) growth hormone
hGHr — growth hormone recombinant

HGPRT — hypoxanthine-guanine phosphoribosyl-transferase
HHS — Department of Health and Human Services
HHT — hydroxyheptadecatrien-oic acid
HI — hemagglutination inhibition
5-HIAA — 5-hydroxyindoleace-tic acid
hi·a·tal
hi·a·tion
hi·a·to·pexy
hi·a·tus
    adductor h.
    h. adductorius
    aortic h.
    h. aorticus
    Breschet's h.
    buccal h.
    esophageal h.
    h. esophageus
    h. of Fallopius
    h. of fallopian canal
    h. fallopii
    false h. of fallopian canal
    h. femoralis
    h. finalis sacralis
    h. interosseus
    h. leukemicus
    h. lumbosacralis
    h. maxillaris
    neural h.
    h. oesophageus
    pleuropericardial h.
    h. pleuroperitonealis
    sacral h.
    h. sacralis
    saphenous h.
    h. saphenus
    Scarpa's h.
    h. of Schwalbe
    semilunar h.
    h. semilunaris
    subarcuate h.
    h. tendineus
    tentorial h.

hi·a·tus *(continued)*
    h. totalis sacralis
    vena caval h.
    h. of Winslow
HIB — *Haemophilus influenzae* type B
Hibbs' operation
hi·ber·na·tion
    artificial h.
hi·ber·no·ma
hic·cough
hic·cup
    epidemic h.
Hicks contractions
Hicks sign
Hicks version
HIDA (hepato-iminodiacetic acid) scan
hide·bound
hi·drad·e·ni·tis
    h. axillaris
    h. suppurativa
hi·drad·e·noid
hi·drad·e·no·ma
    clear cell h.
    eruptive h.
    h. eruptivum
    papillary h.
hid·roa
hid·ro·ad·e·no·ma
hid·ro·cys·to·ma
hid·ro·poi·e·sis
hid·ro·poi·et·ic
hid·ror·rhea
hid·ros·ad·e·ni·tis
hid·ros·che·sis
hi·dro·sis
hi·drot·ic
hi·e·mal
hi·er·ar·chy
    anxiety h.
hi·er·ic
hi·ero·lis·the·sis
high-den·si·ty
high-en·er·gy
High·more's antrum
High·more's body
high-risk

high-spin
high-spi·nal
hi·la
hi·lar
Hil·de·brandt's test
Hil·den·brand's disease
Hil·den·brand's typhus
Hil·gen·rei·ner line
hi·li
hi·li·fuge
hi·li·tis
Hill, Archibald Vivian
Hill coefficient
Hill equation
Hill reaction
Hill's sign
Hil·lis-Mül·ler maneuver
hill·ock
   anal h.
   auricular h's
   axon h.
   Doyère's h.
   ear h's
   facial h.
   germ h.
   germ-bearing h.
   nerve h.
   seminal h.
Hil·ton's law
Hil·ton's line
Hil·ton's muscle
Hil·ton's sac
hi·lum *pl.* hi·la
   h. of caudal olivary nucleus
   h. glandulae suprarenalis
   h. of inferior olivary
     nucleus
   h. lienis
   h. nodi lymphatici
   h. ovarii
   h. pulmonis
   h. renale
   renal h.
   h. of spleen
   h. splenicum
   h. of suprarenal g.
hi·lus *pl.* hi·li
   h. hepatis

hi·lus *(continued)*
   h. of kidney
   h. of lung
   h. of lymph node
   h. lymphoglandulae
   h. nodi lymphatici
   h. ovarii
   h. pulmonis
   h. renalis
hi·man·to·sis
hinch·a·zon
hind·brain
Hin·den·lang's test
hind·foot
hind·gut
hind-kid·ney
hind·wa·ter
Hines-Brown test
   rotating h.
hinge-bow
Hin·ton test
hip
   h. pointer
   snapping h.
Hip·pel's disease
Hip·pe·la·tes
   H. flavipes
   H. pallipes
   H. pusio
Hip·pel-Lin·dau disease
Hip·peu·tis
   H. cantori
Hip·po·bos·ca
   H. rufipes
Hip·po·bos·ci·dae
hip·po·cam·pal
hip·po·cam·pus
   h. major
   h. minor
Hip·poc·ra·tes
hip·po·crat·ic
hip·poc·ra·tism
hip·poc·ra·tist
hip·pom·a·ne
Hip·pu·ran
hip·pu·rate
hip·pu·ria
hip·pu·ric acid

hip·pu·ri·case
hip·pus
Hi·prex
hir·ci
hir·cis·mus
hir·cus *pl.* hir·ci
Hirsch·berg's magnet
Hirsch·berg's method
Hirsch·berg's reflex
Hirsch·feld's canals
Hirsch·feld's disease
Hirsch·sprung's disease
hir·sute
hir·su·ti·es
    h. papillaris penis
hir·sut·ism
    constitutional h.
hi·ru·di·ci·dal
hi·ru·di·cide
hi·ru·din
Hir·u·di·nar·ia
Hir·u·din·ea
hir·u·di·ni·a·sis
    external h.
    internal h.
hir·u·di·ni·za·tion
hi·ru·di·nize
Hi·ru·do
    H. aegyptiaca
    H. japonica
    H. javanica
    H. medicinalis
    H. quinquestriata
    H. sanguisorba
    H. troctina
His — histidine
His' band
His' bundle
His' bursa
His' canal
His' disease
His' duct
His' space
His' spindle
His' zones
His-Held space
His-Pur·kin·je conduction
His-Ta·wa·ra node

His-Wer·ner disease
His·pril
Hiss capsule stain
His·ta·dyl
His·ta·log
his·tam·i·nase
his·ta·mine
    h.$_1$
    h.$_2$
    h. acid phosphate
    h. dihydrochloride
    h. hydrochloride
    h. phosphate
his·tam·i·ne·mia
his·ta·min·er·gic
his·tan·ox·ia
His·ta·span
his·tic
his·ti·dase
his·ti·di·nase
his·ti·dine
    h. decarboxylase
his·ti·dine am·mo·nia-ly·ase
his·ti·din·emia
his·ti·din·uria
his·tio·blast
his·tio·cyte
    cardiac h.
    sea-blue h.
    wandering h's
his·tio·cyt·ic
his·tio·cy·to·ma
    h. cutis
    fibrous h.
    juvenile h.
    lipoid h.
    malignant fibrous h.
his·tio·cy·to·ma·to·sis
his·tio·cy·to·sis
    malignant h.
    nonlipid h.
    pulmonary h.
    sinus h.
    h. X
his·ti·o·gen·ic
his·ti·oid
his·tio·ir·ri·ta·tive
his·ti·o·ma

his·ti·on·ic
his·to·au·to·ra·di·og·ra·phy
his·to·blast
his·to·chem·i·cal
his·to·chem·is·try
his·to·che·mo·ther·a·py
his·to·chro·ma·to·sis
his·to·clas·tic
his·to·clin·i·cal
his·to·com·pa·ti·bil·i·ty
his·to·com·pat·i·ble
his·to·cyte
his·to·di·ag·no·sis
his·to·di·al·y·sis
his·to·dif·fer·en·ti·a·tion
his·to·flu·o·res·cence
his·to·gen·e·sis
his·to·ge·net·ic
his·tog·e·nous
his·tog·e·ny
his·to·gram
his·tog·ra·phy
his·to·hem·a·tog·e·nous
his·to·hy·dria
his·to·hy·pox·ia
his·toid
his·to·in·com·pat·i·bil·i·ty
his·to·in·com·pat·i·ble
his·to·ki·ne·sis
his·to·log·ic, his·to·log·i·cal
his·tol·o·gist
his·tol·o·gy
    normal h.
    pathologic h.
    topographic h.
his·tol·y·sate
his·tol·y·sis
his·to·lyt·ic
his·to·ma
his·to·meta·plas·tic
his·to·mor·phol·o·gy
his·to·mor·pho·met·ric
his·tone
    h. nucleinate
his·to·neu·rol·o·gy
his·ton·o·my
his·ton·uria
his·to·patho·gen·e·sis

his·to·pa·thol·o·gy
his·toph·a·gous
his·to·phys·i·ol·o·gy
His·to·plas·ma
    H. capsulatum
    H. farciminosus
his·to·plas·min
his·to·plas·mo·ma
his·to·plas·mo·sis
    African h.
    ocular h.
his·to·ra·di·og·ra·phy
his·to·re·ten·tion
his·tor·rhex·is
his·to·ry
    case h.
    medical h.
his·to·spec·tros·co·py
his·to·tel·i·o·sis
his·to·ther·a·py
his·to·throm·bin
his·to·tome
his·tot·o·my
his·to·tox·ic
his·to·troph
his·to·troph·ic
his·to·trop·ic
his·to·zo·ic
his·tri·on·ic
his·tri·o·nism
Hit·torf's number
Hit·torf's tube
Hit·zig's girdle
Hit·zig's test
HIV — human
    immunodeficiency virus
hive
hives
HKAFO — hip-knee-ankle-foot-
    orthosis
Hl — latent hyperopia
HLA — human leukocyte
    antigen
Hm — manifest hyperopia
HMG — human menopausal
    gonadotropin
HMM — hexamethylmel-
    amine

HMO — health maintenance organization
HMW-NCF — high-molecular-weight neutrophil chemotactic factor
hnRNA — heterogeneous nuclear RNA
hoarse
hoarse·ness
Ho·bo·ken's nodules
Ho·bo·ken's valves
Hoche's bandelette
Hoch·e·negg's operation
Hoch·sin·ger's phenomenon
Hoch·sin·ger's sign
Hodge's forceps
Hodge's plane
Hodg·en apparatus
Hodg·en splint
Hodg·kin, Alan Lloyd
Hodg·kin's cells
Hodg·kin's cycle
Hodg·kin's disease
Hodg·kin's granuloma
Hodg·kin's sarcoma
Hodg·son's disease
ho·do·graph
ho·dol·o·gy
ho·do·neu·ro·mere
hoe
Hoeh·ne's sign
Hoep·pli's phenomenon
hof
    nuclear h.
Hof·bau·er cells
Hof·fa's disease
Hof·fa's operation
Hof·fa-Lo·renz operation
Hof·fa-Kas·tert disease
Hoff·mann's anodyne
Hoff·mann's atrophy
Hoff·mann's drops
Hoff·mann's duct
Hoff·mann's phenomenon
Hoff·mann's reflex
Hoff·mann's sign
Hoff·mann-Werd·nig syndrome

Hof·mann's bacillus
Hof·mann's violet
Hof·meis·ter's test
Ho·guet maneuver
Hoke's operation
hol·a·gogue
hol·an·dric
hol·ar·thri·tis
Hol·den's line
hold·er
    broach h.
    clamp h.
    needle h.
    rubber dam clamp h.
    sponge h.
hold·fast
Hol·ger Niel·sen method
hol·i·day
    drug h.
hol·ism
ho·lis·tic
Holl's ligament
Hol·lan·der's test
Hol·len·horst bodies
Hol·len·horst plaque
Hol·ley, Robert William
hol·low
    Sebileau's h.
hol·low-back
Holmes, Oliver Wendell
Holmes' degeneration
Holmes operation
Holmes' phenomenon
Holmes' sign
Holmes-Adie syndrome
Holmes-Stew·art phenomenon
Holm·gren's test
Holm·gren-Gol·gi canals
hol·mi·um
holo·acar·di·us
    h. acephalus
    h. acormus
    h. amorphus
holo·an·en·ceph·a·ly
hol·o·an·ti·gen
holo·blast
holo·blas·tic
Hol·o·caine

hol·o·car·box·y·lase syn·the·
  tase deficiency
holo·ce·phal·ic
holo·ceph·a·ly
holo·cor·tex
holo·crine
holo·di·a·stol·ic
holo·en·dem·ic
holo·en·zyme
ho·log·a·my
holo·gas·tros·chi·sis
holo·gen·e·sis
holo·gram
hol·og·ra·phy
  acoustical h.
holo·gyn·ic
holo·mas·ti·gote
holo·me·tab·o·lous
holo·mor·pho·sis
holo·neph·ros
holo·phyt·ic
holo·plex·ia
holo·pros·en·ceph·a·ly
  familial alobar h.
holo·ra·chis·chi·sis
holo·sac·cha·ride
holo·schi·sis
holo·sym·phy·sis
holo·sys·tol·ic
holo·tel·en·ceph·a·ly
holo·thu·rin
holo·thy·rus
holo·to·nia
holo·ton·ic
ho·lot·o·py
ho·lot·ri·chous
holo·type
holo·xen·ic
holo·zo·ic
Holt-Or·am syndrome
Hol·ten's test
Holth's operation
Holt·house's hernia
Holz·knecht's space
hom·a·lo·ceph·a·lus
hom·a·log·ra·phy
Hom·a·lo·my·ia
hom·al·u·ria

Ho·mans' sign
Ho·ma·pin
hom·a·rine
ho·mat·ro·pine
  h. hydrobromide
  h. methylbromide
ho·max·i·al
Home's gland
Home's lobe
Ho·mén's syndrome
ho·meo·chrome
ho·meo·graft
ho·meo·ki·ne·sis
ho·meo·met·ric
ho·meo·mor·phous
ho·meo-os·teo·plas·ty
ho·meo·path
ho·meo·path·ic
ho·me·op·a·thist
ho·me·op·a·thy
ho·meo·pla·sia
ho·meo·plas·tic
ho·me·or·rhe·sis
ho·me·o·sis
ho·meo·sta·sis
  genetic h.
  immunologic h.
ho·meo·stat·ic
ho·meo·ther·a·py
ho·meo·therm
ho·meo·ther·mal
ho·meo·ther·mic
ho·meo·ther·mism
ho·meo·ther·my
ho·meo·tox·ic
ho·meo·tox·in
ho·meo·trans·plant
ho·meo·trans·plan·ta·tion
ho·meo·typ·ic
ho·meo·typ·i·cal
Ho·mer-Wright rosette
hom·er·gic
hom·i·cide
ho·mid·i·um
hom·i·nal
hom·in·i·nox·ious
homme
  h. rouge

ho·mo·ar·te·re·nol hy·dro·
  chlo·ride
Ho·mo·ba·sid·io·my·ce·ti·dae
ho·mo·bio·tin
ho·mo·blas·tic
ho·mo·body
ho·mo·car·no·sin·ase
ho·mo·car·no·sine
ho·mo·car·no·sin·o·sis
ho·mo·cen·tric
ho·moch·ro·nous
ho·mo·cin·cho·nine
ho·mo·clad·ic
ho·mo·cyc·lic
ho·mo·cys·te·ine
ho·mo·cys·te·ine-tet·ra·hy·
  dro·fo·late meth·yl·trans·
  fer·ase
ho·mo·cys·tine
ho·mo·cys·tin·emia
ho·mo·cys·tin·uria
ho·mo·cy·to·trop·ic
ho·mo·des·mot·ic
ho·mo·dont
ho·mod·ro·mous
ho·mo·dy·nam·ic
ho·mo·dy·na·my
ho·moe·ci·ous
ho·moe·o·sis
ho·mo·erot·ic
ho·mo·erot·i·cism
ho·mo·er·o·tism
ho·mo·fer·men·ta·tion
ho·mo·fer·ment·er
ho·mo·gam·ete
ho·mo·ga·met·ic
ho·mog·a·mous
ho·mog·a·my
ho·mog·e·nate
ho·mo·ge·ne·i·ty
ho·mo·ge·ne·iza·tion
ho·mo·ge·ne·ous
ho·mo·gen·e·sis
ho·mo·ge·net·ic
ho·mo·gen·ic
ho·mo·ge·nic·i·ty
ho·mog·e·ni·za·tion
ho·mog·e·nize

ho·mo·ge·note
ho·mog·e·nous
ho·mo·gen·ti·sate
ho·mo·gen·ti·sate 1,2-di·oxy·
  gen·ase
ho·mo·gen·ti·sate ox·i·dase
ho·mo·gen·tis·ic acid
ho·mo·gen·ti·su·ria
ho·mog·e·ny
ho·mo·glan·du·lar
ho·mo·gon·ic
ho·mo·graft
  isogenic h.
ho·moi·op·o·dal
ho·moi·os·mot·ic
ho·moio·tox·in
ho·mo·kary·on
ho·mo·ker·a·to·plas·ty
ho·mo·lac·tic
ho·mo·lat·er·al
ho·mol·o·gen
ho·mol·o·gous
ho·mo·logue
ho·mol·o·gy
  metameric h.
  serial h.
ho·mol·y·sin
ho·mol·y·sis
ho·mo·mor·phic
ho·mo·mor·pho·sis
ho·mon·o·mous
ho·mon·y·mous
ho·mo·phene
ho·mo·phil
ho·mo·phil·ic
ho·mo·plas·tic
ho·mo·plas·ty
ho·mo·poly·mer
ho·mo·poly·sac·cha·ride
hom·or·gan·ic
ho·mo·sal·ate
ho·mo·sce·das·tic·i·ty
ho·mo·ser·ine
ho·mo·sex·u·al
ho·mo·sex·u·al·i·ty
  ego-dystonic h.
  latent h.
  unconscious h.

ho·mo·spore
ho·mos·po·rous
ho·mo·stim·u·lant
ho·mo·stim·u·la·tion
Ho·mo-Tet
ho·mo·thal·lic
ho·mo·thal·lism
ho·mo·therm
ho·mo·ther·mal
ho·mo·ther·mic
ho·mo·ton·ic
ho·mo·top·ic
ho·mo·trans·plant
ho·mo·trans·plan·ta·tion
ho·mot·ro·pism
ho·mo·type
ho·mo·typ·ic
ho·mo·va·nil·lic acid
ho·mox·e·nous
ho·mo·zo·ic
ho·mo·zy·go·sis
ho·mo·zy·gos·i·ty
ho·mo·zy·gote
ho·mo·zy·gous
ho·mun·cu·lus
hon·ey
honk
    precordial h.
hood
    tooth h.
hook
    blunt h.
    Bose's h's
    Braun's h.
    dural h.
    fixation h.
    h. of hamate bone
    Loughnane's h.
    muscle h.
    Pajot's h.
    palate h.
    squint h.
    tracheostomy h.
    Tyrrell's h.
hook·let
hook-up
hook·worm
    American h.

hook·worm (continued)
    European h.
    New World h.
    Old World h.
hoo·la·mite
Hoo·ver's sign
HOP — high oxygen pressure
    hydroxydaunomycin
    (doxorubicin), Oncovin
    (vincristine), and
    prednisone
Hope's sign
Hop·kins, Sir Frederick
    Gowland
Hop·kins-Cole test
Hop·lop·syl·lus anom·a·lus
Hop·mann's papilloma
Hop·mann's polyp
Hoppe-Gold·flam syndrome
Hop·pe-Sey·ler's test
ho·qui·zil hy·dro·chlo·ride
Hor. decub. — L. hora
    decubitus (at bedtime)
hor·de·in
hor·de·nine
hor·de·o·lum
    external h.
    internal h.
hore·hound
Hor·gan's operation
Hor. interm. — L. horis
    intermediis (at the
    intermediate hours)
ho·ri·zon
    Streeter's h's
hor·i·zon·ta·lis
hor·me·sis
hor·mi·on
Hor·mo·car·di·ol
Hor·mo·den·drum
hor·mon·a·gogue
hor·mo·nal
hor·mone
    adaptive h.
    adenohypophysial h.
    adipokinetic h.
    adrenocortical h.
    adrenocorticotropic h.

hor·mone *(continued)*

adrenomedullary h's
androgenic h's
anterior pituitary h.
antidiuretic h.
Aschheim-Zondek h.
chondrotropic h.
chromaffin h.
circulatory h.
conjugated estrogen h's
corpus luteum h.
cortical h.
corticotropin releasing
  hormone (CRH)
diabetogenic h.
estrogenic h's
fat-mobilizing h's
follicle-stimulating h.
  (FSH)
follicle-stimulating h.,
  human
follicle-stimulating
  hormone releasing h.
  (FSH-RH)
follicular h.
galactopoietic h.
gastrointestinal h's
glycoprotein h.
gonadotropic h.
gonadotropic h's, pituitary
gonadotropin releasing h.
  (Gn-RH)
growth h. (GH)
growth hormone release
  inhibiting h. (GH-RIH)
growth hormone releasing
  h. (GH-RH)
gut h.
human (pituitary) growth
  h. (hGH)
hypophysial h.
hypophysiotropic h.
hypothalamic inhibitory h.
hypothalamic releasing h.
inhibiting h's
inhibitory h.
interstitial cell-stimulating
  h.

hor·mone *(continued)*

intestinal h.
intracellular h.
juvenile h.
ketogenic h's
lactation h.
lactogenic h.
lipolytic h's
local h.
luteal h.
luteinizing h.
luteinizing hormone
  releasing h. (LH-RH)
luteotropic h.
melanocyte-stimulating h.
melanocyte stimulating
  hormone inhibiting h.
melanocyte stimulating
  hormone releasing h.
melanophore-stimulating
  h.
morphogenic h.
neurohypophysial h's
ovarian h.
parathyroid h.
placental h's
placental growth h.
plant h.
posterior pituitary h's
preproparathyroid h.
progestational h.
prolactin inhibitory h.
prolactin releasing h.
proparathyroid h.
prothoracicotropic h.
releasing h's
sex h's
somatotrophic h.
somatotropic h.
somatotropin release
  inhibiting h.
somatotropin releasing h.
  (SRH)
steroid h's
testicular h.
testis h.
thyroid h's

hor·mone *(continued)*
    thyroid-stimulating h.
      (TSH)
    thyrotropic h.
    thyrotropin releasing h.
      (TRH)
    tropic h's
hor·mon·ic
hor·mon·o·gen
hor·mo·no·gen·e·sis
hor·mo·no·gen·ic
hor·mo·nol·o·gy
hor·mo·no·poi·e·sis
hor·mo·no·poi·et·ic
hor·mo·no·priv·ia
hor·mo·no·sis
hor·mo·no·ther·a·py
horn
    h. of Ammon
    anterior h. of lateral
      ventricle
    anterior h. of spinal cord
    cicatricial h.
    coccygeal h.
    cutaneous h.
    dorsal h. of spinal cord
    frontal h. of lateral
      ventricle
    gray h's of spinal cord
    greater h. of hyoid bone
    iliac h.
    inferior h. of cerebrum
    inferior h. of falciform
      margin
    inferior h. of lateral
      ventricle
    inferior h. of saphenous
      opening
    inferior h. of thyroid
      cartilage
    lateral h. of coccyx
    lateral h. of hyoid bone
    lateral h. of spinal cord
    lateral h. of uterus
    lesser h. of hyoid bone
    motor h.
    occipital h. of lateral
      ventricle

horn *(continued)*
    posterior h. of lateral
      ventricle
    posterior h. of spinal cord
    h. of pulp
    sacral h.
    sebaceous h.
    superior h. of falciform
      margin
    superior h. of hyoid bone
    superior h. of saphenous
      opening
    superior h. of thymus
    superior h. of thyroid
      cartilage
    temporal h. of lateral
      ventricle
    uterine h.
    ventral h. of spinal cord
    warty h.
Horn's sign
Hor·ner's law
Hor·ner's ptosis
Hor·ner's syndrome
Hor·ner's muscle
Hor·ner-Ber·nard syndrome
horn·i·fi·ca·tion
horny
ho·rop·ter
    Vieth-Müller h.
hor·op·ter·ic
hor·rip·i·la·tion
hor·ror
    h. autotoxicus
    h. fusionis
Hors·ley's operation
Hors·ley's test
Hors·ley's wax
Hor·te·ga cell
Hor·te·ga method
hor·to·be·zoar
Hor·ton's arteritis
Hor·ton's disease
Hor·ton's headache

Hor. un. spatio — L. horae unius spatio (at the end of one hour)

hos·pice

hos·pi·tal
   base h.
   camp h.
   closed h.
   cottage h.
   day h.
   evacuation h.
   field h.
   for-profit h.
   geriatric day h.
   government h.
   lying-in h.
   maternity h.
   mental h.
   mobile army surgical h. (MASH)
   night h.
   open h.
   private h.
   proprietary h.
   psychogeriatric h.
   public h.
   teaching h.
   voluntary h.
   weekend h.

hos·pi·tal·ism

hos·pi·tal·iza·tion
   partial h.

hos·pi·tal·ize

host
   accidental h.
   alternate h.
   dead-end h.
   definitive h.
   final h.
   incidental h.
   intermediate h.
   maintenance h.
   mechanical intermediate h.
   overwintering h.
   paratenic h.
   h. of predilection
   primary h.

host (continued)
   reservoir h.
   secondary h.
   transfer h.
   transport h.

HOT — human old tuberculin

hot-box

hot line

Houns·field, Sir Godfrey Newbold

Houns·field unit

Hous·say, Bernardo Alberto

Hous·say animal

Hous·say phenomenon

Hous·say-Bi·a·sot·ti syndrome

Hous·ton's muscle

Hous·ton's valve

ho·ven

Hov·er·bed

Ho·vi·us' canal

Ho·vi·us' circle

Ho·vi·us' membrane

Ho·vi·us' plexus

How·ard's method

How·ard's test

Howe's silver nitrate

How·el-Ev·ans' syndrome

How·ell's bodies

How·ell's method

How·ell's test

How·ell-Jol·ly bodies

How·ship's lacuna

How·ship-Rom·berg sign

Hoyne's sign

HP — history of present illness
      house physician

Hp — haptoglobin

HPA (hypothalamic-pituitary-adrenal) axis

HPETE — hydroperoxyeicosate-traenoic acid

HPF — high-power field

HPL — human placental lactogen

hPL — human placental lactogen

HPLC — high-performance
liquid chromatography
high-pressure liquid
chromatography
HPRT — hypoxanthine
phosphoribosyltransferase
HRA — health risk appraisal
HRF — histamine releasing
factor
HS — house surgeon
h.s. — L. hora somni (at
bedtime)
HSA — human serum
albumin
HSF — hydrazine-sensitive
factor
HSR — homogeneously
staining regions
5-HT
5-HT — 5-hydroxytryptamine
(serotonin)
Ht — total hyperopia
HTACS — human thyroid
adenylate cyclase stimulators
HTC — homozygous typing
cells
³H-TdR
HTLV — human T-cell
leukemia/lymphoma virus
Hua
    H. ningpoensis
    H. toucheana
Hubbard tank
Hu·bel, David Hunter
Hu·ber's ganglion
Hu·chard's disease
Hu·chard's sign
Hu·chard's symptom
Hud·son's line
Hud·son-Stäh·li line
Hueck's ligament
Hu·ët-Pel·ger nuclear anomaly
Hue·ter's line
Hue·ter's maneuver
Hue·ter's sign
Hug·gins, Charles Brenton
Hug·gins operation
Hughes' reflex

Hu·guen·in's edema
Hu·guier's canal
Hu·guier's circle
Hu·guier's sinus
Huh·ner test
HuIFN — human interferon
hum
    venous h.
Hu·man's sign
Hu·ma·tin
hu·ma·trope
hu·mec·tant
hu·mec·ta·tion
hu·mer·al
hu·meri
hu·mero·ra·di·al
hu·mero·scap·u·lar
hu·mero·ul·nar
hu·mer·us *pl.* hu·meri
    h. varus
hu·mid·i·fi·er
hu·mid·i·ty
    absolute h.
    relative h.
hu·mor *pl.* hu·mors, hu·mo·
res
    aqueous h.
    h. aquosus
    h. cristallinus
    crystalline h.
    ocular h.
    plasmoid h.
    vitreous h.
    h. vitreus
hu·mor·al
hu·mor·al·ism
hu·mor·ism
Hu·mor·sol
hump
    buffalo h.
    dowager's h.
hump·back
Hum·phry's ligament
hu·mus
hunch·back
hunch·backed
Hü·ner·mann's disease
Hung's method

hun·ger
  affect h.
  air h.
  calcium h.
Hun·ner's ulcer
Hunt's atrophy
Hunt's phenomenon
Hunt's method
Hun·ter's canal
Hun·ter's glossitis
Hun·ter's gubernaculum
Hun·ter's ligament
Hun·ter's line
Hun·ter's operation
Hunter's syndrome
Hun·ter-Schre·ger band
hun·ter·i·an
Hun·ting·ton's chorea
Hun·ting·ton's disease
Hup·pert's test
Hur·ler's disease
Hur·ler's syndrome
Hurler-Scheie syndrome
Hurst's disease
Hürth·le cells
Hürth·le cell tumor
Hurt·ley's test
Husch·ke's canal
Husch·ke's foramen
Husch·ke's ligaments
Husch·ke's valve
Hutch·in·son's disease
Hutch·in·son's facies
Hutch·in·son's mask
Hutch·in·son's pupil
Hutch·in·son's sign
Hutch·in·son's triad
Hutch·in·son-Boeck disease
Hutch·in·son-Boeck syndrome
Hutch·in·son-Gil·ford disease
Hutch·in·son-Gil·ford
  syndrome
hutch·in·so·ni·an
Hutch·i·son syndrome
Hutch·i·son type
Hu-Tet
Hu·tin·el's disease
Hux·ley, Andrew Fielding

Hux·ley's layer
Hux·ley's membrane
huy·gen·i·an
Huy·gens (Huy·ghens)
  eyepiece
Huy·gens (Huy·ghens) ocular
Huy·gens (Huy·ghens)
  principle
HV — hyperventilation
  herpes virus
HVA — homovanillic acid
HVL — half-value layer
hy·al
hy·a·lin
  hematogenous h.
hy·a·line
hy·a·lin·iza·tion
  tympanic h.
hy·a·li·no·sis
  h. cutis et mucosae
  tympanic h.
hy·a·lin·u·ria
hy·a·li·tis
  asteroid h.
  punctate h.
  h. punctata
  suppurative h.
  h. suppurativa
hy·al·o·gen
hy·a·loid
hy·a·loid·in
hy·a·loid·itis
hy·a·loi·dop·a·thy
  asteroid h.
hy·a·lo·mere
hy·a·lo·mit·ome
Hy·a·lom·ma
hy·a·lo·mu·coid
hy·a·lo·nyx·is
hy·a·lo·pha·gia
hy·a·loph·a·gy
hy·a·lo·plasm
  nuclear h.
hy·a·lo·se·ro·si·tis
  progressive multiple h.
hy·a·lo·sis
  asteroid h.
  punctate h.

hy·al·o·some
hy·al·o·tome
hy·al·uro·nate
hy·al·uro·nate ly·ase
hy·al·uron·ic acid
hy·al·uron·i·dase
hy·al·urono·glu·co·sa·min·i·dase
hy·al·urono·glu·cu·ron·i·dase
Hy·a·zyme
hy·bar·ox·ia
hy·ben·zate
hy·brid
    F₁ h.
    false h.
    somatic h.
hy·brid·ism
hy·brid·i·ty
hy·brid·iza·tion
    cell h.
    cross h.
    in situ h.
    molecular h.
hy·brid·o·ma
hy·can·thone
    h. mesylate
hy·clate
Hy·co·dan
hy·dan·to·ic acid
hy·dan·to·in
hy·dan·to·in·ate
hy·da·tid
    alveolar h's
    h. of Morgagni
    nonpedunculated h.
    pedunculated h.
    sessile h.
    Virchow's h.
hy·da·tid·i·form
hy·da·tid·o·sis
hy·da·tid·os·to·my
hy·da·tid·uria
Hy·da·tig·ena
hy·da·tism
hy·da·toid
Hy·del·tra
Hy·der·gine
hy·drac·e·tin

hy·drad·e·ni·tis
hy·drad·e·no·ma
hy·draero·peri·to·ne·um
hy·dra·gogue
hy·dral·a·zine hy·dro·chlo·ride
hy·dra·mine
hy·dram·ni·on
hy·dram·ni·os
hy·dran·en·ceph·a·ly
hy·dran·gi·ol·o·gy
hy·drar·gyr·ia
hy·drar·gy·rism
hy·drar·gy·ro·ma·nia
hy·drar·gy·ro·re·laps·ing
hy·drar·gy·ro·sis
hy·drar·thro·di·al
hy·drar·thro·sis
    intermittent h.
hy·drase
hy·dra·tase
hy·drate
hy·drat·ed
hy·dra·tion
hy·drau·lics
hy·dra·zine
hy·dra·zin·ol·y·sis
hy·dra·zone
Hy·drea
hy·dre·mia
hy·dren·ceph·a·lo·cele
hy·dren·ceph·a·lo·me·nin·go·cele
hy·dren·ceph·a·lus
hy·dren·ceph·a·ly
hy·drepi·gas·tri·um
hy·dri·at·ric
hy·dri·at·rics
hy·dric
hy·dride
hy·drin·di·cu·ria
hy·dri·od·ic acid
hy·dri·on
hy·droa
    h. estivale
    h. vacciniforme
hy·dro·adip·sia
hy·dro·ap·pen·dix

Hy·dro·bi·i·dae
Hy·dro·bi·i·nae
hy·dro·bil·i·ru·bin
hy·dro·bleph·a·ron
hy·dro·bro·mic acid
hy·dro·bro·mide
Hy·dro·cal
hy·dro·ca·ly·co·sis
hy·dro·ca·lyx
hy·dro·car·bar·ism
hy·dro·car·bon
  alicyclic h.
  aliphatic h.
  aromatic h.
  carcinogenic h.
  chlorinated h.
  cyclic h.
  fluorinated h.
  halogenated h.
  saturated h.
  unsaturated h.
hy·dro·car·bon·ism
hy·dro·car·dia
hy·dro·cele
  bilocular h.
  cervical h.
  chylous h.
  h. colli
  communicating h.
  congenital h.
  diffused h.
  Dupuytren's h.
  encysted h.
  h. feminae
  filarial h.
  funicular h.
  hernial h.
  inguinal h.
  Maunoir's h.
  h. of neck
  h. renalis
  scrotal h.
  spermatic h.
  h. spinalis
hy·dro·ce·lec·to·my
hy·dro·ce·no·sis
hy·dro·ce·phal·ic
hy·dro·ceph·a·lo·cele

hy·dro·ceph·a·loid
hy·dro·ceph·a·lus
  communicating h.
  compensating h.
  congenital h.
  external h.
  h. ex vacuo
  hypertonic h.
  internal h.
  low-pressure h.
  noncommunicating h.
  normal-pressure h.
  normal-pressure occult h.
  obstructive h.
  occult normal-pressure h.
  otitic h.
  post-traumatic h.
  postmeningitic h.
  primary h.
  secondary h.
  thrombotic h.
  toxic h.
hy·dro·ceph·a·ly
hy·dro·chlo·ric acid
hy·dro·chlo·ride
  oxytetracycline h.
  trifluperidol h.
hy·dro·chlo·ro·thi·a·zide
hy·dro·cho·le·cys·tis
hy·dro·cho·le·re·sis
hy·dro·cho·le·ret·ic
hy·dro·cho·les·ter·ol
hy·dro·cin·chon·i·dine
hy·dro·cir·so·cele
hy·dro·co·done bi·tar·trate
hy·dro·col·li·dine
hy·dro·col·loid
  irreversible h.
  reversible h.
hy·dro·col·po·cele
hy·dro·col·pos
hy·dro·co·ni·on
hy·dro·cor·ta·mate hy·dro·
  chlo·ride
hy·dro·cor·ti·sone
  h. acetate
  h. cyclopentylpropionate
  h. cypionate

hy·dro·cor·ti·sone *(continued)*
   h. hemisuccinate
   h. sodium phosphate
   h. sodium succinate
   h. tertiary-butylacetate
   h. valerate
Hy·dro·cor·tone
hy·dro·cra·nia
hy·dro·cy·an·ic acid
hy·dro·cy·an·ism
hy·dro·cyst
hy·dro·cys·tad·e·no·ma
hy·dro·di·a·scope
hy·dro·dif·fu·sion
hy·dro·dip·sia
hy·dro·dip·so·ma·nia
hy·dro·di·ure·sis
Hy·dro·DI·U·RIL
hy·dro·dy·nam·ics
hy·dro·elec·tric
hy·dro·en·ceph·a·lo·cele
hy·dro·flu·me·thi·a·zide
hy·dro·flu·o·ric acid
hy·dro·gel
hy·dro·gen
   arseniuretted h.
   h. chloride
   h. cyanide
   h. disulfide
   heavy h.
   light h.
   ordinary h.
   h. peroxide
   radioactive h.
   h. selenide
   h. sulfide
   sulfuretted h.
hy·dro·gen·ase
hy·dro·gen·ate
hy·dro·gen·a·tion
hy·dro·gen·ize
hy·drog·e·noid
hy·dro·ge·nol·y·sis
hy·dro·gym·nas·tic
hy·dro·gym·nas·tics
hy·dro·hem·ar·thro·sis
hy·dro·hem·a·to·ne·phro·sis
hy·dro·hem·a·to·sal·pinx

hy·dro·hep·a·to·sis
hy·dro·hy·men·itis
hy·dro·hys·te·ra
hy·dro·ki·ne·si·ther·a·py
hy·dro·ki·net·ic
hy·dro·ki·net·ics
hy·drol
hy·dro·la·bile
hy·dro·la·bil·i·ty
hy·dro·lase
   murein h.
hy·drol·o·gy
Hy·dro·lose
hy·dro-ly·ase
hy·dro·lymph
hy·drol·y·sate
   protein h.
hy·drol·y·sis *pl.* hy·drol·y·ses
   papain h.
hy·dro·lyst
hy·dro·lyte
hy·dro·lyt·ic
hy·dro·lyze
hy·dro·ma
hy·dro·mas·sage
hy·dro·men·in·gi·tis
hy·dro·me·nin·go·cele
hy·drom·e·ter
hy·dro·me·tra
hy·dro·met·ric
hy·dro·me·tro·col·pos
hy·drom·e·try
hy·dro·mi·cro·ceph·a·ly
hy·dro·mor·phone
   h. hydrochloride
Hy·dro·mox
hy·drom·pha·lus
hy·dro·my·e·lia
hy·dro·my·elo·cele
hy·dro·my·elo·me·nin·go·cele
hy·dro·my·o·ma
hy·dro·ne·phro·sis
   closed h.
   congenital h.
   external h.
   infected h.
   intermittent h.
   open h.

hy·dro·ne·phro·sis *(continued)*
   perirenal h.
   subcapsular h.
hy·dro·ne·phrot·ic
hy·dro·ni·um
hy·dro·pan·cre·a·to·sis
hy·dro·para·sal·pinx
hy·dro·par·o·ti·tis
hy·dro·pe·de·sis
hy·dro·pe·nia
hy·dro·pe·nic
hy·dro·peri·car·dit·ic
hy·dro·peri·car·di·tis
hy·dro·peri·car·di·um
hy·dro·peri·ne·phro·sis
hy·dro·per·i·on
hy·dro·peri·to·ne·um
hy·dro·peri·to·nia
hy·dro·per·oxy·ei·co·sa·tet·
  ra·eno·ic acid
hy·dro·pex·ia
hy·dro·pex·ic
hy·dro·pex·is
hy·dro·phago·cy·to·sis
hy·dro·phil
hy·dro·phil·ia
hy·dro·phil·ic
hy·droph·i·lism
hy·droph·i·lous
Hy·droph·i·o·dae
hy·dro·pho·bia
   paralytic h.
hy·dro·pho·bic
hy·dro·pho·ro·graph
hy·droph·thal·mia
hy·droph·thal·mos
   h. anterior
   h. posterior
   h. totalis
hy·droph·thal·mus
hy·dro·phy·so·me·tra
hy·dro·phyte
hy·drop·ic
hy·dro·pig·e·nous
hy·dro·plas·ma
hy·dro·plas·mia
hy·dro·pleu·ra
hy·dro·pneu·ma·to·sis

hy·dro·pneu·mo·go·ny
hy·dro·pneu·mo·peri·car·di·um
hy·dro·pneu·mo·peri·to·ne·um
hy·dro·pneu·mo·tho·rax
Hy·dro·pres
hy·drops
   h. abdominis
   h. ad matulam
   h. amnii
   h. antri
   h. articuli
   Bart's hemoglobin h. fetalis
   endolymphatic h.
   fetal h.
   h. fetalis
   h. folliculi
   hypertensive meningeal h.
   immune h. fetalis
   h. labyrinthi
   labyrinthine h.
   nonimmune h. fetalis
   h. pericardii
   h. spurius
   h. tubae
   h. tubae profluens
   tympanic h.
hy·dro·pyo·ne·phro·sis
hy·dro·quin·one
hy·dro·ra·chis
hy·dro·ra·chi·tis
hy·dror·chis
hy·dror·rhea
   h. gravidarum
   nasal h.
hy·dro·sal·pinx
   h. follicularis
   intermittent h.
   h. simplex
hy·dro·sar·co·cele
hy·dros·cheo·cele
hy·dro·sol
hy·dro·sol·u·ble
hy·dro·sper·ma·to·cele
hy·dro·sphyg·mo·graph
hy·dro·spi·rom·e·ter
hy·dro·sta·bile

hy·dro·stat
hy·dro·stat·ic
hy·dro·stat·ics
hy·dro·sto·mia
hy·dro·sul·fur·ic acid
hy·dro·syn·the·sis
hy·dro·sy·rin·go·my·e·lia
Hy·dro·taea
    H. meteorica
hy·dro·ther·a·peu·tic
hy·dro·tax·is
hy·dro·ther·a·peu·tics
hy·dro·ther·a·py
hy·dro·ther·mic
hy·dro·thio·am·mo·ne·mia
hy·dro·thio·ne·mia
hy·dro·thi·on·uria
hy·dro·tho·rax
    chylous h.
hy·drot·o·my
hy·dro·tox·ic·i·ty
hy·drot·ro·pism
hy·dro·tu·ba·tion
hy·dro·tym·pan·um
hy·dro·ure·ter
hy·dro·ure·tero·neph·ro·sis
hy·dro·ure·ter·o·sis
hy·dro·uria
hy·drous
hy·dro·var·i·um
hy·drox·am·ic acids
hy·drox·ide
hy·droxo·co·bal·a·min
hy·droxy·ac·e·tan·i·lide
3-hy·droxy·ac·yl-CoA de·hy·
    dro·gen·ase
hy·droxy·ac·yl·glu·ta·thi·one
    hy·dro·lase
hy·droxy·am·phet·amine hy·
    dro·bro·mide
11β-hy·droxy·an·dro·stene·
    di·one [11-beta-]
hy·droxy·ap·a·tite
hy·droxy·ben·zene
3-hy·droxy·bu·ty·rate de·hy·
    dro·gen·ase

hy·droxy·bu·tyr·ic acid
    3-h.a.
    4-h.a.
    β-h.a.
    γ-h.a.
hy·droxy·chlo·ro·quine sul·
    fate
25-hy·droxy·cho·le·cal·cif·e·
    rol
17-hy·droxy·cor·ti·co·ster·oid
17-hy·drox·y·cor·ti·co·ster·
    one
25-hy·droxy·di·hy·dro·tach·
    ys·te·rol
hy·droxy·di·one so·di·um suc·
    ci·nate
hy·droxy·ei·co·sa·tet·ra·eno·
    ic acid
25-hy·droxy·er·go·cal·cif·e·
    rol
hy·droxy·es·tra·di·ols
hy·droxy·es·trin ben·zo·ate
hy·droxy·for·mo·ben·zo·yl·ic
    acid
hy·droxy·hep·ta·deca·tri·eno·
    ic acid
5-hy·droxy·in·dole·ace·tic
    acid
3-hy·droxy·iso·bu·ty·ryl-CoA
    hy·dro·lase
11-hy·droxy-17-ke·to·ste·roid
hy·drox·yl
hy·drox·yl·amine
hy·drox·yl·ap·a·tite
hy·drox·y·lase
    11β-h.
    17-h.
    21-h.
    24-h.
hy·droxy·la·tion
hy·drox·y·ly·sine
5-hy·droxy·meth·yl cy·to·sine
hy·droxy·meth·yl·glu·ta·
    ryl-CoA ly·ase
3-hy·drox·y-3-meth·yl·glu·ta·
    ryl CoA (HMG CoA) ly·ase
    deficiency

hy·droxy·meth·yl·glu·ta·
ryl-CoA re·duc·tase
hy·droxy·meth·yl·glu·ta·
ryl-CoA syn·thase
hy·droxy·meth·yl·trans·fer·
ase
hy·droxy·ner·vone
hy·droxy·phen·a·mate
hy·droxy·phen·yl·eth·yl·
amine
4-hy·droxy·phen·yl·py·ru·
vate di·oxy·gen·ase
p-hy·droxy·phen·yl·py·ru·
vate ox·i·dase
hy·droxy·phen·yl·uria
17α-hy·droxy·pro·ges·ter·one
[17-al·pha-]
hy·droxy·pro·ges·ter·one cap·
ro·ate
hy·droxy·pro·line
hy·droxy·pro·lin·emia
hy·droxy·pro·line ox·i·dase
4-hy·droxy-L-pro·line ox·i·
dase deficiency
hy·droxy·pro·lin·uria
hy·droxy·pro·pyl meth·yl·cel·
lu·lose
15-α-hy·droxy pros·ta·glan·
din de·hy·dro·gen·ase
[alpha]
8-hy·droxy·quin·o·line sul·
fate
hy·droxy·ste·a·rin sul·fate
17-hy·droxy·ste·roid
3β-hy·drox·y- Δ⁵-ste·roid de·
hy·dro·gen·ase
hy·droxy·stil·bam·i·dine is·
eth·io·nate
hy·droxy·tet·ra·cy·cline
5-hy·droxy·tryp·ta·mine
5-hy·droxy·tryp·to·phan
hy·droxy·urea
hy·droxy·val·ine
hy·droxy·zine
   h. hydrochloride
   h. pamoate
Hy·dro·zoa
hy·dro·zo·an

hy·dru·ria
hy·dru·ric
hy·e·nan·chin
Hy·geia
hy·gie·ist
hy·giene
   dental h.
   industrial h.
   mouth h.
   occupational h.
   oral h.
   radiation h.
hy·gien·ic
hy·gien·ics
hy·gien·ist
   dental h.
hy·gien·iza·tion
hy·gie·ol·o·gy
hy·gio·gen·e·sis
hy·gi·ol·o·gy
hy·gre·che·ma
hy·gric
hy·gro·ble·phar·ic
hy·gro·ma *pl.* hy·gro·mas, hy·
gro·ma·ta
   h. colli
   cystic h.
   h. cysticum
   h. praepatellare
   subdural h.
hy·gro·ma·tous
hy·grom·e·ter
   hair h.
   Saussure's h.
hy·gro·met·ric
hy·grom·e·try
hy·gro·my·cin
   h. B
hy·gro·scop·ic
Hy·gro·ton
Hy·kin·one
hy·la
Hy·le·my·ia
hy·lo·trop·ic
hy·lot·ro·py
hy·me·cro·mone
hy·men
   annular h.

hy·men *(continued)*
    h. bifenestratus
    h. biforis
    circular h.
    cribriform h.
    denticular h.
    falciform h.
    fenestrated h.
    imperforate h.
    infundibuliform h.
    lunar h.
    persistent h.
    septate h.
    h. septus
    h. subseptus
hy·men·al
hy·men·ec·to·my
hy·men·itis
hy·me·ni·um
hy·me·no·lep·i·a·sis
Hy·me·no·lep·i·di·dae
Hy·me·nol·e·pis
    H. diminuta
    H. fraterna
    H. lanceolata
    H. nana
    H. nana var. *fraterna*
hy·men·ol·o·gy
Hy·me·no·my·ce·tes
Hy·men·op·tera
hy·men·op·ter·an
hy·men·op·ter·ism
hy·men·or·rha·phy
Hy·me·no·sto·ma·tia
Hy·me·no·sto·ma·ti·da
hy·men·ot·o·my
hyo·ba·sio·glos·sus
hyo·epi·glot·tic
hyo·epi·glot·tid·e·an
hyo·glos·sal
hy·oid
hyo·lar·yn·ge·al
hyo·man·dib·u·lar
hyo·men·tal
hyo·scine
hyo·scy·amine
    h. hydrobromide
    h. sulfate

Hyo·scy·a·mus
hy·o·scy·a·mus
hyo·ster·nal
hyo·thy·roid
hyp·ac·i·de·mia
hyp·acu·sia
hyp·acu·sis
hyp·al·bu·min·emia
hyp·al·ge·sia
hyp·al·ge·sic
hyp·al·get·ic
hyp·al·gia
hyp·am·ni·on
hyp·am·ni·os
hyp·ana·ki·ne·sia
hyp·ana·ki·ne·sis
hy·paph·o·rine
hyp·aph·ro·dis·ia
Hy·paque
hyp·ar·te·ri·al
hyp·as·the·nia
hyp·ax·i·al
hyp·azo·tu·ria
hyp·en·chyme
hy·per·ab·sorp·tion
hy·per·ac·an·tho·sis
hy·per·ac·id
hy·per·ac·id·am·in·uria
hy·per·ac·id·i·ty
    gastric h.
hy·per·ac·tive
hy·per·ac·tiv·i·ty
hy·per·acu·i·ty
hy·per·acu·sis
hy·per·acute
hy·per·ad·e·no·sis
hy·per·ad·i·po·sis
hy·per·ad·i·pos·i·ty
hy·per·adre·nal
hy·per·adre·nal·emia
hy·per·adre·nal·ism
hy·per·adre·no·cor·ti·cal
hy·per·adre·no·cor·ti·cism
hy·per·al·bu·min·emia
hy·per·al·bu·min·o·sis
hy·per·al·co·hol·emia
hy·per·al·do·ster·on·emia
hy·per·al·do·ster·on·ism

hy·per·al·do·ster·on·uria
hy·per·al·ge·sia
    auditory h.
    muscular h.
hy·per·al·ge·sic
hy·per·al·get·ic
hy·per·al·gia
hy·per·al·i·men·ta·tion
    parenteral h.
hy·per·al·i·ment·ed
hy·per·al·i·men·to·sis
hy·per·al·ka·les·cence
hy·per·al·ka·lin·i·ty
hy·per·al·lan·to·in·uria
hy·per·al·o·ne·mia
hy·per·al·pha·lipo·pro·tein·emia
hy·per·am·i·no·ac·i·de·mia
hy·per·ami·no·ac·id·uria
hy·per·am·mo·ne·mia
    cerebroatrophic h.
    congenital h., type I
    congenital h., type II
hy·per·am·mo·ni·emia
hy·per·am·mo·nu·ria
hy·per·am·y·las·emia
hy·per·ana·ci·ne·sia
hy·per·ana·ki·ne·sia
hy·per·an·dro·gen·ism
hy·per·aphia
hy·per·aph·ic
hy·per·ar·gin·in·emia
hy·per·arou·sal
hy·per·azo·te·mia
hy·per·azo·tu·ria
hy·per·bar·ic
hy·per·bar·ism
hy·per·baso·phil·ic
hy·per-be·ta-al·a·nin·emia
hy·per·be·ta·lipo·pro·tein·emia
    familial h.
hy·per·bi·car·bo·nat·emia
hy·per·bil·i·ru·bin·emia
    congenital h.
    conjugated h.
    constitutional h.
    h. I

hy·per·bil·i·ru·bin·emia
    (continued)
    hereditary nonhemolytic h.
    neonatal h.
    unconjugated h.
hy·per·blas·to·sis
hy·per·brachy·ce·phal·ic
hy·per·brach·y·ceph·a·ly
hy·per·brady·ki·nin·emia
hy·per·brady·ki·nin·ism
hy·per·cal·ce·mia
    familial hypocalciuric h.
    idiopathic h.
hy·per·cal·ci·ne·mia
hy·per·cal·ci·nu·ria
hy·per·cal·ci·pexy
hy·per·cal·ci·to·nin·emia
hy·per·cal·ci·uria
    absorptive h.
    idiopathic h.
    renal h.
    resorptive h.
    secondary h.
hy·per·cap·nia
hy·per·cap·nic
hy·per·car·bia
hy·per·car·o·ten·emia
hy·per·car·o·tin·emia
hy·per·cat·a·bol·ic
hy·per·ca·tab·o·lism
hy·per·ca·thar·sis
hy·per·ca·thar·tic
hy·per·cel·lu·lar
hy·per·cel·lu·lar·i·ty
    glomerular h.
hy·per·ce·men·to·sis
hy·per·chlor·emia
hy·per·chlor·emic
hy·per·chlor·hy·dria
hy·per·chlo·ri·da·tion
hy·per·chlor·ura·tion
hy·per·chlor·uria
hy·per·cho·les·ter·emia
hy·per·cho·les·ter·emic
hy·per·cho·les·ter·in·emia
hy·per·cho·les·ter·ol·emia
    essential h.
    familial h.

hy·per·cho·les·ter·ol·emic
hy·per·cho·les·ter·ol·ia
hy·per·cho·lia
hy·per·chon·dro·pla·sia
hy·per·chro·maf·fin·ism
hy·per·chro·ma·sia
hy·per·chro·mat·ic
hy·per·chro·ma·tin
hy·per·chro·ma·tism
hy·per·chro·ma·top·sia
hy·per·chro·ma·to·sis
hy·per·chro·me·mia
hy·per·chro·mia
    macrocytic h.
hy·per·chro·mic
hy·per·chro·mic·i·ty
hy·per·chy·lia
hy·per·chy·lo·mi·cron·emia
    familial h.
hy·per·ci·ne·sia
hy·per·ci·tru·ria
hy·per·co·ag·u·la·bil·i·ty
hy·per·co·ag·u·la·ble
hy·per·co·ria
hy·per·cor·ti·cal·ism
hy·per·cor·ti·cism
hy·per·cor·ti·sol·ism
hy·per·cre·a·tin·emia
hy·per·cry·al·ge·sia
hy·per·cry·es·the·sia
hy·per·cu·pre·mia
hy·per·cu·pri·uria
hy·per·cy·a·not·ic
hy·per·cy·e·sis
hy·per·cy·the·mia
hy·per·cy·to·chro·mia
hy·per·cy·to·sis
hy·per·dac·ty·ly
hy·per·di·as·to·le
hy·per·di·crot·ic
hy·per·di·cro·tism
hy·per·dip·loid
hy·per·dip·sia
hy·per·dis·ten·tion
hy·per·di·ure·sis
hy·per·don·tia
hy·per·dy·na·mia
    h. uteri

hy·per·dy·nam·ic
hy·per·ec·cris·ia
hy·per·ec·cri·sis
hy·per·ec·crit·ic
hy·per·eche·ma
hy·per·ech·o·ic
hy·per·elas·tic
hy·per·elec·tro·ly·te·mia
hy·per·em·e·sis
    h. gravidarum
    h. lactentium
hy·per·emet·ic
hy·per·emia
    active h.
    arterial h.
    Bier's passive h.
    collateral h.
    constriction h.
    fluxionary h.
    leptomeningeal h.
    passive h.
    reactive h.
    stauungs h.
    venous h.
hy·per·emic
hy·per·emi·za·tion
hy·per·en·ceph·a·lus
hy·per·en·dem·ic
hy·per·en·do·crin·ism
hy·per·en·er·gia
hy·per·eo·sin·o·phil·ia
    filarial h.
hy·per·epi·neph·rin·emia
hy·per·equi·lib·ri·um
hy·per·er·e·thism
hy·per·er·ga·sia
hy·per·er·gia
hy·per·eryth·ro·cy·the·mia
hy·per·eso·pho·ria
hy·per·es·the·sia
    acoustic h.
    auditory h.
    cerebral h.
    gustatory h.
    muscular h.
    olfactory h.
    oneiric h.
    optic h.

hy·per·es·the·sia *(continued)*
    tactile h.
hy·per·es·thet·ic
hy·per·es·trin·emia
hy·per·es·trin·ism
hy·per·es·tro·gen·emia
hy·per·es·tro·gen·ism
hy·per·es·tro·gen·o·sis
hy·per·eu·ryo·pia
hy·per·evol·u·tism
hy·per·ex·cre·to·ry
hy·per·exo·pho·ria
hy·per·ex·plex·ia
hy·per·ex·ten·sion
hy·per·fer·re·mia
hy·per·fer·re·mic
hy·per·fer·ri·ce·mia
hy·per·fi·bri·no·ge·ne·mia
hy·per·fi·bri·nol·y·sis
    systemic h.
hy·per·fil·tra·tion
hy·per·flex·ion
hy·per·fol·lic·u·lin·ism
hy·per·func·tion
hy·per·func·tion·ing
hy·per·ga·lac·tia
hy·per·gal·ac·to·sis
hy·per·ga·lac·tous
hy·per·gam·ma·glob·u·lin·
  emia
    M-component h.
    monoclonal h.
hy·per·gas·trin·emia
hy·per·gen·e·sis
hy·per·ge·net·ic
hy·per·gen·i·tal·ism
hy·per·geus·es·the·sia
hy·per·geu·sia
hy·per·gia
hy·per·gi·gan·to·so·ma
hy·per·glan·du·lar
hy·per·glob·u·lia
hy·per·glob·u·lin·emia
hy·per·glob·u·lism
hy·per·glu·ca·gon·emia
hy·per·glu·co·neo·gen·e·sis
hy·per·gly·ce·mia
hy·per·gly·ce·mic

hy·per·glyc·er·i·de·mia
hy·per·glyc·er·i·de·mic
hy·per·gly·cin·emia
    ketotic h.
    nonketotic h.
hy·per·gly·cin·uria
hy·per·gly·cis·tia
hy·per·gly·co·gen·ol·y·sis
hy·per·gly·cor·rha·chia
hy·per·gly·co·se·mia
hy·per·gly·cos·uria
hy·per·gly·cys·tia
hy·per·gly·ke·mia
hy·per·gly·ox·yl·emia
hy·per·gno·sis
hy·per·go·nad·ism
hy·per·gon·ad·o·trop·ic
hy·per·go·nia
hy·per·gran·u·la·tion
    juxtaglomerular cell h.
hy·per·guan·i·din·emia
hy·per·he·do·nia
hy·per·he·don·ism
hy·per·he·mo·glo·bin·emia
hy·per·he·mo·lyt·ic
hy·per·hep·a·rin·emia
hy·per·he·pat·ia
hy·per·hi·dro·sis
    axillary h.
    emotional h.
    gustatory h.
    h. unilateralis
    volar h.
hy·per·hi·drot·ic
hy·per·his·ta·min·emia
hy·per·hor·mon·ism
hy·per·hy·dra·tion
hy·per·hy·dro·chlo·ria
hy·per·hy·dro·chlo·rid·ia
hy·per·hy·drox·y·pro·lin·
  emia
hy·per·hyp·no·sis
hy·per·hy·poph·y·sism
hy·per·idro·sis
hy·per·im·id·o·di·pep·tid·
  uria
hy·per·im·mune
hy·per·im·mu·ni·ty

hy·per·im·mu·ni·za·tion
   maternal h.
hy·per·im·mu·no·glob·u·lin·
  emia
   h. E
hy·per·in·di·can·emia
hy·per·in·fla·tion
hy·per·in·ges·tion
hy·per·in·ner·va·tion
hy·per·in·su·lin·ar
hy·per·in·su·lin·emia
hy·per·in·su·lin·ism
   alimentary h.
   functional h.
   iatrogenic h.
hy·per·in·vo·lu·tion
hy·per·io·de·mia
hy·per·ir·ri·ta·bil·i·ty
hy·per·iso·to·nia
hy·per·iso·ton·ic
hy·per·iso·ton·ic·i·ty
hy·per·ka·le·mia
hy·per·kal·i·emia
hy·per·kal·uria
hy·per·ker·a·tin·iza·tion
hy·pe·ker·a·to·sis
   bullous ichthyosiform h.
   h. congenitalis palmaris et
    plantaris
   diffuse congenital h.
   epidermolytic h.
   follicular h.
   h. follicularis in cutem
    penetrans
   h. follicularis et
    parafollicularis in cutem
    penetrans
   h. lacunaris
   h. lacunaris pharyngis
   h. lenticularis perstans
   h. of palms and soles
   h. penetrans
   progressive dystrophic h.
   h. subungualis
hy·per·ke·ton·emia
hy·per·ke·ton·uria
hy·per·ke·to·sis
hy·per·ki·ne·mia

hy·per·ki·ne·mic
hy·per·ki·ne·sia
hy·per·ki·ne·sis
hy·per·ki·net·ic
hy·per·ko·ria
hy·per·lact·ac·i·de·mia
hy·per·lac·ta·tion
hy·per·lac·tic·ac·id·emia
hy·per·lec·i·thin·emia
hy·per·le·thal
hy·per·leu·ko·cy·to·sis
hy·per·ley·dig·ism
hy·per·li·pe·mia
   carbohydrate-induced h.
   combined fat- and
    carbohydrate-induced h.
   familial h., essential
   fat-induced h., familial
   idiopathic h.
   mixed h.
hy·per·lip·id·emia
   combined h., familial
   mixed h.
   multiple lipoprotein-type
    h.
hy·per·li·poid·emia
hy·per·lipo·pro·tein·emia
   acquired h.
   broad-beta h., familial
   combined h., familial
   familial h.
   mixed h.
hy·per·li·po·sis
hy·per·li·the·mia
hy·per·lith·ic
hy·per·li·thu·ria
hy·per·lor·do·sis
hy·per·lu·cen·cy
hy·per·lu·te·in·iza·tion
hy·per·lu·te·mia
hy·per·ly·sin·emia
hy·per·ly·sin·uria
hy·per·mag·ne·se·mia
hy·per·ma·nia
hy·per·mas·tia
hy·per·ma·ture
hy·per·med·i·ca·tion
hy·per·mel·a·no·sis

hy·per·mel·a·not·ic
hy·per·men·or·rhea
hy·per·met·a·bol·ic
hy·per·me·tab·o·lism
    extrathyroidal h.
hy·per·meta·mor·pho·sis
hy·per·meta·pla·sia
hy·per·me·tria
hy·per·met·rope
hy·per·me·tro·pia
hy·per·me·trop·ic
hy·per·mi·cro·so·ma
hy·per·mim·ia
hy·per·min·er·al·iza·tion
hy·perm·ne·sia
hy·perm·ne·sic
hy·per·mo·dal
hy·per·morph
hy·per·mo·til·i·ty
hy·per·myo·to·nia
hy·per·my·ot·ro·phy
hy·per·na·sal·i·ty
hy·per·na·tre·mia
    hypodipsic h.
hy·per·na·tre·mic
hy·per·nat·ron·emia
hy·per·neo·cy·to·sis
hy·per·neph·roid
hy·per·ne·phro·ma
hy·per·ni·da·tion
hy·per·ni·tre·mia
hy·per·nom·ic
hy·per·nor·mal
hy·per·nu·tri·tion
hy·per·oc·clu·sion
hy·per·on·cot·ic
hy·per·onych·ia
hy·per·ope
hy·per·opia
    absolute h.
    axial h.
    curvature h.
    facultative h.
    index h.
    latent h.
    manifest h.
    relative h.
    total h.

hy·per·op·ic
hy·per·or·chi·dism
hy·per·orex·ia
hy·per·or·ni·the·mia
hy·per·or·tho·cy·to·sis
hy·per·os·mia
hy·per·os·mo·lal·i·ty
hy·per·os·mo·lar·i·ty
hy·per·os·mot·ic
hy·per·os·phre·sia
hy·per·os·teo·gen·e·sis
hy·per·os·te·og·e·ny
hy·per·os·to·sis
    calvarial h.
    h. corticalis deformans
     juvenilis
    h. corticalis generalisata
    h. cranii
    flowing h.
    h. frontalis interna
    infantile cortical h.
    Morgagni's h.
    senile ankylosing h. of
     spine
hy·per·os·tot·ic
hy·per·ova·ri·an·ism
hy·per·ova·rism
hy·per·ox·al·uria
    enteric h.
    primary h.
hy·per·ox·emia
hy·per·ox·ia
hy·per·ox·ic
hy·per·ox·i·da·tion
hy·per·pal·les·the·sia
hy·per·pan·cre·or·rhea
hy·per·par·a·site
    second degree h.
hy·per·par·a·sit·ic
hy·per·par·a·sit·ism
hy·per·para·si·toid·ism
hy·per·para·thy·roid·ism
hy·per·path·ia
    thalamic h.
hy·per·pep·sia
hy·per·pep·sin·emia
hy·per·pep·sin·ia
hy·per·pep·sin·uria

hy·per·peri·stal·sis
hy·per·per·me·a·bil·i·ty
hy·per·pex·ia
hy·per·pexy
hy·per·pha·gia
hy·per·pha·gic
hy·per·pha·lan·gia
hy·per·pha·lan·gism
hy·per·phen·yl·al·a·nin·emia
hy·per·pho·ne·sis
hy·per·pho·nia
hy·per·pho·ria
hy·per·phos·pha·ta·se·mia
  chronic congenital
    idiopathic h.
  h. tarda
hy·per·phos·pha·ta·sia
hy·per·phos·pha·te·mia
hy·per·phos·pha·tu·ria
hy·per·phos·pho·re·mia
hy·per·phre·nia
hy·per·pi·esia
hy·per·pi·esis
hy·per·pi·et·ic
hy·per·pig·men·ta·tion
hy·per·pi·ne·al·ism
hy·per·pi·tu·i·ta·rism
  basophilic h.
  eosinophilic h.
hy·per·pla·sia
  adrenal cortical h.
  angiofollicular mediastinal
    lymph node h.
  angiolymphoid h.
  basal cell h.
  benign mediastinal lymph
    node h.
  cementum h.
  chronic perforating pulp h.
  congenital adrenal h.
  congenital adrenocortical
    h.
  congenital sebaceous gland
    h.
  congenital virilizing
    adrenal h.
  cutaneous lymphoid h.
  cystic h. of breasts

hy·per·pla·sia *(continued)*
  cystic-glandular h. of
    endometrium
  denture h.
  Dilantin h.
  endometrial h.
  h. endometrii
  epiphyseal h.
  fibromuscular h.
  fibrous inflammatory h.
  focal adenomyomatous h.
    of gallbladder
  focal nodular h. (FNH)
  giant follicular h.
  gingival h.
  inflammatory h.
  islet cell h.
  juxtaglomerular cell h.
  lipoid h.
  neoplastic h.
  nodular lymphoid h.
  ovarian stromal h.
  polar h.
  polypoid h.
  pseudoepitheliomatous h.
  Schwann h.
  Swiss-cheese h.
  thymic medullary h.
hy·per·plas·mia
hy·per·plas·min·emia
hy·per·plas·tic
hy·per·ploid
hy·per·ploi·dy
hy·per·pnea
hy·per·pne·ic
hy·per·po·lar·iza·tion
hy·per·poly·pep·tid·emia
hy·per·po·ne·sis
hy·per·po·net·ic
hy·per·po·sia
hy·per·po·tas·se·mia
hy·per·pra·gic
hy·per·prax·ia
hy·per·pre·be·ta·lipo·pro·
  tein·emia
    familial h.
hy·per·pres·by·opia
hy·per·pro·ges·te·ron·emia

hy·per·pro·in·su·lin·emia
hy·per·pro·lac·tin·emia
hy·per·pro·lac·tin·emic
hy·per·pro·lac·tin·ism
hy·per·pro·lin·emia
   familial h.
hy·per·pro·ses·sis
hy·per·pro·sex·ia
hy·per·pro·tein·emia
hy·per·pro·te·o·sis
hy·perp·sel·a·phe·sia
hy·per·pty·al·ism
hy·per·py·re·mia
hy·per·py·ret·ic
hy·per·py·rex·ia
   fulminant h.
   heat h.
   malignant h.
hy·per·py·rex·i·al
hy·per·re·ac·tive
hy·per·re·flex·ia
   autonomic h.
   detrusor h.
hy·per·re·nin·emia
hy·per·re·nin·emic
hy·per·res·o·nance
hy·per·sal·emia
hy·per·sa·line
hy·per·sal·i·va·tion
hy·per·sar·co·sin·emia
hy·per·se·cre·tion
   gastric h.
hy·per·seg·men·ta·tion
   hereditary h. of
    neutrophils
hy·per·sen·si·bil·i·ty
hy·per·sen·si·tive
hy·per·sen·si·tiv·i·ty
   atopic h.
   carotid sinus h.
   contact h.
   cutaneous basophil h.
   delayed h. (DH)
   delayed-type h. (DTH)
   immediate h.
   tuberculin-type h.
hy·per·sen·si·ti·za·tion
hy·per·sero·to·ne·mia

hy·per·sex·u·al·i·ty
hy·per·skeo·cy·to·sis
hy·per·so·ma·to·trop·ism
hy·per·so·mia
hy·per·som·nia
   continuous h.
   paroxysmal h.
   periodic h.
hy·per·som·no·lence
hy·per·sphyx·ia
hy·per·sple·nia
hy·per·sple·nism
hy·per·spon·gi·o·sis
Hy·per·stat
hy·per·ste·a·to·sis
hy·per·ster·eo·roent·gen·og·
   ra·phy
hy·per·ster·eo·ski·ag·ra·phy
hy·per·sthe·nia
hy·per·sthen·ic
hy·per·sthen·uria
hy·per·su·pra·re·nal·ism
hy·per·sus·cep·ti·bil·i·ty
hy·per·sym·path·i·co·to·nus
hy·per·ta·rach·ia
hy·per·tau·ro·don·tism
hy·per·telo·rism
   canthal h.
   ocular h.
   orbital h.
Hy·per·ten·sin
hy·per·ten·sin·o·gen
hy·per·ten·sion
   accelerated h.
   adrenal h.
   arterial h.
   benign intracranial h.
   borderline h.
   diastolic h.
   endolymphatic h.
   episodic h.
   essential h.
   gestational h.
   Goldblatt h.
   idiopathic h.
   intracranial h.
   labile h.
   low-renin h.

hy·per·ten·sion *(continued)*
    malignant h.
    neuromuscular h.
    ocular h.
    pale h.
    paroxysmal h.
    pituitary h.
    portal h.
    primary h.
    pulmonary h.
    red h.
    renal h.
    renin-dependent h.
    renoprival h.
    renovascular h.
    secondary h.
    splenoportal h.
    suprarenal h.
    symptomatic h.
    systemic venous h.
    systolic h.
    transient h.
    vascular h.
    venous h.
hy·per·ten·sive
hy·per·ten·sor
hy·per·tes·tos·ter·on·ism
Hy·per-Tet
hy·per·the·co·sis
    testoid h.
hy·per·the·lia
hy·per·ther·mal
hy·per·ther·mal·ge·sia
hy·per·ther·mes·the·sia
hy·per·ther·mia
    h. of anesthesia
    malignant h.
    whole-body h.
hy·per·ther·mo·es·the·sia
hy·per·ther·my
hy·per·throm·bin·emia
hy·per·thy·mia
hy·per·thy·mic
hy·per·thy·mism
hy·per·thy·rea
hy·per·thy·re·o·sis

hy·per·thy·roid
hy·per·thy·roid·ism
    apathetic h.
    factitious h.
    iatrogenic h.
    iodine-induced h.
    masked h.
hy·per·thy·roid·o·sis
hy·per·thy·rox·in·emia
    familial dysalbuminemic h.
hy·per·to·nia
    h. oculi
    h. polycythaemica
hy·per·ton·ic
hy·per·to·nic·i·ty
hy·per·to·nus
hy·per·tox·ic
hy·per·tox·ic·i·ty
hy·per·tri·cho·sis
    h. lanuginosa
    h. pinnae auris
    h. universalis
hy·per·tri·glyc·er·i·de·mia
    alimentary h.
    carbohydrate-induced h.
    endogenous h.
    exogenous h.
    familial fat-induced h.
    familial h.
hy·per·tro·phia
    h. musculorum vera
hy·per·troph·ic
hy·per·tro·phy
    adaptive h.
    adenoid h.
    adult h. of pylorus
    benign h. of pons
    bilateral h. of masseters
    Billroth h.
    biventricular h.
    breast h. of newborn
    cardiac concentric h.
    cicatricial h.
    compensatory h.
    complementary h.
    concentric h.

hy·per·tro·phy *(continued)*
  congenital h. of bladder
    neck
  denture h.
  eccentric h.
  false h.
  fibromuscular h.
  functional h.
  hemangiectatic h.
  hemifacial h.
  juxtaglomerular cell h.
  mammary h.
  Marie's h.
  mulberry h.
  numeric h.
  physiologic h.
  pseudomuscular h.
  quantitative h.
  renal h.
  simple h.
  true h.
  unilateral h.
  ventricular h.
  vicarious h.
hy·per·tro·pia
Hy·per·tus·sis
hy·per·ty·ro·sin·emia
hy·per·ure·sis
hy·per·u·ric·ac·i·de·mia
hy·per·u·ric·ac·i·du·ria
hy·per·uri·ce·mia
  X-linked h.
hy·per·uri·ce·mic
hy·per·u·ric·uria
hy·per·vac·ci·na·tion
hy·per·val·i·ne·mia
hy·per·vas·cu·lar
hy·per·ven·ti·la·tion
  central neurogenic h.
  hysterical h.
hy·per·vis·cos·i·ty
hy·per·vi·ta·min·o·sis
  h. A
  h. D
hy·per·vi·ta·min·ot·ic
hy·per·vo·le·mia
hy·per·vo·le·mic
hy·per·vo·lia

hyp·es·the·sia
hy·pha *pl.* hy·phae
  apical h.
  racquet h.
hy·phal
hyp·he·do·nia
hy·phe·ma
hy·phe·mia
hyp·hid·ro·sis
Hy·pho·my·ces
  H. destruens
hy·pho·my·cete
Hy·pho·my·ce·tes
hy·pho·my·co·sis
  h. destruens equi
hy·phyl·line
hyp·iso·ton·ic
hyp·na·gog·ic
hyp·na·gogue
hyp·nal·gia
hyp·nic
hyp·no·anal·y·sis
hyp·no·an·es·the·sia
hyp·no·cine·mato·graph
hyp·no·cyst
hyp·no·don·tia
hyp·no·don·tics
hyp·no·ge·net·ic
hyp·no·gen·ic
hyp·nog·e·nous
hyp·noid
hyp·noi·dal
hyp·no·lep·sy
hyp·nol·o·gy
hyp·no·pe·dia
hyp·no·pom·pic
hyp·no·sis
hyp·nos·o·phy
hyp·no·ther·a·py
hyp·not·ic
hyp·no·tism
hyp·no·tist
hyp·no·ti·za·tion
hyp·no·tize
hyp·no·tox·in
hyp·no·zo·ite
hy·po
hy·po·ac·id·i·ty

hy·po·ac·tive
hy·po·ac·tiv·i·ty
hy·po·acu·sis
hy·po·ade·nia
hy·po·adren·al·emia
hy·po·adren·a·lism
hy·po·adre·no·cor·ti·cal
hy·po·adre·no·cor·ti·cism
    pituitary h.
    secondary h.
hy·po·aer·a·tion
hy·po·ag·na·thus
hy·po·al·bu·min·emia
hy·po·al·bu·min·o·sis
hy·po·al·do·ster·on·emia
hy·po·al·do·ster·on·ism
    hyporeninemic h.
    isolated h.
hy·po·al·do·ster·on·uria
hy·po·al·ge·sia
hy·po·al·i·men·ta·tion
hy·po·al·ka·line
hy·po·al·ka·lin·i·ty
hy·po·al·ler·gen·ic
hy·po·al·o·ne·mia
hy·po·al·pha·lipo·pro·tein·
  emia
hy·po·am·i·no·ac·i·de·mia
hy·po·an·dro·gen·ism
hy·po·azo·tu·ria
hy·po·bar·ic
hy·po·bar·ism
hy·po·ba·rop·a·thy
hy·po·be·ta·lipo·pro·tein·
  emia
    familial h.
hy·po·bil·i·ru·bin·emia
hy·po·blast
hy·po·blas·tic
hy·po·bran·chi·al
hy·po·bro·mite
hy·po·bro·mous acid
hy·po·cal·ce·mia
    neonatal h.
hy·po·cal·ce·mic
hy·po·cal·cia
hy·po·cal·ci·fi·ca·tion
    enamel h.

hy·po·cal·ci·pec·tic
hy·po·cal·ci·pexy
hy·po·cal·ci·to·nin·emia
hy·po·cal·ci·uria
hy·po·cap·nia
hy·po·cap·nic
hy·po·car·bia
hy·po·cata·la·se·mia
hy·po·cel·lu·lar
hy·po·cel·lu·lar·i·ty
hy·po·ce·ru·lo·plas·min·emia
hy·po·chlor·emia
hy·po·chlor·emic
hy·po·chlor·hy·dria
hy·po·chlo·ri·da·tion
hy·po·chlo·rid·emia
hy·po·chlo·rite
hy·po·chlo·ri·za·tion
hy·po·chlo·rous acid
hy·po·chlor·uria
hy·po·cho·les·te·re·mia
hy·po·cho·les·te·re·mic
hy·po·cho·les·ter·in·emia
hy·po·cho·les·ter·ol·emia
hy·po·cho·les·ter·ol·emic
hy·po·cho·lia
hy·po·chol·uria
hy·po·chon·dria
hy·po·chon·dri·ac
hy·po·chon·dri·a·cal
hy·po·chon·dri·a·sis
hy·po·chon·dri·um *pl.* hy·po·
  chon·dria
hy·po·chon·dro·pla·sia
hy·po·chor·dal
hy·po·chro·ma·sia
hy·po·chro·mat·ic
hy·po·chro·ma·tism
hy·po·chro·ma·to·sis
hy·po·chro·me·mia
    idiopathic h.
hy·po·chro·mia
hy·po·chro·mic
hy·po·chro·mic·i·ty
hy·po·chro·mo·trich·ia
hy·po·chro·sis
hy·po·chy·lia
hy·po·cis·tis

hy·po·ci·tre·mia
hy·po·ci·tru·ria
hy·po·co·ag·u·la·bil·i·ty
hy·po·co·ag·u·la·ble
hy·po·coe·lom
hy·po·com·ple·men·te·mia
hy·po·com·ple·men·te·mic
hy·po·con·dy·lar
hy·po·cone
hy·po·con·id
hy·po·con·u·lid
hy·po·cor·ti·cal·ism
hy·po·cor·ti·cism
hy·po·cot·yl
Hy·po·cre·a·les
hy·po·cu·pre·mia
hy·po·cy·clo·sis
hy·po·cy·the·mia
hy·po·cy·to·sis
hy·po·dac·ty·ly
hy·po·derm
Hy·po·der·ma
    H. bovis
    H. lineatum
hy·po·der·mat·ic
hy·po·der·mato·cly·sis
hy·po·der·mat·o·my
hy·po·der·mi·a·sis
hy·po·der·mic
hy·po·der·mis
hy·po·der·mo·cly·sis
hy·po·der·mo·li·thi·a·sis
hy·po·der·mo·my·co·sis
hy·po·di·a·phrag·mat·ic
hy·po·dip·loid
hy·po·dip·loi·dy
hy·po·ploid
hy·po·ploi·dy
hy·po·dip·sia
hy·po·dip·sic
hy·po·don·tia
hy·po·dy·na·mia
    h. cordis
hy·po·dy·nam·ic
hy·po·ec·cris·ia
hy·po·ec·cri·sis
hy·po·ec·crit·ic
hy·po·echo·ic

hy·po·elec·tro·ly·te·mia
hy·po·eo·sin·o·phil·ia
hy·po·ep·i·neph·rin·emia
hy·po·equi·lib·ri·um
hy·po·er·ga·sia
hy·po·er·gia
hy·po·er·gic
hy·po·er·gy
hy·po·eso·pho·ria
hy·po·es·the·sia
    acoustic h.
    auditory h.
    gustatory h.
    olfactory h.
    tactile h.
hy·po·es·thet·ic
hy·po·es·trin·emia
hy·po·es·tro·gen·emia
hy·po·es·tro·ge·nem·ism
hy·po·evol·u·tism
hy·po·ex·ci·ta·bil·i·ty
hy·po·ex·ci·ta·ble
hy·po·exo·pho·ria
hy·po·fer·re·mia
hy·po·fer·rism
hy·po·fer·tile
hy·po·fer·til·i·ty
hy·po·fi·brin·o·gen·emia
hy·po·func·tion
    convergence h.
    divergence h.
hy·po·ga·lac·tia
hy·po·ga·lac·tous
hy·po·gam·ma·glob·u·lin·emia
    acquired h.
    common variable h.
    congenital h.
    lymphopenic h.
    physiologic h.
    primary h.
    secondary h.
    Swiss-type h.
    transient h. of infancy
    X-linked h.
    X-linked infantile h.
hy·po·gan·gli·o·no·sis
hy·po·gas·tric

hy·po·gas·tri·um
hy·po·gas·trop·a·gus
hy·po·gas·tros·chi·sis
hy·po·gen·e·sis
    polar h.
hy·po·ge·net·ic
hy·po·gen·i·tal·ism
hy·po·geus·es·the·sia
hy·po·geu·sia
hy·po·glan·du·lar
hy·po·glob·u·lia
hy·po·glos·sal
hy·po·glos·sus
hy·po·glot·tis
hy·po·glu·ca·gon·emia
hy·po·gly·ce·mia
    factitial h.
    factitious h.
    fasting h.
    functional h.
    ketotic h.
    leucine-induced h.
    mixed h.
    reactive h.
hy·po·gly·ce·mic
hy·po·gly·ce·mo·sis
hy·po·gly·cine
hy·po·gly·co·gen·ol·y·sis
hy·po·gly·cor·rha·chia
hy·pog·na·thous
hy·pog·na·thus
hy·po·go·nad·al
hy·po·go·nad·ism
    eugonadotropic h.
    familial hypogonadotropic
      h.
    hypergonadotropic h.
    hypogonadotropic h.
    pituitary h.
    primary h.
    secondary h.
hy·po·gon·a·do·trop·ic
hy·po·go·nado·trop·ism
hy·po·gran·u·lo·cy·to·sis
hy·po·he·pat·ia
hy·po·hi·dro·sis
hy·po·hi·drot·ic
hy·po·hor·mo·nal

hy·po·hy·al
hy·po·hy·dra·tion
hy·po·hy·dro·chlo·ria
hy·po·hyp·not·ic
hy·po·hy·poph·y·sism
hy·po·idro·sis
hy·po·in·su·lin·emia
hy·po·in·su·lin·ism
hy·po·io·di·dism
hy·po·iso·ton·ic
hy·po·ka·le·mia
hy·po·ka·le·mic
hy·po·ki·ne·mia
hy·po·ki·ne·sia
hy·po·ki·ne·sis
hy·po·ki·net·ic
hy·po·lac·ta·sia
hy·po·lar·ynx
hy·po·lem·mal
hy·po·le·thal
hy·po·leu·ko·cyt·ic
hy·po·ley·dig·ism
hy·po·li·pe·mia
hy·po·lip·id·emic
hy·po·lipo·pro·tein·emia
hy·po·li·po·sis
hy·po·li·quor·rhea
hy·po·lu·te·mia
hy·po·lym·phe·mia
hy·po·mag·ne·se·mia
hy·po·ma·nia
hy·po·man·ic
hy·po·mas·tia
hy·po·mel·an·cho·lia
hy·po·mel·a·nism
    dominant oculocutaneous
    h.
hy·po·mel·a·no·sis
    hereditary h.
    idiopathic guttate h.
    h. of Ito
hy·po·men·or·rhea
hy·po·mere
hy·po·mery
hy·po·me·so·so·ma
hy·po·met·a·bol·ic
hy·po·me·tab·o·lism
    euthyroid h.

hy·po·me·tria
hy·po·me·tro·pia
hy·po·mi·cron
hy·po·mi·cro·so·ma
hy·po·min·er·al·iza·tion
hy·pom·ne·sis
hy·po·mo·dal
hy·po·morph
hy·po·mo·til·i·ty
hy·po·myo·to·nia
hy·po·myx·ia
hy·po·na·no·so·ma
hy·po·na·sal·i·ty
hy·po·na·tre·mia
    depletional h.
    dilutional h.
    hyperlipemic h.
hy·po·na·tru·ria
hy·po·neo·cy·to·sis
hy·po·ni·tre·mia
hy·po·noia
hy·po·nych·i·al
hy·po·nych·i·um
hy·pon·y·chon
hy·po-on·cot·ic
hy·po-or·chi·dism
hy·po-or·tho·cy·to·sis
hy·po-os·mo·lal·i·ty
hy·po-os·mo·sis
hy·po-os·mot·ic
hy·po-ovar·ia
hy·po-ovar·ri·an·ism
hy·po·pal·les·the·sia
hy·po·pan·cre·a·tism
hy·po·pan·cre·or·rhea
hy·po·para·thy·roid
hy·po·para·thy·roid·ism
    familial h.
hy·po·pep·sia
hy·po·pep·sin·ia
hy·po·per·fu·sion
hy·po·peri·stal·sis
hy·po·peri·stal·tic
hy·po·pex·ia
hy·po·pha·lan·gism
hy·poph·amine
hy·po·pha·ryn·ge·al
hy·po·pha·ryn·go·scope

hy·po·pha·ryn·gos·co·py
hy·po·phar·ynx
hy·po·pho·ne·sis
hy·po·pho·nia
hy·po·pho·ria
hy·po·phos·pha·ta·sia
hy·po·phos·pha·te·mia
    familial h.
    hereditary h.
    renal h.
    X-linked h.
hy·po·phos·pha·te·mic
hy·po·phos·pha·tu·ria
hy·po·phos·phite
    ferric h.
hy·po·phos·pho·re·mia
hy·po·phos·phor·ous acid
hy·po·phre·nia
hy·po·phren·ic
hy·po·phre·ni·um
hy·po·phys·e·al
hy·po·phys·ec·to·mize
hy·po·phys·ec·to·my
    trans-sphenoidal h.
hy·po·phys·i·al
hy·poph·y·sin
hy·po·phys·io·por·tal
hy·po·phys·io·priv·ic
hy·po·phys·i·o·trop·ic
hy·poph·y·sis
    accessory h.
    h. cerebri
    pharyngeal h.
hy·poph·y·si·tis
hy·po·pi·e·sia
hy·po·pi·e·sis
hy·po·pi·et·ic
hy·po·pig·men·ta·tion
hy·po·pig·men·ter
hy·po·pin·e·al·ism
hy·po·pi·tu·i·ta·rism
    postpartum hemorrhagic h.
hy·po·pi·tu·i·tary
hy·po·pla·sia
    cartilage-hair h.
    congenital generalized
      muscular h.
    craniofacial h.

hy·po·pla·sia *(continued)*
  h. cutis congenita
  enamel h.
  focal dermal h.
  granulocytic h.
  hereditary brown h. of
    enamel
  lobular h.
  nasomaxillary h.
  oligomeganephronic renal
    h.
  oligonephronic h.
  pluricystic h.
  thymic h.
  Turner's h.
hy·po·plas·tic
hy·po·plas·ty
hy·po·ploid
hy·po·pnea
hy·po·pne·ic
hy·po·po·ne·sis
hy·po·po·ro·sis
hy·po·po·sia
hy·po·po·tas·se·mia
hy·po·po·tas·se·mic
hy·po·po·ten·tia
hy·po·prax·ia
hy·po·pro·ac·cel·er·in·emia
hy·po·pro·con·ver·tin·emia
  hereditary h.
hy·po·pro·ges·ter·one hex·a·no·ate
hy·po·pros·o·dy
hy·po·pro·tein·emia
  prehepatic h.
hy·po·pro·tein·emic
hy·po·pro·tein·ia
hy·po·pro·tein·ic
hy·po·pro·tein·o·sis
hy·po·pro·throm·bin·emia
hy·pop·sel·a·phe·sia
hy·po·pter·on·o·sis cys·ti·ca
hy·po·pty·al·ism
hy·po·pus
hy·po·py·on
hy·po·re·ac·tive
hy·po·re·flex·ia
hy·po·re·nin·emia
hy·po·re·nin·emic
hy·po·ri·bo·fla·vi·no·sis
hy·por·rhea
hy·po·sa·le·mia
hy·po·sal·i·va·tion
hy·po·sar·ca
hy·pos·che·ot·o·my
hy·po·scle·ral
hy·po·se·cre·tion
hy·po·sen·si·tive
hy·po·sen·si·tiv·i·ty
hy·po·sen·si·ti·za·tion
hy·po·sen·si·tize
hy·po·sex·u·al·i·ty
hy·po·si·a·lo·sis
hy·po·skeo·cy·to·sis
hy·pos·mia
hy·pos·mo·lar·i·ty
hy·pos·mo·sis
hy·po·so·mato·tro·pism
hy·po·so·mia
hy·po·som·nia
hy·po·spa·dia
hy·po·spa·di·ac
hy·po·spa·di·as
  balanic h.
  balanitic h.
  female h.
  glandular h.
  penile h.
  penoscrotal h.
  perineal h.
  pseudovaginal h.
hy·pos·phre·sia
hy·po·splen·ism
hy·pos·ta·sis
hy·po·stat·ic
hy·po·ste·a·tol·y·sis
hy·po·ste·a·to·sis
hy·pos·the·nia
hy·pos·the·ni·ant
hy·pos·then·ic
hy·pos·then·uria
  tubular h.
hy·po·stome
hy·po·sto·mia
hy·po·sto·mi·al
hyp·os·to·sis

hy·po·styp·sis
hy·po·styp·tic
hy·po·sul·fite
hy·po·su·pra·re·nal·ism
hy·po·sym·path·i·co·to·nus
hy·po·syn·er·gia
hy·po·tax·ia
hy·po·telo·rism
    ocular h.
    orbital h.
hy·po·ten·sion
    arterial h.
    chronic orthostatic h.
    controlled h.
    familial orthostatic h.
    idiopathic orthostatic h.
    induced h.
    intracranial h.
    orthostatic h.
    postural h.
    spinal h.
    vascular h.
    ventricular h.
hy·po·ten·sive
hy·po·ten·sor
hy·po·tha·lam·ic
hy·po·thal·a·mot·o·my
hy·po·thal·a·mus
hy·poth·e·nar
hy·po·ther·mal
hy·po·ther·mia
    endogenous h.
    induced h.
    moderate h.
    profound h.
    regional h.
hy·po·ther·mic
hy·poth·e·sis
    alternative h.
    anniversary h.
    biogenic amine h.
    Buergi's h.
    cardionector h.
    catecholamine h.
    chemiosmotic h.
    dopamine h.
    Dreyer and Bennett h.

hy·poth·e·sis *(continued)*
    Gad's h.
    gate h.
    Harrower's h.
    inactive X h.
    insular h.
    intact nephron h.
    jelly roll h.
    lattice h.
    Lyon h.
    Lyon-Russell h.
    Makeham's h.
    master-slave h.
    multiple factor h.
    null h.
    one gene–one enzyme h.
    one gene–one polypeptide
        chain h.
    Orgel's h.
    polarization h.
    polyneme h.
    self-marker h.
    sliding-filament h.
    Starling's h.
    structural h.
    topographic h.
    trade-off h.
    triplet h.
    unineme h.
    unitarian h.
    wobble h.
hy·po·threp·sia
hy·po·throm·bin·emia
hy·po·throm·bo·plas·tin·emia
hy·po·thy·mia
hy·po·thy·mic
hy·po·thy·mism
hy·po·thy·rea
hy·po·thy·re·o·sis
hy·po·thy·roid
hy·po·thy·roi·dea
hy·po·thy·roid·ism
    familial goitrous h.
    hypothalamic h.
    infantile h.
    postoperative h.
    thyroprivic h.
hy·po·thy·ro·sis

hy·po·to·nia
  benign congenital h.
  infantile h.
  h. oculi
hy·po·ton·ic
hy·po·to·nic·i·ty
hy·pot·o·nus
hy·pot·o·ny
hy·po·tox·ic·i·ty
hy·po·trans·fer·rin·emia
hy·po·tri·chi·a·sis
hy·po·tri·cho·sis
hy·po·trich·ous
hy·pot·ro·phy
hy·po·tro·pia
hy·po·tryp·to·phan·ic
hy·po·tym·pa·not·o·my
hy·po·tym·pa·num
hy·po·ure·mia
hy·po·ure·sis
hy·po·uri·ce·mia
hy·po·uri·cu·ria
hy·po·uro·crin·ia
hyp·ovar·i·an·ism
hy·po·va·so·pres·sin·emia
hy·po·ve·nos·i·ty
hy·po·ven·ti·la·tion
  central h.
  chronic alveolar h.
  primary alveolar h.
hy·po·vi·gil·i·ty
hy·po·vi·ta·min·o·sis
hy·po·vo·le·mia
hy·po·vo·le·mic
hy·po·vo·lia
hy·po·xan·thine
hy·po·xan·thine guan·ine phos·pho·ri·bos·yl·trans·fer·ase
hy·po·xan·thine ox·i·dase
hy·po·xan·thine phos·pho·ri·bo·syl·trans·fer·ase (HPRT)
hy·pox·emia
hy·pox·ia
  anemic h.
  circulatory h.
  diffusion h.
  histotoxic h.

hy·pox·ia *(continued)*
  hypoxic h.
  stagnant h.
hy·pox·ic
hy·pox·i·do·sis
Hyp·Rho-D
hyp·sa·rhyth·mia
hyp·sar·rhyth·mia
hyp·si·brachy·ce·phal·ic
hyp·si·ce·phal·ic
hyp·si·ceph·a·ly
hyp·si·con·chous
hyp·si·loid
hyp·si·sta·phyl·ia
hyp·si·steno·ce·phal·ic
hyp·so·ceph·a·lous
hyp·so·chrome
hyp·so·chro·my
hyp·so·dont
hyp·so·ki·ne·sis
hyp·so·no·sus
hyp·so·ther·a·py
hy·pur·gia
Hyrtl's anastomosis
Hyrtl's loop
Hyrtl's recess
Hyrtl's sphincter
hys·te·ral·gia
hys·ter·atre·sia
hys·te·rec·to·my
  abdominal h.
  abdominovaginal h.
  cesarean h.
  complete h.
  partial h.
  Porro h.
  radical h.
  subtotal h.
  total h.
  vaginal h.
hys·ter·em·phy·se·ma
hys·te·re·sis
  protoplasmic h.
hys·ter·eu·ryn·ter
hys·ter·eu·ry·sis
hys·ter·ia
  anxiety h.
  canine h.

hys·ter·ia *(continued)*
    conversion h.
    dissociative h.
    fixation h.
    h. major
hys·ter·ic
hys·ter·i·cal
hys·ter·i·cism
hys·ter·ics
hys·ter·i·form
hys·tero·bu·bono·cele
hys·tero·car·ci·no·ma
hys·tero·cele
hys·tero·clei·sis
hys·tero·col·pec·to·my
hys·tero·col·po·scope
hys·tero·cys·tic
hys·tero·cys·to·clei·sis
hys·ter·odyn·ia
hys·tero·ede·ma
hys·tero·ep·i·lep·sy
hys·tero·gram
hys·tero·graph
hys·ter·og·ra·phy
hys·ter·oid
hys·tero·lith
hys·ter·ol·y·sis
hys·te·rom·e·ter
hys·te·rom·e·try
hys·tero·myo·ma
hys·tero·myo·mec·to·my
hys·tero·my·ot·o·my
hys·tero·neu·ro·sis
hys·te·rop·a·thy
hys·tero·pexy

hys·ter·opia
hys·tero·plas·ty
hys·tero·psy·cho·sis
hys·ter·op·to·sis
hys·ter·or·rha·phy
hys·ter·or·rhex·is
hys·tero·sal·pin·gec·to·my
hys·tero·sal·pin·gog·ra·phy
hys·tero·sal·pin·go-ooph·o·rec·to·my
hys·tero·sal·pin·gos·to·my
hys·tero·sal·pinx
hys·tero·scope
    Baggish h.
    Baloser h.
hys·ter·os·co·py
hys·tero·spasm
hys·tero·stat
hys·ter·os·to·mat·o·my
hys·tero·ther·mom·e·try
hys·tero·tome
hys·ter·ot·o·my
    abdominal h.
    vaginal h.
hys·tero·tra·chel·ec·ta·sia
hys·ter·o·tra·chel·ec·to·my
hys·tero·tra·chelo·plas·ty
hys·tero·tra·chel·or·rha·phy
hys·tero·tra·chel·ot·o·my
hys·tero·tu·bog·ra·phy
hys·tero·vag·i·no-en·tero·cele
Hy·tak·er·ol
Hyz·yd
Hz — hertz
HZV — herpes zoster virus

I — incisor
    inosine
    iodine
I — electric current
    intensity (of radiant
      energy)
    ionic strength
IAEA — International Atomic
    Energy Agency
IAHA — immune adherence
    hemagglutination assay
iam·a·tol·o·gy
ia·tra·lip·tic
ia·tra·lip·tics
ia·treu·si·ol·o·gy
ia·treu·sis
iat·ric
iat·ro·chem·i·cal
iat·ro·chem·is·try
iat·ro·gen·e·sis
iat·ro·gen·ic
ia·trol·o·gy
iat·ro·math·e·mat·i·cal
iat·ro·me·chan·i·cal
iat·ro·phys·i·cal
iat·ro·phys·ics
iat·ro·tech·ni·cal
IB — immune body
    inclusion body
IBC — iron-binding capacity
I-beam
IBF — immunoglobulin-bindin-
  g factor
ibo·ga·ine
ibu·fe·nac
ibu·pro·fen
IC — inspiratory capacity
    intermittent claudication
    internal conversion
ICC — intensive coronary care
ICD — International
  Classification of Diseases
    ischemic coronary disease
ice
    Dry I.
Ice·land disease

ich·no·gram
ichor
ichor·emia
ichor·oid
ichor·ous
ichor·rhea
ichor·rhe·mia
ich·tham·mol
ich·thy·ism
ich·thy·is·mus
ich·thyo·acan·tho·tox·in
ich·thyo·acan·tho·tox·ism
ich·thyo·col·la
ich·thyo·he·mo·tox·in
ich·thyo·he·mo·tox·ism
ich·thy·oid
Ich·thy·ol
ich·thy·ol·sul·fon·ate
ich·thy·oo·tox·in
ich·thy·oo·tox·ism
ich·thyo·pha·gia
ich·thy·oph·a·gous
ich·thyo·sar·co·tox·in
ich·thyo·sar·co·tox·ism
ich·thyo·si·form
ich·thy·o·sis
    acquired i.
    i. congenita
    congenital i.
    i. cornea
    i. fetalis
    i. hystrix
    lamellar i.
    i. linearis circumflexa
    i. palmaris et plantaris
    senile i.
    sex-linked recessive i.
    i. simplex
    i. spinosa
    i. uteri
    i. vulgaris
    X-linked i.
ich·thy·ot·ic
ich·thyo·tox·ic
ich·thyo·tox·i·col·o·gy
ich·thyo·tox·in

ich·thyo·tox·ism
ICN — International Council
of Nurses
ico·sa·no·ic acid
ico·sa·noid
ico·sa·pen·ta·eno·ic acid
ico·sa·tri·eno·ic acid
ICP — intracranial pressure
ICRP — International
Commission on Radiological
Protection
ICRU — International
Commission on Radiological
Units and Measurements
ICS — International College of
Surgeons
ICSH — interstitial
cell–stimulating hormone
(luteinizing hormone)
ICT — inflammation of
connective tissue
insulin coma therapy
ic·tal
ic·ter·ep·a·ti·tis
ic·ter·ic
ic·ter·i·tious
ic·tero·ane·mia
ic·tero·o·gen·ic
ic·tero·ge·nic·i·ty
ic·tero·hem·a·tu·ria
ic·tero·hem·a·tu·ric
ic·tero·he·mo·glob·in·uria
ic·tero·hep·a·ti·tis
ic·ter·oid
ic·ter·us
  chronic familial i.
  congenital familial i.
  congenital hemolytic i.
  epidemic catarrhal i.
  i. gravis
  i. gravis neonatorum
  i. neonatorum
  nuclear i.
  i. praecox
  i. typhoides
ic·to·test
ic·tus pl. ic·tus
  i. cordis

ic·tus (continued)
  i. epilepticus
  i. paralyticus
  i. sanguinis
  i. solis
ICU — intensive care unit
ID — infectious disease
  infective dose
  inside diameter
  intradermal
ID$_{50}$ — median infective dose
Id. — L. idem (the same)
id
IDD — insulin-dependent
diabetes
IDDM — insulin-dependent
diabetes mellitus
idea
  autochthonous i.
  compulsive i.
  dominant i.
  fixed i.
  flight of i's
  imperative i.
  i. of reference
  referential i.
  ruminative i.
ide·al
  ego i.
ide·al·iza·tion
ide·a·tion
ide·a·tion·al
idée
  i. fixe
iden·ti·fi·ca·tion
  cosmic i.
  projective i.
iden·ti·ty
  body i.
  core gender i.
  ego i.
  gender i.
  sexual i.
ideo·ge·net·ic
ide·og·e·nous
ideo·glan·du·lar
ideo·ki·net·ic
ide·ol·o·gy

ideo·meta·bol·ic
ideo·me·tab·o·lism
ideo·mo·tion
ideo·mo·tor
ideo·mus·cu·lar
ideo·vas·cu·lar
id·io·ag·glu·ti·nin
id·io·chro·ma·tin
id·io·chro·mid·ia
id·io·chro·mo·some
id·i·o·cy
    amaurotic i.
    amaurotic familial i.
    athetosic i.
    Aztec i.
    cretinoid i.
    Kalmuk i.
    microcephalic i.
    mongolian i.
    moral i.
    spastic amaurotic axonal i.
    xerodermic i.
id·io·gen·e·sis
id·io·glos·sia
id·io·glot·tic
id·io·gram
id·io·graph·ic
id·io·het·ero·ag·glu·ti·nin
id·io·het·er·ol·y·sin
id·io·hyp·no·tism
id·io-im·be·cile
id·io·iso·ag·glu·ti·nin
id·io·isol·y·sin
id·io·la·lia
id·io·log
id·i·ol·o·gism
id·i·ol·y·sin
id·io·mere
id·io·me·tri·tis
id·io·mi·as·ma
id·io·mus·cu·lar
id·io·no·dal
id·io·pa·thet·ic
id·io·path·ic
id·i·op·a·thy
id·io·re·flex
id·io·ret·i·nal
id·io·some

id·io·spasm
id·io·syn·cra·sy
id·io·syn·crat·ic
id·i·ot
    mongolian i.
    i.-savant
id·io·tope
id·io·topy
id·io·troph·ic
id·i·o·trop·ic
id·io·type
id·io·typ·ic
id·io·var·i·a·tion
id·io·ven·tric·u·lar
idi·tol
L-idi·tol de·hy·dro·ge·nase
IDL — intermediate-density
    lipoprotein
ido·lo·ma·nia
idose
idox·ur·i·dine
IDS — inhibitor of DNA
    synthesis
IDU — idoxuridine
id·uron·ate-2-sul·fa·tase
id·uron·ic acid
id·uron·ic sul·fa·tase
L-id·uron·i·dase
α-L-id·uron·i·dase deficiency
IEM — immune electron
    microscopy
    inborn error of metabolism
IEP — immunoelectrophoresis
    isoelectric point
    isoelectric precipitation
IF — interferon
    interstitial fluid
    intrinsic factor
IFN — interferon
ifos·fa·mide
Ig — immunoglobulin
IgA, IgD, IgE, IgG, IgM —
    immunoglobulin A, etc.
IGF — insulin-like growth
    factor
ig·na·tia
ig·ni·ex·tir·pa·tion
ig·ni·op·er·a·tion

ig·ni·pe·di·tes
ig·ni·punc·ture
ig·ni·sa·tion
IGT — impaired glucose
tolerance
IH — infectious hepatitis
IHSS — idiopathic
hypertrophic subaortic
stenosis
II-para
III-para
IL — interleukin
ILA — insulin-like activity
International Leprosy
Association
Ile — isoleucine
il·e·ac
ile·adel·phus
il·e·al
ile·ec·to·my
il·e·itis
    backwash i.
    distal i.
    regional i.
    terminal i.
il·eo·ce·cal
il·eo·ce·cos·to·my
il·eo·ce·cum
il·eo·col·ic
il·eo·co·li·tis
    tuberculous i.
    i. ulcerosa chronica
il·eo·co·lon·ic
il·eo·co·los·to·my
il·eo·co·lot·o·my
il·eo·cys·to·plas·ty
    Camey i.
    LeDuc-Camey i.
il·eo·cys·tos·to·my
il·eo·ile·os·to·my
il·eo·je·ju·ni·tis
il·eo·pexy
il·eo·proc·tos·to·my
il·eo·rec·tal
il·eo·rec·tos·to·my
il·e·or·rha·phy
il·eo·sig·moid
il·eo·sig·moi·dos·to·my

il·e·os·to·my
    end i.
il·e·ot·o·my
il·eo·trans·vers·os·to·my
il·eo·typh·li·tis
Il·e·tin
    Lente I.
    NPH I.
    protamine, zinc & I.
    regular I.
    Semilente I.
    Ultralente I.
il·e·um
    duplex i.
il·e·us
    adynamic i.
    angiomesenteric i.
    dynamic i.
    hyperdynamic i.
    mechanical i.
    meconium i.
    occlusive i.
    paralytic i.
    i. paralyticus
    spastic i.
    i. subparta
    terminal i.
Ilex
il·ia
il·i·ac
ili·adel·phus
il·i·cin
Il·i·dar
il·io·coc·cyg·e·al
il·io·coc·cyg·e·us
il·io·co·lot·o·my
il·io·cos·tal
il·io·dor·sal
il·io·fem·or·al
il·io·fem·o·ro·plas·ty
il·io·hy·po·gas·tric
il·io·in·gui·nal
il·io·lum·bar
il·io·lum·bo·cos·to·ab·dom·i·
    nal
il·i·om·e·ter
il·i·op·a·gus

il·io·pec·tin·e·al
il·io·pel·vic
il·io·per·o·ne·al
il·io·pso·as
il·io·pu·bic
il·io·sa·cral
il·io·sci·at·ic
il·io·scro·tal
il·io·spi·nal
il·io·tho·ra·cop·a·gus
il·io·tib·i·al
il·io·tro·chan·ter·ic
il·io·xi·phop·a·gus
il·i·um *pl.* il·ia
Il·iz·ar·ov leg-lengthening
   procedure
ill
   föhn i.
il·lac·ri·ma·tion
il·laq·ue·a·tion
il·li·cit
Il·lic·i·um
il·li·ni·tion
ill·ness
   compressed-air i.
   emotional i.
   functional i.
   high-altitude i.
   manic-depressive i.
   mental i.
   psychosomatic i.
   radiation i.
   terminal i.
il·lu·mi·na·tion
   axial i.
   central i.
   contact i.
   critical i.
   darkfield i.
   dark-ground i.
   direct i.
   focal i.
   Köhler i.
   lateral i.
   oblique i.
   orthogonal i.
   surface i.
   through i.

il·lu·mi·na·tor
   Abbe's i.
il·lu·min·ism
il·lu·sion
   autokinetic i.
   epileptic i.
   Fregoli's i.
   optical i.
il·lu·sion·al
il·lu·ta·tion
Il·o·pan
Il·o·sone
Ilo·ty·cin
Il·o·zyme
IM — infectious
   mononucleosis
      internal medicine
      intramuscular
      intramuscularly (by
         intramuscular injection)
ima
im·a·fen hy·dro·chlo·ride
im·age
   accidental i.
   acoustic i.
   auditory i.
   body i.
   direct i.
   double i.
   eidetic i.
   erect i.
   false i.
   gamma i.
   heteronymous i.
   homonymous i.
   incidental i.
   inverted i.
   memory i.
   mental i.
   mirror i.
   motor i.
   negative i.
   optical i.
   pulse echo i.
   Purkinje-Sanson mirror i's
   radioisotope i.
   real i.

im·age *(continued)*
    retinal i.
    Sanson's i's
    sensory i.
    specular i.
    tactile i.
    true i.
    virtual i.
im·ag·ery
imag·i·nes
imag·ing
    digital vascular i. (DVI)
    dynamic i.
    echo-planar i., echo planar
      i.
    electrostatic i.
    Fourier i.
    gated blood pool i.
    line i.
    magnetic resonance i.
      (MRI)
    multiple-gated blood pool i.
    multiple spin echo total
      volume i.
    planar spin i.
    pulse echo i.
    radionuclide i.
    sequential first pass i.
    static i.
    stop-action i.
    three-dimensional i.
    through-transmission i.
    two-dimensional i.
    ventilation perfusion i.
ima·go *pl.* ima·goes, ima·gi·
  nes
ima·go·cide
im·a·pun·ga
im·bal·ance
    autonomic i.
    binocular i.
    gene i.
    sex chromosome i.
    sympathetic i.
    vasomotor i.
im·be·cile
im·be·cil·i·ty
    moral i.

im·bed
im·bi·bi·tion
    hemoglobin i.
im·bri·cate
im·bri·cat·ed
im·bri·ca·tion
im·co·mi·tance
ImD$_{50}$ — median immunizing
  dose
Imers·lund syndrome
Imers·lund-Graes·beck
  syndrome
Imers·lund-Naj·man-Graes·
  beck syndrome
Im·hoff tank
im·id·amine
im·id·az·ole
im·id·azo·lyl·eth·yl·amine
im·ide
imid·o·carb hy·dro·chlo·ride
imi·do·gen
im·in·az·ole
im·ine
im·i·no·gly·cin·uria
    familial renal i.
imi·no·urea
imip·ra·mine hy·dro·chlo·ride
Im·lach's fat plug
im·ma·ture
im·me·di·ate
im·med·i·ca·ble
im·mer·sion
    cold i.
    homogeneous i.
    oil i.
    water i.
im·mi·gra·tion
im·mis·ci·ble
im·mo·bil·i·ty
im·mo·bil·iza·tion
im·mo·bi·lize
im·mune
im·mu·ni·ty
    acquired i.
    active i.
    adoptive i.
    antibacterial i.
    antitoxic i.

im·mu·ni·ty *(continued)*
    antiviral i.
    artificial i.
    cell-mediated i.
    cellular i.
    community i.
    concomitant i.
    cross i.
    familial i.
    functional i.
    genetic i.
    herd i.
    humoral i.
    induced i.
    infection i.
    inherent i.
    inherited i.
    innate i.
    intrauterine i.
    local i.
    maternal i.
    native i.
    natural i.
    nonspecific i.
    passive i.
    phagocytic i.
    placental i.
    preemptive i.
    protective i.
    residual i.
    species i.
    specific i.
    superinfection i.
    T cell–mediated i. (TCMI)
    tissue i.
    transplantation i.
im·mu·ni·za·tion
    active i.
    occult i.
    passive i.
    prophylactic i.
im·mu·nize
im·mu·no·ad·ju·vant
im·mu·no·ad·sor·bent
im·mu·no·ad·sorp·tion
im·mu·no·ag·glu·ti·na·tion
im·mu·no·as·say
    enzyme i.

im·mu·no·as·say *(continued)*
    enzyme multiplied i.
      technique (EMIT)
    nonradioisotopic i.
    radioisotopic i.
im·mu·no·bi·ol·o·gy
im·mu·no·blast
im·mu·no·blas·tic
im·mu·no·chem·i·cal
im·mu·no·chem·is·try
im·mu·no·che·mo·ther·a·py
im·mu·no·com·pe·tence
im·mu·no·com·pe·tent
im·mu·no·com·plex
im·mu·no·com·pro·mised
im·mu·no·con·glu·ti·nin
im·mu·no·cyte
im·mu·no·cy·to·ad·her·ence
im·mu·no·cy·to·chem·is·try
im·mu·no·cy·tol·o·gy
im·mu·no·de·fi·cien·cy
    acquired i. syndrome
      (AIDS)
    acquired primary i.
    combined i.
    common variable i.
    common variable
      unclassifiable i.
    i. with hyper-IgM
    severe combined i.
    i. with short-limbed
      dwarfism
    Swiss-type i.
    i. with thymoma
    thymus-dependent i.
    X-linked i.
im·mu·no·de·fi·cient
im·mu·no·de·pres·sion
im·mu·no·de·pres·sive
im·mu·no·der·ma·tol·o·gy
im·mu·no·de·tec·tion
im·mu·no·de·vi·a·tion
im·mu·no·di·ag·no·sis
im·mu·no·dif·fu·sion
    radial i. (RID)
im·mu·no·dom·i·nance
im·mu·no·dom·i·nant

im·mu·no·elec·tro·pho·re·sis
   counter i.
   countercurrent i.
   crossed i.
   rocket i.
   two-dimensional i.
im·mu·no·fer·ri·tin
im·mu·no·fil·tra·tion
   analytical i.
im·mu·no·flu·o·res·cence
   direct i.
   indirect i.
im·mu·no·gen
im·mu·no·ge·net·ic
im·mu·no·ge·net·ics
im·mu·no·gen·ic
im·mu·no·ge·nic·i·ty
im·mu·no·glob·u·lin
   i. A
   Bence Jones monoclonal i.
   i. D
   i. E
   exocrine i.
   i. G
   i. M
   monoclonal i.
   secretory i. A
   surface i.
   thyroid-binding inhibitory
     i's (TBII)
   thyroid-stimulating i's
     (TSI)
   TSH-binding inhibitory i's
     (TBII)
im·mu·no·glob·u·lin·op·a·
   thy
im·mu·no·hem·a·tol·o·gy
im·mu·no·his·to·chem·i·cal
im·mu·no·his·to·chem·is·try
im·mu·no·his·to·flu·o·res·
   cence
im·mu·no·in·com·pe·tent
im·mu·no·log·ic
im·mu·no·log·i·cal
im·mu·nol·o·gist
im·mu·nol·o·gy
im·mu·no·lym·pho·scin·tig·
   ra·phy

im·mu·no·mod·u·la·tion
im·mu·no·mod·u·la·tor
im·mu·no·par·a·si·tol·o·gy
im·mu·no·patho·gen·e·sis
im·mu·no·patho·log·ic
im·mu·no·pa·thol·o·gy
im·mu·no·per·ox·i·dase
im·mu·no·pho·re·sis
im·mu·no·phys·i·ol·o·gy
im·mu·no·po·ten·cy
im·mu·no·po·ten·ti·a·tion
im·mu·no·po·ten·ti·a·tor
im·mu·no·pre·cip·i·ta·tion
im·mu·no·pre·cip·i·tin
im·mu·no·pro·lif·er·a·tive
im·mu·no·pro·phy·lax·is
im·mu·no·pro·tein
im·mu·no·ra·dio·met·ric
im·mu·no·ra·di·om·e·try
im·mu·no·re·ac·tant
   glucagon i's
im·mu·no·re·ac·tion
im·mu·no·re·ac·tive
im·mu·no·re·ac·tiv·i·ty
   glucagon-like i.
im·mu·no·reg·u·la·tion
im·mu·no·re·spon·sive·ness
im·mu·no·scin·tig·raphy
im·mu·no·se·lec·tion
im·mu·no·se·nes·cence
im·mu·nos·mo·elec·tro·pho·
   re·sis
im·mu·no·sor·bent
   enzyme-linked i. assay
     (ELISA)
im·mu·no·stim·u·lant
im·mu·no·stim·u·la·tion
im·mu·no·sup·pres·sant
im·mu·no·sup·pres·sion
im·mu·no·sup·pres·sive
im·mu·no·sur·veil·lance
im·mu·no·ther·a·py
   adoptive i.
im·mu·no·tol·er·ance
im·mu·no·tol·er·ant
im·mu·no·tox·i·col·o·gy
im·mu·no·tox·in
im·mu·no·trans·fu·sion

Imo·di·um
IMP – inosine monophosphate
IMPA — incisal mandibular
  plane angle
im·pact
im·pact·ed
im·pac·tion
    ceruminal i.
    dental i.
    fecal i.
    food i.
    mucoid i.
im·pac·tor
im·paired
im·pair·ment
    conductive hearing i.
    percentage of i.
im·pal·pa·ble
im·par
im·pari·dig·i·tate
im·pa·ten·cy
im·pa·tent
im·ped·ance
    acoustic i.
    ear i.
im·per·cep·tion
im·per·fo·rate
im·per·fo·ra·tion
im·pe·ri·al·ine
im·per·me·a·ble
im·per·sis·tence
    motor i.
im·per·vi·ous
im·pe·tig·i·ni·za·tion
im·pe·tig·i·nous
im·pe·ti·go
    Bockhart's i.
    i. bullosa
    bullous i.
    chronic symmetric i.
    circinate i.
    i. contagiosa
    i. contagiosa bullosa
    i. herpetiformis
    miliary i.
    i. neonatorum
    i. pityroides
    staphylococcal i.

im·pe·ti·go (continued)
    streptococcal i.
    i. vulgaris
im·pi·la·tion
im·pinge
im·pinge·ment
im·plant
    carcinomatous i's
    cartilaginous i.
    cochlear i.
    dental i.
    deoxycortone acetate i.
    diodontic i.
    dynamic i.
    endodontic i.
    endometrial i's
    endosseous i.
    endosteal i.
    hormone i.
    intraosseous i.
    intraperiosteal i.
    Little intraocular lens
      (IOL) i.
    magnet i.
    needle endosteal i.
    oral i.
    osseointegrated i.
    penile i.
    pin endosteal i.
    subperiosteal i.
    transmandibular i.
im·plan·ta·tion
    central i.
    circumferential i.
    delayed i.
    eccentric i.
    endometrial i.
    hypodermic i.
    interstitial i.
    intrafollicular i.
    juxtafollicular i.
    nerve i.
    periosteal i.
    superficial i.
    teratic i.
    tooth i.
im·plan·to·don·tics
im·plan·to·don·tist

im·plan·to·don·tol·o·gy
im·plan·tol·o·gist
im·plan·tol·o·gy
    dental i.
    oral i.
im·plo·sion
im·po·tence
    functional i.
    organic i.
    orgastic i.
    paretic i.
    psychic i.
    secondary i.
    symptomatic i.
im·po·ten·cy
im·po·ten·tia
    i. coeundi
    i. erigendi
    i. generandi
im·preg·nate
im·preg·na·tion
    artificial i.
im·pres·sio *pl.* im·pres·si·o·nes
    i. cardiaca hepatis
    i. cardiaca pulmonis
    i. colica hepatis
    impressiones digitatae
    i. duodenales hepatis
    i. esophagea hepatis
    i. gastrica hepatis
    i. gastrica renis
    i. gyrorum
    i. hepatica renis
    i. ligamenti
      costoclavicularis
    i. meningealis
    i. muscularis renis
    i. oesophagea hepatis
    i. petrosa pallii
    i. renalis hepatis
    i. suprarenalis hepatis
im·pres·sion
    anatomic i.
    basilar i.
    bridge i.
    cardiac i.
    cleft palate i.

im·pres·sion *(continued)*
    colic i. of liver
    complete denture i.
    composite i.
    copper-ring i.
    costal i's
    i. of costoclavicular
      ligament
    deltoid i. of humerus
    dental i.
    digastric i.
    digital i's
    digitate i's
    direct bone i.
    duodenal i. of liver
    elastic i.
    esophageal i. of liver
    final i.
    fluid wax i.
    functional i.
    gastric i.
    gastric i. of liver
    gyrate i's
    hydrocolloid i.
    lower i.
    mandibular i.
    maxillary i.
    meningeal i.
    mucodisplacement i.
    mucostatic i.
    partial denture i.
    petrous i.
    preliminary i.
    primary i.
    renal i. of liver
    rhomboid i. of clavicle
    secondary i.
    sectional i.
    suprarenal i. of liver
    trigeminal i. of temporal
      bone
    upper i.
im·pres·sio·nes
im·print·ing
im·pro·cre·ance
im·pulse
    apex i.
    apical i.

im·pulse *(continued)*
  cardiac i.
  ectopic i.
  episternal i.
  exteroceptive i's
  interoceptive i's
  involuntary i.
  irresistible i.
  left parasternal i's
  nerve i.
  neural i.
  proprioceptive i's
  right parasternal i's
im·pul·sion
imu
Im·u·ran
imus
IMV — intermittent
mandatory ventilation
INA — International
Neurological Association
in·acid·i·ty
in·ac·ti·vate
in·ac·ti·va·tion
  complement i.
  heat i.
  paternal-X i.
  random-X i.
  X-i.
in·ac·ti·va·tor
  anaphylatoxin i. (AI)
  C3b i. (C3b INA)
in·ac·tose
in·ad·e·qua·cy
in·ag·glu·tin·a·ble
in·al·i·men·tal
in·an·i·mate
in·a·ni·tion
in·ap·pe·tence
In·ap·sine
in·ar·tic·u·late
in ar·tic·u·lo mor·tis
in·as·sim·i·la·ble
in·at·ten·tion
  sensory i.
in·ax·on
in·born
in·bred

in·breed·ing
in·cal·lo·sal
in·can·des·cent
in·can·ous
in·cap·a·ri·na
in·car·cer·at·ed
in·car·cer·a·tion
in·car·na·tio
  i. unguis
in·car·na·tive
in·case·ment
in·cen·di·ar·ism
in·cen·tive
in·cep·tus
in·cer·tae se·dis
in·cest
in·cha·cao
in·ci·dence
in·ci·dent
in·cin·e·ra·tion
in·cip·i·ent
in·ci·sal
in·cised
in·ci·sion
  Battle's i.
  Battle-Jalaguier-Kammerer-i.
  Bevan's i.
  celiotomy i.
  Chernez i.
  chevron i.
  collar i.
  confirmatory i.
  cruciate i.
  curvilinear i.
  Deaver's i.
  decompression i.
  double-Y i.
  Dührssen's i's
  endaural i.
  epigastric i.
  Fergusson's i.
  Gluck's i.
  gridiron i.
  Hayes Martin i.
  hockey stick i.
  Howarth's i.
  Kammerer-Battle i.

in·ci·sion *(continued)*
    Kehr's i.
    Kocher's i.
    LaRoque herniorrhaphy i.
    lateral rectus i.
    lazy S i.
    lazy Z i.
    low transverse abdominal
        i.
    Lynch i.
    MacFee i's
    mastoid i.
    Maylard i.
    McBurney's i.
    median i.
    midline i.
    Munro Kerr i.
    Nagamatsu i.
    paramedian i.
    pararectus i.
    paravaginal i.
    Pfannenstiel's i.
    postauricular i.
    relaxing i.
    relief i.
    Robertson i.
    Rockey-Davis i.
    Ruddy's i.
    Sanders i.
    Schuchardt's i.
    smile
    smiling i.
    Sorensen i.
    subcostal i.
    transverse i.
    Warren's i.
    Weber-Fergusson i.
    Wilde's i.
    Y i.
    Yorke-Mason i.
in·ci·sive
in·ci·so·la·bi·al
in·ci·so·lin·gual
in·ci·so·prox·i·mal
in·ci·sor
    central i.
    first i.
    hawk-bill i's

in·ci·sor *(continued)*
    Hutchinson's i's
    lateral i.
    medial i.
    second i.
    shovel-shaped i's
    winged i.
in·ci·su·ra *pl.* in·ci·su·rae
    i. acetabuli
    anacrotic i.
    i. angularis gastris
    i. angularis ventriculi
    i. anterior auris
    i. apicis cordis
    i. cardiaca
    i. cerebelli anterior
    i. clavicularis sterni
    incisurae costales sterni
    i. fastigii
    i. fibularis tibiae
    i. frontalis
    i. interarytenoidea laryngis
    i. interlobaris hepatis
    i. interlobaris pulmonis
    i. intertragica
    i. ischiadica major
    i. ischiadica minor
    i. ischialis major
    i. ischialis minor
    i. jugularis sterni
    i. lacrimalis maxillae
    i. ligamenti teretis
    i. mandibulae
    i. mastoidea
    i. nasalis maxillae
    i. pancreatis
    i. parietallis
    i. peronea tibiae
    i. preoccipitalis
    i. pterygoidea
    i. radialis ulnae
    i. Rivini
    i. Santorini
    i. scapulae
    i. semilunaris tibiae
    i. semilunaris ulnae
    i. sphenopalatina
    i. supraorbitalis

in·ci·su·ra *(continued)*
    i. temporalis
    i. tentorii cerebelli
    i. terminalis auris
    i. thyroidea inferior
    i. thyroidea superior
    i. tragica
    i. trochlearis ulnae
    i. tympanica [Rivini]
    i. ulnaris radii
    i. umbilicalis
    i. vertebralis inferior
    i. vertebralis superior

in·ci·su·rae

in·ci·su·ral

in·ci·sure
    i. of acetabulum
    angular i.
    i. of apex of heart
    i. of calcaneus
    cardiac i. of left lung
    cardiac i. of stomach
    i. of cerebellum
    clavicular i. of sternum
    costal i's of sternum
    cotyloid i.
    digastric i. of temporal
      bone
    i's of Duverney
    i. of ear, anterior
    i. of ear, terminal
    ethmoidal i. of frontal bone
    falciform i. of fascia lata
    fibular i. of tibia
    frontal i.
    humeral i. of ulna
    iliac i., lesser
    interarytenoid i. of larynx
    interclavicular i.
    intertragic i.
    ischial i., greater
    i. of ischium, greater
    i. of ischium, lesser
    ischial i., lesser
    jugular i. of occipital bone
    jugular i. of sternum
    jugular i. of temporal bone
    lacrimal i. of maxilla

in·ci·sure *(continued)*
    i's of Lanterman
    i's of Lanterman-Schmidt
    lateral i. of sternum
    i. of mandible
    mastoid i. of temporal bone
    maxillary i., inferior
    nasal i. of frontal bone
    nasal i. of maxilla
    obturator i. of pubic bone
    palatine i.
    palatine i. of Henle
    parietal i. of temporal bone
    patellar i. of femur
    peroneal i. of tibia
    popliteal i.
    preoccipital i.
    pterygoid i.
    radial i. of ulna
    Rivinus' i.
    i. of scapula
    Schmidt-Lanterman i's
    semilunar i.
    sigmoid i. of mandible
    sigmoid i. of ulna
    sphenopalatine i. of
      palatine bone
    sternal i.
    supraorbital i.
    suprascapular i.
    i. of talus
    temporal i.
    i. of tentorium of
      cerebellum
    thoracic i.
    thyroid i., inferior
    thyroid i., superior
    trochlear i. of ulna
    tympanic i.
    ulnar i. of radius
    umbilical i.
    vertebral i., greater
    vertebral i., inferior
    vertebral i., lesser
    vertebral i., superior

in·ci·tant

in·ci·to·gram

in·cli·na·tio *pl.* in·cli·na·ti·o·nes
    i. pelvis
in·cli·na·tion
    axial i.
    condylar guidance i.
    condylar guide i.
    lateral condylar i.
    lingual i.
    pelvic i.
    i. of pelvis
in·cli·na·ti·o·nes
in·cline
in·cli·nom·e·ter
in·clu·sion
    cell i.
    dental i.
    fetal i.
    Guaranieri's i's
    intranuclear i's
    leukocyte i's
    Walthard's i's
in·co·ag·u·la·bil·i·ty
in·co·ag·u·la·ble
in·co·her·ent
in·com·pat·i·bil·i·ty
    ABO i.
    chemical i.
    physiologic i.
    Rh i.
    therapeutic i.
in·com·pat·i·ble
in·com·pe·tence
    aortic i.
    i. of the cardiac valves
    ileocecal i.
    ileocolic i.
    relative i.
    valvular i.
    velopharyngeal i.
in·com·pe·ten·cy
in·com·pe·tent
in·com·pres·si·ble
in·con·gru·ence
in·con·ti·nence
    active i.
    fecal i.
    intermittent i.

in·con·ti·nence *(continued)*
    overflow i.
    paradoxical i.
    paralytic i.
    passive i.
    rectal i.
    sphincteric i.
    stress i.
    urge i.
    urgency i.
    urinary i.
in·con·ti·nent
in·con·ti·nen·tia
    i. alvi
    Bloch-Sulzberger i. pigmenti
    Naegeli's i. pigmenti
    i. pigmenti
    i. pigmenti achromians
    i. urinae
in·co·or·di·na·tion
    uterine i.
in·cor·po·ra·tion
in·cos·ta·pe·di·al
in·cre·ment
in·cre·tin
in·cre·tion
in·cross
in·crus·ta·tion
in·cu·bate
in·cu·ba·tion
in·cu·ba·tor
in·cu·bus
in·cu·dal
in·cu·dec·to·my
in·cu·di·form
in·cu·di·us
in·cu·do·mal·le·al
in·cu·do·sta·pe·di·al
in·cu·ne·a·tion
in·cur·a·ble
in·cur·va·tion
in·cus
in·cy·clo·de·vi·a·tion
in·cy·clo·pho·ria
in·cy·clo·tro·pia
in·cy·clo·ver·gence
in d. — L. in dies (daily)

in·da·crin·ic ac·id
in·da·cri·none
in·dane·di·one
in·dem·ni·ty
in·den·iza·tion
in·den·ta·tion
   i. of Hahn
In·der·al
In·der·ide
in·de·ter·mi·nate
in·dex *pl.* in·dex·es, in·di·ces
   absolute refractive i.
   absorbancy i.
   ACH i.
   alpha i.
   altitudinal i.
   alveolar i.
   antitryptic i.
   Arneth i.
   auricular i.
   auriculoparietal i.
   auriculovertical i.
   Ayala i.
   baric i.
   basilar i.
   Becker-Lennhoff i.
   body build i.
   Boedecker's i.
   Bouchard's i.
   brachial i.
   breadth-height i.
   Broders'i.
   Brugsch i.
   calcium i.
   cardiac i.
   cardiothoracic i.
   I.-Catalogue
   centromeric i.
   cephalic i.
   cephalic height i.
   cephalo-orbital i.
   cephalorhachidian i.
   cephalospinal i.
   cerebral i.
   cerebrospinal i.
   chemotherapeutic i.
   coliform i.
   Colour I.

in·dex *(continued)*
   combined thyroid hormone
      i.
   coronofrontal i.
   cranial i.
   Cumulated I. Medicus
   def i.
   degenerative i.
   dental i.
   DMF (decayed, missing,
      and filled) i.
   effective temperature i.
   endemic i.
   erythrocyte indices
   facial i.
   fatigue i.
   femorohumeral i.
   Flower's i.
   forearm-hand i.
   Fourmentin's thoracic i.
   free thyroxin i.
   free triiodothyronine i.
   gnathic i.
   habitus i.
   hair i.
   hand i.
   height i.
   hematopneic i.
   hemophagocytic i.
   hemorenal i.
   hemorenal salt i.
   Hench-Aldrich i.
   high lateral myocardial i.
   intermembral i.
   juxtaglomerular i.
   Kaup i.
   Langelier's i.
   length-breadth i.
   length-height i.
   Lennhoff's i.
   lower leg–foot i.
   Macdonald i.
   maturation i.
   maxilloalveolar i.
   I. Medicus
   Mengert's i.
   metacarpal i.
   mitotic i.

in·dex *(continued)*
  morphological i.
  morphologic face i.
  nasal i.
  nucleoplasmic i.
  obesity i.
  opsonic i.
  optical i.
  orbital i. (of Broca)
  palatal i.
  palatine i.
  palatomaxillary i.
  parasite i.
  pelvic i.
  penile brachial i.
  periodontal i.
  phagocytic i.
  physiognomonic upper face
    i.
  Pignet i.
  Pirquet's i.
  PMA (papilla, gingival
    margin, and attached
    gingiva) i.
  ponderal i.
  Pont's i.
  profunda-popliteal
    collateral i.
  pulsatile i.
  Quarterly Cumulative I.
    Medicus
  radiohumeral i.
  Ramfjord i.
  recession i.
  refractive i.
  Röhrer's i.
  Russell i.
  sacral i.
  salivary urea i.
  saturation i.
  short increment sensitivity
    i. (SISI)
  spleen i.
  splenic i.
  splenometric i.
  stimulation i. (SI)
  tension-time i.
  therapeutic i.

in·dex *(continued)*
  thoracic i.
  tibiofemoral i.
  tibioradial i.
  trunk i.
  urea i.
  uricolytic i.
  vertical i.
  vital i.
  xanthoproteic i.
  Youden's i.
  zygomaticoauricular i.
in·di·can
in·di·can·emia
in·di·can·me·ter
in·di·cano·ra·chia
in·di·cant
in·di·can·uria
in·di·car·mine
in·di·ca·tio
  i. causalis
  i. curativa
  i. morbi
  i. symptomatica
in·di·ca·tion
in·di·ca·tor
  anaerobic i.
  Andrade's i.
  dew point i.
  fluorescent i.
  oxidation-reduction i.
  pH i.
  proportional mortality i.
  radioactive i.
  redox i.
  Schneider's i.
  universal i.
  xylol pulse i.
in·di·co·phose
in·dif·fé·rence
  belle i.
in·dif·fer·ent
in·dig·e·nous
in·di·gest·i·ble
in·di·ges·tion
  acid i.
  fat i.
  gastric i.

in·di·ges·tion *(continued)*
    intestinal i.
    sugar i.
in·dig·i·ta·tion
in·di·glu·cin
in·di·go
in·di·go·gen
in·di·go·pur·pu·rine
in·dig·o·tin
in·di·go·tin·di·sul·fon·ate so·di·um
in·di·rect
in·di·ru·bin
in·di·ru·bin·uria
in·dis·crim·i·nate
in·dis·po·si·tion
in·di·um
    i. 111
    i. 111 DTPA
    i. 111 oxyquinoline
    i. 111 pentetate
    i. 113m
in·di·vid·u·al·iza·tion
in·di·vid·u·a·tion
In·do·cin
In·dok·lon
in·dol·ac·e·tu·ria
in·dol·amine
in·dole
in·dole-3-ace·tic acid
in·do·lent
in·do·log·e·nous
in·dol·uria
in·do·meth·a·cin
in·do·phe·nol
in·do·pro·fen
in·dor·a·min
in·dox·yl
in·dox·yl·emia
in·dox·yl·uria
in·dri·line hy·dro·chlo·ride
in·duced
in·duc·er
in·duc·tance
in·duc·tion
    autonomous i.
    complementary i.
    enzyme i.

in·duc·tion *(continued)*
    i. of labor
    magnetic i.
    Spemann's i.
    spinal i.
in·duc·tor
    gene i.
in·duc·to·ri·um
in·duc·to·therm
in·duc·to·ther·my
in·du·lin
in·du·lin·o·phil
in·du·lin·o·phil·ic
in·du·rat·ed
in·du·ra·tion
    black i.
    brawny i.
    brown i.
    cyanotic i.
    fibroid i.
    Froriep's i.
    granular i.
    gray i.
    laminate i.
    parchment i.
    penile i.
    phlebitic i.
    plastic i.
    red i.
    rigid i. of bladder neck
in·du·ra·tive
in·du·si·um gris·e·um
in·dwell·ing
in·e·bri·ant
in·e·bri·a·tion
in·e·bri·e·ty
in·elas·tic
In·er·mi·cap·si·fer
in·ert
in·er·tia
    colonic i.
    immunological i.
    psychic i.
    i. uteri
    uterine i.
in·ex·ci·ta·ble
in ex·tre·mis
Inf. — L. infunde (pour in)

in·fan·cy
in·fant
    floppy i.
    i. Hercules
    immature i.
    liveborn i.
    low birth weight (LBW) i.
    mature i.
    moderately low birth
        weight (MLBW) i.
    newborn i.
    postmature i.
    post-term i.
    premature i.
    preterm i.
    stillborn i.
    term i.
    very low birth weight
        (VLBW) i.
in·fan·ti·cide
in·fan·tile
in·fan·ti·lism
    Brissaud's i.
    cachetic i.
    celiac i.
    dysthyroidal i.
    hepatic i.
    Herter's i.
    hypophysial i.
    idiopathic i.
    intestinal i.
    Levi-Lorain i.
    Lorain's i.
    lymphatic i.
    myxedematous i.
    pancreatic i.
    partial i.
    pituitary i.
    proportionate i.
    regressive i.
    renal i.
    sexual i.
    symptomatic i.
    thyroid i.
    universal i.
in·farct
    anemic i.
    aseptic i.

in·farct *(continued)*
    bilirubin i's
    bland i.
    bone i.
    Brewer's i's
    calcareous i.
    cerebral i.
    cystic i.
    embolic i.
    hemorrhagic i.
    infected i.
    kidney i.
    mesenteric i.
    pale i.
    placental i.
    pulmonary i.
    red i.
    renal i.
    septic i.
    thrombotic i.
    uric acid i.
    white i.
in·farc·tec·to·my
in·farc·tion
    anterior myocardial i.
    anteroinferior myocardial
        i.
    anterolateral myocardial i.
    anteroseptal myocardial i.
    apical myocardial i.
    atrial i.
    cardiac i.
    cerebral i.
    diaphragmatic myocardial
        i.
    Freiberg's i.
    inferior myocardial i.
    inferolateral myocardial i.
    intestinal i.
    lateral myocardial i.
    mesenteric i.
    myocardial i.
    pituitary i.
    posterior myocardial i.
    posterolateral myocardial
        i.
    pulmonary i.
    renal i.

in·farc·tion *(continued)*
   right ventricular i.
   septal myocardial i.
   silent myocardial i.
   subendocardial i.
   through-and-through
     myocardial i.
   transmural myocardial i.
in·faust
in·fect
in·fec·ti·ble
in·fec·tion
   airborne i.
   apical i.
   autochthonous i.
   colonization i.
   concurrent i.
   contact i.
   covert i.
   cross i.
   cryptogenic i.
   diaplacental i.
   direct i.
   dormant i.
   droplet i.
   dust-borne i.
   ectogenous i.
   endogenous i.
   exogenous i.
   focal i.
   germinal i.
   iatrogenic i.
   inapparent i.
   indirect i.
   intercurrent i.
   invasive burn i.
   latent i.
   local i.
   mass i.
   metastatic i.
   mixed i.
   nonspecific i.
   nosocomial i.
   opportunistic i.
   phycomycotic i.
   puerperal i.
   pyogenic i.
   retrograde i.

in·fec·tion *(continued)*
   secondary i.
   silent i.
   slow i.
   subclinical i.
   vector-borne i.
   Vincent's i.
   water-borne i.
   zoogenic i.
in·fec·ti·os·i·ty
in·fec·tious
in·fec·tious·ness
in·fec·tive
in·fec·tiv·i·ty
in·fe·cun·di·ty
in·fer·ent
in·fe·ri·or
in·fe·ri·or·i·ty
in·fe·ro·fron·tal
in·fe·ro·lat·er·al
in·fe·ro·me·di·al
in·fe·ro·me·di·an
in·fe·ro·na·sal
in·fe·ro·pa·ri·e·tal
in·fe·ro·pos·te·ri·or
in·fe·ro·tem·po·ral
in·fer·tile
in·fer·til·i·tas
in·fer·til·i·ty
   primary i.
   secondary i.
in·fest
in·fes·ta·tion
in·fes·tive
in·fib·u·la·tion
in·fil·trate
   Assmann's tuberculous i.
   leukemic i.
in·fil·tra·tion
   adipose i.
   calcareous i.
   calcium i.
   cellular i.
   epituberculous i.
   fatty i.
   gelatinous i.
   glycogen i.
   gray i.

in·fil·tra·tion *(continued)*
   inflammatory i.
   lymphocytic i. of skin
   paraneural i.
   round cell i.
   sanguineous i.
   serous i.
   tuberculous i.
   urinous i.
in·firm
in·fir·ma·ry
in·fir·mi·ty
in·flamed
in·flam·ma·gen
in·flam·ma·tion
   acute i.
   adhesive i.
   allergic i.
   atrophic i.
   bacterial i.
   catarrhal i.
   chemical i.
   chronic i.
   cirrhotic i.
   croupous i.
   diffuse i.
   disseminated i.
   exudative i.
   fibrinopurulent i.
   fibrinous i.
   fibroid i.
   focal i.
   granulomatous i.
   hyperplastic i.
   hypertrophic i.
   interstitial i.
   metastatic i.
   necrotic i.
   obliterative i.
   parenchymatous i.
   plastic i.
   productive i.
   proliferous i.
   pseudomembranous i.
   purulent i.
   sclerosing i.
   serofibrinous i.
   seroplastic i.

in·flam·ma·tion *(continued)*
   serous i.
   simple i.
   specific i.
   subacute i.
   suppurative i.
   toxic i.
   traumatic i.
   ulcerative i.
in·flam·ma·to·ry
in·fla·tion
in·fla·tor
in·flec·tion
in·flex·ion
in·flexed
in·flo·res·cence
in·flow
in·flu·en·za
   i. A
   Asian i.
   avian i.
   clinical i.
   i. B
   i. C
   endemic i.
   equine i.
   feline i.
   goose i.
   Hong Kong i.
   laryngeal i.
   Russian i.
   Spanish i.
   swine i.
in·flu·en·zal
in·fold
in·fold·ing
in·for·mo·some
in·fra-al·ve·o·lar
in·fra-au·ric·u·lar
in·fra-ax·il·la·ry
in·fra·bulge
in·fra·car·di·ac
in·fra·cer·e·bral
in·fra·cil·i·a·ture
in·fra·class
in·fra·cla·vic·u·lar
in·fra·cli·noid
in·fra·clu·sion

in·fra·con·stric·tor
in·fra·cor·ti·cal
in·fra·cos·tal
in·fra·cot·y·loid
in·frac·tion
    Freiberg's i.
in·frac·ture
in·fra·den·ta·le
in·fra·di·an
in·fra·di·a·phrag·mat·ic
in·fra·duc·tion
in·fra·ge·nic·u·late
in·fra·gen·u·al
in·fra·gle·noid
in·fra·glot·tic
in·fra·hy·oid
in·fra·in·gui·nal
in·fra·mam·il·la·ry
in·fra·mam·ma·ry
in·fra·man·dib·u·lar
in·fra·mar·gin·al
in·fra·max·il·lary
in·fra·nu·cle·ar
in·fra·or·bi·tal
in·fra·pa·tel·lar
in·fra·psy·chic
in·fra·red
    far i.
    near i
in·fra·scap·u·lar
in·fra·son·ic
in·fra·sound
in·fra·spe·cif·ic
in·fra·spi·nous
in·fra·ster·nal
in·fra·struc·ture
    implant i.
in·fra·tem·po·ral
in·fra·ten·to·ri·al
in·fra·tho·rac·ic
in·fra·ton·sil·lar
in·fra·tra·che·al
in·fra·troch·le·ar
in·fra·tu·bal
in·fra·tur·bi·nal
in·fra·um·bil·i·cal
in·fra·ver·gence
in·fra·ver·sion

in·fra·ves·i·cal
in·fra·zy·go·mat·ic
in·fric·tion
in·fun·dib·u·la
in·fun·dib·u·lar
in·fun·dib·u·lec·to·my
    Brock's i.
in·fun·dib·u·li·form
in·fun·dib·u·lo·ma
in·fun·dib·u·lo-ovar·i·an
in·fun·dib·u·lo·pel·vic
in·fun·dib·u·lum *pl.* in·fun·
  dib·u·la
    cardiac i.
    crural i.
    i. crurale
    ethmoidal i.
    i. ethmoidale
    i. of fallopian tube
    i. of frontal sinus
    i. of heart
    i. of hypophysis
    i. hypothalami
    i. of hypothalamus
    infundibula of kidney
    i. nasi
    i. of nose
    i. pulmonis
    i. pulmonum
    infundibula renum
    i. tubae uterinae
    i. of urinary bladder
    i. of uterine tube
In·fuse-a-port
in·fused
in·fu·si·ble
in·fu·sion
    amniotic fluid i.
    cold i.
    meat i.
    saline i.
in·fu·so·de·coc·tion
in·fu·sum
in·ges·ta
in·ges·tant
in·ges·tion
in·ges·tive
in·glu·vi·es

In·gras·sia's apophysis
In·gras·sia's process
In·gras·sia's wings
in·gra·ves·cent
in·growth
    epithelial i.
in·guen *pl.* in·gui·na
in·gui·na
in·gui·nal
in·gui·no·ab·dom·i·nal
in·guino·cele
in·gui·no·cru·ral
in·gui·no·dyn·ia
in·gui·no·la·bi·al
in·gui·no·scro·tal
in·hal·ant
    antifoaming i.
in·ha·la·tion
    isoproterenol sulfate i.
    smoke i.
in·hale
in·hal·er
    Allis'i.
    ether i.
    H. H. i.
    Junker i.
in·her·ent
in·her·i·tance
    alternative i.
    autosomal i.
    biparental i.
    blending i.
    codominant i.
    complemental i.
    cytoplasmic i.
    dominant i.
    extrachromosomal i.
    extranuclear i.
    galtonian i.
    holandric i.
    hologynic i.
    homochronous i.
    homotropic i.
    intermediate i.
    maternal i.
    matrilinear i.
    mendelian i.
    mitochondrial i.

in·her·i·tance *(continued)*
    monofactorial i.
    monogenic i.
    mosaic i.
    multifactorial i.
    particulate i.
    polygenic i.
    quantitative i.
    quasidominant i.
    recessive i.
    sex-linked i.
    unit i.
    X-linked i.
in·her·it·ed
in·hib·in
in·hib·it
in·hi·bi·tion
    allogenic i.
    allosteric i.
    antidromic i.
    autogenous i.
    central i.
    competitive i.
    contact i.
    endproduct i.
    enzyme i.
    feedback i.
    fertility i.
    hemagglutination i. (HI, HAI)
    mixed i.
    motor i.
    noncompetitive i.
    potassium i.
    proactive i.
    reciprocal i.
    recurrent i.
    reflex i.
    Renshaw i.
    retroactive i.
    selective i.
    substrate i.
    uncompetitive i.
    Wedensky i.
in·hib·i·tive
in·hib·i·tor
    active-site-directed
      irreversible i.

in·hib·i·tor *(continued)*
    aldosterone i.
    angiotensin converting
      enzyme (ACE) i's
    C1 i. (C1 INH)
    carbonic anhydrase i.
    C1 esterase i.
    cholesterol i.
    cholinesterase i.
    competitive i.
    irreversible i.
    membrane attack complex
      i. (MAC INH)
    lupus i.
    mitotic i.
    monoamine oxidase i.
      (MAOI)
    noncompetitive i.
    α_2 plasmin i.
    plasminogen activator i.
      (PAI)
    reversible i.
    trypsin i.
in·hib·i·to·ry
in·ho·mo·ge·ne·i·ty
in·ho·mo·ge·neous
in·i·ac
in·i·ad
in·i·al
in·i·en·ceph·a·lus
in·i·en·ceph·a·ly
in·i·od·y·mus
in·i·on
in·i·op·a·gus
in·i·ops
ini·tial
ini·ti·a·tion
in·i·tis
in·ject
in·ject·a·ble
in·ject·ed
in·jec·tion
    anatomical i.
    circumcorneal i.
    coarse i.
    depot i.
    dextrose i.
    endermic i.

in·jec·tion *(continued)*
    epifascial i.
    ethiodized oil i.
    fine i.
    fructose i.
    gaseous i.
    gelatin i.
    hypodermic i.
    insulin i.
    intracutaneous i.
    intradermal i.
    intradermic i.
    intramuscular i.
    intrathecal i.
    intravascular i.
    intravenous i.
    iodinated I 125 albumin i.
    iodinated I 131 albumin i.
    iron dextran i.
    iron sorbitex i.
    jet i.
    opacifying i.
    oxytocin i.
    paraperiosteal i.
    parathyroid i.
    parenchymatous i.
    posterior pituitary i.
    preservative i.
    protamine sulfate i.
    protein hydrolysate i.
    repository i.
    Ringer's i.
    Ringer's i., lactated
    sclerosing i.
    sodium chloride i.
    sodium pertechnate Tc
      99m i.
    sodium radiochromate i.
    subcutaneous i.
    technetium Tc 99m
      albumin aggregated i.
    Teflon i. of vocal cord
    trigger point i.
    vasopressin i.
in·jec·tor
    jet i.
in·jure

in·ju·ry
    air-blast i.
    atmospheric blast i.
    birth i.
    blast i.
    blunt i.
    bucket-handle i.
    bumper i.
    closed head i.
    compression i.
    contrecoup i.
    coup i. of brain
    coup-contrecoup i.
    crush i.
    deceleration i.
    egg-white i.
    Goyrand's i.
    hyperextension-hyperflex-
        ion i.
    immersion blast i.
    internal i.
    neonatal cold i.
    occupational i.
    open head i.
    patterned i.
    shell i.
    soft tissue i.
    steering-wheel i.
    straddle i.
    unintentional i.
    vital i.
    whiplash i.
    wringer i.
in·lay
    bone i.
    epithelial i.
    skin graft i.
in·let
    pelvic i.
    thoracic i.
in·nate
in·ner·vate
in·ner·va·tion
    double i.
    multiple i.
    plurisegmental i.
    polyneuronal i.
    reciprocal i.

in·nid·i·a·tion
in·no·cent
in·noc·u·ous
in·nom·i·na·tal
in·nom·i·nate
in·nom·i·na·tum
In·no·var
in·nox·ious
in·nu·tri·tion
ino·blast
in·oc·ci·pit·ia
ino·chon·dri·tis
in·oc·u·la
in·oc·u·la·bil·i·ty
in·oc·u·la·ble
in·oc·u·late
in·oc·u·la·tion
    protective i.
in·oc·u·la·tive
in·oc·u·lum *pl.* in·oc·u·la
ino·cyte
ino·gen·e·sis
in·og·e·nous
in·og·lia
ino·hy·me·ni·tis
ino·lith
ino·myo·si·tis
in·op·er·a·ble
ino·pex·ia
ino·phrag·ma
in·or·gan·ic
in·or·gan·ic py·ro·phos·pha·
    tase
ino·scle·ro·sis
in·os·co·py
in·os·cu·late
in·os·cu·la·tion
in·ose
in·o·se·mia
in·o·si·nate
in·o·sine
    i. monophosphate (IMP)
in·o·sine phos·pho·ryl·ase
in·o·sin·ic acid
in·o·site
ino·sit·ide
in·o·si·tis

ino·si·tol
    i. niacinate
    i. 1,4,5-triphosphate (InsP$_3$,
    IP$_3$)
in·o·si·tol·uria
in·o·si·tu·ria
in·os·to·sis
in·os·uria
ino·tag·ma
ino·trope
in·o·trop·ic
    negatively i.
    positively i.
in·ot·ro·pism
in ovo
in·pa·tient
in·quest
    coroner's i.
in·qui·line
in·qui·si·tion
in·sac·ca·tion
in·sal·i·va·tion
in·sa·lu·bri·ous
in·sane
    criminally i.
in·san·i·tary
in·san·i·ty
    collective i.
    criminal i.
    double i.
    imposed i.
    induced i.
    moral i.
    partial i.
    puerperal i.
    senile i.
in·scrip·tio *pl.* in·scrip·ti·o·
nes
    i. tendinea
    inscriptiones tendineae
    musculi recti abdominis
in·scrip·tion
    tendinous i.
    tendinous i's of rectus
    abdominis muscle
in·scrip·ti·o·nes
in·sect
In·sec·ta

in·sec·tar·i·um
in·sec·ti·cide
in·sec·ti·fuge
in·sem·i·na·tion
    artificial i.
    donor i.
    heterologous i.
    homologous i.
in·se·nes·cence
in·sen·si·ble
in·sert
    intramucosal i.
    mucosal i.
in·ser·tio
    i. velamentosa
in·ser·tion
    parasol i.
    velamentous i.
in·sheathed
in·sid·i·ous
in·sight
in si·tu
in·so·la·tion
    asphyxial i.
    hyperpyrexial i.
in·sol·u·ble
in·som·nia
in·som·ni·ac
in·som·nic
in·so·nate
in·sorp·tion
InsP$_3$ — inositol
    1,4,5-triphosphate
in·sper·sion
in·spi·rate
in·spi·ra·tion
    crowing i.
in·spi·ra·to·ry
in·spi·rom·e·ter
in·spis·sant
in·spis·sate
in·spis·sat·ed
in·spis·sa·tion
in·spis·sa·tor
in·star
in·step
in·still
in·stil·la·tion

in·stil·la·tor
in·stinct
    aggressive i.
    death i.
    ego i.
    herd i.
    life i.
    mother i.
    sexual i.
in·stinc·tive
in·sti·tu·tion·al·iza·tion
in·sti·tu·tion·al·ize
in·struc·tion
in·stru·ment
    Acufex i.
    hand i.
    plugging i.
    stereotaxic i.
in·stru·men·tal
in·stru·men·tar·i·um
in·stru·men·ta·tion
    Cotrel-Dubousset spinal i.
    Harrington i.
    Luque i.
in·suc·ca·tion
in·su·da·tion
in·suf·fi·cien·cy
    active i.
    adrenal i.
    adrenocortical i.
    anterior pituitary i.
    aortic i.
    basilar i.
    capsular i.
    cardiac i.
    coronary i.
    i. of the externi
    i. of the eyelids
    gastric i.
    gastromotor i.
    hepatic i.
    ileocecal i.
    i. of the interni
    mitral i.
    muscular i.
    myocardial i.
    pancreatic i.
    parathyroid i.

in·suf·fi·cien·cy *(continued)*
    placental i.
    post-traumatic pulmonary i.
    pulmonary i.
    pyloric i.
    renal i.
    thyroid i.
    tricuspid i.
    uterine i.
    valvular i.
    velopharyngeal i.
    venous i.
    vertebral i.
    vertebrobasilar i.
in·suf·flate
in·suf·fla·tion
    cranial i.
    endotracheal i.
    i. of the lungs
    perirenal i.
    presacral i.
    tubal i.
in·suf·fla·tor
in·su·la *pl.* in·su·lae
    insulae of Peyer
    i. of Reil
in·su·lar
in·su·lar·ine
In·su·la·tard NPH
in·su·late
in·su·la·tion
in·su·la·tor
in·su·lin
    beef i.
    beef-pork i.
    dealinated i.
    depot i.
    extended i. zinc suspension
    globin i.
    globin zinc i. injection
    hexamine i.
    human i.
    Humulin i.
    immunoreactive i.
    i. injection
    isophane i. suspension
    Lente i.

in·su·lin *(continued)*
    neutral i.
    Novolin L (N, R) i.
    NPH i.
    pectin i.
    plant i.
    pork i.
    prompt i. zinc suspension
    protamine zinc i.
      suspension
    regular i.
    Semilente i.
    synalbumin i.
    three-to-one i.
    Ultralente i.
    vegetable i.
    i. zinc suspension
in·su·lin·emia
in·su·lin·li·po·dys·tro·phy
in·su·lin·o·gen·e·sis
in·su·lin·o·gen·ic
in·su·lin·oid
in·su·li·no·ma
in·su·lin·o·pe·nia
in·su·lin·o·pe·nic
in·su·lin·o·priv·ic
in·su·lin·o·tar·dic
in·su·lism
in·su·li·tis
in·su·lo·gen·ic
in·su·lo·ma
in·sult
in·sur·ance
    catastrophic health i.
    disability income i.
    health i.
    malpractice i.
    professional liability i.
    supplemental health i.
    Workers' Compensation i.
in·sus·cep·ti·bil·i·ty
in·take
    acceptable daily i. (ADI)
    caloric i.
    conditional daily i.
    fluid i.
    provisional total weekly i.
    unconditional daily i.

In·tal
in·te·gra·tion
    biological i.
    nervous i.
    structural i.
in·te·gra·tor
in·teg·u·ment
    common i.
    spore i.
in·teg·u·men·ta·ry
in·teg·u·men·tum
    i. commune
in te·la
in·tel·lect
in·tel·lec·tu·al·iza·tion
in·tel·li·gence
    artificial i.
    i. quotient
in·tem·per·ance
in·ten·si·fi·ca·tion
    image i.
in·ten·sim·e·ter
in·ten·sio·nom·e·ter
in·ten·si·ty
    i. of electric field
    luminous i.
    pulse average i.
    spatial average i.
    spatial average temporal
      average i.
    spatial peak i.
    spatial peak temporal
      average i.
    temporal average i.
    temporal peak i.
    threshold i.
    intrauterine i.
in·ten·sive
in·ten·siv·ist
in·ten·tion
    first i.
    primary i.
    secondary i.
in·ter·ac·ces·so·ry
in·ter·ac·i·nar
in·ter·ac·i·nous
in·ter·ac·tion
    complementary i.

in·ter·ac·tion *(continued)*
   drug i.
   heme-heme i.
   ion-dipole i.
   primary i.
in·ter·al·ve·o·lar
in·ter·am·ni·os
in·ter·an·gu·lar
in·ter·an·nu·lar
in·ter·apoph·y·se·al
in·ter·ar·tic·u·lar
in·ter·ar·y·te·noid
in·ter·atri·al
in·ter·au·ric·u·lar
in·ter·ax·on·al
in·ter·bands
in·ter·brain
in·ter·ca·lary
in·ter·ca·late
in·ter·can·a·lic·u·lar
in·ter·cap·il·lary
in·ter·ca·rot·ic
in·ter·ca·rot·id
in·ter·car·pal
in·ter·car·ti·lag·i·nous
in·ter·cav·er·nous
in·ter·cel·lu·lar
in·ter·cen·tral
in·ter·cer·e·bral
in·ter·change
   Hamburger i.
in·ter·chon·dral
in·ter·cil·i·um
in·ter·cla·vic·u·lar
in·ter·cli·noid
in·ter·coc·cyg·e·al
in·ter·co·lum·nar
in·ter·con·dy·lar
in·ter·con·dy·loid
in·ter·con·dy·lous
in·ter·cor·nu·al
in·ter·co·ro·noi·de·al
in·ter·cos·tal
in·ter·cos·to·hu·mer·al
in·ter·course
   sexual i.
in·ter·cox·al
in·ter·cri·co·thy·rot·o·my

in·ter·cris·tal
in·ter·cri·ti·cal
in·ter·cross
in·ter·cru·ral
in·ter·cur·rent
in·ter·cus·pal
in·ter·cus·pa·tion
in·ter·cusp·ing
in·ter·def·er·en·tial
in·ter·den·tal
in·ter·den·ta·le
in·ter·den·ti·um
in·ter·dig·it
in·ter·dig·i·tal
in·ter·dig·i·tate
in·ter·dig·i·ta·tion
in·ter·ec·top·ic
in·ter·face
   dermoepidermal i.
   dineric i.
   gamma camera i.
in·ter·fa·cial
in·ter·fas·cic·u·lar
in·ter·fem·o·ral
in·ter·fer·ence
   chiasma i.
   cuspal i.
   initial i.
   interceptive occlusal i.
   interchromosomal i.
   occlusal i's
   premature i.
   proactive i.
   retroactive i.
in·ter·fer·ing
in·ter·fe·rom·e·ter
in·ter·fe·rom·e·try
in·ter·fer·on
   i.-α (IFN-α)
   antigenic i.
   i.-β (IFN-β)
   epithelial i.
   fibroblast i.
   fibroepithelial i.
   i.-γ (IFN-γ)
   immune i.
   immunoreactive i.
   leukocyte i.

in·ter·fer·on *(continued)*
   lymphoblastoid cell i.
   type I i.
   type II i.
in·ter·fi·bril·lar
in·ter·fi·bril·lary
in·ter·fi·brous
in·ter·fil·a·men·tous
in·ter·fi·lar
in·ter·fron·tal
in·ter·fur·ca *pl.* in·ter·fur·cae
in·ter·fur·cae
in·ter·gan·gli·on·ic
in·ter·gem·mal
in·ter·gen·ic
in·ter·glob·u·lar
in·ter·glu·te·al
in·ter·go·ni·al
in·ter·gra·da·tion
in·ter·grade
in·ter·gran·u·lar
in·ter·gy·ral
in·ter·hemi·cer·e·bral
in·ter·hemi·sphe·ric
in·ter·ic·tal
in·te·ri·or
in·ter·is·chi·ad·ic
in·ter·ju·gal
in·ter·ki·ne·sis
in·ter·la·bi·al
in·ter·la·mel·lar
in·ter·leu·kin
   i.-1 (IL-1)
   i.-2 (IL-2)
   i.-3 (IL-3)
in·ter·lig·a·men·ta·ry
in·ter·lig·a·men·tous
in·ter·lo·bar
in·ter·lo·bi·tis
in·ter·lob·u·lar
in·ter·lock·ing
in·ter·mal·ar
in·ter·mal·le·o·lar
in·ter·mam·il·la·ry
in·ter·mam·ma·ry
in·ter·mar·gi·nal
in·ter·mar·riage
in·ter·max·il·lary

in·ter·me·di·ary
in·ter·me·di·ate
in·ter·me·din
in·ter·me·dio·lat·er·al
in·ter·me·dio·me·di·al
in·ter·me·di·us
in·ter·mem·bra·nous
in·ter·me·nin·ge·al
in·ter·men·stru·al
in·ter·men·stru·um
in·ter·meta·car·pal
in·ter·meta·mer·ic
in·ter·meta·tar·sal
in·ter·mis·sion
in·ter·mi·tot·ic
in·ter·mit·tence
in·ter·mit·ten·cy
in·ter·mit·tent
in·ter·mo·lec·u·lar
in·ter·mu·ral
in·ter·mus·cu·lar
in·tern
in·ter·nal
in·ter·nal·iza·tion
in·ter·nar·i·al
in·ter·na·sal
in·ter·na·tal
in·ter·na·tion
In·ter·na·tion·al Clas·si·fi·ca·tion of Dis·eas·es (ICD)
In·ter·na·tion·al Non·pro·pri·e·tary Names
in·terne
in·ter·neu·ral
in·ter·neu·ron
   inhibitory i.
in·ter·neu·ro·nal
in·tern·ist
in·ter·no·dal
in·ter·node
   i. of Ranvier
in·ter·nod·u·lar
in·tern·ship
in·ter·nu·cle·ar
in·ter·nun·ci·al
in·ter·nus
in·ter·oc·clu·sal
in·tero·cep·tion

in·tero·cep·tive
in·tero·cep·tor
in·tero·fec·tion
in·tero·fec·tive
in·tero·in·fe·ri·or·ly
in·ter·ol·i·vary
in·ter·or·bi·tal
in·ter·os·se·al
in·ter·os·se·ous
in·ter·pal·a·tine
in·ter·pal·pe·bral
in·ter·pa·ri·e·tal
in·ter·par·ox·ys·mal
in·ter·pe·dic·u·late
in·ter·pe·dun·cu·lar
in·ter·pha·lan·ge·al
in·ter·phase
in·ter·phy·let·ic
in·ter·pi·al
in·ter·plant
in·ter·pleu·ral
in·ter·pleu·ri·cos·tal
in·ter·po·lar
in·ter·po·lat·ed
in·ter·po·la·tion
in·ter·po·si·tion
in·ter·pos·i·tum
in·ter·pre·ta·tion
in·ter·pret·er
in·ter·pro·to·met·a·mere
in·ter·prox·i·mal
in·ter·pter·y·goid
in·ter·pu·bic
in·ter·pulse
in·ter·pu·pil·lary
in·ter·py·ram·i·dal
in·ter·ra·di·al
in·ter·re·nal
in·ter·rupt·ed
in·ter·sca·pil·i·um
in·ter·scap·u·lar
in·ter·scap·u·lum
in·ter·sci·at·ic
in·ter·sec·tio *pl.* in·ter·sec·ti·o·nes
   i. tendinea
   intersectiones tendineae
     musculi recti abdominis

in·ter·sec·tion
   aponeurotic i.
   tendinous i.
in·ter·sec·ti·o·nes
in·ter·seg·ment
in·ter·seg·men·tal
in·ter·sep·tal
in·ter·sep·tum
in·ter·sex
   female i.
   male i.
   true i.
in·ter·sex·u·al
in·ter·sex·u·al·i·ty
   genital i.
   gonadal i.
in·ter·sig·moid
in·ter·space
   dineric i.
in·ter·spi·nal
in·ter·spi·nous
in·ter·ster·nal
in·ter·stice
in·ter·stim·u·lus
in·ter·sti·tial
in·ter·sti·ti·um
in·ter·tar·sal
in·ter·ten·di·nous
in·ter·trag·ic
in·ter·trans·ver·sal·is
in·ter·trans·verse
in·ter·tri·al
in·ter·trig·i·nous
in·ter·tri·go
   i. labialis
in·ter·tro·chan·ter·ic
in·ter·tu·ber·cu·lar
in·ter·tu·bu·lar
in·ter·ure·ter·al
in·ter·ure·ter·ic
in·ter·utero·pla·cen·tal
in·ter·vag·i·nal
in·ter·val
   a–c i.
   Ae–H i.
   A–H i.
   atrioventricular i.

in·ter·val *(continued)*
    auriculoventricular i.
    A–V i.
    BH i.
    cardioarterial i.
    confidence i.
    coupling i.
    focal i.
    H–Ae i.
    H–V i.
    induction-delivery i.
    interectopic i.
    interstimulus i.
    intertrial i.
    isovolumetric i.
    lucid i.
    P–A i.
    P–J i.
    postmortem i.
    postsphygmic i.
    P–P i.
    P–R i.
    presphygmic i.
    Q–R i.
    QRS i.
    QRST i.
    Q–T i.
    reference i.
    S_2-OS i.
    Sturm's i.
    tolerance i.
in·ter·val·vu·lar
in·ter·vas·cu·lar
in·ter·ven·tion
    crisis i.
in·ter·ven·tric·u·lar
in·ter·ver·te·bral
in·ter·vil·lous
in·ter·zo·nal
in·tes·ti·nal
in·tes·tine
    blind i.
    empty i.
    iced i.
    jejunoileal i.
    large i.
    mesenterial i.
    preoral i.

in·tes·tine *(continued)*
    segmented i.
    small i.
    straight i.
in·tes·ti·no-in·tes·ti·nal
in·tes·ti·num *pl.* in·tes·ti·na
    i. caecum
    i. crassum
    i. ileum
    i. jejunum
    i. rectum
    i. tenue
    i. tenue mesenteriale
in·ti·ma
in·ti·mal
in·ti·mec·to·my
in·ti·mi·tis
In·to·cos·trin
in·toe
in·tol·er·ance
    disaccharide i.
    drug i.
    hereditary fructose i.
    hereditary galactose i.
    lactose i.
    leucine i.
    lysine i.
    lysinuric protein i.
    milk i.
    sucrose i.
in·to·na·tion
    nasal i.
in·tor·sion
in·tort·er
in·tox·i·cant
in·tox·i·ca·tion
    acid i.
    alcohol idiosyncratic i.
    alkaline i.
    anaphylactic i.
    bongkrek i.
    citrate i.
    digitalis i.
    manganese i.
    pathological i.
    roentgen i.
    serum i.
    water i.

in·tra-ab·dom·i·nal
in·tra-ac·i·nous
in·tra-aor·tic
in·tra-ap·pen·dic·u·lar
in·tra-arach·noid
in·tra-ar·te·ri·al
in·tra-ar·tic·u·lar
in·tra-atri·al
in·tra-au·ral
in·tra-au·ric·u·lar
in·tra·bron·chi·al
in·tra·buc·cal
in·tra·cal·i·ce·al
in·tra·can·a·lic·u·lar
in·tra·cap·su·lar
in·tra·car·di·ac
in·tra·car·pal
in·tra·car·ti·lag·i·nous
in·tra·cath·e·ter
in·tra·cav·er·nous
in·tra·cav·i·tary
in·tra·ce·li·al
in·tra·cel·lu·lar
in·tra·ce·phal·ic
in·tra·cer·e·bel·lar
in·tra·cer·e·bral
in·tra·cer·vi·cal
in·tra·change
in·tra·chon·dral
in·tra·chon·dri·al
in·tra·chor·dal
in·tra·cho·ri·on·ic
in·tra·cis·ter·nal
in·tra·col·ic
in·tra·cor·dal
in·tra·co·ro·nal
in·tra·cor·po·ral
in·tra·cor·po·re·al
in·tra·cor·pus·cu·lar
in·tra·cos·tal
in·tra·cra·ni·al
in·tra·cru·re·us
in·trac·ta·ble
in·tra·cu·ta·ne·ous
in·tra·cys·tic
in·tra·cy·to·plas·mic
in·trad
in·tra·der·mal

in·tra·der·mo·re·ac·tion
in·tra·duct
in·tra·duc·tal
in·tra·du·o·de·nal
in·tra·du·ral
in·tra·em·bry·on·ic
in·tra·epi·der·mal
in·tra·ep·i·phys·e·al
in·tra·ep·i·the·li·al
in·tra·eryth·ro·cyt·ic
in·tra·fas·cic·u·lar
in·tra·fat
in·tra·fe·brile
in·tra·fe·ta·tion
in·tra·fi·lar
in·tra·fis·su·ral
in·tra·fis·tu·lar
in·tra·fol·lic·u·lar
in·tra·fu·sal
in·tra·gal·van·iza·tion
in·tra·gas·tric
in·tra·gem·mal
in·tra·gen·ic
in·tra·glan·du·lar
in·tra·glob·u·lar
in·tra·glu·te·al
in·tra·gy·ral
in·tra·he·pat·ic
in·tra·hy·oid
in·tra·ic·tal
in·tra·in·tes·ti·nal
in·tra·jug·u·lar
in·tra·la·mel·lar
in·tra·la·ryn·ge·al
in·tra·le·sion·al
in·tra·leu·ko·cyt·ic
in·tra·lig·a·men·tous
in·tra·lin·gual
In·tra·lip·id
in·tra·lo·bar
in·tra·lob·u·lar
in·tra·loc·u·lar
in·tra·lu·mi·nal
in·tra·mam·ma·ry
in·tra·mar·gin·al
in·tra·mas·toi·di·tis
in·tra·mat·ri·cal
in·tra·med·ul·lary

in·tra·mem·bra·nous
in·tra·me·nin·ge·al
in·tra·men·stru·al
in·tra·mo·lec·u·lar
in·tra·mu·co·sal
in·tra·mu·ral
in·tra·mus·cu·lar
in·tra·myo·car·di·al
in·tra·nar·i·al
in·tra·na·sal
in·tra·na·tal
in·tra·neu·ral
in·tra·nu·cle·ar
in·tra·oc·u·lar
in·tra·op·er·a·tive
in·tra·oral
in·tra·or·bi·tal
in·tra·os·se·ous
in·tra·os·te·al
in·tra·ovar·i·an
in·tra·ov·u·lar
in·tra·pan·cre·at·ic
in·tra·par·en·chym·a·tous
in·tra·pa·ri·e·tal
in·tra·par·tum
in·tra·pel·vic
in·tra·peri·car·di·al
in·tra·per·i·ne·al
in·tra·peri·to·ne·al
in·tra·pi·al
in·tra·pla·cen·tal
in·tra·pleu·ral
in·tra·pon·tine
in·tra·pros·tat·ic
in·tra·pro·to·plas·mic
in·tra·psy·chic
in·tra·pul·mo·nary
in·tra·py·ret·ic
in·tra·ra·chid·i·an
in·tra·rec·tal
in·tra·re·nal
in·tra·ret·i·nal
in·tra·scle·ral
in·tra·scro·tal
in·tra·sel·lar
in·tra·spi·nal
in·tra·spi·nous
in·tra·sple·nic

in·tra·ster·nal
in·tra·sti·tial
in·tra·stro·mal
in·tra·syno·vi·al
in·tra·tar·sal
in·tra·tes·tic·u·lar
in·tra·the·cal
in·tra·the·nar
in·tra·tho·rac·ic
in·tra·ton·sil·lar
in·tra·tra·bec·u·lar
in·tra·tra·che·al
in·tra·tu·bal
in·tra·tu·bu·lar
in·tra·tym·pan·ic
in·tra·ure·ter·al
in·tra·ure·thral
in·tra·uter·ine
in·tra·vag·i·nal
in·trav·a·sa·tion
in·tra·vas·cu·lar
in·tra·ve·na·tion
in·tra·ve·nous
in·tra·ven·tric·u·lar
in·tra·ver·sion
in·tra·ver·te·bral
in·tra·ves·i·cal
in·tra·vil·lous
in·tra·vi·tal
in·tra vi·tam
in·tra·vi·tel·line
in·tra·vit·re·ous
in·tra·zole
in·trin·sic
in·trip·ty·line hy·dro·chlo·ride
in·tro·duc·er
    Littleford-Spector i.
in·tro·fi·er
in·tro·flex·ion
in·tro·gas·tric
in·tro·gres·sion
in·tro·i·tus *pl.* in·tro·i·tus
   i. oesophagi
   i. pelvis
   i. vaginae
in·tro·jec·tion
in·tro·mis·sion

in·tron
In·tro·pin
in·tro·pu·ni·tive
in·tror·sus
in·tro·spec·tion
in·tro·sus·cep·tion
in·tro·ver·sion
in·tro·ver·sion-ex·tro·ver·sion
in·tro·vert
in·tru·sion
in·tu·bate
in·tu·ba·tion
    aqueductal i.
    blind nasal i.
    blind nasotracheal i.
    endotracheal i.
    nasal i.
    nasotracheal i.
    oral i.
    orotracheal i.
in·tu·ba·tion·ist
in·tu·ba·tor
in·tu·i·tion
in·tu·mesce
in·tu·mes·cence
in·tu·mes·cent
in·tu·mes·cen·tia *pl.* in·tu·mes·cen·tiae
    i. cervicalis
    i. ganglioformis
    i. lumbalis
    i. lumbosacralis
    i. tympanica
in·tus·sus·cep·tion
    agonic i.
    appendicular i.
    colic i.
    double i.
    enteric i.
    enterocolic i.
    ileal i.
    ileocecal i.
    ileocolic i.
    jejunogastric i.
    postmortem i.
    retrograde i.
in·tus·sus·cep·tum

in·tus·sus·cip·i·ens
In·u·la
in·u·lase
in·u·lin
in·u·lin·ase
in·u·loid
in·unc·tion
in·unc·tum
    i. mentholis compositum
in utero
in vac·uo
in·vag·i·nate
in·vag·i·na·tion
    basilar i.
    i. of enamel
    mammary i.
in·vag·i·na·tor
in·va·lid
in·va·lid·ism
in·va·sin
in·va·sion
in·va·sive
in·va·sive·ness
in·ven·to·ry
    Maudsley personality i.
    Millon clinical multiaxial i. (MGMI)
    Minnesota Multiphasic Personality I. (MMPI)
in·ver·mi·na·tion
In·ver·sine
in·ver·sion
    i. of bladder
    carbohydrate i.
    chromosome i.
    forced i.
    i. of gradient
    lateral i.
    paracentric i.
    pericentric i.
    sexual i.
    spontaneous i.
    thermic i.
    i. of uterus
    visceral i.
in·ver·sus
in·ver·tase
In·ver·te·bra·ta

in·ver·te·brate
in·ver·tor
in·ver·tose
in·vest
in·vest·ing
    i. the pattern
    vacuum i.
in·vest·ment
    emotional i.
    fibrous i.
    hygroscopic i.
    myelin i.
in·vet·er·ate
in·vis·ca·tion
in vi·tro
in vi·vo
in·vo·lu·crum *pl.* in·vo·lu·cra
in·vol·un·tary
in·vol·un·to·mo·to·ry
in·vo·lute
in·vo·lu·tion
    buccal i.
    pituitary i.
    senile i.
in·vo·lu·tion·al
in·volve·ment
    bifurcation i.
    trifurcation i.
io·ben·zam·ic acid
io·car·mic acid
io·ce·tam·ic acid
iod·al·bu·min
io·da·mide
Iod·amoe·ba beutsch·lii
io·date
iod-Bas·e·dow
io·de·mia
iod·ic acid
io·dide
    ferrous i.
io·dide per·ox·i·dase
io·dim·e·try
io·di·nate
io·din·a·tion
io·dine
    i. 131
    butanol-extractable i.
    imidecyl i.

io·dine *(continued)*
    povidone i.
    protein-bound i.
    radioactive i.
io·dine-fast
io·din·in
io·din·o·phil
io·din·oph·i·lous
io·dip·amide
    i. meglumine
    i. sodium
io·dism
io·dize
io·do·acet·amide
io·do·ace·tic acid
io·do·an·ti·py·rine
io·do·bras·sid
io·do·ca·sein
io·do·chlor·hy·drox·y·quin
io·do·cho·les·ter·ol
5-io·do·de·oxy·uri·dine
io·do·der·ma
io·do·form
io·do·form·ism
io·do·for·mum
io·do·gen·ic
io·do·glob·u·lin
io·do·gor·gon·ine
io·do·gor·gor·ic acid
io·do·hip·pu·rate so·di·um
    i. s. I 123
    i. s. I 131
io·do·log·ra·phy
lo·do·meth·yl·nor·cho·les·ter·ol
io·do·met·ric
io·dom·e·try
io·do·pa·no·ic acid
io·do·phe·nol
io·do·phil
io·do·phil·ia
io·do·phor
io·do·phthal·ein so·di·um
io·do·pro·tein
io·dop·sin
io·do·pyr·a·cet
io·do·quin·ol
io·do·stick

io·do·sul·fate
io·do·ther·a·py
io·do·thio·ura·cil
io·do·thy·ro·glob·u·lin
io·do·thy·ro·nine
io·do·ty·ro·sine
io·do·ty·ro·sine de·hal·o·gen·
    ase
io·do·ty·ro·sine de·io·din·ase
io·do·ven·tric·u·log·ra·phy
io·do·vol·a·til·iza·tion
io·dox·am·ic acid
iod·oxy·quin·o·line·sul·fon·ic
    acid
io·du·ria
io·glic·ic acid
io·gly·cam·ic acid
ion
    dipolar i.
    gram i.
    hydrogen i.
    hydronium i.
Io·na·min
ion·ic
ion·iza·tion
    avalanche i.
    Townsend i.
ion·ize
io·no·col·or·im·e·ter
ion·o·gen
ion·o·gen·ic
ion·om·e·ter
ion·om·e·try
ion·one
ion·o·phore
io·no·phose
ion·o·scope
iono·ther·a·py
ion-pro·tein
ion·ther·a·py
ion·to·pho·re·sis
ion·to·pho·ret·ic
ion·to·quan·tim·e·ter
ion·to·ra·di·om·e·ter
ion·to·ther·a·py
IOP — intraocular pressure
io·pam·i·dol
io·pa·no·ic acid

io·phen·dy·late
io·phen·ox·ic acid
io·py·dol
io·py·done
io·ser·ic acid
io·sul·a·mide meg·lu·mine
io·su·met·ic acid
io·ta
io·ta·cism
io·tet·ric acid
io·thal·a·mate
    i. meglumine
    i. sodium
io·tha·lam·ic acid
io·thio·ura·cil
io·trox·ic acid
IP — intraperitoneally
    isoelectric point
IP$_3$ — inositol
1,4,5-triphosphate
IPAA — International
    Psychoanalytical Association
I-para
IPD — intermittent peritoneal
    dialysis
ip·e·cac
    powdered i.
ipo·date
    i. calcium
    i. sodium
ip·o·mea
Ip·o·moea
IPPB — intermittent positive
    pressure breathing
Ip·ral
ipra·tro·pi·um bro·mide
iprin·dole
ipro·ni·a·zid
ipro·nid·a·zole
iprox·amine hy·dro·chlo·ride
ip·se·fact
ip·si·lat·er·al
IPSP — inhibitory
    postsynaptic potential
IPV — poliovirus vaccine
    inactivated
IQ — intelligence quotient

IRC — inspiratory reserve
capacity
Ir·con
IRI — immunoreactive insulin
iri·dal
iri·dal·gia
ir·id·aux·e·sis
ir·id·avul·sion
iri·dec·ta·sis
iri·dec·tome
iri·dec·to·me·so·di·al·y·sis
iri·dec·to·mize
iri·dec·to·my
    basal i.
    buttonhole i.
    complete i.
    optic i.
    optical i.
    peripheral i.
    preliminary i.
    preparatory i.
    sector i.
    stenopeic i.
    therapeutic i.
    total i.
iri·dec·tro·pi·um
iri·de·mia
iri·den·clei·sis
iri·den·tro·pi·um
iri·de·re·mia
iri·des
iri·des·cence
iri·des·cent
irid·e·sis
iri·di·ag·no·sis
irid·i·al
irid·i·an
irid·ic
irid·is
    rubeosis i.
irid·i·um
iri·di·za·tion
iri·do·avul·sion
iri·do·cap·su·li·tis
iri·do·cap·su·lot·o·my
iri·do·cele
iri·do·cho·roi·di·tis
iri·do·col·o·bo·ma

iri·do·con·stric·tor
iri·do·cor·neo·scle·rec·to·my
iri·do·cy·clec·to·my
iri·do·cy·cli·tis
    heterochromic i.
iri·do·cy·clo·cho·roi·di·tis
iri·do·cys·tec·to·my
iri·do·cyte
iri·dod·e·sis
iri·do·di·ag·no·sis
iri·do·di·al·y·sis
iri·do·di·as·ta·sis
iri·do·di·la·tor
iri·do·do·ne·sis
iri·do·ker·a·ti·tis
iri·do·ki·ne·sia
iri·do·ki·ne·sis
iri·do·ki·net·ic
iri·do·lep·tyn·sis
iri·dol·o·gy
iri·dol·y·sis
iri·do·ma·la·cia
iri·do·me·so·di·al·y·sis
iri·do·mo·tor
iri·don·cus
iri·do·pa·ral·y·sis
iri·dop·a·thy
iri·do·peri·pha·ki·tis
iri·do·ple·gia
    accommodation i.
    complete i.
    reflex i.
    sympathetic i.
iri·dop·to·sis
iri·do·pu·pil·lary
iri·do·rhex·is
iri·dos·chi·sis
iri·do·scle·rot·o·my
iri·do·ste·re·sis
iri·dot·a·sis
iri·do·tome
iri·dot·o·my
iri·do·vi·rus
IRIS — International
Research Information
Service
Iris

iris *pl.* iri·des
    i. bombé
    detached i.
    tremulous i.
    umbrella i.
iri·sin
iris·op·sia
iri·tic
iri·tis
    i. catamenialis
    diabetic i.
    follicular i.
    gouty i.
    i. papulosa
    plastic i.
    purulent i.
    serous i.
    spongy i.
    sympathetic i.
    uratic i.
iri·to·ec·to·my
irit·o·my
ir·i·um
iron
    i. 55
    i. 59
    i. acetate
    i. adenylate
    i. and ammonium sulfate
    i. ascorbate
    available i.
    i. chloride
    i. choline citrate
    i. citrate
    i. dextrin
    i. gluconate
    i. hematoxylin
    i. hypophosphate
    i. lactate
    i. magnesium sulfate
    i. malate
    nonheme i.
    i. oleate
    i. phosphate
    i. protosulfate
    i. pyrophosphate
    Quevenne's i.
    i. and quinine citrate

iron *(continued)*
    radioactive i.
    reduced i.
    i. sorbitex
    i. sulfate
irot·o·my
ir·ra·di·ate
ir·ra·di·a·tion
    interstitial i.
    intracavitary i.
    ultraviolet blood i.
    whole-body i.
ir·re·duc·i·ble
ir·reg·u·lar
ir·reg·u·lar·i·ty
    i. of pulse
ir·re·me·di·al
ir·re·spir·a·ble
ir·re·spon·si·bil·i·ty
    criminal i.
ir·re·sus·ci·ta·ble
ir·re·ver·si·bil·i·ty
    i. of conduction
ir·re·ver·si·ble
ir·ri·gant
ir·ri·gate
ir·ri·ga·tion
    acetic acid i.
    aminoacetic acid i.
    continuous i.
    Ringer's i.
    sodium chloride i.
ir·ri·ga·tor
ir·ri·go·ra·di·os·co·py
ir·ri·gos·co·py
ir·ri·ta·bil·i·ty
    i. of the bladder
    chemical i.
    electric i.
    faradic i.
    galvanic i.
    mechanical i.
    muscular i.
    myotatic i.
    nervous i.
    specific i.
    i. of the stomach
    tactile i.

ir·ri·ta·bil·i·ty *(continued)*
    uterine i.
ir·ri·ta·ble
ir·ri·tant
    primary i.
ir·ri·ta·tion
    cerebral i.
    direct i.
    functional i.
    meningeal i.
    spinal i.
    sympathetic i.
ir·ri·ta·tive
Ir·u·kand·ji sting
IRV — inspiratory reserve
  volume
Ir·vine syndrome
Ir·ving's operation
IS — immune serum
    intercostal space
    intraspinal
ISA — intrinsic
  sympathomimetic activity
Isaacs-Lud·wig arteriole
Isam·bert's disease
isa·mox·ole
isa·tin
is·aux·e·sis
is·che·mia
    brachiocephalic i.
    mesenteric i.
    myocardial i.
    postural i.
    renal i.
    i. retinae
    subendocardial i.
    subepicardial i.
    transient cerebral i.
    vasospasm cerebral i.
is·che·mic
    transient i. attack (TIA)
is·che·sis
is·chia
is·chi·a·del·phus
is·chi·ad·ic
is·chi·al
is·chi·al·gia
is·chi·at·ic

is·chi·dro·sis
is·chi·ec·to·my
is·chio·anal
is·chio·bul·bar
is·chio·cap·su·lar
is·chio·cav·er·nous
is·chio·cele
is·chio·coc·cyg·e·al
is·chio·coc·cyg·e·us
is·chio·did·y·mus
is·chio·dym·ia
is·chio·dyn·ia
is·chio·fem·o·ral
is·chio·fib·u·lar
is·chi·om·e·lus
is·chio·ni·tis
is·chio·pa·gia
is·chi·op·a·gus
    i. parasiticus
    i. tetrapus
    i. tripus
is·chi·op·a·gy
is·chio·pu·bic
is·chio·pu·bis
is·chio·rec·tal
is·chio·sa·cral
is·chio·tho·ra·cop·a·gus
is·chio·vag·i·nal
is·chio·ver·te·bral
is·chi·um *pl.* is·chia
is·cho·gy·ria
is·cho·sper·mia
isch·uret·ic
isch·uria
    i. paradoxa
    i. spastica
ISCP — International Society
  of Comparative Pathology
is·eth·i·o·nate
is·eth·i·o·nic acid
ISGE — International Society
  of Gastro-Enterology
ISH — International Society
  of Hematology
Ish·i·ha·ra's test
isin·glass
    Japanese i.

is·land
  blood i's
  bone i.
  i's of Calleja
  cartilage i's
  i's of Langerhans
  olfactory i's
  i's of pancreas
  Pander's i's
  i. of Reil
  Wolff's i.
is·let
  blood i's
  Calleja's i's
  i's of Langerhans
  pancreatic i's
  Walthard's i's
ISM — International Society
  of Microbiologists
Is·me·lin
ISO — International
  Standards Organization
iso·adre·no·cor·ti·cism
iso·ag·glu·ti·na·tion
iso·ag·glu·ti·nin
iso·al·lele
iso·al·le·lism
iso·al·lox·a·zine
iso·am·yl·amine
iso·am·yl·eth·yl·bar·bi·tu·ric
  acid
iso·am·yl ni·trite
iso·an·dro·ster·one
iso·an·ti·body
iso·an·ti·gen
iso·bar
iso·bar·ic
isob·o·lism
iso·bor·nyl thio·cy·a·no·ac·e·
  tate
iso·bu·caine hy·dro·chlo·ride
iso·bu·tam·ben
iso·but·yl·al·lyl·bar·bit·ur·ic
  acid
iso·ca·lo·ric
iso·car·box·a·zid
iso·cel·lo·bi·ose
iso·cel·lu·lar

iso·cen·ter
iso·cho·les·ter·in
iso·cho·les·ter·ol
iso·chro·mat·ic
iso·chro·mat·o·phil
iso·chro·mo·some
isoch·ro·nal
iso·chro·nia
iso·chron·ic
isoch·ro·nism
isoch·ro·nous
isoch·ro·ous
iso·ci·trate
iso·ci·trate de·hy·dro·gen·ase
  (NAD$^+$)
iso·ci·trate de·hy·dro·gen·ase
  (NADP$^+$)
iso·cit·ric acid
iso·col·loid
iso·com·ple·ment
iso·co·na·zole
iso·co·ria
iso·cor·tex
Iso·crin
iso·cy·a·nate
iso·cy·a·nide
iso·cy·clic
iso·cy·tol·y·sin
iso·cy·to·sis
iso·dac·tyl·ism
iso·des·mo·sine
iso·di·ag·no·sis
iso·di·a·met·ric
iso·dis·per·soid
iso·don·tic
iso·dose
iso·dul·cite
iso·dy·nam·ic
iso·dy·nam·o·gen·ic
iso·echo·ic
iso·ef·fect
iso·elec·tric
iso·elec·tron·ic
iso·en·er·get·ic
iso·en·zyme
  Regan i.
iso·eryth·rol·y·sis
  neonatal i.

iso·eth·a·rine
iso·flu·pre·done ac·e·tate
iso·flu·rane
iso·flu·ro·phate
iso·flu·ro·phos·phate
isog·a·me
iso·gam·ete
iso·ga·met·ic
iso·gam·e·ty
isog·a·mous
isog·a·my
iso·ge·ne·ic
iso·ge·ner·ic
iso·gen·e·sis
iso·gen·ic
isog·e·nous
iso·graft
iso·hem·ag·glu·ti·na·tion
iso·hem·ag·glu·ti·nin
iso·he·mol·y·sin
iso·he·mol·y·sis
iso·he·mo·lyt·ic
iso·hy·dric
iso·hy·dru·ria
iso·ico·nia
iso·icon·ic
iso·im·mu·ni·za·tion
    Rh i.
iso·in·di·ci·al
iso·la·bel·ing
iso·lac·tose
iso·late
iso·lat·er·al
iso·la·tion
    ethologic i.
    sensory i.
iso·la·tor
    surgical i.
iso·lec·i·thal
iso·leu·cine
iso·leu·cyl
iso·leu·ko·ag·glu·ti·nin
isol·o·gous
iso·ly·ser·gic acid
isol·y·sin
isol·y·sis
iso·ly·tic
iso·mal·tase

iso·mal·tose
iso·mas·ti·gote
iso·mer
    cis-trans i.
    conformational i.
    geometric i.
    optical i.
isom·er·ase
    phosphoribose i.
iso·mer·ic
isom·er·ide
isom·e·rism
    chain i.
    cis-trans i.
    configurational i.
    conformational i.
    constitutional i.
    functional group i.
    geometric i.
    optical i.
    position i.
    spatial i.
    stereochemical i.
    structural i.
    substitution i.
isom·er·iza·tion
iso·meth·a·done
iso·meth·ep·tene hy·dro·chlo·
    ride
iso·meth·ep·tene mu·cate
iso·met·ric
iso·met·rics
iso·me·tro·pia
isom·e·try
iso·mi·cro·gam·ete
iso·mor·phic
iso·mor·phism
iso·mor·phous
iso·mus·ca·rine
iso·myl·amine hy·dro·chlo·
    ride
iso·naph·thol
iso·neph·ro·tox·in
iso·ni·a·zid
iso·nic·o·tin·ic acid
    i. a. hydrazide
iso·nic·o·tin·o·yl·hy·dra·zine
iso·nic·o·tin·yl·hy·dra·zine

iso·nip·e·caine
iso·ni·tril
iso·nor·mo·cy·to·sis
iso-on·cot·ic
iso-os·mot·ic
Iso·paque
*Iso·par·or·chis tri·sim·i·li·tu·
    bis*
isop·a·thy
iso·pen·te·nyl di·phos·phate
iso·pen·te·nyl-di·phos·phate
    δ-i·som·er·ase
iso·pen·te·nyl pyro·phos·
    phate
isoph·a·gy
iso·phan
iso·phene
iso·pho·ria
iso·pho·tom·e·ter
Iso·phrin
iso·pia
iso·plas·tic
iso·po·ten·tial
iso·pre·cip·i·tin
iso·preg·ne·none
iso·pren·a·line
iso·prene
iso·pre·noid
Iso·prin·o·sine
iso·pro·pa·mide io·dide
iso·pro·pa·nol
iso·pro·pyl
    i. alcohol
    i. rubbing alcohol
    i. meprobamate
    i. myristate
iso·pro·pyl·ar·te·re·nol
iso·pro·pyl-benz·an·thra·cene
iso·pro·pyl·ep·i·neph·rine
iso·pro·te·re·nol
    i. hydrochloride
    i. sulfate
isop·ter
iso·pyk·nic
iso·pyk·no·sis
iso·pyk·not·ic
Isor·dil
isor·rhea

isor·rhe·ic
iso·rho·de·ose
isor·rhop·ic
iso·rhyth·mic
iso·ri·bo·fla·vin
iso·ru·bin
iso·scope
iso·sen·si·ti·za·tion
iso·sen·si·tize
iso·se·rine
iso·se·ro·ther·a·py
iso·se·rum
iso·sex·u·al
isos·mot·ic
isos·mo·tic·i·ty
iso·sor·bide
    i. dinitrate
Isos·po·ra
    I. belli
    I. hominis
iso·spore
isos·po·ri·a·sis
isos·po·rous
iso·stere
isos·then·uria
iso·tel
iso·the·ba·ine
iso·ther·a·py
iso·ther·mic
iso·ther·mog·no·sia
iso·ther·mo·gno·sis
iso·thi·a·zine hy·dro·chlo·ride
iso·thi·o·cy·a·nate
iso·thi·o·cy·an·ic acid
iso·thi·pen·dyl
iso·throm·bo·ag·glu·ti·nin
iso·tone
iso·to·nia
iso·ton·ic
iso·to·nic·i·ty
iso·tope
    heavy i.
    radioactive i.
    stable i.
iso·to·pol·o·gy
iso·tox·ic
iso·tox·in
iso·trans·plant

iso·trans·plan·ta·tion
iso·tret·i·noin
Isot·ri·cha
iso·tri·mor·phism
iso·tri·mor·phous
iso·tron
iso·trop·ic
isot·ro·py
iso·type
iso·typ·ic
iso·typ·i·cal
iso·ure·tin
iso·va·ler·ic acid
iso·va·ler·ic ac·id CoA de·hy·
 dro·gen·ase deficiency
iso·va·ler·ic·ac·i·de·mia
iso·val·er·yl-CoA de·hy·dro·
 gen·ase
isox·e·pac
isox·i·cam
isox·su·prine hy·dro·chlo·ride
iso·zyme
is·sue
IST — insulin shock therapy
isth·mec·to·my
isth·mi
isth·mi·an
isth·mic
isth·mi·tis
isth·mo·pa·ral·y·sis
isth·mo·ple·gia
isth·mo·spasm
isth·mus *pl.* is·thmi
 anterior i. of fauces
 i. of aorta
 i. aortae
 i. of auditory tube
 i. of cartilage of auricle
 i. cartilaginis auris
 i. of cingulate gyrus
 i. of eustachian tube
 i. of external auditory
  meatus
 i. of fallopian tube
 i. of fauces
 i. faucium
 i. glandulae thyroideae
 gyral i.

isth·mus *(continued)*
 i. gyri cingulatus
 i. gyri cinguli
 i. gyri fornicati
 Haller's i.
 i. hippocampi
 i. of His
 i. of limbic lobe
 oropharyngeal i.
 pharyngo-oral i.
 i. prostatae
 i. rhombencephali
 i. of thyroid gland
 i. tubae auditivae
 i. tubae uterinae
 i. urethrae
 i. uteri
 i. of Vieussens
ISU — International Society
 of Urology
Isu·prel
isu·ria
ITA — International
 Tuberculosis Association
Itard's catheter
Itard-Cho·le·wa sign
itch
 Aujeszky's i.
 bakers'i.
 barbers'i.
 bath i.
 chorioptic i.
 clam diggers'i.
 copra i.
 Cuban i.
 dew i.
 dhobie mark i.
 filarial i.
 grain i.
 grocers' i.
 ground i.
 gym i.
 jock i.
 kabure i.
 mad i.
 Norway i.
 poultryman's i.
 prairie i.

itch *(continued)*
    sarcoptic i.
    Sawah i.
    seven-year i.
    straw i.
    summer i.
    swamp i.
    swimmers' i.
    warehouseman's i.
    water i.
    winter i.
itch·ing
iter
    i. ad infundibulum
    i. chordae anterius
    i. chordae posterius
    i. dentium
    i. of Sylvius
iter·al
it·er·a·tive
it·ero·par·i·ty
it·er·op·a·rous
ith·y·cy·phos
ith·y·lor·do·sis
ith·yo·ky·pho·sis
Ito's nevus
Ito-Reen·stier·na test
ITP — idiopathic
  thrombocytopenic purpura
It·ru·mil
It·sen·ko's disease
IU — immunizing unit
    international unit
    intrauterine
IUCD — intrauterine
  contraceptive device
IUD — intrauterine
  contraceptive device
IUGR — intrauterine growth
  retardation
IV — intervertebral
    intravenous

IV — intervertebral
(continued)
    intravenously (by
      intravenous injection)
Iva·lon
IVC — inferior vena cava
Ive·mark's syndrome
iver·mec·tin
IVP — intravenous pyelogram
    intravenous pyelography
    intraventricular pressure
IVT — intravenous
  transfusion
Ivy's method
Ivy's wiring
Iwan·off's (Iwan·ow's) cysts
Ix·o·des
    I. bicornis
    I. canisuga
    I. cavipalpus
    I. dammini
    I. frequens
    I. hexagonus
    I. holocyclus
    I. pacificus
    I. persulcatus
    I. pilosus
    I. putus
    I. rasus
    I. ricinus
    I. rubicundus
    I. scapularis
    I. spinipalpus
ix·o·di·a·sis
ix·od·ic
ix·o·did
Ix·od·i·dae
Ix·od·i·des
Ix·o·diph·a·gus
    I. caucurtei
ix·o·dism
Ix·o·doi·dea
Izar's reagent

J — joule
jaag·siek·te, jaag·ziek·te
Ja·bou·lay's amputation
Ja·bou·lay's button
Ja·bou·lay's operation
Jac·coud's fever
Jac·coud's sign
jack·et
  Minerva j.
  orthoplast j.
  plaster-of-Paris j.
  porcelain j.
  Risser j.
  strait j.
jack·screw
Jack·son appliance
Jack·son's law
Jack·son's membrane
Jack·son's rule
Jack·son's safety triangle
Jack·son's sign
Jack·son's syndrome
Jack·son's veil
jack·so·ni·an epilepsy
jack·son·ism
Ja·cob, François
Ja·cob's membrane
Ja·cob's ulcer
Jac·o·bae·us operation
ja·co·bine
Ja·cob·son's canal
Ja·cob·son's cartilage
Ja·cob·son's nerve
Ja·cob·son's organ
Ja·cob·son's plexus
Ja·cob·son's retinitis
Ja·cob·son's sulcus
Ja·cobs·thal 's test
Ja·cod syndrome
Ja·cod-Neg·ri syndrome
Jacque·mier's sign
Jacques plexus
Jac·quet's dermatitis
Jac·quet's erythema
jac·ta·tio
  j. capitis nocturna

jac·ta·tion
jac·ti·ta·tion
  periodic j.
jac·u·lif·er·ous
Jad·as·sohn's anetoderma
Jad·as·sohn's sebaceous nevus
Jad·as·sohn's test
Jad·as·sohn-Lew·an·dow·sky
  syndrome
Jad·as·sohn-Pel·li·za·ri
  anetoderma
Jade·lot's furrows
Jade·lot's lines
Jae·ger's test types
Jaf·fe's disease
Jaf·fé's reaction
Jaf·fé's test
Jaf·fe-Lich·ten·stein disease
Jaf·fe-Lich·ten·stein syndrome
Ja·kob's disease
Ja·kob-Creutz·feldt disease
Jaksch's disease
Jaksch's test
jal·ap
ja·mais vu
James fibers
James-Lange-Suth·er·land
  theory
Jam·shi·di needle
Ja·net's disease
Ja·net's test
Jane·way's lesion
Jane·way's
  sphygmoma-nometer
Jane·way's sphygmoma-
  nometer
Jane·way's spots
jan·i·ceps
  j. asymmetros
  j. parasiticus
Ja·nin's tetanus
Ja·no·šík's embryo
Jan·sen's disease
Jan·sen's operation
Jan·sen's test
Jan·sky's classification

Jansky-Bielschowsky disease
Jan·thi·no·so·ma
   J. lutzi
   J. posticata
Ja·quet's apparatus
jar
   bell j.
   Coplin's j.
   Leyden j.
ja·ra·ra·ca
Jar·cho's pressometer
jar·gon
jar·gon·a·pha·sia
Ja·risch-Herx·heim·er
  reaction
Jar·ja·vay's muscle
Jar·ot·zky's (Jarotsky's)
  treatment
Jar·vik heart
Jat·ro·pha
jaun·dice
   acholuric j.
   acholuric familial j.
   anhepatic j.
   anhepatogenous j.
   black j.
   breast milk j.
   cholestatic j.
   chronic acholuric j.
   congenital obliterative j.
   constitutional j.
   Crigler-Najjar j.
   epidemic j.
   familial acholuric j.
   hemolytic j.
   hemorrhagic j.
   hepatocanalicular j.
   hepatocellular j.
   hepatogenic j.
   hepatogenous j.
   homologous serum j.
   human serum j.
   infectious j.
   infective j.
   latent j.
   leptospiral j.
   malignant j.
   mechanical j.

jaun·dice *(continued)*
   j. of the newborn
   nonhemolytic j.
   nonhemolytic j., congenital
   nonhemolytic j., congenital
    familial
   nonhemolytic j., familial
   nonobstructive j.
   nuclear j.
   obstructive j.
   parenchymatous j.
   physiologic j.
   picric acid j.
   regurgitation j.
   retention j.
   Schmorl's j.
   spirochetal j.
   syringe j.
   toxemic j.
   toxic j.
   transfusion j.
Ja·val's ophthalmometer
jaw
   bird-beak j.
   cleft j.
   crackling j.
   Hapsburg j.
   parrot j.
   phossy j.
   pipe j.
   upper j.
jaw·bone
jaw-limb
Ja·wor·ski's bodies
Ja·wor·ski's corpuscles
Ja·wor·ski's test
jaw-wink·ing
Jean·selme's nodules
jec·o·rize
Jec·to·fer
Jef·fer·son fracture
Jef·fer·so·nia
Jef·ron
je·ju·nal
je·ju·nec·to·my
je·ju·ni·tis
je·ju·no·ce·cos·to·my
je·ju·no·co·los·to·my

je·ju·no·gas·tric
je·ju·no·il·e·al
je·ju·no·il·e·itis
je·ju·no·il·e·os·to·my
je·ju·no·il·e·um
je·ju·no·je·ju·nos·to·my
je·ju·no·plas·ty
je·ju·nor·rha·phy
je·ju·nos·to·my
je·ju·not·o·my
je·ju·num
Jel·li·nek's sign
Jel·li·nek's symptom
jel·ly
    cardiac j.
    contraceptive j.
    cyclomethycaine sulfate j.
    electrode j.
    enamel j.
    glycerin j.
    lidocaine hydrochloride j.
    mineral j.
    petroleum j.
    pramoxine hydrochloride j.
    Wharton's j.
Jen·dras·sik's maneuver
Jen·ner, Edward
Jen·ner's stain
jen·ne·ri·an
jen·ner·iza·tion
Jen·sen's choroiditis
Jen·sen's classification
Jen·sen's disease
Jen·sen's sarcoma
Jen·sen's tumor
jerk
    Achilles j.
    ankle j.
    biceps j.
    crossed j.
    elbow j.
    epileptic j.
    finger j.
    jaw j.
    knee j.
    massive myoclonic j.
    nystagmoid j's
    pendular knee j.

jerk *(continued)*
    quadriceps j.
    supinator j.
    tendon j.
    triceps surae j.
Jerne, Niels Kaj
Jer·vell and Lange-Niel·sen
  syndrome
Jes·i·o·nek lamp
jes·sur
Jew·ett's bladder carcinoma
  classification
Jew·ett nail
jig·ger
Job's syndrome
Jo·bert's fossa
Jobst stockings
Joch·mann's test
jod·bas·e·dow
Joest's bodies
Jof·froy's reflex
Jof·froy's sign
Joh·ne's bacillus
Joh·ne's disease
joh·nin
John·son's test
John·son-Ste·vens disease
joint
    acromioclavicular j.
    amphidiarthrodial j.
    ankle j.
    arthrodial j.
    arycorniculate j.
    atlantoaxial j.
    atlanto-occipital j.
    ball-and-socket j.
    biaxial j.
    bicondylar j.
    bilocular j.
    bleeders' j.
    Budin's j.
    calcaneocuboid j.
    capitular j.
    carpal j's
    carpometacarpal j's
    cartilaginous j.
    cartilaginous j's
    Charcot's j.

[handwritten annotation: Johnson-DeMeester Score (GERD)]

joint *(continued)*
- Chopart's j.
- Clutton's j.
- coccygeal j.
- cochlear j.
- composite j.
- compound j.
- condylar j.
- condyloid j.
- costochondral j's
- costotransverse j.
- costovertebral j's
- cotyloid j.
- cricoarytenoid j.
- cricothyroid j.
- Cruveilhier's j.
- cubital j.
- cuboideonavicular j.
- cuneocuboid j.
- cuneometatarsal j.
- cuneonavicular j.
- diarthrodial j.
- dry j.
- elbow j.
- ellipsoidal j.
- enarthrodial j.
- facet j's
- false j.
- femoropatellar j.
- femorotibial j.
- fibrocartilaginous j.
- fibrous j's
- flail j.
- freely movable j.
- fringe j.
- ginglymoid j.
- glenohumeral j.
- gliding j.
- hemophilic j.
- hinge j.
- hip j.
- humeroradial j.
- humeroulnar j.
- immovable j.
- incudomalleolar j.
- incudostapedial j.
- inferior radioulnar j.
- inferior sternal j.

joint *(continued)*
- inferior tibiofibular j.
- interarticular j's
- intercarpal j's
- interchondral j's
- intercuneiform j's
- intermetacarpal j's
- interphalangeal j's
- irritable j.
- knee j.
- ligamentous j.
- Lisfranc's j.
- lumbosacral j.
- j's of Luschka
- mandibular j.
- manubriosternal j.
- mediocarpal j.
- metacarpophalangeal j's
- metatarsophalangeal j's
- midcarpal j.
- midtarsal j.
- mixed j.
- mortise j.
- movable j.
- multiaxial j.
- open j.
- peg-and-socket j.
- pisotriquetral j.
- pivot j.
- plane j.
- polyaxial j.
- radiocarpal j.
- rotary j.
- sacrococcygeal j.
- sacroiliac j.
- saddle j.
- scapuloclavicular j.
- sellar j.
- shoulder j.
- simple j.
- skin j.
- slip j.
- socket j. of tooth
- spheno-occipital j.
- spheroidal j.
- spiral j.
- sternoclavicular j.
- sternocostal j's

joint *(continued)*
    subtalar j.
    superior radioulnar j.
    superior sternal j.
    superior tibiofibular j.
    suture j.
    synarthrodial j's
    synovial j.
    talocalcaneonavicular j.
    talocrural j.
    talonavicular j.
    talotibiofibular j.
    tarsal j., transverse
    tarsometatarsal j's
    temporomandibular j.
    j's of thorax
    through j.
    tibiofibular j.
    trochoid j.
    uniaxial j.
    unilocular j.
    wrist j.
    xiphisternal j.
    zygapophysial j's
Jol·les' test
Jol·ly's bodies
Jol·ly's reaction
Jo·nas symptom
Jones' albumosuria
Jones criteria
Jones' cylinder
Jones' fracture
Jones' position
Jones' protein
Jon·nes·co's fold
Jon·nes·co's fossa
Jonn·son's maneuver
Jon·ston's arc
jo·sa·my·cin
Jo·seph clamp
Jo·seph's disease
Jo·seph knife
Jo·seph rhinoplasty
Jo·sephs-Di·a·mond-Black·fan
    syndrome
joule
ju·ga
ju·gal

ju·ga·le
ju·gate
Ju·glans
jug·lone
ju·go·max·il·lary
jug·u·lar
jug·u·la·tion
jug·u·lo·di·gas·tric
jug·u·lum
ju·gum *pl.* ju·ga
    juga alveolaria mandibulae
    juga alveolaria maxillae
    juga cerebralia ossium
        cranii
    j. sphenoidale
juice
    cancer j.
    cherry j.
    gastric j.
    intestinal j.
    pancreatic j.
    press j.
    raspberry j.
Jukes family
jump·ing
    j. the bite
jump·ing French·men of
    Maine
junc·tion
    adherent j.
    amelodentinal j.
    anorectal j.
    cardioesophageal j.
    cell j.
    cementodentinal j.
    cementoenamel j.
    cervicomedullary j.
    choledochoduodenal j.
    corneoscleral j.
    dentinocemental j.
    dentinoenamel j.
    dentogingival j.
    dermoepidermal j.
    esophagogastric j.
    fibromuscular j.
    gap j.
    gastroesophageal j.
    ileocecal j.

junc·tion *(continued)*
  intermediate j.
  intermembrane j.
  iridociliary j.
  lumbosacral j.
  manubriogladiolar j.
  mucocutaneous j.
  mucogingival j.
  myoneural j.
  myotendinal j.
  neuromuscular j.
  occluding j.
  osseous j's
  pentilaminar j.
  rectosigmoid j.
  root-cord j.
  sclerocorneal j.
  ST j.
  tendinous j's
  tight j.
  tympanostapedial j.
  ureteropelvic j.
  ureterovesical j.
junc·tion·al
junc·tu·ra *pl.* junc·tu·rae
  juncturae cartilagineae
  juncturae fibrosae
  j. lumbosacralis
  juncturae ossium
  j. sacrococcygea
  juncturae synoviales
  juncturae tendinum
  juncturae zygapophyseales

Jung, Carl Gustav
Jung's muscle
Jung·bluth's vasa propria
Jung·bluth's vessels
jun·gi·an
ju·ni·per
Ju·nip·er·us
Jun·ker apparatus
Jun·ker bottle
Jun·ker inhaler
Jür·gen·sen's sign
jur·is·pru·dence
  dental j.
  medical j.
juscul. — L. jusculum (soup or broth)
Jus·ter's reflex
jus·to ma·jor
jus·to mi·nor
ju·van·tia
ju·ve·nile
jux·ta-ar·tic·u·lar
jux·ta·cor·ti·cal
jux·ta·ep·i·phys·e·al
jux·ta·glo·mer·u·lar
jux·tal·lo·cor·tex
jux·tan·gi·na
jux·ta·pap·il·lary
jux·ta·po·si·tion
jux·ta·py·lor·ic
jux·ta·spi·nal
jux·ta·ves·i·cal

K — kelvin
  potassium (L. kalium)
K — equilibrium constant
K_a — acid dissociation constant

K_b — base dissociation constant
K_d — dissociation constant
K_{eq} — equilibrium constant
K_M — Michaelis constant

K_m — Michaelis constant
K_{sp} — solubility product
   constant
K_W — the ion product of water
k — kilo-
k — Boltzmann's constant
   rate constant
κ — kappa, one of the two
   types of immunoglobulin
   light chains
ka·bu·re
Ka·der's operation
Kaes' feltwork
Kaes' line
Kaes-Bekh·ter·ev layer
KAF — conglutinogen
   activating factor (factor I)
ka·fin·do
KAFO — knee-ankle-foot
   orthosis
Ka·fo·cin
Kahl·baum's catatonic stupor
Kahl·baum's syndrome
Kahl·baum-Wer·ni·cke
   syndrome
Kah·ler's disease
Kah·ler's law
kah·we·ol
Kai·ser·ling's fixative
Kai·ser·ling's method
Kai·ser·ling's solution
kai·ser·ling
Kai·ser·stuhl disease
kak·i·dro·sis
kak·ke
kak·o·dyl
kak·os·mia
kak·ot·ro·phy
ka·la-azar
    Mediterranean k.
ka·la·da·na
ka·la·fun·gin
ka·la·gua
ka·le·mia
ka·lig·e·nous
ka·lim·e·ter
ka·lio·pe·nia
ka·lio·pe·nic

Kal·i·scher's disease
ka·li·ure·sis
ka·li·uret·ic
kal·lak
kal·li·din
Kal·li·kak
kal·li·kre·in
   plasma k.
   tissue k.
kal·li·krei·no·gen
Kall·mann syndrome
Kal·mia
Kal·muk idiocy
kal·ure·sis
kal·uret·ic
kam·a·la
Kam·i·ner's reaction
Kam·mer·er-Bat·tle incision
kan·a·my·cin
   k. sulfate
Kan·a·vel's sign
Kan·dori's flock retina
kan·in·lo·ma
Kan·ner's syndrome
Kan·ter sign
Kan·tor's sign
Kan·trex
kan·y·em·ba
Ka·o·chlor
ka·od·ze·ra
ka·o·lin
ka·o·lin·o·sis
Ka·on
Kap·lan's test
Kap·lan-Mei·er method
Kap·lan-Mei·er survival curve
Ka·po·si's sarcoma
Ka·po·si's varicelliform
   eruption
Kap·pa·di·one
Kap·pe·ler's maneuver
ka·ra-kurt
ka·ra·ya
Kar·nof·sky rating scale
Kar·nof·sky status
Kar·nof·sky tumor grading
Kar·plus' sign
Karr's method

Kar·roo syndrome
Kar·ta·gen·er's syndrome
Kar·ta·gen·er's triad
kary·ap·sis
kary·en·chy·ma
karyo·chrome
karyo·chy·le·ma
kary·oc·la·sis
karyo·clas·tic
karyo·cyte
karyo·gam·ic
kary·og·a·my
karyo·gen·e·sis
kar·y·o·gen·ic
karyo·go·nad
karyo·ki·ne·sis
    asymmetrical k.
    hyperchromatic k.
    hypochromatic k.
karyo·ki·net·ic
kary·ok·la·sis
karyo·klas·tic
karyo·lo·bic
karyo·lo·bism
kary·ol·o·gy
karyo·lymph
kary·ol·y·sis
karyo·lyt·ic
karyo·mas·ti·gont
karyo·meg·a·ly
karyo·mere
kary·om·e·try
karyo·mi·cro·some
karyo·mi·to·sis
karyo·mi·tot·ic
karyo·mor·phism
kary·on
kary·on·ide
karyo·phage
karyo·plasm
karyo·plas·mic
karyo·plast
karyo·plas·tin
karyo·pyk·no·sis
karyo·pyk·not·ic
karyo·re·tic·u·lum
kary·or·rhec·tic
kary·or·rhex·is

karyo·some
karyo·sta·sis
karyo·the·ca
karyo·tin
karyo·type
karyo·typ·ic
karyo·zo·ic
Kas·a·bach-Mer·ritt syndrome
ka·sai
ka·sal
Kast syndrome
kat — katal
kata·chro·ma·sis
kata·did·y·mus
kat·al
kata·ther·mom·e·ter
Kat·a·ya·ma disease
Kat·a·ya·ma fever
Kat·a·ya·ma's test
kath·a·rom·e·ter
kath·iso·pho·bia
ka·tine
Ka·to's test
ka·tol·y·sis
kato·pho·ria
kato·tro·pia
Katz, Sir Bernard
Katz formula
kat·zen·jam·mer
ka·va
ka·va·ism
Ka·wa·sa·ki disease
Ka·wa·sa·ki syndrome
Kay Ciel
Kay·ex·a·late
Kay·ser's disease
Kay·ser-Flei·scher ring
Ka·zan·ji·an forceps
Ka·zan·ji·an operation
Kaz·nel·son's syndrome
Kb — kilobase (1000 base
    pairs)
kc — kilocycle
kcal — kilocalorie (Calorie)
kCi — kilocurie
kcps — kilocycles per second
KCT — kathodal (cathodal)
    closure tetanus

Kearns-Sayre syndrome
Keat·ing-Heart treatment
kebo·ceph·a·ly
ked
ke·da·ni
    McNaught k.
Keel·er's polygraph
Keen's operation
Keen's sign
Kef·lex
Kef·lin
Kef·zol
Keg·el exercises
Kehr's incision
Kehr's sign
Kehr·er's reflex
Kehr·er-Adie syndrome
Keith's bundle
Keith's node
Keith's low ionic diet
Keith-Flack node
Keith-Wag·en·er (K-W)
  classification (I-IV)
ke·lec·tome
Kel·ene
Kell blood antibody type
Kell blood group
Kel·ler arthroplasty
Kel·ler operation
Kel·ling's test
Kel·ly's operation
Kel·ly's sign
Kel·ly's speculum
ke·loid
    acne k.
    Addison's k.
    Alibert's k.
    k. of gums
ke·lo·so·mus
ke·lot·o·my
kelp
kel·vin
Kel·vin scale
Kem·a·drin
Kemp·ner diet
Ken·a·cort
Ken·a·log
Ken·dall, Edward Calvin

Ken·dall's method
Ken·dall's rank correlation
  coefficient
Ken·dall's tau
Ken·ne·dy bar
Ken·ne·dy classification
Ken·ne·dy's syndrome
Ken·ny's treatment
ke·no·tox·in
Kent's bundle
Kent-His bundle
ken·tro·ki·ne·sis
ken·tro·ki·net·ic
Ke·pone
Ker·an·del's sign
Ker·an·del's symptom
ker·a·phyl·lo·cele
ker·a·sin
ker·a·tal·gia
ker·a·tan sul·fate
ker·a·tan·sul·fa·tu·ria
ker·a·tec·ta·sia
ker·a·tec·to·my
ker·at·ic
  k. precipitates
ker·a·tin
    α-k.
    alpha k.
    false k.
    hard k.
    soft k.
ker·a·tin·ase
ker·a·tin·iza·tion
ker·a·tin·ize
ke·rat·i·no·cyte
ker·a·tin·oid
ke·rat·i·no·some
ke·rat·i·nous
ker·a·tit·ic
ker·a·ti·tis
    acanthamoeba k.
    acne rosacea k.
    actinic k.
    aerosol k.
    alphabet k.
    anaphylactic k.
    annular k.
    k. arborescens

ker·a·ti·tis *(continued)*
   artificial silk k.
   aspergillus k.
   band k.
   k. bandelette
   band-shaped k.
   k. bullosa
   catarrhal ulcerative k.
   deep k.
   deep pustular k.
   dendriform k.
   dendritic k.
   desiccation k.
   Dimmer's k.
   disciform k.
   k. disciformis
   epithelial diffuse k.
   epithelial punctate k.
   exfoliative k.
   exposure k.
   fascicular k.
   k. filamentosa
   furrow k.
   herpetic k.
   hypopyon k.
   infectious bovine k.
   interstitial k.
   lagophthalmic k.
   lattice k.
   marginal k.
   meta-herpetic k.
   microbial k.
   mycotic k.
   necrogranulomatous k.
   neuroparalytic k.
   neurotrophic k.
   k. nummularis
   parenchymatous k.
   k. petrificans
   phlyctenular k.
   k. profunda
   k. punctata
   k. punctata leprosa
   k. punctata profunda
   k. punctata subepithelialis
   punctate k.
   punctate k., deep
   punctate k., superficial

ker·a·ti·tis *(continued)*
   purulent k.
   k. pustuliformis profunda
   k. ramificata superficialis
   reaper's k.
   reticular k.
   ribbon-like k.
   rosacea k.
   sclerosing k.
   scrofulus k.
   secondary k.
   senile guttate k.
   serpiginous k.
   k. sicca
   striate k.
   superficial punctate k.
   suppurative k.
   trachomatous k.
   trophic k.
   ulcerative k.
   vascular k.
   vesicular k.
   xerotic k.
   zonular k.
ker·a·to·ac·an·tho·ma
ker·a·to·an·gi·o·ma
ker·a·to·cele
ker·a·to·cen·te·sis
ker·a·to·con·junc·ti·vi·tis
   epidemic k.
   flash k.
   phlyctenular k.
   shipyard k.
   k. sicca
   superior limbic k.
   vernal k.
   viral k.
ker·a·to·co·nus
ker·a·to·cyst
ker·a·to·cyte
ker·a·to·der·ma
   k. blennorrhagicum
   k. climactericum
   k. palmare et plantare
   palmoplantar k.
   palmoplantar k., diffuse
   plantar k.
   punctate k.

ker·a·to·der·ma *(continued)*
  symmetric k.
ker·a·to·der·ma·to·cele
ker·a·to·der·mia
  k. plantaris sulcata
ker·a·to·ec·ta·sia
ker·a·to·gen·e·sis
ker·a·to·ge·net·ic
ker·a·tog·e·nous
ker·a·to·glo·bus
ker·a·to·hel·co·sis
ker·a·to·he·mia
ker·a·to·hy·a·lin
ker·a·to·hy·a·line
ker·a·toid
ker·a·toi·di·tis
ker·a·to·ir·i·do·cyc·li·tis
ker·a·to·i·rid·o·scope
ker·a·to·i·ri·tis
  hypopyon k.
ker·a·to·lep·tyn·sis
ker·a·to·leu·ko·ma
ker·a·tol·y·sis
  pitted k.
  k. plantare sulcatum
ker·a·to·lyt·ic
ker·a·to·ma *pl.* ker·a·to·mas,
  ker·a·to·ma·ta
  k. hereditarium mutilans
  k. plantare sulcatum
  k. senile
ker·a·to·ma·la·cia
ker·a·to·ma·ta
ker·a·tome
ker·a·tom·e·ter
ker·a·to·met·ric
ker·a·tom·e·try
ker·a·to·mi·leu·sis
ker·a·to·my·co·sis
  k. linguae
ker·a·ton·o·sus
ker·a·to·nyx·is
ker·a·top·a·thy
  band k.
  band-shaped k.
  bullous k.
  climatic k.
  exposure k.

ker·a·top·a·thy *(continued)*
  filamentary k.
  Labrador k.
  lipid k.
  striate k.
  vesicular k.
ker·a·to·pha·kia
ker·a·to·plas·ty
  autogenous k.
  lamellar k.
  optic k.
  penetrating k.
  refractive k.
  tectonic k.
ker·a·to·pre·cip·i·tates
ker·a·to·pro·tein
ker·a·to·rhex·is, ker·a·tor·
  rhex·is
ker·a·to·scle·ri·tis
ker·a·to·scope
ker·a·tos·co·py
ker·a·to·sis *pl.* ker·a·to·ses
  actinic k.
  arsenic k.
  arsenical k.
  aural k.
  k. blennorrhagica
  k. follicularis
  k. follicularis contagiosa
  k. follicularis decalvans
  inverted follicular k.
  k. labialis
  k. linguae
  k. nigricans
  k. obliterans
  k. obturans
  k. palmaris et plantaris
  k. pharyngea
  k. pilaris
  k. pilaris atrophicans
  k. pilaris rubra
  k. punctata
  roentgen k.
  seborrheic k.
  k. seborrheica
  senile k.
  k. senilis
  solar k.

ker·a·to·sis *(continued)*
 stucco k.
 tar k.
 k. universalis congenita
 wax k.
ker·a·to·sul·fate
ker·a·to·sul·fa·tu·ria
ker·a·tot·ic
ker·a·to·tome
ker·a·tot·o·my
 delimiting k.
 radial k.
ker·a·to·to·rus
Kerck·ring's (Kerk·ring's)
 center
Kerck·ring's (Kerk·ring's) folds
Kerck·ring's (Kerk·ring's)
 ossicle
ke·rec·ta·sis
ke·rec·to·my
Ker·ga·ra·dec's sign
ke·ri·on
ker·ma
Kern
ker·nic·ter·us
Ker·nig's sign
ker·oid
ker·o·sene
Kerr's sign
ker·ril
Ke·shan disease
Kes·ling appliance
Kes·ling spring
Kes·ten·bach-An·der·son
 procedure
Ket·a·ject
ke·tal
Ket·a·lar
keta·mine hy·dro·chlo·ride
Ket·a·set
ke·ta·zo·cine
ke·ta·zo·lam
ke·tene
ke·thox·al
ke·ti·mine
ke·tip·ra·mine fum·a·rate
ke·to ac·id
ke·to ac·id de·car·box·y·lase

ke·to ac·id de·car·box·y·lase
 deficiency
ke·to·ac·i·de·mia
 branched-chain k.
ke·to·ac·i·do·sis
 diabetic k.
ke·to·ac·id·uria
 branched-chain k.
β-ke·to·ac·yl-ACP re·duc·tase
 [beta-]
3-ke·to·ac·yl-CoA thi·o·lase
ke·to-al·de·hyde
ke·to·a·mi·no·ac·i·de·mia
β-ke·to·bu·tyr·ic acid
ke·to·con·a·zole
ke·to·de·oxy·oc·to·nate
Ke·to-Di·a·stix
ke·to·gen·e·sis
ke·to·ge·net·ic
ke·to·gen·ic
2-ke·to·glu·co·nate
α-ke·to·glu·ta·rate
α-ke·to·glu·ta·rate de·hy·
 dro·gen·ase
α-ke·to·glu·ta·rate gly·ox·y·
 late car·bo·li·gase
α-ke·to·glu·tar·ic acid
ke·to·hep·tose
ke·to·hexo·ki·nase
ke·to·hex·ose
ke·to·hy·droxy·es·trin
α-ke·to·iso·val·er·ate de·hy·
 dro·gen·ase
ke·tol
ke·tol-isom·er·ase
ke·tol·y·sis
ke·to·lyt·ic
ke·tone
 dimethyl k.
ke·to·ne·mia
ke·ton·ic
ke·to·ni·za·tion
ke·ton·uria
ke·to·pla·sia
ke·to·plas·tic
ke·to·pro·fen
β-ke·to-re·duc·tase
ke·tose

ke·to·side
ke·to·sis
ke·to·ste·roid
ke·tos·uria
ke·to-tet·ra·hy·dro·phen·an·
   threne
ke·to·tet·rose
3-ke·to·thi·o·lase
β-ke·to·thi·o·lase
ke·tot·ic
ke·to·ti·fen
ke·to·trans·fer·ase
ke·to·urine
ke·tox·ime
keV — kilo electron volt
kev — kilo electron volt
key
   determinative k.
   torquing k.
key·note
Key-Ret·zi·us connective tissue
   sheath
Key-Ret·zi·us foramen
keyway
kg — kilogram
khel·lin
Kho·ra·na, Har Gobind
kHz — kilohertz
ki·bis·i·tome
kick
   atrial k.
   k. counts
Kidd blood antibody type
Kidd blood group
kid·ney
   abdominal k.
   amyloid k.
   arteriosclerotic k.
   artificial k.
   atrophic k.
   cake k.
   cicatricial k.
   clump k.
   congenital double k.
   congested k.
   contracted k.
   crush k.
   cyanotic k.
   cystic k.

kid·ney (continued)
   definite k.
   definitive k.
   disk k.
   doughnut k.
   dystopic k.
   fatty k.
   flea-bitten k.
   floating k.
   Formad's k.
   fused k.
   Goldblatt k.
   gouty k.
   granular k.
   head k.
   hind k.
   horseshoe k.
   hypermobile k.
   infarcted k.
   lardaceous k.
   large red k.
   large white k.
   lumbar k.
   lump k.
   medullary sponge k.
   middle k.
   monopyramidal k.
   mortar k.
   movable k.
   multilobar k.
   mural k.
   myelin k.
   myeloma k.
   palpable k.
   pelvic k.
   polycystic k.
   primitive k.
   primordial k.
   putty k.
   Rokitansky's k.
   Rose-Bradford k.
   sacciform k.
   sclerotic k.
   sigmoid k.
   single k.
   solitary k.
   sponge k.
   sulfa k.

kid·ney *(continued)*
    supernumerary k.
    thoracic k.
    unilateral fused k.
    unilobar k.
    wandering k.
    waxy k.
Kiel classification
Kiel·land's (Kjel·land's)
    forceps
Kien·böck disease
Kien·böck dislocation
Kien·böck phenomenon
Kien·böck unit
Kien·böck-Ad·am·son points
Kier·nan's spaces
kie·sel·guhr
Kies·sel·bach's area
Kies·sel·bach's space
ki·es·te·in
kil
Kil·i·an's line
kil·leen
Kil·li·an's operation
Kil·li·an's test
Kil·li·an-Freer operation
kilo·base
kilo·bec·que·rel
kilo·cal·o·rie
kilo·cu·rie
kilo·cy·cle
kilo·gram
kilo·gram-cal·o·rie
kilo·gram·force
kilo·hertz
Ki·loh-Nev·in syndrome
kil·ohm
ki·lom·e·ter
kilo·pas·cal
kilo·pond
kilo·unit
kilo·volt
Kim·ber·ley horse disease
Kim·mel·stiel-Wil·son
    syndrome
Kimp·ton-Brown tube
kin·an·es·the·sia
ki·nase

kin·dling
kine·mat·ics
ki·ne·mia
ki·ne·mic
kine·plas·tics
kine·plas·ty
kine·sal·gia
kine·scope
ki·ne·sia
    paradoxical k.
ki·ne·si·al·gia
ki·ne·si·at·rics
ki·ne·sics
ki·ne·si-es·the·si·om·e·ter
ki·ne·si·gen·ic
kine·sim·e·ter
ki·ne·si·od·ic
ki·ne·si·ol·o·gy
ki·ne·si·om·e·ter
ki·ne·sio·neu·ro·sis
ki·ne·sio·ther·a·py
ki·ne·sis
ki·ne·si·ther·a·py
kine·sod·ic
kin·es·the·sia
kin·es·the·si·om·e·ter
kin·es·the·sis
kin·es·thet·ic
ki·ne·tia
ki·net·ic
ki·net·i·cist
ki·net·ics
    chemical k.
    first-order k.
    Michaelis k.
    pre–steady-state k.
ki·ne·tin
kine·tism
ki·ne·to·car·dio·gram
ki·ne·to·car·di·og·ra·phy
ki·ne·to·chore
ki·ne·to·des·ma *pl.* ki·ne·to·
    des·ma·ta
ki·ne·to·des·ma·ta
ki·ne·to·des·mos
ki·ne·to·frag·ment
Ki·ne·to·frag·min·o·phor·ea
ki·ne·to·gen·ic

ki·ne·to·graph·ic
ki·ne·tog·ra·phy
ki·ne·to·nu·cle·us
ki·ne·to·plasm
ki·ne·to·plast
ki·ne·to·plas·tid
Ki·ne·to·plas·ti·da
ki·ne·to·scope
ki·ne·tos·co·py
ki·ne·to·sis *pl.* ki·ne·to·ses
ki·ne·to·some
ki·ne·to·ther·a·py
ki·ne·ty *pl.* ki·ne·tia, ki·ne·
    ties
King unit
King-Arm·strong unit
king·dom
King·el·la
    K. denitrificans
    K. indologenes
    K. kingae
Kings·ley appliance
Kings·ley plate
Kings·ley splint
kin·ic acid
ki·nin
    C2 k.
    venom k.
    wasp k.
ki·nin·ase
    k. I
    k. II
ki·nin·o·gen
    high molecular weight k.
    low molecular weight k.
ki·nino·gen·ase
Kin·nier Wil·son disease
ki·no
ki·no·cen·trum
ki·no·cil·ia
ki·no·cil·i·um *pl.* ki·no·cil·ia
ki·no·hapt
ki·nol·o·gy
kino·mere
ki·no·mom·e·ter
kino·plasm
ki·no·sphere
ki·no·tox·in

kin·o·vin
kin·ship
Kin·youn stain
ki·o·tome
ki·ot·o·my
Kirch·ner's diverticulum
Kirk's amputation
kir·ro·my·cin
Kirsch·ner wire
Kir·stein's method
Kisch's reflex
KISS (Kidney Internal
    Splint/Stent) catheter
kit·a·sa·my·cin
Ki·ta·sa·to's filter
kit·ing
ki·tol
Kit·tel's treatment
kj — knee jerk
Kjel·dahl's method
Kjel·dahl's test
Kjel·land forceps
kl — kiloliter
Klapp's creeping treatment
Klau·der syndrome
Klebs-Löf·fler bacillus
Kleb·si·el·la
    K. friedländeri
    K. oxytoca
    K. ozaenae
    K. planticola
    K. pneumoniae
    K. pneumoniae ozaenae
    K. pneumoniae
        rhinoscleromatis
    K. rhinoscleromatis
    K. terrigena
Kleb·si·el·leae
klee·blatt·schä·del
Klei·hau·er test
Kleine-Lev·in syndrome
Kleist's classification
Kleist's phenomenon
Kleist's sign
Klemm's sign
Klemm's tetanus
Klem·per·er's disease
Klem·per·er's tuberculin

klep·to·lag·nia
klep·to·ma·nia
klep·to·ma·ni·ac
Klieg eye
Klig·ler's agar
Klim·ow's test
Kline's test
Kline·fel·ter's syndrome
Klip·pel's disease
Klip·pel-Feil sign
Klip·pel-Feil syndrome
Klippel-Trénaunay-Weber
    syndrome
klis·e·om·e·ter
klis·ma·phil·ia
Klo·nop·in
Klos·si·el·la
Kluge sign
Klump·ke's paralysis
Klump·ke-Dej·er·ine paralysis
Klump·ke-Dej·er·ine
    syndrome
Klü·ver-Bu·cy syndrome
Kluy·vera
Km — Michaelis constant
km — kilometer
Knapp's forceps
Knapp's operation
Knapp's streaks
Knapp's striae
Knapp's test
Knaus rule
knead·ing
knee
    k. of aquaeductus fallopii
    back k.
    beat k.
    Brodie's k.
    conventional single axis k.
    football k.
    housemaid's k.
    hydraulic k.
    k. of internal capsule
    knock k.
    little k. of fascial canal
    locked k.
    rugby k.
    septic k.

knee *(continued)*
    trick k.
    von Willebrandt's k.
knee·cap
kneipp·ism
Knies' sign
knife
    Ballenger swivel k.
    bladebreaker k.
    Blair k.
    buck k.
    button k.
    cataract k.
    cautery k.
    electric k.
    gold k.
    Goldman-Fox k.
    Graefe's k.
    Humby k.
    Joseph k.
    Kirkland k.
    lenticular k.
    Liston's k.
    meniscectomy k.
    Merrifield's k.
    Ramsbotham's sickle k.
    Thiersch k.
Knight brace
Knight-Tay·lor brace
knis·mo·gen·ic
knit·ting
knob
    aortic k.
    basal k.
    embryonic k.
    surfers' k's
    synaptic k's
knock
    pericardial k.
knock-knee
knot
    clove-hitch k.
    double k.
    enamel k.
    false k.
    friction k.
    granny k.
    half-hitch k.

knot *(continued)*
   Hensen's k.
   primitive k.
   protochordal k.
   reef k.
   square k.
   stay k.
   surfers' k's
   surgeons' k.
   surgical k.
   syncytial k's
   true k.
knuck·le
   aortic k.
   cervical aortic k.
knuck·ling
Ko·belt's tubes
Ko·belt's tubules
Ko·ber's test
Ko·bert's test
Köb·ner's effect
Köb·ner's phenomenon
KOC — kathodal (cathodal)
   opening contraction
Koch, Robert
Koch's bacillus
Koch's law
Koch's lymph
Koch's node
Koch's phenomenon
Koch's postulate
Koch's reaction
Koch reservoir
Koch's tuberculin
Koch-Weeks bacillus
Koch·er, Emil Theodor
Koch·er's forceps
Koch·er's incision
Koch·er's maneuver
Koch·er's operation
Koch·er's reflex
Koch·er's sign
Koch·er-De·bré-Se·me·laigne
   syndrome
koch·er·iza·tion
Kocks operation
Koe·ber·lé's forceps
Koeb·ner's phenomenon

Koe·necke's reaction
Koe·necke's test
Koer·ber-Sa·lus-Elsch·nig
   syndrome
Koe·ster's nodule
Ko·goj's pustule
ko·ha
Köh·ler, Alban
Köh·ler's bone disease
Koh·ler-Pel·le·gri·ni-Stie·da
   disease
Kohl·rausch's folds
Kohl·rausch's valves
Kohn's pores
Kohn·stamm's phenomenon
koi·lo·cy·to·sis
koi·lo·cy·tot·ic
koi·lo·nych·ia
koi·lor·rhach·ic
koi·lo·ster·nia
koi·no·nia
ko·jic acid
kok·ti·gen
Ko·lan·tyl
Köl·li·ker's column
Köl·li·ker's granule
Köl·li·ker's membrane
Köl·li·ker's nucleus
Koll·mann's dilator
Kol·mer test
Kol·mo·go·rov-Smir·nov test
ko·ly·pep·tic
Kon·a·ki·on
Kon·do·le·on's operation
Kö·nig's rods
Kö·nig's syndrome
ko·nim·e·ter
ko·nio·cor·tex
ko·ni·ol·o·gy
ko·nom·e·ter
Kon·syl
ko·phe·mia
ko·pi·opia
Kop·lik's sign
Kop·lik's spots
Kopp's asthma
kop·ro·ste·rin
Ko·rán·yi's auscultation

Ko·rán·yi's percussion
Ko·rán·yi's sign
Ko·rán·yi's treatment
Ko·rán·yi-Groc·co triangle
Korff's fibers
Korn·berg, Arthur
ko·ro
ko·ro·ni·on *pl.* ko·ro·nia
ko·ros·co·py
Ko·rot·koff's method
Ko·rot·koff's sounds
Ko·rot·koff's test
Kor·sa·koff's (Kor·sa·kov's) syndrome
Kör·te-Bal·lance operation
ko·sam
Ko·shev·ni·koff's (Ko·schew·ni·kow's, Ko·zhev·ni·kov's) disease
Ko·shev·ni·koff's (Ko·schew·ni·kow's, Ko·zhev·ni·kov's) epilepsy
Kos·sel, Albrecht
Kos·sel's test
Kost·mann's syndrome
Ko·val·ev·sky's canal
Ko·war·sky's test
Koy·ter's muscle
KP — keratitic precipitates keratitis punctata
K-Phos
Krabbe's disease
Krabbe's leukodystrophy
Krae·pe·lin, Emil
krait
Kra·me·ria
Kras·ke's operation
kra·tom
kra·tom·e·ter
krauo·ma·nia
krau·ro·sis
   k. penis
   k. vulvae
Krause's bulbs
Krause's corpuscle
Krause's ligament
Krause's line
Krause's membrane

Krause's operation
Krause's suture
Krause's valve
Krause-Wolfe graft
kre·a·tin
kre·bi·o·zen
Krebs, Sir Hans Adolf
Krebs cycle
Krebs' leukocyte index
kreo·tox·i·con
kreo·tox·in
kreo·tox·ism
kreso·fuch·sin
Kretsch·mann's space
Kretsch·mer types
Kretz's granules
Krey·sig's sign
krimp·siek·te
Kris·hab·er's disease
Kris·tel·ler's expression
Kris·tel·ler's method
Kris·tel·ler's technique
Krogh, Schack August Steenberg
Kro·may·er's burn
Kro·may·er's lamp
Krom·pech·er's carcinoma
Krom·pech·er's tumor
krom·skop
Kro·neck·er's center
Kro·neck·er's puncture
Krö·nig's area
Krö·nig's field
Krö·nig's isthmus
Krön·lein's hernia
Krön·lein's operation
Kru·ken·berg's arm
Kru·ken·berg's hand
Kru·ken·berg's spindle
Kru·ken·berg's tumor
Kru·ken·berg's veins
Krum·wiede agar
Kruse's brush
kry·os·co·py
kryp·ton
   k. 85
KSC — kathodal (cathodal) closing contraction

KST — kathodal (cathodal) closing tetanus
KUB — kidney, ureter, and bladder \
ku·bis·a·ga·ri, ku·bis·ga·ri
Kufs' disease
Ku·gel·berg-Wel·an·der disease
Kuhl·mann's test
Kuhn's mask
Kuhn's tube
Küh·ne's methylene blue
Küh·ne's muscular phenomenon
Küh·ne's spindle
Küh·ne's terminal plates
Kuhnt's illusion
Kuhnt-Ju·ni·us degeneration
Kuhnt-Ju·ni·us disease
Kuhnt-Szy·ma·now·ski operation
Kuhnt-Szy·ma·now·ski procedure
Kul·chit·sky's cells
Ku·len·kampff's anesthesia
Külz's cast
Külz's cylinder
Külz's test
Küm·mell's disease
Küm·mell's spondylitis
Küm·mell-Ver·neuil disease
Kun·kel's syndrome
Künt·scher nail
Kupf·fer's cells
ku·pra·mite
Ku·pres·soff's center
Ku·rie plot
Kur·loff's (Kur·lov's) bodies
Kur·thia
kur·to·sis
ku·ru
Küss' experiment
Kuss·maul's aphasia
Kuss·maul's paralysis
Kuss·maul's pulse
Kuss·maul's respiration
Kuss·maul's sign
Kuss·maul-Kien respiration
Kuss·maul-Lan·dry paralysis

Kuss·maul-Mai·er disease
Küst·ner's law
Küst·ner's sign
Ku·trol
kut·taro·some
kV — kilovolt
Kveim antigen
Kveim reaction
Kveim test
KVO — keep vein open
kVp — kilovolts peak
kW — kilowatt
kwash·i·or·kor
    marasmic k.
kwa·ski
kW-hr — kilowatt-hour
Ky·a·na·sur For·est disease
ky·es·te·in
kyl·lo·sis
ky·ma·tism
ky·mo·cy·clo·graph
ky·mo·gram
ky·mo·graph
    x-ray k.
ky·mog·ra·phy
    roentgen k.
Ky·nex
ky·no·ceph·a·lus
kyn·uren·ic acid
kyn·ure·nin
kyn·uren·i·nase
kyn·ure·nine
kyn·ure·nine 3-hy·drox·y·lase
kyn·ure·nine 3-mono·oxy·gen·ase
ky·phec·to·my
ky·pho·ra·chi·tis
ky·phos
ky·pho·sco·li·o·sis
ky·pho·sis
    angular k.
    k. dorsalis juvenilis
    juvenile k.
    post-traumatic k.
    Scheuermann's k.
ky·phot·ic
Kyrle's disease
kyr·tor·rhach·ic

L — lambert
   left
   light chain (of
     immunoglobulins)
   liter
   lumbar vertebra (L1–L5)
   lung
L — luminance
   self-inductance
L_0 — limes nul
$L+$ — limes tod
l — liter
l. — L. ligamentum (ligament)
l — length
l- — levorotatory (enantiomer)
L0 — limes nul
L & A — light and
   accommodation (reaction of
   pupils)
La·bar·raque's solution
Lab·bé's triangle
Lab·bé's vein
la·bel
   radioactive l.
la·bel·ing
   affinity l.
   ferritin l.
   isotope l.
   peroxidase l.
   pulse l.
   spin l.
la·bet·a·lol
la·bia
   inert l.
   l. majora
   l. minora
la·bi·al
la·bi·a·lism
la·bi·al·ly
la·bi·cho·rea
Lab·i·dog·na·tha
la·bile
   heat l.
la·bil·i·ty
la·bio·al·ve·o·lar
la·bio·ax·io·gin·gi·val

la·bio·cer·vi·cal
la·bio·cho·rea
la·bio·cli·na·tion
la·bio·den·tal
la·bio·gin·gi·val
la·bio·glos·so·la·ryn·ge·al
la·bio·glos·so·pha·ryn·ge·al
la·bio·graph
la·bio·in·ci·sal
la·bio·lin·gual
la·bi·o·log·ic
la·bi·ol·o·gy
la·bio·men·tal
la·bio·my·co·sis
la·bio·na·sal
la·bio·pal·a·tine
la·bio·place·ment
la·bio·plas·ty
la·bio·te·nac·u·lum
la·bio·ver·sion
la·bi·um *pl.* la·bia
   l. anterius
   l. cerebri
   l. externum cristae iliacae
   l. inferius oris
   l. majus pudendi
   l. mandibulare
   l. maxillare
   l. minus pudendi
   labia oris
   l. posterius
   l. superius oris
   l. urethrae
   l. vocale
la·bor
   active l.
   arrested l.
   artificial l.
   atonic l.
   complicated l.
   delayed l.
   dry l.
   false l.
   immature l.
   induced l.
   instrumental l.

la·bor *(continued)*
    mimetic l.
    missed l.
    multiple l.
    obstructed l.
    postmature l.
    postponed l.
    precipitate l.
    premature l.
    premature l., habitual
    prolonged l.
    protracted l.
    spontaneous l.
    spurious l.
    stages of l.
    trial of l.
lab·o·ra·to·ri·an
lab·o·ra·to·ry
    clinical l.
La·borde's forceps
La·borde's method
La·borde's sign
La·borde's test
la·bra
la·bra·le
    l. inferius
    l. superius
lab·ro·cyte
la·brum *pl.* la·bra
    l. acetabulare
    l. glenoidale
lab·y·rinth
    acoustic l.
    bony l.
    cochlear l.
    cortical l.
    endolymphatic l.
    l. of ethmoid
    ethmoidal l.
    Ludwig's l's
    membranous l.
    nonacoustic l.
    olfactory l.
    osseous l.
    perilymphatic l.
    renal l.
    Santorini's l.
    statokinetic l.

lab·y·rinth *(continued)*
    vestibular l.
lab·y·rin·thec·to·my
    membranous l.
    transtympanic l.
    ultrasonic l.
lab·y·rin·thi
lab·y·rin·thine
lab·y·rin·thi·tis
    circumscribed l.
    serous l.
    suppurative l.
    traumatic l.
lab·y·rin·thot·o·my
lab·y·rin·thus *pl.* lab·y·rin·
   thi
    l. cochlearis
    l. ethmoidalis
    l. membranaceus
    l. osseus
    l. vestibularis
lac *pl.* lac·ta
    l. femininum
    l. vaccinum
Lac·ci·fer
lac·er·a·ble
lac·er·ate
lac·er·at·ed
lac·er·a·tion
    dicing l.
    first-degree obstetric l.
la·cer·tus
    l. cordis
    l. fibrosus musculi bicipitis
    brachii
    l. medius Weitbrechtii
    l. medius Wrisbergii
    l. musculi recti lateralis
    bulbi
Lach·e·sis
Lach·man test
Lach·no·spi·ra
lac·ri·ma *pl.* lac·ri·mae
lac·ri·mal
lac·ri·ma·tion
lac·ri·ma·tor
lac·ri·ma·to·ry
lac·ri·mo·na·sal

lac·ri·mo·tome
lac·ri·mot·o·my
lac·ta
lac·tac·i·de·mia
lac·tac·i·din
lac·ta·cid·o·gen
lac·tac·id·uria
lac·ta·gogue
lac·tal·bu·min
lac·tam
β-lac·ta·mase
lac·tam·ide
Lac·ta·ri·us
lac·tase
lac·tate
 ferrous l.
 lactic acid l.
 l. racemase
 Ringer's l.
L-lac·tate de·hy·dro·gen·ase
 (LDH)
lac·ta·tion
lac·ta·tion·al
lac·te·al
 central l.
lac·tein
lac·te·nin
lac·tes·cence
lac·tes·cent
lac·tic
lac·tic acid
lac·tic·ac·i·de·mia
lac·ti·ce·mia
lac·tif·er·ous
lac·ti·fuge
lac·tig·e·nous
lac·tig·er·ous
lac·tim
lac·tin
lac·ti·nat·ed
lac·tiv·o·rous
Lac·to·bac·il·la·ceae
Lac·to·bac·il·leae
lac·to·bac·il·li
Lac·to·bac·il·lus
 L. acidophilus
 L. bifidus
 L. bulgaricus

Lac·to·bac·il·lus (continued)
 L. salivarius
lac·to·bac·il·lus *pl.* lac·to·ba·
 cil·li
 l. of Boas-Oppler
Lac·to·bac·te·ri·a·ceae
lac·to·bu·ty·rom·e·ter
lac·to·cele
lac·to·crit
lac·to·den·sim·e·ter
lac·to·far·i·na·ceous
lac·to·fer·rin
lac·to·fla·vin
lac·to·gen
 human placental l.
lac·to·gen·e·sis
lac·to·gen·ic
lac·to·glob·u·lin
lac·to·lin
lac·tom·e·ter
lac·tone
 homoserine l.
lac·to·per·ox·i·dase
lac·to-ovo·ve·ge·ta·ri·an
lac·to·phos·phate
lac·to·pre·cip·i·tin
lac·to·pro·tein
lac·tor·rhea
lac·to·sa·zone
lac·to·scope
lac·tose
 beta l.
lac·to·se·rum
lac·to·side
 ceramide l.
lac·to·si·do·sis *pl.* lac·to·si·
 do·ses
 ceramide l.
lac·to·sum
lac·tos·uria
lac·to·syl cer·am·i·dase
lac·to·syl·cer·a·mide
lac·to·syl·cer·a·mide ga·lac·
 to·syl hy·dro·lase
lac·to·syl·cer·a·mi·do·sis
lac·to·tox·in
lac·to·trope
lac·to·tro·pin

lac·to·ve·ge·ta·ri·an
lac·to·yl·glu·ta·thi·one ly·ase
lac·tu·lose
lac·tu·lum un·guis
la·cu·na *pl.* la·cu·nae
   absorption l.
   air l.
   Blessig's l.
   blood l.
   bone l.
   cartilage l.
   cerebral lacunae
   great l. of urethra
   Howship l.
   intervillous l.
   lacunae laterales
   lateral lacunae
   l. magna
   lacunae of Morgagni
   lacunae Morgagnii
     urethrae muliebris
   l. of muscles
   l. musculorum
   osseous l.
   parasinoidal l's
   l. pharyngis
   resorption l.
   trophoblastic l.
   lacunae of urethra
   urethral lacunae
   urethral lacunae of
     Morgagni
   lacunae urethrales
   l. vasorum
   l. of vessels
la·cu·nar
la·cu·nu·la
la·cu·nule
la·cus *pl.* la·cus
   l. lacrimalis
LAD — left anterior
  descending (coronary artery)
Ladd-Frank·lin theory
La·den·dorff's test
La·din's sign
Lae·laps
Laën·nec's catarrh
Laën·nec's cirrhosis

Laën·nec's disease
Laën·nec's pearl
Laën·nec's sign
La·e·trile
lae·ve
LAF — lymphocyte activating
  factor
La·fo·ra's bodies
La·fo·ra's disease
La·fo·ra's sign
Lag. — L. lagena (a flask)
lag
   anaphase l.
   eyelid l.
   globe l.
   lid l.
   nitrogen l.
   phenomic l.
   phenotypic l.
la·ge·na
la·gen·i·form
lag·no·sis
Lag·o·chi·las·ca·ris mi·nor
lag·oph·thal·mos
La·grange's operation
lai·ose
lake
   capillary l.
   lacrimal l.
   marginal l's
   subchorial l.
   venous l.
Laki-Lor·and factor
la·li·a·try
lal·la·tion
Lal·le·mand's bodies
Lal·le·mand-Trous·seau bodies
lal·og·no·sis
lalo·pa·thol·o·gy
la·lop·a·thy
lalo·pho·bia
lalo·ple·gia
lal·or·rhea
La·lou·ette's pyramid
La·marck's theory
La·maze method
lamb·da
lamb·da·cism

lamb·da·cis·mus
lamb·doid
lam·bert
Lam·bert's cosine law
Lam·bert-Ea·ton syndrome
Lam·blia
    L. intestinalis
lam·bli·a·sis
lam·bli·o·sis
lame
lame fo·li·a·cée
lam·el
la·mel·la *pl.* la·mel·lae
    annulate lamellae
    articular l.
    basic l.
    circumferential l.
    concentric l.
    cornoid l.
    elastic l.
    enamel lamellae
    endosteal l.
    ground l.
    haversian l.
    intermediate l.
    interstitial l.
    osseous l.
    periosteal l.
    peripheral l.
    photoreceptor l.
    posterior border l. of Fuchs
    triangular l.
    vitreous l.
la·mel·lae
la·mel·lar
la·mel·li·form
la·mel·li·po·di·um *pl.* la·mel·li·po·dia
lamin
lam·i·na *pl.* lam·i·nae
    l. affixa
    alar l.
    l. alaris
    laminae albae cerebelli
    anterior limiting l.
    l. anterior vaginae musculi
        recti abdominis
    l. arcus vertebrae

lam·i·na *(continued)*
    basal l.
    l. basalis
    basement l.
    bony spiral l.
    buccal l.
    buccogingival l.
    Bowman's l.
    l. cartilaginis
    l. choriocapillaris
    l. chorioidea
    l. choroidocapillaris
    cribriform l.
    l. cribrosa
    l. densa
    dental l.
    l. dentalis
    l. dentata
    dentogingival l.
    l. dura
    elastic l., external
    elastic l., internal
    l. elastica anterior
        [Bowmani]
    l. elastica posterior
        [Demoursi, Descemeti]
    episcleral l.
    l. episcleralis
    epithelial l.
    l. epithelialis
    l. externa cranii
    l. fibrocartilaginea
        interpubica
    l. fibroreticularis
    fibrous nuclear l.
    foliate l.
    l. fusca sclerae
    hepatic l.
    l. interna cranii
    interpubic l.,
        fibrocartilaginous
    labial l.
    labiodental l.
    labiogingival l.
    l. lucida
    laminae mediastinales
    l. membranacea tubae
        auditivae

lam·i·na *(continued)*
    membranous l. of auditory
      tube
    l. mesenterii propria
    l. modioli
    l. molecularis corticis
      cerebri
    l. multiformis corticis
      cerebri
    l. muscularis mucosae
    nuclear l.
    orbital l.
    palatine l. of maxilla
    l. papyracea
    l. parietalis pericardii
    periclaustral l.
    l. plexiformis corticis
      cerebri
    posterior limiting l.
    l. profunda
    l. propria mucosae
    l. quadrigemina
    l. rara
    l. rara externa
    l. rara interna
    reticular l.
    l. reticularis
    Rexed's laminae
    rostral l.
    l. rostralis
    l. septi pellucidi
    l. of septum pellucidum
    spiral l., bony
    spiral l., secondary
    l. spiralis ossea
    l. spiralis secundaria
    submucous l. of stomach
    l. superficialis
    suprachoroid l.
    l. suprachoroidea
    l. supraneuroporica
    tectal l. of mesencephalon
    l. of tectum of
      mesencephalon
    l. tecti mesencephali
    terminal l. of
      hypothalamus
    l. terminalis hypothalami

lam·i·na *(continued)*
    l. tragi
    l. tragica
    ungual l.
    vascular l. of choroid
    vascular l. of stomach
    l. vasculosa choroideae
    l. of vertebra
    l. of vertebral arch
    vestibular l.
    l. visceralis pericardii
    l. vitrea
    vitreal l.
    vitreous l.
    zonal l.
    l. zonalis of cerebellum
lam·i·nae
lam·i·na·gram
lam·i·na·graph
lam·i·nag·ra·phy
lam·i·na·plas·ty
lam·i·nar
Lam·i·na·ria
lam·i·na·rin
    l. sulfate
lam·i·na·tion
lam·i·nec·to·my
lam·i·ni·tis
lam·i·no·gram
lam·i·nog·ra·phy
lam·i·no·plas·ty
lam·i·not·o·my
lamp
    annealing l.
    arc l.
    carbon arc l.
    cold quartz mercury vapor
      l.
    diagnostic l.
    Eldridge-Green l.
    Finsen l.
    Finsen-Reya l.
    Gullstrand's slit l.
    high pressure mercury arc
      l.
    hot quartz l.
    Jesionek l.
    Kromayer's l.

lamp *(continued)*
    Lortet l.
    low pressure mercury arc l.
    mercury vapor l.
    mignon l.
    quartz l.
    Simpson l.
    slit l.
    sun l.
    ultraviolet l.
    Wood's l.
    xenon arc l.
lam·pas
lam·pro·pho·nia
lam·pro·phon·ic
La·mus
lam·ziek·te
la·na
la·nat·o·side C
lan·au·rin
lance
Lance·field classification
lan·ce·o·late
Lan·ce·reau-Ma·thieu disease
lan·cet
    abscess l.
    acne l.
    gingival l.
    gum l.
    spring l.
    thumb l.
Lan·cet coefficient
lan·ci·nat·ing
Lan·ci·si's nerves
Lan·ci·si's stria
Lan·dau reflex
land·mark
Lan·dolt's bodies
Lan·dolt's operation
Lan·dou·zy's disease
Lan·dou·zy's dystrophy
Lan·dou·zy's type
Lan·dou·zy-De·je·rine atrophy
Lan·dou·zy-De·je·rine dystrophy
Lan·dou·zy-De·je·rine type
Lan·dou·zy-Gras·set law
Lan·dry's disease

Lan·dry's palsy
Lan·dry's paralysis
Lan·dry's syndrome
Land·stei·ner, Karl
Land·ström's muscle
Land·zert's fossa
Lane's band
Lane's disease
Lane's kink
Lane's operation
Lane's plate
Lang·don Down's disease
Lange's reaction
Lange's solution
Lange's test
Lan·gen·beck's amputation
Lan·gen·beck's flap
Lan·gen·beck's triangle
Lan·gen·dorff's method
Lan·gen·dorff's preparation
Lan·ger's axillary arch
Lan·ger's lines
Lan·ger's muscle
Lan·ger·hans' cells
Lan·ger·hans' granules
Lan·ger·hans' islands
Lan·ger·hans' islets
Lang·hans' cells
Lang·hans' layer
Lang·hans' stria
Lang·ley's ganglion
Lang·ley's granules
Lang·ley's nerves
Lang·muir trough
lan·i·ary
Lan·ne·longue's foramen
lan·o·lin
    anhydrous l.
la·nos·ter·ol
La·nox·in
Lan·ter·man's clefts
Lan·ter·man's incisures
Lan·ter·man-Schmidt incisures
lan·than·ic
lan·tha·nin
lan·tha·num
lan·tho·pine

la·nu·gi·nous
la·nu·go
Lanz's point
LAP — leucine
  aminopeptidase
    leukocyte alkaline
      phosphatase
la·pac·tic
lap·a·rec·to·my
lap·a·ro·cele
lap·a·ro·cho·le·cys·tot·o·my
lap·a·ro·co·lec·to·my
lap·a·ro·co·los·to·my
lap·a·ro·co·lot·o·my
lap·a·ro·cys·tec·to·my
lap·a·ro·cys·ti·dot·o·my
lap·a·ro·cys·tot·o·my
lap·a·ro·en·ter·os·to·my
lap·a·ro·en·ter·ot·o·my
lap·a·ro·gas·tros·co·py
lap·a·ro·gas·tros·to·my
lap·a·ro·gas·trot·o·my
lap·a·ro·hep·a·tot·o·my
lap·a·ro·hys·ter·ec·to·my
lap·a·ro·hys·tero-ooph·o·rec·
  to·my
lap·a·ro·hys·tero·sal·pin·
  go-ooph·o·rec·to·my
lap·a·ro·hys·ter·ot·o·my
lap·a·ro·il·e·ot·o·my
lap·a·ro·mono·did·y·mus
lap·a·ro·my·itis
lap·a·ro·myo·mec·to·my
lap·a·ro·myo·my·ot·o·my
lap·a·ro·ne·phrec·to·my
lap·a·ror·rha·phy
lap·a·ro·sal·pin·gec·to·my
lap·a·ro·sal·pin·go-ooph·o·
  rec·to·my
lap·a·ro·sal·pin·got·o·my
lap·a·ro·scope
lap·a·ros·co·py
lap·a·ro·sple·nec·to·my
lap·a·ro·sple·not·o·my
lap·a·rot·o·ma·phil·ia
lap·a·ro·tome
lap·a·rot·o·my
  second-look l.

lap·a·ro·typh·lot·o·my
lap·a·thin
La·picque's constant
La·picque's law
Lap·i·dus operation
lap·in·iza·tion
lap·in·ize
La·place law
La·place-Gauss distribution
lap·sus
  l. calami
  l. linguae
  l. memoriae
la·pyr·i·um chlo·ride
La·rat's treatment
lard
  benzoinated l.
lar·da·ce·in
lar·da·ceous
Lar·gon
lar·i·at
la·rith·mics
la·rix·in
lark·spur
Lar·mor equation
Lar·mor frequency
Lar·o·do·pa
La·ron dwarf
La·Roque herniorrhaphy
  incision
Lar·rey's amputation
Lar·rey's cleft
Lar·rey's operation
Lar·rey's spaces
Lar·rey-Weil disease
Lar·sen's disease
Lar·sen syndrome
Lar·sen-Jo·hans·son disease
lar·va *pl.* lar·vae
  l. currens
  filariform l.
  l. migrans
  rat-tailed l.
lar·va·ceous
lar·val
lar·vate
lar·vi·cide
lar·vip·a·rous

lar·vi·pha·gic
lar·vi·po·si·tion
lar·viv·o·rous
lar·yn·gal·gia
lar·yn·ge·al
lar·yn·gec·to·mee
lar·yn·gec·to·my
    frontolateral partial l.
    lateral partial l.
    supraglottic l.
    total l.
la·ryn·ges
lar·yn·gis·mal
lar·yn·gis·mus
    l. paralyticus
    l. stridulus
lar·yn·git·ic
lar·yn·gi·tis
    acute catarrhal l.
    acute spasmodic l.
    atrophic l.
    chronic catarrhal l.
    chronic hyperplastic l.
    chronic nonspecific l.
    croupous l.
    diphtheritic l.
    edematous l.
    membranous l.
    necrotic l.
    phlegmonous l.
    l. sicca
    simple l.
    l. stridulosa
    subglottic l.
    supraglottic l.
    syphilitic l.
    tuberculous l.
    vestibular l.
la·ryn·go·cele
    external l.
    internal l.
    ventricular l.
la·ryn·go·cen·te·sis
la·ryn·go·fis·sure
la·ryn·go·gram
lar·yn·gog·ra·phy
la·ryn·go·hy·po·phar·ynx
lar·yn·gol·o·gist

lar·yn·gol·o·gy
la·ryn·go·ma·la·cia
lar·yn·gom·e·try
la·ryn·go·pa·ral·y·sis
lar·yn·gop·a·thy
la·ryn·go·pha·ryn·ge·al
la·ryn·go·phar·yn·gec·to·my
la·ryn·go·pha·ryn·ge·us
la·ryn·go·phar·yn·gi·tis
la·ryn·go·phar·ynx
lar·yn·goph·o·ny
lar·yn·goph·thi·sis
la·ryn·go·plas·ty
la·ryn·go·ple·gia
la·ryn·go·pto·sis
la·ryn·go·pyo·cele
la·ryn·go·rhi·nol·o·gy
lar·yn·gor·rha·gia
lar·yn·gor·rha·phy
la·ryn·gor·rhea
la·ryn·go·scle·ro·ma
la·ryn·go·scope
    Dedo-Pilling l.
    Jako l.
    Sanders l.
la·ryn·go·scop·ic
lar·yn·gos·co·pist
lar·yn·gos·co·py
    direct l.
    fiberoptic l.
    indirect l.
    mirror l.
    suspension l.
la·ryn·go·spasm
la·ryn·go·sta·sis
la·ryn·go·stat
la·ryn·go·ste·no·sis
lar·yn·gos·to·my
la·ryn·go·stro·bo·scope
la·ryn·go·tome
lar·yn·got·o·my
    complete l.
    inferior l.
    median l.
    subhyoid l.
    superior l.
    thyrohyoid l.
la·ryn·go·tra·che·al

la·ryn·go·tra·che·itis
la·ryn·go·tra·cheo·bron·chi·tis
la·ryn·go·tra·cheo·bron·chos·co·py
la·ryn·go·tra·che·os·co·py
la·ryn·go·tra·che·ot·o·my
la·ryn·go·ves·tib·u·li·tis
la·ryn·go·xe·ro·sis
lar·ynx *pl.* la·ryn·ges
    artificial l.
la·sal·o·cid
La·sègue's sign
la·ser
    argon l.
    carbon-dioxide l.
    dye l.
    helium-neon l.
    Hruby l.
    ion l.
    krypton l.
    neodymium: yttrium-alu-minum-garnet (Nd:YAG) l.
    Sharplan 733 CO_2 l.
    Visulas Nd:YAG l.
Las·io·he·lea
La·six
Lassa fever
Lassa virus
Las·sar's betanaphthol paste
Las·sar's paste
Las·sar's plain zinc paste
las·si·tude
la·tah
Lat·ar·jet's nerve
Lat·ar·jet's vein
Lat. dol. — L. lateri dolenti (to the painful side)
lat·e·bra
la·ten·cy
    absolute l.
    reducible l.
    total reflex l.
la·tent
la·ten·ti·a·tion
lat·er·ad
lat·er·al

lat·er·al·de·tru·sion
lat·er·a·lis
lat·er·al·i·ty
    crossed l.
    dominant l.
    mixed l.
lat·er·al·iza·tion
    sound l.
lat·er·i·ceous
lat·eri·cum·bent
lat·er·i·tious
lat·ero·ab·do·mi·nal
lat·ero·de·vi·a·tion
lat·ero·dor·sal
lat·ero·duc·tion
lat·ero·flex·ion
lat·ero·gnath·ism
lat·ero·mar·gin·al
lat·ero·po·si·tion
lat·ero·pul·sion
lat·ero·re·tru·sive
lat·ero·sel·lar
lat·ero·tor·sion
lat·ero·tru·sion
lat·ero·ver·sion
la·tex
La·tham's circle
lath·y·rism
lath·y·rit·ic
lath·y·ro·gen
lath·y·ro·gen·ic
la·tis·si·mo·con·dy·lar·is
la·tis·si·mus
lat·ro·dec·tism
Lat·ro·dec·tus
    L. mactans
LATS — long-acting thyroid stimulator
LATS-p — LATS protector
lat·tice
la·tus (la·ta, la·tum)
la·tus *pl.* lat·e·ra
Latz·ko's cesarean section
Lau·ber's disease
laud·a·ble
lau·da·num
laugh
    canine l.

laugh *(continued)*
    sardonic l.
laugh·ter
    compulsive l.
    forced l.
    obsessive l.
Lau·gier's hernia
Lau·gier's sign
Lau·mo·nier's ganglion
Lau·nois-Clé·ret syndrome
Lau·rence-Bie·dl syndrome
Lau·rence-Moon-Bie·dl
    syndrome
Lau·rens operation
lau·reth 9
lau·ric acid
Lauth's canal
Lauth's ligament
Lauth's sinus
Lauth's violet
LAV — lymphadenopathy-asso-
    ciated virus
la·vage
    bronchoalveolar l.
    gastric l.
    intestinal l.
    peritoneal l.
    pleural l.
La·van·du·la
la·va·tion
La·ve·ma
La·ve·ran, Charles Louis
    Alphonse
La·ve·ran's bodies
La·ve·ran's corpuscles
La·ve·ra·nia fal·cip·a·ra
la·veur
law
    Adrian-Bronk l.
    Allen's paradoxic l.
    all-or-none l.
    Angström's l.
    antisubstitution l.
    Aran's l.
    Arndt's l.
    Arndt-Schulz l.
    l's of articulation
    l. of avalanche

law *(continued)*
    l. of average localization
    Avogadro's l.
    Babinski's l.
    Baer's l.
    Barfurth's l.
    Baruch's l.
    Bastian's l.
    Bastian-Bruns l.
    Baume's l.
    Beer's l.
    Beer-Lambert l.
    Behring's l.
    Bell's l.
    Bell-Magendie l.
    Bergonié-Tribondeau l.
    biogenetic l.
    Bowditch's l.
    Boyle's l.
    Breton's l.
    Brigg's l.
    Broadbent's l.
    Buhl-Dittrich l.
    Bunge's l.
    Bunsen-Roscoe l.
    Camerer's l.
    Cannon's l. of denervation
    Charles' l.
    Colles l.
    Collin's l.
    l. of conservation of energy
    l. of conservation of matter
    l. of contrary innervation
    Cope's l.
    Coulomb's l.
    Courvoisier's l.
    Coutard's l.
    Curie's l.
    Cushing's l.
    Dale-Feldberg l.
    Dalton's l.
    Dalton-Henry l.
    Deiter's l.
    l. of definite proportions
    l. of denervation
    Descartes' l.
    Desmarres' l.
    l. of diffusion

law *(continued)*

Dollo's l.
Donders' l.
Draper's l.
DuBois-Reymond's l.
Dulong and Petit's l.
Edinger's l.
Einstein-Starck l.
Einthoven l.
Elliott's l.
Ewald's l.
l. of excitation
l. of exponential decay
l. of facilitation
Faget's l.
Fajans' l.
Faraday's l.
Farr's l.
l. of fatigue
Fechner's l.
Ferry-Porter l.
Fick's first l. of diffusion
l. of filial regression
first l. of thermodynamics
Fitz l.
Flatau's l.
Flechsig's myelogenetic l.
Flint's l.
Flourens' l.
Froriep's l.
Fuerbringer's
  (Fürbringer's) l.
Galton's l.
Galton's l. of regression
gas l.
Gay-Lussac's l.
Geiger-Nuttall l.
Gerhardt-Semon l.
Giraud-Teulon l.
Godélier's l.
Golgi's l.
Gompertz l.
Goodell's l.
Good Samaritan l.
Graham's l.
Grasset's l.
l. of gravitation
Grotthus' l.

law *(continued)*

Gudden's l.
Guldberg and Waage's l.
Gull-Toynbee l.
Gullstrand's l.
Gunn's l.
Haeckel's l.
Haldane's l.
Hanau's l's of articulation
Hardy-Weinberg l.
l. of the heart
Hecker's l.
Heidenhain's l.
Hellin's l.
Hellin-Zeleny l.
Henry's l.
Hering's l.
Heyman's l.
Hilton's l.
Hoff's l.
Hoorweg's l.
Horner's l.
Houghton's l.
ideal gas l.
l. of independent
  assortment
l. of initial value
inverse square l.
l. of isochronism
isodynamic l.
l. of isolated conduction
Jackson's l.
Kahler's l.
Knapp's l.
Koch's l.
Küstner's l.
Lambert's cosine l.
Lambert-Holzknecht l.
Landouzy-Grasset l.
Lapicque's l.
Laplace's l.
Leopold's l.
Levret's l.
Listing's l.
Lossen's l.
Louis' l.
Magendie's l.
malthusian l.

law *(continued)*
Marey's l.
Mariotte's l.
mass l.
l. of mass action
Maxwell-Boltzmann
distribution l.
Meltzer's l.
Mendel's laws
Mendeléeff's l.
mendelian l.
Meyer's l.
Minot's l.
Müller's l.
Müller-Haeckel l.
l. of multiple variants
myelogenetic l.
Naegeli's l.
Nernst's l.
Neumann's l.
Newland's l.
Newton's l.
Nysten's l.
Ohm's l.
Ollier's l.
Pajot's l.
l. of parsimony
Pascal's l.
periodic l.
Petit's l.
Pflüger's l.
Poiseuille's l.
Prévost's l.
Profeta's l.
Proust's l.
psychophysical l.
Raoult's l.
Rayleigh scattering l.
l. of reciprocal proportions
l. of referred pain
l. of refraction
l. of refreshment
l. of regression
l. of relativity
Ricco's l.
Ritter-Valli l.
Rosa's l.
Rosenbach's l.

law *(continued)*
Rubner's l.
Schroeder van der Kolk's l.
second l. of
thermodynamics
l. of segregation
Semon's l.
Semon-Rosenbach l.
Sherrington's l.
l. of similars
l. of sines
Snell's l.
Spallanzani's l.
l. of specific energies
l. of specific irritability
l. of specificity of bacteria
Starling's l.
Stokes' l.
surface l.
Talbot's l.
Teevan's l.
l's of thermodynamics
third l. of thermodynamics
Toynbee's l.
Valli-Ritter l.
van der Kolk's l.
van't Hoff's l.
Virchow's l.
l. of von Baer
Vulpian's l.
Waller's l.
wallerian l.
Walton's l.
Weber's l.
Weber-Fechner l.
Weigert's l.
Wien's l.
Wilder's l. of initial value
Wolff's l.
Wundt-Lamansky l.
zeroth l. of
thermodynamics
lawn
bacterial l.
Law·rence-Seip syndrome
law·ren·ci·um
Law·son Tait
law·sone

Law·so·nia
lax·a·tion
lax·a·tive
   bulk l.
lax·a·tor
   l. tympani major
   l. tympani minor
lax·i·ty
lay·er
   adamantine l.
   ambiguous l.
   ameloblastic l.
   anterior elastic l.
   anterior limiting l. of iris
   bacillary l.
   Baillarger's l.
   basal l.
   basal l. of epidermis
   basement l.
   Bekhterev's l.
   Bernard's glandular l.
   blastodermic l.
   Bowman's l.
   Bruch's l.
   cerebral l. of retina
   Chievitz l.
   choriocapillary l.
   claustral l.
   clear l. of epidermis
   columnar l.
   compact l.
   cortical l.
   l's of cranial colliculus
   cremasteric l.
   cutaneous l. of tympanic
     membrane
   cuticular l.
   dense l.
   dermic l.
   Dobie's l.
   enamel l., inner
   enamel l., outer
   ependymal l.
   epitrichial l.
   external granular l. of
     cerebrum
   external pyramidal l.
   fatty l. of perineum

lay·er *(continued)*
   fibrous l. of articular
     capsule
   Floegel's l.
   functional l.
   fusiform l. of cerebral
     cortex
   ganglion cell l.
   ganglionic l.
   Gennari's l.
   germ l.
   germinative l.
   granular l.
   granular-cell l.
   granular l. of Tomes
   granule l.
   gray l.
   half-value l.
   Haller's l.
   Henle's l.
   Henle's fiber l.
   Henle's nervous l.
   horny l. of epidermis
   horny l. of nail
   Huxley's l.
   inferior l. of pelvic
     diaphragm
   infragranular l.
   inner neuroblastic l.
   inner nuclear l.
   internal pyramidal l.
   Kaes-Bekhterev l.
   keratohyaline l.
   Kölliker's l.
   Langhans' l.
   lateral cartilaginous l.
   limiting l., internal
   malpighian l.
   mantle l.
   marginal l.
   medial cartilaginous l.
   medullary l's of thalamus,
     internal and external
   membranous l. of
     perineum
   Meynert's l.
   molecular l.
   monomolecular l.

lay·er *(continued)*

mucous l.

multiform l. of cerebral cortex

nerve fiber l.

nervous l. of retina

neuroepidermal l.

neuroepithelial l. of retina

Nitabuch's l.

nuclear l.

odontoblastic l.

Oehl's l.

osteoblastic l.

Ollier's l.

osteogenetic l.

outer neuroblastic l.

outer nuclear l.

outer plexiform l. of retina

palisade l.

Pander's l.

papillary l. of corium

papillary l. of dermis

parietal l.

perforated l. of sclera

pericyte l.

peripheral l.

pigmented l.

piriform neuronal l.

plexiform l.

Polyak l.

polymorphic l. of cerebral cortex

pretracheal l.

prickle cell l.

primitive l.

Purkinje l.

Purkinje cell l.

pyramidal l. of cerebral cortex, external

radiate l. of tympanic membrane

Rauber's l.

Renaut's l.

reticular l.

l. of rods and cones

Rohr's l.

Sattler's l.

sclerotogenous l.

lay·er *(continued)*

skeletogenous l.

second half-value l.

sluggish l.

somatic l.

spindle-celled l.

spinous l. of epidermis

splanchnic l.

spongy l.

subcallosal l.

subcutaneous l.

subendocardial l.

subendothelial l.

subepicardial l.

submantle l.

submucous l.

subodontoblastic l.

subpapillary l.

subserous l.

superficial l. of fascia of perineum

suprachorioid l.

supragranular l.

synovial l. of articular capsule

Tomes' granular l.

trophic l.

vascular l. of choroid

vascular l. of testis

vegetative l.

Waldeyer's l.

Weil's basal l.

white l's

Zeissel's l.

zonal l.

laz·a·ret·to

lb — L. *libra* (pound)

LBBB — left bundle branch block

LBW — low birth weight

LCAT — lecithin-cholesterol acyltransferase

LCF — left circumflex (coronary artery)

LCT — liquid crystal thermogram

liquid crystal thermography

LD — lethal dose
   light difference
LD_{50} — median lethal dose
LDA — left descending artery
   left dorsoanterior
LDH — lactate dehydrogenase
LDL — low-density
  lipoproteins
L-dopa
LDP — left dorsoposterior
LE — left eye
   lupus erythematosus
leach·ing
lead
   l. acetate
   black l.
   l. chloride
   l. monoxide
   l. nitrate
   l. oxide
   radioactive l.
   l. subacetate
   tetra-ethyl l.
lead
   l. I
   l. II
   l. III
   aV_F l.
   aV_L l.
   aV_R l.
   bipolar l.
   CF l.
   chest l.
   CL l.
   CM l.
   CR l.
   electrocardiogram (EKG) l.
   electroencephalographic l.
   esophageal l.
   limb l's
   precordial l's
   standard l.
   unipolar l.
   V l's
   Wilson's l's
Lead·bet·ter maneuver
Lead·bet·ter-Pol·i·ta·no
  ureterovesicoplasty

lead zir·con·ate ti·tan·ate
leaf
   anterior mesodermal l.
   digitalis l.
leaf·let
   aortic l.
   mitral valve l.
learn·ing
   avoidance l.
   conditioning l.
   discriminative l.
   escape l.
   immunologic l.
   incidental l.
   insight l.
   latent l.
   motor l.
   perceptual l.
   programmed l.
   state-dependent l.
leash
Le·ber's atrophy
Le·ber's congenital amaurosis
Le·ber's corpuscle
Le·ber's disease
Le·ber's plexus
Le·bis·tes
   L. reticulatus
Le·boy·er method
Le·boy·er technique
lec·an·op·a·gus
le·ca·no·so·ma·top·a·gus
Le·cat's gulf
le·che de hi·gue·rón
lech·o·py·ra
lec·i·thal
lec·i·thal·bu·min
lec·i·thid
   cobra l.
lec·i·thin
lec·i·thin·ase
   l. A
   l. B
   l. C
   l. D
lec·i·thin-cho·les·ter·ol ac·yl·
  trans·fer·ase (LCAT)
lec·i·thin·emia

lec·i·tho·blast
lec·i·tho·pro·tein
lec·i·tho·vi·tel·lin
Le·clan·ché cell
lec·tin
lec·to·type
lec·ture·scope
led·bän·der
Le Den·tu's suture
Led·er stain
Led·er·berg, Joshua
Led·er·cil·lin
Led·er·er's anemia
Le·duc's current
Le·Duc-Camey ileocystoplasty
Lee's ganglion
leech
    American l.
    artificial l.
    horse l.
    land l.
    medicinal l.
leech·ing
Leede-Rum·pel phenomenon
Leeu·wen·hoek's canal
Leeu·wen·hoe·kia aus·tra·li·
    en·sis
Le Fort amputation
Le Fort fracture
Le Fort operation
Le Fort sound
Le Fort suture
left-hand·ed
leg
    badger l.
    baker l.
    bandy l.
    Barbados l.
    bayonet l.
    black l.
    bow l.
    cross l.
    elephant l.
    game l.
    jimmy l's
    jitter l's
    milk l.
    restless l's

leg *(continued)*
    rider's l.
    scissor l.
    tennis l.
    white l.
Le·gal's disease
Le·gal's test
Le Gen·dre (Le·gen·dre) sign
Legg's disease
Legg-Cal·vé-Per·thes disease
Le·gio·nel·la
    L. bozemanii
    L. dumoffii
    L. feeleii
    L. gormanii
    L. jordanis
    L. longbeachae
    L. micdadei
    L. pittsburgensis
    L. pneumophila
    L. wadsworthii
le·gio·nel·la *pl.* le·gio·nel·lae
Le·gio·nel·la·ceae
le·gion·el·lae
le·gion·el·lo·sis
le·gion·naires' disease
le·gume
leg·u·me·lin
le·gu·min
le·gu·mi·niv·o·rous
lei·as·the·nia
Leich·ten·stern's encephalitis
Leich·ten·stern's phenomenon
Leich·ten·stern's sign
Leich·ten·stern's type
Leif·son flagella stain
Leigh disease
Leigh syndrome
Lei·ner's disease
Lei·ner's test
leio·der·mia
leio·dys·to·nia
Lei·og·na·thus ba·co·ti
leio·myo·blas·to·ma
leio·myo·fi·bro·ma
leio·myo·ma
    bizarre l.
    l. cutis

leio·myo·ma *(continued)*
   epithelioid l.
   multiple cutaneous l.
   parasitic l.
   l. uteri
   vascular l.
   Zenker's l.
leio·myo·ma·ta
leio·myo·ma·to·sis
leio·myo·ma·tous
leio·myo·sar·co·ma
Leish·man's cells
Leish·man's stain
Leish·man-Don·o·van body
Leish·ma·nia
   L. aethiopica
   L. brasiliensis
   L. braziliensis
   L. braziliensis braziliensis
   L. braziliensis guyanensis
   L. braziliensis panamensis
   L. donovani
   L. donovani chagasi
   L. donovani donovani
   L. donovani infantum
   L. enrietti
   L. garnhami
   L. infantum
   L. major
   L. mexicana
   L. mexicana amazonensis
   L. mexicana mexicana
   L. mexicana pifanoi
   L. nilotica
   L. peruviana
   L. pifanoi
   L. tropica
   L. tropica aethiopica
   L. tropica major
   L. tropica minor
   L. tropica tropica
leish·ma·nia
leish·ma·ni·al
leish·ma·ni·a·sis
   American l.
   anergic l.
   anergic cutaneous l.
   cutaneous l.

leish·ma·ni·a·sis *(continued)*
   diffuse cutaneous l.
   infantile l.
   lupoid   l.
   mucocutaneous l.
   New World l.
   Old World l.
   post–kala-azar dermal l.
   l. recidivans
   rural l.
   l. tegmentaria diffusa
   urban l.
   visceral l.
leish·man·i·ci·dal
leish·man·id
leish·ma·nin
leish·man·i·o·sis
leish·ma·noid
   dermal l.
   post–kala-azar dermal l.
Leit·ner syndrome
Le·jeune's syndrome
le·ma
Lem·bert's suture
le·me·mia
lem·ma
lem·mo·blast
lem·mo·blas·tic
lem·mo·cyte
lem·nis·ci
lem·nis·cus *pl.* lem·nis·ci
   lateral l.
   l. lateralis
   medial l.
   l. medialis
   optic l.
   l. sensitivus
   sensory l.
   spinal l.
   l. spinalis
   trigeminal l.
   l. trigeminalis
lem·on
le·mo·pa·ral·y·sis
le·mo·ste·no·sis
Lem·pert's fenestration
   operation
Lem·u·roi·dea

Len·ard rays
Len·drum inclusion body stain
Len·e·tran
length
    arch l.
    basialveolar l.
    basinasal l.
    cranial l.
    crown-heel l.
    crown-rump l.
    dental l.
    focal l.
    foot l.
    greatest l.
    sitting l.
    stem l.
    wave l.
Len·hos·sek's fibers
len·i·quin·sin
len·i·tive
Lenn·hoff's index
Lenn·hoff's sign
Len·nox syndrome
Len·nox-Gas·taut syndrome
Le·noir facet
Len·ox Hill brace
len·per·one
lens
    achromatic l.
    acoustic l.
    acrylic l.
    adherent l.
    anastigmatic l.
    aniseikonic l.
    anterior chamber
      intraocular l. (IOL)
    aplanatic l.
    apochromatic l.
    astigmatic l.
    Bagolini l.
    bandage l.
    biconcave l.
    biconvex l.
    bicylindrical l.
    bifocal l.
    bispherical l.
    Brücke l.
    cataract l.

lens *(continued)*
    compound l.
    concave l.
    concavoconcave l.
    concavoconvex l.
    condensing l.
    contact l.
    contact l., corneal
    contact l., gas permeable
    contact l., hard
    contact l., hydrophilic
    contact l., hydrophobic
    contact l., non–gas
      permeable hard
    contact l., PMMA
    contact l., rigid
    contact l., scleral
    contact l., soft
    converging l.
    convex l.
    convexoconcave l.
    corneal l.
    Crookes' l.
    crossed l.
    l. crystallina
    crystalline l.
    cylindrical l.
    decentered l.
    dispersing l.
    diverging l.
    electron l.
    flat l.
    Fresnel l.
    honey bee l.
    Hruby l.
    immersion l.
    intraocular l. (IOL)
    iridocapsular l.
    iris plane l.
    iseikonic l.
    Lieb and Guerry cataract
      implant l.
    meniscus l.
    meniscus l., converging
    meniscus l., diverging
    meniscus l., negative
    meniscus l., positive
    meter l.

lens *(continued)*
    minus l.
    omnifocal l.
    orthoscopic l.
    periscopic l.
    periscopic concave l.
    periscopic convex l.
    photochromic l.
    photosensitive l.
    plane l.
    plano l.
    planoconcave l.
    planoconvex l.
    plus l.
    posterior chamber
      intraocular l. (IOL)
    progressive l.
    punktal l.
    safety l.
    size l.
    spherical l.
    spherocylindrical l.
    stigmatic l.
    toric l.
    trial l.
    trifocal l.
lens·om·e·ter
Len·tard
len·tec·to·my
len·ti·cel
len·ti·co·nus
len·tic·u·la
len·tic·u·lar
len·tic·u·lo-op·tic
len·tic·u·lo·stri·ate
len·tic·u·lo·tha·lam·ic
len·ti·form
len·tig·i·nes
len·tig·i·no·sis
    progressive
      cardiomyopathic l.
len·tig·i·nous
len·ti·glo·bus
len·ti·go *pl.* len·ti·gi·nes
    l. aestiva
    Hutchinson's malignant l.
    l. maligna
    nevoid l.

len·ti·go *(continued)*
    senile l.
    l. senilis
    l. simplex
    solar l.
len·ti·go·mel·a·no·ma
len·ti·go·mel·a·no·sis
len·ti·tis
len·ti·vi·rus
len·tu·la
len·tu·lo
Leo's test
Leo·nar·do's band
le·on·ti·a·sis
    l. ossea
    l. ossea generalisata
    l. ossium
Le·o·pold's law
le·o·trop·ic
lep·er
le·pid·ic
Lep·i·dop·tera
Lé·pine-Froin syndrome
Lep·ley-Ernst tube
lepo·cyte
lepo·thrix
lep·ra
lep·re·chaun·ism
lep·rid
lep·rol·o·gist
lep·rol·o·gy
lep·ro·ma
lep·ro·ma·tous
lep·ro·min
lep·ro·sa·ri·um
lep·ro·sary
lep·ro·stat·ic
lep·ro·sy
    borderline l.
    borderline lepromatous l.
    borderline tuberculous l.
    cutaneous l.
    diffuse l. of Lucio
    dimorphous l.
    histoid l.
    indeterminate l.
    intermediate l.
    lazarine l.

lep·ro·sy *(continued)*
   lepromatous l.
   Lucio l.
   macular l.
   polar lepromatous l.
   pure neural l.
   reactional l.
   spotted l.
   subpolar lepromatous l.
   tuberculoid l.
   uncharacteristic l.
   virchowian l.
   water-buffalo l.
lep·rot·ic
lep·rous
lep·ta·zol
lep·to·ce·phal·ic
lep·to·ceph·a·lous
lep·to·ceph·a·lus
lep·to·ceph·a·ly
lep·to·chro·mat·ic
Lep·to·ci·mex
   L. boueti
Lep·to·co·nops
lep·to·cyte
lep·to·cyt·ic
lep·to·cy·to·sis
lep·to·dac·ty·lous
lep·to·dac·ty·ly
Lep·to·dera pel·lio
lep·to·don·tous
lep·to·kur·tic
lep·to·me·nin·ge·al
lep·to·me·nin·ges *sing.* lep·to·men·inx
lep·to·me·nin·gi·o·ma
lep·to·me·nin·gi·tis
   l. interna
   sarcomatous l.
lep·to·men·in·gop·a·thy
lep·to·men·inx
Lep·tom·i·tus
lep·to·mo·nad
Lep·to·mo·nas
lep·to·mo·nas
Lep·to·myx·i·da
lep·to·ne·ma
lep·to·no·mor·phol·o·gy

lep·to·pel·lic
lep·to·pho·nia
lep·to·phon·ic
lep·top·ro·sope
lep·to·pro·so·pia
lep·to·pro·so·pic
Lep·to·psyl·la
   L. musculi
   L. segnis
lep·tor·rhine
lep·to·scope
lep·to·so·mat·ic
Lep·to·spi·ra
   L. australis
   L. autumnalis
   L. bataviae
   L. biflexa
   L. canicola
   L. grippotyphosa
   L. hebdomidis
   L. hyos
   L. icterohaemorrhagiae
   L. illini
   L. interrogans
   L. interrogans serogroup *australis*
   L. interrogans serogroup *autumnalis*
   L. interrogans serogroup *bataviae*
   L. interrogans serogroup *canicola*
   L. interrogans serogroup *grippotyphosa*
   L. interrogans serogroup *hebdomidis*
   L. interrogans serogroup *icterohaemorrhagiae*
   L. interrogans serogroup *pomona*
   L. interrogans serogroup *pyrogenes*
   L. pomona
   L. pyrogenes
lep·to·spi·ra
Lep·to·spi·ra·ceae
lep·to·spi·ral
lep·to·spire

lep·to·spi·ro·sis
  anicteric l.
  benign l.
  l. hebdomadis
  icteric l.
  l. icterohaemorrhagica
lep·to·spir·uria
lep·to·staph·y·line
lep·to·tene
lep·to·thri·co·sis
Lep·to·thrix
lep·to·thrix
Lep·to·trich·ia
lep·to·tri·cho·sis
  l. conjunctivae
Lep·to·trom·bid·i·um
Lep·tus
  L. akamushi
  L. irritans
Lerch's percussion
ler·go·trile
  l. mesylate
Le·ri's sign
Lé·ri-Weill syndrome
Le·riche's disease
Le·riche's syndrome
Ler·i·tine
Ler·mo·yez's syndrome
les — local excitatory state
les·bi·an
les·bi·an·ism
Lesch-Ny·han syndrome
Le·ser-Tré·lat sign
Les·gaft's space
Les·gaft's triangle
le·sion
  Armanni-Ebstein l.
  Baehr-Löhlein l.
  benign lymphoepithelial l.
  birds' nest l.
  Blumenthal l.
  Bracht-Wächter l.
  Brown-Séquard l.
  bull's eye l.
  capsular drop l.
  caviar l.
  central l.
  coin l.

le·sion *(continued)*
  complement l.
  compressive l. of
    lumbosacral region
  Councilman l.
  dendritic l.
  desmoid l.
  destructive l.
  diffuse l.
  discharging l.
  DREZ (dorsal root entry
    zone) l.
  Duret's l.
  Ebstein's l.
  focal l.
  frondy l.
  functional l.
  Ghon's primary l.
  gross l.
  hepatic veno-occlusive l.
  herpetiform l. of Cole
  histologic l.
  hyaline l.
  impaction l.
  indiscriminate l.
  initial syphilitic l.
  irritative l.
  Janeway l.
  jet l.
  Kimmelstiel-Wilson l.
  local l.
  Löhlein-Baehr l.
  local glomerular l.
  lower motor neuron l.
  macroscopic l.
  mass l.
  molecular l.
  onion scale l.
  onionskin l.
  organic l.
  partial l.
  peripheral l.
  phlyctenule l.
  pinguecula l.
  precancerous l.
  primary l.
  retrocochlear l.
  ring-wall l.

le·sion *(continued)*
    satellite l.
    Scheibe l.
    shagreen l.
    structural l.
    swan-neck tubular l.
    systemic l.
    target l.
    total l.
    trophic l.
    wire-loop l.
Les·ser's test
Les·shaft's space
Les·shaft's triangle
Les·ter Mar·tin procedure
LET — linear energy transfer
let-down
le·thal
le·thal·i·ty
le·thar·go·gen·ic
leth·ar·gy
    African l.
    hypnotic l.
    hysteric l.
    induced l.
    lucid l.
let·i·mide hy·dro·chlo·ride
Let·ter
Let·ter·er-Si·we disease
Leu — leucine
leu·ce·mia
leu·cine
leu·cine am·i·no-pep·ti·dase
leu·cin·im·ide
leu·ci·no·sis
leu·cin·uria
leu·ci·tis
leu·co·cyte
leu·co·cy·to·sis
leu·co·flu·o·res·ce·in
Leu·co·i·um
leu·co·my·cin
Leu·co·nos·toc
    L. citrovorum
    L. cremoris
    L. dextranicum
    L. lactis
    L. mesenteroides

Leu·co·nos·toc (continued)
    L. oenos
leu·cop·ter·in
leu·co·sin
leu·cot·o·my
leu·co·vo·rin
    l. calcium
    l. rescue
leu·cyl
Leud·et's bruit
Leud·et's sign
Leud·et's tinnitus
leu-en·keph·a·lin
leuk·ag·glu·ti·nin
leu·ka·phe·re·sis
leu·ke·mia
    acute lymphoblastic l.
     (ALL)
    acute monoblastic l.
     (AMOL)
    acute myeloblastic l. (AML)
    acute myelomonoblastic l.
     (AMMOL)
    acute nonlymphocytic l.
     (ANLL)
    acute promyelocytic l.
    adult T-cell l.
    aleukemic l.
    aleukocythemic l.
    basophilic l.
    blast cell l.
    chronic granulocytic l.
    chronic lymphocytic l.
     (CLL)
    chronic myelocytic l.
    l. cutis
    embryonal l.
    eosinophilic l.
    granulocytic l.
    hairy-cell l.
    hemoblastic l.
    hemocytoblastic l.
    histiocytic l.
    leukopenic l.
    lymphatic l.
    lymphoblastic l.
    lymphocytic l.
    lymphogenous l.

leu·ke·mia *(continued)*
  lymphoid l.
  lymphosarcoma cell l.
  mast cell l.
  mature cell l.
  medullary l.
  megakaryocytic l.
  micromyeloblastic l.
  monoblastic l.
  monocytic l.
  myeloblastic l.
  myelocytic l.
  myelogenous l.
  myeloid l.
  myeloid granulocytic l.
  myelomonocytic l.
  Naegeli l.
  neutrophilic l.
  null cell lymphoblastic l.
  plasma cell l.
  plasmacytic l.
  polymorphocytic l.
  progranulocytic l.
  promyelocytic l.
  Rieder cell l.
  Schilling's l.
  splenic l.
  splenomyelogenous l.
  stem cell l.
  subleukemic l.
  undifferentiated cell l.
leu·ke·mic
leu·ke·mid
leu·ke·mo·gen
leu·ke·mo·gen·e·sis
leu·ke·mo·gen·ic
leu·ke·moid
leuk·en·ceph·a·li·tis
Leu·ker·an
leu·kex·o·sis
leu·kin
leu·ko·ag·glu·ti·nin
leu·ko·blast
  granular l.
leu·ko·blas·to·sis
leu·ko·ci·din
  Neisser-Wechsberg l.
  Panton-Valentine (P-V) l.

leu·ko·crit
leu·ko·cy·tal
leu·ko·cyte
  acidophilic l.
  agranular l's
  basophilic l.
  cystinotic l.
  endothelial l.
  eosinophilic l.
  globular l.
  granular l's (granulocytes)
  heterophilic l's
  hyaline l.
  lymphoid l's
  mast l.
  motile l.
  neutrophilic l.
  nonfilament
    polymorphonuclear l.
  nongranular l's
  nonmotile l.
  polymorphonuclear l.
  polynuclear neutrophilic l.
  l.-poor red blood cells
  Türk's irritation l.
leu·ko·cyte-poor
leu·ko·cy·the·mia
leu·ko·cyt·ic
leu·ko·cy·to·blast
leu·ko·cy·to·gen·e·sis
leu·ko·cy·toid
leu·ko·cy·tol·o·gy
leu·ko·cy·tol·y·sin
leu·ko·cy·tol·y·sis
  venom l.
leu·ko·cy·to·lyt·ic
leu·ko·cy·to·ma
leu·ko·cy·tom·e·ter
leu·ko·cy·to·pe·nia
leu·ko·cy·toph·a·gy
leu·ko·cy·to·pla·nia
leu·ko·cy·to·poi·e·sis
leu·ko·cy·to·sis
  absolute l.
  agonal l.
  basophilic l.
  digestive l.
  eosinophilic l.

leu·ko·cy·to·sis *(continued)*
  lymphocytic l.
  mononuclear l.
  neutrophilic l.
  l. of the newborn
  pathologic l.
  physiologic l.
  pure l.
  relative l.
  terminal l.
  toxic l.
leu·ko·cy·to·tac·tic
leu·ko·cy·to·tax·is
leu·ko·cy·to·ther·a·py
leu·ko·cy·to·tox·ic·i·ty
leu·ko·cy·to·tox·in
leu·ko·cy·to·trop·ic
leu·ko·cy·tu·ria
leu·ko·de·riv·a·tive
leu·ko·der·ma
  l. acquisitum centrifugum
  l. colli
  genital l.
  occupational l.
  postinflammatory l.
  syphilitic l.
leu·ko·der·ma·tous
leu·ko·der·mic
leu·ko·dex·trin
leu·ko·dys·tro·phia cer·e·bri
  pro·gres·si·va
leu·ko·dys·tro·phy
  cerebral l.
  demyelinogenic l.
  globoid l.
  globoid cell l.
  hereditary cerebral l.
  Krabbe's l.
  melanodermic l.
  metachromatic l.
  progressive cerebral l.
  spongiform l.
  sudanophilic l.
leu·ko·ede·ma
leu·ko·en·ceph·a·li·tis
  acute hemorrhagic l.
  concentric periaxial l.
  l. periaxialis concentrica

leu·ko·en·ceph·a·li·tis
  (continued)
  Scholz metachromatic l.
  subacute sclerosing l.
  van Bogaert's sclerosing l.
leu·ko·en·ceph·a·lop·a·thy
  acute hemorrhagic l.
  acute necrotizing
    hemorrhagic l.
  metachromatic l.
  multifocal progressive l.
  progressive multifocal l.
  subacute sclerosing l.
leu·ko·en·ceph·a·ly
  metachromatic l.
leu·ko·eryth·ro·blas·to·sis
leu·ko·gram
leu·ko·ker·a·to·sis
  congenital oral l.
leu·ko·ki·ne·sis
leu·ko·ki·net·ic
leu·ko·ki·net·ics
leu·ko·ki·nin
leu·ko·ko·ria
leu·ko·krau·ro·sis
leu·ko·lym·pho·sar·co·ma
leu·kol·y·sin
leu·kol·y·sis
leu·ko·lyt·ic
leu·ko·ma
  adherent l.
  l. adhaerens
leu·ko·maine
leu·ko·main·emia
leu·ko·main·ic
leu·ko·ma·ta
leu·ko·ma·tous
leu·ko·mel·a·no·der·ma
leu·ko·mono·cyte
leu·ko·my·eli·tis
leu·ko·my·elop·a·thy
leu·ko·my·o·ma
leu·kon
leu·ko·ne·cro·sis
leu·ko·nych·ia
leu·ko·path·ia
  l. punctata reticularis
    symmetrica

leu·ko·path·ia *(continued)*
  l. unguium
leu·kop·a·thy
  symmetric progressive l.
leu·ko·pe·de·sis
leu·ko·pe·nia
  basophil l.
  basophilic l.
  congenital l.
  eosinophilic l.
  lymphocytic l.
  malignant l.
  monocytic l.
  neutrophilic l.
  pernicious l.
leu·ko·pe·nic
leu·ko·phago·cy·to·sis
leu·ko·pla·kia
  l. buccalis
  l. lingualis
  oral l.
  oral hairy l.
  speckled l.
  l. vulvae
leu·ko·pla·kic
leu·ko·poi·e·sis
leu·ko·poi·et·ic
leu·ko·poi·e·tin
leu·ko-poor
leu·ko·pre·cip·i·tin
leu·kop·sin
leu·kor·rha·gia
leu·kor·rhea
  menstrual l.
  periodic l.
leu·kor·rhe·al
leu·ko·sar·co·ma
leu·ko·sar·co·ma·to·sis
leu·ko·scope
leu·ko·sis *pl.* leu·ko·ses
  acute l.
  lymphoid l.
  myeloblastic l.
  myelocytic l.
  skin l.
leu·ko·tac·tic
leu·ko·tax·is
leu·ko·ther·a·py

leu·ko·ther·a·py
  preventive l.
Leu·ko·thrix
leu·ko·throm·bin
leu·kot·ic
leu·ko·tome
leu·kot·o·my
  transorbital l.
leu·ko·tox·ic
leu·ko·tox·ic·i·ty
leu·ko·tox·in
leu·ko·trich·ia
leu·ko·tri·ene
leu·ko·uro·bi·lin
leu·ko·vi·rus
leu·pro·lide
Lev·a·di·ti's stain
lev·al·lor·phan tar·trate
le·vam·fet·amine
  l. succinate
le·vam·i·sole hy·dro·chlo·ride
le·vam·phet·amine
lev·an
lev·an·su·crase
lev·ar·te·re·nol
  l. bitartrate
le·va·tor *pl.* le·va·to·res
  l. claviculae
lev·a·to·res
Le·Veen valve
lev·el
  α l.
  air-fluid l.
  l. of anesthesia
  bone conduction hearing l.
  l's of brightness
  cidal l.
  confidence l.
  l's of consciousness
  continuous noise l.
  developmental l.
  isoelectric l.
  loudness discomfort l.
  masking zero reference l.
  noise emission l.
  sensation l.
  sensorineural acuity l.

lev·el *(continued)*
    significance l., l. of
      significance
    sound pressure l.
    threshold l.
    tonal l.
lev·el·ing
Lé·vi-Lo·rain type
lev·i·cel·lu·lar
le·vid·u·lin·ose
lev·i·ga·tion
Le·vin's tube
Le·vine's agar
Le·vine's clenched-fist sign
Le·vine's eosin-ethylene blue
lev·i·ta·tion
le·vo·an·gio·car·di·og·ra·phy
le·vo·car·dia
    isolated l.
    mixed l.
le·vo·car·dio·gram
le·vo·cli·na·tion
le·vo·con·dyl·ism
le·vo·cy·clo·duc·tion
le·vo·cy·clo·ver·sion
le·vo·do·pa
Le·vo-Dro·mo·ran
le·vo·duc·tion
le·vo·fur·al·ta·done
levo·gram
le·vo·gy·ral
le·vo·gy·ra·tion
Le·void
le·vo·me·pro·ma·zine
le·vo·meth·a·dyl ac·e·tate
le·vo·nor·de·frin
Lev·o·phed
Le·vo·prome
le·vo·pro·poxy·phene nap·sy·late
le·vo·pro·pyl·cil·lin po·tas·si·um
le·vo·ro·ta·ry
le·vo·ro·ta·tion
le·vo·ro·ta·to·ry
lev·or·pha·nol tar·trate
le·vo·sin
le·vo·thy·rox·ine so·di·um

le·vo·tor·sion
le·vo·ver·sion
le·vox·a·drol hy·dro·chlo·ride
Lev·ret's forceps
Lev·ret's law
Lev·u·gen
lev·u·lan
lev·u·lin
lev·u·lin·ate
lev·u·lin·ic acid
lev·u·lo·san
lev·u·lo·sa·zone
lev·u·lose
lev·u·los·emia
lev·u·los·uria
Lé·vy-Rous·sy syndrome
Le·vy, Rown·tree, and Mar·ri·ott method
Le·wan·dow·sky nev·us
Le·wan·dow·sky-Lutz disease
Lew·is acid
Lew·is base
Lew·is blood group
Lew·is and Pic·ker·ing test
lew·i·site
Lew·i·sohn's method
Le·wy bodies
Ley·den's ataxia
Ley·den's crystals
Ley·den's disease
Ley·den jar
Ley·den-Mö·bi·us dystrophy
Ley·den-Mö·bi·us type
Ley·dig's cells
Ley·dig's cylinders
Ley·dig's duct
ley·dig·ar·che
Le·zak's Malingering Test
Lf — limit flocculation
LFA — left frontoanterior
L-form
LFP — left frontoposterior
LFT — left frontotransverse
    liver function test
LGV — lymphogranuloma
    venereum
LH — luteinizing hormone
Lher·mitte's sign

LH-RF — luteinizing hormone releasing factor

LH-RH — luteinizing hormone–releasing hormone

LIA — leukemia-associated inhibitory activity

lia·bil·i·ty
    professional l.

lib·ero·mo·tor

li·bid·i·nal

li·bid·i·nous

li·bi·do *pl.* li·bi·di·nes
    ego l.
    object l.

Libman's sign

Lib·man-Sacks disease

Lib·man-Sacks syndrome

li·bra *pl.* li·brae

li·brary
    gene l.

Lib·ri·um

lice

li·cense

li·cen·ti·ate

Lich-Gre·goire repair

li·chen
    l. albus
    l. amyloidosus
    l. axillaris
    l. corneus hypertrophicus
    l. fibromucinoidosus
    follicular l. planus
    hypertrophic l. planus
    l. myxedematosus
    l. nitidus
    l. obtusus corneus
    l. pilaris
    l. planopilaris
    l. planus
    l. planus actinicus
    l. planus annularis
    l. planus atrophicus
    l. planus, bullous
    l. planus erythematosus
    l. planus follicularis
    l. planus hypertrophicus
    l. planus morpheicus
    l. planus subtropicum

li·chen *(continued)*
    l. planus tropicum
    l. planus verrucosus
    l. planus, vesiculobullous
    l. ruber moniliformis
    l. ruber planus
    l. ruber verrucosus
    l. sclerosus
    l. sclerosus et atrophicus
    l. scrofulosorum
    l. scrofulosus
    l. simplex chronicus
    l. spinulosus
    l. striatus
    l. tropicus
    l. urticatus
    Wilson's l.

li·chen·i·fi·ca·tion

li·chen·i·form·in

li·chen·oid

Lich·ten·stein hernia repair

Licht·heim's aphasia

Licht·heim's disease

Licht·heim's plaque

Licht·heim's sign

Licht·heim's syndrome

Licht·heim's tests

lic·o·rice

lid
    granular l's
    tucked l. of Collier

Li·da-Man·tle

li·dam·i·dine

li·da·mine

Lid·dell and Sher·ring·ton reflex

Li·dex

li·do·caine
    l. hydrochloride

li·do·fen·in

li·do·fil·con

li·do·fla·zine

lie
    longitudinal l.
    oblique l.
    transverse l.

Lieb and Guer·ry cataract implant lens

Lie·ben's reaction
Lie·ben's test
Lie·ber·kühn's ampulla
Lie·ber·kühn's crypts
Lie·ber·kühn's follicles
Lie·ber·kühn's glands
Lie·ber·mann's test
Lie·ber·mann-Bur·chard
　reaction
Lie·ber·mann-Bur·chard test
Lie·ber·meis·ter's furrows
Lie·ber·meis·ter's grooves
Lie·ber·meis·ter's rule
Lie·big's test
Lie·big's theory
li·en
　　l. accessorius
　　l. mobilis
li·enal
li·en·cu·lus
li·en·ec·to·my
li·eni·tis
li·eno·cele
li·en·og·ra·phy
li·eno·ma·la·cia
li·eno·med·ul·lary
li·eno·my·elog·e·nous
li·eno·my·elo·ma·la·cia
li·eno·pan·cre·at·ic
li·en·op·a·thy
li·eno·re·nal
li·eno·tox·in
li·en·ter·ic
li·en·tery
li·en·un·cu·lus
Liep·mann's apraxia
Lie·se·gang's phenomenon
Lie·se·gang's striae
Lie·se·gang's waves
Lieu·taud's body
Lieu·taud's luette
Lieu·taud's triangle
Lieu·taud's uvula
LIF　—　left iliac fossa
　　leukocyte inhibitory factor
life
　　antenatal l.
　　embryonic l.

life *(continued)*
　　fetal l.
　　intrauterine l.
　　mean l.
　　potential years of l. lost
　　uterine l.
life·time
li·fi·brate
lig.　—　ligament
　　ligamentum
lig·a·ment
　　accessory l.
　　accessory atlantoaxial l.
　　acromioclavicular l.
　　acromiocoracoid l.
　　adipose l. of knee (of
　　　Cruveilhier)
　　alar l's
　　alveolodental l.
　　annular l.
　　anococcygeal l.
　　l. of antibrachium (of
　　　Weitbrecht)
　　apical dental l.
　　apical odontoid l.
　　appendiculo-ovarian l.
　　Arantius' l.
　　arcuate l's
　　Arnold's l.
　　articular l. of vertebrae
　　arytenoepiglottic l.
　　atlantooccipital l.
　　auricular l.
　　Barkow's l.
　　Bellini's l.
　　Bérard's l.
　　Berry's l.
　　Bertin's l.
　　Bichat's l.
　　bifurcate l.
　　Bigelow's l.
　　bigeminate l's of Arnold
　　l. of Botallo
　　Bourgery's l.
　　brachiocubital l.
　　brachioradial l.
　　broad l. of liver
　　broad l. of lung

lig·a·ment *(continued)*
broad l. of uterus
Brodie's l.
Burns' l.
calcaneocuboid l.
calcaneofibular l.
calcaneonavicular l.
calcaneotibial l.
Caldani's l.
Campbell's l.
Camper's l.
canthal l's
capitular l., volar
capsular l's
Carcassonne's l.
cardinal l.
caroticoclinoid l.
carpal l.
carpometacarpal l's
Casser's l.
casserian l.
caudal l. of common
  integument
cemental l.
ceratocricoid l.
cervical l.
cervicobasilar l.
check l's of axis
chondrosternal l.,
  interarticular
chondroxiphoid l's
l. of Chopart
l. of Civinini
Clado's l.
Cleland's l.
Cloquet's l.
coccygeal l., superior
collateral l.
Colles' l.
l's of colon
conoid l.
conus l.
Cooper's l.
Cooper's suspensory l's
coracoacromial l.
coracoclavicular l.
coracohumeral l.
coracoid l. of scapula

lig·a·ment *(continued)*
cordiform l. of diaphragm
corniculopharyngeal l.
coronary l. of knee
coronary l. of liver
coronary l. of radius
costocentral l.
costoclavicular l.
costocolic l.
costocoracoid l.
costopericardiac l.
costosternal l's, radiate
costotransverse l.
costovertebral l.
costoxiphoid l's
cotyloid l.
Cowper's l.
cricoarytenoid l., posterior
cricopharyngeal l.
cricosantorinian l.
cricothyroarytenoid l.
cricothyroid l.
cricotracheal l.
cruciate l.
cruciform l.
crural l.
Cruveilhier's l's
cubitoradial l.
cubitoulnar l.
cuboideometatarsal l's
cuboideonavicular l.
cubonavicular l.
cuboscaphoid l., plantar
cuneocuboid l.
cuneometatarsal l's
cutaneophalangeal l's
cysticoduodenal l.
deltoid l.
Denonvilliers l.
dental l.
dentate l. of spinal cord
denticulate l.
Denucé's l.
diaphragmatic l.
digital vaginal l's
Douglas' l.
l. of ductus venosus
duodenohepatic l.

lig·a·ment *(continued)*
  duodenorenal l.
  epihyal l.
  external l's of Barkow,
    plantar
  extracapsular accessory l's
  fabellofibular l.
  falciform l.
  fallopian l.
  l. of Fallopius
  false l.
  Ferrein's l.
  fibrous l.
  fibular collateral l.
  flaval l's
  Flood's l.
  gastrocolic l.
  gastrohepatic l.
  gastrolienal l.
  gastropancreatic l's of
    Huschke
  gastrophrenic l.
  gastrosplenic l.
  genitoinguinal l.
  Gerdy's l.
  Gillette suspensory l.
  Gimbernat's l.
  gingivodental l.
  glenohumeral l's
  glenoid l.
  Grayson's l.
  Günz's l.
  hamatometacarpal l.
  hammock l.
  Helmholtz's l.
  l's of Helvetius
  Henle's l.
  Hensing's l.
  hepatic l's
  hepatocolic l.
  hepatocystocolic l.
  hepatoduodenal l.
  hepatoesophageal l.
  hepatogastric l.
  hepatogastroduodenal l.
  hepatorenal l.
  hepatoumbilical l.
  Hesselbach's l.

lig·a·ment *(continued)*
  Hey's l.
  Holl's l.
  Hueck's l.
  Humphry's l.
  Hunter's l.
  Huschke's l's
  hyaloideocapsular l.
  hyoepiglottic l.
  hypsiloid l.
  iliocostal l.
  iliofemoral l.
  iliolumbar l.
  iliopectineal l.
  iliopubic l.
  iliosacral l's
  iliotibial l. of Maissiat
  iliotrochanteric l.
  infundibulo-ovarian l.
  infundibulopelvic l.
  inguinal l.
  interarticular l.
  intercarpal l's
  interchondral l.
  interclavicular l.
  interclinoid l.
  intercornual l.
  intercostal l's
  intercuneiform l's
  interfoveolar l.
  interlaminar l's
  intermaxillary l.
  intermetacarpal l's
  intermetatarsal l's
  intermuscular l.
  interosseous l.
  interosseous l. of pubis (of
    Winslow)
  interprocess l.
  interpubic l.
  interspinal l's
  interspinous l's
  intertarsal l's
  intertransverse l's
  interureteral l.
  intervertebral l.
  intraarticular
    costovertebral l.

lig·a·ment *(continued)*

  intraarticular sternocostal
    l.
  intrinsic l.
  ischiocapsular l.
  ischiofemoral l.
  ischioprostatic l.
  ischiosacral l's
  Jarjavay's l.
  Krause's l.
  laciniate l.
  lacunar l.
  lacunar l. of Gimbernat
  lambdoid l.
  Lannelongue's l.
  lateral l. of colon
  lateral l. of knee
  lateral l's of liver
  lateral l. of malleus
  lateral meniscofemoral l.
  Lauth's l.
  lienophrenic l.
  lienorenal l.
  Lisfranc's l.
  Lockwood's l.
  longitudinal l. of abdomen
  lumbocostal l.
  l's of Luschka
  Mackenrodt's l.
  l. of Maissiat
  Mauchart's l's
  maxillary l.
  l. of Mayer
  Meckel's l.
  medial l. of elbow joint
  medial l. of temporo-
    mandibular articulation
  medial l. of wrist
  meniscofemoral l.
  mesocolic l. of colon
  metacarpal l's
  metacarpophalangeal l's
  metatarsal l.
  metatarsophalangeal l's,
    inferior
  mucous l.
  l. of nape
  natatory l.

lig·a·ment *(continued)*

  navicularicuneiform l's,
    plantar
  nephrocolic l.
  nuchal l.
  oblique l. of Cooper
  oblique l. of forearm
  oblique l's of knee
  obturator l.,
    atlantooccipital
  obturator l. of atlas
  obturator l. of pelvis
  occipitoaxial l.
  occipitoodontoid l's
  odontoid l., middle
  odontoid l's of axis
  orbicular l. of radius
  ovarian l.
  palmar l's
  palpebral l., lateral
  palpebral l., medial
  patellar l.
  pectinal l. of iris
  pectineal l.
  pectineal l. of Cooper
  pericardiovertebral l.
  perineal l. of Carcassone
  periodontal l.
  peritoneal l.
  Petit's l.
  Pétrequin's l.
  petrosphenoid l.
  pharyngeal l.
  phrenicocolic l.
  phrenicolienal l.
  phrenicosplenic l.
  phrenocolic l.
  pisimetacarpal l.
  pisohamate l.
  pisometacarpal l.
  pisounciform l.
  pisouncinate l.
  plantar l's
  popliteal l., arcuate
  popliteal l., external
  popliteal l., oblique
  posterior false l. of bladder
  Poupart's l.

lig·a·ment *(continued)*

preurethral l. of Waldeyer
prismatic l. of Weitbrecht
proper l.
pterygomandibular l.
pterygomaxillary l.
pterygospinal l.
pubic l., inferior
pubic l., superior
pubic l. of Cowper
pubic l. of Cruveilhier,
  anterior
pubocapsular l.
pubofemoral l.
puboprostatic l.
puborectal l.
pubovesical l.
pulmonary l.
quadrate l.
quadrate l. of Denucé
radial l., lateral
radiate l.
radiocarpal l.
radiocarpal l., anterior
rectouterine l.
reflected l.
reflex l. of Gimbernat
reinforcing l's
Retzius' l.
rhomboid l. of clavicle
rhomboid l. of wrist
ring l. of hip joint
Robert's l.
round l. of acetabulum
round l. of Cloquet
round l. of femur
round l. of forearm
round l. of liver
round l. of uterus
sacciform l.
sacrococcygeal l.
sacroiliac l's
sacrosciatic l.
sacrospinal l.
sacrospinous l.
sacrotuberal l.
sacrotuberous l.
salpingopharyngeal l.

lig·a·ment *(continued)*

Santorini's l.
Sappey's l.
l. of Scarpa
Schlemm's l's
Sebileau suspensory l's
serous l.
Soemmering's l.
sphenoideotarsal l's
sphenomandibular l.
spinoglenoid l.
spinosacral l.
spiral l. of cochlea
splenogastric l.
splenophrenic l.
splenorenal l.
spring l.
Stanley's cervical l.
stapedial l.
stellate l., anterior
sternoclavicular l.
sternocostal l's
sternopericardiac l's
l. of Struthers
stylohyoid l.
stylomandibular l.
stylomaxillary l.
stylomylohyoid l.
subflaval l.
subpubic l.
suprascapular l.
supraspinal l's
supraspinous l's
suspensory l.
sutural l.
synovial l.
talocalcaneal l.
l. of talocrural joint
talofibular l.
talonavicular l.
talotibial l.
tarsal l., anterior
tarsometatarsal l's
temporomandibular l.
tendinotrochanteric l.
tensor l.
Teutleben's l's
Thompson's l.

lig·a·ment *(continued)*
  thyroepiglottic l.
  thyrohyoid l.
  tibiocalcaneal l.
  tibiofibular l.
  tibionavicular l.
  Toldt's l.
  Toynbee's l.
  tracheal l's
  trapezoid l.
  l. of Treitz
  triangular l. of Colles
  trigeminate l's of Arnold
  triquetral l.
  trochlear l.
  tuberososacral l.
  tubopharyngeal l. of
    Rauber
  Tuffier's inferior l.
  ulnar l. of carpus
  ulnar l., lateral
  ulnocarpal l., palmar
  umbilical l., lateral
  umbilical l., medial
  umbilical l., median
  utero-ovarian l.
  uteropelvic l's
  uterosacral l.
  uterovesical l.
  l's of Valsalva
  venous l. of liver
  ventricular l. of larynx
  vertebropelvic l.
  vertebropericardial l.
  vertebropleural l.
  l. of Vesalius
  vesical l., lateral
  vesicopubic l.
  vesicoumbilical l.
  vesicouterine l.
  vestibular l.
  vocal l.
  Walther's oblique l.
  Weitbrecht's l.
  Whitnall's l.
  Winslow's l.
  Wrisberg's l.
  xiphicostal l's of Macalister

lig·a·ment *(continued)*
  xiphoid l's
  Y l.
  yellow l's
  l. of Zaglas
  Zinn's l.
  zonal l. of thigh
  zonular l.
lig·a·men·ta
lig·a·men·to·pexy
lig·a·men·tous
lig·a·men·tum *pl.* lig·a·men·ta
  l. acromioclaviculare
  ligamenta alaria
  l. anococcygeum
  l. arcuatum laterale
  l. arcuatum mediale
  l. arcuatum medianum
  l. arcuatum pubis
  l. arteriosum
  ligamenta auricularia
    [Valsalvae]
  l. basium
  l. bifurcatum
  l. calcaneocuboideum
  l. calcaneofibulare
  l. calcaneonaviculare
  l. calcaneotibiale
  ligamenta capsularia
  l. caudale integumenti
    communis
  l. ceratocricoideum
  l. collateralia
  l. colli costae
  l. conoideum
  l. coracoacromiale
  l. coracoclaviculare
  l. coracohumerale
  l. coronarium hepatis
  l. costoclaviculare
  l. costotransversarium
  ligamenta costoxiphoidea
  l. cricoarytenoideum
    posterius
  l. cricopharyngeum
  l. cricothyroideum
    medianum

lig·a·men·tum *(continued)*
l. cricotracheale
l. cruciatum anterius genus
l. cruciatum atlantis
l. cruciatum cruris
ligamenta cruciata genus
l. cruciatum posterius
  genus
l. cruciforme atlantis
l. cuboideonaviculare
  dorsale
l. cuboideonaviculare
  plantare
l. cuneocuboideum dorsale
l. cuneocuboideum
  interosseum
l. cuneocuboideum
  plantare
l. deltoideum
l. denticulatum
l. duodenorenale
ligamenta extracapsularia
l. falciforme hepatis
ligamenta flava
l. gastrocolicum
l. gastrolienale
l. gastrophrenicum
l. gastrosplenicum
l. genitoinguinale
ligamenta glenohumeralia
ligamenta hepatis
l. hepatocolicum
l. hepatoduodenale
l. hepatogastricum
l. hepatorenale
l. hyoepiglotticum
l. iliofemorale
l. iliolumbale
l. iliopectineale
l. inguinale
l. inguinale [Pouparti]
l. inguinale reflexum
  [Collesi]
ligamenta intercarpalia
  dorsalia
ligamenta intercarpalia
  interossea

lig·a·men·tum *(continued)*
ligamenta intercarpalia
  palmaria
l. interclaviculare
ligamenta intercostalia
ligamenta
  intercuneiformia
l. interfoveolare
l. interfoveolare
  [Hesselbachi]
ligamenta interspinalia
ligamenta
  intertransversaria
ligamenta intracapsularia
l. ischiocapsulare
l. ischiofemorale
l. laciniatum
l. lacunare
l. lacunare [Gimbernati]
l. latum uteri
l. lienorenale
l. lumbocostale
l. meniscofemorale
  anterius
l. meniscofemorale
  posterius
l. nuchae
l. ovarii proprium
l. palpebrale laterale
l. palpebrale mediale
l. patellae
l. pectinatum anguli
  iridocornealis
l. pectinatum iridis
l. pectineale
l. phrenicocolicum
l. phrenicolienale
l. phrenicosplenicum
l. pisohamatum
l. pisometacarpeum
l. plantare longum
l. popliteum arcuatum
l. popliteum obliquum
l. pterygospinale
l. pterygospinosum
l. pubicum superius
l. pubocapsulare
l. pubofemorale

lig·a·men·tum *(continued)*
l. puboprostaticum
l. pubovesicale
l. pubovesicale laterale
l. pubovesicale medium
l. pulmonale
l. quadratum
l. radiocarpale dorsale
l. radiocarpeum dorsale
l. radiocarpale palmare
l. radiocarpeum palmare
l. reflexum
l. sacrococcygeum anterius
l. sacrococcygeum laterale
l. sacrococcygeum posterius
    profundum
l. sacrococcygeum posterius
    superficiale
l. sacrococcygeum ventrale
ligamenta sacrospinalia
l. sacrotuberale
l. serosum
l. sphenomandibulare
l. spirale cochleae
l. splenorenale
l. sternoclaviculare
l. sternoclaviculare
    anterius
l. sternoclaviculare
    posterius
l. sternocostale
    interarticulare
l. sternocostale
    intra-articulare
ligamenta sternocostalia
    radiata
ligamenta
    sternopericardiaca
l. stylohyoideum
l. stylomandibulare
l. supraspinale
l. suspensorium clitoridis
ligamenta suspensoria
    mammae
l. suspensorium ovarii
l. suspensorium penis
l. talocalcaneare
    interosseum

lig·a·men·tum *(continued)*
l. talocalcaneare laterale
l. talocalcaneare mediale
l. talofibulare anterius
l. talofibulare posterius
l. talonaviculare
ligamenta tarsi dorsalia
ligamenta tarsi interossea
ligamenta tarsi plantaria
l. teres femoris
l. teres hepatis
l. teres uteri
l. testis
l. thyreoepiglotticum
l. thyroepiglotticum
l. thyrohyoideum laterale
l. thyrohyoideum
    medianum
l. tibiofibulare anterius
l. tibiofibulare posterius
l. tibionaviculare
ligamenta trachealia
l. transversum acetabuli
l. transversum atlantis
l. transversum cruris
l. transversum genus
l. transversum pelvis
l. transversum perinei
l. trapezoideum
l. triangulare sinistrum
    hepatis
l. umbilicale laterale
l. umbilicale mediale
l. vaginale
l. venae cavae sinistrae
l. venosum
l. venosum [Arantii]
l. ventriculare
l. vestibulare
l. vocale
li·gand
li·gase
li·gate
li·ga·tion
    Barron l.
    proximal l.
    quadruple l.
    rubber band l.

li·ga·tion *(continued)*
    surgical l.
    teeth l.
    tubal l.
lig·a·tor
lig·a·ture
    l. in continuity
    double l.
    elastic l.
    grass-line l.
    interlacing l.
    interlocking l.
    lateral l.
    occluding l.
    provisional l.
    soluble l.
    Stannius l.
    suboccluding l.
    terminal l.
    thread-elastic l.
ligg. — ligaments
    ligamenta
light
    actinic l.
    axial l.
    central l.
    l. chaos
    coherent l.
    cold l.
    l. difference
    diffused l.
    Finsen l.
    idioretinal l.
    infrared l.
    intrinsic l.
    Landeker-Steinberg l.
    l. minimum
    Minin l.
    monochromatic l.
    neon l.
    oblique l.
    polarized l.
    reflected l.
    refracted l.
    Simpson l.
    transmitted l.
    Tyndall l.
    ultraviolet l.

light *(continued)*
    white l.
    Wood's l.
light·en·ing
Light·wood syndrome
Lig·nac's disease
Lig·nac-Fan·co·ni syndrome
lig·ne·ous
lig·no·caine
lig·no·cer·ic acid
lig·num
    l. sanctum
    l. vitae
lig·ro·in
lig·u·la
Lil·i·en·thal's probe
Lilie·quist's membrane
limb
    anacrotic l.
    aneurogenic l.
    l's of anthelix
    ascending l.
    catacrotic l.
    descending l.
    l. of incus, long
    l. of incus, short
    inferior l.
    l. of internal capsule,
      anterior
    l. of internal capsule,
      posterior
    lower l.
    pectoral l.
    pelvic l.
    phantom l.
    l. of stapes, anterior
    l. of stapes, posterior
    superior l.
    thick ascending l.
    thick descending l.
    thick l. of loop of Henle
    thoracic l.
    upper l.
lim·bal
Lim·berg flap
lim·ber·neck
lim·bi
lim·bic

Lim·bi·trol
lim·bous
lim·bus *pl.* lim·bi
    l. acetabuli
    alveolar l. of mandible
    alveolar l. of maxilla
    l. alveolaris mandibulae
    l. alveolaris maxillae
    l. angulosus
    l. chorioideus
    l. conjunctivae
    l. of cornea
    l. corneae
    l. corticalis
    l. foraminis ovalis
    l. fossae ovalis
    l. fossae ovalis [Vieussenii]
    l. luteus retinae
    l. medullaris
    l. membranae tympani
    l. of sclera
    l. of sphenoid bone
    spiral l.
    l. of Vieussens
lime
    barium hydroxide l.
    chlorinated l.
    slaked l.
    soda l.
li·men *pl.* li·mi·na
    difference l.
    l. of insula
    l. insulae
    l. nasi
    l. of twoness
li·mes
    l. dose
    l. nul dose
    l. zero
lim·i·na
lim·i·nal
lim·i·nom·e·ter
lim·it
    Anstie's l.
    assimilation l.
    audibility l.
    elastic l.
    l. of flocculation

lim·it *(continued)*
    l. of perception
    quantum l.
    saturation l.
lim·i·tans
lim·i·ta·tion
    eccentric l.
lim·it dex·trin·ase
lim·i·troph·ic
Lim·na·tis
    L. nilotica
lim·o·nene
li·moph·thi·sis
li·mo·sis
li·mo·ther·a·py
Lin·a·cre, Thomas
lin·a·ma·rin
Lin·co·cin
lin·co·my·cin
    l. hydrochloride
linc·ture
linc·tus
lin·dane
Lin·dau's disease
Lin·dau-von Hip·pel disease
Lind·bergh pump
Linde·mann method
Lind·ner bodies
line
    abdominal l.
    absorption l's
    acanthiomeatal l.
    accretion l's
    adrenal l.
    ala-tragal l.
    Aldrich-Mees l's
    alveolobasilar l.
    Amberg's l.
    l. of Amici
    angular l.
    anococcygeal l., white
    anocutaneous l.
    anorectal l.
    arcuate l.
    Arlt's l.
    arterial l. (A-line)
    atropic l.
    auriculobregmatic l.

line *(continued)*
  axial l.
  axillary l.
  l's of Baillarger
  base l.
  base-apex l.
  basinasal l.
  basiobregmatic l.
  Baudelocque's l.
  Beau's l's
  biauricular l.
  bi-iliac l.
  bismuth l.
  blood l.
  blue l.
  Borsieri's l.
  Brödel's white l.
  Brücke's l's
  Bryant's l.
  bufylline
  Burton's l.
  calcification l's
  Camper's l.
  cell l.
  cement l.
  cervical l.
  Chamberlain's l.
  Chaussier's l.
  chorionic plate l.
  Clapton's l.
  clavicular l.
  cleavage l's
  Conradi's l.
  contour l's
  copper l.
  Correra's l.
  Corrigan's l.
  costoarticular l.
  costoclavicular l.
  costophrenic septal l's
  Crampton's l.
  cricoclavicular l.
  cruciate l.
  curved l. of ilium
  curved l. of occipital bone
  Czermak's l's
  Daubenton's l.
  dentate l.

line *(continued)*
  De Salle's l.
  developmental l's
  Dobie's l.
  l. of Douglas
  Duhot's l.
  dynamic l's
  Eberth's l's
  l's of Ebner
  ectental l.
  Egger's l.
  Ellis' l.
  Ellis-Garland l.
  embryonic l.
  epiphyseal l.
  established cell l.
  l's of expression
  external oblique l.
  facial l.
  Farre's white l.
  Feiss' l.
  finish l.
  fissural l.
  l. of fixation
  Fleischner's l.
  flexure l.
  focal l., anterior
  focal l., posterior
  Fränkel's l.
  Frommann's l's
  fulcrum l.
  fulcrum l., retentive
  fulcrum l., stabilizing
  Gant's l.
  gas density l.
  genal l.
  l. of Gennari
  germ l.
  gingival l.
  gluteal l., anterior
  gluteal l., inferior
  gluteal l., posterior
  Gottinger's l.
  Granger l.
  gray l.
  growth arrest l.
  Gubler's l.
  gum l.

line *(continued)*
    Haller's l.
    Hampton l.
    Harris l's
    health l.
    heave l.
    Helmholtz's l.
    Hensen's l.
    Hilgenreiner's l.
    Hilton's white l.
    Holden's l.
    hot l.
    Hudson's l.
    Hudson-Stähli l.
    Hueter's l.
    Hunter's l.
    iliopectineal l.
    imbrication l's of
      cementum
    imbrication l's of Pickerill
    incremental l's
    inflating l.
    infracostal l.
    infrascapular l.
    intercondylar l.
    intercondyloid l.
    intermediate l. of iliac crest
    interspinal l.
    intertrochanteric l.
    intertuberal l.
    intertubercular l.
    intraperiod l's
    isoeffect l's
    isoelectric l.
    Jadelot's l's
    l. of Kaes
    Kerley's l's
    Kilian's l.
    Krause's l.
    labial l.
    Langer's l's
    Lanz l.
    lateral l.
    lateral sinus l.
    lateral sternal l.
    lead l.
    lip l.
    lip l., high

line *(continued)*
    lip l., low
    Lorentzian l.
    lower lung l.
    McKee's l.
    magnetic l's of force
    major dense l's
    major period l's
    mamillary l.
    mammary l.
    median l.
    medioclavicular l.
    Mees' l's
    mercurial l.
    mesenteric l.
    Meyer's l.
    midaxillary l.
    midclavicular l.
    midspinal l.
    midsternal l.
    milk l.
    l's of minimal tension
    Monro's l.
    Monro-Richter l.
    Morgan's l.
    Moyer's l.
    mucogingival l.
    Muercke's l's
    muscular l's of scapula
    mylohyoid l. of mandible
    mylohyoidean l.
    nasal l.
    nasobasal l.
    nasobasilar l.
    nasolabial l.
    nasosubnasal l.
    Nélaton's l.
    neonatal l.
    nigra l.
    nipple l.
    nuchal l., highest
    nuchal l., inferior
    nuchal l., median
    nuchal l., superior
    nuchal l., supreme
    Obersteiner-Redlich l.
    oblique l.
    obturator l.

line *(continued)*
  l. of occlusion
  oculozygomatic l.
  Ogston's l.
  omphalospinous l.
  orthostatic l's
  Ouchterlony l.
  l's of Owen
  papillary l.
  pararectal l.
  parasternal l.
  paravertebral l.
  Pastia's l's
  pectinate l.
  pectineal l.
  pelvic pain l.
  period l's
  Pickerill's imbrication l's
  pigmented l. of the cornea
  pleuroesophageal l.
  Poirier's l.
  popliteal l. of femur
  popliteal l. of tibia
  postaxillary l.
  Poupart's l.
  preaxillary l.
  precentral l.
  primitive l.
  profile l.
  protrusive l.
  pupillary l.
  quadrate l.
  radial longitudinal l.
  recessional l's
  regression l.
  Reid's base l.
  relaxed skin tension l's
  Retzius' l's
  Richter-Monro l.
  Robson's l.
  Rolando's l.
  Roser's l.
  rough l. of femur
  Salter's l's
  scapular l.
  Schoemaker's l.
  l's of Schreger
  Schwalbe's l.

line *(continued)*
  segmental l's
  semicircular l. of Douglas
  semilunar l.
  semilunar l. of Spieghel
  septal l.
  Sergent's white adrenal l.
  Shenton's l.
  simian l.
  Skinner's l.
  soleal l. of tibia
  Spieghel's l.
  Spigelius' l.
  spiral l. of femur
  Stähli's l.
  Stähli's pigment l.
  sternal l.
  sternal l., lateral
  sternomastoid l.
  subcostal l.
  subscapular l's
  superficial l. of the cornea
  supracondylar l. of femur,
    lateral
  supracondylar l. of femur,
    medial
  supracrestal l.
  supraorbital l.
  survey l.
  suture l.
  Sydney l.
  sylvian l.
  temporal l.
  Thompson's l.
  thyroid red l.
  Toldt's l.
  Topinard's l.
  tram l's
  transverse l. of sacrum
  trapezoid l.
  triradiate l's
  Trümmerfeld l.
  Ullmann's l.
  umbilicoiliac l.
  l. of Venus
  vertebral l.
  Veslingius' l.
  vibrating l.

line *(continued)*
  Virchow's l.
  visual l.
  Voigt's l's
  Wagner's l.
  Weiger's l.
  white l.
  white l. of Fränkel
  Wimberger's l.
  Wrisberg's l's
  Y l.
  Z l.
  l's of Zahn
  Zöllner's l's.
lin·ea *pl.* lin·eae
  l. alba
  l. epiphysialis
  l. fusca
  l. iliopectinea
  l. innominata
  l. intertrochanterica
  l. mamillaris
  l. nigra
  l. pararectalis
  l. para-sternalis
  l. paravertebralis
  l. pectinea femoris
  l. poplitea tibiae
  l. scapularis
  l. semilunaris
  l. semilunaris [Spigeli]
  l. spiralis
  l. sternalis
  l. trapezoidea
  l. vertebralis
lin·eae
lin·e·age
  cell l.
lin·e·al
lin·e·ar
line·breed·ing
lin·er
  cavity l.
  soft l.
Line·weav·er-Burk equation
Line·weav·er-Burk plot
Ling's methods

lin·gua *pl.* lin·guae
  l. cerebelli
  l. frenata
  l. geographica
  l. nigra
  l. plicata
  l. villosa nigra
lin·guae
lin·gual
lin·gua·le
lin·gua·lis *pl.* lin·gua·les
lin·gual·ly
Lin·guat·u·la
  L. rhinaria
  L. serrata
lin·guat·u·li·a·sis
lin·guat·u·lid
Lin·gua·tu·li·dae
lin·guat·u·lo·sis
lin·gui·form
lin·gu·la *pl.* lin·gu·lae
  l. cerebelli
  l. of cerebellum
  l. of left lung
  l. of lower jaw
  l. of mandible
  l. mandibulae
  l. pulmonis sinistri
  l. of sphenoid
  sphenoidal l.
  l. of sphenoidalis
lin·gu·lae
lin·gu·lar
lin·gu·late
lin·gu·lec·to·my
lin·guo·ax·i·al
lin·guo·ax·io·gin·gi·val
lin·guo·cer·vi·cal
lin·guo·cli·na·tion
lin·guo·clu·sion
lin·guo·den·tal
lin·guo·dis·tal
lin·guo·gin·gi·val
lin·guo·in·ci·sal
lin·guo·me·si·al
lin·guo-oc·clu·sal
lin·guo·pap·il·li·tis

lin·guo·place·ment
lin·guo·plate
lin·guo·pul·pal
lin·guo·ver·sion
lin·i·ment
    camphor l.
    medicinal soft soap l.
lin·i·men·tum
    l. camphorae
    l. saponis mollis
li·nin
li·ni·tis
    l. plastica
link·age
    sex l.
    Y l.
linked
lin·nae·an
lin·ne·an
Lin·o·dil
Lin·og·na·thus
lin·o·le·ic acid
lin·o·le·in
lin·o·len·ic acid
lin·o·lic acid
lin·seed
Lin·ser method
Lin·sto·wi·i·dae
lint
lin·tin
Lin·ton procedure
li·num
Lin·zen·meier test
Li·or·e·sal
li·o·thy·ro·nine
    l. sodium
li·o·trix
LIP — lymphocytic interstitial pneumonitis
lip
    acetabular l.
    articular l.
    cleft l.
    dorsal l. of blastophore
    double l.
    glenoid l.
    greater l. of pudendum
    Hapsburg l.

lip *(continued)*
    inferior l.
    lower l.
    rhombic l.
    superior l.
    tapir l's
    upper l.
lip·ac·i·de·mia
lip·ac·i·du·ria
lip·aro·cele
lip·a·ro·dysp·nea
li·par·om·pha·lus
lip·ase
    acid l.
    pancreatic l.
li·pa·sic
lip·as·uria
li·pec·to·my
    submental l.
    suction l.
lip·ede·ma
li·pe·mia
    alimentary l.
    diabetic l.
    postprandial l.
    l. retinalis
li·pe·mic
lip·fan·o·gen
lip·id
    l. A
    Gaucher l.
    Niemann-Pick l.
    skin surface l.
lip·i·dase
lip·i·de·mia
lip·id·ic
lip·i·dol
lip·i·dol·y·sis
lip·i·do·lyt·ic
lip·i·do·sis
    cerebral l.
    cerebroside l.
    galactosylceramide l.
    ganglioside l.
    glucosylceramide l.
    hereditary dystopic l.
    neurovisceral l.
    sphingomyelin l.

lip·i·do·sis *(continued)*
    sulfatide l.
lip·id·temns
lip·i·du·ria
Lip·io·dol
Lip·mann, Fritz Albert
lipo·ad·e·no·ma
lipo·am·ide
lipo·ar·thri·tis
lipo·at·ro·phy
    insulin l.
lipo·blast
lipo·blas·to·ma
lipo·blas·to·ma·to·sis
lipo·ca·ic
lipo·car·di·ac
lipo·cata·bol·ic
lipo·cele
lipo·cel·lu·lose
lipo·cer·a·tous
lipo·cere
lipo·chon·dro·ma
lipo·chrome
lipo·chro·me·mia
lip·o·chro·mo·gen
lipo·cla·sis
lipo·clas·tic
lipo·cor·ti·coid
lipo·cy·a·nine
lipo·cyte
lipo·der·ma·to·scle·ro·sis
lipo·di·er·e·sis
lipo·di·er·et·ic
lipo·dys·tro·phia
    l. intestinalis
    l. progressiva
lipo·dys·tro·phy
    acquired generalized l.
    acquired partial l.
    cephalothoracic l.
    congenital progressive l.
    familial l. of limbs and
      trunks
    generalized l.
    inferior l.
    insulin l.
    intestinal l.
    partial l.

lipo·dys·tro·phy *(continued)*
    progressive l.
    progressive congenital l.
    progressive partial l.
    reverse partial l.
    total l.
    total l. and acromegaloid
      gigantism
    trochanteric l.
li·pof·er·ous
lipo·fi·bro·ma
lipo·fus·cin
lipo·fus·cin·o·sis
    neuronal ceroid l.
lipo·gen·e·sis
lipo·ge·net·ic
lip·o·gen·ic
li·pog·e·nous
lipo·gran·u·lo·ma
lipo·gran·u·lo·ma·to·sis
    Farber's l.
lipo·hem·ar·thro·sis
lipo·he·mia
Lipo-Hep·in
lipo·his·tio·di·er·e·sis
lipo·hy·a·lin
lipo·hy·per·tro·phy
    insulin l.
lipo·ic acid
lip·oid
    anisotropic l.
    Forssman's l.
lip·oi·dal
lip·oi·de·mia
li·poi·dic
li·poi·do·lyt·ic
lip·oi·do·sis
    arterial l.
    cerebroside l.
    cholesterol l.
    l. cutis et mucosae
    renal l.
lip·oid·pro·tein·o·sis
lip·oid·sid·e·ro·sis
lip·oi·du·ria
lipo·lip·oi·do·sis
Lipo-Lu·tin
li·pol·y·sis

lipo·lyt·ic
li·po·ma
    l. annulare colli
    l. arborescens
    calcified l.
    l. capsulare
    l. cavernosum
    l. of corpus callosum
    diffuse l.
    diffuse symmetrical l's of
      neck
    l. diffusum renis
    l. dolorosa
    fat cell l., fetal
    l. fibrosum
    intradural l.
    intramuscular l.
    l. myxomatodes
    nevoid l.
    l. ossificans
    renal l.
    l. sarcomatodes
    l. of spermatic cord
    spinal l.
    telangiectatic l.
    l. telangiectodes
li·po·ma·toid
li·po·ma·to·sis
    l. atrophicans
    congenital l. of pancreas
    diffuse l.
    l.   dolorosa
    l. gigantea
    medullary l.
    l. neurotica
    nodular circumscribed l.
    renal l.
    l. renis
    replacement l. of kidney
    symmetrical l.
li·po·ma·tous
lipo·me·nin·go·cele
li·po·me·ria
lipo·meta·bol·ic
lipo·me·tab·o·lism
lipo·mi·cron
li·pom·pha·lus

lipo·mu·co·poly·sac·cha·ri·
    do·sis
lipo·myo·he·man·gi·o·ma
lipo·my·o·ma
lipo·myx·o·ma
lipo·myxo·sar·co·ma
lipo·ne·phro·sis
Lipo·nys·soi·des
li·pop·a·thy
lipo·pec·tic
lipo·pe·nia
lipo·pe·nic
lipo·pep·tid
lipo·pex·ia
lipo·pex·ic
lipo·phage
lipo·pha·gia
    l. granulomatosis
lipo·pha·gic
li·poph·a·gy
lipo·phan·e·ro·sis
lipo·phil
lipo·phil·ia
lipo·phil·ic
lipo·phore
lipo·plas·tic
lipo·poly·sac·cha·ride
lipo·pro·tein
    high-density l. (HDL)
    intermediate-density l.
      (IDL)
    low-density l. (LDL)
    Lp(a) l.
    plasma l.
    very low-density l. (VLDL)
    l. X
lipo·pro·tein·emia
lipo·pro·tein lip·ase
lipo·pro·tein·o·sis
lipo·rho·din
lipo·sar·co·ma
    myxoid l.
lip·ose
li·po·sis
lipo·sol·u·ble
lipo·some
li·pos·to·my
Lip·o·syn

lipo·tei·choic acid
lipo·thy·mia
lipo·troph
lipo·troph·ic
li·pot·ro·phy
lipo·trop·ic
β-lipo·tro·pin
li·pot·ro·pism
li·pot·ro·py
lipo·tu·ber·cu·lin
lipo·vac·cine
lipo·vi·tel·lin
lipo·xan·thine
li·pox·en·ous
li·pox·e·ny
li·pox·i·dase
li·poxy·ge·nase
lip·ox·ysm
lipo·yl trans·acet·y·lase
lip·pa
Lip·pes loop
lip·ping
lip·pi·tude
Lip·schütz bodies
Lip·schütz disease
Lip·schütz ulcer
li·pu·ria
li·pu·ric
Li·qua·mar
liq·ue·fa·cient
liq·ue·fac·tion
    gas l.
liq·ue·fac·tive
li·que·fy
li·ques·cent
liq·uid
    Altmann's l.
    Fleming's l.
    Müller's l.
    Thoma's l.
liq·ui·form
liq·uo·gel
li·quor *pl.* li·quors, li·quo·res
    l. amnii
    l. cerebrospinalis
    l. chorii
    l. cotunnii
    l. entericus

li·quor *(continued)*
    l. folliculi
    l. gastricus
    mother l.
    l. pancreaticus
    l. pericardii
    l. prostaticus
    l. puris
    l. sanguinis
    l. of Scarpa
    l. scarpae
    l. seminis
li·quo·res
Lis·a·cort
Lis·franc's amputation
Lis·franc's joint
Lis·franc's ligament
Lis·franc's tubercle
lisp·ing
Lis·sau·er's column
Lis·sau·er's marginal zone
Lis·sau·er's paralysis
Lis·sau·er's tract
Lis·sen·ceph·a·la
lis·sen·ce·phal·ic
lis·sen·ceph·a·ly
lis·sive
lis·ten·ing
    dichotic l.
Lis·ter, Baron Joseph
Lis·ter's tubercle
Lis·ter·el·la
lis·ter·el·lo·sis
Lis·te·ria
    L. monocytogenes
lis·te·ri·al
lis·ter·i·o·sis
lis·ter·ism
Lis·ting's law
Lis·ting's plane
list·ing gait
Lis·ton's knives
Lis·ton's operation
li·ter
lith·a·gog·ec·ta·sia
lith·a·gogue
Lith·ane
lith·an·gi·uria

lith·arge
lith·ate
li·thec·bo·le
li·thec·ta·sy
li·thec·to·my
li·the·mia
li·the·mic
lith·ia
lith·i·as·ic
li·thi·a·sis
    appendicular l.
    l. conjunctivae
    pancreatic l.
    renal l.
lith·ic
lith·ic acid
lith·i·co·sis
lith·i·um
    l. carbonate
    l. citrate
litho·ce·no·sis
litho·cho·late
litho·cho·lic acid
litho·cho·lyl·gly·cine
litho·cho·lyl·tau·rine
litho·clast
litho·cys·tot·o·my
litho·di·al·y·sis
litho·gen·e·sis
lith·o·gen·ic
li·thog·e·nous
litho·kel·y·pho·pe·di·on
litho·kel·y·phos
litho·labe
li·thol·a·paxy
li·thol·o·gy
li·thol·y·sis
litho·lyte
litho·lyt·ic
li·thom·e·ter
litho·mos·cus
litho·myl
litho·ne·phri·tis
litho·ne·phrot·o·my
litho·pe·di·on
litho·scope
li·tho·sis
Lith·o·stat

litho·tome
li·thot·o·mist
li·thot·o·my
    bilateral l.
    high l.
    lateral l.
    marian l.
    median l.
    mediolateral l.
    perineal l.
    prerectal l.
    rectal l.
    rectovesical l.
    suprapubic l.
    vaginal l.
    vesicovaginal l.
li·thot·o·ny
litho·tre·sis
    ultrasonic l.
litho·trip·sy
    electrohydraulic l.
    extracorporeal shock wave
      l.
litho·trip·tic
litho·trip·ter
litho·trip·tor
    Dornier gallstone l.
litho·trip·to·scope
litho·trip·tos·co·py
litho·trite
    cystoscopic l.
    electrohydraulic l.
li·thot·ri·ty
litho·troph
lith·ous
lith·ox·i·du·ria
lith·ure·sis
lith·ure·te·ria
lith·uria
lit·mo·ci·din
lit·mus
Lit·ten's diaphragm
Lit·ten's phenomenon
Lit·ten's sign
lit·ter
Lit·tle's area
Lit·tle's disease

Lit·tle intraocular lens (IOL)
   implant
Lit·tre's crypts
Lit·tre's glands
Lit·tre's hernia
lit·tri·tis
Litz·mann's obliquity
li·ve·do
   l. annularis
   l. calorica
   l. racemosa
   l. reticularis
   l. telangiectatica
liv·e·doid
liv·er
   albuminoid l.
   amyloid l.
   biliary cirrhotic l.
   brimstone l.
   bronze l.
   cirrhotic l.
   degraded l.
   desiccated l.
   fatty l.
   floating l.
   foamy l.
   frosted l.
   hobnail l.
   icing l.
   infantile l.
   iron l.
   lardaceous l.
   nutmeg l.
   pigmented l.
   polycystic l.
   sago l.
   stasis l.
   sugar-icing l.
   wandering l.
   waxy l.
li·ve·tin
Li·vi's index
liv·id
li·vid·i·ty
   cadaveric l.
   postmortem l.
Li·vi·e·ra·to's sign
Liv·ing·ston's triangle

li·vor pl. li·vo·res
   l. mortis
Lix·am·i·nol
lix·iv·i·a·tion
lix·iv·i·um
Li·zars' operation
LLL — left lower lobe (of the
   lung)
Lloyd syndrome
LLQ — left lower quadrant
LLS — lazy leukocyte
   syndrome
LM — light minimum
   linguomesial
LMA — left mentoanterior
LMF — lymphocyte mitogenic
   factor
LMP — left mentoposterior
LMR — localized magnetic
   resonance
LMT — left mentotransverse
LNPF — lymph node
   permeability factor
LOA — left occipitoanterior
Loa
   L. loa
load
   occlusal l.
load·ing
lo·a·i·a·sis
lo·bar
lo·bate
lo·ba·tion
   renal l.
lobe
   ansiform l.
   appendicular l.
   azygos l.
   caudate l. of cerebrum
   caudate l. of liver
   cuneate l.
   cuneiform l.
   flocculonodular l.
   frontal l.
   gracile l. of cerebellum
   grand l. limbique of Broca
   hepatic l's

lobe *(continued)*
 Home's l.
 inferior crescentic l. of
  cerebellum
 limbic l.
 linguiform l.
 neural l.
 occipital l.
 olfactory l.
 optic l's
 parietal l.
 piriform l.
 polyalveolar l.
 prefrontal l.
 l's of prostate
 pulmonary l's
 pyriform l.
 pyramidal l. of thyroid
  gland
 quadrangular l. of
  cerebellum
 quadrate l. of cerebral
  hemisphere
 quadrate l. of liver
 renal l's
 Riedel's l.
 semilunar l., inferior
 semilunar l., superior
 spigelian l.
 temporal l.
 vagal l.
 vermiform l.
 visceral l.
lo·bec·to·my
 sleeve l.
lo·be·lia
lob·e·line
lo·be·lism
lo·ben·da·zole
lo·bi
lo·bite
lo·bi·tis
Lo·bo's disease
Lo·boa lo·boi
lo·bo·cyte
lo·bo·my·co·sis
lo·bo·po·di·um *pl.* lo·bo·po·
 dia

lob·ose
Lo·bo·sea
lo·bot·o·my
 frontal l.
 prefrontal l.
 transorbital l.
Lob·stein's disease
Lob·stein's ganglion
Lob·stein's syndrome
lob·u·lar
lob·u·lat·ed
lob·u·la·tion
 fetal l.
 portal l.
lob·ule
 ansiform l.
 anterior lunate l.
 l. of auricle
 l. of azygos vein
 biventral l.
 central l. of cerebellum
 cerebellar l.
 cortical l's of kidney
 digastric l.
 ear l.
 floccular l.
 fusiform l.
 glandular l.
 glomerular l.
 gracile l.
 hepatic l's
 paracentral l.
 paramedian l.
 parietal l., inferior
 parietal l., superior
 portal l.
 primary l. of lung
 quadrangular l. of
  cerebellum
 quadrate l.
 renal l.
 respiratory l.
 secondary l. of lung
 semilunar l., caudal
 semilunar l., cranial
 semilunar l., inferior
 semilunar l., superior
 spermatic l's

lob·u·lette
lob·u·li
lob·u·li·za·tion
lob·u·lose
lob·u·lous
lob·u·lus *pl.* lob·u·li
  l. auriculae
  l. biventer
  l. centralis cerebelli
  l. clivi
  lobuli corticales renis
  l. culminis
  l. cuneiformis
  lobuli epididymidis
  l. folii
  lobuli glandulae
    mammariae
  lobuli glandulae thyroideae
  l. gracilis cerebelli
  lobuli hepatis
  lobuli mammae
  l. pancreatis
  l. paracentralis
  l. paramedianus cerebelli
  l. parietalis inferior
  l. parietalis superior
  lobuli pulmonum
  l. quadrangularis cerebelli
  l. semilunaris caudalis
  l. semilunaris cranialis
  l. semilunaris inferior
  l. semilunaris rostralis
  l. semilunaris superior
  l. simplex cerebelli
  lobuli testis
  lobuli thymi
lo·bus *pl.* lo·bi
  l. anterior cerebelli
  l. anterior hypophyseos
  l. caudalis cerebelli
  l. caudatus
  l. caudatus hepatis
  l. caudatus [Spigeli]
  l. centralis
  lobi cerebri
  l. clivi
  l. cranialis cerebelli
  l. falciformis

lo·bus *(continued)*
  l. flocculonodularis
  l. frontalis
  lobi glandulae mammariae
  lobi hepatis
  l. hepatis dexter
  l. hepatis sinister
  l. inferior pulmonis dextri
  l. inferior pulmonis sinistri
  l. insularis
  lobi mammae
  l. medius prostatae
  l. medius pulmonis dextri
  l. nervosus hypophyseos
  l. nervosus
    neurohypophyseos
  l. occipitalis
  l. olfactorius
  l. parietalis
  lobi placentae
  l. posterior cerebelli
  l. posterior hypophyseos
  l. prostatae dexter/sinister
  l. pyramidalis glandulae
    thyroideae
  l. quadratus hepatis
  lobi renales
  l. rostralis cerebelli
  l. spigelii
  l. superior pulmonis dextri
  l. superior pulmonis
    sinistri
  l. temporalis
  l. thymi [dexter/sinister]
  l. vagi
lo·cal
lo·cal·iza·tion
  cerebral l.
  germinal l.
  pneumotaxic l.
  selective l.
  spatial l.
lo·cal·ized
lo·cal·iz·er
lo·ca·tor
  abutment l.
  Berman-Moorhead l.
  electroacoustic l.

lo·ca·tor *(continued)*
Moorhead foreign body l.
Loc. dol. — L. loco dolenti (to the painful spot)
lo·chia
l. alba
l. cruenta
l. purulenta
l. rubra
l. sanguinolenta
l. serosa
lo·chi·al
lo·chio·col·pos
lo·chio·cyte
lo·chio·me·tra
lo·chio·me·tri·tis
lo·chi·or·rha·gia
lo·chi·or·rhea
lo·chi·os·che·sis
lo·chi·os·ta·sis
lo·cho·me·tri·tis
lo·ci
lock
friction l.
heparin l.
transfer l.
Locke's fluid
Locke's solution
Locke-Rin·ger solution
lock·ing
head l.
lock·jaw
Lock·wood's ligament
lo·co
lo·co·ism
lo·co·mo·tion
brachial l.
fictive l.
lo·co·mo·tive
lo·co·mo·tor
lo·co·mo·to·ri·al
lo·co·mo·to·ri·um
lo·co·mo·to·ry
Lo·cor·ten
loc·u·lar
loc·u·late
loc·u·la·tion
loc·u·li
loc·u·lus *pl.* loc·u·li

lo·cum
l. tenens
lo·cus *pl.* lo·ci, lo·ca
l. caeruleus
l. ceruleus
l. cinereus
l. coeruleus
complex l.
l. ferrugineus
H-2 l.
heteromorphic l.
histocompatibility l.
l. minoris resistentiae
l. niger
operator l.
l. perforatus anticus
l. perforatus posticus
PTC (phenylthiocarbamide) l.
l. ruber
lo·dox·a·mide tro·meth·amine
Loeb's deciduoma
Loeb's reaction
loef·fler·ia
loem·pe
Loe·nen sign
Loe·vit's cell
Loe·wi, Otto
Loe·wi's reaction
Loe·wi's symptom
Loe·wi's test
Löff·ler's agar
Löff·ler's blood serum
Löff·ler's culture medium
Löff·ler's disease
Löff·ler's endocarditis
Löff·ler's eosinophilia
Löff·ler's stain
Löff·ler's syndrome
log·a·dec·to·my
log·ag·no·sia
log·a·graph·ia
log·am·ne·sia
Lo·gan's bow
log·a·pha·sia
log·as·the·nia

loge
    l. de Guyon
Log Etron·ics
log·e·tron·og·ra·phy
log·it
logo·clo·nia
logo·gram
logo·ko·pho·sis
logo·ma·nia
log·op·a·thy
logo·pe·dia
logo·pe·dics
logo·ple·gia
log·or·rhea
    jargon aphasic l.
logo·scope
lo·gos·co·py
logo·spasm
Loh·mann's reaction
Lohn·stein's saccharimeter
lo·i·a·sis
loli·ism
Lo·lip·id
Lom·bard's test
Lom·bar·di's sign
lo·met·ra·line hy·dro·chlo·ride
lo·mo·fun·gin
lo·mo·some
Lo·mo·til
lo·mus·tine
Lon·cho·car·pus
Long's coefficient
Long's formula
lon·gev·i·ty
lon·gi·lin·e·al
lon·gi·man·ous
lon·gi·pe·date
lon·gi·ra·di·ate
lon·gis·si·mus
lon·gi·tu·di·nal
lon·gi·tu·di·na·lis
lon·gi·typ·i·cal
long·sight·ed·ness
lon·gus
loop
    Axenfeld's nerve l.
    Bricker l.

loop *(continued)*
    capillary l's
    cervical l.
    closed l.
    Cordonnier ureteroileal l.
    cutting l.
    gamma l.
    Gerdy's interauricular l.
    Granit l.
    Henle's l.
    l. of hypoglossal nerve
    Hyrtl's l.
    intestinal l.
    lenticular l.
    Lippes l.
    Meyer's l.
    nephronic l.
    open l.
    P l.
    l. of pectoral nerves
    peduncular l.
    platinum l.
    primitive intestinal l.
    QRS l.
    l. of recurrent laryngeal nerve
    regulatory feedback l.
    Roux-en-Y l.
    sentinel l.
    Silastic l's
    l's of spinal nerves
    Stoerck's l.
    subclavian l.
    vector l.
    ventricular l.
    l. of Vieussens
loop·ful
loop·o·gram
loo·sen·ing
Loo·ser's transformation zones
Loo·ser-Milk·man syndrome
LOP — left occipitoposterior
lo·per·amide hy·dro·chlo·ride
loph·odont
Lo·phoph·o·ra
    L. williamsii
lo·phoph·o·rine
lo·phot·ri·chous

Lo·pid
Lo·pres·sor
Lo·pur·in
Lo·rain's disease
Lo·rain's infantilism
Lo·rain's type
Lo·rain-Le·vi dwarf
lor·aj·mine hy·dro·chlo·ride
lor·a·ze·pam
lor·ba·mate
lor·cai·nide hy·dro·chlo·ride
lor·do·sco·li·o·sis
lor·do·sis
    compensatory l.
    dorsal l.
lor·dot·ic
Lo·rent·zi·an line
Lor·enz, Konrad Zacharias
Lor·enz's operation
Lor·enz's osteotomy
Lor·fan
lo·ri·ca *pl.* lo·ri·cae
lor·i·cate
Lor·i·dine
loss
    anaphase lag l.
    autoimmune sensorineural
      hearing l.
    birth l.
    coincidence l.
    conductive hearing l.
    congenital hearing l.
    dissociated sensory l.
    evaporative water l.
    hearing l.
    noise-induced hearing l.
    nonorganic hearing l.
    ototoxic hearing l.
    profound hearing l.
    saddle sensory l.
    sensorineural hearing l.
Los·sen's law
Los·sen's rule
LOT — left occipitotransverse
Lot. — L. lotio (lotion)
Lo·theis·sen's operation
lo·tio
    l. alba

lo·tio *(continued)*
    l. sulfurata
Lo·tio·blanc
lo·tion
    amphotericin B l.
    benzyl benzoate l.
    benzyl benzoate-
      chlorophenothane-benzo-
      caine l.
    betamethasone
      dipropionate l.
    betamethasone valerate l.
    calamine l.
    dimethisoquin
      hydrochloride l.
    flurandrenolide l.
    gamma benzene
      hexachloride l.
    Goulard's l.
    hydrocortisone l.
    lindane l.
    methylbenzethonium
      chloride l.
    nystatin l.
    selenium sulfide l.
    white l.
Lo·trim·in
Lo·tu·sate
Lou·is's angle
Lou·is's law
Lou·is-Bar syndrome
loupe
louse *pl.* lice
    biting l.
    body l.
    chicken l.
    clothes l.
    crab l.
    goat l.
    head l.
    horse l.
    pubic l.
    sucking l.
lous·i·cide
lov·a·sta·tin
Lo·ven reflex
Løv·set's method
Low-Beers projection

low-cer·vi·cal
Lo·we's disease
Lö·we's ring
Lo·we's syndrome
Lö·wen·berg's canal
Lö·wen·berg's forceps
Lö·wen·berg's scala
Lö·wen·stein-Jen·sen agar
Lö·wen·thal's tract
low·er·ing
 vapor pressure l.
Low·er's rings
Low·er's tubercle
Lö·witt's bodies
Lö·witt's lymphocytes
Low·man balance board
Lown-Gan·ong-Le·vine
 syndrome
lox·a·pine
 l. succinate
lox·ar·thron
lox·ar·thro·sis
lox·ia
Lox·i·tane
lox·oph·thal·mus
Lox·os·ce·les
 L. laeta
 L. reclusa
Lox·os·cel·i·dae
lox·os·ce·lism
 viscerocutaneous l.
lox·ot·o·my
loz·enge
LP — lumbar puncture
LPF — low-power field
 lymphocytosis-promoting
  factor
LPH — lipotropic hormone
LPL — lipoprotein lipase
LPN — licensed practical
 nurse
LPS — lipopolysaccharide
LRF — luteinizing hormone
 releasing factor
L/S — lecithin/sphingomyelin
 (ratio)
LSA — left sacroanterior

LSA — left sacroanterior
 Licentiate of Society of
  Apothecaries
LScA — left scapuloanterior
LScP — left scapuloposterior
LSD — lysergic acid
 diethylamide
LSH — lutein-stimulating
 hormone
LSO — lumbosacral orthosis
LSP — left sacroposterior
LST — left sacrotransverse
LT — lymphotoxin
LTB_4, LTC_4, etc. — symbols
 for various leukotrienes
LTF — lymphocyte
 transforming factor
LTH — luteotropic hormone
LTR — long terminal repeat
Lu·barsch's crystals
lubb
lubb-dupp
lu·bri·cant
Luc's operation
lu·can·thone hy·dro·chlo·ride
Lu·cas' sign
lu·cent
Lu·ci·ani's triad
lu·cid
lu·cid·i·ty
lu·cif·er·ase
lu·cif·er·in
lu·cif·u·gal
Lu·cil·ia
 L. caesar
 L. cuprina
 L. illustris
 L. regina
 L. sericata
Lu·cio leprosy
Lu·cio phenomenon
lu·cip·e·tal
Lücke's test
Lucké's virus
lück·en·schä·del
Luck·ett's operation
lu·co·ther·a·py
Lu·der-Shel·don syndrome

Lu·di·o·mil
Lud·loff's sign
Lud·wig's angina
Lud·wig's angle
Lud·wig's ganglion
Lud·wig's theory
Lu·er's syringe
lu·es
lu·et·ic
lu·ette
    Lieutaud's l.
lug
    occlusal l.
    retention l.
Lu·gol's caustic
Lu·gol's solution
Luhr maxillofacial system
Lukes-Col·lins classification
LUL — left upper lobe (of
   lungs)
lu·li·ber·in
lum·ba·go
    ischemic l.
lum·bar
lum·bar·iza·tion
lum·bo·ab·dom·i·nal
lum·bo·co·los·to·my
lum·bo·co·lot·o·my
lum·bo·cos·tal
lum·bo·cru·ral
lum·bo·dor·sal
lum·bo·dyn·ia
lum·bo·il·i·ac
lum·bo·in·gui·nal
lum·bo·sa·cral
lum·bri·cal
lum·bri·ci
lum·bri·cide
lum·bri·coid
lum·bri·co·sis
Lum·bri·cus
lum·bri·cus *pl.* lum·bri·ci
lum·bus
lu·men *pl.* lu·mi·na
    residual l.
lu·men-sec·ond
lu·mi·chrome
lu·mi·fla·vin

lu·mi·na
Lu·mi·nal
lu·mi·nal
lu·mi·nes·cence
lu·mi·nif·er·ous
lu·mi·no·phore
lu·mino·scope
lu·mi·nous
lu·mi·rho·dop·sin
lu·mi·some
lum·pec·to·my
Lums·den's center
lu·na·cy
lu·nar
lu·na·re
lu·nate
lu·na·tic
lu·na·to·ma·la·cia
lung
    arc-welder l.
    artificial l.
    bird-breeder's l.
    bird-fancier's l.
    black l.
    brown l.
    cardiac l.
    coal-miner's l.
    colliers' l.
    drowned l.
    eosinophilic l.
    farmer's l.
    fibroid l.
    fluid l.
    harvester's l.
    honeycomb l.
    hyperlucent l.
    iron l.
    masons' l.
    miners' l.
    mushroom workers' l.
    pigeon-breeder's l.
    postperfusion l.
    shock l.
    silo-filler's l.
    thresher's l.
    traumatic wet l.
    uremic l.
    vanishing l.

lung *(continued)*
   Vietnam l.
   wet l.
   white l.
lung·mo·tor
lung·worm
lu·nu·la *pl.* lu·nu·lae
   lunulae of aortic valves
   l. of nail
   lunulae of pulmonary
     trunk valves
   l. of scapula
   lunulae of semilunar
     valves
   l. unguis
lu·pi·form
lu·pi·nine
lu·pin·o·sis
lu·poid
lu·po·ma
lu·pus
   butterfly l.
   chilblain l.
   disseminated l.
     erythematosus
   disseminated follicular l.
   drug-induced l.
   l. endemicus
   l. erythematosus (LE)
   l. erythematosus, chilblain
   l. erythematosus,
     cutaneous
   l. erythematosus, discoid
     (DLE)
   l. erythematosus,
     hypertrophic
   l. erythematosus, systemic
     (SLE)
   l. erythematosus migrans
   l. erythematosus profundus
   l. erythematosus tumidus
   l. fibrosus
   hydralazine l.
   l. hypertrophicus
   laryngeal l.
   l. miliaris disseminatus
     faciei
   neonatal l.

lu·pus *(continued)*
   l. nephritis
   l. pernio
   postexanthematic l.
   l. profundus
   l. sclerosus
   l. serpiginosus
   transient neonatal
     systemic l. erythematosus
   l. tumidus
   l. verrucosus
   l. vulgaris
   l. vulgaris fibromatosus
   warty l.
LUQ — left upper quadrant
Lur·ia, Salvador Edward
Lu·ride
Lusch·ka's bursa
Lusch·ka's crypts
Lusch·ka's duct
Lusch·ka's gland
Lusch·ka's joint
Lusch·ka's muscle
Lusch·ka's nerve
Lus·tig-Gal·e·ot·ti vaccine
lu·te·al
lu·te·ec·to·my
lu·te·in
   serum l.
lu·te·in·ic
lu·te·in·iza·tion
lu·te·in·ize
Lu·tem·bach·er's complex
Lu·tem·bach·er's disease
Lu·tem·bach·er's syndrome
lu·teo·gen·ic
lu·teo·hor·mone
lu·te·oid
lu·te·ol·y·sin
   uterine l.
lu·te·ol·y·sis
lu·te·o·ma
lu·teo·troph
lu·teo·troph·ic
lu·teo·tro·phin
lu·teo·trop·ic
lu·teo·tro·pin
lu·te·ti·um

Lu·ther·an blood group
Lu·trex·in
Lu·tro·mone
lu·tu·trin
Lutz-Splen·dore-Al·mei·da
  disease
Lut·zo·my·ia
  L. *flaviscutellata*
  L. *intermedia*
  L. *longipalpis*
  L. *noguchu*
  L. *olmeca*
  L. *peruensis*
  L. *pessoai*
  L. *trapidoi*
  L. *verrucarum*
  L. *umbratilis*
lux
lux·a·tio
  l. coxae congenita
  l. erecta
  l. imperfecta
  l. perinealis
lux·a·tion
  Malgaigne's l.
lux·u·ri·ant
lux·us
Luys' body
Luys' body syndrome
Luys' nucleus
LVE — left ventricular
  diastolic pressure
LVH — left ventricular
  hypertrophy
LVN — licensed vocational
  nurse
Lwoff, André Michael
ly·ase
  heparin l.
  isocitrate l.
ly·can·thro·py
ly·ce·ta·mine
Lych·nis gith·a·go
ly·cine
ly·co·pene
ly·co·pe·ne·mia
Ly·co·per·da·les
Ly·co·per·don

ly·co·per·do·no·sis
Ly·co·po·di·um
ly·co·po·di·um
lyco·rine
Lyc·o·ris
Ly·co·sa ta·ren·tu·la
lyd·i·my·cin
lye
Ly·ell's disease
Ly·ell's syndrome
Ly·gran·um
ly·ing-in
Lyme disease
Lym·naea
lymph
  aplastic l.
  corpuscular l.
  croupous l.
  euplastic l.
  fibrinous l.
  inflammatory l.
  intercellular l.
  intravascular l.
  plastic l.
  tissue l.
lym·pha
lym·pha·den
lym·phad·e·nec·ta·sis
lym·phad·e·nec·to·my
lym·phad·en·hy·per·tro·phy
lym·pha·de·nia
lym·phad·e·ni·tis
  acute suppurative l.
  caseous l.
  mesenteric l.
  nonbacterial regional l.
  paratuberculous l.
  regional l.
  tuberculoid l.
  tuberculous l.
  venereal suppurative
    benign l.
lym·phad·e·no·cele
lym·phad·e·no·cyst
lym·phad·e·no·gram
lym·phad·e·nog·ra·phy
lym·phad·e·noid

lym·phad·e·no·leu·ko·poi·e·
sis
lym·phad·e·no·ma
   malignant l.
   multipole l.
lymph·ad·e·no·ma·to·sis
lymph·ad·e·nom·a·tous
lym·phad·e·nop·a·thy
   angioimmunoblastic l.
   angioimmunoblastic l. with
     dysproteinemia (AILD)
   dermatopathic l.
   giant follicular l.
   immunoblastic l.
   tuberculous l.
lym·phad·e·no·sis
   acute epidemic l.
   aleukemic l.
   benign l.
   l. benigna cutis
   leukemic l.
   malignant l.
lym·phad·e·not·o·my
lym·phad·e·no·va·rix
lym·pha·gogue
lym·phan·ge·itis
lym·phan·gi·al
lym·phan·gi·ec·ta·sia
   intestinal l.
lym·phan·gi·ec·ta·sis
   cystic l.
   pericaliceal l.
   pulmonary l.
lym·phan·gi·ec·tat·ic
lym·phan·gi·ec·to·des
lym·phan·gi·ec·to·my
lym·phan·gi·itis
lym·phan·gio·ad·e·nog·ra·
phy
lym·phan·gio·en·do·the·li·o·
ma
lym·phan·gio·fi·bro·ma
lym·phan·gio·gram
lym·phan·gi·og·ra·phy
   pedal l.
lym·phan·gio·leio·my·o·ma·
to·sis
lym·phan·gi·ol·o·gy

lym·phan·gi·o·ma
   capillary l.
   l. capsulare varicosum
   l. cavernosum
   cavernous l.
   l. circumscriptum
   cystic l.
   l. cysticum
   fissural l.
   simple l.
   l. simplex
   l. xanthelasmoideum
lym·phan·gi·om·a·tous
lym·phan·gio·my·o·ma
lym·phan·gio·my·o·ma·to·sis
lym·phan·gio·phle·bi·tis
lym·phan·gio·plas·ty
   Handley's l.
lym·phan·gio·sar·co·ma
lym·phan·gi·ot·o·my
lym·phan·gi·tis
   l. carcinomatosa
   carcinomatous l.
   l. epizootica
   gummatous l.
   nonvenereal sclerosing l.
   ulcerative l.
   l. ulcerosa pseudofarcinosa
lym·pha·phe·re·sis
lym·phat·ic
   afferent l.
   efferent l.
   gluteal l's
   ischial l's
   obturator l's
lym·phat·i·co·splen·ic
lym·phat·i·cos·to·my
lym·pha·tism
lym·pha·ti·tis
lym·pha·tog·e·nous
lym·pha·tol·o·gy
lym·pha·tol·y·sis
lym·pha·to·lyt·ic
lym·phec·ta·sia
lym·phe·de·ma
   congenital l.
   filarial l.

lym·phe·de·ma *(continued)*
  l. praecox
  l. tarda
lymph·en·do·the·li·o·ma
lym·phen·ter·itis
lymph·epi·the·li·o·ma
lym·phi·za·tion
lymph·no·di·tis
lym·pho·blast
lym·pho·blas·tic
lym·pho·blas·to·ma
lym·pho·blas·to·sis
lym·pho·cele
lym·pho·ce·ras·tism
lym·pho·ci·ne·sia
lym·pho·cys·to·sis
lym·pho·cy·ta·phe·re·sis
lym·pho·cyte
  amplifier T-l.
  atypical l.
  B l's
  cytotoxic T l's (CTL)
  educated T l.
  helper T l.
  killer l.
  large granular l's
  NUL l.
  primed l.
  Rieder's l.
  small l.
  suppressor T l.
  T l's
  thymus-dependent l's
  thymus-independent l's
  variant
    thymus-independent l.
lym·pho·cyt·ic
lym·pho·cy·to·blast
lym·pho·cy·to·ma
  benign cutaneous l.
  l. cutis
lym·pho·cy·to·pe·nia
lym·pho·cy·to·phe·re·sis
lym·pho·cy·to·poi·e·sis
lym·pho·cy·to·poi·et·ic
lym·pho·cy·tor·rhex·is
lym·pho·cy·to·sis
  acute infectious l.

lym·pho·cy·to·sis *(continued)*
  relative l.
lym·pho·cy·tot·ic
lym·pho·cy·to·tox·ic·i·ty
lym·pho·cy·to·tox·in
lym·pho·duct
lym·pho·epi·the·li·o·ma
lym·pho·gen·e·sis
lym·phog·e·nous
lym·pho·glan·du·la *pl.* lym·pho·glan·du·lae
lym·pho·gram
lym·pho·gran·u·lo·ma
  l. benignum
  l. inguinale
  l. malignum
  l. venereum
lym·pho·gran·u·lo·ma·to·sis
  benign l.
  l. cutis
  l. inguinalis
  l. maligna
lym·phog·ra·phy
lym·pho·his·tio·cyt·ic
lym·pho·his·tio·plas·ma·cyt·ic
lym·phoid
lym·phoi·dec·to·my
lym·phoi·do·cyte
lym·pho·ken·tric
lym·pho·kine
lym·pho·ki·ne·sis
lym·phol·o·gy
lym·phol·y·sis
  cell-mediated l. (CML)
lym·pho·lyt·ic
lym·pho·ma
  African l.
  B cell l.
  Burkitt's l.
  centroblastic l.
  centrocytic l.
  convoluted l.
  cutaneous T cell l.
  l. cutis
  diffuse l.
  fascicular l.
  follicular l.

lym·pho·ma *(continued)*
   follicular center cell l.
   giant follicle l.
   giant follicular l.
   histiocytic l.
   Hodgkin's l.
   immunoblastic l.
   intestinal l.
   Lennert's l.
   lymphoblastic l.
   lymphocytic l. of
     intermediate
     differentiation
   lymphocytic l.,
     plasmacytoid
   lymphocytic l., poorly
     differentiated
   lymphocytic l.,
     well-differentiated
   lymphoepithelioid cell l.
   lymphoplasmacytic l.
   malignant l.
   malignant l. of cattle
   Mediterranean l.
   mixed
     lymphocytic-histiocytic l.
   nodular l.
   non-Hodgkin's l's
   null type non-Hodgkin's l.
   pleomorphic l.
   prolymphocytic l.
   sclerosing l.
   signet-ring cell l.
   small B-cell l.
   stem cell l.
   T-cell l's.
   T-cell l., convoluted
   T-cell l., cutaneous
   T-cell l., small lymphocytic
   U-cell (undefined) l.
   undifferentiated l.
lym·pho·ma·toid
lym·pho·ma·to·sis
   neural l.
   ocular l.
   osteopetrotic l.
   visceral l.
lym·pho·ma·tous

lym·pho·myx·o·ma
lym·pho·no·di
lym·pho·nod·u·li
lym·pho·nod·u·lus *pl.* lym·pho·nod·u·li
   lymphonoduli splenici
lym·pho·no·dus *pl.* lym·pho·no·di
lym·pho·path·ia
   l. venereum
lym·phop·a·thy
   ataxic l.
lym·pho·pe·nia
lym·pho·pla·sia
   cutaneous l.
lym·pho·plasm
lym·pho·plas·ma·phe·re·sis
lym·pho·poi·e·sis
lym·pho·poi·et·ic
lym·pho·poi·e·tin
lym·pho·pro·lif·er·a·tive
lym·pho·re·tic·u·lar
lym·pho·re·tic·u·lo·sis
   benign l.
lym·phor·rhage
lym·phor·rha·gia
lym·phor·rhea
lymph·or·rhoid
lym·pho·sar·co·leu·ke·mia
lym·pho·sar·co·ma
   fascicular l.
   Murphy-Sturm l.
   poorly differentiated l.
   sclerosing l.
lym·pho·sar·co·ma·to·sis
lym·pho·sar·com·a·tous
lym·pho·scin·tig·ra·phy
   radiocolloid l.
lym·pho·scro·tum
lym·pho·spo·rid·i·o·sis
lym·phos·ta·sis
lym·pho·tax·is
lym·pho·tism
lym·pho·tox·ic
lym·pho·tox·in
lym·pho·troph·ic
lym·phot·ro·phy
lym·pho·trop·ic

lym·phous
lymph·uria
    filarial l.
lymph-vas·cu·lar
Lyn·chia mau·ra
Ly·nen, Feodor
lyn·es·tre·nol
Lyn·or·al
lyo·chrome
lyo·gel
Ly·on hypothesis
Ly·on-Rus·sell hypothesis
ly·on·iza·tion
ly·on·ized
lyo·phil
lyo·phile
lyo·phil·ic
ly·oph·i·li·za·tion
ly·oph·i·lize
lyo·phobe
lyo·pho·bic
ly·o·sol
lyo·sorp·tion
lyo·trop·ic
Ly·per·o·sia ir·ri·tans
Ly·po·nys·sus
ly·pres·sin
ly·ra
lyre
Lys — lysine
ly·sate
lyse
ly·se·mia
ly·ser·gic acid
    l. a. diethylamide (LSD)
ly·ser·gide
lys·i·din
    l. bitartrate
ly·sim·e·ter
ly·sin
    beta l.
    hot-cold l.
    immune l.
    sperm l.
ly·sine
ly·sine de·hy·dro·gen·ase

ly·sine ke·to·glu·ta·rate re·duc·tase
L-ly·sine:NAD ox·i·do·re·duc·tase
ly·sin·o·gen
lys·i·no·sis
ly·sis
    bone l.
    hot-cold l.
    immune l.
    osmotic l.
ly·so·ceph·a·lin
ly·so·chrome
ly·so·cy·thin
Ly·so·dren
ly·so·gen
ly·so·gen·e·sis
ly·so·gen·ic
ly·so·ge·nic·i·ty
ly·so·gen·iza·tion
ly·sog·e·ny
ly·so·ki·nase
ly·so·lec·i·thin
ly·so·phos·pha·tide
ly·so·phos·pha·tid·ic acid
ly·so·phos·pha·ti·dyl·cho·line
ly·so·phos·pho·li·pase
ly·so·so·mal
ly·so·some
ly·so·staph·in
ly·so·type
ly·so·zyme
ly·so·zy·mu·ria
lys·sa
Lys·sa·vi·rus
lys·sic
lys·soid
lys·so·pho·bia
Lys·ter tube
ly·syl
ly·syl hy·drox·y·lase
ly·syl ox·i·dase
ly·te·ri·an
lyt·ic
Lyt·ta
    L. vesicatoria
lyx·ose

M — mega-
M. — L. misce (mix)
   L. mistura (mixture)
M — molar (concentration)
   molar mass
   mutual inductance
M_r — relative molecular mass
m — median
   meter
   milli-
m. — minim
   molal
   L. musculus (muscle)
m- — meta-
μ — electrophoretic mobility
   the heavy chain of IgM
   linear attenuation
     coefficient
   micro-
   micron
   population mean
MA — Master of Arts
   mental age
   meter angle
mA — milliampere
μA — microampere
MAC — maximum allowable
  concentration
   membrane attack complex
   minimal alveolar
     concentration
Mac. — L. macerare
  (macerate)
Ma·ca·ca
   M. cynomulgus
   M. mulatta
Mc·Ar·dle's disease
Mc·Ar·dle's syndrome
Mc·Bride operation
Mc·Bur·ney's incision
Mc·Bur·ney's operation
Mc·Bur·ney's point
Mc·Bur·ney's sign
Mac·Cal·lum's patch
Mc·Carey-Kauf·man (M-K)
  medium

Mc·Car·thy's reflex
Mc·Clin·tock, Barbara
Mc·Clin·tock sign
Mac·Con·key's agar
Mc·Cort sign
Mc·Cune-Al·bright syndrome
Mac·don·ald index
Mc·Don·ald maneuver
Mc·Don·ald rule
Mac·dow·el's frenulum
Mac·dow·el's frenum
Mace
mac·er·ate
mac·er·a·tion
mac·er·a·tive
Mac·ew·en's operation
Mac·ew·en's sign
Mac·ew·en's triangle
Mc·Gaw pump
Mc·Ginn-White sign
Mc·Goon technique
Ma·cha·do-Jo·seph disease
Mache unit
ma·chine
   Cybex m.
   heart-lung m.
   Holtz m.
   Stryker Surgilav m.
   Surgitron m.
   Van de Graaff m.
   Wimshurst m.
Mac·ho·ver test
ma·cies
MAC INH — membrane
  attack complex inhibitor
Mc·In·tire
  aspiration-irrigation system
Mac·Kay-Marg electronic
  tonometer
Mc·Kee line
Mc·Kee-Far·rar acetabular
  cup
Mc·Kee-Far·rar hip
  arthroplasty
Mc·Kee-Far·rar prosthesis
Mack·en·rodt's ligament

Mac·ken·zie's disease
Mac·ken·zie's syndrome
Mc·Kin·non test
Mc·Krae herpes virus
Mac·lag·an's thymol turbidity
   test
Mc·Lean's formula
Mc·Lean's index
Mac·Lean-Max·well disease
Mac·leod, John James Rickard
Mc·Leod blood phenotype
Mac·Leod's capsular
   rheumatism
Mac·leod's syndrome
Mac·Munn's test
Mc·Mur·ray's sign
Mc·Mur·ray's test
Mc·Ne·mar test
Mc·Phee·ters' treatment
mac·rad·e·nous
mac·ren·ce·pha·lia
mac·ren·ceph·a·ly
mac·ro·ag·gre·gate
mac·ro·aleu·rio·spore
mac·ro·am·y·lase
mac·ro·am·yl·a·se·mia
mac·ro·am·yl·a·se·mic
mac·ro·anal·y·sis
Mac·rob·del·la
   M. decora
mac·ro·bi·o·ta
mac·ro·bi·ot·ic
mac·ro·blast
   m. of Naegeli
mac·ro·ble·pha·ria
mac·ro·bra·chia
mac·ro·car·dia
mac·ro·car·di·us
mac·ro·ce·phal·ic
mac·ro·ceph·a·lous
mac·ro·ceph·a·lus
mac·ro·ceph·a·ly
mac·ro·chei·lia
mac·ro·chei·ria
mac·ro·chem·i·cal
mac·ro·chem·is·try
mac·ro·chy·lo·mi·cron
mac·ro·chy·lo·mi·cron·emia

mac·ro·clit·o·ris
mac·ro·cne·mia
mac·ro·co·lon
mac·ro·co·nid·i·um *pl.* mac·
   ro·co·nid·ia
mac·ro·cor·nea
mac·ro·cra·nia
mac·ro·cryo·glob·u·lin·emia
mac·ro·cyst
mac·ro·cyte
mac·ro·cyt·ic
mac·ro·cy·the·mia
mac·ro·cy·to·sis
mac·ro·dac·ty·ly
Mac·ro·dan·tin
mac·ro·dont
mac·ro·don·tia
mac·ro·don·tic
mac·ro·don·tism
mac·ro·dys·tro·phia
   m. lipomatosa progressiva
mac·ro·el·e·ment
mac·ro·en·ceph·a·ly
mac·ro·e·ryth·ro·blast
mac·ro·es·the·sia
mac·ro·fau·na
mac·ro·flo·ra
mac·ro·gam·ete
mac·ro·ga·me·to·cyte
mac·ro·gam·ont
mac·ro·gen·e·sis
mac·ro·gen·ia
mac·ro·gen·i·to·so·mia
   m. precox
mac·ro·gin·gi·vae
mac·rog·lia
mac·ro·gli·al
mac·ro·glob·u·lin
   α_2-m.
mac·ro·glob·u·lin·emia
   Waldenström's m.
mac·ro·glos·sia
mac·ro·gna·thia
mac·ro·gol
   m. 400
   m. 4000
mac·ro·gra·phia
mac·rog·ra·phy

mac·ro·gy·ria
mac·ro·la·bia
mac·ro·lec·i·thal
mac·ro·leu·ko·blast
mac·ro·lide
mac·ro·lym·pho·cyte
mac·ro·lym·pho·cy·to·sis
mac·ro·mas·tia
mac·ro·ma·zia
mac·ro·me·lia
mac·rom·e·lus
mac·ro·mere
mac·ro·meth·od
mac·ro·mo·lec·u·lar
mac·ro·mol·e·cule
mac·ro·mono·cyte
mac·ro·my·elo·blast
mac·ro·nod·u·lar
mac·ro·nor·mo·blast
mac·ro·nu·cle·us
mac·ro·nu·tri·ent
mac·ro·nych·ia
mac·ro-or·chi·dism
mac·ro·par·a·site
mac·ro·pa·thol·o·gy
mac·ro·pe·nis
mac·ro·phage
   alveolar m.
   armed m.'s
   fixed m.
   free m.
   inflammatory m.
   tingible-body m.
mac·ro·phago·cyte
mac·ro·phago·cy·to·sis
ma·croph·a·gus
mac·ro·phal·lus
mac·roph·thal·mia
mac·roph·thal·mous
mac·ro·pla·sia
mac·ro·plas·tia
mac·ro·po·dia
mac·ro·poly·cyte
mac·ro·pro·lac·ti·no·ma
mac·ro·pro·my·elo·cyte
mac·ro·pro·so·pia
ma·crop·sia
mac·ro·rhin·ia

mac·ro·sce·lia
mac·ro·scop·ic
mac·ro·scop·i·cal
ma·cros·co·py
mac·ro·sig·moid
mac·ro·sis
mac·ros·mat·ic
mac·ro·so·ma·tia
   m. adiposa congenita
mac·ro·so·mia
mac·ro·spore
mac·ro·ste·reo·gno·sia
mac·ro·sto·mia
mac·ro·struc·tur·al
mac·ro·tia
mac·ro·tome
mac·ro·tooth *pl.* mac·ro·teeth
mac·u·la *pl.* mac·u·lae
   acoustic maculae
   maculae acusticae
   m. acustica sacculi
   m. acustica utriculi
   m. adherens
   maculae albidae
   maculae atrophicae
   cerebral m.
   maculae ceruleae
   m. communis
   m. corneae
   maculae cribrosae
   m. cribrosa inferior
   m. cribrosa media
   m. cribrosa superior
   m. densa
   false m.
   m. flava laryngis
   m. flava retinae
   m. folliculi
   m. germinativa
   m. gonorrhoeica
   maculae lacteae
   m. lutea retinae
   maculae of membranous
     labyrinth
   mongolian m.
   m. neglecta
   m. retinae
   m. retinae occludens

mac·u·la *(continued)*
  m. sacculi
  Saenger's m.
  m. solaris
  maculae tendineae
  m. utriculi
mac·u·lae
mac·u·lar
mac·u·late
mac·ule
mac·u·lo·cer·e·bral
mac·u·lo·pap·u·lar
mac·u·lo·ve·sic·u·lar
Mc·Vay operation
Mac·Wil·liam's test
mad·a·ro·sis
MADD — multiple acyl CoA
  dehydrogenation deficiency
Mad·den technique
mad·der
Mad·dox prism
Mad·dox rods
Mad·e·lung's deformity
Mad·e·lung's neck
Mad·len·er operation
Mad·u·rel·la
ma·du·ro·my·co·sis
mae·di
MAF — macrophage
  activating factor
maf·en·ide
  m. acetate
  m. hydrochloride
Maf·fuc·ci's syndrome
ma·fil·con A
Mag. — L. magnus (large)
mag·al·drate
Mag·an
ma·gen·bla·se
Ma·gen·die's foramen
Ma·gen·die's law
Ma·gen·die's sign
Ma·gen·die's solution
Ma·gen·die's space
Ma·gen·die's symptom
Ma·gen·die-Hert·wig sign
ma·gen·stras·se

ma·gen·ta
  m. 0
  m. I
  m. II
  m. III
  acid m.
  basic m.
  m. O
mag·got
  Congo floor m.
  rat-tail m.
mag·is·tery
mag·is·tral
mag·ma
  bentonite m.
  bismuth m.
  dihydroxyaluminum
    aminoacetate m.
  magnesia m.
  m. reticulare
Mag·na·cort
Mag·nan's movement
Mag·nan's sign
Mag·nan's symptom
mag·nes·emia
mag·ne·sia
  citrate of m.
  milk of m.
mag·ne·si·um
  m. aluminum silicate
  m. carbonate
  m. chloride
  m. citrate
  m. hydroxide
  m. oxide
  m. peroxide
  m. phosphate
  m. salicylate
  m. stearate
  m. sulfate
  m. sulfate, exsiccated
  m. trisilicate
mag·net
  denture m.
  Grüning's m.
  Haab's m.
  Hirschberg's m.

---

mag·ne·tism
   animal m.
mag·ne·ti·za·tion
   longitudinal m.
mag·ne·to·car·dio·graph
mag·ne·to·elec·tric·i·ty
mag·ne·to·en·ceph·a·lo·graph
mag·ne·tol·o·gy
mag·ne·tom·e·ter
mag·ne·to·ther·a·py
mag·ne·tron
mag·net·ro·pism
mag·ni·cel·lu·lar
mag·ni·fi·ca·tion
mag·ni·fy
mag·no·cel·lu·lar
Mag·no·lia
mag·no·lia
mag·num
Mag·nus and de Kleijn neck reflex
Mag·nu·son-Stack shoulder arthrotomy
Ma·haim bundle
Ma·her's disease
Mah·ler's sign
ma huang
MAI — *Mycobacterium avium-intracellulare*
Mai·er's sinus
maim
Mai·mon·i·des
main
   m. d'accoucheur
   m. en crochet
   m. fourché
   m. en griffe
   m. en lorgnette
   m. en pince
   m. en singe
   m. en squelette
   m. succulente
   m. de tranchées
main·tain·er
   space m.
main·te·nance

Mainz pouch urinary reservoir
mai·sin
Mai·son·neuve's amputation
Mai·son·neuve's bandage
Mai·son·neuve's urethrotome
Mais·siat's band
Mais·siat's ligament
Mais·siat's tract
maize
Ma·joc·chi's disease
Ma·joc·chi's purpura
ma·joon
Make·ham hypothesis
Mak·kas operation
mal
   m. de caderas
   m. de Cayenne
   m. comitial
   grand m.
   haut m.
   m. de Meleda
   m. de mer
   m. morado
   petit m.
   m. del pinto
   m. rouge
ma·la
mal·ab·sorp·tion
   congenital lactose m.
   glucose-galactose m., familial
   sucrose-isomaltose m., congenital
Mal·a·carne's antrum
Mal·a·carne's pyramid
Mal·a·carne's space
ma·la·cia
   m. cordis
   metaplastic m.
   myeloplastic m.
   porotic m.
   m. traumatica
ma·la·cic
mal·a·co·ma
mal·a·co·pla·kia
   m. vesicae
mal·a·co·sar·co·sis
mal·a·co·sis

mal·a·cos·te·on
mal·a·cot·ic
mal·a·cot·o·my
ma·lac·tic
mal·a·die
    m. des jambes
    m. de plongeurs
    m. de Roger
    m. du sommeil
    m. des tics
mal·ad·just·ment
mal·a·dy
ma·lag·ma
mal·aise
mal·a·ko·pla·kia
mal·align·ment
ma·lar
ma·lar·ia
    algid m.
    autochthonous m.
    benign subtertian m.
    benign tertian m.
    bilious remittent m.
    bovine m.
    cerebral m.
    double tertian m.
    dysenteric m.
    estivoautumnal m.
    falciparum m.
    gastric m.
    hemolytic m.
    hemorrhagic m.
    induced m.
    intermittent m.
    malariae m.
    malignant tertian m.
    nonan m.
    ovale m.
    pernicious m.
    quartan m.
    quintan m.
    quotidian m.
    recrudescent m.
    relapsing m.
    remittent m.
    subtertian m.
    tertian m.
    therapeutic m.

ma·lar·ia *(continued)*
    transfusion m.
    vivax m.
ma·lar·ia·ci·dal
ma·lar·i·al
ma·lar·ia·ther·a·py
ma·lar·i·ol·o·gist
ma·lar·i·ol·o·gy
ma·lar·io·ther·a·py
ma·lar·i·ous
ma·la·ris
mal·ar·tic·u·la·tion
Mal·as·sez's disease
Mal·as·sez's rests
Mal·as·se·zia
    M. furfur
    M. macfadyani
    M. ovalis
    M. tropica
mal·as·sim·i·la·tion
ma·late
ma·late de·hy·dro·gen·ase
ma·late-NAD de·hy·dro·gen·ase
ma·late-NADPH de·hy·dro·gen·ase
mal·a·thi·on
mal·ax·ate
mal·ax·a·tion
Mal·co·tran
mal·de·vel·op·ment
mal·di·ges·tion
male
mal·e·ate
ma·le·ic acid
ma·le·ic hy·dra·zide
mal·emis·sion
Ma·ler·ba's test
mal·erup·tion
mal·eth·a·mer
ma·le·yl·ace·to·ac·e·tate isom·er·ase
mal·for·ma·tion
    Arnold-Chiari m.
    arteriovenous m. (AVM)
    atrioventricular m. (AVM)
    cystic adenomatoid m.
    Ebstein's m.

mal·for·ma·tion *(continued)*
  Klippel-Feil m.
  Mondini m.
  Taussig-Bing m.
  vascular m.
mal·func·tion
  eustachian tube m.
Mal·gaigne's amputation
Mal·gaigne's luxation
Mal·gaigne's triangle
Mal·herbe's calcifying
  epithelioma
mal·i·as·mus
mal·ic acid
mal·ic en·zyme
ma·lig·nan·cy
ma·lig·nant
ma·lig·nin
ma·li-ma·li
ma·lin·ger·er
ma·lin·ger·ing
mal·in·ter·dig·i·ta·tion
Mall's formula
mal·le·a·bil·i·ty
mal·le·a·ble
mal·le·al
mal·le·ar
mal·le·a·tion
mal·lei·form
mal·le·in
mal·leo·in·cu·dal
mal·le·o·lar
mal·le·o·li
mal·le·o·lus *pl.* mal·le·o·li
  external m.
  m. externus
  m. fibulae
  fibular m.
  inner m.
  internal m.
  m. internus
  lateral m.
  lateral m. of fibula
  m. lateralis
  m. lateralis fibulae
  medial m.
  medial m. of tibia
  m. medialis

mal·le·o·lus *(continued)*
  m. medialis tibiae
  outer m.
  radial m.
  m. radialis
  m. tibiae
  tibial m.
  ulnar m.
  m. ulnaris
mal·le·ot·o·my
mal·le·us
mal·lo·cho·ri·on
Mal·loph·a·ga
Mal·lo·ry's bodies
Mal·lo·ry's stain
Mal·lory-Azan stain
Mal·lory-Weiss syndrome
mal·lo·tox·in
mal·low
mal·nu·tri·tion
  malignant m.
  protein m.
  protein-calorie m.
mal·oc·clu·sion
  closed-bite m.
  open-bite m.
malo·max·il·lary
mal·on·al
ma·lon·ic acid
mal·o·nyl
mal·o·nyl-ACP
mal·o·nyl co·en·zyme A
mal·o·nyl·u·rea
Mal·pi·ghi's pyramids
Mal·pi·ghi's vesicles
mal·pi·ghi·an bodies
mal·pi·ghi·an capsule
mal·pi·ghi·an cell
mal·pi·ghi·an corpuscle
mal·pi·ghi·an glomerulus
mal·pi·ghi·an layer
mal·pi·ghi·an rete
mal·pi·ghi·an stigma
mal·pi·ghi·an tubule
mal·pi·ghi·an tuft
mal·posed
mal·po·si·tion
mal·prac·tice

mal·pres·en·ta·tion
mal·ro·ta·tion
malt
mal·tase
mal·thu·si·an law
mal·to·bi·ose
mal·to·dex·trin
mal·tol
mal·to·sa·zone
mal·tose
mal·to·side
mal·tos·uria
mal·to·tri·ose
mal·turned
Mal·u·ci·din
ma·lum
    m. articulorum senilis
    m. senile
    m. vertebrale suboccipitale
mal·un·ion
Mal·va
mal·var·ia
Ma·ly's test
mam·ba
mam·e·lon
ma·mil·la *pl.* ma·mil·lae
ma·mil·lae
mam·il·lary
mam·il·lat·ed
mam·il·la·tion
ma·mil·li·form
ma·mil·li·plas·ty
mam·il·li·tis
mam·il·lo·pe·dun·cu·lar
mam·ma *pl.* mam·mae
    mammae accessoriae
      [femininae et masculinae]
    accessory mammae
    m. areolata
    m. masculina
    supernumerary mammae
    m. virilis
mam·mae
mam·mal
mam·mal·gia
Mam·ma·lia
mam·mal·o·gy

mam·ma·plas·ty
    Aries-Pitanguy m.
    augmentation m.
    Biesenberger m.
    Conway m.
    reduction m.
    Strömbeck m.
mam·ma·ry
mam·ma·troph
mam·mec·to·my
mam·mi·form
mam·mil·la
mam·mil·lary
mam·mil·lat·ed
mam·mil·la·tion
mam·mil·li·form
mam·mil·li·tis
    bovine ulcerative m.
mam·mi·pla·sia
mam·mi·tis
mam·mo·gen
mam·mo·gen·e·sis
mam·mo·gram
mam·mog·ra·phy
mam·mo·pla·sia
    adolescent m.
mam·mo·plas·ty
    augmentation m.
    Goulian m.
    reduction m.
mam·mose
mam·mot·o·my
mam·mo·troph
mam·mo·trop·ic
mam·mot·ro·pin
Man. — L. manipulus (a
    handful)
Man·ches·ter operation
man·chette
man·chi·neel
Man·ci·ni plates
Man·del·amine
man·del·ic acid
man·di·ble
man·dib·u·la *pl.* man·dib·u·
    lae
man·dib·u·lar

man·dib·u·lec·to·my
man·dib·u·lo·fa·cial
man·dib·u·lo·glos·sus
man·dib·u·lo·mar·gi·nal·is
man·dib·u·lo·pha·ryn·ge·al
Man·drag·o·ra
man·drake
man·drel
man·dril
man·drin
ma·neu·ver
    Adson's m.
    Allen m.
    Bracht's m.
    Brandt-Andrews m.
    Bruhat m.
    Chassard-Lapiné m.
    Credé's m.
    DeLee's m.
    Duecollement m.
    Engel-Lysholm m.
    forward-bending m.
    Fowler m.
    Gowers' m.
    Halstead m.
    Hampton's maneuver
    Heimlich m.
    hippocratic m.
    Hodge m.
    Hoguet's m.
    Hueter's m.
    Jendrassik's m.
    Jonnson's m.
    key-in-lock m.
    Kocher m.
    Kristeller's m.
    Lasègue's m.
    Leadbetter m.
    Leopold's m's
    Levret m.
    Lovset's m.
    McDonald m.
    McMurray's circumduction
      m.
    Mattox m.
    Mauriceau m.
    Mauriceau-Smellie-Veit m.
    Müller's m.

ma·neu·ver *(continued)*
    Müller-Hillis m.
    Munro Kerr m.
    Nylen-Bárány m.
    Pajot's m.
    Phalen's m.
    Pinard's m.
    Prague m.
    Proust-Lichtheim m.
    Queckenstedt m.
    Ritgen m.
    Roos m.
    Saxtorph's m.
    Scanzoni m.
    Schatz m.
    Schreiber's m.
    Sellick m.
    Smellie-Veit m.
    Thorn m.
    Toynbee m.
    Valsalva's m.
    Van Hoorn's m.
    Westphal m.
    Wigand's m.
    Wigand-Martin m.
man·ga·nese
    m. hypophosphite
    m. sulfate
man·gan·ic
man·ga·nism
man·ga·nous
mange
ma·nia
    m. à potu
    religious m.
    unproductive m.
ma·ni·ac
ma·ni·a·cal
man·ic
man·ic-de·pres·sive
man·i·fes·ta·tion
man·i·kin
ma·nil·o·quism
Manip. — L. manipulus (a
  handful)
man·i·pha·lanx
ma·nip·u·la·tion
    conjoined m.

ma·nip·u·la·tion *(continued)*
    Hippocrates' m.
Mann's sign
Mann-Boll·man fistula
Mann-Wil·liam·son ulcer
man·na
man·nan
man·nans
man·ner
    m. of death
man·ner·ism
man·ni·no·tri·ose
man·ni·tan
man·nite
man·ni·tol
    m. hexanitrate
man·ni·tose
Mann·kopf's sign
man·no·caro·lose
man·no·hy·dra·zone
man·no·py·ra·nose
man·no·san
man·nose
man·nose-6-phos·phate isom·
    er·ase
α-man·no·si·dase
man·no·side
man·no·si·do·sis
man·no·sido·strep·to·my·cin
man·no·so·cel·lu·lose
Mann-Whit·ney test
ma·nom·e·ter
    airway pressure m.
    aneroid m.
    Dinamap ultrasound blood
     pressure m.
    Honan m.
    Koenig's m.
mano·met·ric
ma·nom·e·try
    Cartesian diver m.
man·op·to·scope
man·os·co·py
Man. pr. — L. mane primo
   (early in the morning)
man·quea
man·sa
Man·sil

man·slaught·er
Man·son's disease
Man·son's hemoptysis
Man·son's schistosomiasis
Man·son·el·la
    M. ozzardi
    M. perstans
    M. streptocerca
man·so·nel·li·a·sis
man·so·nel·lo·sis
Man·so·nia
    M. annulifera
Man·so·ni·oi·des
    M. annulifera
man·tle
    blue m's of Manasse
    brain m.
    chordomesodermal m.
    myoepicardial m.
Man·toux reaction
Man·toux test
man·u·al
ma·nu·bria
ma·nu·bri·al
ma·nu·brio·ster·nal
ma·nu·bri·um *pl.* ma·nu·bria
    m. mallei
    m. of malleus
    m. sterni
    m. of sternum
man·u·duc·tion
manu·dy·na·mom·e·ter
ma·nus *pl.* ma·nus
    m. cava
    m. extensa
    m. flexa
    m. plana
    m. superextensa
    m. valga
    m. vara
many·plies
Manz's glands
man·za·ni·ta
Man·zul·lo's test
MAO — monoamine oxidase
MAOI — monoamine oxidase
   inhibitor
Ma·o·late

MAP — mean arterial
  pressure
map
    chromosome m.
    cognitive m.
    cytogenetic m.
    fate m.
    gene m.
    genetic m.
    linkage m.
map·ping
    cytologic m.
    deletion m.
    fine structure genetic m.
ma·pro·ti·line
Ma·quet technique
Mar·a·glas
Ma·ra·gli·a·no tuberculin
Ma·ra·ñón sign
Ma·ran·ta
ma·ran·tic
mar·as·mat·ic
ma·ras·mic
ma·ras·moid
ma·ras·mus
    enzootic m.
    nutritional m.
mar·ble·iza·tion
Mar·burg disease
Mar·burg hemorrhagic fever
Mar·burg's triad
Mar·burg virus
marc
Mar·caine
march
    jacksonian m.
Mar·chand's adrenals
Mar·chand's organs
Mar·chant's detachable zone
marche à pe·tits pas
Mar·che·sa·ni syndrome
Mar·chi's balls
Mar·chi's globule
Mar·chi's method
Mar·chi's reaction
Mar·chi's tract
Mar·chi·a·fa·va-Bi·gna·mi
  disease

Mar·chi·a·fa·va-Mi·che·li
  disease
Mar·chi·a·fa·va-Mi·che·li
  syndrome
Mar·cus Gunn dots
Mar·cus Gunn phenomenon
Mar·cus Gunn pupillary
  phenomenon
Mar·cus Gunn sign
Mar·cus Gunn syndrome
mar·cy
Mar·é·chal's test
Mar·é·chal-Ro·sin test
ma·ren·nin
Ma·rey reflex
Mar·e·zine
Mar·fan's sign
Mar·fan's syndrome
mar·fan·oid
mar·gar·ic acid
mar·gar·i·to·ma
mar·gar·one
mar·gin
    m. of acetabulum
    alveolar m. of mandible
    alveolar m. of maxilla
    axillary m. of scapula
    cartilaginous m. of
      acetabulum
    cervical m.
    ciliary m. of iris
    convex m. of testis
    coronal m. of frontal bone
    coronal m. of parietal bone
    crenate m. of spleen
    cristate m. of spleen
    dentate m.
    falciform m. of fascia lata
    falciform m. of saphenus
      hiatus
    m. of fibula, anterior
    m. of fibula, posterior
    m. of foot, fibular
    m. of foot, lateral
    m. of foot, medial
    free m. of eyelid
    free gingival m.
    free gum m.

mar·gin *(continued)*

    free m. of ovary
    frontal m. of parietal bone
    gingival m.
    gum m.
    hidden m. of nail
    m. of humerus, lateral
    m. of humerus, medial
    incisal m.
    inferior m. of liver
    infraorbital m. of maxilla
    infraorbital m. of orbit
    interosseous m. of fibula
    interosseous m. of tibia
    interosseous m. of ulna
    m. of kidney, lateral
    m. of kidney, medial
    lacrimal m. of maxilla
    lambdoid m. of occipital
      bone
    lambdoid m. of parietal
      bone
    lateral margin of orbit
    m. of lung, anterior
    m. of lung, inferior
    malar m.
    mamillary m.
    mastoid m. of occipital
      bone
    mastoid m. of parietal bone
    medial m. of orbit
    mesovarial m. of ovary
    m. of nail, free
    m. of nail, hidden
    m. of nail, lateral
    nasal m. of frontal bone
    obtuse m. of spleen
    occipital m. of parietal
      bone
    occipital m. of temporal
      bone
    orbital m.
    m. of pancreas, superior
    parietal m. of frontal bone
    parietal m. of occipital
      bone
    parietal m. of parietal bone

mar·gin *(continued)*

    parietal m. of temporal
      bone
    m. of parietal bone,
      anterior
    m. of parietal bone, frontal
    m. of parietal bone, sagittal
    m. of parietal bone,
      superior
    pupillary m. of iris
    radial m. of forearm
    m. of radius, dorsal
    red m.
    sagittal m. of parietal bone
    m. of scapula, anterior
    m. of scapula, external
    m. of scapula, lateral
    m. of scapula, superior
    sphenoidal m. of parietal
      bone
    sphenoidal m. of temporal
      bone
    sphenotemporal m. of
      parietal bone
    m. of spleen, anterior
    m. of spleen, inferior
    m. of spleen, posterior
    m. of spleen, superior
    squamous m. of parietal
      bone
    straight m. of testis
    supraorbital m. of frontal
      bone
    supraorbital m. of orbit
    m. of suprarenal gland,
      inferior
    m. of suprarenal gland,
      medial
    m. of suprarenal gland,
      superior
    temporal m. of parietal
      bone
    m. of testis, anterior
    m. of testis, external
    m. of testis, internal
    m. of testis, posterior
    m. of tibia, anterior
    m. of tibia, medial

mar·gin *(continued)*
 tibial m. of foot
 m. of tongue
 m. of tongue, lateral
 m. of ulna, anterior
 m. of ulna, dorsal
 m. of ulna, posterior
 ulnar m's of fingers
 ulnar m. of forearm
 m. of uterus, lateral
 m. of uterus, left
 m. of uterus, right
 vertebral m. of scapula
 volar m. of radius
 volar m. of ulna
mar·gi·nal
mar·gi·na·tion
mar·gi·nes
mar·gino·plas·ty
mar·go *pl.* mar·gi·nes
 m. acetabuli
 m. alveolaris
 m. anterior fibulae
 m. anterior hepatis
 m. anterior lienis
 m. anterior pancreatis
 m. anterior pulmonis
 m. anterior radii
 m. anterior testis
 m. anterior tibiae
 m. anterior ulnae
 m. axillaris scapulae
 m. ciliaris iridis
 m. dexter cordis
 m. dorsalis radii
 m. dorsalis ulnae
 m. falciformis fasciae latae
 m. falciformis hiatus
  saphenus
 m. fibularis pedis
 m. frontalis alae magnae
 m. frontalis alae majoris
 m. frontalis ossis parietalis
 m. gingivalis
 m. incisalis
 m. inferior cerebri
 m. inferior hepatis
 m. inferior lienis

mar·go *(continued)*
 m. inferior pancreatis
 m. inferior pulmonis
 m. inferior splenis
 m. inferolateralis cerebri
 m. inferomedialis cerebri
 m. infraglenoidalis tibiae
 m. infraorbitalis maxillae
 m. infraorbitalis orbitae
 m. interosseus fibulae
 m. interosseus radii
 m. interosseus tibiae
 m. interosseus ulnae
 m. lacrimalis maxillae
 m. lateralis antebrachii
 m. lateralis humeri
 m. lateralis [linguae]
 m. lateralis orbitae
 m. lateralis pedis
 m. lateralis renis
 m. lateralis scapulae
 m. lateralis unguis
 m. lateralis uteri
 m. liber ovarii
 m. liber unguis
 m. linguae
 m. medialis antebrachii
 m. medialis cerebri
 m. medialis glandulae
  suprarenalis
 m. medialis humeri
 m. medialis orbitae
 m. medialis pedis
 m. medialis renis
 m. medialis scapulae
 m. medialis tibiae
 m. mesovaricus ovarii
 m. nasalis
 m. nasalis ossis frontalis
 m. nasi
 m. occultus unguis
 m. orbitalis
 m. palpebrae
 m. parietalis alae majoris
 m. parietalis ossis frontalis
 m. parietalis ossis
  temporalis

mar·go *(continued)*
    m. parietalis squamae
      temporalis
    m. pedis lateralis
    m. pedis medialis
    m. posterior fibulae
    m. posterior lienis
    m. posterior pancreatis
    m. posterior radii
    m. posterior testis
    m. posterior ulnae
    m. pupillaris iridis
    m. radialis antebrachii
    m. radialis antibrachii
    m. radialis humeri
    m. sphenoidalis ossis
      temporalis
    m. sphenoidalis squamae
      temporalis
    m. squamosus alae magnae
    m. squamosus alae majoris
    m. squamosus ossis
      parietalis
    m. superior cerebri
    m. superior glandulae
      suprarenalis
    m. superior lienis
    m. superior pancreatis
    m. superior scapulae
    m. superior splenis
    m. superomedialis cerebri
    m. supraorbitalis orbitae
    m. supraorbitalis ossis
      frontalis
    m. tibialis pedis
    m. ulnaris antebrachii
    m. ulnaris antibrachii
    m. ulnaris humeri
    m. uteri dexter/sinister
    m. vertebralis scapulae
    m. volaris radii
    m. volaris ulnae
Ma·rie's ataxia
Ma·rie's disease
Ma·rie's hypertrophy
Ma·rie's sign
Ma·rie-Bam·ber·ger disease
Ma·rie-Foix sign

Ma·rie-Strüm·pell disease
Ma·rie-Strüm·pell syndrome
Ma·rie-Tooth disease
mar·i·jua·na
Ma·rin Amat phenomenon
Ma·ri·nes·co's sign
Ma·ri·nes·co's succulent hand
Ma·ri·nes·co-Ra·do·vici reflex
Ma·ri·nes·co-Sjö·gren-Gar·
    land syndrome
mar·i·no·bu·fa·gin
Mar·i·on's disease
Mar·i·otte's experiment
Mar·i·otte's law
Mar·i·otte's spot
mar·i·po·sia
mar·i·to·nu·cle·us
Mar·jo·lin's ulcer
mark
    beauty m.
    birth m.
    current m.
    hesitation m's
    lightning m.
    mulberry m.
    pock m.
    Pohl's m.
    port-wine m.
    quillon m.
    raspberry m.
    strawberry m.
mark·er
    Amsler's m.
    cell-surface m.
    Crane-Kaplan pocket m.
    D'Assumpção rhytidoplasty
      m.
    Freeman "cookie-cutter"
      areola m.
    genetic m.
mark·ing
    Fontana's m's
    interstitial m.
    pulmonary vascular m.
Mar·lex
Mar·low's test
mar·mo·ra·tion
mar·mo·re·al

mar·mot
Ma·ro·teaux-La·my syndrome
Mar·plan
Mar·ri·ott's method
mar·row
    bone m.
    bone m., red
    bone m., yellow
    depressed m.
    fat m.
    gelatinous m.
    red m.
    spinal m.
    yellow m.
Marsh's disease
Mar·shall's fold
Mar·shall's syndrome
Mar·shall's vein
Mar·shall Hall's method
Mar·shall-Mar·chet·ti
  operation
Mar·shall-Mar·chet·ti-Krantz
  operation
Mar·shall and Tan·ner
  pubertal staging
mar·su·pia
mar·su·pi·al
Mar·su·pi·a·lia
mar·su·pi·al·iza·tion
mar·su·pi·um *pl.* mar·su·pia
  marsupia patellaris
Mar·tei·li·i·da
Mar·tin's bandage
Mar·tin's disease
Mar·tin pelvimeter
Mar·ti·not·ti's cells
Mar·ti·us yellow
Mar·tor·ell syndrome
masc — mass concentration
mas·chal·ad·e·ni·tis
mas·chal·on·cus
mas·cu·la·tion
mas·cu·line
mas·cu·lin·i·ty
mas·cu·lin·iza·tion
mas·cu·li·nize
mas·cu·lin·iz·ing
mas·cu·lin·ovo·blas·to·ma

ma·ser
MASH — mobile army
  surgical unit
mask
    Bili m.
    BLB m.
    Boothby's m.
    Bulbulian m.
    death m.
    ecchymotic m.
    m. facies
    full-face m.
    Hutchinson's m.
    luetic m.
    meter m.
    nonrebreathing m.
    Parkinson's m.
    partial rebreathing m.
    m. of pregnancy
    tabetic m.
    tracheostomy m.
    Venturi m.
    Wanscher's m.
mask·er
    central m.
    tinnitus m.
maso·chism
maso·chist
maso·chis·tic
Ma·son gastroplasty
Mas. pil. — L. massa
  pilularum (pill mass)
mass
    achromatic m.
    appendiceal m.
    appendix m.
    atomic m.
    blue m.
    body cell m.
    electronic m.
    fibrillar m. of Flemming
    injection m.
    inner cell m.
    intermediate m.
    intermediate cell m.
    lateral m. of atlas
    lateral m's of ethmoid bone
    lateral m. of occipital bone

mass *(continued)*
    lateral m. of sacrum
    lateral m. of vertebrae
    lean body m.
    molecular m.
    muscle m.
    physical atomic m.
    pill m.
    pilular m.
    relative atomic m.
    relative molecular m.
    relativistic m.
    sarcoplasmic m's
    Stent's m.
    tigroid m's
    total red cell m.
    ventrolateral m.
mas·sa *pl.* mas·sae
    m. innominata
    m. intermedia
    m. lateralis atlantis
    massae laterales ossis
      ethmoidalis
    m. lateralis ossis sacri
    m. lateralis vertebrae
mas·sage
    cardiac m.
    carotid sinus m.
    Cederschiöld's m.
    douche m.
    electrovibratory m.
    gingival m.
    heart m.
    hydropneumatic m.
    nerve-point m.
    spray m.
    tremolo m.
    trigger point m.
    vapor m.
    vibratory m.
Mas·se·lon's spectacles
Mas·set's test
mas·se·ter
mas·se·ter·ic
mas·seur
mas·seuse
mas·si·cot
mas·sive

Mas·son stain
mas·so·ther·a·py
MAST — military (medical)
    anti-shock trousers
mas·tad·e·ni·tis
mas·tad·e·no·ma
mas·tad·e·no·vi·rus
mas·tal·gia
mas·ta·tro·phia
mas·tat·ro·phy
mas·tauxe
mast·ec·chy·mo·sis
mas·tec·to·my
    Auchincloss modified
      radical m.
    extended radical m.
    Halsted m.
    Meyer m.
    modified radical m.
    partial m.
    radical m.
    segmental m.
    simple m.
    subcutaneous m.
    total m.
Mas·ter "2-step" exercise test
mast·hel·co·sis
mas·tic
mas·ti·cate
mas·ti·ca·tion
mas·ti·ca·to·ry
mas·ti·che
mas·ti·gont
Mas·ti·goph·o·ra
mas·ti·goph·o·ran
mas·ti·goph·o·rous
mas·ti·gote
mas·ti·tis
    chronic cystic m.
    gargantuan m.
    glandular m.
    interstitial m.
    m. neonatorum
    parenchymatous m.
    periductal m.
    phlegmonous m.
    plasma cell m.
    puerperal m.

mas·ti·tis *(continued)*
   retromammary m.
   stagnation m.
   submammary m.
   suppurative m.
mas·to·car·ci·no·ma
mas·toc·cip·i·tal
mas·to·chon·dro·ma
mas·to·chon·dro·sis
mas·to·cyte
mas·to·cy·to·gen·e·sis
mas·to·cy·to·ma
mas·to·cy·to·sis
   diffuse m.
   diffuse cutaneous m.
   malignant m.
   systemic m.
mas·to·dyn·ia
mas·to·gram
mas·tog·ra·phy
mas·toid
   acellular m.
   diploic m.
   ivory m.
   pneumatized m.
   sclerotic m.
mas·toid·al
mas·toi·da·le
mas·toid·al·gia
mas·toi·dea
mas·toid·ec·to·my
   Bondy m.
   combined approach m.
   conservative m.
   cortical m.
   modified radical m.
   radical m.
   Schwartze's m.
   simple m.
mas·toi·deo·cen·te·sis
mas·toi·de·um
mas·toid·itis
   Bezold's m.
   coalescent m.
   m. externa
   m. interna
   masked m.
   sclerosing m.

mas·toid·itis *(continued)*
   silent m.
   tuberculous m.
   zygomatic m.
mas·toid·ot·o·my
mas·toi·do·tym·pa·nec·to·my
mas·to·me·nia
Mas·to·mys nat·a·len·sis
mas·ton·cus
mas·to-oc·cip·i·tal
mas·to·pa·ri·e·tal
mas·to·path·ia
   m. cystica
mas·top·a·thy
   cystic m.
mas·to·pexy
   endotheliomatous m.
   fibrous m.
   hemangioblastic m.
   hemangiopericytic m.
   meningothelial m.
   meningotheliomatous m.
   myxomatous m.
   parasagittal m.
   psammomatous m.
   syncytial m.
   transitional m.
Mas·toph·o·ra
   M. gasteracanthoides
mas·to·pla·sia
mas·to·plas·ty
mas·to·pto·sis
mas·tor·rha·gia
mas·to·scir·rhus
mas·to·sis *pl.* mas·to·ses
mas·to·squa·mous
mas·tos·to·my
mas·to·syr·inx
mas·tot·ic
mas·tot·o·my
mas·tur·ba·tion
Ma·su·gi's nephritis
Mat·as' band
Mat·as' operation
Mat·as' test
match·ing
   cross m.
ma·té

Má·té·fy's reaction
ma·ter
    dura m.
    pia m.
ma·te·ria
    m. alba
    m. dentica
    m. medica
ma·te·ri·al
    baseplate m.
    cross-reacting m. (CRM)
    dental m.
    genetic m.
    impression m.
    tissue equivalent m.
ma·te·ri·es
ma·ter·nal
ma·ter·ni·ty
ma·ter·no·he·mo·ther·a·py
Math·i·eu's disease
mat·ing
    assortative m.
    assorted m.
    assortive m.
    backcross m.
    nonrandom m.
    random m.
mat·rass
mat·ri·cal
Mat·ri·ca·ria
ma·tri·cec·to·my
ma·tri·ces
ma·tri·cial
mat·ri·cli·nous
ma·tri·lin·e·al
ma·trix *pl.* ma·tri·ces
    amalgam m.
    bone m.
    capsular m.
    cartilage m.
    cartilaginous m.
    cytoplasmic m.
    functional m.
    hair m.
    interterritorial m.
    mesangial m.
    mitochondrial m.
    nail m.

ma·trix *(continued)*
    nuclear m.
    sarcoplasmic m.
    territorial m.
    m. unguis
mat·ro·cli·nous
mat·ro·cli·ny
Mats·ner median episiotomy
  and repair
Mat·son operation
matt, matte
mat·ter
    gelatinous m.
    gray m. of nervous system
    radiant m.
    white m. of nervous system
Mat·tox maneuver
mat·tress
    alternating pressure m.
    divided m.
    egg-crate m.
    ripple m.
Mat·u·lane
mat·u·rant
mat·u·rate
mat·u·ra·tion
ma·ture
ma·tur·i·ty
Matut. — L. matutinus (in the
  morning)
ma·tu·ti·nal
Mau·chart's ligament
Mau·me·né's test
Mau·noir's hy·dro·cele
Mau·rer's clefts
Mau·rer's dots
Mau·rer's spots
Mau·rer's stippling
Mau·ri·ac's syndrome
Mau·ri·ceau's lance
Mau·ri·ceau's maneuver
Mau·ri·ceau-Smel·lie-Veit
  maneuver
Mauth·ner's cell
Mauth·ner's fiber
Mauth·ner's membrane
Mauth·ner's sheath
Mauth·ner's test

mau·ve·in
MAVIS — mobile artery and
vein imaging system
Max·ib·o·lin
max·il·la *pl.* max·il·lae, max·
il·las
inferior m.
max·il·lary
max·il·lec·to·my
max·il·li·tis
max·il·lo·den·tal
max·il·lo·eth·moi·dec·to·my
max·il·lo·fa·cial
max·il·lo·ju·gal
max·il·lo·la·bi·al
max·il·lo·man·dib·u·lar
max·il·lo·pal·a·tine
max·il·lo·pha·ryn·ge·al
max·il·lot·o·my
max·i·ma
max·i·mal
Max·i·mow's method
Max·i·mow's stain
max·i·mum *pl.* max·i·ma
excretory tubular
transport m.
glucose transport m.
reabsorptive tubular
transport m.
transport m.
tubular m.
tubular reabsorption m.
Max·i·pen
Max·i·tate
max·well
Max·well's ring
Max·well's spot
May·dl's operation
may·er
May·er's hemalum
May·er's muchematein
May·er's pessary
May·er's reagent
May·er's reflex
May·er's test
may·fly
May-Grün·wald stain
May-Heg·glin anomaly

Ma·yo's operation
Ma·yo's sign
Ma·yo Rob·son's line
Ma·yo Rob·son's point
Ma·yo Rob·son's position
May·or's scarf
may·tan·sine
maze
ma·zin·dol
ma·zo·dyn·ia
ma·zo·pexy
ma·zo·pla·sia
Maz·zi·ni's test
Maz·zo·ni's corpuscle
MB — L. Medicinae
Baccalaureus (Bachelor of
Medicine)
m.b. — L. misce bene (mix
well)
MBC — maximum breathing
capacity
MBD — minimal brain
dysfunction
MBP — mean blood pressure
myelin basic protein
MBq — megabecquerel
mbun·du
MC — L. Magister Chirurgiae
(Master of Surgery)
Medical Corps
Mc — megacycle
Mc- — *see* Mac-
mC — millicoulomb
μC — microcoulomb
MCA — 3-methylcholanthrene-
MCF — macrophage
chemotactic factor
mcg — microgram
MCH — mean corpuscular
hemoglobin
MCHC — mean corpuscular
hemoglobin concentration
MCHg — mean corpuscular
hemoglobin
MCi — megacurie
mCi — millicurie
μCi — microcurie
mCi-hr — millicurie-hour

μCi-hr — microcurie-hour
MCL — midclavicular line
MCMI — Millon clinical
multiaxial inventory
Mcps — megacycles per
second
MCT — mean circulation time
medium-chain triglyceride
MCTD — mixed connective
tissue disease
MCV — mean corpuscular
volume
MD — L. Medicinae Doctor
(Doctor of Medicine)
MDA — motor discriminative
acuity
MDP — methylene
diphosphonate
L. mento-dextra posterior
(right mentoposterior)
MDR — minimum daily
requirement
MDT — L. mento-dextra
transversa (right
mentotransverse)
Me — methyl
MEA — multiple endocrine
abnormalities
multiple endocrine
adenomatosis
multiple endocrine
adenopathies
meal
barium m.
Boyden m.
butter m.
opaque m.
Oslo m.
retention m.
test m.
mean
arithmetic m.
geometric m.
population m.
sample m.
Mean's sign
mea·sles
atypical m.

mea·sles *(continued)*
black m.
German m.
hemorrhagic m.
three-day m.
mea·sly
meas·ure
meas·ure·ment
Hirschberg m.
Krimsky m.
OFC (occipitofrontal
circumference) m.
real-time m.
skinfold m's
SNA (sella, nasion, point
A) m.
SNB (sella, nasion, point B)
m.
torr m.
Van Herick m.
me·a·tal
mea·ti·tis
ulcerative m.
me·a·tome
me·a·tom·e·ter
me·a·to·plas·ty
Stacke's m.
me·a·tor·rha·phy
me·ato·scope
me·a·tos·co·py
ureteral m.
me·ato·tome
me·a·tot·o·my
me·a·tus *pl.* me·a·tus
acoustic m., external
acoustic m., external, bony
acoustic m., external
cartilaginous
acoustic m., internal
acoustic m., internal, bony
m. acusticus externus
m. acusticus externus
cartilagineus
m. acusticus externus
osseus
m. acusticus internus
m. acusticus internus
osseus

me·a·tus *(continued)*
    m. auditorius externus
    m. auditorius internus
    auditory m., external
    auditory m., external, bony
    auditory m., external,
      cartilaginous
    auditory m., internal
    auditory m., internal, bony
    fish-mouth m.
    nasal m., common, bony
    nasal m., inferior
    nasal m., inferior, bony
    nasal m., middle
    nasal m., middle, bony
    nasal m., superior
    nasal m., superior, bony
    m. nasi communis
    m. nasi communis osseus
    m. nasi inferior
    m. nasi inferior osseus
    m. nasi medius
    m. nasi medius osseus
    m. nasi superior
    m. nasi superior osseus
    nasopharyngeal m.
    m. nasopharyngeus
    m's of nose
    m. of nose, bony, common
    m. of nose, common
    m. of nose, inferior
    m. of nose, inferior, bony
    m. of nose, middle
    m. of nose, middle, osseous
    m. of nose, superior
    m. of nose, superior,
      osseous
    m. urinarius
    urinary m.
Meb·a·ral
me·ben·da·zole
me·bev·er·ine hy·dro·chlo·ride
me·bu·ta·mate
mec·amine
mec·a·myl·amine hy·dro·chlo·ride
MeCbl — methylcobalamin

me·chan·i·cal
me·chan·i·co·re·cep·tor
me·chan·i·co·ther·a·peu·tics
me·chan·i·co·ther·a·py
me·chan·ics
    animal m.
    body m.
    developmental m.
mech·a·nism
    coping m.
    countercurrent m.
    defense m.
    double-displacement m.
    Douglas m.
    Duncan m.
    Frank-Starling m.
    ion-exchange m.
    m. of labor
    mental m.
    middle-ear transformer m.
    mote-beam m.
    oculogyric m.
    pinchcock m.
    ping-pong m.
    pressoreceptive m.
    re-entrant m.
    scapegoat m.
    Schultze m.
    suspensory m.
mech·a·nist
mech·a·no·cyte
mech·a·nol·o·gy
mech·a·no·re·cep·tor
mech·a·no·ther·a·py
mech·a·no·ther·my
mech·lor·eth·amine
me·cil·li·nam
me·cism
me·cis·to·ce·phal·ic
me·cis·to·ceph·a·lous
Me·cis·to·cir·rhus
    M. digitatus
Meck·el's band
Meck·el's cartilage
Meck·el's cavity
Meck·el's diverticulum
Meck·el's ganglion
Meck·el's ligament

Meck·el's plane
Meck·el's rod
Meck·el's space
Meck·el's syndrome
meck·el·ec·to·my
mec·li·zine hy·dro·chlo·ride
mec·lo·cy·cline
me·clo·fen·am·ate
me·clo·fen·am·ic acid
me·clo·fen·ox·ate
Me·clo·men
mec·lo·qua·lone
me·co·bal·amine
me·co·ce·phal·ic
me·co·nal·gia
meco·nate
me·con·ic acid
me·co·ni·or·rhea
me·con·ism
me·co·ni·um
me·cry·late
me·cys·ta·sis
MED — minimal effective
  dose
    minimal erythema dose
me·dal·lion
Med·a·war, Peter Brian
me·daz·e·pam hy·dro·chlo·
  ride
Med·ex
me·dia
me·di·ad
me·di·al
me·di·a·lec·i·thal
me·di·a·lis
me·di·an
me·di·a·nus
me·di·a·om·e·ter
me·di·as·ti·na
me·di·as·ti·nal
me·di·as·ti·ni·tis
    fibrous m.
    indurative m.
me·di·as·ti·nog·ra·phy
    gas m.
    opaque m.
me·di·as·ti·no·gram
me·di·as·ti·no·peri·car·di·tis

me·di·a·sti·no·scope
me·di·as·ti·no·scop·ic
me·di·as·ti·nos·co·py
me·di·as·ti·not·o·my
me·di·as·ti·num *pl.* me·di·as·
  ti·na
    anterior m.
    m. anterius
    inferior m.
    m. inferius
    m. medium
    middle m.
    posterior m.
    m. posterius
    superior m.
    m. superius
    m. testis
me·di·ate
me·di·a·tion
    chemical m.
me·di·a·tor
med·i·ca·ble
Med·i·caid
med·i·cal
med·i·ca·ment
med·i·ca·men·to·sus
med·i·ca·men·tous
Med·i·care
med·i·cate
med·i·cat·ed
med·i·ca·tion
    conservative m.
    dialytic m.
    hypodermatic m.
    ionic m.
    preanesthetic m.
    prophylactic m.
    sublingual m.
    substitutive m.
    transduodenal m.
med·i·ca·tor
me·di·ce·phal·ic
me·di·cer·e·bral
me·dic·i·nal
med·i·cine
    adolescent m.
    aerospace m.
    aviation m.

med·i·cine *(continued)*
    behavioral m.
    clinical m.
    community m.
    comparative m.
    compound m.
    domestic m.
    dosimetric m.
    emergency m.
    environmental m.
    experimental m.
    family m.
    fetal-maternal m.
    folk m.
    forensic m.
    galenic m.
    geographic m.
    geriatric m.
    group m.
    hermetic m.
    holistic m.
    hyperbaric m.
    industrial m.
    internal m.
    ionic m.
    laboratory animal m.
    legal m.
    manipulative m.
    neo-hippocratic m.
    neonatal m.
    nuclear m.
    occupational m.
    oral m.
    osteopathic m.
    patent m.
    perinatal m.
    physical m.
    preclinical m.
    preventive m.
    proprietary m.
    psychological m.
    psychosomatic m.
    rational m.
    rehabilitation m.
    social m.
    socialized m.
    space m.
    spagyric m.

med·i·cine *(continued)*
    sports m.
    state m.
    tropical m.
    veterinary m.
med·i·co·chi·rur·gic
med·i·co·den·tal
med·i·co·le·gal
med·i·co·me·chan·i·cal
med·i·co·phys·ics
med·i·co·so·cial
med·i·co·topo·graph·i·cal
med·i·co·zoo·log·i·cal
me·di·fron·tal
Me·din's disease
me·dio·car·pal
me·di·oc·cip·i·tal
me·dio·lat·er·al
me·dio·ne·cro·sis
    m. of aorta
me·dio·pon·tine
me·dio·syl·vi·an
me·dio·tar·sal
me·dio·tem·po·ral
me·dio·tru·sion
Med·i·Port vascular access
  device
me·di·sca·le·nus
me·di·sect
med·i·ta·tion
    transcendental m.
me·di·um *pl.* me·dia, me·di·
ums
    active m.
    Bavister's m.
    brain-heart infusion m.
    Bruns' glucose m.
    Cary-Blair transport m.
    clearing m.
    complete m.
    contrast m.
    culture m.
    deoxycholate-citrate m.
    dioptric media
    disperse m.
    dispersion m.
    dispersive m.
    Dubos m.

me·di·um *(continued)*
  HAT m.
  Löwenstein-Jensen m.
  McCarey-Kaufman (M-K)
    m.
  meglumine diatrizoate m.
  metrizamide m.
  motility test m.
  mounting m.
  NNN m.
  Novy, McNeal and Nicolle
    m.
  nutrient m.
  radiolucent m.
  radiopaque m.
  refracting media
  Sabouraud's m.
  separating m.
  Stuart transport m.
  Thayer-Martin m.
  Wickersheimer's m.
me·di·us
med·or·rhea
med·phal·an
med·ro·ges·tone
Med·rol
med·ro·nate di·so·di·um
med·roxy·pro·ges·ter·one ac·
  e·tate
med·ry·sone
me·dul·la *pl.* me·dul·lae
  adrenal m.
  m. of bone
  m. glandulae suprarenalis
  m. of kidney
  m. of lymph node
  m. nephrica
  m. nodi lymphatici
  m. oblongata
  m. ossium
  m. ossium flava
  m. ossium rubra
  m. ovarii
  m. of ovary
  m. renis
  m. renalis
  spinal m.
  m. spinalis

me·dul·la *(continued)*
  suprarenal m.
  m. of suprarenal gland
  m. thymi
  m. of thymus
me·dul·lae
med·ul·lar·is
  conus m.
med·ul·lary
med·ul·lat·ed
med·ul·la·tion
med·ul·lec·to·my
me·dul·li·adre·nal
med·ul·li·spi·nal
med·ul·li·tis
med·ul·li·za·tion
me·dul·lo·adre·nal
me·dul·lo·ar·thri·tis
me·dul·lo·blast
me·dul·lo·blas·to·ma
  desmoplastic m.
me·dul·lo·en·ce·phal·ic
me·dul·lo·epi·the·li·o·ma
me·dul·lo·su·pra·re·no·ma
me·dul·lo·ther·a·py
me·du·sa
me·du·so·con·ges·tin
Mees' lines
me·fe·nam·ic acid
me·fen·o·rex hy·dro·chlo·ride
me·fex·amide
mef·lo·quine
mef·ru·side
MEG — magnetoencaphalo-
  graph
mega·bec·que·rel
mega·blad·der
mega·cal·y·co·sis
mega·car·dia
Me·gace
mega·ce·cum
mega·cho·led·o·chus
mega·co·lon
  acquired m.
  acquired functional m.
  acute m.
  aganglionic m.
  congenital m.

mega·co·lon *(continued)*
   m. congenitum
   idiopathic m.
   toxic m.
mega·cu·rie
mega·cy·cle
mega·dont
mega·don·tia
mega·du·o·de·num
mega·dyne
mega·elec·tron·volt (MeV, Mev)
mega·esoph·a·gus
mega·ga·me·to·phyte
mega·hertz
mega·karyo·blast
mega·karyo·cyte
mega·karyo·cy·to·pe·nia
mega·karyo·cy·to·poi·e·sis
mega·karyo·cy·to·sis
mega·lec·i·thal
meg·al·en·ceph·a·lon
meg·al·en·ceph·a·ly
meg·al·er·y·the·ma
meg·al·gia
meg·a·lo·blast
   m. of Sabin
meg·a·lo·blas·tic
meg·a·lo·blas·toid
meg·a·lo·blas·to·sis
meg·a·lo·bul·bus
meg·a·lo·car·dia
meg·a·lo·ce·phal·ic
meg·a·lo·ceph·a·ly
meg·a·loc·e·ros
meg·a·lo·chei·ria
meg·a·lo·clit·o·ris
meg·a·lo·cor·nea
meg·a·lo·cys·tis
meg·a·lo·cyte
meg·a·lo·cy·to·sis
meg·a·lo·dac·ty·lism
meg·a·lo·dac·ty·lous
meg·a·lo·dac·ty·ly
meg·a·lo·don·tia
meg·a·lo·en·ce·phal·ic
meg·a·lo·en·ter·on
meg·a·lo·esoph·a·gus

meg·a·lo·gas·tria
meg·a·lo·glos·sia
meg·a·lo·gra·phia
meg·a·lo·he·pat·ia
meg·a·lo·kar·y·o·cyte
meg·a·lo·ma·nia
meg·a·lo·ma·ni·ac
meg·a·lo·me·lia
meg·a·lo·mi·cin po·tas·si·um phos·phate
meg·a·lo·nych·ia
meg·a·lo·pe·nis
meg·a·loph·thal·mos
   anterior m.
meg·a·lo·pia
meg·a·lo·po·dia
meg·a·lop·sia
Meg·a·lo·pyge
   M. opercularis
meg·a·lo·sple·nia
meg·a·lo·spore
Meg·a·los·po·ron
meg·a·los·po·ron *pl.* meg·a·los·po·ra
meg·a·lo·syn·dac·ty·ly
meg·a·lo·thy·mus
meg·a·lo·ure·ter
   congenital m.
   primary m.
   reflux m.
meg·a·lo·ure·thra
mega·pros·o·pous
mega·rec·tum
Mega·rhi·ni·ni
Mega·rhi·nus
mega·roent·gen (MR)
Mega·sel·ia sca·lar·is
mega·seme
mega·sig·moid
mega·so·ma
mega·so·mia
Mega·sphae·ra
mega·spo·ran·gi·um *pl.* mega·spo·ran·gia
mega·spore
Mega·tri·cho·phy·ton
Mega·tryp·a·num
mega·unit

mega·vi·ta·min
mega·volt
mega·vol·tage
me·ges·trol ac·e·tate
Meg·i·mide
Mé·glin's point
meg·lu·mine
meg·lu·tol
meg·ohm
meg·oph·thal·mos
me·grim
mehl·nähr·scha·den
mei·bo·mi·an cyst
mei·bo·mi·an foramen
mei·bo·mi·an glands
mei·bo·mi·an stye
mei·bo·mi·a·ni·tis
mei·bo·mi·tis
Meige's disease
Meigs' capillaries
Meigs' syndrome
Meigs' test
Mei·ni·cke reaction
Mei·ni·cke test
mei·o·gen·ic
mei·o·sis
mei·ot·ic
Mei·row·sky phenomenon
Meiss·ner's corpuscles
Meiss·ner's ganglion
Meiss·ner's plexus
mel
mel·ag·ra
mel·al·gia
mel·an·cho·lia
   m. agitata
   agitated m.
   involutional m.
mel·an·chol·ic
mel·an·choly
mel·an·ede·ma
mel·a·nem·e·sis
mel·a·ne·mia
mel·a·nic·ter·us
mel·a·nif·er·ous
mel·a·nin
   artificial m.
   factitious m.

mel·a·nism
   industrial m.
   metallic m.
mel·a·nis·tic
mel·a·no·ac·an·tho·ma
mel·a·no·a·melo·blas·to·ma
mel·a·no·blast
   amelanotic m.
mel·a·no·blas·to·ma
mel·a·no·blas·to·sis
mel·a·no·car·ci·no·ma
mel·a·no·cyte
   dendritic m.
mel·a·no·cyt·ic
mel·a·no·cy·to·ma
   compound m.
   dermal m.
mel·a·no·cy·to·sis
   oculodermal m.
mel·a·no·der·ma
   parasitic m.
   senile m.
mel·a·no·der·ma·ti·tis
   m. toxica lichenoides
me·lan·o·gen
mel·a·no·gen·emia
mel·a·no·gen·e·sis
mel·a·no·gen·ic
mel·a·no·glos·sia
mel·a·noid
Mel·a·no·les·tes
   M. picipes
mel·a·no·leu·ko·der·ma
   m. colli
mel·a·no·ma
   acral-lentiginous m.
   amelanotic m.
   benign juvenile m.
   Cloudman's m. S91
   Harding-Passey m.
   juvenile m.
   lentigo maligna m.
   malignant m.
   nodular m.
   spindle cell m.
   subungual m.
   superficial spreading m.

mel·a·no·ma·to·sis
mel·a·no·ma·tous
mel·a·no·nych·ia
mel·a·no·phage
mel·a·no·phore
mel·a·noph·o·rin
mel·a·no·pla·kia
mel·a·no·pre·cip·i·ta·tion
mel·a·nop·ty·sis
mel·a·no·sis
   m. bulbi
   circumscribed
     precancerous m. of
     Dubreuilh
   m. coli
   Dubreuilh's precancerous
     m.
   m. iridis
   m. of the iris
   m. lenticularis progressiva
   m. oculi
   oculocutaneous m.
   Riehl's m.
   m. sclerae
   tar m.
mel·a·no·some
   compound m.
mel·a·not·ic
mel·a·no·trich·ia
   m. linguae
mel·a·no·troph
mel·a·no·trop·ic
mel·a·no·tro·pin
mel·an·thin
mel·an·u·re·sis
mel·an·uria
mel·an·uric
mel·ar·so·prol
me·las·ma
   m. addisonnii
   m. gravidarum
   m. suprarenale
mel·a·to·nin
Me·le·da disease
me·le·na
   m. neonatorum
   m. spuria
   m. vera

Me·le·ney's chronic
   undermining ulcer
Me·le·ney's synergistic
   gangrene
Me·le·ney's ulcer
mel·en·ges·trol ac·e·tate
me·le·nic
mel·e·tin
me·lez·i·tose
meli·bi·ase
meli·bi·ose
mel·i·ce·ra
mel·i·ce·ris
me·lic·i·tose
mel·i·lo·tox·in
me·li·oi·do·sis
Me·lis·sa
me·lis·sic acid
me·lis·so·ther·a·py
mel·i·tin
me·li·tis
mel·i·to·pty·a·lism
mel·i·to·pty·a·lon
mel·i·tose
mel·i·tra·cen hy·dro·chlo·ride
me·lit·ri·ose
mel·i·tu·ria
   m. inosita
mel·i·tu·ric
mel·i·zame
me·liz·i·tose
Mel·kers·son's syndrome
Mel·kers·son-Ro·sen·thal
   syndrome
Mel·la·ril
mel·li·tum *pl.* mel·li·ti
mel·li·tu·ria
Mel·nick-Nee·dles syndrome
melo·did·y·mus
melo·melia
me·lom·e·lus
me·lon·cus
me·lono·plas·ty
Me·loph·a·gus
   M. ovinus
melo·plas·tic
melo·plas·ty
melo·rhe·os·to·sis

melo·sal·gia
me·los·chi·sis
me·lo·tia
Me·lotte's metal
mel·pha·lan
Melt·zer's anesthesia
Melt·zer's law
Melt·zer's method
Melt·zer-Ly·on test
mem·ber·ment
mem·bra
mem·bra·na *pl.* mem·bra·nae
  m. abdominis
  m. adamantina
  m. adventitia
  m. agnina
  m. atlanto-occipitalis
    anterior
  m. atlanto-occipitalis
    posterior
  m. basalis
  m. basalis ductus
    semicircularis
  m. basilaris ductus
    cochlearis
  m. caduca
  m. capsularis
  m. capsulopupillaris
  m. choriocapillaris
  m. cricovalis
  membranae deciduae
  m. elastica laryngis
  m. epipapillaris
  m. fibroelastica laryngis
  m. fibrosa capsulae
    articularis
  m. flaccida
  m. fusca
  m. germinativa
  m. gliae superficialis
  m. granulosa
  m. granulosa externa
  m. granulosa interna
  m. hyaloidea
  m. hyothyreoidea
  m. intercostalis externa
  m. intercostalis interna
  m. interossea antebrachii

mem·bra·na *(continued)*
  m. interossea antibrachii
  m. interossea cruris
  m. limitans
  m. mucosa nasi
  m. mucosa vesicae felleae
  m. nictitans
  m. obturatoria
  m. obturatoria [stapedis]
  m. obturatrix
  m. perforata
  m. perinei
  m. pituitosa
  m. preformativa
  m. propria
  m. propria ductus
    semicircularis
  m. pupillaris
  m. quadrangularis
  m. reticularis ductus
    cochlearis
  m. reticulata
  m. ruyschiana
  m. sacciformis
  m. serosa
  m. serotina
  m. spiralis ductus
    cochlearis
  m. stapedis
  m. statoconiorum
    macularum
  m. sterni
  m. succingens
  m. suprapleuralis
  m. synovialis capsulae
    articularis
  m. synovialis inferior
  m. synovialis superior
  m. tectoria
  m. tectoria ductus
    cochlearis
  m. tensa
  m. thyrohyoidea
  m. tympani
  m. tympani, metatarsal
  m. tympani secundaria
  m. versicolor of Fielding
  m. vestibularis

mem·bra·na *(continued)*
    m. vestibularis [Reissneri]
    m. vibrans
    m. vitellina
    m. vitrea
mem·bra·na·ceous
mem·bra·nae
mem·bra·nate
mem·brane
    abdominal m.
    accidental m.
    adamantine m.
    allantoid m.
    alveolocapillary m.
    alveolodental m.
    anal m.
    animal m.
    aponeurotic m.
    arachnoid m.
    Ascherson's m.
    asphyxial m.
    atlanto-occipital m.,
      anterior
    atlanto-occipital m.,
      posterior
    basal m. of semicircular
      duct
    basement m.
    basilar m. of cochlear duct
    Bichat's m.
    birth m's
    Bogros serous m.
    Bowman's m.
    brood m.
    Bruch's m.
    Brunn's m.
    bucconasal m.
    buccopharyngeal m.
    capsular m.
    capsulopupillary m.
    cell m.
    chorioallantoic m.
    chromatic m.
    cloacal m.
    complex m.
    compound m.
    Corti's m.
    costocoracoid m.

mem·brane *(continued)*
    cribriform m.
    cricothyroid m.
    cricotracheal m.
    cricovocal m.
    croupous m.
    crural interosseous m.
    cyclitic m.
    cytoplasmic m.
    Debove's m.
    decidual m's
    deciduous m's
    Demours m.
    dentinoenamel m.
    Descemet's m.
    dialysis m.
    diphtheritic m.
    drum m.
    Duddell's m.
    egg m.
    elastic m.
    elastic m., external
    elastic m., internal
    enamel m.
    endoneural m.
    endoral m.
    excitable m.
    exocoelomic m.
    extraembryonic m's
    false m.
    fenestrated m.
    fertilization m.
    fetal m's
    fibroelastic m. of larynx
    fibrous m. of articular
      capsule
    Fielding's m.
    flaccid m. of Shrapnell
    germinal m.
    glassy m.
    glomerular m.
    gradocol m's
    ground m.
    Haller's m.
    Hannover's intermediate
      m.
    Held's limiting m.
    hemodialyzer m.

mem·brane *(continued)*
  Henle's m.
  Henle's elastic m.
  Henle's fenestrated m.
  Heuser's m.
  homogeneous m.
  Hovius' m.
  Huxley's m.
  hyaline m.
  hyaloid m.
  hymenal m.
  hyoglossal m.
  hyothyroid m.
  intercostal m., external
  intercostal m., internal
  interosseous m. of forearm
  interosseous m., radioulnar
  interosseous m. of leg
  interspinal m's
  intersutural m.
  ion-selective m.
  Jackson's m.
  Jacob's m.
  keratogenous m.
  Kölliker's m.
  Krause's m.
  ligamentous m.
  Liliequist's m.
  limiting m.
  limiting m., external
  limiting m., inner
  limiting m., internal
  limiting m., outer
  Mauthner's m.
  medullary m.
  mucocutaneous m.
  mucous m.
  mucous m., proper
  mucous m. of colon
  mucous m. of esophagus
  mucous m. of gallbladder
  mucous m. of mouth
  mucous m. of pharynx
  mucous m. of rectum
  mucous m. of small
    intestine
  mucous m. of stomach
  mucous m. of tongue

mem·brane *(continued)*
  mucous m. of ureter
  mucous m. of urinary
    bladder
  Nasmyth's m.
  nictitating m.
  m. of Nitabuch
  nuclear m.
  oblique m. of forearm
  obturator m.
  obturator m. of atlas,
    anterior
  obturator m. of atlas,
    posterior
  obturator m. of larynx
  occipitoaxial m., long
  olfactory m.
  oral m.
  oronasal m.
  oropharyngeal m.
  otolithic m.
  ovular m.
  palatine m.
  pansporoblastic m.
  paroral m.
  pericolic m.
  pericolonic m.
  peridental m.
  perineal m.
  m. of perineum
  periodontal m.
  periorbital m.
  peritrophic m.
  pharyngeal m.
  pharyngobasilar m.
  pial-glial m.
  pituitary m. of nose
  placental m.
  plasma m.
  platelet demarcation m.
  pleuropericardial m.
  pleuroperitoneal m.
  postsynaptic m.
  presynaptic m.
  proligerous m.
  proper m. of semicircular
    duct
  prophylactic m.

mem·brane *(continued)*
    pseudoserous m.
    pulmonary hyaline m.
    pupillary m.
    pyogenic m.
    pyophylactic m.
    quadrangular m.
    Ranvier's m.
    Reichert's m.
    Reissner's m.
    respiratory m.
    reticular m.
    reticulated m.
    Rivinus' m.
    ruffle m.
    Ruysch's m.
    ruyschian m.
    Scarpa's m.
    schneiderian m.
    Schwann's m.
    semipermeable m.
    serous m.
    serous m. of epididymis
    shell m.
    Shrapnell's m.
    m. of Slavianski
    slit m.
    spiral m. of cochlear duct
    stapedial m.
    statoconic m. of maculae
    sternal m.
    m. of sternum
    striated m.
    subepithelial m.
    submucous m.
    submucous m. of stomach
    subzonal m.
    suprapleural m.
    sutural m.
    synaptic m.
    synovial m., inferior
    synovial m., superior
    synovial m. of articular
      capsule
    tarsal m.
    tectorial m.
    tendinous m.
    Tenon's m.

mem·brane *(continued)*
    thyreohyoid m.
    Toldt's m.
    Traube's m.
    tympanic m.
    tympanic m., secondary
    undulating m.
    unit m.
    urogenital m.
    urorectal m.
    vascular m. of viscera
    vernix m.
    vestibular m. of cochlear
      duct
    virginal m.
    vitelline m.
    vitreous m.
    Volkmann's m.
    Wachendorf's m.
    yolk m.
    Zinn's m.
mem·bra·nec·to·my
mem·bra·nelle
    adoral zone of m's
mem·bra·ni·form
mem·bra·nin
mem·bra·no·car·ti·lag·i·nous
mem·bra·noid
mem·bran·ol·y·sis
mem·bra·nous
mem·brum *pl.* mem·bra
    m. inferius
    m. muliebre
    m. superius
    m. virile
Me·mo·ri·al Sloan-Ket·ter·ing
    protocol
mem·o·ry
    anterograde m.
    echoic m.
    eye m.
    iconic m.
    immediate m.
    immunologic m.
    kinesthetic m.
    long-term m.
    recent m.
    remote m.

mem·o·ry *(continued)*
    retrograde m.
    rote m.
    screen m.
    short-term m.
    virtual m.
    visual m.
mem·o·tine hy·dro·chlo·ride
MEN — multiple endocrine neoplasia
me·nac·me
men·a·di·ol so·di·um di·phos·phate
men·a·di·one
    m. sodium bisulfite
Men·a·gen
men·al·gia
men·aph·thone
men·a·quin·one
me·nar·chal
me·nar·che
me·nar·che·al, me·nar·chi·al
Men·del's law
Men·del's reflex
Men·del's test
Men·del-Bekh·ter·ev reflex
Men·del-Bekh·ter·ev sign
men·de·le·vi·um
men·de·li·an
men·del·ism
men·del·iz·ing
Men·del·sohn's test
Men·del·son's syndrome
Men·doc·u·tes
Men·do·sic·u·tes
Men·est
Mé·né·trier's disease
Men·for·mon
Menge's pessary
Men·gert's index
men·gin·go·ra·dic·u·lo·my·eli·tis
men·hi·dro·sis
men·id·ro·sis
Men·i·ere's disease
Men·i·ere's syndrome
me·nin·ge·al
me·nin·gem·a·to·ma

me·nin·geo·cor·ti·cal
me·nin·ge·o·ma
me·nin·ge·or·rha·phy
me·nin·ges
me·ning·hem·a·to·ma
me·nin·gi·o·ma
    anaplastic m.
    angioblastic m.
    angiomatous m.
    arachnotheliomatous m.
me·nin·gi·o·ma·to·sis
me·nin·gism
men·in·gis·mus
men·in·git·ic
men·in·gi·tis *pl.* men·in·git·i·des
    acute aseptic m.
    acute septic m.
    aseptic m.
    basal m.
    m. of the base
    basilar m.
    benign lymphocytic m.
    benign recurrent endothelioleukocytic m.
    m. carcinomatosa
    cerebral m.
    cerebrospinal m.
    chronic posterior basic m.
    m. circumscripta spinalis
    eosinophilic m.
    epidemic cerebrospinal m.
    external m.
    granulomatous m.
    gummatous m.
    internal m.
    lymphocytic m.
    meningococcal m.
    Mollaret's m.
    mumps m.
    m. necrotoxica reactiva
    occlusive m.
    m. ossificans
    otitic m.
    otogenic m.
    parameningococcus m.
    plague m.
    posterior m.

men·in·gi·tis *(continued)*
  posterior basic m.
  purulent m.
  pyogenic m.
  Quincke's m.
  rheumatic m.
  sarcoid m.
  septicemic m.
  m. serosa
  m. serosa circumscripta
  m. serosa circumscripta
    cystica
  serous m.
  simple m.
  spinal m.
  sterile m.
  suppurative m.
  m. sympathica
  torula m.
  torular m.
  tubercular m.
  tuberculous m.
  viral m.
  Wallgren's aseptic m.
  yeast m.
me·nin·go·ar·ter·i·tis
me·nin·go·blast
me·nin·go·blas·to·ma
me·nin·go·cele
  spurious m.
  traumatic m.
me·nin·go·ceph·a·li·tis
me·nin·go·cer·e·bri·tis
me·nin·go·coc·ce·mia
  acute fulminating m.
me·nin·go·coc·ci
me·nin·go·coc·cin
me·nin·go·coc·co·sis
me·nin·go·coc·cus *pl.* me·nin·
  go·coc·ci
me·nin·go·cor·ti·cal
me·nin·go·cyte
me·nin·go·en·ceph·a·li·tis
  biundulant m.
  eosinophilic m.
  mumps m.
  primary amebic m.
  syphilitic m.

me·nin·go·en·ceph·a·li·tis
  (continued)
  trypanosomal m.
  Tüga's m.
me·nin·go·en·ceph·a·lo·my·
  eli·tis
me·nin·go·en·ceph·a·lo·my·
  elop·a·thy
me·nin·go·en·ceph·a·lo·my·
  elo·ra·dic·u·lo·neu·ri·tis
me·nin·go·en·ceph·a·lop·a·
  thy
me·nin·go·fi·bro·blas·to·ma
me·nin·go·gen·ic
me·nin·go·ma
me·nin·go·ma·la·cia
me·nin·go·my·eli·tis
  blastomycotic m.
  sporotrichotic m.
  torular m.
me·nin·go·my·elo·cele
me·nin·go·my·elo·en·ceph·a·
  li·tis
me·nin·go·my·elo·ra·dic·u·
  li·tis
me·nin·go-os·teo·phle·bi·tis
me·nin·gop·a·thy
me·nin·go·pneu·mo·ni·tis
me·nin·go·ra·chid·i·an
me·nin·go·ra·dic·u·lar
me·nin·go·ra·dic·u·li·tis
me·nin·go·re·cur·rence
me·nin·gor·rha·gia
me·nin·gor·rhea
me·nin·go·sis
me·nin·go·the·li·o·ma
me·nin·go·the·li·um
me·nin·go·trop·ism
me·nin·go·vas·cu·lar
men·in·gu·ria
me·ninx *pl.* me·nin·ges
me·nis·cal
men·is·cec·to·my
  arthroscopic m.
men·is·che·sis
me·nis·ci
men·is·ci·tis
me·nis·co·cyte

me·nis·co·cy·to·sis
me·nis·cop·a·thy
me·nis·co·pexy
me·nis·co·syn·o·vi·al
me·nis·cot·o·my
me·nis·cus *pl.* me·nis·ci
    m. of acromioclavicular
      joint
    articular m.
    m. articularis
    converging m.
    discoid m.
    discoid lateral m.
    diverging m.
    m. of inferior radioulnar
      joint
    joint m.
    Kuhnt's m.
    lateral m. of knee joint
    m. lateralis articulationis
      genus
    medial m. of knee joint
    m. medialis articulationis
      genus
    negative m.
    positive m.
    m. of sternoclavicular joint
    tactile menisci
    menisci tactus
    m. of temporomaxillary
      joint
meni·sper·mine
Men·i·sper·mum
Men·kes disease
meno·lip·sis
meno·met·ror·rha·gia
meno·pau·sal
meno·pause
    artificial m.
    male m.
    m. praecox
    premature m.
meno·pla·nia
men·or·rha·gia
    functional m.
men·or·rhal·gia
men·or·rhea
men·or·rhe·al

me·nos·che·sis
men·o·sta·sia
men·o·sta·sis
meno·stax·is
meno·tro·pins
men·ses
men·stru·al
men·stru·ant
men·stru·ate
men·stru·a·tion
    anovular m.
    anovulatory m.
    delayed m.
    difficult m.
    infrequent m.
    nonovulational m.
    profuse m.
    regurgitant m.
    retained m.
    retrograde m.
    scanty m.
    supplementary m.
    suppressed m.
    vicarious m.
men·stru·ous
men·stru·um
    Pitkin m.
men·su·al
men·su·ra·tion
men·ta·groph·y·ton
men·tal
men·ta·lis
men·tal·i·ty
men·ta·tion
Men·tha
    M. canadensis
    M. cardiaca
    M. piperita
    M. pulegium
    M. spicata
    M. viridis
men·thol
men·thyl
men·ti·cide
men·to·an·te·ri·or
men·to·la·bi·al
men·ton
men·to·plas·ty

men·to·pos·te·ri·or
men·to·trans·verse
men·tum
Men·y·an·thes
me·o·ben·tine sul·fate
Me·o·nine
MEP — motor evoked
  potential
    multimodality evoked
      potential
mep·a·crine hy·dro·chlo·ride
me·par·fy·nol
me·par·tri·cin
mep·a·zine ac·e·tate
me·pen·zo·late bro·mide
me·per·i·dine hy·dro·chlo·
  ride
me·phen·amine
me·phen·e·sin
meph·en·ox·a·lone
me·phen·ter·mine sul·fate
me·phen·y·to·in
me·phit·ic
me·phi·tis
meph·o·bar·bi·tal
Meph·y·ton
me·piv·a·caine hy·dro·chlo·
  ride
Me·prane
me·pred·ni·sone
me·pro·ba·mate
    isopropyl m.
Me·pro·span
Me·pro·tabs
mep·ryl·caine hy·dro·chlo·
  ride
me·pyr·amine mal·e·ate
me·py·ra·pone
mEq — milliequivalent
meq — milliequivalent
meq·ui·dox
MER — methanol extraction
  residue
mer·ac·ti·no·my·cin
mer·a·le·in so·di·um
me·ral·gia
    m. paresthetica
me·ral·lu·ride

mer·bro·min
mer·cap·tal·bu·min
mer·cap·tan
mer·cap·tide
mer·cap·to·eth·a·nol
mer·cap·to·eth·yl·amine
2-mer·cap·to·im·id·az·ole
mer·cap·tol
mer·cap·to·mer·in
6-mer·cap·to·pur·ine
mer·cap·tur·ic acid
6-MP — 6-mercaptopurine
Mer·cier's bar
Mer·cier's valve
mer·co·cre·sols
mer·cu·pu·rin
mer·cur·amide
mer·cur·am·mo·ni·um
    m. chloride
mer·cu·ri·al
mer·cu·ri·al·ism
p-mer·cu·ri·ben·zo·ate
  [para-]
mer·cur·ic
    m. chloride
    m. oxide, yellow
    interzonal m.
Mer·cu·ro·chrome
mer·cu·ro·phyl·line
mer·cu·rous
    m. chloride
mer·cu·ry
    ammoniated m.
    m. bichloride
    m. with chalk
    m. chloride, mild
    methyl m.
    m. oleate
    m. perchloride
Mer·cu·zan·thin
mer·e·thox·yl·line pro·caine
Mer·en·di·no's technique
me·rid·i·an
    m. of cornea
    m's of eyeball
    horizontal m.
    vertical m.
me·rid·i·a·ni

me·rid·i·a·nus *pl.* me·rid·i·a·
ni
 meridiani bulbi oculi
me·rid·i·o·nal
mer·i·sis
mer·ism
meri·spore
mer·i·stem
mer·i·ste·mat·ic
mer·is·tic
Mer·kel's cells
Mer·kel's corpuscles
Mer·kel's disks
Mer·kel's filtrum
Mer·kel's muscle
Mer·kel's tactile cells
Mer·kel-Ran·vier cells
mer·mi·thid
Mer·mith·i·dae
Mer·mith·oi·dea
mero·acra·nia
mero·an·en·ceph·a·ly
mero·blas·tic
mero·cele
me·ro·cox·al·gia
mero·crine
mero·cyst
mero·cyte
mero·di·a·stol·ic
mero·en·ceph·a·ly
me·rog·a·my
mero·gas·tru·la
mero·gen·e·sis
mero·ge·net·ic
mer·o·gen·ic
mero·gon·ic
me·rog·o·ny
 diploid m.
 parthenogenetic m.
mero·me·lia
mero·mi·cro·so·mia
mero·mor·pho·sis
mer·o·my·a·ri·al
mer·o·my·a·ri·an
mero·myo·sin
me·ro·nec·ro·bi·o·sis
me·ro·ne·cro·sis
mer·ont

me·ro·pia
me·ro·ra·chis·chi·sis
me·ros
me·ros·mia
mer·os·tot·ic
me·rot·o·my
mero·zo·ite
mero·zy·gote
mer·pha·lan
Mer·phen·yl
mer·sa·lyl
Mer·se·burg triad
Mer·si·lene suture
Mer·thi·o·late
mer·y·cism
mer·y·cis·mus
Merz·bach·er-Pel·i·zae·us
 disease
me·sad
me·sal
mes·an·gi·al
mes·an·gio·cap·il·lary
mes·an·gi·ol·y·sis
mes·an·gi·um
Me·san·to·in
mes·a·ra·ic
mes·ar·ter·itis
 Mönckeberg's m.
me·sati·ce·phal·ic
me·sati·ker·kic
me·sati·pel·lic
me·sati·pel·vic
mes·ax·on
mes·cal
mes·ca·line
mes·cal·ism
me·sec·la·zone
mes·ec·to·blast
mes·ec·to·derm
mes·en·ce·phal·ic
mes·en·ceph·a·li·tis
mes·en·ceph·a·lo·hy·po·
 phys·e·al
mes·en·ceph·a·lon
mes·en·ceph·a·lot·o·my
mes·en·chy·ma
mes·en·chy·mal
mes·en·chyme

mes·en·chy·mo·ma
   benign m.
   malignant m.
mes·en·ter·ec·to·my
mes·en·ter·ic
mes·en·ter·i·o·lum
   m. appendicis vermiformis
   m. processus vermiformis
mes·en·ter·io·pexy
mes·en·ter·i·or·rha·phy
mes·en·ter·i·pli·ca·tion
mes·en·ter·itis
   retractile m.
mes·en·te·ri·um
   m. commune
   m. dorsale commune
mes·en·ter·on
mes·en·tery
   m. of ascending part of
     colon
   caval m.
   common m.
   common m., dorsal
   m. of descending part of
     colon
   dorsal m.
   persistent common m.
   primitive m.
   m. of rectum
   m. of sigmoid colon
   m. of transverse part of
     colon
   ventral m.
   m. of vermiform appendix
me·sen·to·derm
me·sen·to·mere
mes·en·tor·rha·phy
mes·epi·the·li·um
mesh
   Dexon m.
   Marlex m.
   tantalum m.
   Teflon m.
   wire m.
meshwork
   trabecular m.
me·si·ad
me·si·al
me·si·al·ly

me·si·en
me·sio·buc·cal
me·sio·buc·co-oc·clu·sal
me·sio·buc·co·pul·pal
me·sio·cer·vi·cal
me·sio·cli·na·tion
me·sio·clu·sion
me·sio·dens *pl.* me·sio·den·tes
me·sio·den·tes
me·sio·dis·tal
me·sio·gin·gi·val
me·sio·in·ci·so·dis·tal
me·sio·la·bi·al
me·sio·la·bio·in·ci·sal
me·sio·lin·gual
me·sio·lin·guo·in·ci·sal
me·sio·lin·guo-oc·clu·sal
me·sio·lin·guo·pul·pal
me·si·on
me·si·o-oc·clu·sal
me·si·o-oc·clu·so·dis·tal
me·sio·pul·pal
me·sio·pul·po·la·bi·al
me·sio·pul·po·lin·gual
me·sio·ver·sion
mes·it·y·lene

Mes·mer, Franz (Friedrich)
   Anton

mes·mer·ism
meso-aor·ti·tis
   m. syphilitica
meso·ap·pen·di·ci·tis
meso·ap·pen·dix
meso·ar·i·al
meso·ar·i·um
meso·bi·lin
meso·bil·i·ru·bin
mes·o·bil·i·ru·bin·o·gen
meso·bil·i·vi·o·lin
meso·blast
meso·blas·te·ma
meso·blas·tic
meso·bron·chi·tis
meso·car·dia
meso·car·di·um
   arterial m.
   dorsal m.
   lateral m.

meso·car·di·um *(continued)*
   venous m.
   ventral m.
meso·car·pal
meso·ca·val
meso·ce·cal
meso·ce·cum
meso·ce·phal·ic
meso·ceph·a·lon
meso·ceph·a·ly
meso·ces·toi·des
meso·ces·toi·di·dae
meso·chon·dri·um
meso·cho·roi·dea
meso·col·ic
meso·co·lon
   m. ascendens
   ascending m.
   m. descendens
   descending m.
   iliac m.
   left m.
   pelvic m.
   right m.
   sigmoid m.
   m. sigmoideum
   transverse m.
   m. transversum
meso·co·lo·pexy
meso·co·lo·pli·ca·tion
meso·cord
meso·cor·nea
meso·cra·nic
Meso·cri·ce·tus
meso·cu·nei·form
meso·cyst
meso·cy·to·ma
meso·derm
   extraembryonic m.
   gastral m.
   head m.
   intermediate m.
   intraembryonic m.
   lateral m.
   paraxial m.
   peristomal m.
   prochordal m.
   secondary m.

meso·derm *(continued)*
   somatic m.
   splanchnic m.
meso·der·mal
meso·der·mic
meso·di·a·stol·ic
mes·odont
mes·odon·tic
mes·odon·tism
meso·du·o·de·nal
meso·duo·de·ni·tis
meso·du·o·de·num
meso·epi·did·y·mis
meso·esoph·a·gus
meso·gas·ter
meso·gas·tric
meso·gas·tri·um
   dorsal m.
   ventral m.
meso·glea
mes·og·lia
meso·gli·o·ma
meso·glu·te·al
meso·glu·te·us
mes·og·nath·ic
meso·gnath·i·on
me·sog·na·thous
meso·hy·lo·ma
meso·hy·po·blast
meso·ile·um
meso-ino·si·tol
meso·je·ju·num
meso·lec·i·thal
me·sol·o·gy
meso·me·lia
meso·mel·ic
meso·mere
meso·mer·ic
me·som·er·ism
meso·me·tri·um
meso·morph
meso·mor·phic
meso·mor·phy
meso·mu·cin·ase
me·som·u·la
meso·na·sal
meso·neph·ric
meso·neph·roi

meso·ne·phro·ma
meso·neph·ron
meso·neph·ros *pl.* meso·neph·roi
meso-omen·tum
meso·pal·li·um
meso·pexy
meso·phile
meso·phil·ic
meso·phle·bi·tis
meso·phrag·ma
me·soph·ry·on
meso·phyll
mes·o·pia
mes·op·ic
Mes·o·pin
meso·pneu·mon
meso·por·phy·rin
meso·pro·sop·ic
meso·pul·mo·num
meso·ra·chis·chi·sis
me·sor·chi·al
me·sor·chi·um
meso·rec·tum
meso·rid·a·zine
   m. besylate
meso·rop·ter
mes·or·rha·phy
mes·or·rhine
meso·sal·pinx
meso·scap·u·la
meso·seme
meso·sig·moid
meso·sig·moi·di·tis
meso·sig·moido·pexy
meso·some
meso·staph·y·line
meso·ste·ni·um
meso·ster·num
meso·stro·ma
meso·sys·tol·ic
meso·tar·sal
meso·tau·ro·don·tism
meso·ten·din·e·um
meso·ten·don
meso·ten·on
meso·tes·tis

meso·the·li·al
meso·the·li·o·ma
   pleural m.
meso·the·li·um
mes·oth·e·nar
mes·o·trop·ic
meso·tym·pa·num
mes·o·var·i·um
mes·ox·a·lyl urea
mes·sen·ger
   second m.
mes·ter·o·lone
Mes·ti·non
mes·tra·nol
mes·u·prine hy·dro·chlo·ride
mes·uran·ic
mes·y·late
Met — methionine
met
meta-analysis
meta-ar·thrit·ic
me·tab·a·sis
meta·bi·o·sis
met·a·bol·ic
met·a·bo·lim·e·ter
met·a·bo·lim·e·try
me·tab·o·lism
   acid-base m.
   aerobic m.
   ammonotelic m.
   basal m.
   endergonic m.
   endogenous m.
   energy m.
   excess m. of exercise
   exergonic m.
   exogenous m.
   inborn error of m.
   intermediary m.
   ureotelic m.
   uricotelic m.
me·tab·o·lite
   essential m.
   secondary m.
me·tab·o·liz·a·ble
me·tab·o·lize
meta·brom·sa·lan

meta·bu·teth·amine hy·dro·chlo·ride
meta·bu·toxy·caine hy·dro·chlo·ride
meta·car·pal
meta·car·pec·to·my
meta·car·po·pha·lan·ge·al
meta·car·pus
meta·cele
meta·cen·tric
meta·cer·ca·ria *pl.* meta·cer·ca·riae
meta·chro·ma·sia
meta·chro·mat·ic
meta·chro·ma·tin
meta·chro·ma·tism
meta·chro·mato·phil
meta·chro·mia
meta·chro·mic
meta·chro·mo·phil
meta·chro·mo·phile
meta·chro·mo·some
me·tach·ro·nous
meta·chro·sis
meta·coele
meta·coe·lo·ma
meta·cone
meta·con·id
meta·con·ule
meta·cor·tan·dra·cin
meta·cor·tan·dra·lone
meta·cre·sol
    m. purple
    m. sulfonphthalein
meta·cryp·to·zo·ite
meta·cy·e·sis
meta·du·o·den·um
meta·fe·male
meta·gas·ter
meta·gas·tru·la
meta·gel·a·tin
meta·gen·e·sis
meta·glob·u·lin
meta·go·ni·mi·a·sis
Meta·gon·i·mus
    M. ovatus
    M. yokogawai
meta·gran·u·lo·cyte

meta·he·mo·glo·bin
meta·hy·drin
meta·ic·ter·ic
meta·in·fec·tive
meta·io·do·ben·zyl·gua·ni·dine
meta·ki·ne·sis
met·al
    alkali m.
    alkaline earth m's
    Babbitt m.
    bell m.
    colloidal m.
    fusible m.
    heavy m.
    Melotte's m.
    Wood's m.
met·al·bu·min
met·al·de·hyde
me·tal·lic
met·al·lized
met·al·liz·ing
me·tal·lo·cy·a·nide
me·tal·lo·en·zyme
met·al·lo·fla·vo·de·hy·dro·gen·ase
me·tal·lo·fla·vo·pro·tein
met·al·loid
met·al·lo·phil
me·tal·lo·phil·ic
me·tal·lo·por·phy·rin
met·al·lo·pro·tein
met·al·los·co·py
me·tal·lo·ther·a·py
met·al·lo·thio·nein
met·al-sol
meta·mer
meta·mere
meta·mer·ic
me·tam·er·ism
    cutaneous m.
Met·a·mine
meta·mo·nad
meta·mor·phop·sia
meta·mor·pho·sis
    fatty m.
    ovulational m.
    platelet m.

meta·mor·pho·sis *(continued)*
    retrograde m.
    retrogressive m.
    revisionary m.
    structural m.
    tissue m.
    viscous m.
meta·mor·phot·ic
Met·a·mu·cil
meta·my·elo·cyte
meta·my·xo·vi·rus
Me·tan·dren
meta·neph·ric
meta·neph·rine
met·a·neph·ro·gen·ic
meta·neph·roi
meta·neph·ros *pl.* meta·neph·roi
meta·neu·tro·phil
met·a·nil yel·low
meta·nu·cle·us
meta·phase
Met·a·phed·rin
Met·a·phen
meta·phos·phate
meta·phos·phor·ic acid
meta·phys·e·al
me·taph·y·ses
meta·phys·i·al
me·taph·y·sis *pl.* me·taph·y·ses
meta·phys·itis
meta·pla·sia
    apocrine m.
    intestinal m.
    myeloid m.
    myeloid m., agnogenic
    primary myeloid m.
    pseudopyloric m.
    m. of pulp
    squamous m.
me·tap·la·sis
meta·plasm
meta·plas·tic
meta·pneu·mon·ic
meta·po·di·a·lia
meta·poph·y·sis
Met·a·prel

meta·pro·tein
meta·pro·ter·e·nol sul·fate
meta·psy·chol·o·gy
meta·py·rone
meta·ram·i·nol
    m. bitartrate
met·ar·chon
meta·rho·dop·sin
met·ar·te·ri·ole
meta·ru·bri·cyte
meta·sac·cha·ric acid
meta·so·ma·tome
meta·sta·ble
me·tas·ta·ses
me·tas·ta·sis
    biochemical m.
    calcareous m.
    cannonball m.
    contact m.
    cotton-ball m.
    crossed m.
    direct m.
    implantation m.
    osteoblastic m.
    osteolytic m.
    osteoplastic m.
    paradoxical m.
    retrograde m.
    transplantation m.
me·tas·ta·size
meta·stat·ic
meta·ster·num
meta·stron·gyl·i·dae
Meta·stron·gy·lus
meta·sy·nap·sis
meta·syn·cri·sis
meta·syn·de·sis
meta·tar·sal
meta·tar·sal·gia
meta·tar·sec·to·my
meta·tar·so·pha·lan·ge·al
meta·tar·sus
    m. adductocavus
    m. adductovarus
    m. adductus
    m. atavicus
    m. brevis
    m. latus

meta·tar·sus *(continued)*
    m. primus varus
    m. varus
Met·a·ten·sin
meta·thal·a·mus
meta·the·ria
meta·the·ri·an
me·tath·e·sis
meta·thet·ic
meta·throm·bin
meta·troph
meta·tro·phia
meta·troph·ic
met·at·ro·phy
meta·typ·ic
meta·typ·i·cal
meta·van·a·date
    sodium m.
me·tax·a·lone
meta·xe·nia
me·tax·e·ny
Meta·zoa
met·a·zoa
meta·zo·al
meta·zo·an
meta·zo·nal
meta·zo·on *pl.* meta·zoa
meta·zoo·no·sis
Metch·ni·koff, Elie
Metch·ni·koff's theory
Metch·ni·ko·vel·li·da
me·te·cious
met·en·ce·phal·ic
met·en·ceph·a·lon
met·en·ceph·a·lo·spi·nal
met-en·keph·a·lin
me·te·or·ism
me·te·o·rol·o·gy
me·te·oro·pa·thol·o·gy
me·te·orop·a·thy
me·te·oro·re·sis·tant
me·te·oro·sen·si·tive
me·te·oro·trop·ic
me·te·orot·ro·pism
met·ep·en·ceph·a·lon
me·ter
    counting-rate m.
    dosage m.

me·ter *(continued)*
    dose-rate m.
    electronic pH m.
    integrating dose m.
    light m.
    peak flow m.
    potential acuity m.
    rate m.
    zero-crossing m.
met·er·ga·sis
met·for·min
meth·ac·e·tin
meth·a·cho·line
    m. bromide
    m. chloride
meth·ac·ry·late
meth·a·cryl·ic acid
meth·a·cy·cline
    m. hydrochloride
meth·a·done hy·dro·chlo·ride
meth·a·dyl ac·e·tate
meth·al·le·nes·tril
meth·al·li·bure
meth·am·phet·amine
    m. hydrochloride
meth·an·dri·ol
meth·an·dro·sten·o·lone
meth·ane
meth·ane·sul·fo·nate
meth·ane·sul·fon·ic acid
Meth·a·no·bac·te·ri·a·ceae
Meth·a·no·bac·te·ri·um
Meth·a·no·coc·cus
meth·a·no·gen
meth·a·no·gen·ic
meth·a·nol
meth·a·nol·y·sis
Meth·a·no·sar·ci·na
me·than·the·line bro·mide
meth·a·pyr·i·lene
    m. fumarate
    m. hydrochloride
me·tha·qua·lone
    m. hydrochloride
me·thar·bi·tal
meth·a·zo·la·mide
meth·di·la·zine
    m. hydrochloride

met·hem·al·bu·min
met·hem·al·bu·min·emia
met·heme
met·he·mo·glo·bin
met·he·mo·glo·bin·emia
    enterogenous m.
    toxic m.
met·he·mo·glo·bin·emic
met·he·mo·glo·bin re·duc·
tase (NADPH)
met·he·mo·glo·bin·uria
meth·en·amine
    m. hippurate
    m. mandelate
    m. silver
meth·ene
me·then·o·lone
    m. acetate
    m. enanthate
Meth·er·gine
meth·es·trol di·pro·pri·o·nate
me·thet·o·in
meth·ex·e·nyl
meth·i·cil·lin so·di·um
meth·im·a·zole
meth·ine
meth·io·dal so·di·um
me·thi·o·nine
me·thi·o·nine syn·thase
me·thi·o·nyl
me·this·a·zone
Meth·i·um
me·thix·ene hy·dro·chlo·ride
meth·o·car·ba·mol
Meth·o·cel
meth·od
    Abbott's m.
    A.B.C. (alum, blood, clay)
      m.
    Abell-Kendall m.
    absorption m.
    acid hematin m.
    Addis m.
    agar diffusion m.
    Altmann-Gersh m.
    aniline-fuchsin-methyl
      green m.
    Arnold and Gunning's m.

meth·od *(continued)*
    Aronson's m.
    Ashby m.
    Askenstedt's m.
    Astrup m.
    Austin and Van Slyke's m.
    Autenrieth and Funk's m.
    autoclave m.
    auxanographic m.
    back pressure–arm lift m.
    Baer's m.
    Bang's m.
    Bangerter's m.
    Barger's m.
    Barraquer's m.
    Bass m.
    bathophenanthroline m.
    Beck's m.
    Bell m.
    bench m.
    Benedict's m.
    Benedict and Newton m.
    Bergonie m.
    Bethea's m.
    Bielschowsky's m.
    Bivine's m.
    Black's m.
    Bliss m.
    Bloch's m. for dopa oxidase
    Bloor, Pelkan, and Allen's
      m.
    Bock and Benedict's m.
    Bodian m.
    Bogg's m.
    Born m.
    Brandt-Andrews m.
    breath alcohol m.
    Brehmer's m.
    Breslau's m.
    brine flotation m.
    bromcresol green m.
    Brunn's m.
    Cajal m.
    caliper m.
    Callahan m.
    Carrel's m.
    Castaneda's m.
    Castel m.

meth·od *(continued)*
    Cathelin's m.
    centric heterochromatin m.
    Chandler's m.
    Charter's m.
    Cherry-Crandall m.
    Chervin's m.
    chest pressure–arm lift m.
    Chick-Martin m.
    chloropercha m.
    Ciaccio's m.
    Clark-Collip m.
    Clausen's m.
    closed-plaster m.
    Converse m.
    Conway m.
    Coons fluorescent antibody
        m.
    Copenhagen m.
    copper sulfate m.
    Corley and Denis' m.
    Corning's m.
    Corri's m.
    Couette m.
    coupling m.
    Coutard's m.
    Crane m.
    Credé's m.
    Cronin m.
    cross-sectional m.
    Cuignet's m.
    cup plate m.
    cyanmethemoglobin m.
    Dakin-Carrel m.
    Davenport's alcoholic
        silver nitrate m.
    definitive m.
    Dehn and Clark's m.
    deletion m.
    Denis' m.
    Denis and Leche's m.
    Denman's m.
    Dick's m.
    Dickinson m.
    differential agglutination
        m.
    direct m.
    direct aeration m.

meth·od *(continued)*
    direct centrifugal flotation
        m.
    disk diffusion m.
    disk sensitivity m.
    Domagk's m.
    Douglas' m.
    Duke's m.
    Eggleston's m.
    Eicken's m.
    Ellinger's m.
    Emmet-Studdiford m.
    Epstein's m.
    Erlangen m.
    Esbach's m.
    Fahraeus m.
    falling drop m.
    Faust's m.
    Feulgen m.
    Fichera's m.
    Fick m.
    Fishberg's m.
    Fiske's m.
    Fiske and Subbarow's m.
    Fitz Gerald m.
    flash m.
    flotation m.
    flush m.
    Folin's m.
    Folin, Benedict, and
        Myers's m.
    Folin and Svedberg m.
    Folin and Wu's m.
    Fone's m.
    Freiburg m.
    Frey and Gigon's m.
    Fridericia's m.
    Fülleborn's m.
    gasometric m.
    Gerota's m.
    Giemsa m.
    Girard's m.
    Given's m.
    glucose oxidase m.
    gold number m.
    Golgi's m.
    Gomori's m.
    Gordon and Sweet m.

meth·od *(continued)*
   Graff m.
   Gram's m.
   Greenwald's m.
   Greenwald and Lewman's
     m.
   Greenwood-Yule m.
   Griffith's m.
   Gross's m.
   Guinard's m.
   Habel's m.
   Hagedorn and Jensen's m.
   Hall's m.
   Hamilton's m.
   Hammerschlag's m.
   Handley's m.
   Hartel's m.
   Heintz's m.
   hematoxylin-safranin m.
   Henriques and Sörensen's
     m.
   Herter and Foster's m.
   Heublein m.
   hexokinase m.
   Hirschberg's m.
   Hirschfeld's m.
   Hoffa's tendon shortening
     m.
   holding m.
   Holger Nielsen m.
   horizontal scrub m.
   Hortega m.
   Hotchkiss m.
   Howard's m.
   Howell's m.
   Hung's m.
   Hunt's m.
   Hunter and Given's m.
   impedance m.
   India ink m.
   indirect m.
   introspective m.
   Ionescu m.
   Ivy's m.
   Jenckel's chloecysto-
     duodenostomy m.
   Johnson m.
   Johnston's m.

meth·od *(continued)*
   Kaiserling's m.
   Kaplan-Meier m.
   Karr's m.
   Kendall's m.
   Kenny's m.
   Kety-Schmidt m.
   Kirstein's m.
   Kittrich m.
   Kjeldahl's m.
   Klüver-Barrera m.
   Koch and McMeekin's m.
   Korotkoff's m.
   Kramer and Gittleman's
     m.
   Kramer and Tisdall's m.
   Kristeller's m.
   Krogh's m.
   Krueger and Schmidt's m.
   Kwilecki's m.
   Laborde's m.
   Lamaze m.
   Lane m.
   Lange tendon lengthening
     m.
   Langendorff's m.
   lateral condensation m.
   m. of least squares
   Leboyer m.
   Leipert's m.
   Letonoff and Reinhold m.
   Levanditi's m.
   Levy, Rowntree, and
     Marriott's m.
   Lewis and Benedict's m.
   Lewisohn's m.
   lime m.
   Lindemann's m.
   Ling's m.
   Linser's m.
   Lister's m.
   longitudinal m.
   Looney and Dyer m.
   Lorenz m.
   Løvset's m.
   Lown and Woolf m.
   Lyman's m.
   McCrudden's m.

meth·od *(continued)*
 macro-Kjeldahl m.
 McLean and Van Slyke's
  m.
 Majorstrüm m.
 Malfatti's m.
 Malloy-Evelyn m.
 Manchester m.
 Mann's m.
 Mantel-Haenszel m.
 Marchi's m.
 Marfan's m.
 Marriott's m.
 Marshall's m.
 Masson's trichrome m.
 Mauriceau-Smellie-Veit m.
 Maximow's m.
 Meltzer's m.
 Messinger and Huppert's
  m.
 Mett's m.
 Meulengracht's m.
 Meyer's m.
 micro-Astrup m.
 micro-Kjeldahl m.
 Millard m.
 Minkowski's m.
 Moerner-Sjöqvist m.
 Mohr's m.
 Mosley m.
 mouth-to-mouth m.
 multiple cone m.
 Murphy m.
 Myers' m.
 Myers and Wardell's m.
 Naunyn-Minkowski m.
 Nègre and Bretey m.
 Neumann's m.
 Nielsen m.
 nigrosin m.
 Nikiforoff's m.
 Nimeh's m.
 Nirenstein and Schiff's m.
 Nissi's m.
 no-touch m.
 nutritional table m.
 Oberst's m.
 Ogata's m.

meth·od *(continued)*
 Ogino-Knaus m.
 Oliver-Rosalki m.
 Ombrédanne m.
 optical density m.
 Orr m.
 Orsi-Grocco m.
 Osborne and Folin's m.
 ovulation m.
 Pachon's m.
 panoptic m.
 Pap's silver m.
 Paracelsian m.
 parallax m.
 Parker's m.
 Parker-Kerr m.
 Partipilo m.
 Pavlov's m.
 Payr's m.
 Perdrau's m.
 Peter's m.
 Pfeiffer-Comberg m.
 Pfiffner and Myers'm.
 piggybacking m.
 Plimmer and Skelton's m.
 point source m.
 Power and Wilder's m.
 Price-Jones m.
 probit m.
 projective m.
 Pryce slide-culture m.
 psychometric m.
 psychophysical m.
 pulse reflection m.
 Purdy's m.
 Purmann's m.
 quinacrine fluorescent m.
 radioactive balloon m.
 Raiziss and Dubin's m.
 recall m.
 recognition m.
 Reed and Muench m.
 reference m.
 Regaud's (Regaut's) m.
 Rehfuss'm.
 Reichert's m.
 retrofilling m.
 Reverdin's m.

meth·od *(continued)*
    reverse Giemsa m.
    rhythm m.
    Rideal-Walker m.
    Ritchie's formol-ether m.
    Ritgen's m.
    Roaf's m.
    roll m.
    Romanovsky's
      (Romanowsky's) m.
    Rosenheim and
      Drummond's m.
    Roughton-Scholander m.
    Ruhemann's uricometer m.
    Sahli's m.
    Salkowski's m.
    Salkowski and Arnstein's
      m.
    Salkowski, Autenrieth, and
      Barth's m.
    Satterthwaite's m.
    savings m.
    Sayre's m.
    Schafer m.
    Scherer's m.
    Schlossmann's m.
    Schüller's m.
    Schweninger's m.
    Scott and Wilson's m.
    sectional m.
    segmentation m.
    Shaffer's m.
    Shaffer-Hartmann m.
    Shaffer and Marriott's m.
    Shohl and Pedley's m.
    Siffert m.
    Sigma m.
    silver point (cone) m.
    Silvester m.
    single cone m.
    Sippy m.
    Sjöqvist's m.
    Skoog's m.
    Sluder m.
    Smellie's m.
    Smellie-Veit m.
    Somogyi m.
    Sörensen's m.

meth·od *(continued)*
    split cast m.
    Staffieri's m.
    Stamm m.
    Stammer's m.
    Stas-Otto m.
    Stehle's m.
    Stillman's m.
    Stockholm and Koch's m.
    Stoll's m.
    m. of successive
      approximations
    suction m.
    Sumner's m.
    suspension m.
    symptothermal m.
    syringe-capillary m.
    Taylor and Hulton's m.
    Thane's m.
    thick-film m.
    Thom flap m.
    Tisdall's m.
    Torkildsen shunt m.
    Tracy and Welker's m.
    Trillat's m.
    Trueta m.
    Tswett's m.
    turbidity m.
    uranium acetate m.
    van Gehuchten's m.
    Van Slyke's m.
    Van Slyke and Cullen's m.
    Van Slyke and Fitz's m.
    Van Slyke and Meyer's m.
    Van Slyke and Neill m.
    Van Slyke and Palmer's m.
    vertical condensation m.
    Volhard and Arnold's m.
    Volhard and Harvey's m.
    von Fürth and Charnass'
      m.
    Wade's m.
    Wade-Fite m.
    Wade-Fite-Faraco m.
    Walgren's m.
    Walker's m.
    Wallace and Diamond's m.

meth·od *(continued)*
   Wallhauser and
     Whitehead's m.
   Wardill's m.
   Wardill four-flap m.
   Wardill two-flap m.
   Waring's m.
   Weber's m.
   Weed-McKibben m.
   Weigert-Pal m.
   Weil-Hallé m.
   Welcker's m.
   Welker's m.
   Westergren m.
   Whipple's m.
   Whitehorn's m.
   Wiechowski and
     Handorsky's m.
   Wilson's m.
   Wintrobe m.
   Wintrobe and Landsberg's
     m.
   Wolter's m.
   Wroblewski m.
   Wynn m.
   Ziehl-Neelsen m.
   Zsigmondy's gold number
     m.
meth·od·ism
Meth·od·ist
meth·od·ol·o·gy
meth·o·hex·i·tal
   m. sodium
meth·o·pho·line
meth·o·pro·ma·zine mal·e·ate
meth·o·trex·ate
meth·o·tri·mep·ra·zine
me·thox·amine hy·dro·chlo·ride
me·thox·sa·len
me·thoxy ac·et·an·i·lide
me·thoxy·chlor
meth·oxy·flu·rane
me·thox·y·in·doles
me·thox·yl
me·thoxy·phen·amine hy·dro·chlo·ride

me·thoxy·pro·ma·zine mal·e·ate
8-me·thoxy·psor·a·len
meth·phen·oxy·di·ol
meth·sco·pol·amine bro·mide
meth·sux·i·mide
meth·y·clo·thi·a·zide
meth·yl
   m. amylketone
   m. anthranilate
   m. benzene
   m. chloride
   m. ethyl-maleicimid
   m. ethyl-pyrrole
   m. hydride
   m. hydroxy-furfurol
   m. iodide
   m. isobutyl ketone
   m. methacrylate
   m. salicylate
   m. sulfonate
α-meth·yl·a·ce·to·ac·e·tyl CoA-β-ke·to·thi·o·lase
meth·yl·al
meth·yl·amine
meth·yl·as·par·tate am·mo·nia-ly·ase
meth·yl·ate
meth·yl·at·ed
meth·yl·a·tion
meth·yl·at·ro·pine hy·dro·bro·mide
meth·yl·at·ro·pine ni·trate
meth·yl·az·oxy·meth·a·nol
meth·yl·ben·ze·tho·ni·um chlo·ride
meth·yl·cat·e·chol
meth·yl·cel·lu·lose
   hydroxypropyl m.
meth·yl·chlo·ro·for·mate
3-meth·yl·cho·lan·threne
meth·yl·cre·o·sol
meth·yl·cro·ton·o·yl-CoA car·box·y·lase
3-meth·yl·cro·to·nyl CoA car·box·y·lase deficiency
β-meth·yl·cro·to·nyl·gly·cin·uria

meth·yl·cy·to·sine
meth·yl·di·chlor·ar·sin
meth·yl·di·hy·dro·mor·phi·none
meth·yl·do·pa
meth·yl·do·pate hy·dro·chlo·ride
meth·y·lene
    m. bichloride
    m. blue
    m. chloride
    m. dichloride
meth·yl·ene·tet·ra·hy·dro·fol·ate (THF) de·hy·dro·gen·ase
5,10-meth·yl·ene·tet·ra·hy·dro·fo·late re·duc·tase (FADH$_2$)
meth·yl·ene·tet·ra·hy·dro·fo·late (THF) re·duc·tase deficiency
meth·y·len·o·phil
meth·yl·en·oph·i·lous
meth·yl·er·go·no·vine mal·e·ate
meth·yl·glu·ca·mine
meth·yl·gly·ox·a·lase
meth·yl·gly·ox·a·li·din
meth·yl·guan·i·dine
meth·yl·gua·no·sine
meth·yl·hex·amine
meth·yl·hex·ane·amine
meth·yl·hy·dan·to·in
me·thyl·ic
me·thyl·i·dyne
meth·yl·in·dol
meth·yl·ino·sine
meth·yl·ma·lon·ic acid
meth·yl·ma·lon·ic·ac·i·du·ria
meth·yl·mal·o·nyl-CoA epim·er·ase
meth·yl·mal·o·nyl-CoA mu·tase
meth·yl·mal·o·nyl-CoA ra·ce·mase
meth·yl·mer·cap·tan
meth·yl·mor·phine
meth·yl·par·a·ben

meth·yl·par·a·fy·nol
meth·yl·pen·tose
meth·yl·pen·ty·nol
meth·yl·phen·i·date hy·dro·chlo·ride
meth·yl·phen·yl lev·u·lo·sa·zone
meth·yl·phen·yl·hy·dra·zine
meth·yl·pred·nis·o·lone
    m. acetate
    m. hemisuccinate
    m. sodium phosphate
    m. sodium succinate
meth·yl·pu·rine
meth·yl·py·ra·pone
meth·yl·py·ri·dine
meth·yl·ro·san·i·line chlo·ride
meth·yl·tes·tos·ter·one
5-meth·yl·te·tra·hy·dro·fo·late-ho·mo·cys·teine meth·yl·trans·fer·ase
meth·yl·the·o·bro·mine
meth·yl·thi·o·nine chlo·ride
meth·yl·thio·ura·cil
meth·yl·trans·fer·ase
meth·yl·uram·ine
5-meth·yl·ura·cil
meth·yl·xan·thine
me·thyn·o·di·ol di·ac·e·tate
meth·y·pry·lon
meth·y·ser·gide
    m. maleate
me·ti·amide
me·ti·a·pine
Met·i·cor·te·lone
Met·i·cor·ten
me·tiz·o·line hy·dro·chlo·ride
met·myo·glo·bin
met·o·clo·pra·mide hy·dro·chlo·ride
met·o·cu·rine io·dide
met·o·gest
me·tol·a·zone
    methyl m.
me·ton·y·my
me·top·a·gus
me·top·ic

met·o·pim·a·zine
me·to·pi·on
Met·o·pi·rone
met·o·pism
met·op·odyn·ia
me·to·pon
met·o·pop·a·gus
me·topo·plas·ty
met·o·prine
me·to·pro·lol
Met·or·chis
met·o·ser·pate hy·dro·chlo·
   ride
me·tox·e·nous
me·tox·e·ny
me·tra
me·tral·gia
me·tra·nas·trophe
me·tra·term
me·trat·o·my
me·tra·to·nia
me·tra·tro·phia
Met·ra·zol
met·re·chos·co·py
me·trec·ta·sia
me·trec·to·my
me·trec·to·pia
Met·re·ton
me·treu·ryn·ter
me·treu·ry·sis
me·tria
met·ric
met·ri·fo·nate
met·rio·ce·phal·ic
met·ri·pho·nate
me·tri·tic
me·tri·tis
   m. dissecans
   dissecting m.
   puerperal m.
me·triz·a·mide
met·ri·zo·ate so·di·um
me·tri·zo·ic acid
me·tro·car·ci·no·ma
me·tro·cele
me·tro·col·po·cele
me·tro·cys·to·sis
me·tro·cyte

me·tro·dyn·ia
me·tro·en·do·me·tri·tis
me·tro·fi·bro·ma
me·trog·e·nous
me·trog·ra·phy
me·tro·leu·kor·rhea
me·trol·o·gy
me·tro·lym·phan·gi·tis
me·tro·ma·la·cia
me·tro·mal·a·co·ma
me·tro·men·or·rha·gia
me·tro·na·nia
me·tro·ni·da·zole
me·trono·scope
me·tro·pa·ral·y·sis
me·tro·path·ia
   m. hemorrhagica
me·tro·path·ic
me·trop·a·thy
   syncytiotrophoblastic m.
me·tro·peri·to·ne·al
me·tro·peri·to·ni·tis
me·tro·pexy
me·tro·phle·bi·tis
Me·tro·pine
me·tro·plas·ty
me·trop·o·lis
me·trop·to·sis
me·tror·rha·gia
   m. myopathica
me·tror·rhea
me·tror·rhex·is
me·tro·sal·pin·gi·tis
me·tro·sal·pin·gog·ra·phy
me·tro·sal·pinx
me·tro·scope
me·tros·ta·sis
me·tro·stax·is
me·tro·ste·no·sis
me·tro·ther·a·py
me·trot·o·my
me·tro·tu·bog·ra·phy
M. et sig. — L. misce et signa
   (mix and write a label)
Mett's (Mette) method
Mett's (Mette) test tubes
Me·tu·bine
met·ure·de·pa

me·tyr·a·pone
   m. tartrate
me·ty·ro·sine
Meu·len·gracht's diet
Meu·len·gracht's method
Meu·nier sign
MeV — megaelectron volt
Mev — megaelectron volt
me·val·o·nate
me·va·lon·ic acid
me·vino·lin
Mex·ate
mex·il·e·tine
mex·ren·o·ate po·tas·si·um
Mey·en·burg's complexes
Mey·er's disease
Mey·er's line
Mey·er's loop
Mey·er's operation
Mey·er's organ
Mey·er's sinus
Mey·er's system
Mey·er's theory
Mey·er-Betz disease
Mey·er-Over·ton theory
Mey·er·hof, Otto Fritz
Mey·nert's bundle
Mey·nert's cell
Mey·nert's commissure
Mey·nert's fasciculus
Mey·nert's tract
Mey·net's nodes
me·ze·re·um
mez·lo·cil·lin
MF — microscopic factor
   mycosis fungoides
μF — microfarad
MFD — minimal fatal dose
M. flac. — L. membrana
   flaccida (pars flaccida
   membranae tympani)
M. ft. — L. mistura fiat (let a
   mixture be made)
mg — milligram
mγ — milligamma
   (nanogram)
μg — microgram
$\mu\gamma$ — microgamma (picogram)

mgm — milligram
MHA — microhemagglutina-
   tion
MHA-TP — microhemagglutination assay–*Treponema*
   pallidum
MHC — major
   histocompatibility complex
MHD — minimum hemolytic
   dose
MHz — megahertz
Mi·an·eh bug
mi·an·ser·in hy·dro·chlo·ride
mi·as·ma
mi·as·mat·ic
Mi·bel·li's porokeratosis
MIBG — metaiodobenzylguanid-
   ine
mi·bol·er·one
mi·ca
mi·ca·ceous
Mi·ca·Tin
mi·ca·tion
mi·ca·to·sis
mi·cel·la
mi·celle
Mi·chae·lis constant
Mi·chae·lis's rhomboid
Mi·chae·lis stain
Mi·chae·lis-Gut·mann bodies
Mi·chae·lis-Men·ten equation
Mi·chel deformity
mi·con·a·zole ni·trate
mi·cra
mi·cran·at·o·my
mi·cran·gi·um
mi·cran·thine
mi·cren·ceph·a·lon
mi·cren·ceph·a·lous
mi·cren·ceph·a·ly
mi·cro·ab·scess
   Munro m.
   Pautrier's m.
mi·cro·ad·e·no·ma
mi·cro·ad·e·nop·a·thy
mi·cro·aero·phile
mi·cro·aero·phil·ic
mi·cro·aer·oph·i·lous

mi·cro·aer·o·sol
mi·cro·aero·to·nom·e·ter
mi·cro·ag·gre·gate
mi·cro·al·bu·min·uria
mi·cro·aleu·rio·spore
mi·cro·am·me·ter
mi·cro·am·pere
mi·cro·anal·y·sis
mi·cro·an·as·to·mo·sis
mi·cro·anat·o·mist
mi·cro·anat·o·my
mi·cro·an·eu·rysm
mi·cro·an·gi·og·ra·phy
mi·cro·an·gio·path·ic
mi·cro·an·gi·op·a·thy
    diabetic m.
    thrombotic m.
mi·cro·an·gi·os·co·py
mi·cro·bac·te·ria
Mi·cro·bac·te·ri·um
    M. *flavum*
    M. *lacticum*
mi·cro·bac·te·ri·um *pl.* mi·
    cro·bac·te·ria
mi·cro·bal·ance
mi·cro·bar
mi·crobe
mi·cro·be·mia
mi·cro·bi·al
mi·cro·bi·an
mi·cro·bic
mi·cro·bi·ci·dal
mi·cro·bid
mi·cro·bi·emia
mi·cro·bi·cide
mi·cro·bio·as·say
mi·cro·bi·o·log·i·cal
mi·cro·bi·ol·o·gist
mi·cro·bi·ol·o·gy
mi·cro·bio·pho·tom·e·ter
mi·cro·bi·o·ta
mi·cro·bi·ot·ic
mi·cro·bism
mi·cro·blast
mi·cro·ble·pha·ria
mi·cro·bleph·a·rism
mi·cro·bleph·a·ry
mi·cro·body

mi·cro·bra·chia
mi·cro·bra·chi·us
mi·cro·bren·ner
mi·cro·bu·ret
mi·cro·ca·lix
mi·cro·cal·o·rie
mi·cro·cal·cu·lus
mi·cro·cal·o·rim·e·try
mi·cro·cap·sule
mi·cro·car·dia
mi·cro·car·ri·er
mi·cro·cau·lia
mi·cro·cen·trum
mi·cro·ce·phal·ic
mi·cro·ceph·a·lism
mi·cro·ceph·a·lous
mi·cro·ceph·a·lus
mi·cro·ceph·a·ly
    encephaloclastic m.
    schizencephalic m.
mi·cro·chei·lia
mi·cro·chei·ria
mi·cro·chem·i·cal
mi·cro·chem·is·try
mi·cro·cin·e·ma·tog·ra·phy
mi·cro·cir·cu·la·tion
mi·cro·cir·cu·la·to·ry
mi·cro·cli·mate
mi·cro·cne·mia
Mi·cro·coc·ca·ceae
mi·cro·coc·ci
Mi·cro·coc·cus
mi·cro·coc·cus *pl.* mi·cro·coc·
    ci
mi·cro·co·lon
mi·cro·col·o·ny
mi·cro·con·cen·tra·tion
mi·cro·co·nid·ia
mi·cro·co·nid·i·um *pl.* mi·
    cro·co·nid·ia
mi·cro·co·ria
mi·cro·cor·nea
mi·cro·cou·lomb
mi·cro·cra·nia
mi·cro·crys·tal
mi·cro·crys·tal·line
mi·cro·cu·rie
mi·cro·cu·rie-hour

mi·cro·cyst
mi·cro·cys·tom·e·ter
mi·cro·cyte
mi·cro·cy·the·mia
mi·cro·cy·to·sis
mi·cro·cy·to·tox·ic·i·ty
mi·cro·dac·tyl·ia
mi·cro·dac·ty·ly
mi·cro·dens·i·tom·e·ter
mi·cro·den·tism
mi·cro·der·ma·tome
mi·cro·de·ter·mi·na·tion
mi·cro·dis·sec·tion
mi·cro·dont
mi·cro·don·tia
mi·cro·don·tic
mi·cro·don·tism
mi·cro·do·sage
mi·cro·dose
mi·cro·drep·a·no·cyt·ic
mi·cro·drep·a·no·cy·to·sis
mi·cro·ecol·o·gy
mi·cro·eco·sys·tem
mi·cro·elec·trode
mi·cro·elec·tro·pho·re·sis
mi·cro·elec·tro·pho·ret·ic
mi·cro·em·bo·lus *pl.* mi·cro·em·bo·li
mi·cro·en·ceph·a·ly
mi·cro·en·vi·ron·ment
mi·cro·eryth·ro·cyte
mi·cro·es·the·sia
mi·cro·es·ti·ma·tion
mi·cro·far·ad
mi·cro·fau·na
mi·cro·fi·bril
mi·cro·fil·a·ment
mi·cro·fil·a·re·mia
mi·cro·fi·la·ria
   m. bancrofti
   m. diurna
   m. loa
   sheathed m.
   m. streptocerca
   m. volvulus
mi·cro·fil·i·a·ri·a·sis
mi·cro·film
mi·cro·flo·ra

mi·cro·flu·or·om·e·try
mi·cro·fol·lic·u·lar
mi·cro·frac·ture
mi·cro·fun·gus
mi·cro·gam·ete
mi·cro·ga·me·to·cyte
mi·cro·ga·me·to·phyte
mi·cro·gam·ma
mi·cro·gam·ont
mi·crog·a·my
mi·cro·gas·tria
mi·cro·gen·e·sis
mi·cro·gen·ia
mi·cro·gen·i·tal·ism
mi·crog·lia
mi·crog·li·al
mi·crog·lio·cyte
mi·cro·gli·o·ma
mi·cro·gli·o·ma·to·sis
   m. cerebri
mi·cro·gli·o·sis
mi·cro·glob·u·lin
β_2-mi·cro·glob·u·lin
mi·cro·glos·sia
mi·cro·glos·sic
mi·cro·gna·thia
mi·cro·go·nio·scope
mi·cro·gram
mi·cro·graph
   acoustic m.
   electron m.
mi·cro·gra·phia
mi·crog·ra·phy
mi·cro·grav·i·ty
mi·cro·gy·ri
mi·cro·gyr·ia
mi·cro·gy·rus *pl.* mi·cro·gy·ri
mi·cro·he·ma·to·crit
mi·cro·he·pat·ia
mi·cro·het·ero·ge·ne·i·ty
mi·cro·his·tol·o·gy
mi·cro·in·cin·er·a·tion
mi·cro·in·ci·sion
mi·cro·in·farct
mi·cro·in·jec·tion
mi·cro·in·jec·tor
mi·cro·in·va·sion
mi·cro·in·va·sive

mi·cro·kat·al
mi·cro·kin·e·ma·tog·ra·phy
mi·cro·lar·yn·gos·co·py
mi·cro·lec·i·thal
mi·cro·len·tia
mi·cro·le·sion
mi·cro·leu·ko·blast
mi·cro·li·ter
mi·cro·lith
mi·cro·li·thi·a·sis
    m. alveolaris pulmonum
    pulmonary alveolar m.
mi·crol·o·gy
mi·cro·lym·phoido·cyte
mi·cro·man·di·ble
mi·cro·ma·nip·u·la·tion
mi·cro·ma·nip·u·la·tor
mi·cro·ma·nom·e·ter
mi·cro·mano·met·ric
mi·cro·mas·tia
mi·cro·max·il·la
mi·cro·ma·zia
mi·cro·meg·a·lop·sia
mi·cro·me·lia
    rhizomelic m.
mi·crom·e·lus
mi·cro·mere
mi·cro·me·tab·o·lism
mi·cro·me·tas·ta·sis
mi·crom·e·ter
    eyepiece m.
    filar m.
    ocular m.
    stage m.
mi·cro·me·ter
mi·cro·meth·od
mi·crom·e·try
mi·cro·mo·lar
mi·cro·mo·lec·u·lar
Mi·cro·mo·nos·po·ra
    M. inyoensis
    M. keratolyticum
    M. purpurea
Mi·cro·mo·nos·po·ra·ceae
mi·cro·my·e·lia
mi·cro·my·elo·blast
mi·cro·my·elo·lym·pho·cyte
mi·cron *pl.* mi·cra, mi·crons

mi·cro·nee·dle
mi·cro·neme
mi·cro·neu·ro·sur·gery
mi·cro·nize
mi·cro·nod·u·lar
mi·cro·nor·mo·blast
mi·cro·nu·cle·us
mi·cro·nu·tri·ent
mi·cro·nych·ia
mi·cro·nys·tag·mus
mi·cro-or·chid·ia
mi·cro-or·chi·dism
mi·cro·or·gan·ic
mi·cro·or·gan·ism
mi·cro·or·gan·is·mal
mi·cro·par·a·site
mi·cro·pa·thol·o·gy
mi·cro·pe·nis
mi·cro·per·fu·sion
mi·cro·phage
mi·cro·phago·cyte
mi·cro·pha·kia
mi·cro·phal·lus
mi·cro·phone
    cardiac catheter-m.
mi·cro·pho·nia
mi·cro·phon·ic
    cochlear m's
mi·cro·pho·no·graph
mi·cro·pho·to·graph
mi·croph·thal·mia
mi·croph·thal·mic
mi·croph·thal·mos
mi·croph·thal·mo·scope
mi·cro·phyte
mi·cro·pi·no·cy·to·sis
mi·cro·pi·pet
mi·cro·pi·tu·i·cyte
mi·cro·pla·sia
mi·cro·pleth·ys·mog·ra·phy
mi·cro·pli·cae
mi·cro·po·dia
mi·cro·po·lar·i·scope
mi·cro·poly·gy·ria
Mi·cro·poly·spo·ra
    M. faeni
mi·cro·pore
mi·cro·pre·cip·i·ta·tion

mi·cro·pre·da·tion
mi·cro·pred·a·tor
mi·cro·probe
 laser m.
mi·cro·pro·jec·tion
mi·cro·pro·jec·tor
mi·cro·pro·lac·ti·no·ma
mi·cro·pro·so·pus
mi·crop·sia
mi·crop·tic
mi·cro·punc·ture
mi·cro·pus
mi·cro·pyk·nom·e·ter
mi·cro·pyle
mi·cro·quan·ti·ty
mi·cro·ra·dio·gram
mi·cro·ra·dio·graph
mi·cro·ra·di·og·ra·phy
mi·cror·chid·ia
mi·cro·re·frac·tom·e·ter
mi·cro·res·pi·rom·e·ter
Mo·rel-Wil·di syndrome
mi·cro·rhin·ia
Mor·er·as·tron·gyl·us cos·tar·
 i·cen·sis
mi·cro·roent·gen
mi·cros·ce·lous
mi·cro·scler
mi·cro·scope
 acoustic m.
 beta ray m.
 binocular m.
 capillary m.
 centrifuge m.
 color-contrast m.
 comparison m.
 compound m.
 corneal m.
 darkfield m.
 dissecting m.
 electron m.
 fluorescence m.
 flying spot m.
 hypodermic m.
 infrared m.
 integrating m.
 interference m.
 ion m.

mi·cro·scope *(continued)*
 laser m.
 light m.
 ocular m.
 Omni operating m.
 opaque m.
 operating m.
 optical m.
 phase m.
 phase-contrast m.
 polarizing m.
 polarizing m., rectified
 projection x-ray m.
 reflecting m.
 Rheinberg m.
 scanning m.
 scanning electron m.
 schlieren m.
 simple m.
 slit lamp m.
 stereoscopic m.
 stroboscopic m.
 surgical m.
 trinocular m.
 ultra-m.
 ultrapaque m.
 ultrasonic m.
 ultraviolet m.
 Wild operating m.
 x-ray m.
mi·cro·scop·ic
mi·cro·scop·i·cal
mi·cros·co·pist
mi·cros·co·py
 bright-field m.
 clinical m.
 darkfield m.
 electron m.
 fluorescence m.
 fundus m.
 immersion m.
 immunofluorescence m.
 phase-contrast m.
 scanning transmission
  electron m.
 television m.
mi·cro·sec·ond
mi·cro·sec·tion

mi·cro·seme
mi·cro·slide
mi·cros·mat·ic
mi·cro·so·ma
mi·cro·so·mal
mi·cro·some
mi·cro·so·mia
   m. fetalis
mi·cro·spec·trog·ra·phy
mi·cro·spec·tro·pho·tom·e·
   ter
mi·cro·spec·tro·pho·tom·e·
   try
mi·cro·spec·tro·scope
mi·cro·sphere
mi·cro·sphe·ro·cyte
mi·cro·sphero·cy·to·sis
mi·cro·sphero·lith
mi·cro·spher·u·la·tion
mi·cro·sphyg·mia
mi·cro·sphyg·my
mi·cro·splanch·nia
mi·cro·splanch·nic
mi·cro·sple·nia
mi·cro·sple·nic
Mi·cros·po·ra
mi·cro·spo·ran·gia
mi·cro·spo·ran·gi·um *pl.* mi·
   cro·spo·ran·gia
mi·cro·spore
Mi·cro·spor·ea
mi·cro·spo·rid
Mi·cro·spor·i·da
mi·cro·spor·i·dan
mi·cro·spo·rid·i·an
mi·cro·spo·ro·sis
Mi·cros·po·rum
   M. audouinii
   M. canis
   M. felineum
   M. fulvum
   M. furfur
   M. gypseum
   M. lanosum
mi·cro·ster·e·og·no·sia
mi·cro·steth·o·phone
Mi·cro·stix-3

mi·cro·sto·mia
mi·cro·stra·bis·mus
mi·cro·sur·gery
mi·cro·su·ture
mi·cro·syr·inge
mi·cro·tech·nic
mi·cro·the·lia
mi·cro·throm·bo·sis
mi·cro·throm·bus *pl.* mi·cro·
   throm·bi
mi·cro·tia
mi·cro·ti·ter
mi·cro·tome
   freezing m.
   rocking m.
   rotary m.
   sliding m.
   Stadie-Riggs m.
mi·cro·tom·iza·tion
mi·cro·to·mog·ra·phy
mi·crot·o·my
mi·cro·to·nom·e·ter
mi·cro·trans·fu·sion
mi·cro·trau·ma
mi·cro·trich·ia
*Mi·cro·trom·bid·i·um ak·a·
   mu·shi*
mi·cro·tro·pia
mi·cro·tu·bule
   chromsomal m.
   kinetochore m.
   spindle m.
   subpellicular m.
Mi·cro·tus
   M. montebelli
mi·cro·tus
mi·cro·unit
mi·cro·vas·cu·lar
mi·cro·vas·cu·la·ture
mi·cro·vil·lus *pl.* mi·cro·vil·li
   placental m.
mi·cro·vis·co·sim·e·ter
mi·cro·viv·i·sec·tion
mi·cro·volt
mi·cro·vol·tom·e·ter
mi·cro·watt
mi·cro·wave
mi·croxy·cyte

mi·croxy·phil
mi·cro·zoa
mi·cro·zo·on *pl.* mi·cro·zoa
mi·crur·gic
mi·crur·gy
Mi·cru·roi·des
Mi·cru·rus
mic·tion
mic·tu·rate
mic·tu·ri·tion
MID — minimum infective
  dose
    minimum inhibiting dose
mi·da·flur
Mi·da·mor
mid·ax·il·la
mid·az·o·lam mal·e·ate
mid·body
mid·brain
mid·car·pal
mid·cla·vic·u·lar
mid·dle·piece
mid·epi·gas·tric
mid·foot
mid·fron·tal
midge
    owl m.
mid·get
mid·gut
mid·head
Mid·i·cel
mid·line
mid·oc·cip·i·tal
mid·pain
mid·pe·riph·e·ry
mid·pha·lan·ge·al
mid·plane
mid·riff
mid·sec·tion
mid·ster·num
mid·tar·sal
mid·teg·men·tum
mid·ven·tral
mid·ves·i·cal
mid·wife
mid·wi·fery
Miege syndrome
Mier·ze·jew·ski effect

Mie·scher's tube
Mie·scher's tubule
MIF — melanocyte-stimulating hormone inhibiting factor
mi·graine
    abdominal m.
    acute confusional m.
    complicated m.
    epileptic m.
    facioplegic m.
    fulgurating m.
    hemiplegic m.
    menstrual m.
    ophthalmic m.
    ophthalmoplegic m.
mi·grain·eur
mi·grain·oid
mi·grain·ous
mi·gra·tion
    anodic m.
    cathodic m.
    external m.
    internal m.
    m. of leukocytes
    m. of ovum
    retrograde m.
    tooth m., pathologic
    tooth m., physiologic
    transperitoneal m.
Mi·gu·la's classification
Mi·ked·i·mide
Mik·u·licz's angle
Mik·u·licz's aphthae
Mik·u·licz's cells
Mik·u·licz's clamp
Mik·u·licz's disease
Mik·u·licz's drain
Mik·u·licz's operation
Mik·u·licz's pad
Mik·u·licz's procedure
Mik·u·licz's pyloroplasty
Mik·u·licz's syndrome
Mik·u·licz-Ra·de·cki
  syndrome
Mik·u·licz-Sjö·gren syndrome
mil·am·me·ter
mil·dew
mi·len·pe·rone

Miles' operation
mile·stone
    developmental m's
mil·ia
Mil·i·an's erythema
mil·i·a·ria
    m. alba
    apocrine m.
    m. crystallina
    m. papulosa
    m. profunda
    m. propria
    pustular m.
    m. rubra
    m. vesiculosa
mil·i·ary
Mil·i·bis
mi·lieu
    m. extérieur
    m. intérieur
mil·i·per·tine
mil·i·um *pl.* mil·ia
    colloid m.
    m. neonatorum
milk
    acidophilus m.
    adapted m.
    after-m.
    albumin m.
    m. of bismuth
    bitter m.
    blue m.
    breast m.
    Bulgarian m.
    bulgaricus m.
    cancer m.
    casein m.
    certified m.
    condensed m.
    diabetic m.
    dialyzed m.
    dried m.
    evaporated m.
    fat m.
    fore-m.
    fortified m.
    grade A m.
    grade B m.

milk *(continued)*
    hind m.
    homogenized m.
    humanized m.
    laboratory m.
    lactic acid m.
    litmus m.
    m. of magnesia
    modified m.
    pasteurized m.
    protein m.
    roller-dried m.
    Schloss m.
    skimmed m.
    sour m.
    sterilized m.
    m. of sulfur
    tuberculin-tested m.
    uterine m.
    uviol m.
    vegetable m.
    vitamin D m.
    witch's m.
    yeast m.
milk·ing
milk-leg
Milk·man's syndrome
milk·pox
milk sick
Mil·lar's asthma
Mil·lard's test
Mil·lard-Gub·ler paralysis
Mil·lard-Gub·ler syndrome
Mil·len technique
Mil·ler-Ab·bott tube
mil·li·am·me·ter
mil·li·am·pere
mil·li·bar
mil·li·cou·lomb
mil·li·cu·rie
mil·li·cu·rie-hour
mil·li·equiv·a·lent
mil·li·gram
mil·li·gray
mil·li·herz
mil·li·joule
Mil·li·kan rays
mil·li·kat·al

mil·li·lam·bert
mil·li·li·ter
mil·li·me·ter
mil·li·mi·cro·cu·rie
mil·li·mo·lar
mil·li·mole
mill·ing-in
mil·lions
mil·li·os·mol, mil·li·os·mole
mil·li·pede
mil·li·rad
mil·li·rem
mil·li·roent·gen
mil·li·sec·ond
mil·li·unit
mil·li·volt
Mil·lon's reaction
Mil·lon's reagent
Mil·lon's test
Mills' disease
Mills-Rein·cke phenomenon
Mi·lon·tin
mil·ox·an·trone
Mil·path
mil·pho·sis
mil·ri·none
Mil·roy's disease
Mil·roy's edema
Mil·ton's disease
Mil·ton's edema
Mil·town
Mi·ma pol·y·mor·pha
mim·bane hy·dro·chlo·ride
mi·me·sis
mi·met·ic
mim·ic
mim·ic·ry
mim·ma·tion
mi·mo·sis
min. — L. minimum (minim)
Min·a·ma·ta disease
Min·card
mind
Min·der·e·rus, spirit of
min·er·al
    trace m's
min·er·al·i·za·tion
min·er·alo·cor·ti·coid

Min·er·va jac·ket
mini-arou·sals
mini·cell
mini·film
min·i·fy
mini·lap·a·rot·o·my
Mini-Lix
min·im
min·i·ma
min·i·mal
min·i·mum *pl.* min·i·ma
    m. audibile
    m. audible
    m. cognoscibile
    m. legibile
    light m.
    m. sensibile
    m. separabile
    m. visibile
Min·in light
mini·pill
mini·plate
mini·pol·y·my·o·clo·nus
mini·press
mini·spor·i·da
mini·zide
Min·kow·ski's figure
Min·kow·ski-Chauf·fard
  syndrome
Min·ne·so·ta Mul·ti·pha·sic
  Per·so·nal·i·ty In·ven·tory
  (MMPI)
Min·ne·so·ta tube
Mi·no·cin
mi·no·cy·cline
    m. hydrochloride
Mi·nor's disease
Mi·nor's sign
Mi·not, George Richards
Mi·not-Mur·phy diet
Mi·not-Mur·phy treatment
mi·nox·i·dil
mint
    mountain m.
    wild m.
Min·te·zol
min·u·the·sis

MIO — minimal identifiable odor
mio·car·dia
Mio·chol
mio·did·y·mus
mio·lec·i·thal
mio·phone
mio·pra·gia
mi·o·pus
mi·o·sis
   irritative m.
   paralytic m.
   spastic m.
   spinal m.
mi·ot·ic
mi·ra·cid·ia
mi·ra·cid·i·um *pl.* mi·ra·cid·ia
mir·ac·u·lin
Mir·a·don
mire
mir·in·ca·my·cin hy·dro·chlo·ride
mir·ror
   concave m.
   convex m.
   dental m.
   frontal m.
   head m.
   Glatzel m.
   laryngeal m.
   mouth m.
   nasographic m.
   nasopharyngeal m.
   plane m.
   van Helmont's m.
mir·ror·ing
mir·y·a·chit
mis·an·thro·py
mis·car·riage
mis·ce
mis·ceg·e·na·tion
mis·ci·ble
mis·er·e·re mei
mis·i·den·ti·fi·ca·tion
   delusional m.
mis·match
   acoustic m.

mi·sog·a·my
mi·sog·y·ny
mi·so·nid·a·zole
mist. — L. mistura (mixture)
mis·tle·toe
mis·tu·ra
   m. cretae
   m. pectoralis
MIT — monoiodotyrosine
Mit. — L. mitte (send)
mit·ap·sis
Mitch·ell's disease
Mitch·ell's treatment
Mitch·ell operation
mitch·el·la
mite
   auricular m.
   beetle m.
   bird m.
   burrowing m.
   cheese m.
   chicken m.
   chigger m.
   clover m.
   coolie-itch m.
   copra m.
   depluming m.
   face m.
   flour m.
   follicle m.
   food m.
   fowl m.
   grain itch m.
   hair follicle m.
   harvest m.
   house dust m.
   itch m.
   kedani m.
   louse m.
   mange m.
   meal m.
   mouse m.
   mower's m.
   Northern fowl m.
   onion m.
   poultry m.
   rat m.
   red m.

mite *(continued)*
    scab m.
    spider m.
    spinning m.
    straw m.
    tropical fowl m.
    tropical rat m.
mi·tel·la
Mith·ra·cin
mith·ra·my·cin
mith·ri·da·tism
mi·ti·ci·dal
mi·ti·cide
mit·i·gate
mi·tis
mi·to·car·cin
mi·to·chon·dri·al
mi·to·chon·dri·on
    giant m.
    m. of hemoflagellates
mi·to·cro·min
mi·to·gen
    pokeweed m.
mi·to·ge·ne·sia
mi·to·gen·e·sis
mi·to·ge·net·ic
mi·to·gen·ic
mi·to·ki·net·ic
mi·to·mal·cin
mi·tome
mi·to·my·cin
mi·to·plasm
mi·tos·chi·sis
mi·to·ses
mi·to·sin
mi·to·sis *pl.* mi·to·ses
    anastral m.
    astral m.
    asymmetrical m.
    heterotypic m.
    homeotypic m.
    multicentric m.
    multipolar m.
    pathologic m.
    pluripolar m.
mi·to·some
mi·to·sper
mi·to·spore

mi·to·tane
mi·tot·ic
mi·tral
mi·tral·ism
mi·tral·iza·tion
mi·troid
Mit·su·da antigen
Mit·su·da reaction
Mit·su·da test
mit·tel·schmerz
Mit·ten·dorf dot
mit·tor
mix·i·dine
mixo·sco·pia
mixo·troph
mixo·troph·ic
Mix·tard
mix·ture
    A.C.E. m.
    Basham's m.
    Biedert's cream m.
    Brompton m.
    Chabaud's m.
    chalk m.
    compound m. of senna
    expectorant m.
    extemporaneous m.
    Gunning's m.
    kaolin m. with pectin
    magnesium hydroxide m.
    Mayer's glycerin-albumin
      m.
    pectoral m.
    racemic m.
    Ringer's m.
    Tellyesniczky's m.
    toxin-antitoxin m.
    Vincent's m.
Mi·ya·ga·wa bodies
Mi·ya·ga·wa·nel·la
MK — monkey lung (cell
   culture)
ml — milliliter
μl — microliter
MLA — L. mento-laeva
   anterior (left mentoanterior)
     Medical Library
       Association

MLBW — moderately low
birth weight
MLC — mixed lymphocyte
culture
MLD — median lethal dose
minimum lethal dose
MLNS — mucocutaneous
lymph node syndrome
MLP — L. mento-laeva
posterior (left
mentoposterior)
MLR — mixed lymphocyte
reaction
MLT — L. mento-laeva
transversa (left
mentotransverse)
MM — mucous membranes
mM — millimolar
mm — millimeter
mm^2 — square millimeter
mm^3 — cubic millimeter
mμ — millimicron
μM — micromolar
μm — micrometer
mμCi — millimicrocurie
(nanocurie)
$\mu\mu$Ci — micromicrocurie
(picocurie)
MMEF — maximum
midexpiratory flow rate
mm Hg — millimeters of
mercury
MMIHS — megacystis-microcolon–intestinal hypoperistalsis
syndrome
M-mode echo·car·dio·gram
MMPI — Minnesota
Multiphasic Personality
Inventory
mmpp — millimeters partial
pressure
MMR — measles-mumps-rubel-
la (vaccine)
MMTV — mouse mammary
tumor virus
M'Nagh·ten (Mc·Naugh·ten)
rule
mne·mic

mne·mon·ic
mne·mon·ics
MO — Medical Officer
mesio-occlusal
Mo·ban
Mo·bi·li·na
mo·bil·i·ty
electrophoretic m.
mo·bi·li·za·tion
chromosome m.
stapes m.
mo·bil·i·zer
patient m.
mo·bil·om·e·ter
Mo·bitz (I, II) AV heart block
Mö·bi·us' disease
Mö·bi·us' sign
Mö·bi·us' syndrome
moc·ca·sin
cottonmouth water m.
MOD — mesio-occlusodistal
mo·dal·i·ty
mode
A m.
B m.
isocontour m.
list m.
M m.
radial m.
TM m.
mod·el
animal m.
Danielli-Davson m.
Hassell-Varley m.
Watson-Crick m.
mod·el·ing
Mod·er·il
mod·i·fi·ca·tion
behavior m.
racemic m.
mod·i·fi·er
mo·di·o·li·form
mo·di·o·lus
m. labii
Mod. praesc. — L. modo
praescripto (in the way
directed)

mod·u·la·tion
    amplitude m.
    antigenic m.
    frequency m.
    intensity m.
mod·u·la·tor
mod·u·lus
    m. of elasticity
    Young's m.
Mod·uret·ic
MODY — maturity-onset
  diabetes of youth
Moe plate
Moel·ler's glossitis
Moel·ler-Bar·low disease
Moer·ner-Sjöq·vist method
Moer·ner-Sjöq·vist test
Moersch-Wolt·man syndrome
mogi·ar·thria
mogi·la·lia
mogi·pho·nia
Mohr's test
Moh·ren·heim's fossa
Moh·ren·heim's triangle
Mohs' chemosurgery
Mohs' surgery
Mohs' technique
moi·e·ty
    carbohydrate m.
    corrin m.
mo·lal
mo·lal·i·ty
mo·lar
    dome-shaped m.
    Moon's m's
    mulberry m.
    sixth-year m.
    supernumerary m.
    third m.
    twelfth-year m.
mo·lar·i·form
mo·la·ris
    m. tertius
mol·ar·i·ty
mo·las·ses
    sugar-house m.
    West India m.
molc — molar concentration

mold
    slime m.
    white m.
mold·ing
    border m.
    compression m.
    injection m.
    tissue m.
mole
    blood m.
    Breus'm.
    carneous m.
    cystic m.
    false m.
    fleshy m.
    grape m.
    hairy m.
    hemorrhagic m.
    hydatid m.
    hydatidiform m.
    invasive m.
    malignant m.
    metastasizing m.
    maternal m.
    pigmented m.
    placental m.
    stone m.
    true m.
    tubal m.
    tuberous m.
    vesicular m.
    warty m.
mo·lec·u·lar
mol·e·cule
    cell interaction (CI) m's
    CI m's
    diatomic m.
    effector m.
    hexatomic m.
    monatomic m.
    nonpolar m.
    polar m.
    tetratomic m.
    triatomic m.
moli·la·lia
mo·li·men *pl.* mo·lim·i·na
    menstrual m.

mo·lim·i·na
mo·lin·done hy·dro·chlo·ride
Mol-Iron
Mo·lisch's reaction
Mo·lisch's test
Moll's glands
Mol·lar·et's meningitis
mol·les·cuse
Mol·li·cu·tes
mol·lin
mol·li·ti·es
    m. ossium
    m. unguium
Mol·lus·ca
mol·lusc·a·ci·dal
mol·lusc·a·cide
mol·lus·can
mol·lusc·i·cide
mol·lus·cous
mol·lus·cum
    m. contagiosum
    m. giganteum
    m. verrucosum
mol·lusk
Mo·lo·ney reaction
Mo·lo·ney test
molt·ing
Mol wt — molecular weight
mo·lyb·date
mo·lyb·de·no·sis
mo·lyb·den·um
    stainless steel with m.
    (SMo)
mo·lyb·dic
mo·lyb·dic acid
mo·lyb·do·pro·tein
mo·lyb·dous
mo·ment
    m. of death
    magnetic m.
mo·men·tum
    angular m.
mon·ac·id
mon·aco·liln K
mon·ad
    springing m.
Mo·na·kow's bundle
Mo·na·kow's fasciculus

Mo·na·kow's syndrome
Mo·na·kow's theory
Mo·na·kow's tract
mon·an·gle
mon·ar·thric
mon·ar·thri·tis
    m. deformans
    traumatic deforming m.
mon·ar·tic·u·lar
mon·as·ter
mon·ath·e·to·sis
mon·atom·ic
mon·auch·e·nos
mon·au·ral
mon·avi·ta·min·o·sis
mon·ax·i·al
mon·ax·on
mon·ax·on·ic
Mön·cke·berg's arteriosclerosis
Mon·di·ni's dysplasia
Mon·do·ne·si reflex
Mon·dor's disease
mo·nel·lin
mo·nen·sin
Mo·ne·ra
mo·ner·u·la *pl.* mo·ner·u·lae
mon·es·thet·ic
mon·es·trous
Mon·ge's disease
mon·go·li·an
mon·go·lism
    translocation m.
mon·go·loid
mon·il·at·ed
mo·nil·e·thrix
Mo·nil·ia
Mo·nil·i·a·ceae
mo·nil·i·al
Mo·nil·i·a·les
mon·i·li·a·sis
mo·nil·i·form
Mo·nili·for·mis
mo·nil·i·id
mo·nil·i·o·sis
Mo·ni·stat
mon·i·tor
    apnea m.
    Doplette m.

mon·i·tor *(continued)*
  Doppler m.
  Doptone m.
  Holter m.
  ICP (intracranial pressure) m.
  Jako facial nerve m.
  tumescence m.
mon·i·tor·ing
  biological m.
  cardiac m.
  electronic fetal m.
  wound m.
Mo·niz, Antonio Caetano de Abreu Friere Egas
mon·key paw
mon·key·pox
Mon·ne·ret's pulse
mono·am·ide
mono·amine
mono·amine ox·i·dase
mono·am·in·er·gic
mono·ami·no acid
mono·ami·no·di·phos·pha·tide
mono·ami·no·mono·phos·pha·tide
mono·am·ni·ot·ic
mono·an·es·the·sia
mono·ar·tic·u·lar
mono·auric·u·lar
mono·bac·te·ri·al
mono·bal·lism
mono·ba·sic
mono·ben·zone
mono·blast
mono·blas·to·ma
mono·blep·sia
mono·bra·chia
mono·bra·chi·us
mono·bro·mat·ed
mono·cal·cic
mono·car·box·yl·ic
mono·car·di·an
mono·celled
mono·cel·lu·lar
mono·cen·tric

mono·ceph·a·lus
  m. tetrapus dibrachius
  m. tripus dibrachius
mono·chlo·ro·thy·mol
mono·chord
  Schultze m.
mono·cho·rea
mono·cho·ri·al
mono·cho·ri·on·ic
mono·chro·ic
mono·chro·ma·sy
mono·chro·mat
mono·chro·mat·ic
mono·chro·ma·tism
  cone m.
  rod m.
mono·chro·mato·phil
mono·chro·ma·to·phil·ic
mono·chro·ma·tor
mono·chro·mo·phil·ic
mono·clin·ic
mono·clo·nal
mono·con·tam·i·nat·ed
mono·con·tam·i·na·tion
mono·cor·di·tis
mono·cra·ni·us
mono·crot·ic
mo·noc·ro·tism
mon·oc·u·lar
mon·oc·u·lus
mono·cy·clic
mono·cy·e·sis
mono·cyte
mono·cyt·ic
mono·cy·toid
mono·cy·to·ma
mono·cy·to·pe·nia
mono·cy·to·poi·e·sis
mono·cy·to·sis
Mo·nod, Jacques Lucien
mono·dac·tyl·ia
mono·dac·tyl·ism
mono·dac·ty·ly
mono·dal
mono·der·mo·ma
mono·did·y·mus
mono·di·plo·pia

mono·dis·perse
Mono·dral bro·mide
mo·noe·cious
mono·es·ter·ase
mono·eth·a·nol·amine
mono·fac·tor·i·al
mono·fil·a·ment
mono·film
mo·nog·a·mous
mo·nog·a·my
mono·gan·gli·al
mono·gas·tric
mono·gen
mono·gen·e·sis
mono·ge·net·ic
mono·gen·ic
mo·nog·e·nous
mono·ger·mi·nal
mono·glyc·er·ide
mono·graph
mono·hy·brid
mono·hy·drate
mono·hy·drat·ed
mono·hy·dric
mono·in·fec·tion
mono·io·do·ty·ro·sine
mono·kary·on
mono·kary·ote
mono·kary·ot·ic
mono·kine
mono·lay·er
mono·lep·sis
mono·lob·u·lar
mono·loc·u·lar
mono·ma·nia
mono·mas·ti·gote
mono·max·il·lary
mono·mel·ic
mono·mer
    fibrin m.
mono·mer·ic
mono·me·tal·lic
mono·meth·yl·mor·phine
mono·mi·cro·bic
mono·mo·lec·u·lar
mono·mor·phic
mono·mor·phism
mono·mor·phous

mon·om·pha·lus
mono·myo·ple·gia
mono·myo·si·tis
Mo·non·chus
mono·neph·rous
mono·neu·ral
mono·neu·ral·gia
mono·neu·ric
mono·neu·ri·tis
    m. multiplex
mono·neu·rop·a·thy
    cranial m.
mono·nu·cle·ar
mono·nu·cle·ate
mono·nu·cle·o·sis
    cytomegalovirus m.
    infectious m.
    post-transfusion m.
mono·nu·cle·o·tide
    isoalloxazine m.
mono-os·te·it·ic
mono-ov·u·lar
mono·oxy·gen·ase
    unspecific m.
mono·par·e·sis
mono·par·es·the·sia
mo·nop·a·thy
mono·pe·nia
mono·pha·gia
mo·noph·a·gism
mono·pha·sia
mono·pha·sic
mono·phe·nol mono·oxy·gen·ase
mono·phen·yl ox·i·dase
mono·phos·phate
mon·oph·thal·mus
mono·phy·let·ic
mono·phy·le·tism
mono·phy·le·tist
mono·phy·odont
mon·o·pia
mono·plas·mat·ic
mono·plast
mono·plas·tic
mono·ple·gia
mono·ple·gic
mono·ploid

mono·po·dia
mono·po·di·al
mono·poi·e·sis
mono·po·lar
mon·ops
Mono·psyl·lus
  M. anisus
mono·pty·chi·al
mono·pus
mon·or·chia
mon·or·chid
mon·or·chid·ic
mon·or·chid·ism
mon·or·chis
mon·or·chism
Mon·or·cho·tre·ma
mono·rhin·ic
mono·sac·cha·ride
mono·sac·cha·rose
mon·ose
mono·sex·u·al
mono·so·di·um glu·ta·mate
mono·some
mono·so·mic
mono·so·my
mono·spasm
mono·spe·cif·ic
mono·sper·my
Mono·spo·ri·um
  M. apiospermum
Mono·spot test
Mono·sto·ma
Mono·sto·mum
mon·os·tot·ic
mono·stra·tal
mono·strat·i·fied
mono·sub·sti·tut·ed
mono·symp·tom
mono·symp·to·mat·ic
mono·syn·ap·tic
Mono·tard
mono·ter·mi·nal
mono·ter·pene
mono·ther·a·py
mono·ther·mia
mono·thet·ic
mono·thio·glyc·er·ol
mon·o·tic

mo·not·o·cous
mono·treme
mono·trich·ic
mon·ot·ri·chous
mon·o·trop·ic
mono·ure·ide
mono·va·lent
mon·ov·u·lar
mon·ov·u·la·to·ry
mono·xen·ic
mo·nox·e·nous
mon·ox·e·ny
mon·ox·ide
mon·oxy·gen·ase
mono·zy·gos·i·ty
mono·zy·got·ic
mono·zy·gous
Mon·ro's bursa
Mon·ro's fissure
Mon·ro's foramen
Mon·ro's line
Mon·ro's sulcus
Mon·ro-Rich·ter line
mons *pl.* mon·tes
  m. pubis
  m. ureteris
  m. veneris
Mon·son's curve
Mon·so·nia
mon·ster
  acardiac m.
  acraniate m.
  autositic m.
  celosomian m.
  compound m.
  cyclopic m.
  diaxial m.
  double m.
  emmenic m.
  endocymic m.
  Gila m.
  hair m.
  monoaxial m.
  parasitic m.
  polysomatous m.
  single m.
  sirenoform m.
  triplet m.

mon·ster *(continued)*
    twin m.
mon·stra
mon·stri·cide
mon·stros·i·ty
mon·strum *pl.* mon·stra
    m. abundans
    m. deficiens
    m. per defectum
    m. per excessum
    m. per fabricam alienam
    m. sirenoforme
Mon·teg·gia's dislocation
Mon·teg·gia's fracture
mon·tes
Mon·te·vi·deo units
Mont·gom·ery's cups
Mont·gom·ery's follicles
Mont·gom·ery's glands
Mont·gom·ery's tubercles
mon·tic·u·lus *pl.* mon·ti·cu·li
    m. cerebelli
mood
mood-con·gru·ent
mood-in·con·gru·ent
Moon's molars
Moon's teeth
moon face
moon fa·ci·es
Moore's fracture
Moore's syndrome
Moore's test
Moor·en's ulcer
Moor·head foreign body locator
Mor·and's foot
Mor·and's foramen
Mor·and's spur
mo·ran·tel tar·trate
Mor·a·witz theory
Mor·ax-Ax·en·feld bacillus
Mor·ax-Ax·en·feld
    conjunctivitis
Mor·ax-Ax·en·feld diplococcus
Mo·rax·el·la
    M. (Branhamella)
        catarrhalis
    M. (Moraxella) lacunata
mor·bid

mor·bid·i·ty
    puerperal m.
mor·bif·ic
mor·big·e·nous
mor·bil·li
mor·bil·li·form
Mor·bil·li·vi·rus
mor·bil·lous
mor·bus
    coxae senilis
    m. moniliformis
MORC — Medical Officers
    Reserve Corps
mor·cel
mor·cel·la·tion
mor·celle·ment
mor·dant
Mor. dict. — L. more dicto (in
    the manner directed)
Mo·rel ear
Mo·rel syndrome
Mo·rel·li's reaction
Mo·rel·li's test
mo·res
Mo·ret·ti's test
Mor·ga·gni's appendix
Mor·ga·gni's caruncle
Mor·ga·gni's foramen
Mor·ga·gni's fossa
Mor·ga·gni's globule
Mor·ga·gni's hernia
Mor·ga·gni's lacuna
Mor·ga·gni's prolapse
Mor·ga·gni's tubercle
Mor·ga·gni-Ad·ams-Stokes
    syndrome
mor·gag·ni·an
Mor·gan, Thomas Hunt
Mor·gan's bacillus
mor·gan
Mor·ga·nel·la
    M. morganii
morgue
mo·ria
mor·i·bund
Mo·rin·ga
    M. pterygosperma

Mor·i·son's pouch
Mo·ri·ta therapy
Mo·ritz reaction
Mo·ritz test
Mör·ner's body
Mör·ner's reagent
Mör·ner's test
Mor·ni·dine
Mo·ro's embrace reflex
Mo·ro's test
mo·ron
mor·phal·lac·tic
mor·phal·lax·is
mor·phea
    acroteric m.
    generalized m.
    guttate m.
    linear m.
    m. linearis
    m. pigmentosa
mor·pheme
mor·phine
    dimethyl m.
    m. hydrochloride
    m. sulfate
mor·phin·ic
mor·phin·ism
mor·phin·iza·tion
mor·pho·cy·tol·o·gy
mor·pho·dif·fer·en·ti·a·tion
mor·pho·gen
mor·pho·ge·ne·sia
mor·pho·gen·e·sis
mor·pho·ge·net·ic
mor·phog·e·ny
mor·pho·log·i·cal
mor·phol·o·gy
mor·phol·y·sis
mor·phom·e·try
mor·phon
mor·phoph·y·ly
mor·pho·phys·ics
mor·pho·plasm
mor·pho·sis
mor·pho·syn·the·sis
mor·phot·ic
Mor·quio's disease
Mor·quio's syndrome

Mor·quio-Brails·ford syndrome
Mor·quio-Ull·rich disease
mor·rhua
mor·rhu·ate
    m. sodium
mor·rhu·in
Mor·ris syndrome
mors
    m. thymica
mor·sal
mor·sel·ize
mor·si·ca·tio buc·car·um
Mor. sol. — L. more solito (in
    the usual way)
mor·su·lus
mor·sus
    m. diaboli
    m. humanus
mor·tal
mor·tal·i·ty
    fetal m.
    neonatal m.
    perinatal m.
    postnatal m.
    postneonatal m.
    proportionate m.
    reproductive m.
mor·tar
mor·ti·cian
Mor·ti·e·rel·la
mor·ti·fi·ca·tion
Mor·ti·mer's disease
mor·ti·na·tal·i·ty
mor·tise
    ankle m.
Mor·ton's cough
Mor·ton's current
Mor·ton's disease
Mor·ton's foot
Mor·ton's neuralgia
Mor·ton's test
Mor·ton's toe
mor·tu·ary
mor·u·la
mor·u·lar
mor·u·la·tion
mor·u·loid
mor·u·lus

Mor·van's chorea
Mor·van's disease
Mor·van's syndrome
mo·sa·ic
    chromsomal m.
mo·sa·i·cism
    erythrocyte m.
    gonadal m.
    haploid-diploid m.
    Turner's m.
Mosch·co·witz's disease
Mosch·co·witz's sign
Mosch·co·witz's test
Mo·sen·thal's test
Mos·et·ig-Moor·hof bone wax
Mos·et·ig-Moor·hof filling
Mosh·er air cells
Mosler's sign
Mos·ley method
mOsm — milliosmol
mos·qui·to pl. mos·qui·toes
    anautogenous m.
    arygamous m.
    autogenous m.
    house m.
    steyogamous m.
    tiger m.
mos·qui·to·ci·dal
mos·qui·to·cide
moss
    Ceylon m.
    Irish m.
    juniper m.
    pearl m.
    salt rock m.
Moss' classification
Mosse's syndrome
Mos·so's ergograph
Mos·so's sphygmomanometer
Mo·tais' operation
moth
    brown-tail m.
    flannel m.
    io m.
    meal m.
    tussock m.
moth·er
    Colles m.

moth·er *(continued)*
    expectant m.
    phallic m.
    schizophrenogenic m.
    surrogate m.
mo·tile
mo·til·in
mo·til·i·ty
    automatic m.
    segmental m.
    voluntary m.
motion
    active range of m.
    continuous passive m.
     (CPM)
    range of m.
    systolic anterior m. (SAM)
mo·ti·va·tion
mo·tive
    achievement m.
    aroused m.
mo·to·cep·tor
mo·to·fa·cient
mo·to·neu·ron
    alpha m's
    beta m's
    gamma m's
    heteronymous m's
    homonymous m's
    lower m's
    peripheral m's
    upper m's
mo·tor
    air m.
    club m.
    loop m.
    plastic m.
mo·tor·graph·ic
mo·tor·ic·i·ty
mo·to·ri·us
mo·toro·ger·mi·na·tive
Mo·trin
MOTT — mycobacteria other
    than tubercle bacilli
Mott's law of anticipation
mot·tling
Mou·chet's disease
mou·lage

mould
mould·ing
   anal m.
mound·ing
mount
   wet m.
Mount-Re·back syndrome
mount·ant
mount·ing
   split cast m.
mourn·ing
mouse
   B m.
   BALB
   CBA m.
   C.F.W. m.
   deprived m.
   joint m.
   nude m.
   nu/nu m.
   NZB (New Zealand black)
    mice
   peritoneal m.
   pleural m.
   Snell-Bagg m.
mouse·pox
mouth
   Ceylon sore m.
   denture sore m.
   dry m.
   glass-blowers'm.
   parrot m.
   sore m.
   tapir m.
   trench m.
   white m.
mouth·wash
move·ment
   active m.
   adversive m.
   ameboid m.
   angular m.
   associated contralateral m.
   associated m.
   athetoid m's
   automatic m.
   Bennett m.
   bodily m.

move·ment *(continued)*
   border m.
   border tissue m's
   brownian m.
   Brownian-Zsigmondy m.
   brunonian m.
   cardinal m's
   choreic m's
   choreiform m's
   ciliary m.
   circus m.
   contralateral associated m.
   curtain m.
   cytoplasmic m.
   delta m.
   dystonic m.
   euglenoid m.
   excursive m's
   fetal m.
   forced m.
   free mandibular m.
   Frenkel's m's
   gliding m.
   hinge m.
   index m.
   intermediary m's
   intermediate m's
   involuntary m.
   jaw m.
   Magnan's m.
   mandibular m.
   mandibular m., free
   mandibular m's, functional
   masticatory m's
   mirror m.
   molecular m.
   morphogenetic m.
   nucleopetal m.
   opening m.
   opening m., posterior
   passive m.
   pedal m.
   pendular m.
   percussion m's
   protoplasmic m.
   rapid eye m. (REM)
   reflex m.
   resistive m.

move·ment *(continued)*
 rolling m.
 running m.
 saccadic m.
 scissors m.
 segmentation m.
 spontaneous m.
 stepping m's
 streaming m.
 Swedish m.
 synkinetic m's
 tipping m.
 vermicular m's
 voluntary m.
mov·er
 prime m.
moxa
mox·a·lac·tam
 m. disodium
mox·a·zo·cine
mox·i·bus·tion
mox·nid·a·zole
Moy·na·han's syndrome
Moy·ni·han's cream
Moy·ni·han's test
6-MP — 6-mercaptopurine
mp — melting point
MPD — maximum permissible dose
MPH — Master of Public Health
MPHR — maximum predicted heart rate
MPO — myeloperoxidase
MPS — mononuclear phagocyte system
 mucopolysaccharidosis
MR — megaroentgen
mR — milliroentgen
μR — microroentgen
MRA — Medical Record Administrator
MRACP — Member of Royal Australasian College of Physicians
mrad — millirad
MRC — Medical Reserve Corps

MRCP — Member of the Royal College of Physicians
MRCPE — Member of the Royal College of Physicians of Edinburgh
MRCP (Glasg) — Member of the Royal College of Physicians and Surgeons of Glasgow *qua* Physician
MRCPI — Member of the Royal College of Physicians of Ireland
MRCS — Member of the Royal College of Surgeons
MRCSE — Member of the Royal College of Surgeons of Edinburgh
MRCSI — Member of the Royal College of Surgeons of Ireland
MRCVS — Member of the Royal College of Veterinary Surgeons
MRD — minimum reacting dose
mrem — millirem
MRF — melanocyte-stimulating hormone releasing factor
MRI — magnetic resonance imaging
MRL — Medical Record Librarian (now Medical Record Administrator)
mRNA — messenger RNA
MS — Master of Surgery
 mitral stenosis
 morphine sulfate
 multiple sclerosis
ms — millisecond
μs — microsecond
msec — millisecond
μsec — microsecond
MSG — monosodium glutamate
MSH — melanocyte-stimulating hormone

MSH-IF — melanocyte-stimulating hormone inhibiting factor

MSH-RF — melanocyte-stimulating hormone releasing factor

MSL — midsternal line

MSUD — maple syrup urine disease

MT — Medical Technologist
Medical Transcriptionist
membrana tympani

MTU — methylthiouracil

MTX — methotrexate

Mu — Mache unit

mU — milliunit

m.u. — mouse unit

μU — microunit

MUAP — motor unit action potential

Muc. — L. mucilago (mucilage)

Much's granules

Mu·cha's disease

Mu·cha-Ha·ber·mann disease

mu·ci·car·mine

mu·ci·car·mi·no·phil·ic

mu·cif·er·ous

mu·ci·fi·ca·tion

mu·ci·form

mu·ci·gen

mu·cig·e·nous

mu·ci·gogue

mu·ci·hem·a·te·in
Mayer's m.

mu·ci·lage
acacia m.
tragacanth m.

mu·ci·lag·i·nous

mu·ci·la·go
m. acaciae
m. tragacanthae

mu·cil·loid
psyllium hydrophilic m.

mu·cin

mu·cin·ase

mu·cin·emia

mu·cino·blast

mu·cin·o·gen

mu·ci·noid

mu·ci·no·lyt·ic

mu·ci·no·sis
follicular m.
papular m.

mu·ci·nous

mu·cin·uria

mu·cip·a·rous

mu·ci·tis

mu·civ·or·ous

Muck·le-Wells syndrome

mu·co·al·bu·min·ous

mu·co·an·ti·body

mu·co·buc·cal

mu·co·car·ti·lage

mu·co·cele
ethmoid sinus m.
frontal sinus m.
frontoethmoid m.
lacrimal m.
maxillary sinus m.
paranasal sinus m.
suppurating m.

mu·co·cla·sis

mu·co·co·li·tis

mu·co·col·pos

mu·co·cu·ta·ne·ous

mu·co·cyst

mu·co·cyte

mu·co·derm

mu·co·en·ter·itis

mu·co·ep·i·der·moid

mu·co·fi·brous

mu·co·floc·cu·lent

mu·co·gin·gi·val

mu·co·glob·u·lin

mu·co·hem·or·rhag·ic

mu·coid

mu·co·i·tin sul·fate

mu·co·lem·ma

mu·co·lip·id

mu·co·lip·i·do·sis
m. I
m. II
m. III
m. IV

mu·co·lyt·ic

mu·co·mem·bra·nous
Mu·co·myst
mu·co·pep·tide
mu·co·peri·chon·dri·al
mu·co·peri·chon·dri·um
mu·co·peri·os·te·al
mu·co·peri·os·te·um
mu·co·poi·e·sis
mu·co·poly·sac·cha·ri·dase
mu·co·poly·sac·cha·ride
mu·co·poly·sac·cha·ri·do·sis
   m. I
   m. H
   m. IH/S
   m. IS
   m. II
   m. III
   m. IV
   m. V
   m. VI
   m. VII
mu·co·poly·sac·cha·ri·du·ria
mu·co·pro·tein
   Tamm-Horsfall m.
mu·co·pu·ru·lent
mu·co·pus
Mu·cor
   M. corymbifer
   M. mucedo
   M. pusillus
   M. racemosus
   M. ramosus
   M. rhizopodiformis
Mu·co·ra·ceae
mu·co·ra·ceous
Mu·cor·a·les
mu·co·rin
mu·cor·my·co·sis
mu·co·sa
   alveolar m.
   buccal m.
   endocervical m.
   labial m.
   laryngeal m.
   masticatory m.
   muscular m.
   olfactory m.
   oral m.

mu·co·sa *(continued)*
   pharyngeal m.
   respiratory m.
   tracheal m.
mu·co·sal
mu·co·sal·pinx
mu·co·san·guin·e·ous
mu·co·sed·a·tive
mu·co·se·rous
mu·co·sin
mu·co·si·tis
   m. necroticans
     agranulocytica
mu·co·so·cu·ta·ne·ous
mu·co·stat·ic
mu·co·sul·fa·ti·do·sis
mu·co·tome
mu·cous
mu·co·vis·ci·do·sis
mu·cro *pl.* mu·cro·nes
   m. baseos cartilaginis
     arytaenoideae
   m. cordis
   m. sterni
mu·cro·nate
mu·cron·i·form
Mu·cu·na
mu·cus
Muer·cke's lines
muf·fle
MUGA (multiple gaited
  acquisition) scan
Muir·head's treatment
Mul·der's angle
Mul·der's test
Mules' operation
mu·li·e·bria
mu·li·eb·ris
mu·li·eb·ri·ty
mu·li·to·cos·tate
mull
   plaster m.
Mul·ler, Hermann Joseph
Mül·ler, Paul Herrmann
Mül·ler's canal
Mül·ler's capsule
Mül·ler's cells
Mül·ler's duct

[handwritten annotation: Confluent mucositis]

Mül·ler's fibers
Mül·ler's fluid
Mül·ler's liquid
Mül·ler's maneuver
Mül·ler's muscle
Mül·ler's radial cells
Mül·ler's sign
Mül·ler-Haeck·el law
Mül·ler-Hil·lis maneuver
mull·er
mül·le·ri·an
mül·le·ri·a·no·ma
Mül·le·ri·us
    M. capillaris
mull·ing
mul·tan·gu·lar
mul·ti·al·lel·ic
mul·ti·ar·tic·u·lar
mul·ti·bac·il·lary
mul·ti·cap·su·lar
mul·ti·cell
mul·ti·cel·lu·lar
mul·ti·cel·lu·lar·i·ty
mul·ti·cen·tric
mul·ti·cen·tric·i·ty
Mul·ti·ceps
    M. multiceps
    M. serialis
mul·ti·cip·i·tal
mul·ti·clo·nal
mul·ti·con·tam·i·nat·ed
mul·ti·core
    m's in muscle
mul·ti·cus·pid
mul·ti·cus·pi·date
mul·ti·cys·tic
mul·ti·den·tate
mul·ti·de·ter·mi·na·tion
mul·ti·dig·i·tate
mul·ti·fac·to·ri·al
mul·tif·e·ta·tion
mul·ti·fid
mul·tif·i·dus
mul·ti·fla·gel·late
mul·ti·fo·cal
mul·ti·form
mul·ti·gan·glio·nate
mul·ti·gan·gli·on·ic

mul·ti·ges·ta
mul·ti·glan·du·lar
mul·ti·grav·i·da
    grand m.
mul·ti·hal·lu·cal·ism
mul·ti·hal·lu·cism
mul·ti·hem·a·tin·ic
mul·ti·in·farct
mul·ti·in·fec·tion
mul·ti·lo·bar
mul·ti·lob·u·lar
mul·ti·loc·u·lar
mul·ti·mam·mae
mul·ti·mer
mul·ti·mo·dal
mul·ti·no·dal
mul·ti·nod·u·lar
mul·ti·nu·cle·ar
mul·ti·nu·cle·ate
mul·tip·a·ra
    grand m.
mul·ti·par·i·ty
mul·tip·a·rous
mul·ti·par·tite
mul·ti·pen·nate
mul·ti·pha·sic
mul·ti·pla·nar
mul·ti·ple
mul·ti·plex·er
mul·ti·plic·i·tas
    m. cordis
mul·ti·po·lar
mul·ti·pol·li·cal·ism
mul·ti·pol·li·cism
mul·ti·root·ed
mul·ti·sen·si·tiv·i·ty
mul·ti·syn·ap·tic
mul·ti·sys·tem
mul·ti·ter·mi·nal
mul·ti·tu·ber·cu·late
mul·ti·va·lent
mul·ti·va·ri·ate
mul·ti·vi·ta·min
mum·mi·fi·ca·tion
    fetal m.
    m. of pulp
mumps
    iodine m.

mumps *(continued)*
  m. meningoencephalitis
  metastatic m.
mu·mu
Mün·chau·sen's syndrome
Münch·mey·er's disease
Munk's disease
mu·ni·ty
Mun·ro's abscess
Mun·ro's microabscess
Mun·ro's point
Mun·ro Kerr cesarean section
Mun·ro Kerr incision
Mun·ro Kerr maneuver
MUP — motor unit potential
mu·ral
mu·ram·ic acid
mu·ram·i·dase
Mu·rat sign
Mur·chi·son-Pel-Eb·stein
  fever
mu·rein
Mu·rel
Mu·rex
  M. purpurea
mu·rex·ide
mu·rex·ine
mu·ri·at·ic acid
mu·ri·form
mu·rine
mu·ri·vi·rus
mur·mur
  accidental m.
  amphoric m.
  anemic m.
  aneurysmal m.
  aortic m.
  apex m.
  apical diastolic m's
  arterial m.
  atriosystolic m.
  attrition m.
  Austin Flint m.
  basal diastolic m's
  Baumgarten's m.
  bellows m.
  blood m.
  brain m.

mur·mur *(continued)*
  bronchial m.
  cardiac m.
  cardiopulmonary m.
  cardiorespiratory m.
  Carey Coombs m.
  continuous m.
  cooing m.
  crescendo m.
  crescendo-decrescendo m.
  Cruveilhier-Baumgarten
    m.
  deglutition m.
  diamond-shaped m.
  diastolic m.
  Docke's m.
  Duroziez's m.
  ejection m.
  exocardial m.
  expiratory m.
  extracardiac m.
  Flint's m.
  friction m.
  functional m.
  Gibson m.
  Graham Steell's m.
  Hamman's m.
  heart m.
  hemic m.
  holodiastolic m.
  holosystolic m.
  hourglass m.
  humming-top m.
  incidental m.
  innocent m.
  late systolic m.
  machinery m.
  mid-diastolic m.
  mill-house m.
  mill wheel m.
  mitral m.
  musical m.
  organic m.
  outflow tract m.
  pansystolic m.
  pericardial m.
  physiologic m.
  pleuropericardial m.

mur·mur *(continued)*
   prediastolic m.
   presystolic m.
   pulmonic m.
   regurgitant m.
   Roger's m.
   sea-gull m.
   seesaw m.
   short systolic m.
   Steell's m.
   stenosal m.
   Still's m.
   subclavicular m.
   systolic m.
   to-and-fro m.
   transmitted m.
   Traube's m.
   tricuspid m.
   vascular m.
   venous m.
   vesicular m.
   waterwheel m.
Mur·phy, William Parry
Mur·phy button
Mur·phy method
Mur·phy percussion
Mur·phy sign
Mur·phy tests
Mur·phy-Sturm
   lymphosarcoma
Mur·ray Val·ley encephalitis
Mur·ray Val·ley disease
Mur·ray Val·ley virus
Mur·ri's disease
Mus
   M. alexandrinus
   M. decumanus
   M. musculus
   M. norvegicus
   M. rattus rattus
Mus·ca
   M. autumnalis
   M. domestica
   M. domestica nebulo
   M. domestica vicina
   M. luteola
   M. sorbens
   M. vomitoria

mus·ca *pl.* mus·cae
   muscae hispanicae
   muscae volitantes
mus·ca·cide
mus·cae
mus·car·dine
mus·ca·rine
mus·ca·rin·ic
mus·ca·rin·ism
mus·ce·ge·net·ic
mus·ci·cide
Mus·ci·dae
Mus·ci·na
mus·cio·lep·sy
mus·cle
   abducent m.
   abductor m. of great toe
   abductor m. of little finger
   abductor m. of little toe
   abductor m. of thumb, long
   abductor m. of thumb,
     short
   adductor m., great
   adductor m., long
   adductor m., short
   adductor m., smallest
   adductor m. of great toe
   adductor m. of thumb
   accessory m.
   accessory flexor m.
   accessory m's of respiration
   Aeby's m.
   agonistic m.
   Albinus' m.
   anconeus m.
   anconeus m., lateral
   anconeus m., medial
   anconeus m., short
   antagonistic m.
   antigravity m's
   m. of antitragus
   appendicular m's
   arrector m's of hair
   articular m.
   articular m. of elbow
   articular m. of knee
   aryepiglottic m.

mus·cle *(continued)*

  arytenoid m., oblique
  arytenoid m., transverse
  aryvocalis m. of Ludwig
  m's of auditory ossicles
  auricular m's
  axial m.
  Bell's m.
  biceps m. of arm
  biceps m. of thigh
  bicipital m.
  bipennate m.
  bipenniform m.
  Bowman's m.
  brachial m.
  brachioradial m.
  Braune's m.
  bronchoesophageal m.
  Brücke's m.
  buccinator m.
  buccopharyngeal m.
  bulbar m's
  bulbocavernous m.
  canine m.
  cardiac m.
  Casser's m.
  casserian m.
  ceratocricoid m.
  ceratopharyngeal m.
  Chassaignac's axillary m.
  cheek m.
  chondroglossus m.
  chondropharyngeal m.
  ciliary m.
  circumpennate m.
  coccygeal m's
  Coiter's m.
  compressor m. of naris
  congenerous m's
  constrictor m's of pharynx
  coracobrachial m.
  costocervicalis m.
  Crampton's m.
  cremaster m.
  cricoarytenoid m., lateral
  cricoarytenoid m., posterior
  cricopharyngeal m.

mus·cle *(continued)*

  cricothyroid m.
  cruciate m.
  cutaneous m.
  dartos m.
  deltoid m.
  depressor m., superciliary
  depressor m. of angle of mouth
  depressor m. of lower lip
  depressor m. of septum of nose
  dermal m.
  detrusor m. of bladder
  detrusor urinae muscle
  diaphragmatic m.
  digastric m.
  dilator m. of naris
  dilator m. of pupil
  dorsal m's
  Dupré's m.
  Duverney's m.
  emergency m's
  epicranial m.
  epimeric m.
  epitrochleoanconeus m.
  erector m. of penis
  erector m. of spine
  eustachian m.
  extensor m. of digits, common
  extensor m. of fingers
  extensor m. of fifth digit, proper
  extensor m. of great toe, long
  extensor m. of great toe, short
  extensor m. of index finger
  extensor m. of little finger
  extensor m. of thumb, long
  extensor m. of thumb, short
  extensor m. of toes, long
  extensor m. of toes, short
  extraocular m's
  extrinsic m.
  m's of eye

mus·cle *(continued)*
    facial m's
    m's of facial expression
    facial and masticatory m's
    fast m.
    m's of fauces
    femoral m.
    fibular m., long
    fibular m., short
    fibular m., third
    fixation m's
    fixator m's
    fixator m. of base of stapes
    flexor m., accessory
    flexor m. of fingers, deep
    flexor m. of fingers,
      superficial
    flexor m. of great toe, long
    flexor m. of great toe, short
    flexor m. of little finger,
      short
    flexor m. of little toe, short
    flexor m. of thumb, long
    flexor m. of thumb, short
    flexor m. of toes, long
    flexor m. of toes, short
    flexor m. of wrist, radial
    flexor m. of wrist, ulnar
    Folius' m.
    frontal m.
    frontalis m.
    fusiform m.
    gastrocnemius m.
    Gavard's m.
    gemellus m., inferior
    gemellus m., superior
    genioglossus m.
    geniohyoid m.
    glossopalatine m.
    glossopharyngeal m.
    gluteal m., greatest
    gluteal m., least
    gracilis m.
    Guthrie's m.
    hamstring m's
    m. of Henle
    Hilton's m.
    Horner's m.

mus·cle *(continued)*
    Houston's m.
    hyoglossal m.
    hyoglossus m.
    hypaxial m's
    hypomeric m.
    iliac m.
    iliococcygeal m.
    iliocostal m's
    iliopsoas m.
    incisive m's
    infrahyoid m's
    infraspinous m.
    inspiratory m's
    interarytenoid m's
    intercostal m's, external
    intercostal m's, innermost
    intercostal m's, internal
    interfoveolar m.
    interosseous m's, palmar
    interosseous m's, plantar
    interosseous m's, volar
    interspinal m's
    intertransverse m's
    intraauricular m's
    intraocular m's
    intratympanic m.
    intrinsic m.
    involuntary m.
    iridic m's
    ischiocavernous m.
    Jarjavay's m.
    Jung's m.
    Koyter's m.
    Landström's m.
    Langer's m.
    lateral straight m.
    latissimus dorsi m.
    levator m. of angle of
      mouth
    levator ani m.
    levator m. of prostate
    levator m's of ribs
    levator m. of scapula
    levator m. of thyroid gland
    levator m. of upper eyelid
    levator m. of upper lip

mus·cle *(continued)*

    levator muscle of velum palatini
    lingual m's
    long m. of head
    long m. of neck
    longissimus m.
    longissimus m. of back
    longissimus m. of head
    longissimus m. of neck
    longissimus m. of thorax
    longitudinal m. of tongue, inferior
    longitudinal m. of tongue, superior
    Ludwig's m.
    lumbrical m's of foot
    lumbrical m's of hand
    Luschka's m's
    masseter m.
    m's of mastication
    masticatory m's
    Merkel's m.
    mesothenar m.
    Müller's m.
    multicipital m.
    multifidus m's
    multipennate m.
    multi-unit m.
    mylohyoid m.
    mylopharyngeal m.
    nasal m.
    m's of neck
    nonstriated m.
    oblique m. of abdomen, external
    oblique m. of abdomen, internal
    oblique m. of auricle
    oblique m. of eyeball, inferior
    oblique m. of eyeball, superior
    oblique m. of head, inferior
    oblique m. of head, superior
    obturator m., external
    obturator m., internal

mus·cle *(continued)*

    occipital m.
    occipitofrontal m.
    Ochsner's m.
    ocular m's
    oculorotatory m's
    Oddi's m.
    omohyoid m.
    opposing m. of little finger
    opposing m. of thumb
    orbicular m.
    orbicular m. of eye
    orbicular m. of mouth
    orbital m.
    organic m.
    m's of palate and fauces
    palatine m's
    palatoglossus m.
    palatopharyngeal m.
    palmar m., long
    palmar m., short
    papillary m's
    pectinate m's
    pectineal m.
    pectoral m., greater
    pectoral m., smaller
    pectorodorsalis m.
    pennate m.
    penniform m.
    perineal m's
    m's of perineum
    peroneal m., long
    peroneal m., short
    peroneal m., third
    pharyngopalatine m.
    Phillips'm.
    piriform m.
    plantar m.
    platysma m.
    pleuroesophageal m.
    popliteal m.
    postaxial m.
    postural m's
    preaxial m.
    prevertebral m's
    procerus m.
    pronator m., quadrate
    pronator m., round

mus·cle *(continued)*
  psoas m., greater
  psoas m., smaller
  pterygoid m., external
  pterygoid m., internal
  pterygoid m., lateral
  pterygoid m., medial
  pterygopharyngeal m.
  pubicoperitoneal m.
  pubococcygeal m.
  puboprostatic m.
  puborectal m.
  pubovaginal m.
  pubovesical m.
  pyloric sphincter m.
  pyramidal m.
  pyramidal m. of auricle
  quadrate m.
  quadrate m. of lower lip
  quadrate pronator m.
  quadrate m. of sole
  quadrate m. of thigh
  quadrate m. of upper lip
  quadriceps femoris m.
  quadriceps m. of thigh
  radial flexor m. of wrist
  rectococcygeus m.
  rectourethral m.
  rectouterine m.
  rectovesical m.
  red m.
  Reisseisen's m's
  rhomboid m., greater
  rhomboid m., lesser
  ribbon m's
  rider's m's
  Riolan's m.
  risorius m.
  rotator m's
  rotator m's, long
  rotator m's, short
  Ruysch's m.
  sacrococcygeal m., anterior
  sacrococcygeal m., dorsal
  sacrococcygeal m., posterior
  sacrococcygeal m., ventral
  sacrospinal m.

mus·cle *(continued)*
  salpingopharyngeal m.
  Santorini's m.
  Santorini's m's, circular
  m. of Sappey
  sartorius m.
  scalene m., anterior
  scalene m., middle
  scalene m., posterior
  scalene m., smallest
  Sebileau's m.
  semimembranous m.
  semispinal m.
  semispinal m. of head
  semispinal m. of neck
  semispinal m. of thorax
  semitendinous m.
  serratus m., anterior
  serratus m., posterior, inferior
  serratus m., posterior, superior
  shunt m's
  Sibson's m.
  skeletal m's
  slow m.
  smooth m.,
  Soemmering's m.
  soleus m.
  somatic m's
  sphincter m.
  sphincter m. of anus, external
  sphincter m. of anus, internal
  sphincter m. of bile duct
  sphincter m. of hepatopancreatic ampulla
  sphincter m. of membranous urethra
  sphincter m. of pupil
  sphincter m. of pylorus
  sphincter m. of urethra
  sphincter m. of urinary bladder
  spinal m.
  splenius m. of head

mus·cle *(continued)*
  splenius m. of neck
  spurt m's
  stapedius m.
  sternal m.
  sternocleidomastoid m.
  sternohyoid m.
  sternomastoid m.
  sternothyroid m.
  strap m's
  striated m.
  striped m.
  styloglossus m.
  stylohyoid m.
  stylopharyngeus m.
  subanconeus m.
  subclavius m.
  subcostal m's
  suboccipital m's
  subscapular m.
  subvertebral m's
  superciliary corrugator m.
  superciliary depressor m.
  supinator m.
  suprahyoid m's
  supraspinous m.
  suspensory m. of
   duodenum
  synergic m's
  synergistic m's
  tarsal m., inferior
  tarsal m., superior
  temporal m.
  temporoparietal m.
  tensor m. of fascia lata
  tensor tympani m.
  tensor m. of tympanic
   membrane
  tensor m. of tympanum
  tensor m. of velum palatini
  tensor veli palatini m.
  teres major m.
  teres minor m.
  thenar m's
  thyroarytenoid m.
  thyroepiglottic m.
  thyrohyoid m.
  thyropharyngeal m.

mus·cle *(continued)*
  tibial m., anterior
  tibial m., posterior
  Tod's m.
  m's of tongue
  tonic m.
  tracheal m.
  trachelomastoid m.
  m. of tragus
  transverse m. of abdomen
  transverse m. of auricle
  transverse m. of chin
  transverse m. of nape
  transverse m. of perineum,
   deep
  transverse m. of perineum,
   superficial
  transverse m. of thorax
  transverse m. of tongue
  transversospinal m.
  transversus abdominis m.
  trapezius m.
  m. of Treitz
  triangular m.
  triceps m. of arm
  triceps m. of calf
  tricipital m.
  twitch m.
  ulnar flexor m. of wrist
  unipennate m.
  unitary m.
  unstriated m.
  m. of uvula
  Valsalva's m.
  vertical m. of tongue
  vestigial m.
  visceral m.
  vocal m.
  voluntary m.
  white m.
  Wilson's m.
  yoked m's
  zygomatic m.
  zygomatic m., greater
  zygomatic m., lesser
mus·cle phos·phor·y·lase
mus·cle-trim·ming
mus·coid

mus·cu·lam·ine
mus·cu·lar
mus·cu·la·ris
   m. mucosae
mus·cu·lar·i·ty
mus·cu·lar·ize
mus·cu·la·tion
mus·cu·la·ture
mus·cu·li
mus·cu·lo·apo·neu·rot·ic
mus·cu·lo·cu·ta·ne·ous
mus·cu·lo·der·mic
mus·cu·lo·elas·tic
mus·cu·lo·fas·ci·al
mus·cu·lo·fi·brous
mus·cu·lo·in·tes·ti·nal
mus·cu·lo·mem·bra·nous
mus·cu·lo·phren·ic
mus·cu·lo·ra·chid·i·an
mus·cu·lo·skel·e·tal
mus·cu·lo·spi·ral
mus·cu·lo·spi·ra·lis
mus·cu·lo·teg·u·men·ta·ry
mus·cu·lo·ten·di·nous
mus·cu·lo·ton·ic
mus·cu·lo·trop·ic
mus·cu·lus *pl.* mus·cu·li
   m. antitragicus
   musculi arrectores pilorum
   m. articularis
   m. biceps brachii
   m. biceps femoris
   m. brachialis
   m. brachioradialis
   m. buccopharyngeus
   m. bulbocavernosus
   m. bulbospongiosus
   m. chondroglossus
   m. ciliaris
   m. corrugator supercilii
   m. cricopharyngeus
   m. dartos
   m. erector spinae
   m. gastrocnemius
   m. genioglossus
   m. geniohyoideus
   m. glossopalatinus
   m. glossopharyngeus

mus·cu·lus *(continued)*
   m. gluteus maximus
   m. gluteus medius
   m. gluteus minimus
   m. gracilis
   m. hyoglossus
   m. iliopsoas
   m. infraspinatus
   m. latissimus dorsi
   m. levator ani
   musculi linguae
   m. longissimus
   m. longus capitis
   m. longus colli
   m. masseter
   m. omohyoideus
   m. orbicularis oculi
   m. orbicularis oris
   m. pectoralis major
   m. pectoralis minor
   m. peroneus brevis
   m. peroneus longus
   m. piriformis
   m. popliteus
   m. pronator quadratus
   m. pronator teres
   m. psoas major
   m. psoas minor
   m. quadratus femoris
   m. quadriceps femoris
   m. rectus abdominis
   m. rectus femoris
   m. rhomboideus major
   m. rhomboideus minor
   m. risorius
   m. sacrospinalis
   m. sartorius
   m. scalenus anterior
   m. scalenus medius
   m. scalenus minimus
   m. scalenus posterior
   m. semispinalis
   m. semitendinosus
   m. serratus anterior
   m. serratus posterior
    inferior
   m. serratus posterior
    superior

mus·cu·lus *(continued)*
   m. soleus
   m. sphincter pupillae
   m. sphincter pylori
   m. sphincter pyloricus
   m. sphincter urethrae
   m. spinalis
   m. stapedius
   m. sternohyoideus
   m. styloglossus
   m. stylohyoideus
   m. stylopharyngeus
   m. subclavius
   m. subscapularis
   m. supinator
   m. supraspinatus
   m. temporalis
   m. tensor fasciae latae
   m. tensor tympani
   m. tensor veli palatini
   m. teres major
   m. teres minor
   m. thyroepiglotticus
   m. thyrohyoideus
   m. tibialis anterior
   m. tibialis posterior
   m. tragicus
   m. trapezius
   m. triangularis
   m. triceps brachii
   m. triceps surae
   m. vastus intermedius
   m. vastus lateralis
   m. vastus medialis
   m. zygomaticus major
   m. zygomaticus minor
mush·room
mu·si·co·gen·ic
mu·si·co·ther·a·py
Mus·set's sign
mus·si·ta·tion
mus·tard
   nitrogen m.
   L-phenylalanine m.
   uracil m.
Mus·tarde flap otoplasty
Mus·tard operation
Mus·tar·gen

mu·ta·cism
mu·ta·gen
mu·ta·gen·e·sis
   directed m.
   insertional m.
mu·ta·gen·ic
mu·ta·ge·nic·i·ty
mu·ta·gen·ize
Mu·ta·my·cin
mu·tant
   amber m.
   auxotrophic m.
   cryptic m.
   leaky m.
   polarity m.
   R m.
   rough m.
   temperature-sensitive m.
mu·ta·ro·tase
mu·ta·ro·ta·tion
mu·tase
mu·ta·tion
   allelic m's
   amber m.
   auxotrophic m.
   back m.
   biochemical m.
   chromosomal m.
   clear plaque m.
   cold-sensitive m.
   conditional m.
   conditional lethal m.
   constitutive m.
   forward m.
   frameshift m.
   genomic m.
   germinal m.
   heat-sensitive m.
   homoeotic m.
   induced m.
   lethal m.
   missense m.
   natural m.
   neutral m.
   nonsense m.
   nutritional m.
   ochre m.
   opal m.

mu·ta·tion *(continued)*
    point m.
    polar m.
    reading frameshift m.
    reverse m.
    silent m.
    somatic m.
    spontaneous m's
    suppressor m.
    temperature-sensitive (t-s)
      m.
    umber m.
    visible m.
mu·ta·tion·al
mute
    deaf m.
mu·te·in
mu·ti·late
mu·ti·la·tion
Mu·tis·ia
    M. viciaefolia
mu·tism
    akinetic m.
    deaf m.
    elective m.
mu·tu·al·ism
mu·tu·al·ist
mu·zo·li·mine
MV — L. Medicus
  Veterinarius (veterinary
  physician)
    megavolt
MVV — maximum voluntary
  ventilation
mV — millivolt
μV — microvolt
MW — megawatt
    molecular weight
mW — milliwatt
μW — microwatt
Mx — Medex
My — myopia
my — mayer
my·al·gia
    m. abdominis
    m. capitis
    m. cervicalis
    epidemic m.

my·al·gia *(continued)*
    lumbar m.
    spastic m.
My·am·bu·tol
My·an·e·sin
my·a·sis
my·as·the·nia
    angiosclerotic m.
    carcinomatous m.
    m. gastrica
    m. gravis
    m. gravis pseudoparalytica
    m. laryngis
    neonatal m.
my·as·then·ic
my·a·to·nia
    m. congenita
my·at·o·ny
my·at·ro·phy
my·au·ton·o·my
my·ce·li·al
my·ce·li·an
my·ce·li·oid
my·ce·li·um *pl.* my·ce·lia
my·cete
my·ce·the·mia
my·ce·tism
my·ce·tis·mus
    m. cerebris
    m. choleriformis
    m. gastrointestinalis
    m. nervosus
    m. sanguinarius
my·ce·to·gen·ic
my·ce·tog·e·nous
my·ce·toid
my·ce·to·ma
    actinomycotic m.
    Carter's m.
    eumycotic m.
My·ce·to·zoa
My·ce·to·zoi·da
my·cid
My·cif·ra·din
my·co·bac·te·ria
My·co·bac·te·ri·a·ceae
my·co·bac·te·ri·o·sis

My·co·bac·te·ri·um
   M. *abscessus*
   M. *africanum*
   M. *aquae*
   M. *avium–intracellulare*
   M. *balnei*
   M. *borstelense*
   M. *bovis*
   M. *brunense*
   M. *buruli*
   M. *chelonei*
   M. *flavescens*
   M. *fortuitum*
   M. *gastri*
   M. *giae*
   M. *gordonae*
   M. *habana*
   M. *haemophilum*
   M. *intracellulare*
   M. *kansasii*
   M. *leprae*
   M. *lepraemurium*
   M. *littorale*
   M. *luciflavum*
   M. *malmoense*
   M. *marianum*
   M. *marinum*
   M. *microti*
   M. *minetti*
   M. *moelleri*
   M. *nonchromogenicum*
   M. *paraffinicum*
   M. *paratuberculosis*
   M. *phlei*
   M. *platypoecilus*
   M. *ranae*
   M. *scrofulaceum*
   M. *simiae*
   M. *smegmatis*
   M. *szulgai*
   M. *terrae*
   M. *triviale*
   M. *tuberculosis*
   M. *tuberculosis* var. *avium*
   M. *tuberculosis* var. *bovis*
   M. *tuberculosis* var.
     hominis
   M. *tuberculosis* var. *muris*

My·co·bac·te·ri·um
(continued)
   M. *ulcerans*
   M. *vaccae*
   M. *xenopi*
my·co·bac·te·ri·um *pl.* my·
  co·bac·te·ria
   anonymous mycobacteria
   atypical mycobacteria
   Group I–IV mycobacteria
   nontuberculous
    mycobacteria
my·co·bac·tin
my·co·ci·din
my·co·der·ma
my·co·der·ma·ti·tis
my·co·flo·ra
my·co·he·mia
my·coid
my·co·lic acids
my·col·o·gist
my·col·o·gy
my·co·myr·in·gi·tis
my·co·pa·thol·o·gy
my·co·phage
my·coph·a·gy
My·co·plas·ma
   M. *faucium*
   M. *fermentans*
   M. *hominis*
   M. *orale*
   M. *pneumoniae*
   M. *salivarium*
my·co·plas·ma *pl.* my·co·plas·
  mas, my·co·plas·ma·ta
   T-strain m.
my·co·plas·mal
My·co·plas·ma·ta·ceae
My·co·plas·ma·ta·les
my·co·plas·mo·sis
my·co·pre·cip·i·tin
my·co·pus
my·cose
my·co·side
my·co·sis
   cutaneous m.
   m. fungoides
   m. fungoides d'emblée

my·co·sis *(continued)*
    m. fungoides en plaques
    Gilchrist's m.
    m leptothrica
    Posada m.
    splenic m.
my·cos·ta·sis
my·co·stat
My·co·stat·in
my·cos·ter·ol
my·cot·ic
My·co·tor·u·loi·des
my·co·tox·i·col·o·gy
my·co·tox·i·co·sis
my·co·tox·in
my·co·tox·in·iza·tion
myc·ter·ic
myc·tero·xe·ro·sis
my·da·le·ine
my·da·tox·ine
My·dri·a·cyl
my·dri·a·sis
    alternating m.
    bounding m.
    paralytic m.
    spasmodic m.
    spastic m.
    spinal m.
    springing m.
myd·ri·at·ic
my·ec·to·my
my·ec·to·pia
my·ec·to·py
my·el·aceph·a·lus
my·el·al·gia
my·el·ap·o·plexy
my·el·ate·lia
my·el·at·ro·phy
my·el·auxe
my·el·emia
my·el·en·ceph·a·li·tis
my·el·en·ceph·a·lon
my·el·en·ceph·a·lo·spi·nal
my·el·et·er·o·sis
my·elic
my·elin
my·eli·nat·ed
my·eli·na·tion

my·elin·ic
my·eli·ni·za·tion
my·eli·noc·la·sis
    acute perivascular m.
    central pontine m.
    postinfection perivenous m.
my·elino·gen·e·sis
    dystopic cortical m.
my·elino·ge·net·ic
my·eli·nog·e·ny
my·eli·nol·y·sis
    central pontine m.
my·eli·nop·a·thy
my·eli·no·sis
    pontine m.
my·elino·tox·ic
my·elino·tox·ic·i·ty
my·elit·ic
my·eli·tis
    acute m.
    acute syphilitic m.
    amyotrophic syphilitic m.
    angiohypertrophic spinal
        m.
    apoplectiform m.
    ascending m.
    bulbar m.
    cavitary m.
    central m.
    chronic m.
    compression m.
    concussion m.
    cornual m.
    descending m.
    diffuse m.
    disseminated m.
    focal m.
    foudroyant m.
    funicular m.
    hemorrhagic m.
    interstitial m.
    metastatic m.
    neuro-optic m.
    parenchymatous m.
    periependymal m.
    postvaccinal m.
    pressure m.
    pseudotumoral m.

my·eli·tis *(continued)*
   radiation m.
   sclerosing m.
   subacute necrotic m.
   systemic m.
   transverse m.
   traumatic m.
   tuberculous m.
   m. vaccinia
my·elo·ar·chi·tec·ture
my·elo·blast
my·elo·blas·te·mia
my·elo·blas·tic
my·elo·blas·to·ma
my·elo·blas·to·ma·to·sis
my·elo·blas·to·sis
my·elo·cele
my·elo·clast
my·elo·coele
my·elo·cyst
my·elo·cys·tic
my·elo·cys·to·cele
my·elo·cys·tog·ra·phy
my·elo·cys·to·me·nin·go·cele
my·elo·cyte
my·elo·cy·the·mia
my·elo·cyt·ic
my·elo·cy·to·ma
my·elo·cy·to·ma·to·sis
my·elo·cy·to·sis
my·elo·di·as·ta·sis
my·elo·dys·pla·sia
my·elo·en·ce·phal·ic
my·elo·en·ceph·a·li·tis
   eosinophilic m.
   epidemic m.
my·elo·fi·bro·sis
   osteosclerosis m.
my·elof·u·gal
my·elo·gen·e·sis
my·elo·gen·ic
my·elog·e·nous
my·elog·e·ny
my·elo·gone
my·elo·gon·ic
my·elo·go·ni·um
my·elo·gram

my·elog·ra·phy
   air m.
   oxygen m.
my·eloid
my·eloi·din
my·eloi·do·sis
my·elo·ken·tric
my·elo·leu·ke·mia
my·elo·li·po·ma
my·elo·lym·phan·gi·o·ma
my·elo·ly·sis
my·elo·lyt·ic
my·elo·ma
   endothelial m.
   extramedullary m.
   giant cell m.
   indolent m.
   localized m.
   multiple m.
   plasma cell m.
   solitary m.
my·elo·ma·la·cia
my·elo·ma·toid
my·elo·ma·to·sis
my·elo·me·nia
my·elo·men·in·gi·tis
my·elo·me·nin·go·cele
my·elo·mere
my·elo·mono·cyte
my·elom·y·ces
my·elo·neu·ri·tis
my·elo-op·ti·co·neu·rop·a·thy
   subacute m.
my·elo·path·ic
my·elop·a·thy
   apoplectiform m.
   arteriosclerotic m.
   ascending m.
   cervical m.
   compression m.
   concussion m.
   descending m.
   diabetic m.
   focal m.
   funicular m.
   hemorrhagic m.
   interstitial m.

my·elop·a·thy *(continued)*
  ischemic m.
  necrotic m.
  parenchymatous m.
  radiation m.
  sclerosing m.
  spondylotic cervical m.
  systemic m.
  toxic m.
  transverse m.
  traumatic m.
my·e·lo·per·ox·i·dase (MPO)
my·elop·e·tal
my·elo·phage
my·elo·phthi·sis
my·elo·plaque
my·elo·plasm
my·elo·plast
my·elo·plax
my·elo·ple·gia
my·elo·poi·e·sis
  ectopic m.
  extramedullary m.
my·elo·pore
my·elo·pro·lif·er·a·tive
my·elop·ti·co·neu·rop·a·thy
my·elo·ra·dic·u·li·tis
my·elo·ra·dic·u·lo·dys·pla·sia
my·elo·ra·dic·u·lop·a·thy
my·elo·ra·dic·u·lo·poly·neu·ro·ni·tis
my·elor·rha·gia
my·elo·sar·co·ma
  erythroblastic m.
my·elo·sar·co·ma·to·sis
my·elos·chi·sis
my·elo·scin·to·gram
my·elo·scle·ro·sis
my·el·o·sis
  aleukemic m.
  aplastic m.
  chronic nonleukemic m.
  erythremic m.
  funicular m.
  nonleukemic m.
my·elo·spon·gi·um
my·elo·sup·pres·sion

my·elo·sup·pres·sive
my·elo·syph·i·lis
my·elo·syph·i·lo·sis
my·elo·ther·a·py
my·elo·tome
my·elot·o·my
  Bischof's m.
  commissural m.
  midline m.
my·elo·tox·ic
my·elo·tox·ic·i·ty
my·elo·tox·in
my·elo·trop·ic
my·en·ter·ic
my·en·ter·on
My·ers method
My·er·son's sign
my·es·the·sia
my·ia·sis
  aural m.
  creeping m.
  cutaneous m.
  dermal m.
  m. dermatosa
  intestinal m.
  m. linearis
  nasal m.
  ocular m.
  subcutaneous m.
  traumatic m.
my·io·des·op·sia
my·io·sis
my·itis
My·lax·en
Myl·er·an
My·li·con
my·lo·hy·oid
myo·ad·en·yl·ate de·am·i·nase
myo·ad·en·yl·ate (AMP) de·am·i·nase deficiency
myo·al·bu·min
myo·ar·chi·tec·ton·ic
myo·at·ro·phy
myo·blast
myo·blas·tic
myo·blas·to·ma
  granular cell m.

myo·blas·to·my·o·ma
myo·bra·dia
myo·car·di·ac
myo·car·di·al
myo·car·dio·gram
myo·car·dio·graph
myo·car·di·ol·y·sis
myo·car·di·op·a·thy
    alcoholic m.
    chagasic m.
myo·car·di·or·rha·phy
myo·car·di·o·sis
myo·car·dit·ic
myo·car·di·tis
    acute bacterial m.
    acute isolated m.
    Chagas m.
    chronic m.
    Coxsackie m.
    diphtheritic m.
    fibrous m.
    Fiedler's m.
    fragmentation m.
    giant cell m.
    idiopathic m.
    interstitial m.
    local m.
    nutritional m.
    parenchymatous m.
    rheumatic m.
    suppurative m.
    syphilitic m.
    toxic m.
    tuberculoid m.
    tuberculous m.
    virus m.
myo·car·di·um
myo·car·do·sis
myo·cele
myo·ce·li·al·gia
myo·ce·li·tis
myo·cel·lu·li·tis
myo·cep·tor
myo·ce·ro·sis
myo·chor·di·tis
myo·chrome
myo·chry·sine
myo·cine·sim·e·ter

myo·clo·nia
    m. epileptica
    m. fibrillaris multiplex
    fibrillary m.
    infectious m.
    pseudoglottic m.
    Unverricht's m.
myo·clon·ic
my·oc·lo·nus
    action m.
    diaphragmatic m.
    encephalitic m.
    epileptic m.
    hereditary essential m.
    intention m.
    m. multiplex
    massive epileptic m.
    nocturnal m.
    palatal m.
    palatopharyngolaryngeal
      m.
    petit mal m.
    postural m.
    spinal m.
    startle m.
myo·coele
myo·col·pi·tis
myo·com·ma
myo·cris·mus
my·oc·to·nine
my·oc·u·la·tor
myo·cu·ta·ne·ous
myo·cyst
myo·cyte
    Anichkov's m.
myo·cy·tol·y·sis
    coagulative m.
    focal m. of heart
myo·cy·to·ma
myo·de·gen·er·a·tion
myo·de·mia
myo·des·op·sia
myo·di·as·ta·sis
myo·di·op·ter
myo·dy·nam·ic
myo·dy·nam·ics
myo·dy·na·mom·e·ter

my·odyn·ia
myo·dys·pla·sia
   m. fibrosa multiplex
myo·dys·to·nia
myo·dys·tro·phia
   m. fetalis
myo·dys·tro·phy
myo·ede·ma
myo·elas·tic
myo·elec·tric
myo·elec·tri·cal
myo·en·do·car·di·tis
myo·epi·the·li·al
myo·epi·the·li·o·ma
myo·epi·the·li·um
myo·fas·ci·al
myo·fas·ci·tis
myo·fi·ber
myo·fi·bril
myo·fi·bril·la *pl.* myo·fi·bril·
  lae
myo·fi·bril·lar
myo·fi·bro·blast
myo·fi·bro·ma
   infantile m.
myo·fi·bro·sis
   m. cordis
myo·fi·bro·si·tis
myo·fila·ment
myo·func·tion·al
myo·gas·ter
myo·ge·lo·sis
my·o·gen
myo·gen·e·sis
myo·ge·net·ic
my·o·gen·ic
my·og·e·nous
my·og·lia
myo·glo·bin
myo·glo·bin·emia
myo·glo·bin·uria
   familial m.
   idiopathic m.
   paroxysmal m.
   traumatic m.
myo·glob·u·lin
myo·glob·u·lin·uria
my·og·na·thus

myo·gram
myo·graph
myo·graph·ic
my·og·ra·phy
myo·he·ma·tin
myo·he·mo·glo·bin
myo·hy·per·tro·phia
   m. kymoparalytica
my·oid
   visual cell m.
my·oi·de·um
my·oid·ism
*myo·*ino·si·tol
myo·is·che·mia
myo·ke·ro·sis
myo·ki·nase
myo·kine·sim·e·ter
myo·ki·ne·sio·gram
myo·ki·ne·sis
myo·ki·net·ic
myo·kym·ia
   facial m.
   hereditary m.
myo·lem·ma
myo·li·po·ma
myo·lo·gia
my·ol·o·gy
my·ol·y·sis
   m. cardio-toxica
my·o·ma *pl.* my·o·mas, my·o·
  ma·ta
   ball m.
   myoblastic m.
   m. previum
   m. sarcomatodes
   m. striocellulare
   m. telangiectodes
my·o·ma·gen·e·sis
my·o·ma·la·cia
   m. cordis
my·o·ma·ta
my·o·ma·tec·to·my
my·o·ma·to·sis
my·o·ma·tous
my·o·mec·to·my
   abdominal m.
   vaginal m.
myo·mel·a·no·sis

myo·mere
my·om·e·ter
myo·me·tri·tis
myo·me·tri·um
myo·mi·to·chon·drion
myo·mo·hys·ter·ec·to·my
myo·mot·o·my
my·on
myo·ne·cro·sis
    clostridial m.
myo·neme
myo·neph·ro·pexy
myo·neu·ral
myo·neu·ral·gia
myo·neur·as·the·nia
myo·neure
myo·neu·ro·ma
my·on·o·sus
my·on·y·my
myo·pa·chyn·sis
myo·pal·mus
myo·pa·ral·y·sis
myo·par·e·sis
myo·path·ia
    m. cordis
    m. infraspinata
myo·path·ic
my·op·a·thy
    acromegalic m.
    ACTH m.
    acute thyrotoxic m.
    alcoholic m.
    arachnodactyly nemaline
      m.
    carcinomatous m.
    centronuclear m.
    Cushing's disease m.
    diabetic m.
    distal m.
    Duchenne's m.
    fingerprint body m.
    granulomatous m.
    hypermetabolic m.
    hyperparathyroid m.
    hypothyroid m.
    Kiloh-Nevin m.
    Landouzy-Dejerine m.
    megaconial m.

my·op·a·thy *(continued)*
    metabolic m.
    mitochondrial m.
    myogranular m.
    myotonic m.
    myotubular m.
    myxedematous m.
    nemaline m.
    ocular m.
    pleoconial m.
    rod m.
    sarcoid m.
    scapuloperoneal m.
    steroid m.
    thyrotoxic m.
    uremic m.
    Welander's m.
my·ope
myo·peri·car·di·tis
myo·phage
myo·pha·gia
my·oph·a·gism
myo·phone
my·o·pia
    curvature m.
    index m.
    malignant m.
    pernicious m.
    primary m.
    prodromal m.
    progressive m.
    simple m.
my·op·ic
myo·plasm
myo·plas·tic
myo·plas·ty
myo·po·lar
myo·pro·tein
my·op·sis
myo·re·cep·tor
my·or·rha·phy
my·or·rhex·is
my·or·rhyth·mia
myo·sal·gia
myo·sal·pin·gi·tis
myo·sal·pinx
my·o·san
myo·sar·co·ma

myo·schwan·no·ma
myo·scle·ro·sis
myo·scope
myo·seism
myo·sep·tum
myo·se·rum
my·o·sin
my·o·sin ATPase
my·o·sin·o·gen
my·o·sin·uria
my·o·sis
    endolymphatic stromal m.
myo·sit·ic
myo·si·tis
    acute disseminated m.
    acute progressive m.
    Coxsackie m.
    epidemic m.
    m. a frigore
    m. fibrosa
    generalized m. ossificans
    infectious m.
    interstitial m.
    multiple m.
    orbital m.
    m. ossificans
    m. ossificans circumscripta
    m. ossificans progressiva
    m. ossificans traumatica
    parenchymatous m.
    primary multiple m.
    progressive ossifying m.
    m. purulenta
    m. purulenta tropica
    rheumatoid m.
    m. serosa
    spontaneous bacterial m.
    suppurative m.
    trichinous m.
    tropical m.
myo·spa·sia
myo·spasm
myo·spas·mia
myo·sta·sis
myo·stat·ic
my·os·te·o·ma
my·os·then·ic
my·os·then·om·e·ter

myo·stro·ma
myo·stro·min
myo·su·ria
myo·su·ture
myo·syn·i·ze·sis
myo·tac·tic
my·ot·a·sis
myo·tat·ic
myo·ten·di·ni·tis
myo·ten·di·nous
myo·ten·on·to·plas·ty
myo·teno·si·tis
myo·te·not·o·my
myo·ther·mic
my·ot·ic
myo·til·i·ty
myo·tome
myo·tom·ic
my·ot·o·my
    cricopharyngeal m.
    Heller's m.
    Livadatis' circular m.
myo·ton·a·chol
myo·tone
myo·to·nia
    m. acquisita
    m. atrophica
    chondrodystrophic m.
    m. congenita
    m. hereditaria
    m. congenita intermittens
    congenital m.
    m. dystrophica
    m. paradoxa
    Schwartz-Jampel m.
myo·ton·ic
my·ot·o·noid
myo·to·nom·e·ter
my·ot·o·nus
my·ot·o·ny
myo·troph·ic
my·ot·ro·phy
my·o·trop·ic
myo·tube
myo·tu·bu·lar
myo·tu·bule
myo·vas·cu·lar
myr·cene

myr·ia·pod
Myr·i·ap·o·da
myr·i·cin
myr·i·cyl
my·rin·ga
my·rin·gec·to·my
my·rin·gi·tis
    m. bullosa
    bullous m.
    m. bullosa hemorrhagica
my·rin·go·dec·to·my
my·rin·go·der·ma·ti·tis
my·rin·go·my·co·sis
    m. aspergillina
my·rin·go·plas·ty
    inlay m.
    onlay m.
    underlay m.
my·rin·go·rup·ture
my·rin·go·sta·pe·dio·pexy
my·rin·go·tome
my·rin·got·o·my
my·rinx
myr·is·tate
    isopropyl m.
my·ris·tic acid
My·ris·ti·ca
my·ris·ti·ca
my·ris·ti·cene
myr·is·ti·cin
my·ris·ti·col
my·ris·tin
myrrh
myrrh·o·lin
myr·te·nol
Myr·tus
    M. communis
My·so·line
my·so·phil·ia
my·so·pho·bia
my·so·pho·bic
my·ta·cism
My·te·lase
mytho·ma·nia
mytho·pho·bia
myx·ad·e·ni·tis
    m. labialis
myx·ad·e·no·ma

myx·ame·ba
myx·an·gi·tis
myx·an·go·itis
myx·as·the·nia
myx·ede·ma
    circumscribed m.
    circumscribed plane m.
    hypothalamic m.
    infantile m.
    nodular m.
    operative m.
    papular m.
    pituitary m.
    pretibial m.
    tuberous m.
myx·edem·a·toid
myx·edem·a·tous
myx·i·o·sis
myxo·ad·e·no·ma
myxo·blas·to·ma
myxo·chon·dro·fi·bro·sar·co·ma
myxo·chon·dro·ma
myxo·chon·dro·sar·co·ma
myxo·cys·ti·tis
myxo·cys·to·ma
myxo·cyte
myxo·en·chon·dro·ma
myxo·en·do·the·li·o·ma
myxo·fi·bro·ma
myxo·fi·bro·sar·co·ma
myxo·gli·o·ma
myxo·glob·u·lo·sis
myx·oid
myxo·lipo·fi·bro·sar·co·ma
myxo·li·po·ma
myxo·lipo·sar·co·ma
myx·o·ma *pl.* myx·o·mas,
  myx·o·ma·ta
    atrial m.
    cystic m.
    enchondromatous m.
    erectile m.
    m. fibrosum
    giant mammary m.
    m. of heart
    infectious m.
    lipomatous m.

myx·o·ma *(continued)*
   odontogenic m.
   m. sarcomatosum
   vascular m.
myx·o·ma·to·sis
   m. cuniculi
   infectious m.
myx·o·ma·tous
myxo·my·o·ma
myxo·pap·il·lo·ma
myxo·poi·e·sis
myx·or·rhea

myx·or·rhea
   m. intestinalis
myxo·sar·co·ma
myxo·sar·co·ma·tous
Myx·o·so·ma
myxo·spor·an
myxo·spor·ea
myxo·vi·rus
myxo·zoa
myxo·zo·an
My·zo·my·ia

N

N — newton
   nitrogen
   normal (solution)
N — Avogadro's number
   neutron number
   normal
   number
   population size
N_A — Avogadro's number
   neutron
   refractive index
n. — L. nervus (nerve)
n — (haploid) chromosome
   number
   refractive index
   sample size
n- — normal
n_D — refractive index
ν — degrees of freedom
   frequency
   kinematic viscosity
   neutrino
NA — Nomina Anatomica
   numerical aperture
nab·i·drox
nab·i·lone
Na·both's cysts

Na·both's follicles
Na·both's glands
Na·both's ovules
Na·both's vesicles
na·bo·thi·an
na·cre·ous
Nac·ton
NAD — nicotinamide-adenine
   dinucleotide
   no appreciable disease
   nothing abnormal detected
NAD^+ — the oxidized form of
   NAD
Nad·bath akinesia
NADH — the reduced form of
   NAD
NADH cy·to·chrome b_5 re·
   duc·tase
NADH de·hy·dro·ge·nase
   (ubi·quin·one)
NADH-met·he·mo·glo·bin re·
   duc·tase
NADH ox·i·dase
na·dide
NAD ki·nase
na·do·lol

NADP — nicotinamide-adenine-dinucleotide phosphate
NADP⁺ — the oxidized form of NADP
NADPH — the reduced form of NADP
NADPH-cy·to·chrome re·duc·tase
NADPH dia·phor·ase
NADPH-fer·ri·he·mo·pro·tein re·duc·tase
NADPH met·he·mo·glo·bin re·duc·tase
NADPH ox·i·dase
Nae·ge·li's leukemia
Nae·ge·li's syndrome
Nae·gle·ria
    N. fowleri
nae·gle·ri·a·sis
nae·paine
naf·cil·lin
na·fen·o·pin
Naff·zig·er's operation
Naff·zig·er's syndrome
naf·o·mine mal·ate
naf·ox·i·dine hy·dro·chlo·ride
naf·ro·nyl ox·a·late
naf·ta·lo·fos
na·ga·na
nag·a·nol
Na·gel's test
Nä·ge·le's obliquity
Nä·ge·le's pelvis
Nä·ge·le's rule
Nage·otte bracelets
Nage·otte cell
Nager's acrofacial dysostosis
Nager's syndrome
Nager-De Reynier syndrome
Na·gler effect
Na·gler's reaction
Na·gler's test
nai·ad
nail
    cloverleaf n.
    eggshell n.
    fracture n.
    hippocratic n.

nail *(continued)*
    ingrown n.
    Jewett n.
    Küntscher n.
    Neufeld n.
    parrot beak n.
    pitted n's
    racket n.
    n. en raquette
    reedy n.
    Smith-Petersen n.
    spoon n.
    Thornton n.
    turtle-back n.
    watch-crystal n.
nail·ing
    intramedullary n.
    marrow n.
    medullary n.
na·ja
Nak·a·ya·ma's reagent
Nak·a·ya·ma's test
nal·bu·phine hy·dro·chlo·ride
Nal·fon
nal·i·dix·ate so·di·um
nal·i·dix·ic acid
Nal·line
nal·mex·one hy·dro·chlo·ride
nal·or·phine
    n. hydrochloride
nal·ox·one hy·dro·chlo·ride
nal·trex·one
name
    British Approved N.
    generic n.
    International Nonproprietary N.
    nonproprietary n.
    proprietary n.
    semisystematic n.
    semitrivial n.
    systematic n.
    trivial n.
    United States Adopted N.
NAN — *N*-acetylneuraminic acid
nan·dro·lone
    n. cyclotate

nan·dro·lone *(continued)*
   n. decanoate
   n. phenpropionate
na·nism
   mulibrey n.
   pituitary n.
   renal n.
   senile n.
   symptomatic n.
Nan·niz·zia
Nan·no·mo·nas
nano·ce·pha·lia
nano·ceph·a·lous
nano·ceph·a·ly
na·no·cor·mia
na·no·cu·rie
na·no·gram
na·noid
na·no·li·ter
na·no·me·lia
na·nom·e·lous
na·nom·e·lus
na·no·me·ter
na·noph·thal·mia
na·noph·thal·mos
Na·no·phy·e·tus sal·min·co·la
na·no·plank·ton
na·no·sec·ond
na·no·so·ma
na·no·so·mia
na·no·unit
na·nous
na·nu·ka·ya·mi
na·nus
NAP — nasion, point A, pogonion
na·pex
naph·az·o·line hy·dro·chlo·ride
naph·tha
   wood n.
naph·tha·lene
naph·tha·mine
naph·thol
   β-n.
   beta-n.
naph·tho·late

naph·thol·ism
naph·tho·re·sor·cine
naph·thyl
   n. alcohol
   n. phenol
naph·thyl·para·ro·san·i·line
na·pi·form
NAPNES — National Association for Practical Nurse Education and Services
nap·ra·path
na·prap·a·thy
Na·pro·syn
na·prox·en
na·prox·ol
nap·sy·late
nap·tho·qui·none
nap·thyl·amine
Na·qua
Na·qui·val
nar·a·nol hy·dro·chlo·ride
nar·a·sin
Nar·can
nar·cism
nar·cis·sine
nar·cis·sism
nar·cis·sis·tic
nar·co·anal·y·sis
nar·co·hyp·nia
nar·co·hyp·no·sis
nar·co·lep·sy
nar·co·lep·tic
nar·co·ma
nar·cose
nar·co·sine
nar·co·sis
   basal n.
   basis n.
   carbon dioxide n.
   insufflation n.
   intravenous n.
   medullary n.
   nitrogen n.
   Nussbaum's n.
nar·co·stim·u·lant
nar·co·syn·the·sis
nar·cot·ic

nar·cot·i·co-ac·rid
nar·cot·i·co-ir·ri·tant
nar·co·tile
nar·co·tine
nar·co·tize
nar·cous
Nar·di test
Nar·dil
na·res
na·ris *pl.* na·res
    anterior n.
    external n.
    internal nares
    posterior nares
Nar·one
na·sal
na·sa·lis
na·sal·i·ty
nas·cent
na·sio·in·i·ac
na·si·on
na·si·tis
Nas·myth's membrane
NAS-NRC — National
  Academy of
  Sciences–National Research
  Council
na·so·an·tral
na·so·an·tri·tis
na·so·an·tros·to·my
na·so·bron·chi·al
na·so·buc·cal
na·so·buc·co·pha·ryn·ge·al
na·so·cil·i·ary
na·soc·u·lar
na·so·en·do·scope
na·so·en·dos·co·py
na·so-eth·moi·dal
na·so·fa·cial
na·so·fron·tal
na·so·gas·tric
na·so·je·ju·nal
na·so·la·bi·al
na·so·lac·ri·mal
na·so·ma·nom·e·ter
na·so·max·il·lary
na·sonne·ment
na·so-oc·cip·i·tal

na·so-oral
na·so·pal·a·tine
na·so·pha·ryn·ge·al
na·so·pha·ryn·gi·tis
na·so·pha·ryn·go·la·ryn·go·
  scope
na·so·pha·ryn·go·scope
na·so·pha·ryn·gos·co·py
na·so·phar·ynx
na·so·ros·tral
na·so·scope
na·so·sep·tal
na·so·sep·ti·tis
na·so·si·nu·si·tis
na·so·spi·na·le
na·so·tur·bi·nal
na·sus
  n. externus
  n. osseus
na·tal
na·tal·i·ty
nat·a·my·cin
na·ta·tory
na·tes
Na·thans, Daniel
na·ti·mor·tal·i·ty
Na·tion·al For·mu·lary
na·tis
na·tive
Nat·o·lone
na·tre·mia
na·tri·ure·sis
na·tri·uret·ic
na·ture-nur·ture
Nat·ure·tin
na·turo·path
na·turo·path·ic
na·tur·op·a·thy
Nau·heim bath
Nau·heim treatment
Nau·nyn-Min·kow·ski method
nau·sea
  n. epidemica
  n. gravidarum
nau·se·ant
nau·se·ate
nau·seous
Nav·ane

na·vel
  blue n.
  enamel n.
na·vic·u·la
na·vic·u·lar
na·vic·u·lar·thri·tis
na·vic·u·lo·cu·boid
NBS — National Bureau of Standards
NBT — nitroblue tetrazolium
NCA — neurocirculatory asthenia
  nonspecific cross-reacting antigen
NCF — neutrophil chemotactic factor
NCHS — National Center Health Statistics
NCI — National Cancer Institute
nCi — nanocurie
NCMH — National Committee Mental Hygiene
NCN — National Council of Nurses
NCRP — National Committee on Radiation Protection and Measurements
NCV — nerve conduction velocity
  noncholera vibrios
NDA — National Dental Association
NDV — Newcastle disease virus
ne·al·o·gy
near-sight
near·sight·ed
near·sight·ed·ness
ne·ar·thro·sis
ne·ben·kern
neb·ra·my·cin
neb·u·la pl. neb·u·lae
neb·u·lar·ine
neb·u·li·za·tion
neb·u·liz·er
  ultrasonic n.

NEC — necrotizing enterocolitis
Ne·ca·tor
  N. americanus
ne·ca·to·ri·a·sis
ne·ces·si·ty
  pharmaceutic n.
  pharmaceutical n.
neck
  anatomical n. of humerus
  n. of ankle bone
  bladder n.
  buffalo n.
  bull n.
  n. of condyloid process of mandible
  dental n.
  n. of dorsal head of spinal cord
  false n. of humerus
  n. of femur
  n. of fibula
  n. of gallbladder
  n. of glans penis
  n. of hair follicle
  n. of humerus
  lateral n. of vertebra
  Madelung's n.
  n. of malleus
  n. of mandible
  n. of pancreas
  n. of posterior horn of spinal cord
  n. of radius
  n. of rib
  n. of scapula
  n. of spermatozoon
  stiff n.
  surgical n. of humerus
  n. of talus
  n. of tooth
  true n. of humerus
  turkey gobbler n.
  n. of urinary bladder
  uterine n.
  n. of uterus
  n. of vertebra
  n. of vertebral arch

neck *(continued)*
    webbed n.
    wry n.
neck·lace
    Casal's n.
nec·rec·to·my
nec·ren·ceph·a·lus
nec·ro·bac·il·lo·sis
nec·ro·bi·o·sis
    n. lipoidica
    n. lipoidica diabeticorum
nec·ro·bi·ot·ic
nec·ro·cy·to·sis
nec·ro·cy·to·tox·in
nec·ro·gen·ic
ne·crog·e·nous
nec·ro·log·ic
ne·crol·o·gist
ne·crol·o·gy
ne·crol·y·sis
    toxic epidermal n.
nec·ro·ma·nia
ne·crom·e·ter
nec·ro·mi·me·sis
nec·ro·nec·to·my
ne·croph·a·gous
nec·ro·phil·ia
nec·ro·phil·ic
ne·croph·i·lism
ne·croph·i·lous
ne·croph·i·ly
nec·ro·pho·bia
nec·ro·pneu·mo·nia
nec·rop·sy
nec·ro·sa·dism
ne·cros·co·py
nec·rose
nec·ro·ses
ne·cro·sis *pl.* ne·cro·ses
    acute tubular n.
    arteriolar n.
    aseptic n.
    avascular n.
    bacillary n.
    Balser's fatty n.
    bilateral renal cortical n.
    bland n.
    bridging n.

ne·cro·sis *(continued)*
    caseous n.
    central n.
    cerebrocortical n.
    cheesy n.
    chemical n.
    coagulation n.
    colliquative n.
    contraction band n.
    cortical n.
    coumarin n.
    cystic medial n.
    diphtheritic n.
    dry n.
    embolic n.
    epiphyseal ischemic n.
    Erdheim's cystic medial n.
    exanthematous n.
    fat n.
    fibrinoid n.
    focal n.
    gangrenous n.
    gangrenous pulp n.
    glomerular n.
    gummatous n.
    hyaline n.
    ischemic n.
    labial n. of rabbits
    laminar cortical n.
    liquefaction n.
    mandibular n.
    massive hepatic n.
    mechanical n.
    medial n.
    mercurial n.
    moist n.
    mummification n.
    nephrotoxic tubule n.
    Paget's quiet n.
    papillary n.
    peripheral n.
    phosphorus n.
    physical n.
    piecemeal n.
    postpartum pituitary n.
    pressure n.
    n. progrediens

ne·cro·sis *(continued)*
  progressive
    emphysematous n.
  quiet n.
  radiation n.
  radium n.
  renal coagulation n.
  n. of renal papillae
  renal papillary n.
  septic n.
  simple n.
  spontaneous n.
  subacute hepatic n.
  subcutaneous fat n.
  subendocardial n.
  submassive hepatic n.
  superficial n.
  syphilitic n.
  total n.
  transmural n.
  tubular n.
  n. ustilaginea
  Zenker's n.
nec·ro·sper·mia
nec·ro·sper·mic
ne·crot·ic
nec·ro·tize
nec·ro·tiz·ing
ne·crot·o·my
  osteoplastic n.
nec·ro·tox·in
nec·ro·zoo·sper·mia
Nec·tu·rus
NED — no evidence of disease
nee·dle
  Abrams' n.
  aneurysm n.
  aspirating n.
  atraumatic n.
  biopsy n.
  butterfly n.
  cataract n.
  Chiba n.
  Cibis ski n.
  Cope's n.
  cutting n.
  Deschamps' n.
  discission n.

nee·dle *(continued)*
  docking n.
  electrosurgical n.
  fascia n.
  fine n.
  Hagedorn's n's
  hypodermic n.
  Jamshidi n.
  knife n.
  ligature n.
  lumbar puncture n.
  Menghini n.
  milliner's n.
  pop-off n.
  radium n.
  Reverdin's n.
  side-cutting spatulated n.
  Silverman n.
  skinny n.
  spinal n.
  stop n.
  swaged n.
  Tru-Cut n.
  ventriculopuncture n.
  Verres n.
  vicat n.
  Vim-Silverman n.
  Voorhees n.
nee·dle-hold·er
Neef's hammer
Neel·sen, Karl Adolf
ne·en·ceph·a·lon
NEEP — negative
  end-expiratory pressure
NEFA — nonesterified fatty
  acids
ne·flu·o·ro·pho·tom·e·ter
nef·o·pam hy·dro·chlo·ride
Neg·a·tan
neg·a·tiv·ism
neg·a·tol
neg·a·to·scope
neg·a·tron
Neg·Gram
neg·li·gence
  comparative n.
  contributory n.
Ne·gri bodies

Ne·gro's phenomenon
Neg·us dilator
Neg·us esophagoscope
Neg·us tube
neigh·bor·wise
Neill-Moo·ser bodies
Neill-Moo·ser reaction
Neis·ser's diplococcus
Neis·ser's syringe
Neis·ser-Wechs·berg
   phenomenon
Neis·se·ria
   N. catarrhalis
   N. flavescens
   N. gonorrhoeae
   N. lactamica
   N. meningitidis
   N. mucosa
   N. sicca
   N. subflava
Neis·se·ri·a·ceae
neis·se·ri·al
ne·la·vane
Nel·son syndrome
Né·la·ton's catheter
Né·la·ton's line
Né·la·ton's operation
Né·la·ton's probe
Né·la·ton's sphincter
Ne·ma
ne·ma
nem·a·line
nem·a·thel·minth
Nem·a·thel·min·thes
nem·a·thel·min·thi·a·sis
ne·mat·i·cide
nem·a·ti·za·tion
nem·a·to·blast
Nem·a·toc·era
nem·a·to·cide
nem·a·to·cyst
Nem·a·to·da
nem·a·tode
nem·a·to·des·ma *pl.* nem·a·
   to·des·ma·ta
nem·a·to·di·a·sis
   nonpatent n.
nem·a·toid

nem·a·tol·o·gist
nem·a·tol·o·gy
Nem·a·to·mor·pha
nem·a·to·sis
nem·a·to·sper·mia
Nem·bu·tal
nem·ic
Nen·cki's test
Neo-An·ter·gan
neo·an·ti·gen
neo·ar·thro·sis
neo·bio·gen·e·sis
Neo·bi·ot·ic
neo·blas·tic
Neo-Cal·glu·con
neo·cer·e·bel·lum
neo·ci·net·ic
Neo-Cob·e·frin
neo·cor·tex
neo·cys·tos·to·my
   ureteral n.
   ureteroileal n.
neo·cy·to·sis
neo·dar·win·ism
neo·dec·a·dron
neo·di·a·ther·my
Neo-Di·lo·derm
neo·dym·i·um
neo·en·ceph·a·lon
neo·fe·tal
neo·fe·tus
neo·for·ma·tion
neo·for·ma·tive
Neo·frakt
ne·og·a·la
neo·gen·e·sis
neo·ge·net·ic
neo·ger·mi·trine
neo·glot·tic
neo·glot·tis
   phonatory n.
neo·gly·co·gen·e·sis
neo·he·tra·mine
neo-hip·poc·ra·tism
Neo-Hom·bre·ol
neo·hy·men
neo·ki·net·ic
ne·o·lal·ia

ne·o·lal·ism
ne·ol·o·gism
Ne·o·loid
neo·mal·thu·si·an·ism
neo·mem·brane
ne·o·min
neo·morph
neo·mor·phism
neo·my·cin
    n. palmitate
    n. sulfate
ne·on
neo·na·tal
neo·nate
neo·na·tol·o·gist
neo·na·tol·o·gy
neo-ol·ive
neo·pal·li·um
neo·pha·sia
neo·pla·sia
    multiple endocrine n.
     (MEN)
neo·plasm
    benign n.
    histoid n.
    malignant n.
    metastatic n.
    organoid n.
    trophoblastic n.
neo·plas·tic
ne·o·plas·ti·gen·ic
Ne·op·syl·la
neo·quas·sin
Neo·rick·ett·sia
Neo·schoen·gas·tia
    N. americana
neo·sti·bo·san
neo·stig·mine
    n. bromide
    n. methylsulfate
ne·os·to·my
neo·stri·a·tum
neo·stro·phin·gic
Neo-Sy·neph·rine
ne·ot·e·ny
neo·thal·a·mus
neo·thyl·line
Ne·ot·o·ma

Ne·ot·o·ma
    N. lepida
neo·tri·zine
neo·type
neo·vas·cu·lar
neo·vas·cu·lar·iza·tion
ne·pen·thic
Nep·e·ta
nep·e·ta·lac·tone
neph·e·lom·e·ter
    photoelectric n.
neph·e·lom·e·try
neph·rad·e·no·ma
ne·phral·gia
ne·phral·gic
Neph·ra·mine
neph·ra·pos·ta·sis
neph·ra·ton·ia
neph·rauxe
neph·rec·ta·sia
ne·phrec·ta·sis
ne·phrec·ta·sy
ne·phrec·to·mize
ne·phrec·to·my
    abdominal n.
    anterior n.
    lumbar n.
    paraperitoneal n.
    posterior n.
    radical n.
    simple n.
    transthoracic n.
neph·re·de·ma
neph·rel·co·sis
ne·phre·mia
neph·ric
ne·phrid·i·um
ne·phrit·ic
ne·phrit·i·des
ne·phri·tis *pl.* ne·phrit·i·des
    acute n.
    acute focal n.
    acute serum sickness n.
    allergic n.
    anaphylactoid purpura n.
    antiglomerular basement
     membrane antibody n.
    arteriosclerotic n.

ne·phri·tis *(continued)*
  azotemic n.
  bacterial n.
  Balkan n.
  capsular n.
  n. caseosa
  caseous n.
  cheesy n.
  chloro-azotemic n.
  chronic n.
  chronic interstitial n.
  congenital n.
  croupous n.
  degenerative n.
  diffuse suppurative n.
  n. dolorosa
  dropsical n.
  embolic n.
  epidemic n.
  exudative n.
  familial hemorrhagic n.
  fibrolipomatous n.
  fibrous n.
  focal embolic n.
  glomerular n.
  glomerulocapsular n.
  n. gravidarum
  hemorrhagic n.
  hereditary n.
  Heymann's n.
  hydremic n.
  hydropigenous n.
  indurative n.
  interstitial n.
  interstitial granulomatous
    n.
  interstitial nonsuppurative
    n.
  interstitial scarlatinal n.
  interstitial syphilitic n.
  Lancereaux's n.
  latent n.
  leptospiral n.
  Löhlein's n.
  lipomatous n.
  lupus n.
  Masugi n.
  nephrotoxic serum n.

ne·phri·tis *(continued)*
  parenchymatous n.
  parenchymatous n.,
    chronic
  pneumococcus n.
  post-streptococcal n.
  potassium-losing n.
  n. of pregnancy
  productive n.
  radiation n.
  n. repens
  salt-losing n.
  saturnine n.
  scarlatinal n.
  Schönlein-Henoch purpura
    n.
  shunt n.
  Steblay n.
  subacute n.
  suppurative n.
  suppurative cortical n.
  syphilitic n.
  transfusion n.
  tubal n.
  tubular n.
  tuberculous n.
  tubulointerstitial n.
  vascular n.
  water-losing n.
ne·phrit·o·gen·ic
neph·ro·ab·dom·i·nal
neph·ro·an·gio·scle·ro·sis
neph·ro·blas·to·ma
neph·ro·cal·ci·no·sis
neph·ro·cap·sec·to·my
neph·ro·cap·su·lec·to·my
neph·ro·cap·su·lot·o·my
neph·ro·car·di·ac
neph·ro·cele
neph·ro·col·ic
neph·ro·col·o·pexy
neph·ro·co·lop·to·sis
neph·ro·cyst·anas·to·mo·sis
neph·ro·cys·ti·tis
neph·ro·cys·to·sis
neph·ro·er·y·sip·e·las
neph·ro·gas·tric
neph·ro·gen·e·sis

neph·ro·gen·ic
ne·phrog·e·nous
neph·ro·gram
ne·phrog·ra·phy
    isotope n.
neph·ro·he·mia
neph·ro·hy·dro·sis
neph·ro·hy·per·tro·phy
neph·roid
neph·ro·lith
neph·ro·li·thi·a·sis
    uric acid n.
neph·ro·li·thot·o·my
neph·ro·log·ic
ne·phrol·o·gist
ne·phrol·o·gy
ne·phrol·y·sis
neph·ro·lyt·ic
ne·phro·ma
    embryonal n.
    malignant n.
    mesoblastic n.
    multilocular cystic n.
neph·ro·ma·la·cia
neph·ro·meg·a·ly
neph·ro·mere
neph·ron
    lower n.
neph·ron·cus
neph·ron·oph·thi·sis
    familial juvenile n.
neph·ro-omen·to·pexy
neph·ro·path·ia
    n. epidermica
neph·ro·path·ic
ne·phrop·a·thy
    acute hypokalemic n.
    acute urate n.
    amphotericin B n.
    analgesic n.
    Balkan n.
    chronic hypokalemic n.
    diabetic n.
    dropsical n.
    epidemic n.
    familial n.
    gouty n.
    hypazoturic n.

ne·phrop·a·thy *(continued)*
    hypercalcemic n.
    hypochloruric n.
    hypokalemic n.
    IgA n.
    kaliopenic n.
    kanamycin n.
    malarial n.
    membranous n.
    mesangial n.
    obstructive n.
    oxalate n.
    phenacetin n.
    polymyxin n.
    potassium-losing n.
    reflux n.
    salt-losing n.
    streptomycin n.
    sulfonamide n.
    thin-basement-membrane
      n.
    toxic n.
    tubular n.
    urate n.
    vascular n.
neph·ro·pexy
neph·ro·pha·gi·a·sis
ne·phroph·thi·sis
neph·ro·poi·et·ic
neph·rop·to·sis
neph·ro·py·eli·tis
neph·ro·py·elog·ra·phy
neph·ro·py·elo·li·thot·o·my
neph·ro·py·elo·plas·ty
neph·ro·py·o·sis
neph·ror·rha·gia
neph·ror·rha·phy
neph·ro·scle·ria
neph·ro·scle·ro·sis
    arterial n.
    arteriolar n.
    benign n.
    congenital n.
    hyaline arteriolar n.
    hyperplastic arteriolar n.
    intercapillary n.
    malignant n.
    senile n.

neph·ro·scle·rot·ic
neph·ro·scope
neph·ros·co·py
ne·phro·ses
ne·phro·sis *pl.* ne·phro·ses
   acute n.
   amyloid n.
   avian n.
   cholemic n.
   chronic n.
   congenital n.
   Epstein's n.
   glycogen n.
   Haymann's n.
   hydropic n.
   hypokalemic n.
   infectious avian n.
   larval n.
   lipid n.
   lipoid n.
   lower nephron n.
   mercurial n.
   necrotizing n.
   osmotic n.
   pure n.
   toxic n.
   vacuolar n.
neph·ro·so·ne·phri·tis
   hemorrhagic n.
   Korean hemorrhagic n.
neph·ro·so·nog·ra·phy
neph·ro·spas·is
neph·ro·sple·no·pexy
neph·ros·to·gram
neph·ro·sto·li·thot·o·my
   percutaneous n. (PCNL)
ne·phros·to·ma
neph·ro·stome
ne·phros·to·my
   percutaneous n.
ne·phrot·ic
neph·ro·tome
neph·ro·to·mo·gram
neph·ro·to·mog·ra·phy
ne·phrot·o·my
   abdominal n.
   anatrophic n.
   lumbar n.

neph·ro·tox·ic
neph·ro·tox·ic·i·ty
   salicylate n.
neph·ro·tox·in
neph·ro·troph·ic
neph·ro·trop·ic
neph·ro·tu·ber·cu·lo·sis
neph·ro·ure·ter·ec·to·my
neph·ro·ure·tero·cys·tec·to·my
neph·ry·dro·sis
neph·ry·drot·ic
Nep·ta·zane
nep·tu·ni·um
ne·quin·ate
Neri sign
Ne·ri·um
Nernst equation
Nernst potential
ne·rol
ner·o·li
nerve
   abducent n.
   accelerator n's
   accessory n.
   accessory n., spinal
   accessory n., vagal
   acoustic n.
   adrenergic n.
   afferent n.
   alveolar n.
   ampullar n.
   anabolic n.
   anal n's, inferior
   Andersch's n.
   anococcygeal n's
   anterior crural n.
   anterior vagal n.
   aortic n.
   Arnold's n.
   articular n.
   auditory n.
   augmentor n's
   auricular n's
   auriculotemporal n.
   autonomic n.
   axillary n.
   Bell's n.

nerve *(continued)*
    Bock's n.
    buccal n.
    buccinator n.
    cardiac n.
    caroticotympanic n's
    carotid n's
    cavernous n's of clitoris
    cavernous n's of penis
    celiac n's
    centrifugal n.
    centripetal n.
    cerebral n's
    cervical n's
    cholinergic n's
    chorda tympani n.
    ciliary n's, long
    ciliary n's, short
    circumflex n.
    circumflex humeral n.
    clunial n's
    coccygeal n.
    cochlear n.
    n. of Cotunnius
    cranial n's (I-XII)
    crotaphitic n.
    cubital n.
    cutaneous n.
    Cyon's n.
    dental n., inferior
    depressor n.
    descending diaphragmatic
      n.
    diaphragmatic n.
    digastric n.
    digital n's
    dorsal n. of clitoris
    dorsal n. of penis
    dorsal n. of scapula
    efferent n.
    encephalic n's
    esodic n.
    ethmoidal n., anterior
    ethmoidal n., posterior
    exciter n.
    excitoreflex n.
    exodic n.

nerve *(continued)*
    n. of external acoustic
      meatus
    external respiratory n. of
      Bell
    facial n.
    facial n., temporal
    femoral n.
    fibular n., common
    fibular n., deep
    fibular n., superficial
    frontal n.
    furcal n.
    fusimotor n's
    Galen's n.
    gangliated n.
    gastric n's
    genitofemoral n.
    glossopalatine n.
    glossopharyngeal n.
    gluteal n's
    great sciatic n.
    hemorrhoidal n's, inferior
    Hering's n.
    hypogastric n.
    hypoglossal n.
    iliohypogastric n.
    ilioinguinal n.
    infraoccipital n.
    infraorbital n.
    infratrochlear n.
    inhibitory n.
    intercostal n's
    intercostobrachial n's
    intermediary n.
    intermediate n.
    interosseous n.
    ischiadic n.
    Jacobson's n.
    jugular n.
    labial n's, anterior
    labial n's, posterior
    lacrimal n.
    n's of Lancisi
    Langley's n's
    laryngeal n., inferior
    laryngeal n., recurrent
    laryngeal n., superior

nerve *(continued)*
  laryngeal n., superior,
    internal
  Latarjet's n.
  lingual n.
  longitudinal n's of Lancisi
  Ludwig's n.
  lumbar n's
  lumboinguinal n.
  n. of Luschka
  mandibular n.
  masseteric n.
  maxillary n.
  median n.
  medullated n.
  meningeal n.
  mental n.
  mixed n.
  motor n.
  motor n. of tongue
  musculocutaneous n.
  musculospiral n.
  myelinated n.
  mylohyoid n.
  nasociliary n.
  nasopalatine n.
  nonmedullated n.
  obturator n.
  occipital n., least
  occipital n., lesser
  occipital n., third
  oculomotor n.
  olfactory n's
  ophthalmic n.
  optic n.
  pain n.
  palatine n's
  parasympathetic n.
  parotid n's
  pectoral n., lateral
  pectoral n., medial
  perineal n's
  peripheral n.
  peroneal n.
  petrosal n.
  phrenic n.
  phrenicoabdominal n's
  pilomotor n's

nerve *(continued)*
  piriform n.
  plantar n.
  pneumogastric n.
  popliteal n.
  post-trematic n.
  presacral n.
  pressor n.
  pretrematic n.
  pterygoid n.
  n. of pterygoid canal
  pterygopalatine n's,
  pudendal n.
  pudic n.
  n. of quadrate muscle of
    thigh
  radial n.
  rectal n's, inferior
  recurrent n.
  renal n.
  saccular n.
  sacral n's
  saphenous n.
  Scarpa's n.
  sciatic n.
  sciatic n., small
  scrotal n's
  secretomotor n's
  secretory n.
  segmental n.
  sensorimotor n.
  sensory n.
  seventh n.
  sinus n.
  sinu-vertebral n.
  Soemmering's n.
  somatic n's
  somitic n.
  spermatic n., external
  spinal n's
  Spitz n.
  splanchnic n's
  stapedial n.
  stapedius n.
  stylohyoid n.
  stylopharyngeal n.
  subclavian n.
  subcostal n.

nerve *(continued)*
    subcutaneous temporal n's
    sublingual n.
    submaxillary n's
    suboccipital n.
    subscapular n's
    sudomotor n's
    supraclavicular n's
    supraorbital n.
    suprascapular n.
    supratrochlear n.
    sural n.
    sympathetic n.
    temporal n's, deep
    temporal n's, subcutaneous
    n. of tensor tympani
    n. of tensor veli palatini
    tenth n.
    tentorial n.
    terminal n's
    third n.
    thoracic n's
    thoracodorsal n.
    tibial n.
    Tiedemann's n.
    tonsillar n's
    transverse n. of neck
    trifacial n.
    trigeminal n.
    trochlear n.
    trophic n.
    tympanic n.
    ulnar n.
    ulnar collateral n. of
      Krause
    unmyelinated n.
    uterine n's
    utricular n.
    utriculoampullar n.
    vaginal n's
    vagus n.
    vascular n's
    vasoconstrictor n.
    vasodilator n.
    vasomotor n.
    vasosensory n.
    vertebral n.
    vestibular n.

nerve *(continued)*
    vestibulocochlear n.
    vidian n.
    visceral n.
    volar interosseous n.
    n. of Willis
    Wrisberg's n.
    zygomatic n.
    zygomaticofacial n.
    zygomaticotemporal n.
ner·vi
ner·vi·mo·til·i·ty
ner·vi·mo·tion
ner·vi·mo·tor
ner·vi·mus·cu·lar
ner·vo·mus·cu·lar
ner·vone
ner·von·ic acid
ner·vous
ner·vous break·down
ner·vous·ness
ner·vous sys·tem
ner·vus *pl.* ner·vi
    n. abducens
    n. accessorius
    n. acusticus
    n. buccalis
    n. celiaci
    nervi cerebrales
    nervi cervicales
    nervi ciliares breves
    nervi ciliares longi
    n. coccygeus
    n. cutaneus
    n. dorsalis clitoridis
    n. dorsalis penis
    n. dorsalis scapulae
    n. facialis
    n. femoralis
    n. glossopharyngeus
    n. gluteus inferior
    n. gluteus superior
    n. hypoglossus
    n. intermedius
    n. ischiadicus
    n. jugularis
    n. lacrimalis
    nervi lumbales

ner·vus *(continued)*
    n. medianus
    n. pudendus
    n. quadratus femoris
    n. radialis
    n. recurrens
    n. tensoris tympani
    n. tensoris veli palatini
    n. transversus colli
    nervi vasorum
Nes·a·caine
ne·sid·i·ec·to·my
ne·sid·io·blast
ne·sid·io·blas·to·ma
    malignant n.
ne·sid·io·blas·to·sis
Ness·ler's reagent
Ness·ler's solution
Ness·ler's test
ness·ler·iza·tion
ness·ler·ize
nest
    birds' n's
    Brunn's epithelial n's
    cancer n's
    cell n.
    swallow's n.
    Walthard's cell n's
    Walthard cell n's
nes·ti·os·to·my
net
    achromatic n.
    Chiari's n.
    chromidial n.
    nerve n.
    Trolard's n.
neth·a·lide
Neth·er·ton's syndrome
net·il·mi·cin sul·fate
net·tle
Net·tle·ship-Falls type ocular
   albinism
net·work
    acromial n.
    arterial n.
    calcanean n.
    cell n.
    Chiari's n.

net·work *(continued)*
    Gerlach's n.
    n. of Gesvelst
    idiotype–anti-idiotype n.
    lateral malleolar n.
    medial malleolar n.
    neurofibrillar n.
    peritarsal n.
    Purkinje's n.
    subpapillary n.
    trabecular n.
    venous n.
    weighting n.
Neu·bau·er's artery
Neu·bau·er-Fisch·er test
Neu·berg ester
Neu·feld nail
Neu·feld's reaction
Neu·feld's test
Neu·mann's cells
Neu·mann's law
Neu·mann's method
Neu·mann's sheath
neu·rag·mia
neu·ral
neu·ral·gia
    atypical facial n.
    auriculotemporal n.
    brachial n.
    cervical n.
    cervicobrachial n.
    ciliary n.
    cervico-occipital n.
    cranial n.
    n. facialis vera
    femoral n.
    Fothergill's n.
    geniculate n.
    glossopharyngeal n.
    hallucinatory n.
    Harris' migrainous n.
    herpetic n.
    Hunt's n.
    idiopathic n.
    intercostal n.
    mammary n.
    mandibular joint n.
    migrainous n.

neu·ral·gia *(continued)*
    Morton's n.
    nasociliary n.
    obturator n.
    otic n.
    Parsonage and Turner
      amyotrophic n.
    peripheral n.
    posterior auricular n.
    postherpetic n.
    pudendal plexus n.
    red n.
    reminiscent n.
    sciatic n.
    Sluder's n.
    sphenopalatine n.
    stump n.
    supraorbital n.
    symptomatic trigeminal n.
    trifacial n.
    trigeminal n.
    vidian n.
    Wartenberg's paresthetic
      n.
neu·ral·gic
neu·ral·gi·form
neu·ra·min·ic acid
neu·ra·min·i·dase
neu·rana·gen·e·sis
neur·an·gi·o·sis
neu·ra·poph·y·sis
neu·ra·prax·ia
neu·rar·chy
neu·rar·throp·a·thy
neu·ras·the·nia
neu·ra·tro·phia
neu·ra·troph·ic
neu·rat·ro·phy
neu·rax·i·al
neu·rax·is
neu·rec·ta·sia
neur·ec·to·derm
neu·rec·to·my
    gastric n.
    presacral n.
    retrogasserian n.
    tympanic n.
neu·rec·to·pia

neu·rec·to·py
neu·ren·ter·ic
neur·epi·the·li·al
neur·epi·the·li·um
neu·rer·gic
neur·ex·er·e·sis
neu·ri·a·try
neu·ri·ci·ty
neu·ri·dine
neu·ri·lem·ma
neu·ri·lem·mal
neu·ri·lem·mi·tis
neu·ri·lem·mo·sar·co·ma
neu·ri·le·mo·ma
    acoustic n.
    malignant n.
neu·ril·i·ty
neu·ri·mo·til·i·ty
neu·ri·mo·tor
neu·rine
neu·ri·no·ma
    acoustic n.
    malignant n.
neu·rit·ic
neu·ri·tis
    adventitial n.
    alcoholic n.
    amyloid n.
    arsenical n.
    ascending n.
    brachial n.
    central n.
    compression n.
    degenerative n.
    descending n.
    dietetic n.
    diphtheric n.
    disseminated n.
    endemic n.
    fallopian n.
    femoral n.
    Gombault's n.
    influenzal n.
    interstitial n.
    interstitial hypertrophic n.
    intraocular n.
    ischemic n.
    jake n.

neu·ri·tis *(continued)*
    latent n.
    lead n.
    leprous n.
    malarial n.
    malarial multiple n.
    n. migrans
    migrating n.
    multiple n.
    n. multiplex endemica
    n. nodosa
    optic n.
    orbital optic n.
    paralytic brachial n.
    parenchymatous n.
    periaxial n.
    peripheral n.
    porphyric n.
    postfebrile n.
    postocular n.
    pressure n.
    n. puerperalis traumatica
    radiation n.
    radicular n.
    retrobulbar n.
    rheumatic n.
    n. saturnina
    sciatic n.
    segmental n.
    senile n.
    serum n.
    shoulder-girdle n.
    syphilitic n.
    tabetic n.
    toxic n.
    traumatic n.
neu·ro·al·ler·gy
neu·ro·am·e·bi·a·sis
neu·ro·anas·to·mo·sis
neu·ro·anat·o·my
neu·ro·ar·throp·a·thy
neu·ro·as·tro·cy·to·ma
neu·ro·avi·ta·min·o·sis
neu·ro·be·hav·ior·al
neu·ro·bi·ol·o·gist
neu·ro·bi·ol·o·gy
neu·ro·bio·tax·is
neu·ro·blast

neu·ro·blast
    sympathetic n.
neu·ro·blas·to·ma
    olfactory n.
    Pepper type n.
neu·ro·ca·nal
neu·ro·car·di·ac
neu·ro·cen·tral
neu·ro·cen·trum
neu·ro·cep·tor
neu·ro·chem·is·try
neu·ro·chi·tin
neu·ro·chon·drite
neu·ro·cho·rio·ret·i·ni·tis
neu·ro·cho·roi·di·tis
neu·ro·cir·cu·la·to·ry
neu·roc·la·dism
neu·ro·clon·ic
neu·ro·com·mu·ni·ca·tions
neu·ro·cra·ni·al
neu·ro·cra·ni·um
neu·ro·crine
neu·ro·crin·ia
neu·ro·cris·top·a·thy
neu·ro·cu·ta·ne·ous
neu·ro·cyte
neu·ro·cy·tol·o·gy
neu·ro·cy·tol·y·sin
neu·ro·cy·tol·y·sis
neu·ro·cy·to·ma
    olfactory n.
neu·ro·de·al·gia
neu·ro·de·atro·phia
neu·ro·de·gen·er·a·tive
neu·ro·den·drite
neu·ro·den·dron
neu·ro·derm
neu·ro·der·ma·ti·tis
    circumscribed n.
    disseminated n.
    exudative n.
    localized n.
    nummular n.
neu·ro·der·ma·to·myo·si·tis
neu·ro·di·ag·no·sis
neu·ro·din
neu·ro·dyn·ia
neu·ro·ec·to·derm

neu·ro·ec·to·der·mal
neu·ro·ef·fec·tor
neu·ro·elec·tric·i·ty
neu·ro·en·ceph·a·lo·my·elop·a·thy
   optic n.
neu·ro·en·do·crine
neu·ro·en·do·cri·nol·o·gy
neu·ro·en·ter·ic
neu·ro·epi·der·mal
neu·ro·epi·the·li·al
neu·ro·epi·the·li·o·ma
neu·ro·epi·the·li·um
   n. of ampullary crest
   n. cristae ampullaris
   n. of maculae
   n. macularum
neu·ro·fi·ber
   afferent n's
   association n's
   commissural n's
   efferent n's
   postganglionic n's
   preganglionic n's
   projection n's
   somatic n's
   tangential n's
   visceral n's
neu·ro·fi·bra *pl.* neu·ro·fi·brae
neu·ro·fi·bril
neu·ro·fi·bril·la *pl.* neu·ro·fi·bril·lae
neu·ro·fi·bril·lar
neu·ro·fi·bro·ma
   acoustic n.
   dumbbell n.
   n. gangliocellulare
   n. ganglionare
   granular cell n.
   malignant n.
   symmetrical bundle n's
neu·ro·fi·bro·ma·to·sis
neu·ro·fi·bro·myx·o·ma
neu·ro·fi·bro·sar·co·ma
neu·ro·fil·a·ment
neu·ro·gan·gli·itis
neu·ro·gan·gli·o·ma

neu·ro·gan·gli·on
neu·ro·gan·gli·on·itis
neu·ro·gas·tric
neu·ro·gen
neu·ro·gen·e·sis
neu·ro·ge·net·ic
neu·ro·gen·ic
neu·rog·e·nous
neu·rog·lia
   interfascicular n.
   peripheral n.
   protoplasmic n.
neu·rog·li·al
neu·rog·li·ar
neu·ro·glio·cyte
neu·ro·glio·cy·to·ma
neu·ro·gli·o·ma
   n. ganglionare
neu·ro·gli·o·ma·to·sis
neu·ro·gli·o·sis
neu·ro·gly·co·pe·nia
neu·ro·gram
neu·rog·ra·phy
neu·ro·he·mal
neu·ro·his·tol·o·gy
neu·ro·hor·mo·nal
neu·ro·hor·mone
neu·ro·hu·mor
neu·ro·hu·mor·al
neu·ro·hu·mor·al·ism
neu·ro·hy·po·phys·e·al
neu·ro·hy·po·phys·ec·to·my
neu·ro·hy·po·phys·i·al
neu·ro·hy·poph·y·sis
neu·roid
neu·ro·im·mu·no·log·ic
neu·ro·im·mu·nol·o·gy
neu·ro·ker·a·tin
neu·ro·lab·y·rin·thi·tis
neu·ro·lath·y·rism
neu·ro·lem·ma
neu·ro·lem·mi·tis
neu·ro·lem·mo·ma
neu·ro·lep·tan·al·ge·sia
neu·ro·lep·tan·al·ge·sic
neu·ro·lep·tan·es·the·sia
neu·ro·lep·tan·es·thet·ic
neu·ro·lep·tic

neu·ro·li·po·ma·to·sis
   n. dolorosa
neu·ro·lo·gia
neu·ro·log·ic
neu·rol·o·gist
neu·rol·o·gy
   clinical n.
neu·ro·lymph
neu·ro·lym·pho·ma·to·sis
   n. gallinarum
neu·rol·y·sin
neu·rol·y·sis
neu·ro·lyt·ic
neu·ro·ma
   acoustic n.
   amputation n.
   amyelinic n.
   appendiceal n.
   n. cutis
   cystic n.
   false n.
   fascicular n.
   medullated n.
   ganglionar n.
   ganglionated n.
   ganglionic n.
   malignant n.
   Morton's n.
   multiple n.
   myelinic n.
   nevoid n.
   plexiform n.
   post-traumatic n.
   n. telangiectodes
   traumatic n.
   true n.
   Verneuil's n.
   n. verum
neu·ro·ma·la·cia
neu·ro·ma·to·sis
neu·rom·a·tous
neu·ro·mech·a·nism
neu·ro·mel·a·nin
neu·ro·men·in·ge·al
neu·ro·mere
neu·ro·mi·me·sis
neu·ro·mi·met·ic
neu·ro·mit·tor

neu·ro·mod·u·la·tion
neu·ro·mod·u·la·tor
neu·ro·mo·tor
neu·ro·mus·cu·lar
neu·ro·my·al
neu·ro·my·as·the·nia
neu·ro·my·eli·tis
   n. hyperalbuminotica
   n. optica
neu·ro·my·ic
neu·ro·myo·car·di·um
neu·ro·myo·path·ic
neu·ro·my·op·a·thy
   carcinomatous n.
neu·ro·myo·si·tis
neu·ro·myo·to·nia
neu·ron
   afferent n.
   alpha motor n.
   bipolar n.
   central n.
   connector n.
   correlation n.
   effector n.
   efferent n.
   exciter n.
   first-order n.
   gamma motor n.
   Golgi type I n's
   Golgi type II n's
   horizontal n's
   intercalary n.
   internuncial n.
   long n.
   Martinotti n.
   motor n.
   multiform n.
   multipolar n.
   peripheral motor n.
   peripheral sensory n.
   phasic motor n.
   polymorphic n.
   postganglionic n's
   preganglionic n's
   premotor n.
   primary n.
   primary sensory n.
   projection n.

neu·ron *(continued)*
    pseudounipolar n.
    pyramidal n.
    second-order n.
    sensory n.
    short n.
    superior motor n.
    tonic motor n.
    unipolar n.
    upper motor n.
neu·rona·gen·e·sis
neu·ro·nal
neu·rone
neu·ro·neph·ric
neu·ro·ne·vus
neu·ron·ic
neu·ro·ni·tis
    myoclonic spinal n.
    vestibular n.
neu·ron·og·ra·phy
    strychnine n.
neu·rono·phage
neu·rono·pha·gia
neu·ron·oph·a·gy
neu·ro·no·sis
neu·ro·no·trop·ic
neu·ron·y·my
neu·ro-oph·thal·mol·o·gy
neu·ro-otol·o·gy
neu·ro·pace·mak·er
neu·ro·pap·il·li·tis
neu·ro·para·site
neu·ro·path·ic
neu·ro·patho·gen·e·sis
neu·ro·patho·ge·nic·i·ty
neu·ro·pa·thol·o·gy
neu·rop·a·thy
    abetalipoproteinemic n.
    acrodystrophic n.
    acute autonomic n.
    alcoholic n.
    amyloid n.
    Andrade type amyloid n.
    ascending n.
    axonal n.
    carcinomatous n.
    Denny-Brown sensory n.
    descending n.

neu·rop·a·thy *(continued)*
    diabetic n.
    dying-back n.
    entrapment n.
    giant axonal n.
    glue-sniffers' n.
    hereditary hypertrophic
      interstitial n.
    hereditary sensorimotor n.
     (types I–III)
    hereditary sensory
      radicular n.
    hypertrophic n.
    Indiana type amyloid n.
    intercostal n.
    Iowa type amyloid n.
    ischemic n.
    isoniazid n.
    Jamaican n.
    lead n.
    myxedematous n.
    periaxial n.
    plexus n.
    Portugese type amyloid n.
    pressure n.
    progressive hypertrophic
      interstitial n.
    radiation n.
    segmental (demyelination)
     n.
    sensorimotor n.
    sensory n.
    serum n.
    serum sickness n.
    topical ataxic n.
    trigeminal n.
    triorthocresyl phosphate n.
    uremic n.
neu·ro·pep·tide
neu·ro·phage
neu·ro·phar·ma·co·log·i·cal
neu·ro·phar·ma·col·o·gy
neu·ro·phil
neu·ro·phil·ic
neu·ro·pho·nia
neu·ro·phre·nia
neu·roph·thal·mol·o·gy
neu·roph·thi·sis

neuropraxia

neu·ro·phy·sin
neu·ro·phys·i·ol·o·gy
neu·ro·pil
neu·ro·plasm
neu·ro·plas·mic
neu·ro·plas·ty
neu·ro·plex·us
neu·ro·po·dia
neu·ro·po·di·um *pl.* neu·ro·
   po·dia
neu·ro·pore
    anterior n.
    posterior n.
neu·ro·pro·ba·sia
neu·ro·pros·the·sis
neu·ro·psy·chi·a·trist
neu·ro·psy·chi·a·try
neu·ro·psy·chol·o·gy
neu·ro·psy·chop·a·thy
neu·ro·psy·cho·phar·ma·col·
   o·gy
neu·ro·ra·di·ol·o·gy
neu·ro·reg·u·la·tion
neu·ro·ret·i·ni·tis
neu·ro·ret·i·nop·a·thy
    hypertensive n.
neu·ro·roent·gen·og·ra·phy
neu·ror·rha·phy
neu·ro·sar·co·clei·sis
neu·ro·sar·co·ma
neu·ro·sci·ence
neu·ro·scle·ro·sis
neu·ro·se·cre·tion
neu·ro·se·cre·to·ry
neu·ro·seg·men·tal
neu·ro·sen·so·ry
neu·ro·ses
neu·ro·sis *pl.* neu·ro·ses
    actual n.
    anankastic n.
    anxiety n.
    artificial n.
    association n.
    cardiac n.
    character n.
    combat n.
    compensation n.
    compulsion n.

neu·ro·sis *(continued)*
    conversion n.
    defense n.
    depersonalization n.
    depressive n.
    expectation n.
    experimental n.
    fright n.
    housewife's n.
    hypochondriacal n.
    hysterical n.
    obsessional n.
    obsessive-compulsive n.
    occupational n.
    organ n.
    pension n.
    phobic n.
    phobic anxiety-deper-
      sonalization n.
    professional n.
    pseudoschizophrenic n.
    sphenopalatine ganglion n.
    substitution n.
    transference n.
    traumatic n.
    vagabond n.
    vegetative n.
    war n.
neu·ro·skel·e·tal
neu·ro·skel·e·ton
neu·ro·some
neu·ro·spasm
neu·ro·splanch·nic
neu·ro·spon·gi·o·ma
neu·ro·spon·gi·um
Neu·ros·po·ra
neu·ro·sta·tus
neu·ro·stim·u·la·tor
neu·ro·sur·geon
neu·ro·sur·gery
    functional n.
neu·ro·su·ture
neu·ro·syph·i·lid
neu·ro·syph·i·lis
    asymptomatic n.
    juvenile n.
    latent n.
    meningeal n.

neu·ro·syph·i·lis *(continued)*
    meningovascular n.
    parenchymatous s.
    paretic n.
    tabetic n.
neu·ro·ta·bes
neu·ro·tag·ma
neu·ro·ten·di·nous
neu·ro·ten·sin
neu·ro·ter·mi·nal
neu·ro·thele
neu·rot·ic
neu·rot·i·cism
neu·rot·i·gen·ic
neu·rot·iza·tion
neu·rot·me·sis
neu·ro·tol·o·gy
neu·ro·tome
neu·ro·to·mog·ra·phy
neu·rot·o·my
    radiofrequency n.
    retrogasserian n.
neu·rot·o·ny
neu·ro·tox·ic
neu·ro·tox·ic·i·ty
neu·ro·tox·in
neu·ro·trans·duc·er
neu·ro·trans·mis·sion
neu·ro·trans·mit·ter
    false n.
neu·ro·trau·ma
neu·ro·troph·ic
neu·rot·ro·phy
neu·ro·trop·ic
neu·rot·ro·pism
neu·rot·ro·py
neu·ro·tro·sis
neu·ro·tu·bule
neu·ro·vac·cine
neu·ro·var·i·co·sis
neu·ro·va·ri·o·la
neu·ro·vas·cu·lar
neu·ro·veg·e·ta·tive
neu·ro·vir·u·lence
neu·ro·vir·u·lent
neu·ro·vi·rus
neu·ro·vis·cer·al
neu·ru·la

neu·ru·la·tion
neu·rur·gic
Neus·ser's granules
neu·tral
neu·tral·ism
neu·tral·i·ty
neu·tral·iza·tion
    viral n.
neu·tral·ize
neu·tra·my·cin
Neu·tra·pen
Neu·tra-Phos-K
neu·tri·no
neu·tro·clu·sion
neu·tro·cyte
neu·tro·cy·to·pe·nia
neu·tro·cy·to·phil·ia
neu·tro·cy·to·sis
neu·tro·fla·vine
neu·tron
    epithermal n.
    fast n.
    intermediate n.
    slow n.
    thermal n.
neu·tron·ther·a·py
neu·tro·pe·nia
    chronic benign n. of
      childhood
    chronic hypoplastic n.
    congenital n.
    cyclic n.
    familial benign chronic n.
    hypersplenic n.
    idiopathic n.
    Kostmann n.
    malignant n.
    neonatal n., transitory
    periodic n.
    peripheral n.
    primary splenic n.
    toxic n.
    transitory neonatal n.
neu·tro·phil
    band n.
    filamented n.
    giant n.
    hypersegmented n.

neu·tro·phil *(continued)*
   immature n.
   juvenile n.
   mature n.
   nonfilamented n.
   rod n.
   segmented n.
   stab n.
neu·tro·phil·ia
neu·tro·phil·ic
neu·tro·pism
neu·tro·tax·is
ne·vi
Nev·ille prosthesis
ne·vo·blast
ne·vo·cyte
ne·vo·cyt·ic
ne·void
ne·vo·li·po·ma
ne·vo·xan·tho·en·do·the·li·o·ma
ne·vus *pl.* ne·vi
   achromic n.
   n. acneiformis unilateris
   amelanotic n.
   n. anemicus
   angiomatous n.
   n. arachnoideus
   n. araneosus
   n. araneus
   balloon cell n.
   basal cell n.
   bathing trunk n.
   Becker's n.
   blue n.
   blue rubber bleb n.
   capillary n.
   cellular n.
   cellular blue n.
   chromatophore n. of
     Naegeli
   comedo n.
   n. comedonicus
   compound n.
   connective tissue n.
   n. depigmentosus
   dermal n.
   dysplastic n.

ne·vus *(continued)*
   n. elasticus
   n. elasticus of
     Lewandowsky
   epidermal n.
   epithelial n.
   n. epitheliomato-
     cylindromatosus
   erectile n.
   fatty n.
   n. flammeus
   n. follicularis
   n. fragarius
   n. fuscoceruleus
     acromiodeltoideus
   n. fuscoceruleus
     ophthalmomaxillaris
   giant congenital pigmented
     n.
   giant hairy n.
   giant pigmented n.
   hair follicle n.
   halo n.
   hard n.
   honeycomb n.
   hepatic n.
   intradermal n.
   n. of Ito
   Jadassohn-Tièche n.
   junction n.
   junctional n.
   Lewandowsky n.
   n. lipomatodes superficialis
   n. lipomatosus
   l. lipomatosus cutaneus
     superficialis
   lymphatic n.
   n. maculosus
   malignant blue n.
   marginal n.
   melanocytic n.
   mixed n.
   n. molluscum
   n. morus
   multiplex n.
   neural n.
   neuroid n.
   n. nervosus

ne·vus *(continued)*
  nevocellular n.
  nevocytic n.
  nevus cell n.
  nodular connective tissue n.
  nonpigmented n.
  nuchal n.
  oral epithelial n.
  n. of Ota
  pigmented n.
  pigmented hairy epidermal n.
  n. pigmentosus
  n. pilosus
  plane n.
  port-wine n.
  n. profundus
  raspberry n.
  sebaceous n.
  n. sebaceus of Jadassohn
  segmental n.
  soft n.
  spider n.
  n. spilus
  n. spilus tardus
  spindle and epithelioid cell n.
  Spitz n.
  n. spongiosus albus mucosae
  stellar n.
  straight hair n.
  strawberry n.
  subcutaneous n.
  Sutton's n.
  n. syringocystadenosus papilliferus
  n. tardus
  n. unilateralis comedonicus
  n. unius lateris
  Unna's n.
  vascular n.
  n. vascularis
  n. vascularis fungosus
  n. vasculosus
  n. venosus
  venous n.

ne·vus *(continued)*
  verrucous n.
  white sponge n.
  zoniform n.
new·born
New·cas·tle disease
New·ton's law
New·ton's rings
new·ton
new·ton-me·ter
nex·er·i·dine hy·dro·chlo·ride
nex·in
nex·us *pl.* nex·us
Ney·man's bias
Nez·lof's syndrome
NF — National Formulary
NFLPN — National Federation of Licensed Practical Nurses
ng — nanogram
NGF — nerve growth factor
ngm — nanogram
NHC — National Health Council
  neonatal hypocalcemia
NHL — non-Hodgkin's lymphoma
NHLI — National Heart and Lung Institute
NHMRC — National Health and Medical Research Council
NHS — National Health Service (British)
NH₂-ter·mi·nal
ni·a·cin
ni·a·cin·amide
ni·a·cin·am·i·do·sis
NIAID — National Institute of Allergy and Infectious Diseases
ni·al·amide
NIAMD — National Institute of Arthritis and Metabolic Diseases
Ni·a·mid
nib
ni·brox·ane

Nic·a·lex
ni·car·di·pine
ni·cer·go·line
niche
    Barclay's n.
    ecologic n.
    enamel n.
    Haudek's n.
    n. of round window
NICHHD — National
  Institute of Child Health and
  Human Development
Nich·ol procedure
nick·el
    n. carbonyl
nick·ing
    AV n.
nick·krampf
ni·clo·sa·mide
Nic·ol prism
Ni·co·la·do·ni's sign
Nic·o·las-Fa·vre disease
Ni·coll bone graft
Ni·colle, Charles Jules Henri
Ni·co·nyl
Nic·o·rette
Nic·o·ti·a·na
nic·o·tin·a·mide
    n. adenine dinucleotide
      (NAD)
    n. adenine dinucleotide
      phosphate (NADP)
    n. mononucleotide (NMN)
nic·o·tine
    n. polacrilex
nic·o·tin·ic
nic·o·tin·ic acid
nic·o·tin·ism
nic·o·tino·lyt·ic
nico·tin·uric acid
β-nic·o·ty·rine
ni·cou·ma·lone
Nic·o·zide
nic·ta·tio spas·ti·ca
nic·ta·tion
nic·ti·tate
nic·ti·ta·tion

NIDA — National Institute on
  Drug Abuse
ni·dal
ni·da·tion
NIDD — non–insulin-dependen-
  t diabetes
NIDDM — non-insulin-depende-
  nt diabetes mellitus
NIDR — National Institute of
  Dental Research
ni·dus *pl.* ni·di
    n. avis
    n. hirundinis
Nie·bau·er prosthesis
Niel·sen method
Nie·mann's disease
Nie·mann's splenomegaly
Nie·mann-Pick cells
Nie·mann-Pick disease
Nie·wen·glow·ski's ray
ni·fed·i·pine
ni·fun·gin
ni·fur·a·dene
ni·fur·al·de·zone
ni·fur·a·tel
ni·fur·a·trone
ni·fur·da·zil
ni·fur·i·mide
ni·fur·mer·one
ni·fur·ox·ime
ni·fur·pir·i·nol
ni·fur·quin·a·zol
ni·fur·sem·i·zone
ni·fur·sol
ni·fur·ti·mox
night·mare
night·shade
    deadly n.
NIGMS — National Institute
  of General Medical Sciences
ni·gra
ni·gral
ni·gri·cans
ni·gri·ti·es
    n. linguae
ni·gro·sin
ni·gro·stri·a·tal

NIH — National Institutes of Health

ni·hil·ism

    therapeutic n.

ni·keth·a·mide

Ni·ki·for·off's method

Ni·kol·sky's sign

Ni·le·var

nim·a·zone

Ni·meh's method

NIMH — National Institute of Mental Health

nim·i·dane

nimo·di·pine

NINDB — National Institute of Neurological Diseases and Blindness

Nin·hy·drin

ni·o·bi·um

Ni·o·nate

NIOSH — National Institute of Occupational Safety and Health

ni·per·yt

nipha·blep·sia

nip·pers

nip·ple

    crackled n.

    crater n.

    herniated n.

    inverted n.

    retracted n.

Nip·po·stron·gy·lus

Nip·ride

Nir·en·berg, Marshall Warren

ni·rid·a·zole

nis·bu·te·rol mes·y·late

Ni·sen·til

ni·sin

ni·so·ba·mate

ni·sox·e·tine

Nis·sen operation

Nis·sl bodies

Nis·sl degeneration

Nis·sl granules

Nis·sl method of staining

Nis·sl substance

ni·ster·ime ac·e·tate

ni·sus

nit

Nit·a·buch's layer

Nit·a·buch'stria

Nit·a·buch's zone

ni·tar·sone

ni·ta·vi·rus

ni·thi·amide

ni·tram·ine

ni·tram·i·sole hy·dro·chlo·ride

ni·tra·tase

ni·trate

ni·trate re·duc·tase

ni·tra·ze·pam

ni·tre

    cubic n.

ni·tre·mia

ni·tric

ni·tric acid

ni·tri·da·tion

ni·tride

ni·tri·fi·ca·tion

ni·tri·fi·er

ni·tri·fy·ing

ni·trile

ni·trite

ni·tri·toid

ni·tri·tu·ria

ni·tro-amine

Ni·tro·bac·te·ra·ceae

ni·tro·bac·te·ria

ni·tro·bac·te·ri·um *pl.* ni·tro·bac·te·ria

ni·tro·ben·zene

ni·tro·ben·zol

ni·tro·blue te·tra·zo·li·um

ni·tro·cel·lu·lose

ni·tro·cy·cline

ni·tro·fu·ran

ni·tro·fu·ran·to·in

ni·tro·fu·ra·zone

ni·tro·gen

    amide n.

    blood urea n. (BUN)

    n. dioxide

    Kjeldahl n.

    n. monoxide

ni·tro·gen *(continued)*
    n. mustards
    nomadic n.
    nonprotein n.
    n. pentoxide
    n. peroxide
    rest n.
    n. tetroxide
    urea n.
ni·tro·gen·ase
ni·tro·gen-fix·ing
ni·trog·e·nous
ni·tro·glyc·er·in
Ni·tro·glyn
ni·tro·hy·dro·chlo·ric acid
Ni·trol
ni·tro·man·nite
ni·tro·mer·sol
ni·trom·e·ter
ni·tro·mi·fene cit·rate
ni·tro·naph·tha·lene
ni·tro·phe·nol
p-ni·tro·phen·yl phos·phate
ni·tro·pro·tein
ni·tro·prus·side
ni·tro·sac·cha·rose
ni·tros·amine
ni·tro·sate
ni·tro·sa·tion
ni·tro·scan·ate
ni·trose
ni·tro·si·fi·ca·tion
ni·tro·si·fy·ing
ni·tro·so·bac·te·ria
ni·tro·so·bac·te·ri·um *pl.* ni·tro·so·bac·te·ria
ni·tro·so·in·dol
ni·tro·so·sub·sti·tu·tion
ni·tro·so·urea
Ni·tro·stat
ni·tro·sug·ars
p-ni·tro·sul·fa·thi·a·zole
ni·tro·syl
ni·trous
    n. oxide
ni·trous acid
Ni·tro·vas
ni·tro·xan·thic acid

ni·trox·yl
ni·tryl
ni·va·zol
niv·e·my·cin
ni·vi·me·done so·di·um
nl — nanoliter
NLN — National League for Nursing
NLP — neurolinguistic programming
    no light perception
NM — neuromuscular
    nuclear medicine
Nm. — L. nux moschata (nutmeg)
nm — nanometer
NMA — National Medical Association
NMN — nicotinamide mononucleotide
NMR — nuclear magnetic resonance
NMRI — Naval Medical Research Institute
N-Mul·ti·stix
nn. — L. nervi (nerves)
NND — neonatal death
No. — L. numero (to the number of)
No·bel prize
no·be·li·um
No·ble's position
No·car·dia
    N. asteroides
    N. brasiliensis
    N. caviae
    N. coeliaca
    N. farcinica
    N. lutea
    N. madurae
    N. otitidis-caviarum
No·car·di·a·ceae
no·car·di·al
no·car·di·a·sis
no·car·din
No·car·di·op·sis
no·car·di·o·sis
    granulomatous n.

no·ci·as·so·ci·a·tion
no·ci·cep·tion
no·ci·cep·tive
no·ci·cep·tor
    polymodal n.
no·ci·fen·sor
no·ci-in·flu·ence
no·ci·per·cep·tion
no·co·da·zole
Noct. — L. nocte (at night)
noc·tal·bu·min·uria
noc·tam·bu·la·tion
noc·tam·bu·lic
Noc·tec
noc·ti·pho·bia
Noct. maneq. — L. nocte maneque (at night and in the morning)
noc·tu·ria
noc·tur·nal
noc·u·ous
    bishop's n.
no·dal
node
    abdominal lymph n's, parietal
    abdominal lymph n's, visceral
    anorectal lymph n's
    anterior cecal lymph n's
    anterior vesical lymph n's
    aortic lymph n's
    apical lymph n's
    appendicular lymph n's
    Aschoff's n.
    n. of Aschoff and Tawara
    atrioventricular n.
    Auerbach's n.
    AV n.
    axillary lymph n's
    Babès' n's
    biliary lymph n's
    Bouchard's n's
    brachial lymph n's
    bronchopulmonary lymph n's
    buccal lymph n.
    buccinator lymph n.

node *(continued)*
    caval lymph n's, lateral
    cecoappendicular lymph n's
    celiac lymph n's
    central lymph n's
    central superior n's
    cervical lymph n's, anterior
    cervical lymph n's, anterior superficial
    cervical lymph n's, deep anterior
    cervical lymph n's, deep lateral
    cervical lymph n's, prelaryngeal
    cervical lymph n's, superficial lateral
    Cloquet's n.
    colic lymph n's
    colic lymph n's, intermediate
    colic lymph n's, left
    colic lymph n's, middle
    colic lymph n's, right
    colic lymph n's, terminal
    coronary n.
    cubital lymph n's
    cystic n.
    Delphian n.
    deltoideopectoral n's
    diaphragmatic lymph n's
    Dürck's n's
    epicolic lymph n's
    epigastric lymph n's, inferior
    n. of epiploic foramen
    epitrochlear lymph n's
    Ewald's n.
    facial lymph n's
    femoral lymph n's
    Féréol's n's
    fibular n.
    Flack's n.
    foraminal n.
    gastric lymph n's, left
    gastric lymph n's, right

node *(continued)*

gastroepiploic lymph n's, left

gastroepiploic lymph n's, right

gastro-omental lymph n's, left

gastro-omental lymph n's, right

gluteal lymph n's, inferior

gluteal lymph n's, superior

gouty n.

Haygarth's n's

Heberden's n's

hemal n's

hemolymph n's

Hensen's n.

hepatic lymph n's

hilar lymph n's

His-Tawara n.

ileocolic lymph n's

iliac circumflex lymph n's

iliac lymph n's, circumflex

iliac lymph n's, common

iliac lymph n's, external

iliac lymph n's, intermediate common

iliac lymph n's, intermediate external

iliac lymph n's, internal

iliac lymph n's, lateral common

iliac lymph n's, lateral external

iliac lymph n's, medial common

iliac lymph n's, medial external

iliac lymph n's, promontory common

iliac lymph n's, subaortic common

infraclavicular n's

infraclavicular lymph n's

infrahyoid lymph n's

inguinal lymph n's, deep

inguinal lymph n's, inferior

node *(continued)*

inguinal lymph n's, superficial

inguinal lymph n's, superolateral

inguinal lymph n's, superomedial

intercostal lymph n's

interiliac lymph n's

internal thoracic lymph n's

interpectoral lymph n's

jugular lymph n's, anterior

jugular lymph n's, lateral

jugulodigastric lymph n.

jugulo-omohyoid lymph n.

juxta-articular n.

juxtaintestinal n's

Keith's n.

Keith-Flack n.

Koch's n.

lacunar n., intermediate

lacunar n., lateral

lacunar n., medial

n. of ligamentum arteriosum

lingual lymph n's

lumbar lymph n's

lumbar lymph n's, intermediate

lumbar lymph n's, left

lumbar lymph n's, right

lymph n.

malar lymph n.

mandibular lymph n.

mastoid lymph n's

mediastinal lymph n's, anterior

mediastinal lymph n's, posterior

mesenteric lymph n's

mesenteric lymph n's, inferior

mesenteric lymph n's, superior

mesocolic lymph n's

Meynet's n's

milker's n's

nasolabial lymph n.

node *(continued)*
n. of neck of gallbladder
obturator lymph n's
occipital lymph n's
Osler's n's
pancreatic lymph n's
pancreaticoduodenal
  lymph n's, inferior
pancreaticoduodenal
  lymph n's, superior
pancreaticolienal lymph
  n's
pancreaticosplenic lymph
  n's
paracardial lymph n's
paracolic lymph n's
paramammary lymph n's
pararectal lymph n's
parasternal lymph n's
paratracheal lymph n's
parauterine lymph n's
paravaginal lymph n's
paravesicular lymph n's
parotid lymph n's, deep
parotid lymph n's,
  infra-auricular deep
parotid lymph n's,
  intraglandular deep
parotid lymph n's,
  preauricular deep
parotid lymph n's,
  superficial
Parrot's n.
pectoral axillary n's
pectoral lymph n's
pelvic lymph n's, parietal
pelvic lymph n's, visceral
pericardial lymph n's,
  lateral
peritracheal lymph n's
peroneal n.
phrenic lymph n's, inferior
phrenic lymph n's,
  superior
popliteal lymph n's
popliteal lymph n's, deep
popliteal lymph n's,
  superficial

node *(continued)*
postaortic lymph n's
postcaval lymph n's
postvesicular lymph n's
preaortic lymph n's
preauricular lymph n's
pulmonary juxta-
  esophageal lymph n's
precaval lymph n's
prececal lymph n's
prelaryngeal n.
prepericardial lymph n's
pretracheal n.
pretracheal lymph n's
prevertebral lymph n's
prevesicular lymph n's
primitive n.
pulmonary
  juxtaesophageal lymph
  n's
pulmonary lymph n's
pyloric lymph n's
n's of Ranvier
rectal lymph n's, superior
retroaortic lymph n's
retroauricular lymph n's
retrocaval lymph n's
retrocecal lymph n's
retropharyngeal lymph n's
retropyloric n's
Rosenmüller's n.
Rotter's n's
n. of Rouvière
sacral lymph n's
Schmidt's n.
Schmorl's n.
sentinel n.
signal n.
shotty n.
sigmoid lymph n's
singer's n.
sinoatrial n.
sinus n.
Sister Mary Joseph n.
splenic lymph n's
sternal lymph n's
submandibular lymph n's
submental lymph n's

node *(continued)*
 subpyloric n's
 subscapular lymph n's
 supraclavicular lymph n's
 suprapyloric n.
 supratrochlear lymph n's
 syphilitic n.
 n. of Tawara
 teacher's n.
 thyroid lymph n's
 tibial n., anterior
 tibial n., posterior
 tracheal lymph n's
 tracheobronchial lymph
  n's, inferior
 tracheobronchial lymph
  n's, superior
 triticeous n.
 Troisier's n.
 Virchow's n.
 vesicular lymph n's, lateral
 vital n.
 vocal n's
no·di
no·dose
no·dos·i·ty
 Haygarth's n's
nod·u·lar
nod·u·lat·ed
nod·u·la·tion
nod·ule
 accessory thymic n's
 aggregate n's
 Albini's n's
 n's of aortic valve
 apple jelly n's
 n's of Arantius
 Aschoff's n's
 Babès' n's
 Bianchi's n's
 Bohn's n's
 Bouchard's n's
 Busacca n's
 Caplan's n's
 cold n.
 n. of cerebellum
 cortical n's
 Cruveilhier's n's

nod·ule *(continued)*
 Dalen-Fuchs n's
 enamel n.
 Fraenkel's n's
 Gamna n's
 Gandy-Gamna n's
 Hoboken's n's
 hot n.
 Jeanselme's n's
 juxta-articular n's
 n's of Kerckring
 Koeppe n's
 Koester's n.
 Leishman's n's
 lumbar-sacral n's
 Lutz-Jeanselme n's
 lymphatic n's
 lymphatic n's of stomach
 malpighian n.
 milkers' n's
 Morgagni's n's
 pearly n.
 periosteal n's
 primary n.
 pulmonary n's
 pulp n.
 rabic n's
 rheumatic n's
 Schmorl's n.
 secondary n.
 siderotic n's
 singers' n.
 Sister Joseph's n.
 splenic lymph n's
 subcutaneous n.
 surfers'n's
 n's tabac
 teachers' n.
 triticeous n.
 tubal lymphatic n's
 typhoid n.
 typhus n's
 n. of vermis
 vestigial n.
 vocal n.
 warm n.
nod·u·lous

nod·u·lus *pl.* nod·u·li
    n. cerebelli
    n. lymphaticus
    n. primarius
    noduli valvularum aortae
    noduli valvularum
      semilunarium
    noduli valvularum
      semilunarium [Arantii]
    n. vermis
no·dus *pl.* no·di
    n. atrioventricularis
    n. lymphaticus
    nodi sigmoidei
    n. sinuatrialis
    nodi subpylorici
    nodi superiores centrales
    n. suprapyloricus
    n. tibialis anterior
    n. tibialis posterior
no·e·ma·tacho·graph
no·e·ma·ta·chom·e·ter
no·e·mat·ic
no·e·sis
no·et·ic
    n. vital
No·gu·chi's reagent
No·gu·chi's test
noise
    transient n.
    white n.
no·lin·i·um bro·mide
no·ma
    n. vulvae
no·mad·ic
no·men·cla·ture
    binomial n.
no·mi·fen·sine mal·e·ate
No·mi·na An·a·tom·i·ca
no·mo·gen·e·sis
no·mo·gram
    blood volume n.
no·mo·graph
nomo·thet·ic
no·mo·top·ic
no·na
non·ac·cess
non·ad·her·ent

no·nan
non·an·ti·gen·ic
non·a·pep·tide
non·ar·tic·u·lar
non·cho·le·cys·to·ki·nin
non·chro·maf·fin
non·co·mi·tance
non·com·pli·ance
non com·pos men·tis
non·con·duc·tor
non·de·po·lar·iz·er
non·dis·junc·tion
non·elec·tro·lyte
non·en·cap·su·lat·ed
non·gran·u·lo·cyte
non·heme
non·ho·mo·ge·ne·i·ty
non·homo·logues
no·ni·grav·i·da
non·in·fec·tious
non·in·va·sive
non·in·vo·lu·tion
non·ion·ic
no·nip·a·ra
non·lam·el·lar
non·med·ul·lat·ed
non·met·al
non·my·eli·nat·ed
Non·ne's syndrome
Non·ne's test
Non·ne-Apelt phase
Non·ne-Apelt reaction
Non·ne-Apelt test
Non·ne-Mil·roy-Meige
    syndrome
non-neu·ro·nal
non-nu·cle·at·ed
non·oc·clu·sion
non·ol·i·gu·ric
non·on·co·gen·ic
non·opaque
non·ose
non·ovu·la·tory
no·nox·y·nol
    n. 9
non·para·met·ric
non·par·ous
non·pen·e·trant

non·per·mis·sive
non·pho·to·chro·mo·gen
non·po·lar
non repetat. — L. non
    repetatur (do not repeat)
non·ro·ta·tion
    n. of the intestine
non·se·cre·tor
non·self
non·sep·tate
non·spe·cif·ic
non·sur·gi·cal
non·tast·er
non·union
    established n.
non·va·lent
non·vi·a·ble
non·vis·u·al·iza·tion
no·nyl
Noo·nan's syndrome
Noor·den treatment
noo·trop·ic
no·pal·in G
NOPHN — National
    Organization for Public
    Health Nursing
nor·adren·a·line
nor·adren·er·gic
nor·an·dro·sten·o·lone
Nor·cu·ron
nor·def·rin hy·dro·chlo·ride
nor·epi·neph·rine
    n. bitartrate
nor·eth·an·dro·lone
nor·eth·in·drone
    n. acetate
nor·eth·is·ter·one
nor·ethy·no·drel
Nor·flex
nor·flox·a·cin
nor·flu·rane
nor·ges·ti·mate
nor·ges·to·met
nor·ges·trel
nor·hyo·scy·amine
Nor·iso·drine
Nor·land-Cam·er·on photon
    densitometry

nor·leu·cine
Nor·lu·tate
Nor·lu·tin
norm
nor·ma
    n. anterior
    n. basilaris
    n. facialis
    n. frontalis
    n. inferior
    n. lateralis
    n. occipitalis
    n. posterior
    n. sagittalis
    n. superior
    n. temporalis
    n. ventralis
    n. verticalis
nor·mal
nor·mal·i·ty
nor·mal·iza·tion
nor·mal·ize
Nor·man-Wood syndrome
nor·meta·neph·rine
nor·mo·blast
    acidophilic n.
    basophilic n.
    early n.
    eosinophilic n.
    intermediate n.
    late n.
    orthochromatic n.
    oxyphilic n.
    polychromatic n.
    polychromatophilic n.
nor·mo·blas·tic
nor·mo·blas·to·sis
nor·mo·cal·ce·mia
nor·mo·cal·ce·mic
nor·mo·cap·nia
nor·mo·cap·nic
nor·mo·cho·les·ter·ol·emia
nor·mo·cho·les·ter·ol·emic
nor·mo·chro·ma·sia
nor·mo·chro·mat·ic
nor·mo·chro·mia
nor·mo·chro·mic
nor·mo·crin·ic

nor·mo·cyte
nor·mo·cyt·ic
Nor·mo·cy·tin
nor·mo·cy·to·sis
Nor·mo·dyne
nor·mo·eryth·ro·cyte
nor·mo·gly·ce·mia
nor·mo·gly·ce·mic
nor·mo·ka·le·mia
nor·mo·ka·le·mic
nor·mo·re·flex·ia
nor·mo-or·tho·cy·to·sis
nor·mo·skeo·cy·to·sis
nor·mo·sper·mic
nor·mo·sthen·uria
nor·mo·ten·sion
nor·mo·ten·sive
nor·mo·ther·mia
nor·mo·ther·mic
nor·mo·to·nia
nor·mo·ton·ic
nor·mo·troph·ic
nor·mo·uri·ce·mia
nor·mo·uri·ce·mic
nor·mo·uri·cu·ria
nor·mo·uri·cu·ric
nor·mo·vo·le·mia
nor·mo·vo·le·mic
nor·nico·tine
Nor·o·din
Nor·pace
Nor·pram·in
nor·pseu·do·ephed·rine
Nor·rie's disease
Nor·ris' corpuscles
North·rop, John Howard
nor·trip·ty·line hy·dro·chlo·ride
nos·az·on·tol·o·gy
nos·ca·pine
   n. hydrochloride
nose
   cleft n.
   copper n.
   external n.
   familial hump n.
   potato n.
   rabbit n.

nose *(continued)*
   saddle n.
   saddle-back n.
   swayback n.
   strawberry n.
   Swedish n.
   telescope n.
   whiskey n.
nose·bleed
nose·gay
   Riolan's n.
No·se·ma
no·se·ma·to·sis
nos·en·ceph·a·lus
nose·piece
   quick-change n.
   rotating n.
nos·eti·ol·o·gy
no·si·hep·tide
nos·och·tho·nog·ra·phy
noso·co·mi·al
noso·gen·e·sis
nos·o·gen·ic
no·sog·e·ny
noso·ge·og·ra·phy
no·sog·ra·phy
noso·log·ic
no·sol·o·gy
   psychiatric n.
noso·ma·nia
no·som·e·try
noso·my·co·sis
no·son·o·my
noso·para·site
noso·phil·ia
noso·pho·bia
noso·phyte
noso·poi·et·ic
Noso·psyl·lus
   N. fasciatus
noso·taxy
noso·ther·a·py
noso·tox·ic
noso·tox·ic·i·ty
noso·tox·i·co·sis
noso·tox·in
no·sot·ro·phy
nos·o·trop·ic

nos·to·ma·nia
nos·trate
nos·tril
nos·trum
Nos·tyn
no·tal
no·tal·gia
    n. paresthetica
no·tan·ce·pha·lia
no·tan·en·ce·pha·lia
notch
    acetabular n.
    anacrotic n.
    angular n. of stomach
    antegonial n.
    anterior n. of ear
    aortic n.
    auricular n.
    cardiac n. of left lung
    cardiac n. of stomach
    catacrotic n.
    cerebellar n., anterior
    cerebellar n., posterior
    clavicular n. of sternum
    coracoid n.
    costal n's of sternum
    cotyloid n.
    craniofacial n.
    dicrotic n.
    digastric n.
    ethmoidal n. of frontal
      bone
    fibular n.
    fibular n. of tibia
    frontal n.
    n. of gallbladder
    gastric n.
    hamular n.
    Hutchinson's crescentic n.
    interarytenoid n.
    interclavicular n.
    intercondylar n. of femur
    interlobar n.
    intertragic n.
    intervertebral n.
    ischial n., greater
    ischial n., lesser
    jugular n. of occipital bone

notch (continued)
    jugular n. of sternum
    jugular n. of temporal bone
    Kernohan n.
    lacrimal n. of maxilla
    n. of ligamentum teres
    mandibular n.
    marsupial n.
    mastoid n.
    nasal n. of maxilla
    median prostatic n.
    palatine n.
    palatine n. of palatine bone
    pancreatic n.
    parietal n. of temporal
      bone
    parotid n.
    popliteal n.
    preoccipital n.
    presternal n.
    pterygoid n.
    radial n.
    rivinian n.
    n. of Rivinus
    sacrosciatic n., greater
    sacrosciatic n., lesser
    scapular n.
    sciatic n., greater
    sciatic n., lesser
    semilunar n. of mandible
    semilunar n. of scapula
    Sibson's n.
    sigmoid n.
    sphenopalatine n. of
      palatine bone
    spinoglenoid n.
    sternal n.
    supraorbital n.
    suprascapular n.
    suprasternal n.
    tentorial n.
    thyroid n., inferior
    thyroid n., superior
    trigeminal n.
    trochlear n. of ulna
    tympanic n.
    ulnar n.
    umbilical n.

notch *(continued)*
    vertebral n., inferior
    vertebral n., superior
note
    bell n.
    cracked-pot n.
    percussion n.
No·tech·is
no·ten·ceph·a·lo·cele
no·ten·ceph·a·lus
Noth·na·gel's bodies
Noth·na·gel's syndrome
Noth·na·gel's type
no·ti·fi·able
no·tif·i·ca·tion of birth
no·to·chord
no·to·chor·do·ma
No·to·ed·res
    N. cati
no·to·gen·e·sis
no·tom·e·lus
no·to·my·eli·tis
not-self
no·tum
nou·me·nal
No·val·din
no·vau·ran·tia
no·vo·bio·cin
    n. calcium
    n. sodium
No·vo·cain
no·vo·scope
Nov·rad
No·vy's rat disease
Novy, Mc·Neal, and Ni·colle
    culture medium
noxa *pl.* noxae
nox·ious
NPA — National Perinatal
    Association
NPH — neutral protamine
    Hagedorn (insulin)
        normal pressure
            hydrocephalus
NPN — nonprotein nitrogen
NPO — L. nil per os (nothing
    by mouth)

NRC — normal retinal
    correspondence
NREM — non-rapid eye
    movements
NS — normal saline
ns — nanosecond
    not significant
NSAIA — nonsteroidal
    antiinflammatory analgesic
NSAID — nonsteroidal
    antiinflammatory drug
nsec — nanosecond
NSHD — nodular sclerosing
    Hodgkin's disease
NSILA — nonsuppressible
    insulin-like activity
NSNA — National Student
    Nurse Association
NSR — normal sinus rhythm
NST — nonstress test
NSVD — normal spontaneous
    vaginal delivery
N-ter·min·al
NTP — normal temperature
    and pressure
nU — nanounit
nu·bec·u·la
nu·bil·i·ty
nu·cha
nu·chal
Nuck's canal
Nuck's diverticulum
Nuck's hydrocele
nu·cle·ar
nu·cle·ase
nu·cle·at·ed
nu·cle·a·tion
nu·clec·to·my
nu·clei
nu·cle·ic acid
    infectious n. a.
nu·cle·ide
nu·cle·i·form
nu·cle·in
nu·cle·in·ic acid
nu·cleo·cap·sid
nu·cleo·chy·le·ma
nu·cleo·chyme

nu·cleo·cy·to·plas·mic
nu·cle·of·u·gal
nu·cleo·glu·co·pro·tein
nu·cle·og·ra·phy
nu·cleo·his·tone
nu·cleo·hy·a·lo·plasm
nu·cle·oid
nu·cleo·ker·a·tin
nu·cle·o·lar
nu·cle·o·li
nu·cle·o·li·form
nu·cle·o·lin
nu·cle·o·li·nus
nu·cle·o·loid
nu·cle·ol·o·lus
nu·cleo·lo·ne·ma
nu·cleo·lo·neme
nu·cleo·lo·nu·cle·us
nu·cle·o·lus *pl.* nu·cle·o·li
    chromatin n.
    false n.
    nucleinic n.
    secondary n.
nu·cleo·lymph
nu·cleo·mi·cro·some
nu·cle·on
nu·cle·on·ic
nu·cle·on·ics
nu·cle·op·e·tal
nu·cleo·phago·cy·to·sis
nu·cleo·phile
nu·cleo·phil·ic
nu·cleo·phos·pha·tase
nu·cleo·plasm
nu·cleo·pro·tein
    deoxyribose n.
    ribose n.
nu·cleo·re·tic·u·lum
nu·cle·or·rhex·is
nu·cleo·si·dase
nu·cleo·side
nu·cleo·side de·am·i·nase
nu·cleo·side di·phos·phate
nu·cleo·side di·phos·phate ki·nase
nu·cleo·side mono·phos·phate ki·nase
nu·cleo·side phos·phate

nu·cle·o·side phos·phor·y·lase
nu·cleo·side tri·phos·phate
nu·cleo·side·di·phos·pha·tase
nu·cle·o·sis
nu·cleo·some
nu·cleo·spin·dle
nu·cleo·ti·dase
5′-nu·cle·o·ti·dase
nu·cleo·tide
    cyclic n's
nu·cleo·tide cy·clase
nu·cleo·tide pol·ym·er·ase
nu·cleo·tide py·ro·phos·pha·tase
nu·cleo·tid·yl
nu·cleo·tid·yl·exo·trans·fer·ase
nu·cleo·tid·yl·trans·fer·ase
nu·cleo·tox·in
nu·cleo·trop·ic
nu·cle·us *pl.* nu·clei
    n. abducens
    n. of abducens nerve
    n. accessorius
    accessory n.
    accessory oculomotor n.
    n. of accessory nerve
    n. accumbens septi
    acetabular n.
    acoustic nuclei
    n. alae cinereae
    ambiguous n.
    ambiguous n. of Quain
    n. ambiguus
    n. amygdalae
    n. amygdaliformis of J. Stilling
    amygdaloid n.
    n. angularis
    n. ansae lenticularis
    n. of ansa lenticularis
    anterior median n.
    anterior olfactory n.
    n. anterodorsalis
    n. anteromedialis
    n. anteroventralis
    n. arcuatus
    nuclei areae

nu·cle·us *(continued)*
atomic n.
auditory nuclei
nuclei of auditory nerve
auditory n., large cell
autonomic n.
n. autonomicus
Balbiani's n.
basal n.
n. basalis
basal nuclei
nuclei basales
Béclard's n.
basal olfactory n.
Bekhterev's n.
Blumenau's n.
n. of Burdach's column
n. caeruleus (ceruleus, coeruleus)
n. of caudal colliculus
caudal vestibular n.
n. caudalis centralis
caudate n.
n. caudatus
cell n.
central caudal n.
centrodorsal n.
n. of cerebellum, dentate
n. of cerebellum, medullary
cervical n.
cholane n.
Clarke's n.
Clarke-Monakow n.
cleavage n.
cochlear nuclei
nuclei cochleares
n. colliculi caudalis
n. colliculi inferioris
commissural n.
n. commissuralis
compact n.
conjugation n.
cortical n. of amygdala
nuclei of cranial nerves
cuneate n.
n. cuneatus
n. cuneatus accessorius
Darkshevich's n.

nu·cle·us *(continued)*
daughter n.
Deiters' n.
dental n.
dentate n.
n. dentatus
n. dentatus cerebelli
descending vestibular n.
diploid n.
dorsal n. (of Clarke)
n. dorsalis
dorsolateral n.
n. dorsolateralis
dorsomedial n.
n. dorsomedialis
droplet nuclei
drumstick n.
Duval's n.
Edinger's n.
Edinger-Westphal n.
emboliform n.
n. emboliformis cerebelli
end nuclei
entopeduncular n.
n. entopeduncularis
external cuneate n.
n. facialis
n. of facial nerve
fastigial n.
n. fastigii
fertilization n.
free n.
n. funiculi cuneati
n. funiculi gracilis
gametic n.
n. gelatinosus
geniculate n., lateral
geniculate n., medial
n. geniculatus lateralis
n. geniculatus medialis
germ n.
germinal n.
gingival n.
globose n.
n. globosus cerebelli
n. of Goll's column
gonad n.
n. gracilis

nu·cle·us *(continued)*
  gray n.
  n. of Gudden
  nuclei of habenula
  nuclei habenulae
  habenular nuclei
  haploid n.
  hypoglossal n.
  n. hypoglossalis
  hypothalamic nuclei
  n. of inferior colliculus
  infundibular n.
  n. infundibularis
  n. intercalatus
  intermediolateral n.
  n. intermediolateralis
  intermediomedial n.
  n. intermediomedialis
  n. of internal geniculate
    body
  interpeduncular n.
  n. interpeduncularis
  interstitial n.
  interstitial n. of Cajal
  n. interstitialis
  intracerebellar nuclei
  Kaiser's nuclei
  Kölliker's n.
  n. lacrimalis
  laryngeal n.
  n. of lateral geniculate
    body
  n. of lateral lemniscus
  n. lateralis of Le Gros
    Clark
  n. lemnisci lateralis
  n. of lens
  lenticular n.
  n. lenticularis
  n. lentiformis
  n. lentis
  n. of Luys
  n. magnocellularis
  magnocellular n.
  n. of medial geniculate
    body
  nuclei mediales thalami
  nuclei of median raphe

nu·cle·us *(continued)*
  nuclei mediani thalami
  n. mediodorsalis
  n. medullaris cerebelli
  metastable n.
  n. of Meynert
  Monakow's n.
  motor n.
  motor n. of trigeminal
    nerve
  n. motorius nervi trigemini
  n. motorius trigeminalis
  n. oculomotorius
  n. oculomotorius
    accessorius
  n. oculomotorius
    autonomicus
  oculomotor n.
  n. of olfactory tract
  n. olivaris
  n. olivaris accessorius
    dorsalis
  n. olivaris accessorius
    medialis
  n olivaris accessorius
    posterior
  n. olivaris caudalis
  n. olivaris cranialis
  n. olivaris inferior
  n. olivaris rostralis
  n. olivaris superior
  n. olivaris superioris
  olivary n.
  olivary n., caudal
  olivary n., inferior
  olivary n., medial accessory
  olivary n., posterior
    accessory
  olivary n., rostral
  olivary n., superior
  ootid n.
  nuclei of origin
  nuclei originis
  Pander's n.
  parabducent n.
  parabigeminal n.
  paramedian n., dorsal
  paramedian n., posterior

nu·cle·us *(continued)*
  paramedian reticular n.
  n. paramedianus dorsalis
  n. paramedianus posterior
  n. parasolitarius
  parasolitary n.
  nuclei parasympathici
    sacrales
  perihypoglossal n.
  n. periventricularis
    posterior
  Perlia's n.
  phenanthrene n.
  n. of phrenic nerve
  n. pigmentosus pontis
  polymorphic n.
  nuclei of pons
  pontine nuclei
  nuclei pontis
  pontine n. of trigeminal
    nerve
  n. pontinus nervi trigemini
  pontobulbar n.
  posterior periventricular n.
  nuclei posteriores thalami
  posteromarginal n.
  premamillary n.
  preolivary n.
  preoptic nuclei
  n. prepositus
  n. of prerubral field
  pretectal n.
  n. pretectalis
  n. proprius
  n. pulposus
  pulvinar n.
  nuclei pulvinares thalami
  pyknotic n.
  pyramidal n.
  rapheal nuclei
  red n.
  reproductive n.
  reticular n., lateral
  reticular n. of subthalamus
  reticular n. of thalamus
  n. reticularis tegmenti
  n. reticularis thalami
  reticulotegmental n.

nu·cle·us *(continued)*
  n. reuniens thalami
  n. rhomboidalis thalami
  Roller's n.
  roof nuclei
  n. of Rose
  n. ruber
  sacral parasympathetic
    nuclei
  n. salivatorius caudalis
  n. salivatorius cranialis
  n. salivatorius inferior
  n. salivatorius rostralis
  n. salivatorius superior
  salivatory n., caudal
  salivatory n., cranial
  salivatory n., inferior
  n. of Sappey
  Schwalbe's n.
  Schwann's n.
  secondary n.
  segmentation n.
  semilunar n.
  sensory n.
  septal n.
  Setchenow's (Sechenoff's)
    nuclei
  shadow n.
  Siemerling's n.
  n. solitarius
  solitary n.
  n. of solitary tract
  somatic n.
  sperm n.
  spherical n.
  spinal n.
  n. spinalis
  spinocerebellar n.
  Spitzka's n.
  Staderini's n.
  steroid n.
  Stilling's n.
  striate n.
  n. subcaeruleus
    (subceruleus,
    subcoeruleus)
  subependymal n.
  sublingual n.

nu·cle·us *(continued)*
  submedial n. of thalamus
  subthalamic n.
  n. subthalamicus
  superior n.
  n. of superior olive
  suprachiasmatic n.
  suprageniculate n.
  supramamillary n.
  n. supraopticus
    hypothalami
  supraspinal n.
  n. sympathicus lateralis
  n. taeniaeformis
  n. tecti
  tectoral n.
  tegmental nuclei
  nuclei tegmentales
  n. of tegmental field
  tegmental n. of Gudden
  nuclei tegmenti
  terminal nuclei
  nuclei terminationis
  nuclei of thalamus,
    anterior
  nuclei of thalamus,
    intralaminar
  nuclei of thalamus, lateral
  nuclei of thalamus, medial
  nuclei of thalamus, median
  n. of thalamus,
    parafasicular
  nuclei of thalamus,
    paraventricular
  n. of thalamus, reticular
  n. of thalamus, rhomboid
  nuclei of thalamus,
    ventrolateral
  thoracic n.
  n. thoracicus
  n. of tongue, fibrous
  n. tractus solitarii
  n. of trapezoid body, dorsal
  n. of trapezoid body,
    ventral
  triangular n.
  n. triangularis

nu·cle·us *(continued)*
  trigeminal mesencephalic
    n.
  n. trochlearis
  trochlear n.
  n. of trochlear nerve
  trophic n.
  tuberal nuclei
  tuberal nuclei, lateral
  nuclei tuberales
  nuclei tuberis lateralis
  vagal n., dorsal
  n. vagalis dorsalis
  vagoglossopharyngeal n.
  n. of vagus nerve, dorsal
  vegetative n.
  n. ventrales thalami
  n. ventrobasolateralis
  nuclei ventrolaterales
    thalami
  n. ventromedialis
  vesicular n.
  vestibular nuclei
  nuclei vestibulares
  vestibulocochlear nuclei
  Voit's n.
  Westphal's n.
  yolk n.
  zygote n.
nu·clide
  radioactive n.
nu·do·pho·bia
Nu·el's space
nu·fe·nox·ole
NUG — necrotizing ulcerative
    gingivitis
Nuhn's glands
nui·sance
nul·li·grav·id
nul·li·grav·i·da
nul·lip·a·ra
nul·li·par·i·ty
nul·lip·a·rous
nul·li·som·ic
num·ber
  acetyl n.
  acid n.
  atomic n.

num·ber *(continued)*
    Avogadro's n.
    Brinell hardness n.
    chromosome n.
    CT n's
    dibucaine n.
    haploid n.
    hardness n.
    Hehner n.
    Hittorf n.
    Hübl n.
    hydrogen n.
    iodine n.
    isotopic n.
    Knoop hardness n.
    linking n.
    Loschmidt's n.
    mass n.
    Mohs hardness n.
    monoploid n.
    oxidation n.
    polar n.
    Polenske n.
    random n.
    Reichert-Meissl n.
    Reynold's n.
    Rockwell hardness n.
    saponification n.
    transport n.
    turnover n.
    viable n.
    Vickers hardness n.
    wave n.
    winding n.
numb·ness
    waking n.
num·mu·lar
Nu·mor·phan
nun·na·tion
Nu·per·cain·al
Nu·per·caine
nup·tial·i·ty
N-Uri·stix
nurse
    charge n.
    clinical n. specialist
    n. clinician
    community n.

nurse *(continued)*
    community health n.
    district n.
    general duty n.
    graduate n.
    head n.
    hospital n.
    licensed practical n.
    licensed vocational n.
    monthly n.
    occupational health n.
    office n.
    operating room n.
    practical n.
    n. practitioner
    private n.
    private duty n.
    probationer n.
    public health n.
    Queen's n.
    registered n.
    school n.
    scrub n.
    special n.
    n. specialist
    student n.
    theater n.
    trained n.
    visiting n.
    wet n.
nurse-an·es·thet·ist
nurse-mid·wife
nurse-mid·wi·fery
nurse-prac·ti·tion·er
nur·se·ry
    day n.
    day care n.
nurs·ing
    foster n.
Nuss·baum's experiment
Nuss·baum's narcosis
nut
    betel n.
nu·ta·tion
nu·ta·to·ry
nut·gall
nut·meg

nu·tri·ent
   essential n's
   secondary n.
   trace n.
nu·tri·lite
nu·tri·ment
nu·tri·ol·o·gy
nu·tri·tion
   adequate n.
   high n.
   total enteral n.
   total parenteral n.
nu·tri·tion·al
nu·tri·tion·gram
nu·tri·tion·ist
nu·tri·tious
nu·tri·tive
nu·tri·ture
nu·trose
nux
   n. moschata
   n. vomica
ny·a·cyne
ny·ad
nyc·tal·gia
nyc·ta·lope
nyc·ta·lo·pia
nyc·ta·pho·nia
nyc·ter·ine
nyc·tero·hem·er·al
nyc·to·hem·er·al
nyc·to·phil·ia
nyc·to·pho·bia
nyc·to·pho·nia
nyc·to·typh·lo·sis
nyc·tu·ria
NYD — not yet diagnosed
Ny·dra·zid
Ny·len-Bá·rá·ny maneuver
ny·les·tri·ol
nyl·i·drin hy·dro·chlo·ride
ny·lon
nymph
nym·pha *pl.* nym·phae
   n. of Krause
nym·phal
nym·phec·to·my
nym·phi·tis

nym·pho·ca·run·cu·lar
nym·pho·hy·me·ne·al
nym·phoid
nym·pho·ma·nia
nym·pho·ma·ni·ac
nym·phon·cus
nym·phot·o·my
Nysso·rhyn·chus
nys·tag·mic
nys·tag·mi·form
nys·tag·mo·graph
nys·tag·mog·ra·phy
nys·tag·moid
nys·tag·mus
   amaurotic n.
   amblyopic n.
   ataxic n.
   aural n.
   benign positional n.
   caloric n.
   central n.
   cervical torsion n.
   Cheyne's n.
   Cheyne-Stokes n.
   congenital n.
   congenital hereditary n.
   convergence n.
   deviational n.
   disjunctive n.
   dissociated n.
   downbeat n.
   electrical n.
   end-point n.
   end-position n.
   fixation n.
   galvanic n.
   gaze n.
   incongruent n.
   jerk n.
   jerky n.
   labyrinthine n.
   latent n.
   lateral n.
   miner's n.
   monocular n.
   occupational n.
   ocular n.
   opticokinetic n.

nys·tag·mus *(continued)*
    optokinetic n.
    oscillating n.
    palatal n.
    paretic n.
    pendular n.
    periodic alternating n.
    phasic n.
    positional n.
    postrotational n.
    postural n.
    provocation n.
    railroad n.
    resilient n.
    retraction n.
    n. retractorius
    rhythmical n.
    rotatory n.

nys·tag·mus *(continued)*
    secondary n.
    see-saw n.
    spontaneous n.
    train-dispatchers' n.
    undulatory n.
    unilateral n.
    upbeat n.
    vertical n.
    vestibular n.
    vibratory n.
    visual n.
    voluntary n.
nys·tag·mus-my·oc·lo·nus
nys·ta·tin
nys·tax·is
Ny·sten's law
nyx·is

O

O — occiput
    ohne Hauch
    oxygen
O. — L. oculus (eye)
O₂ — diatomic (molecular)
    oxygen
O₃ — ozone
OA — ocular albinism
OA1 — ocular albinism type 1
OA2 — ocular albinism type 2
OAF — osteoclast activating
    factor
oak
    poison o.
oa·sis *pl.* oa·ses
OAT — ornithine
    aminotransferase
oath
    o. of Hippocrates
    hippocratic o.
OB — obstetrics

ob·ce·ca·tion
ob·du·cent
ob·duc·tion
O'Beirne's sphincter
obe·li·ac
obe·li·ad
obe·li·on
Ober's operation
Ober's sign
Ober's test
Ober·may·er's test
Ober·mül·ler's test
Oberst's method
Ober·stei·ner-Red·lich area
Ober·stei·ner-Red·lich zone
obese
obes·i·ty
    adrenocortical o.
    adult-onset o.
    alimentary o.
    centripetal o.

obes·i·ty *(continued)*
   endocrine o.
   endogenous o.
   exogenous o.
   hyperinsulinar o.
   hyperinterrenal o.
   hyperplasmic o.
   hyperplastic-hypertrophic
     o.
   hypertrophic o.
   hypogonad o.
   hypoplasmic o.
   hypothalamic o.
   hypothyroid o.
   lifelong o.
   morbid o.
   plethoric o.
   simple o.
obes·og·e·nous
Obe·sum·bac·te·ri·um
obex
obi·dox·ime chlo·ride
ob·ject
   transitional o.
ob·jec·tive
   achromatic o.
   apochromatic o.
   binocular o's
   dry o.
   flat field o.
   fluorite o.
   immersion o.
   oil-immersion o.
   semiapochromatic o.
ob·li·gate
oblique
obliq·ui·ty
   biparietal o.
   Litzmann's o.
   Nägele's o.
   o. of pelvis
   Roederer's o.
obli·quus
oblit·er·a·tion
   cortical o.
ob·lon·ga·ta
ob·lon·ga·tal
ob·nu·bi·la·tion

O'Bri·en akinesia
OBS — organic brain
  syndrome
ob·ses·sion
ob·ses·sive
ob·ses·sive-com·pul·sive
ob·so·les·cence
ob·stet·ric
ob·stet·ri·cal
ob·ste·tri·cian
ob·stet·rics
ob·sti·pa·tion
ob·struc·tion
   false colonic o.
   intestinal o.
   renal pelvic o.
   ureteral o.
   ureterovesical o.
   uteropelvic o.
ob·struc·tive
ob·stru·ent
ob·tund
ob·tun·da·tion
ob·tun·dent
ob·tun·di·ty
ob·tu·ra·tion
   canal o.
ob·tu·ra·tor
   buccofacial o.
ob·tu·sion
OCA — oculocutaneous
  albinism
Oc·cam's razor
oc·cip·i·tal
oc·cip·i·ta·lis
oc·cip·i·tal·iza·tion
oc·cip·i·to·an·te·ri·or
oc·cip·i·to·at·loid
oc·cip·i·to·ax·oid
oc·cip·i·to·bas·i·lar
oc·cip·i·to·breg·mat·ic
oc·cip·i·to·cal·car·ine
oc·cip·i·to·cer·vi·cal
oc·cip·i·to·fa·cial
oc·cip·i·to·fron·tal
oc·cip·i·to·fron·ta·lis
oc·cip·i·to·mas·toid
oc·cip·i·to·men·tal

oc·cip·i·to·pa·ri·e·tal
oc·cip·i·to·pon·tine
oc·cip·i·to·pos·te·ri·or
oc·cip·i·to·tem·po·ral
oc·cip·i·to·tha·lam·ic
oc·ci·put
oc·clude
oc·clu·dens
   zonula o.
oc·clud·er
oc·clu·sal
oc·clu·sion
   abnormal o.
   acentric o.
   anatomic o.
   anterior o.
   balanced o.
   buccal o.
   centric o.
   convenience o.
   coronary o.
   distal o.
   dynamic o.
   eccentric o.
   edge-to-edge o.
   end-to-end o.
   enteromesenteric o.
   equilibrated o.
   functional o.
   gliding o.
   habitual o.
   hyperfunctional o.
   ideal o.
   labial o.
   lateral o.
   lingual o.
   locked o.
   mechanically balanced o.
   mesial o.
   neutral o.
   normal o.
   pathogenic o.
   physiologically balanced o.
   posterior o.
   postnormal o.
   prenormal o.
   protrusive o.
   retrusive o.

oc·clu·sion *(continued)*
   spherical form of o.
   terminal o.
   traumatic o.
   traumatogenic o.
   working o.
oc·clu·sive
oc·clu·so·cer·vi·cal
oc·clu·som·e·ter
oc·clu·so·re·ha·bil·i·ta·tion
oc·cult
oc·cu·pan·cy
ocel·lus
OCG — oral cholecystogram
och·le·sis
Ochoa, Severo
ochrom·e·ter
Ochro·my·ia
ochro·no·sis
   exogenous o.
   ocular o.
ochro·no·sus
ochro·not·ic
Ochs·ner's muscle
Ochs·ner's ring
Ochs·ner's treatment
oc·ry·late
OCT — ornithine
  carbamoyltransferase
   oxytocin challenge test
oc·ta·ben·zone
oc·ta·co·sa·nol
oc·ta·dec·a·no·ate
oc·ta·he·dral
oc·ta·he·dron
oc·ta·meth·yl pyro·phos·
  phor·amide
oc·tam·y·lose
oc·tan
oc·tane
oc·ta·no·ic acid
oc·ta·pep·tide
oc·tar·i·us
oc·ta·va·lent
oc·ta·za·mide
oc·tet
oc·ti·ci·zer
oc·ti·grav·i·da

Oc·tin
oc·tip·a·ra
oc·to·drine
oc·to·fol·lin
oc·to·mi·tus hom·in·is
Oc·to·my·ces
     O. etiennei
oc·to·pam·ine
oc·tose
oc·tox·y·nol 9
oc·trip·ty·line phos·phate
oc·tyl gal·late
oc·tyl·phe·noxy poly·eth·oxy·
   eth·a·nol
oc·u·fil·con
oc·u·lar
     Huygens (Huyghens) o.
     wide-field o.
oc·u·len·tum *pl.* oc·u·len·ta
oc·u·li
oc·u·list
oc·u·lis·tics
oc·u·lo·ce·phal·ic
oc·u·lo·ceph·a·lo·gyr·ic
oc·u·lo·cu·ta·ne·ous
oc·u·lo·fa·cial
oc·u·lo·gy·ra·tion
oc·u·lo·gy·ric
oc·u·lo·met·ro·scope
oc·u·lo·mo·tor
oc·u·lo·mo·to·ri·us
oc·u·lo·my·co·sis
oc·u·lo·na·sal
oc·u·lop·a·thy
oc·u·lo·ple·thys·mog·ra·phy
oc·u·lo·pneu·mo·ple·thys·
   mog·ra·phy
oc·u·lo·pu·pil·lary
oc·u·lo·sen·so·ry
oc·u·lo·spi·nal
oc·u·lo·zy·go·mat·ic
oc·u·lus *pl.* oc·u·li
     o. caesius
     o. dexter (OD)
     fundus oculi
     o. laevus (OL)
     o. leporinus
     o. sinister (OS)

Oc·u·sert
OD — Doctor of Optometry
     L. oculus dexter (right eye)
     optical density
     outside diameter
     overdose
ODA — L. occipito-dextra
   anterior (right
   occipito-anterior)
odax·es·mus
odax·et·ic
ODC — orotidine 5′-phosphate
   decarboxylase
Od·di's muscle
Od·di's sphincter
od·di·tis
odo·gen·e·sis
odon·tal·gia
odon·tal·gic
odon·tec·to·my
odon·ter·ism
odon·tex·e·sis
odon·ti·at·ro·gen·ic
odon·tic
odon·to·am·e·lo·blas·to·ma
odon·to·at·lan·tal
odon·to·blast
odon·to·blas·to·ma
odon·to·both·ri·on
odon·to·both·ri·tis
odon·to·cla·mis
odon·to·clast
odon·to·dys·pla·sia
odon·to·gen
odon·to·gen·e·sis
     o. imperfecta
odon·to·ge·net·ic
odon·to·gen·ic
odon·tog·e·nous
odon·to·gram
odon·to·graph
odon·tog·ra·phy
odon·to·iat·ria
odon·toid
odon·to·lith
odon·to·li·thi·a·sis
odon·tol·o·gist
odon·tol·o·gy

odon·tol·o·gy
    forensic o.
odon·tol·y·sis
odon·to·ma
    o. adamantinum
    ameloblastic o.
    calcified o.
    complex o.
    composite o.
    composite o., complex
    composite o., compound
    compound o.
    coronal o.
    coronary o.
    cystic o.
    dilated composite o.
    dilated o.
    embryoplastic o.
    epithelial o.
    fibrous o.
    gestant o.
    mixed o.
    radicular o.
odon·ton·o·my
odon·to·par·al·lax·is
odon·to·path·ic
odon·top·a·thy
odon·to·peri·os·te·um
odon·to·pho·bia
odon·to·plas·ty
odon·to·pri·sis
odon·to·ra·dio·graph
odon·to·sar·co·ma
    ameloblastic o.
odon·to·schism
odon·tos·co·py
odon·to·sei·sis
odon·to·sis
odon·to·the·ca
odon·tot·o·my
odon·to·trip·sis
odor
    minimal identifiable o.
odor·ant
odor·a·tism
odor·if·er·ous
odor·im·e·ter
odor·im·e·try

odor·i·phore
odor·i·vec·tor
odoro·gram
odor·og·ra·phy
odor·ous
ODP — L. occipito-dextra
    posterior (right
    occipitoposterior)
ODT — L. occipito-dextra
    transversa (right
    occipitotransverse)
odyn·acu·sis
odyn·om·e·ter
od·y·no·pha·gia
odyn·uria
Oeci·a·cus
oed·i·pism
Oed·i·pus complex
Oeh·ler's symptom
oenan·thol
Oer·tel's treatment
oesoph·a·go·sto·mi·a·sis
Oesoph·a·gos·to·mum
    Oe. apiostomum
    Oe. bifurcum
    Oe. brevicaudum
    Oe. brumpti
    Oe. columbianum
    Oe. dentatum
    Oe. inflatum
    Oe. longicaudum
    Oe. radiatum
    Oe. stephanostomum
    Oe. suis
Oest·rei·cher's reaction
oes·tri·a·sis
Oes·tri·dae
Oes·trus
    O. hominis
    O. ovis
OFC — occipitofrontal
    circumference
OFD — oral-facial-digital
    (syndrome)
of·fi·cial
of·fic·i·nal
oflox·a·cin
Oga·ta's method

Ogen
Og·il·vie syndrome
Ogi·no-Knaus method
Og·ston's line
Og·ston-Luc operation
Ogu·chi's disease
Ohara's disease
OH-Cbl — hydroxocobalamin
Ohl·mach·er solution
ohm
    reciprocal o.
Ohm's law
ohm·am·me·ter
ohm·me·ter
ohne Hauch
OI — osteogenesis imperfecta
OIC — osteogenesis
  imperfecta congenita
oid·i·o·my·co·sis
oid·i·o·my·cot·ic
Oid·i·um
OIH — orthoiodohippurate
oil
    almond o.
    almond o., bitter
    almond o., expressed
    almond o., sweet
    anise o.
    apricot kernel o.
    arachis o.
    argemone o.
    Benne o.
    bergamot o.
    betula o.
    bhilawanol o.
    birch o., sweet
    birch tar o., rectified
    cade o.
    o. of cajuput
    camphorated o.
    caraway o.
    cardamom o.
    cassia o.
    castor o.
    castor o., aromatic
    cedar o.
    chenopodium o.
    chloriodized o.

oil *(continued)*
    cinnamon o.
    citronella o.
    clove o.
    coconut o.
    cod liver o.
    cod liver o.,
      nondestearinated
    coriander o.
    corn o.
    cottonseed o.
    croton o.
    o. of dill
    distilled o.
    drying o.
    empyreumatic o.
    essential o.
    ethereal o.
    ethiodized o.
    eucalyptus o.
    expressed o.
    fatty o.
    fennel o.
    fixed o.
    flaxseed o.
    gaultheria o.
    gingili o.
    groundnut o.
    Haarlem o.
    halibut liver o.
    immersion o.
    iodized o.
    juniper o.
    lavender o.
    lavender flowers o.
    lemon o.
    linseed o.
    raw linseed o.
    o. of male fern
    mineral o.
    mineral o. light
    mineral o., light white
    mineral o., white
    o. of mirbane
    o. of mustard
    myristica o.
    neroli o.
    nutmeg o.

oil *(continued)*
  olive o.
  orange o.
  orange o., bitter
  orange o., sweet
  orange flower o.
  o. of Palma Christi
  peach kernel o.
  peanut o.
  peppermint o.
  persic o.
  pine o.
  pine needle o.
  pine needle o., dwarf
  ricinus o.
  rose o.
  rosemary o.
  safflower o.
  sandalwood o.
  santal o.
  sassafras o.
  savin o.
  sesame o.
  spearmint o.
  o. of spike
  o. of spruce
  sweet o.
  tangan-tangan o.
  tar o., rectified
  teel o.
  theobroma o.
  thyme o.
  turpentine o.
  turpentine o., rectified
  volatile o.
  wheat-germ o.
  wintergreen o.
  wormseed o., American
oint·ment
  ammoniated mercury o.
  anthralin o.
  bacitracin o.
  bacitracin ophthalmic o.
  belladonna o.
  benzocaine o.
  benzoic and salicylic acids
    o.
  betamethasone valerate o.

oint·ment *(continued)*
  boric acid o.
  calamine o.
  candicidin o.
  carbolic acid o.
  chloramphenicol
    ophthalmic o.
  chrysarobin o.
  coal tar o.
  Credé's o.
  cyclomethycaine sulfate o.
  dexamethasone sodium
    phosphate ophthalmic o.
  dibucaine o.
  dimethisoquin
    hydrochloride o.
  diperodon o.
  emulsifying o.
  erythromycin o.
  erythromycin ophthalmic
    o.
  eserine o.
  ethyl aminobenzoate o.
  fluocinolone acetonide o.
  flurandrenolide o.
  gentamicin sulfate o.
  gentamicin sulfate
    ophthalmic o.
  golden o.
  hydrocortisone o.
  hydrocortisone acetate o.
  hydrocortisone acetate
    ophthalmic o.
  hydrophilic o.
  hydroquinone o.
  ichthammol o.
  idoxuridine ophthalmic o.
  iodine o.
  iodochlorhydroxyquin o.
  iodochlorhydroxyquin and
    hydrocortisone o.
  isoflurophate ophthalmic o.
  lanolin o.
  lidocaine o.
  mercuric oxide ophthalmic
    o., yellow
  methyl salicylate o.

oint·ment *(continued)*
  methylbenzethonium
    chloride o.
  monobenzone o.
  neomycin sulfate o.
  neomycin and polymyxin B
    sulfates, and bacitracin
    zinc o.
  nitrofurazone o.
  Nitrol o.
  nystatin o.
  Pagenstecher's o.
  paraffin o.
  penicillin o.
  phenol o.
  physostigmine o.
  pine tar o.
  polyethylene glycol o.
  polymyxin B sulfate o.
  resorcinol o., compound
  rose water o.
  rose water o., petrolatum
  scarlet red o.
  simple o.
  sulfacetamide sodium
    ophthalmic o.
  sulfisoxazole diolamine
    ophthalmic s.
  sulfur o.
  tar o., compound
  tetracaine o.
  tetracaine ophthalmic o.
  triamcinolone acetonide o.
  triclobisonium chloride o.
  undecylenic acid o.,
    compound
  white o.
  white precipitate o.
  Whitfield's o.
  wintergreen o.
  yellow o.
  zinc o.
  zinc oxide o.
  zinc undecenoate o.
Oken's body
Oken's canal
Oken's corpus

OKN — opticokinetic
  nystagmus
OL — L. oculus laevus (left
  eye)
Ol. — L. oleum (oil)
OLA — L. occipito-laeva
  anterior (left
  occipito-anterior)
ol·amine
Olea
olea
ole·ag·i·nous
ole·an·der
ole·an·do·my·cin phos·phate
ole·an·drin
ole·an·drism
ole·a·nol
ole·as·ter
ole·ate
olec·ra·nal
ole·cra·nar·thri·tis
ole·cra·nar·throc·a·ce
ole·cra·nar·throp·a·thy
olec·ra·noid
olec·ra·non
ole·fin
ole·ic acid
ole·in
olen·itis
oleo·chryso·ther·a·py
oleo·cre·o·sote
oleo·gran·u·lo·ma
oleo·in·fu·sion
ole·o·ma
oleo·mar·ga·rine
ole·om·e·ter
oleo·nu·cleo·pro·tein
oleo·pal·mi·tate
oleo·peri·to·ne·og·ra·phy
oleo·res·in
  aspidium o.
  capsicum o.
oleo·sac·cha·rum
oleo·ste·ar·ate
oleo·sus
oleo·ther·a·py
oleo·vi·ta·min
  o. A

oleo·vi·ta·min *(continued)*
   o. A and D
   o. D, synthetic
   o. D$_2$
   o. D$_3$
ole·um *pl.* olea
ol·fact
ol·fac·tion
ol·fac·tism
ol·fac·tol·o·gy
ol·fac·tom·e·ter
   blast o.
   Proetz o.
ol·fac·tom·e·try
ol·fac·to·ry
ol·fac·tus
ol·i·gak·i·su·ria
ol·i·ge·mia
ol·i·ge·mic
ol·i·go·am·ni·os
ol·i·go·arth·ri·tis
ol·i·go·as·tro·cy·to·ma
ol·i·go·blast
ol·i·go·car·dia
ol·i·go·chro·ma·sia
ol·i·go·chro·me·mia
ol·i·go·clo·nal
ol·i·go·cys·tic
ol·i·go·cy·the·mia
ol·i·go·cy·them·ic
ol·i·go·cy·to·sis
ol·i·go·dac·ty·ly
ol·i·go·den·dria
ol·i·go·den·dro·blast
ol·i·go·den·dro·blas·to·ma
ol·i·go·den·dro·cyte
ol·i·go·den·drog·lia
ol·i·go·den·dro·gli·o·ma
ol·i·go·den·dro·glio·ma·to·sis
   o. cerebri
ol·i·go·dip·sia
ol·i·go·don·tia
ol·i·go·dy·nam·ic
ol·i·go·en·ceph·a·lon
ol·i·go·ga·lac·tia
ol·i·go·gen·ic
ol·i·gog·lia
   interfascicular o.

ol·i·go-1,6-glu·co·si·dase
ol·i·go·he·mia
ol·i·go·hi·dro·sis
ol·i·go·hy·dram·ni·os
ol·i·go·hy·dru·ria
Ol·i·go·hy·me·no·phor·ea
ol·i·go·hy·per·men·or·rhea
ol·i·go·hy·po·men·or·rhea
ol·i·go·lec·i·thal
ol·i·go·leu·ko·cy·the·mia
ol·i·go·leu·ko·cy·to·sis
ol·i·go·meg·a·ne·phro·nia
ol·i·go·meg·a·neph·ron·ic
ol·i·go·men·or·rhea
ol·i·go·mer
ol·i·go·mer·ic
ol·i·go·me·tal·lic
ol·i·go·mor·phic
ol·i·go·my·cin
ol·i·go·nec·ro·sper·mia
ol·i·go·ni·tro·phil·ic
ol·i·go·nu·cle·o·tide
ol·i·go-ov·u·la·tion
ol·i·go·pep·tide
ol·i·go·phos·pha·tu·ria
ol·i·go·phre·nia
ol·i·go·phren·ic
ol·i·go·plas·mia
ol·i·go·plas·tic
ol·i·gop·nea
ol·i·go·py·rene
ol·i·go·py·rous
ol·i·go·sac·cha·ride
ol·i·go·sid·er·emia
ol·i·go·sper·mat·ic
ol·i·go·sper·ma·tism
ol·i·go·sper·mia
ol·i·go·stea·to·sis
ol·i·go·symp·to·mat·ic
ol·i·go·syn·ap·tic
ol·i·go·tro·phia
ol·i·go·troph·ic
ol·i·got·ro·phy
ol·i·go·zo·o·sper·ma·tism
ol·i·go·zo·o·sper·mia
ol·i·gu·re·sis
ol·i·gu·ria
ol·i·gu·ric

olis·thero·chro·ma·tin
olis·thy
oli·va *pl.* oli·vae
    o. cerebellaris
ol·i·vary
ol·ive
    inferior o.
    medullary o.
    spurge o.
    superior o.
Ol·i·ver's sign
Ol·i·ver's test
Ol·i·ver-Ro·sal·ki method
ol·i·vif·u·gal
ol·i·vip·e·tal
ol·i·vo·cere·bel·lar
ol·i·vo·cor·ti·cal
ol·i·vo·nu·cle·ar
ol·i·vo·pon·to·cer·e·bel·lar
ol·i·vo·spi·nal
Ol·lier's disease
Ol·lier's law
Ol·lier's layer
Ol·lier-Thiersch graft
Ol. oliv. — L. oleum olivae
    (olive oil)
olo·pho·nia
OLP — L. occipito-laeva
    posterior (left
    occipitoposterior)
Ol·pi·trich·um
Ols·hau·sen's operation
Ol·shev·sky tube
OLT — L. occipito-laeva
    transversa (left
    occipitotransverse)
Olym·pus scopes
OM — obtuse marginal
    (coronary artery)
    otitis media
    outer membrane
o.m. — L. omni mane (every
    morning)
oma·ceph·a·lus
oma·gra
omal·gia
omar·thri·tis
oma·si·tis

oma·sum
Om·bré·danne's operation
om·bro·phore
omen·ta
omen·tal
omen·tec·to·my
omen·ti·tis
omen·to·fix·a·tion
omen·to·pexy
omen·to·plas·ty
omen·to·por·tog·ra·phy
omen·tor·rha·phy
omen·to·sple·no·pexy
omen·tot·o·my
omen·to·vol·vu·lus
omen·tum *pl.* omen·ta
    colic o.
    gastrocolic o.
    gastric o.
    gastrohepatic o.
    gastrosplenic o.
    greater o.
    lesser o.
    o. majus
    o. minus
    pancreaticosplenic o.
    splenogastric o.
omen·tum·ec·to·my
om·i·cron
omi·tis
om·ma·tid·i·um *pl.* om·ma·
    tid·ia
Om·ma·ya reservoir
Omn. bih. — L. omni bihora
    (every two hours)
Omn. hor. — L. omni hora
    (every hour)
Om·ni·pen
om·nip·o·tence of thought
om·niv·o·rous
Omn. noct. — L. omni nocte
    (every night)
omo·ceph·a·lus
omo·cer·vi·ca·lis
omo·cla·vic·u·lar
omo·dyn·ia
omo·hy·oid
omo·pha·gia

omo·plata
omo·ster·num
omo·thy·roid
OMPA — octamethyl
    pyrophosphoramide
om·pha·lec·to·my
om·phal·el·co·sis
om·phal·ic
om·pha·li·tis
om·pha·lo·an·gi·op·a·gous
om·pha·lo·an·gi·op·a·gus
om·pha·lo·cele
om·pha·lo·cho·ri·on
om·pha·lo·did·y·mus
om·pha·lo·gen·e·sis
om·pha·lo·is·chi·op·a·gus
om·pha·lo·ma
om·pha·lo·mes·a·ra·ic
om·pha·lo·mes·en·ter·ic
om·pha·lon·cus
om·pha·lop·a·gus
om·pha·lo·phle·bi·tis
om·pha·lor·rha·gia
om·pha·lor·rhea
om·pha·lor·rhex·is
om·pha·lo·site
om·pha·lot·o·my
om·pha·lus
Om. quar. hor. — L. omni
    quadrante hora (every
    quarter of an hour)
o.n. — L. omni nocte (every
    night)
ona·ye
On·cho·cer·ca
    O. caecutiens
    O. volvulus
on·cho·cer·ci·a·sis
    ocular o.
on·cho·cer·cid
On·cho·cer·ci·dae
on·cho·cer·co·ma
on·cho·cer·co·sis
on·cho·der·ma·ti·tis
On·ci·o·lo
on·co·cyte
on·co·cyt·ic
on·co·cy·to·ma

on·co·cy·to·sis
on·cod·na·vi·rus
on·co·fe·tal
on·co·gene
on·co·gen·e·sis
on·co·ge·net·ic
on·co·gen·ic
on·co·ge·nic·i·ty
on·cog·e·nous
on·coi·des
on·co·log·ic
on·col·o·gist
on·col·o·gy
on·col·y·sate
on·col·y·sis
on·co·lyt·ic
on·co·ma
On·co·me·la·nia
on·com·e·ter
on·cor·na·vir·i·nae
on·cor·na·vi·rus
on·co·sis
on·co·sphere
on·co·ther·a·py
on·co·thlip·sis
on·cot·ic
on·cot·o·my
on·co·trop·ic
On·co·vin
on·co·vi·rus
On·dine's curse
onei·ric
onei·rism
onei·ro·de·lir·i·um
onei·ro·dyn·ia
onei·ro·gen·ic
onei·rog·mus
onei·roid
onei·rol·o·gy
onei·ro·phre·nia
onei·ros·co·py
oni·um
on·kino·cele
on·lay
    epithelial o.
on·o·mato·ma·nia
on·o·mato·pho·bia
on·o·mato·poi·e·sis

on·to·gen·e·sis
on·to·ge·net·ic
on·to·gen·ic
on·tog·e·ny
ony·al·ai, ony·al·ia
on·y·cha·tro·phia
on·y·chat·ro·phy
on·y·chaux·is
on·y·chec·to·my
onych·ia
    o. lateralis
    monilial o.
    o. periungualis
    o. sicca
    syphilitic o.
on·y·chi·tis
on·y·choc·la·sis
on·y·cho·cryp·to·sis
on·y·cho·dys·tro·phy
on·y·cho·gen·ic
on·y·cho·gram
on·y·cho·graph
on·y·chog·ra·phy
on·y·cho·gry·pho·sis
on·y·cho·gry·po·sis
on·y·cho·het·ero·to·pia
on·y·chol·o·gy
on·y·chol·y·sis
on·y·cho·ma·de·sis
on·y·cho·ma·la·cia
on·y·cho·my·co·sis
    dermatophytic o.
onych·opac·i·ty
on·y·cho·os·teo·dys·pla·sia
on·y·cho·path·ic
on·y·cho·pa·thol·o·gy
on·y·chop·a·thy
on·y·cho·pha·gia
on·y·choph·a·gy
on·y·cho·pho·sis
on·y·chop·to·sis
on·y·chor·rhex·is
on·y·cho·schi·zia
on·y·cho·sis
on·y·cho·stro·ma
on·y·cho·til·lo·ma·nia
on·y·chot·o·my
O'nyong-nyong

on·yx
on·yx·is
oo·blast
oo·ceph·a·lus
oo·ci·ne·sia
oo·cy·e·sis
oo·cyst
oo·cyte
    primary o.
    secondary o.
oog·a·mous
oog·a·my
oo·gen·e·sis
oo·ge·net·ic
oo·gen·ic
oo·go·ni·um *pl.* oo·go·nia
oo·ki·ne·sis
oo·ki·nete
oo·lem·ma
Oo·my·ce·tes
oo·pha·gia
ooph·a·gy
ooph·or·al·gia
ooph·o·rec·to·mize
ooph·o·rec·to·my
ooph·o·ri·tis
    o. parotidea
ooph·o·ro·cys·tec·to·my
ooph·o·ro·cys·to·sis
ooph·o·rog·e·nous
ooph·o·ro·hys·ter·ec·to·my
ooph·o·ro·ma
    o. folliculare
ooph·o·ron
ooph·o·rop·a·thy
ooph·o·ro·pexy
ooph·o·ro·plas·ty
ooph·o·ro·sal·pin·gec·to·my
ooph·o·ro·sal·pin·gi·tis
ooph·o·ros·to·my
ooph·o·rot·o·my
ooph·or·rha·gia
oo·phyte
oo·plasm
oo·some
oo·sperm
oo·sphere
oo·spo·ran·gi·um

oo·spore
oo·the·ca
oo·the·cos·to·my
oo·thec·to·my
oo·thec·to·sal·pin·gec·to·my
oo·tid
oot·o·my
oo·type
oo·zo·oid
opac·i·fi·ca·tion
opac·i·fy
opac·i·ty
    snowball o's
opal·es·cent
opal·gia
opa·line
opa·lin·id
Opal·ski cell
opaque
OPD — outpatient
  department
open·ing
    aortic o.
    cardiac o.
    cutaneous o. of male
      urethra
    duodenal o. of stomach
    ileocecal o.
    orbital o.
    piriform o.
    pyloric o.
    saphenous o.
    semilunar o. of ethmoid
      bone
    tendinous o.
    vesicourethral o.
op·er·a·bil·i·ty
op·er·a·ble
op·er·ant
op·er·ate
op·er·a·tion
    Abbe o.
    Abbe-Estlander o.
    Adams' o.
    Adelmann's o.
    Akin o.
    Albee's o.
    Albee-Delbet o.

op·er·a·tion *(continued)*
    Albert's o.
    Aldridge o.
    Alexander's o.
    Alexander-Adams o.
    Allarton's o.
    Alouette's o.
    Ammon's o.
    Amussat's o.
    Anagnostakis' o.
    anastomotic o.
    Anderson's o.
    Annandale's o.
    Aries-Pitanguy o.
    Arlt's o.
    Asch o.
    Auchincloss o.
    Aufranc-Turner o.
    Babcock's o.
    Badal's o.
    Baldy's o.
    Baldy-Webster o.
    Barkan's o.
    Barker's o.
    Barraquer's o.
    Barsky's o.
    Barton's o.
    Barwell's o.
    Basset's o.
    Bassini's o.
    Battle's o.
    Beck (I, II) o.
    Beer's o.
    Belfield's o.
    Belsey Mark IV o.
    Bent's o.
    Berger's o.
    Berke o.
    Bernard's o.
    Bevan's o.
    Bier's o.
    Biesenberger's o.
    Bigelow's o.
    Billroth's o.
    Blair-Brown o.
    Blalock's o.
    Blalock-Hanlon o.
    Blalock-Taussig o.

op·er·a·tion *(continued)*
- Blaskovics o.
- bloodless o.
- Boari's o.
- Bondy o.
- Borthen's o.
- bottle o.
- Bozeman's o.
- Brailey's o.
- Bricker's o.
- Brock's o.
- Brophy's o.
- Browne o.
- Brunschwig's o.
- Buck's o.
- (von) Burow's o.
- buttonhole o.
- Caldwell-Luc o.
- Calot's o.
- capital o.
- Carnochan's o.
- Carpue's o.
- Cecil's o.
- celsian o.
- Charles o.
- Chopart's o.
- cinch o.
- Civiale's o.
- Codivilla's o.
- Colonna's o.
- Commando's o.
- Conway o.
- cosmetic o.
- Cotte's o.
- Cotting's o.
- crescent o.
- Critchett's o.
- Cushing's o.
- Dana's o.
- Daviel's o.
- decompression o.
- Denis Browne o.
- Denker's o.
- Denonvilliers' o.
- Dieffenbach's o.
- Dittel's o.
- Dohlman's o.
- Doléris' o.

op·er·a·tion *(continued)*
- Dorrance o.
- Doyen's o.
- Duhamel o.
- Dührssen's o.
- Duplay's o.
- Dupuy-Dutemps o.
- Dupuytren's o.
- Eagleton's o.
- Elliot's o.
- Emmet's o.
- equilibrating o.
- Esser's o.
- Estes' o.
- Estlander's o.
- Eversbusch's o.
- exploratory o.
- Fasanella-Servat o.
- Fergusson's o.
- Fick o.
- filtering o.
- Finney's o.
- Finzi-Harmer o.
- flap o.
- Förster's o.
- Fontan's o.
- forceps o.
- Fothergill o.
- Fothergill-Donald o.
- Franco's o.
- Frank's o.
- Frazier-Spiller o.
- Freckner's o.
- Fredet-Ramstedt o.
- Freund's o.
- Freyer's o.
- Frost-Lang o.
- Fukala's o.
- Fuller's o.
- Gifford's o.
- Gigli's o.
- Gill's o.
- Gilliam's o.
- Gillies o.
- Girdlestone o.
- Glenn o.
- Gonin's o.
- Graefe's o.

op·er·a·tion *(continued)*
  Gritti's o.
  Grondahl-Finney o.
  Guyon's o.
  Hajek's o.
  Halsted's o.
  Hancock's o.
  Hartmann's o.
  Hartley-Krause o.
  Haultain's o.
  Heath's o.
  Heine's o.
  Heineke's o.
  Heineke-Mikulicz o.
  Heller's o.
  Herbert's o.
  Hey's o.
  Hibbs' o.
  high forceps o.
  Hochenegg's o.
  Hoffa's o.
  Hoffa-Lorenz o.
  Hofmeister's o.
  Hoke's o.
  Holmes o.
  Holth's o.
  Horgan's o.
  Horsley's o.
  Horton-Devine o.
  Huggins' o.
  Hunter's o.
  Huntington's o.
  Indian o.
  interposition o.
  interval o.
  iris inclusion o.
  Irving's o.
  Irving's sterilization o.
  Italian o.
  Jaboulay's o.
  Jackson-Babcock o.
  Jacobaeus o.
  Jewett o.
  Jonnesco's o.
  Joseph's o.
  Kader's o.
  Kasai o.
  Kazanjian's o.

op·er·a·tion *(continued)*
  Keller o.
  Kelly's o.
  Killian's o.
  Killian-Freer o.
  King's o.
  Knapp's o.
  Kocher's o.
  Kocks o.
  Kondoleon o.
  König's o.
  Körte-Ballance o.
  Kraske's o.
  Krause's o.
  Krimer's o.
  Krönlein's o.
  Kuhnt-Szymanowski o.
  Küstner o.
  Lagrange's o.
  Landolt's o.
  Lane's o.
  Lapidus o.
  Larrey's o.
  laryngeal drop o.
  Latzko's o.
  Laurens o.
  Lawson's o.
  Le Fort's o.
  Le Fort-Neugebauer o.
  Lempert's fenestration o.
  Lisfranc's o.
  Liston's o.
  Lizars' o.
  Lorenz's o.
  Lotheissen's o.
  low forceps o.
  Lowsley's o.
  Luc's o.
  Luckett's o.
  Ludloff's o.
  McBride o.
  McBurney's o.
  Macewen's o.
  Mackenrodt's o.
  MacVay's o.
  McGill's o.
  McKissock's o.
  Madlener o.

op·er·a·tion *(continued)*
    magnet o.
    major o.
    Makkas o.
    Manchester o.
    Marshall-Marchetti o.
    Marshall-Marchetti-Krantz-
        o.
    mastoid o.
    Matas' o.
    Matson's o.
    Maydl's o.
    Mayo's o.
    Meller's o.
    Meyer's o.
    midforceps o.
    mika o.
    Mikulicz's o.
    Miles' o.
    Millard o.
    Millin-Read o.
    minor o.
    Mitchell o.
    Moschcowitz's o.
    Motais' o.
    Mules' o.
    Müller's o.
    Mustard o.
    Naffziger's o.
    Nissen o.
    Ober's o.
    Ollier's o.
    Olshausen's o.
    Ombrédanne's o.
    open o.
    palatal pushback o.
    Partsch's o.
    Patey's o.
    Péan's o.
    Peet's o.
    Pereyra o.
    Phelps' o.
    Phemister o.
    plastic o.
    Pollock's o.
    Polya's o.
    Pomeroy's o.
    Portmann interposition o.

op·er·a·tion *(continued)*
    Potts o.
    Potts-Smith-Gibson o.
    Puussepp's o.
    radical o.
    Ramadier's o.
    Ramstedt's o.
    Rashkind o.
    Rastelli's o.
    reconstructive o.
    Regnoli's o.
    Reverdin's o.
    Ridell o.
    Ripstein o.
    Rose-Thompson o.
    Roux-en-Y o.
    Royle's o.
    saccus o.
    Saemisch's o.
    Sayre's o.
    Scanzoni's o.
    Schauta's o.
    Schauta-Amreich vaginal
        o.
    Schauta-Wertheim o.
    Schede's o.
    Scheie's o.
    Schönbein's o.
    Schwartze's o.
    Sédillot's o.
    Senning o.
    Serre's o.
    seton o.
    shelving o.
    Shirodkar o.
    Silver o.
    Sistrunk o.
    Sjöquist's o.
    Skoog's o.
    Smith's o.
    Smith-Gibson o.
    Smith-Robinson o.
    Smithwick's o.
    Soave o.
    Socin's o.
    Spinelli's o.
    Ssabanejew-Frank o.
    Stacke's o.

op·er·a·tion *(continued)*
  State o.
  Stein o.
  Steindler o.
  Stokes' o.
  Stookey-Scarff o.
  string o.
  Strömbeck o.
  Sturmdorf's o.
  Swenson's o.
  Syme's o.
  Szymanowski's o.
  Taarnhøj's o.
  tack o.
  tagliacotian o.
  Talma's o.
  Tanner's o.
  Tansini's o.
  Tanzer's o.
  Teale's o.
  Tennison-Randall o.
  Tessier's o.
  Thiersch's o.
  Thiersch-Duplay o.
  Torek o.
  Torkildsen's o.
  Toti's o.
  Trendelenburg's o.
  Turner-Warwick o.
  uterine suspension o.
  vacuum extraction o.
  van Hook's o.
  Verhoeff's o.
  Vineberg o.
  Vladimiroff o.
  von Langenbeck's o.
  Waters' o.
  Waterston o.
  Watkins' o.
  Webster's o.
  Weir's o.
  Wertheim's o.
  Wertheim-Schauta o.
  Whipple's o.
  White's o.
  Whitehead's o.
  Whitman's o.
  Wier's o.

op·er·a·tion *(continued)*
  Witzel's o.
  Wölfler's o.
  Woodman's o.
  Young's o.
  Ziegler's o.
op·er·a·tive
op·er·a·tor
  gene o.
oper·cle
oper·cu·la
oper·cu·lar
oper·cu·lat·ed
oper·cu·lec·to·my
oper·cu·li·tis
oper·cu·lum *pl.* oper·cu·la
  cartilaginous o.
  cortical o.
  dental o.
  frontal o.
  o. frontale
  frontoparietal o.
  o. frontoparietale
  opercula of insula
  o. insulae
  occipital o.
  o. orbitale
  parietal o.
  temporal o.
  o. temporale
  trophoblastic o.
op·er·on
  lack o.
OPG/CPA — oculoplethys-
  mography/carotid
  phonoangiography
ophi·a·sis
Ophid·ia
ophi·di·a·sis
ophid·ic
ophi·dism
Oph·i·oph·a·gus han·nah
ophi·o·tox·emia
ophi·tox·emia
Oph·ry·o·gle·ni·na
oph·ry·on
oph·ry·o·sis
Oph·thaine

oph·thal·mag·ra
oph·thal·mal·gia
oph·thal·ma·tro·phia
oph·thal·mec·to·my
oph·thal·men·ceph·a·lon
oph·thal·mia
    actinic ray o.
    Brazilian o.
    catarrhal o.
    caterpillar o.
    o. eczematosa
    Egyptian o.
    electric o.
    flash o.
    gonorrheal o.
    granular o.
    hepatic o.
    jequirity o.
    metastatic o.
    migratory o.
    mucous o.
    o. neonatorum
    neuroparalytic o.
    o. nivialis
    o. nodosa
    periodic o.
    phlyctenular o.
    purulent o.
    scrofulous o.
    solar o.
    spring o.
    strumous o.
    sympathetic o.
    transferred o.
    ultraviolet ray o.
    varicose o.
oph·thal·mi·ac
oph·thal·mi·at·rics
oph·thal·mic
oph·thal·mic acid
oph·thal·mit·ic
oph·thal·mi·tis
    sympathetic o.
oph·thal·mo·blen·nor·rhea
oph·thal·mo·cele
oph·thal·mo·co·pia
oph·thal·mo·des·mi·tis

oph·thal·mo·di·a·phan·o·
  scope
oph·thal·mo·di·as·tim·e·ter
oph·thal·mo·do·ne·sis
oph·thal·mo·dy·na·mom·e·
  ter
oph·thal·mo·dy·na·mom·e·
  try
oph·thal·mo·dyn·ia
oph·thal·mo·ei·ko·nom·e·ter
oph·thal·mo·graph
oph·thal·mog·ra·phy
oph·thal·mo·gy·ric
oph·thal·mo·leu·ko·scope
oph·thal·mo·lith
oph·thal·mo·log·ic
oph·thal·mol·o·gist
oph·thal·mol·o·gy
oph·thal·mo·ma·la·cia
oph·thal·mom·e·ter
oph·thal·mo·met·ro·scope
oph·thal·mom·e·try
oph·thal·mo·my·co·sis
oph·thal·mo·my·ia·sis
oph·thal·mo·my·itis
oph·thal·mo·myo·si·tis
oph·thal·mo·my·ot·o·my
oph·thal·mo·neu·ri·tis
oph·thal·mo·neu·ro·my·eli·
  tis
oph·thal·mo·pa·ral·y·sis
oph·thal·mop·a·thy
    dysthyroid o.
    endocrine o.
    external o.
    hyperthyroid o.
    infiltrative o.
    internal o.
    thyrotoxic o.
oph·thal·mo·pha·com·e·ter
oph·thal·mo·phan·tom
oph·thal·mo·phle·bot·o·my
oph·thal·moph·thi·sis
oph·thal·mo·plas·ty
oph·thal·mo·ple·gia
    basal o.
    congenital o.
    diabetic o.

oph·thal·mo·ple·gia
  (continued)
    exophthalmic o.
    external o.
    fascicular o.
    hyperthyroid o.
    internal o.
    internuclear o.
    nuclear o.
    orbital o.
    painful o.
    Parinaud's o.
    partial o.
    progressive external o.
    relapsing o.
    Sauvineau's o.
    sensorimotor o.
    thyrotoxic o.
    total o.
    o. totalis
oph·thal·mo·ple·gic
oph·thal·mop·to·sis
oph·thal·mo·re·ac·tion
oph·thal·mor·rha·gia
oph·thal·mor·rhea
oph·thal·mor·rhex·is
oph·thal·mo·scope
    binocular o.
    direct o.
    indirect o.
oph·thal·mos·co·py
    direct o.
    indirect o.
    medical o.
    metric o.
oph·thal·mo·spec·tro·scope
oph·thal·mo·spec·tros·co·py
oph·thal·mos·ta·sis
oph·thal·mo·stat
oph·thal·mo·sta·tom·e·ter
oph·thal·mo·ste·re·sis
oph·thal·mo·syn·chy·sis
oph·thal·mo·ther·mom·e·ter
oph·thal·mot·o·my
oph·thal·mo·to·nom·e·ter
oph·thal·mo·to·nom·e·try
oph·thal·mo·tox·in
oph·thal·mo·trope

oph·thal·mo·tro·pom·e·ter
oph·thal·mo·tro·pom·e·try
oph·thal·mo·vas·cu·lar
oph·thal·mo·xe·ro·sis
oph·thal·mox·ys·ter
Oph·thet·ic
Oph·tho·chlor
opi·an
opi·a·nine
opi·ate
Opie paradox
opi·oid
opip·ra·mol hy·dro·chlo·ride
Opi·so·cros·tis
    O. bruneri
opis·the
opis·the·nar
opis·then·ceph·a·lon
opis·thi·o·ba·si·al
opis·thi·on
opis·thio·na·si·al
opis·tho·cra·ni·on
opis·tho·ge·nia
opis·thog·ly·phic
opis·thog·na·thism
opis·tho·mas·ti·gote
opis·tho·po·reia
opis·thor·chi·a·sis
opis·thor·chid
Opis·thor·chis
    O. felineus
    O. noverca
    O. sinensis
    O. tenuicollis
    O. viverrini
opis·thor·cho·sis
opis·thot·ic
opis·thot·o·noid
opis·thot·o·nos
    o. fetalis
Opitz's disease
Opitz's syndrome
opi·um
    crude o.
    denarcotized o.
    o. deodoratum
    deodorized o.
    granulated o.

opi·um *(continued)*
  o. granulatum
  gum o.
  powdered o.
  o. pulveratum
opo·ceph·a·lus
opo·did·y·mus
opod·y·mus
opos·sum
Op·pen·heim's disease
Op·pen·heim's reflex
Op·pen·heim's sign
Op·pen·heim's syndrome
op·po·nens
op·por·tu·nis·tic
op·po·si·tion
op·pos·i·ti·po·lar
OPRT — orotate
  phosphoribosyltransferase
op·si·al·gia
op·sin
op·sin·og·e·nous
op·si·om·e·ter
op·si·uria
op·so·clo·nia
op·so·clo·nus
op·son·ic
op·so·ni·fi·ca·tion
op·so·nin
  immune o.
op·so·ni·za·tion
op·so·nize
op·so·no·cy·to·phag·ic
op·so·no·phil·ia
op·so·no·phil·ic
Op·tef
op·tes·the·sia
op·tic
op·ti·cal
op·ti·cian
op·ti·cian·ry
op·ti·co·ag·no·sia
  Wernicke's subcortical o.
op·ti·co·chi·as·mat·ic
op·ti·co·cil·i·ary
op·ti·co·ki·net·ic
op·ti·co·na·si·on
op·ti·co·pu·pil·lary

op·tics
  fiber o.
op·ti·cus
op·ti·mal
op·tim·e·ter
op·tim·ism
  therapeutic o.
op·ti·mi·za·tion
op·ti·mize
op·ti·mum
op·to·chi·as·mic
op·to·gram
op·to·ki·net·ic
op·to·me·ninx
op·tom·e·ter
op·tom·e·trist
op·tom·e·try
op·to·my·om·e·ter
op·to·phone
op·to·type
Opun·tia
  Mitchell's o.
OPV — poliovirus vaccine live
  oral
OR — operating room
ora *pl.* orae
  o. serrata retinae
Or·a·bi·lex
orad
orae
Or·a·graf·in
oral
ora·le
oral·i·ty
oral·o·gy
or·ange
  o. II
  o. III
  acid o. 10
  acridine o.
  ethyl o.
  o. G
  gold o.
  methyl o.
  Poirrier's o.
  victoria o.
  wool o.

or·an·ge·o·phil
orang·u·tan
Or·a·nix·on
Ora-Tes·tryl
Or·be·li effect
Or·be·li phenomenon
or·bic·u·lar
or·bic·u·la·re
or·bic·u·lar·is
    o. oris
or·bic·u·li
or·bic·u·lus *pl.* or·bic·u·li
    o. ciliaris
or·bit
or·bi·ta *pl.* or·bi·tae
or·bi·tal
or·bi·ta·le
or·bi·ta·lis
or·bi·to·na·sal
or·bi·to·nom·e·ter
or·bi·to·nom·e·try
or·bi·top·a·gus
or·bi·top·a·thy
    dysthyroid o.
    Graves' o.
or·bi·to·stat
or·bi·to·tem·po·ral
or·bi·tot·o·my
or·bi·vi·rus
or·ce·in
or·chec·to·my
or·chel·la
or·chi·al·gia
or·chic
or·chi·cho·rea
or·chi·dal·gia
or·chi·dec·to·my
or·chid·ic
or·chi·di·tis
or·chi·do·epi·did·y·mec·to·my
or·chi·dom·e·ter
    Prader o.
or·chi·don·cus
or·chi·dop·a·thy
or·chi·do·pexy
or·chi·do·plas·ty
or·chi·dop·to·sis

or·chi·dor·rha·phy
or·chi·dot·o·my
or·chi·ec·to·my
or·chi·en·ceph·a·lo·ma
or·chi·epi·did·y·mi·tis
or·chi·lyt·ic
or·chio·ca·tab·a·sis
or·chio·cele
or·chio·dyn·ia
or·chio·my·elo·ma
or·chi·on·cus
or·chio·neu·ral·gia
or·chio·op·a·thy
or·chio·pexy
or·chio·plas·ty
or·chi·or·rha·phy
or·chi·os·cheo·cele
or·chio·scir·rhus
or·chi·ot·o·my
Or·chis
or·chis
or·chit·ic
or·chi·tis
    metastatic o.
    mumps o.
    o. parotidea
    spermatogenic
      granulomatous o.
    traumatic o.
    o. variolosa
or·chi·to·lyt·ic
or·chot·o·my
or·cin
or·ci·nol
ORD — optical rotatory
  dispersion
or·der
    birth o.
    form-o.
or·der·ly
or·di·nate
ore·o·se·li·num
Oret·ic
Oret·i·cyl
Or·e·ton
orex·i·gen·ic
or·gan
    absorbent o.

or·gan *(continued)*
    accessory o's of eye
    acoustic o.
    adipose o.
    Bidder's o.
    cell o.
    cement o.
    Chievitz's o.
    o. of Corti
    critical o.
    cutaneous sense o's
    digestive o's
    effector o.
    enamel o.
    end o.
    essential o. of thalamus
    extraperitoneal o.
    genital o's
    o. of Giraldés
    Golgi tendon o.
    gustatory o.
    intromittent o.
    Jacobson's o.
    lateral line o's
    Marchand's o.
    o's of mastication
    Meyer's o.
    neurotendinous o.
    olfactory o.
    parapineal o.
    parenchymal o.
    parenchymatous o.
    parietal o.
    pineal o.
    primitive fat o.
    reproductive o's
    retroperitoneal o.
    Rosenmüller's o.
    rudimentary o.
    o. of Ruffini
    segmental o.
    sense o's
    sensory o's
    shock o.
    o's of special sense
    spiral o.
    subcommissural o.
    subfornical o.

or·gan *(continued)*
    target o.
    tendon o.
    terminal o.
    urinary o's
    vestibular o.
    vestibulocochlear o's
    vestigial o.
    o. of vision
    visual o.
    vomeronasal o.
    Weber's o.
    o's of Zuckerkandl
or·ga·na
or·ga·nel·la *pl.* or·ga·nel·lae
or·ga·nelle
    paired o.
or·gan·ic
or·gan·i·cism
or·gan·i·cist
Or·gan·i·din
or·ga·nism
    consumer o's
    nitrifying o's
    nitrosifying o's
    pleuropneumonia-like o's
or·gan·i·za·tion
    health maintenance o.
      (HMO)
    preferred provider o. (PPO)
or·ga·nize
or·ga·niz·er
    mesodermic o.
    nucleolar o.
    nucleolus o.
    primary o.
    procentriole o.
    secondary o.
    tertiary o.
or·ga·no·chlo·rine
or·ga·no·fac·tion
or·ga·no·fer·ric
or·ga·no·gel
or·ga·no·gen·e·sis
or·ga·no·ge·net·ic
or·ga·no·gen·ic
or·ga·nog·e·ny
or·ga·nog·ra·phy

or·ga·noid
or·ga·no·lep·tic
or·ga·nol·o·gy
or·ga·no·ma
or·ga·no·meg·a·ly
or·ga·no·mer·cu·ri·al
or·ga·no·me·tal·lic
or·ga·non *pl.* or·ga·na
    o. auditus
    o. parenchymatosum
or·ga·nop·a·thy
or·ga·no·pexy
or·ga·no·phil·ic
or·ga·noph·i·lism
or·ga·no·phos·phate
or·ga·no·phos·pho·rus
or·ga·no·tax·is
or·ga·no·ther·a·py
    heterologous o.
    homologous o.
or·ga·no·trope
or·ga·no·troph·ic
or·ga·no·trop·ic
or·ga·not·ro·pism
or·ga·not·ro·py
or·gan-spe·cif·ic
or·gan·ule
or·ga·num *pl.* or·ga·na
    o. extraperitoneale
    organa genitalia
    o. gustatorium
    o. gustus
    o. olfactorium
    o. olfactus
    o. retroperitoneale
    organa sensoria
    organa sensuum
    o. spirale
    o. subcommissurale
    o. subfornicale
    organa urinaria
    organa uropoëtica
    o. vestibulocochleare
    o. visuale
    o. visus
    o. vomeronasale
or·gasm
    inhibited male o.

or·go·tein
Or·i·ba·si·us
ori·en·ta·tion
    coronal o.
    double o.
    reality o.
    sagittal o.
    transverse o.
or·i·ent·ed
ORIF — open reduction and
  internal fixation
or·i·fice
    aortic o.
    atrioventricular o.
    auriculoventricular o.
    buccal o.
    cardiac o.
    epiploic o.
    esophagogastric o.
    gastroduodenal o.
    golf-hole ureteral o.
    hymenal o.
    mitral o.
    pilosebaceous o's
    pulmonary o.
    pyloric o.
    tricuspid o.
    vaginal o.
    vesicourethral o.
    o. of Vieussens
or·i·fi·cial
ori·fi·ci·um *pl.* ori·fi·cia
    o. externum isthmi
    o. externum uteri
    o. hymenis
    o. internum isthmi
    o. internum uteri
    o. ureteris
    o. urethrae internum
    o. vaginae
or·i·form
or·i·gin
Or·i·mune
Or·i·nase
ori·no·ther·a·py
or·met·o·prim
Or·mond's disease
Orn — ornithine

or·nid·a·zole
or·ni·thine
or·ni·thine am·i·no·trans·fer·
   ase
or·ni·thine car·bam·oyl·
   trans·fer·ase
or·ni·thine de·car·box·y·lase
or·ni·thine-ke·to-ac·id am·i·
   no·trans·fer·ase
or·ni·thin·emia
or·ni·thine trans·car·ba·mo·
   yl·ase
Or·ni·thod·o·ros
   O. coriaceus
   O. hermsi
   O. parkeri
   O. rudis
   O. talaje
   O. turicata
Or·ni·tho·nys·sus
   O. bacoti
   O. bursa
   O. sylviarum
or·ni·tho·sis
oro·an·tral
oro·lin·gual
oro·max·il·lary
oro·men·in·gi·tis
oro·na·sal
oro·phar·ynx
Orop·syl·la
   O. idahoensis
   O. montana
   O. silantiewi
or·o·so·mu·coid
or·o·tate phos·pho·ri·bo·syl·
   trans·fer·ase (OPRT)
orot·ic acid
orot·ic·ac·i·du·ria
orot·i·dine 5′-phos·phate de·
   car·boxy·lase
oro·ti·dine 5′-phos·phate py·
   ro·phos·pho·ryl·ase
orot·i·dyl·ate de·car·box·y·
   lase
oro·ti·dyl·ic acid
Oro·ya fever
or·pa·nox·in

or·phen·a·drine
   o. citrate
   o. hydrochloride
Orr method
Orr technic
Orr treatment
Orr-Loygue technique
or·rho·men·in·gi·tis
or·ris
Or·si-Groc·co method
Orth solution
Orth stain
or·ther·ga·sia
or·the·sis *pl.* or·the·ses
or·thet·ic
or·thet·ics
or·the·tist
or·tho-ac·id
or·tho·ar·te·ri·ot·o·ny
or·tho·bi·o·sis
or·tho·car·di·ac
or·tho·ce·phal·ic
or·tho·ceph·a·lous
or·tho·cho·rea
or·tho·chro·mat·ic
or·tho·chro·mia
or·tho·chro·mic
or·tho·chro·mo·phil
or·tho·cre·sol
or·tho·cy·to·sis
or·tho·dac·ty·lous
or·tho·den·tin
or·tho·de·ox·ia
or·tho·dia·graph
or·tho·di·ag·ra·phy
or·tho·di·chlo·ro·ben·zene
or·tho·dig·i·ta
or·tho·don·tia
or·tho·don·tic
or·tho·don·tics
   corrective o.
   interceptive o.
   preventive o.
   prophylactic o.
   surgical o.
or·tho·don·tist
or·tho·don·tol·o·gy

or·tho·drom·ic
or·tho·gen·e·sis
or·tho·gen·ics
or·tho·gly·ce·mic
Or·thog·na·tha
or·thog·nath·ia
or·thog·na·thic
or·thog·na·thous
or·thog·o·nal
or·tho·grade
or·tho·ker·a·to·sis
or·tho·ki·net·ics
or·tho·mel·ic
or·thom·e·ter
or·tho·mo·lec·u·lar
or·tho·mor·phia
Or·tho·myxo·vi·ri·dae
or·tho·myxo·vi·rus
or·tho·neu·tro·phil
or·tho·pae·dic
or·tho·pae·dics
or·tho·pan·to·graph
Or·tho·pan·to·mo·graph
or·tho·pe·dic
or·tho·pe·dics
    dentofacial o.
    functional jaw o.
or·tho·pe·dist
or·tho·per·cus·sion
or·tho·phe·nan·thro·line
or·thoph·o·ny
or·tho·pho·ria
or·tho·phor·ic
or·tho·phos·phate
or·tho·phos·phor·ic acid
or·tho·phre·nia
or·tho·pia
or·tho·plast
or·tho·ples·sim·e·ter
or·thop·nea
    three-pillow o.
    two-pillow o.
or·thop·ne·ic
or·tho·pod
Or·tho·pox·vi·rus
or·tho·pox·vi·rus
or·tho·prax·is
or·tho·praxy

or·tho·psy·chi·a·try
Or·thop·tera
or·thop·tic
or·thop·tics
or·thop·tist
or·thop·to·scope
or·tho·ra·di·os·co·py
or·tho·rhom·bic
or·tho·roent·ge·nog·ra·phy
or·thor·rhach·ic
or·tho·scope
or·tho·scop·ic
or·thos·co·py
or·tho·sis *pl.* or·tho·ses
    balanced forearm o.
    dynamic o.
    Engen extension o.
    inductive o.
    lively o.
or·tho·stat·ic
or·tho·stat·ism
or·tho·ste·reo·scope
or·tho·sym·pa·thet·ic
or·tho·ther·a·py
or·thot·ic
or·thot·ics
or·thot·ist
or·tho-tol·u·eno-azo-
  be·ta-naph·thol
or·thot·o·nos
or·tho·top·ic
or·tho·vol·tage
Or·thox·ine
or·thu·ria
Or·to·la·ni's click
Or·to·la·ni's sign
Ory·za
ory·ze·nin
OS — L. oculus sinister (left
  eye)
os *pl.* ora
    o. externum uteri
    incompetent cervical o.
    Scanzoni second o.
    o. of uterus, external
os *pl.* os·sa
    o. acetabuli
    o. acromiale

os *(continued)*
- o. acromiale secondarium
- o. basilare
- o. breve
- o. calcis
- o. capitatum
- ossa carpalia
- ossa carpi
- o. centrale
- o. coccygis
- o. coronae
- o. costae
- o. costale
- o. coxae
- ossa cranialia
- ossa cranii
- o. cuboideum
- o. cuneiforme
- o. epitympanicum
- o. ethmoidale
- o. femorale
- ossa fonticulorum
- o. frontale
- o. hamatum
- o. hyoideum
- o. ilii
- o. incae
- o. incisivum
- o. innominatum
- o. intercuneiforme
- o. interfrontale
- o. intermedium
- o. intermetatarseum
- o. interparietale
- o. irregulare
- o. ischii
- o. japonicum
- o. lacrimale
- o. longum
- o. lunatum
- o. magnum
- o. mastoideum
- ossa metacarpalia
- o. multangulum majus
- o. multangulum minus
- o. nasale
- o. naviculare
- o. novum

os *(continued)*
- o. occipitale
- o. odontoideum
- o. orbiculare
- os in os
- o. palatinum
- o. parietale
- o. pedis
- o. pelvicum
- o. penis
- o. peroneum
- o. pisiforme
- o. planum
- o. pneumaticum
- o. priapi
- o. pubis
- o. purum
- o. radiale
- o. sacrale
- o. sacrum
- o. scaphoideum
- o. sedentarium
- ossa sesamoidea manus
- ossa sesamoidea pedis
- o. sphenoidale
- o. styloideum
- o. subtibiale
- ossa suprasternalia
- ossa suturalia
- ossa tarsalia
- ossa tarsi
- o. tarsi fibulare
- o. tarsi tibiale
- o. temporale
- ossa thoracis
- o. tibiale externum
- o. tibiale posterius
- o. trapezium
- o. trapezoideum
- o. triangulare
- o. tribasilare
- o. trigonum tarsi
- o. triquetrum
- o. unguis
- o. vesalianum pedis
- ossa Wormi
- o. zygomaticum

os·amine

OSAS — obstructive sleep
    apnea syndrome
osa·zone
Os·bil
os·ce·do
os·chea
os·che·al
os·che·itis
osch·el·e·phan·ti·a·sis
os·cheo·cele
os·cheo·hy·dro·cele
os·cheo·lith
os·che·o·ma
os·che·on·cus
os·cheo·plas·ty
os·chi·tis
os·cil·la·tion
    bradykinetic o.
    damped o.
os·cil·la·tor
os·cil·lo·gram
os·cil·lo·graph
os·cil·lom·e·ter
os·cil·lo·met·ric
os·cil·lom·e·try
os·cil·lop·sia
os·cil·lo·scope
Os·ci·nis pal·li·pes
os·ci·tate
os·ci·ta·tion
os·cu·lum *pl.* os·cu·la
Os·good-Has·kins test
Os·good-Schlat·ter disease
OSHA — Occupational Safety
    and Health Administration
Os·i·an·der sign
os·la·din
Os·ler's disease
Os·ler's nodes
Os·ler's sign
Os·ler's triad
Os·ler-Va·quez disease
Os·ler-We·ber-Ren·du disease
Os·lo breakfast
Os·lo meal
os·mate
os·mat·ic
os·me·sis

os·mes·the·sia
os·mic
os·mic acid
os·mi·cate
os·mics
os·mi·dro·sis
os·mi·fi·ca·tion
os·mi·oph·i·lic
os·mio·pho·bic
os·mi·um
    o. tetroxide
os·mo·cep·tor
os·mo·con·form·er
os·mol
os·mo·lal
os·mo·lal·i·ty
    calculated serum o.
    urine o.
os·mo·lar
os·mo·lar·i·ty
os·mole
os·mol·o·gy
os·mo·lute
os·mom·e·ter
    freezing-point o.
    Hepp o.
    membrane o.
os·mom·e·try
os·mo·no·sol·o·gy
os·mo·phil·ic
os·mo·pho·bia
os·mo·phore
os·mo·re·cep·tor
os·mo·reg·u·la·tion
os·mo·reg·u·la·tor
os·mo·reg·u·la·to·ry
os·mo·scope
os·mose
os·mo·sis
    reverse o.
os·mo·sol·o·gy
os·mo·stat
os·mo·tax·is
os·mo·ther·a·py
os·mot·ic
osone
os·phre·si·ol·o·gy
os·phre·si·om·e·ter

os·phre·sis
os·phret·ic
os·phy·ar·thro·sis
os·phyo·my·eli·tis
os·phy·ot·o·my
os·sa
os·sa·ture
os·se·in
os·se·let
os·seo·al·bu·moid
os·seo·apo·neu·rot·ic
os·seo·car·ti·lag·i·nous
os·seo·fi·brous
os·seo·in·te·gra·tion
os·seo·lig·a·ment·ous
os·seo·mu·cin
os·seo·mu·coid
os·seo·so·nom·e·ter
os·seo·so·nom·e·try
os·se·ous
os·si·cle
    Andernach's o's
    auditory o's
    o's of Bertin
    epactal o's
    episternal o's
    intercalcar o's
    Kerckring's o.
    pterion o.
    Riolan's o's
    sphenoturbinal o's
    wormian o's
os·sic·u·la
os·sic·u·lar
os·sic·u·lec·to·my
os·sic·u·lo·plas·ty
os·si·cu·lot·o·my
os·sic·u·lum *pl.* os·sic·u·la
    ossicula auditus
os·si·des·mo·sis
os·sif·er·ous
os·sif·ic
os·si·fi·ca·tion
    cartilaginous o.
    ectopic o.
    endochondral o.
    heterotopic o.
    intramembranous o.

os·si·fi·ca·tion *(continued)*
    membranous o.
    metaplastic o.
    perichondral o.
    periosteal o.
os·sif·lu·ence
os·si·form
os·si·fy
os·si·fy·ing
os·si·phone
os·tal·gia
os·tar·thri·tis
os·te·al
os·te·al·bu·moid
os·te·al·gia
os·te·ana·bro·sis
os·te·ana·gen·e·sis
os·te·anaph·y·sis
os·te·ar·thri·tis
os·te·ar·throt·o·my
os·tec·to·my
os·te·in
os·te·ite
os·te·it·ic
os·te·itis
    acute o.
    o. albuminosa
    alveolar o.
    apical o.
    carious o.
    o. carnosa
    caseous o.
    central o.
    chronic o.
    chronic nonsuppurative o.
    o. condensans
    o. condensans generalisata
    o. condensans ilii
    condensing o.
    cortical o.
    o. deformans
    fibrocystic o.
    o. fibrosa circumscripta
    o. fibrosa cystica
    o. fibrosa cystica
      generalisata
    o. fibrosa disseminata
    o. fibrosa localisata

os·te·itis *(continued)*
o. fibrosa osteoplastica
formative o.
o. fragilitans
o. fungosa
Garré's o.
o. granulosa
gummatous o.
hematogenous o.
multifocal o. fibrosa
necrotic o.
o. ossificans
pagetoid o.
parathyroid o.
pedal o.
polycystic o.
productive o.
o. pubis
rarefying o.
sclerosing o.
secondary hyperplastic o.
o. tuberculosa cystica
o. tuberculosa multiplex
   cystoides
typhoid o.
vascular o.
os·te·ma
os·tem·bry·on
os·tem·py·e·sis
Os·ten·sin
os·teo·acu·sis
os·teo·ana·gen·e·sis
os·teo·an·es·the·sia
os·teo·an·eu·rysm
os·teo·ar·threc·to·my
os·teo·ar·thrit·ic
os·teo·ar·thri·tis
o. deformans
o. deformans endemica
endemic o.
erosive o.
hyperplastic o.
hypertrophic o.
interphalangeal o.
ochronotic o.
os·teo·ar·throp·a·thy
familial o. of fingers
hypertrophic o., idiopathic

os·teo·ar·throp·a·thy
(continued)
hypertrophic o., primary
hypertrophic pneumic o.
hypertrophic pulmonary o.
pneumogenic o.
pulmonary o.
secondary hypertrophic o.
tabetic o.
os·teo·ar·thro·sis
o. juvenilis
os·teo·ar·throt·o·my
os·teo·ar·tic·u·lar
os·teo·blast
os·teo·blas·tic
os·teo·blas·to·ma
os·teo·ca·chec·tic
os·teo·ca·chex·ia
os·teo·camp·sia
os·teo·car·ti·lag·i·nous
os·teo·cele
os·teo·ce·men·tum
os·teo·chon·dral
os·teo·chon·dri·tis
adolescent o.
calcaneal o.
o. deformans juvenilis
o. deformans juvenilis dorsi
o. dissecans
o. ischiopubica
juvenile deforming
   metatarsophalangeal o.
o. necroticans
o. ossis metacarpi et
   metatarsi
syphilitic o.
os·teo·chon·dro·ar·throp·a·
thy
os·teo·chon·dro·dys·pla·sia
os·teo·chon·dro·dys·tro·phy
o. deformans
os·te·o·chon·dro·dys·tro·phy
familial o.
os·teo·chon·dro·fi·bro·ma
os·teo·chon·drol·y·sis
os·teo·chon·dro·ma
fibrosing o.

os·teo·chon·dro·ma·to·sis
    Ollier's o.
    synovial o.
os·teo·chon·dro·myx·o·ma
os·teo·chon·dro·path·ia
    o. cretinoidea
os·teo·chon·drop·a·thy
    polyglucose (dextran)
      sulfate–induced o.
os·teo·chon·dro·phyte
os·teo·chon·dro·sar·co·ma
os·teo·chon·dro·sis
    o. deformans tibiae
    o. dissecans
os·teo·chon·drous
os·teo·cla·sia
os·te·oc·la·sis
os·teo·clast
    Collin's o.
os·teo·clas·tic
os·teo·clas·to·ma
os·teo·com·ma
os·teo·cope
os·teo·cop·ic
os·teo·cra·ni·um
os·teo·cys·to·ma
os·teo·cyte
os·teo·den·tin
os·teo·den·ti·no·ma
os·teo·der·mia
os·teo·des·mo·sis
os·teo·di·as·ta·sis
os·te·odyn·ia
os·teo·dys·pla·sia
os·teo·dys·plas·ty
    o. of Melnick and Needles
os·teo·dys·tro·phia
    o. cystica
    o. fibrosa
os·teo·dys·tro·phy
    Albright's hereditary o.
    azotemic o.
    parathyroid o.
    renal o.
os·teo·ec·ta·sia
    familial o.
os·teo·en·chon·dro·ma
os·teo·epiph·y·sis

os·teo·fi·bro·chon·dro·sar·co·ma
os·teo·fi·bro·ma
os·teo·fi·bro·ma·to·sis
    cystic o.
os·teo·fi·bro·sis
os·teo·flu·o·ro·sis
os·teo·gen
os·teo·gen·e·sis
    endochondral o.
    o. imperfecta (OI)
    o. imperfecta congenita
    o. imperfecta cystica
    periosteal o.
os·teo·ge·net·ic
os·te·o·gen·ic
os·te·og·e·nous
os·te·og·e·ny
os·teo·gram
os·te·og·ra·phy
os·teo·ha·lis·ter·e·sis
os·teo·hema·chro·ma·to·sis
os·teo·hy·da·tid·o·sis
os·teo·hy·per·troph·ic
os·te·oid
os·teo·in·duc·tion
os·teo·lath·y·rism
os·teo·lipo·chon·dro·ma
os·teo·li·po·ma
os·teo·lith
os·teo·lo·gia
os·te·ol·o·gist
os·te·ol·o·gy
os·te·ol·y·sis
os·teo·lyt·ic
os·te·o·ma
    cavalryman's o.
    compact o.
    o. cutis
    o. durum
    o. eburneum
    ethmoid sinus o.
    frontal sinus o.
    giant osteoid o.
    ivory o.
    maxillary o.
    o. medullare
    osteoid o.

os·te·o·ma *(continued)*
  o. sarcomatosum
  sphenoidal sinus o.
  o. spongiosum
os·teo·ma·la·cia
  antacid-induced o.
  anticonvulsant o.
  familial hypophosphatemic
    o.
  hepatic o.
  infantile o.
  juvenile o.
  osteogenic o.
  puerperal o.
  renal tubular o.
  senile o.
os·teo·ma·la·cic
os·teo·mal·a·co·sis
os·teo·ma·toid
os·teo·ma·to·sis
os·teo·mere
os·te·om·e·try
os·teo·mi·o·sis
os·teo·my·elit·ic
os·teo·my·eli·tis
  chronic hemorrhagic o.
  chronic sclerosing o.
  conchiolin o.
  diffuse sclerosing o.
  focal sclerosing o.
  Garré's o.
  salmonella o.
  sclerosing nonsuppurative
    o.
  tuberculous spinal o.
  typhoid o.
  o. variolosa
os·teo·my·elo·dys·pla·sia
os·teo·my·elog·ra·phy
os·teo·my·elo·scle·ro·sis
os·teo·myxo·chon·dro·ma
os·te·on
os·teo·ne·cro·sis
os·teo·nec·tin
os·teo·neu·ral·gia
os·te·on·o·sus
os·teo-odon·to·ma

os·teo·path
os·teo·path·ia
  o. condensans
  o. condensans disseminata
  o. condensans generalisata
  o. hemorrhagica infantum
  o. hyperostotica congenita
  o. hyperostotica multiplex
    infantilis
  o. striata
os·teo·path·ic
os·teo·pa·thol·o·gy
os·te·op·a·thy
  alimentary o.
  disseminated condensing o.
  hunger o.
  myelogenic o.
  scorbutic o.
  starvation o.
os·teo·pe·cil·ia
os·teo·pe·di·on
os·teo·pe·nia
  hyperthyroid o.
os·teo·pen·ic
os·teo·peri·os·te·al
os·teo·peri·os·ti·tis
  alveolodental o.
os·teo·pe·tro·sis
  o. gallinarum
os·teo·phage
os·teo·pha·gia
os·teo·phle·bi·tis
os·te·oph·o·ny
os·teo·phy·ma
os·teo·phyte
  bridging o's
os·teo·phy·to·sis
  spinal o.
  subperiosteal o.
os·teo·plaque
os·teo·pla·sia
os·teo·plast
os·teo·plas·tic
os·teo·plas·ti·ca
os·teo·plas·ty
os·teo·poi·ki·lo·sis
os·teo·poi·ki·lot·ic

os·teo·po·ro·sis
   o. circumscripta cranii
   o. of disuse
   postmenopausal o.
   post-traumatic o.
   senile o.
os·teo·po·rot·ic
os·te·op·sath·y·ro·sis
os·teo·ra·dio·ne·cro·sis
os·te·or·rha·gia
os·te·or·rha·phy
os·teo·sar·co·ma
   juxtacortical o.
   parosteal o.
   telangiectatic o.
os·teo·sar·co·ma·tous
os·teo·scle·ro·sis
   o. congenita
   o. fragilis
   o. fragilis generalisata
   o. myelofibrosis
os·teo·scle·rot·ic
os·teo·scope
os·teo·sep·tum
os·te·o·sis
   o. cutis
   o. eburnisans monomelica
   ivory o.
   parathyroid o.
   renal o.
os·teo·su·ture
os·teo·syn·o·vi·tis
os·teo·syn·the·sis
os·teo·ta·bes
os·teo·te·lan·gi·ec·ta·sia
os·teo·throm·bo·phle·bi·tis
os·teo·throm·bo·sis
os·teo·tome
os·te·ot·o·my
   angulation o.
   block o.
   chevron o.
   cuneiform o.
   cup-and-ball o.
   displacement o.
   dome o.
   hinge o.
   innominate o.

os·te·ot·o·my *(continued)*
   intertrochanteric o.
   Le Fort o.
   Le Fort I o.
   linear o.
   Lorenz's o.
   Macewen's o.
   pelvic o.
   sagittal ramus o.
   sagittal split o.
   Salter o.
   sandwich o.
   segmental alveolar o.
   Southwick o.
   step o.
   subtrochanteric o.
   total maxillary o.
   transtrochanteric o.
   vertical ramus o.
   visor o.
   visor/sandwich o.
os·te·o·tribe
os·te·o·trite
os·te·ot·ro·phy
os·te·ot·y·lus
os·teo·tym·pan·ic
os·tia
os·ti·al
os·ti·tis
os·ti·um *pl.* os·tia
   o. aorticum
   o. appendicis vermiformis
   o. arteriosum cordis
   o. atrioventriculare
     dextrum
   o. atrioventriculare
     sinistrum
   o. cardiacum
   o. commune
   coronary o.
   o. ileocaecale
   o. internum uteri
   o. maxillare
   persistent o. primum
   o. primum
   o. pyloricum
   o. secundum
   o. sinus coronarii

os·ti·um *(continued)*
   sinusoidal o.
   sphenoidal o.
   o. trunci pulmonalis
   o. ureteris
   o. urethrae internum
   o. uteri
   o. vaginae
   o. valvae ilealis
   o. venosum cordis
os·to·mate
os·to·my
os·to·sis
os·tra·ceous
os·tra·co·sis
os·treo·tox·ism
os·treo·tox·is·mus
Os·trum-Furst syndrome
Ost·wald's coefficient
Os·wal·do·cru·zia
OT — occupational therapy
   old term (in anatomy)
   original tuberculin
otag·ra
otal·gia
   o. dentalis
   geniculate o.
   o. intermittens
   referred o.
   reflex o.
   tabetic o.
otal·gic
OTC — over the counter
   ornithine
     transcarbamoylase
     (ornithine
     carbamoyltrans-
     ferase)
OTD — organ tolerance dose
otic
otio·bio·sis
otit·ic
oti·tis
   aviation o.
   barotraumatic o.
   catarrhal o.
   o. crouposa
   o. desquamativa

oti·tis *(continued)*
   o. diphtheritica
   o. externa
   o. externa circumscripta
   o. externa diffusa
   o. externa furunculosa
   o. externa hemorrhagica
   o. externa, malignant
   o. externa mycotica
   exudative o. media
   furuncular o.
   influenzal o.
   o. interna
   o. labyrinthica
   malignant o. externa
   o. mastoidea
   o. media
   o. media, adhesive
   o. media, secretory
   o. media, serous
   o. media catarrhalis acuta
   o. media catarrhalis
     chronica
   o. media purulenta acuta
   o. media purulenta
     chronica
   o. media sclerotica
   o. media serosa
   o. media suppurativa
   o. media vasomotorica
   mucosis o.
   mucosus o.
   mycotic o. externa
   o. mycotica
   necrotizing o. externa
   necrotizing o. media
   parasitic o.
   pneumococcal o. media
   o. sclerotica
   traumatic o.
   tuberculous o. media
oto·ac·a·ri·a·sis
oto·an·tri·tis
oto·bi·o·sis
Oto·bi·us
oto·blen·nor·rhea
oto·ca·ri·a·sis
oto·ceph·a·lus

oto·ceph·a·ly
oto·cer·e·bri·tis
oto·clei·sis
oto·co·nia
otoc·o·nite
oto·co·ni·um
oto·cra·ni·al
oto·cra·ni·um
oto·cyst
Oto·dec·tes
oto·dyn·ia
oto·en·ceph·a·li·tis
oto·gan·gli·on
oto·gen·ic
otog·e·nous
otog·ra·phy
oto·lar·yn·gol·o·gist
oto·lar·yn·gol·o·gy
oto·lith
oto·li·thi·a·sis
oto·log·ic
otol·o·gist
otol·o·gy
oto·mas·toid·itis
oto·mu·cor·my·co·sis
oto·my·as·the·nia
Oto·my·ces
    O. hageni
    O. purpureus
oto·my·co·sis
    o. aspergillina
oto·my·ia·sis
oto·neu·ral·gia
oto·neu·ro·log·ic
oto·neu·rol·o·gy
otop·a·thy
oto·pha·ryn·ge·al
oto·plas·ty
    Crikelair o.
    Mustarde flap o.
oto·poly·pus
oto·py·or·rhea
oto·py·o·sis
oto·rhi·no·lar·yn·gol·o·gist
oto·rhi·no·lar·yn·gol·o·gy
oto·rhi·nol·o·gy
otor·rha·gia
otor·rhea

otor·rhea
    cerebrospinal fluid o.
oto·sal·pinx
oto·scle·ro·sis
    clinical o.
    cochlear o.
    obliterative o.
oto·scle·rot·ic
oto·scope
    Brunton's o.
    Siegle's o.
    Toynbee's o.
otos·co·py
oto·sis
oto·spon·gi·o·sis
    o. otosclerosis syndrome
otos·te·ons
oto·tox·ic
oto·tox·ic·i·ty
Otri·vin
Ott's test
Ot·to disease
Ot·to pelvis
OU — L. oculus uterque (each eye)
oua·ba·in
Ouch·ter·lo·ny technique
Ou·din current
Ou·din resonator
oulec·to·my
ouli·tis
ounce
    apothecary's o. (oz. ap.)
    o. avoirdupois (oz.)
    fluid o.
    o. troy (oz. t.)
out·break
out·breed·ing
out·cross
Out·er·bridge's ridge
Out·er·bridge's scale
out·flow
    craniosacral o.
    thoracolumbar o.
out·frac·ture
out·let
    pelvic o.
    thoracic o.

out·li·er
out·limb
out·pa·tient
out·pock·et
out·pock·et·ing
out·pouch·ing
out·put
    cardiac o.
    energy o.
    insensible fluid o.
    stroke o.
    urinary o.
ova
oval
ov·al·bu·min
ova·lo·cy·tary
ovalo·cyte
ovalo·cy·to·sis
ovar·i·al·gia
ovar·i·an
ovar·i·ec·to·my
ovar·io·cele
ovar·io·cen·te·sis
ovar·io·cy·e·sis
ovar·io·dys·neu·ria
ovar·io·ep·i·lep·sy
ovar·i·o·gen·ic
ovar·io·hys·ter·ec·to·my
ovar·io·lyt·ic
ovar·i·op·a·thy
ovar·io·pexy
ovar·i·or·rhex·is
ovar·io·sal·pin·gec·to·my
ovar·io·ste·re·sis
ovar·i·os·to·my
ovar·io·tes·tis
ovar·i·ot·o·my
    abdominal o.
    vaginal o.
ovar·io·tu·bal
ova·ri·tis
ova·ri·um *pl.* ova·ria
    o. bipartitum
    o. gyratum
    o. lobatum
    o. masculinum
ova·ry
    adenocystic o.

ova·ry *(continued)*
    embryonic o.
    oyster o's
    polycystic o.
OVD — occlusal vertical
  dimension
over·bite
    deep o.
    horizontal o.
    vertical o.
over·breath·ing
over·clo·sure
    reduced interarch distance
    o.
over·com·pen·sa·tion
over·cor·rec·tion
over·den·ture
over·de·ter·mi·na·tion
over·dom·i·nance
over·dose
over·do·sage
over·drive
over·erup·tion
over·ex·ten·sion
over·flex·ion
over·flow
over·graft
over·graft·ing
over·growth
over·hang
over·hy·dra·tion
over·in·fla·tion
    nonobstructive pulmonary
    o.
    obstructive pulmonary o.
over·jet
over·jut
over·lap
    horizontal o.
    vertical o.
over·lay
    emotional o.
    psychogenic o.
over·load
    aortic o.
    circulatory o.
    iron o.
over·nu·tri·tion

over·pro·tec·tion
    maternal o.
over·reach·ing
over·re·sponse
over·rid·ing
over·stain
over·stim·u·la·tion
over·strain
over·stress
over·toe
over·tone
    psychic o.
over·trans·fu·sion
over·tube
    Christopher-Williams o.
over·ven·ti·la·tion
over·weight
ovi·cide
ovi·du·cal
ovi·duct
ovi·duc·tal
ovif·er·ous
ovi·form
ovi·gen·e·sis
ovi·ge·net·ic
ovi·gen·ic
ovig·e·nous
ovi·germ
ovig·er·ous
ovi·par·i·ty
ovip·a·rous
ovi·po·si·tion
ovi·pos·i·tor
ovi·sac
ovist
ovi·um
ovo·cyte
ovo·fla·vin
ovo·gen·e·sis
ovo·glob·u·lin
ovo·go·ni·um
ovoid
    fetal o.
    Manchester o.
ovo·lyt·ic
ovo·mu·cin
ovo·mu·coid
ovo·plasm

ovo·tes·tis
ovo·trans·fer·rin
ovo·vi·tel·lin
ovo·vivi·par·i·ty
ovo·vi·vip·a·rous
Ov·rette
ov·u·la
ovu·lar
ovu·la·tion
    amenstrual o.
    anestrous o.
    paracyclic o.
    supplementary o.
ov·u·la·to·ry
ovule
    graafian o's
    Naboth's o's
    primitive o.
    primordial o.
ovu·log·e·nous
ov·u·lum *pl.* ov·u·la
    ovula nabothi
ovum *pl.* ova
    alecithal o.
    blighted o.
    Bryce-Teacher o.
    centrolecithal o.
    cleidoic o.
    ectolecithal o.
    fertilized o.
    Hertig-Rock ova
    holoblastic o.
    isolecithal o.
    macrolecithal o.
    Mateer-Streeter o.
    medialecithal o.
    megalecithal o.
    meroblastic o.
    mesolecithal o.
    microlecithal o.
    Miller o.
    miolecithal o.
    oligolecithal o.
    permanent o.
    Peters' o.
    primitive o.
    primordial o.
    Rock's ova

ovum *(continued)*
    telolecithal o.
    unfertilized o.
Owen's lines
Ow·ren's deficiency
Ow·ren's disease
ox·ac·id
ox·a·cil·lin so·di·um
Ox·aine
ox·al·al·de·hyde
ox·a·late
    ammonium o.
    balanced o.
    calcium o.
    potassium o.
ox·a·lat·ed
ox·a·la·tion
ox·a·le·mia
ox·al·ic acid
Ox·a·lid
ox·al·ism
ox·a·lo·ac·e·tate
ox·a·lo·ace·tic acid
ox·a·lo·sis
ox·a·lo·suc·cin·ate
ox·a·lo·suc·cin·ic acid
ox·al·uria
ox·al·ur·ic acid
ox·a·lyl
ox·a·lyl·urea
ox·am·ide
ox·am·ni·quine
ox·an·amide
ox·an·dro·lone
ox·an·tel pam·o·ate
ox·a·pro·zin
ox·ar·ba·zole
ox·a·to·mide
ox·az·e·pam
ox·eth·a·zaine
ox·et·o·rone fu·mar·ate
ox·fen·da·zole
ox·i·ben·da·zole
ox·i·dant
ox·i·dase
    direct o.
    indirect o.

ox·i·dase *(continued)*
    primary o.
ox·i·da·tion
    aerobic o.
    anaerobic o.
    beta o.
    biological o.
    coupled o.
    omega o.
ox·i·da·tion-re·duc·tion
ox·i·da·tive
ox·ide
    arsenous o.
    diethyl o.
    stannic o.
ox·i·di·za·ble
ox·i·dize
ox·i·do·pa·mine
ox·i·do·re·duc·tase
ox·i·do·re·duc·tion
ox·i·do·sis
ox·i·fun·gin hy·dro·chlo·ride
ox·il·or·phan
ox·ime
ox·im·e·ter
    ear o.
    finger o.
    intracardiac o.
    pulse o.
    whole blood o.
ox·im·e·try
ox·i·per·o·mide
ox·ir·amide
ox·i·sur·an
ox·met·i·dine mes·y·late
oxo acid
oxo-ac·id-ly·ase
3-oxo·ac·yl-ACP re·duc·tase
3-oxo·ac·yl-ACP syn·thase
oxo·ges·tone phen·pro·pi·o·nate
oxo·glu·ta·rate de·hy·dro·gen·ase
2-oxo·glu·tar·ic acid
2-oxo·iso·val·er·ate de·hy·dro·gen·ase (lipoamide)
oxo·lin·ic acid
oxo·ni·um

oxo·phen·ar·sine hy·dro·chlo·ride
5-oxo·pro·li·nase (ATP hydrolyzing)
5-oxo·pro·line
5-oxo·pro·lin·uria
ox·pen·tif·yl·line
ox·pren·o·lol hy·dro·chlo·ride
Ox·sor·a·len
ox·triph·yl·line
oxy·achres·tia
oxy·ac·id
oxy·ben·zene
oxy·ben·zo·ic acid
oxy·ben·zone
oxy·blep·sia
oxy·bu·ty·nin chlo·ride
oxy·bu·tyr·ia
oxy·bu·tyr·ic·ac·i·de·mia
oxy·cal·o·rim·e·ter
Oxy·cel
oxy·ce·phal·ic
oxy·ceph·a·lous
oxy·ceph·a·ly
oxy·chlo·ride
oxy·chlo·ro·sene
 o. sodium
oxy·cho·line
oxy·chro·mat·ic
oxy·chro·ma·tin
oxy·ci·ne·sia
oxy·co·done hy·dro·chlo·ride
oxy·cy·a·nide
oxy·den·dron
oxy·ecoia
oxy·es·the·sia
oxy·ethero·ther·a·py
ox·y·gen
 blow-by o.
 excess o.
 heavy o.
 high pressure o.
 hyperbaric o.
 molecular o.
 singlet o.
 T-piece o.
ox·y·ge·nase
ox·y·ge·nate

ox·y·gen·at·ed
ox·y·ge·na·tion
 apneic o.
 extracorporeal membrane o. (ECMO)
 hyperbaric o.
ox·y·ge·na·tor
 bubble o.
 disk o.
 film o.
 membrane o.
 pump-o.
 rotating disk o.
 screen o.
ox·y·gen·ic
oxy·geu·sia
oxy·he·ma·tin
oxy·hem·a·to·por·phy·rin
oxy·heme
oxy·he·mo·chro·mo·gen
oxy·he·mo·cy·a·nine
oxy·he·mo·glo·bin
oxy·hy·dro·ceph·a·lus
oxy·hy·per·gly·ce·mia
oxy·io·dide
oxy·lal·ia
Oxy·lone
oxy·met·az·o·line hy·dro·chlo·ride
oxy·meth·o·lone
ox·ym·e·try
oxy·mor·phone hy·dro·chlo·ride
oxy·myo·glo·bin
oxy·myo·he·ma·tin
oxy·ner·von
oxy·neu·rine
ox·yn·tic
oxy·opia
oxy·op·ter
oxy·o·sis
oxy·os·mia
oxy·os·phre·sia
oxy·para·plas·tin
oxy·pa·thia
ox·yp·a·thy
oxy·per·tine
oxy·phen·bu·ta·zone

oxy·phen·cy·cli·mine hy·dro·
  chlo·ride
oxy·phe·ni·sa·tin
    o. acetate
oxy·phe·no·ni·um bro·mide
oxy·phen·yl·eth·yl·amine
oxy·phil
oxy·phil·ic
ox·yph·i·lous
oxy·pho·nia
Oxy·pho·to·bac·te·ria
oxy·plasm
oxy·pu·rine
oxy·pur·i·nol
oxy·quin·o·line sul·fate
oxy·rhine
oxy·salt
oxy·san·to·nin
oxy·spore
ox·yt·a·lan
ox·yt·a·lan·ol·y·sis
oxy·tet·ra·cy·cline
    o. calcium
    o. hydrochloride
oxy·to·cia
oxy·to·cic

oxy·to·cin
    arginine o.
    o. citrate
oxy·to·ci·nase
ox·yt·ro·pism
oxy·uria
oxy·uri·a·sis
oxy·uri·cide
oxy·urid
oxy·uri·fuge
oxy·uri·o·sis
Ox·y·u·ris
    O. incognita
oxy·uroid
Oxy·uroi·dea
oz — ounce
oza·min
oze·na
    o. laryngis
oze·nous
ozo·li·none
ozone
ozo·nom·e·ter
ozo·no·phore
ozo·sto·mia

P

P — para
    peta-
    phosphate group
    phosphorus
    poise
    posterior
    premolar
    pupil
    plasma
P — power
    pressure
    probability
P_1 — parental generation

P_2 — pulmonic second sound
P_{CO_2} — carbon dioxide partial
    pressure (tension)
P_i — orthophosphate
P_{O_2} — oxygen partial pressure
    (tension)
p — pico-
    proton
    short arm of a chromosome
p — momentum
    probability
p- — para-
π — osmotic pressure

PA — pernicious anemia
    physician assistant
    posteroanterior
    pulmonary artery
Pa — pascal
    protactinium
P&A — percussion and
    auscultation
Paas' disease
PAB — para-aminobenzoic
    acid
PABA — para-aminobenzoic
    acid
Pab·a·nol
pab·u·lar
pab·u·lin
pab·u·lum
PAC — papular
    achrodermatitis of childhood
    premature atrial
      contraction
Pac·chi·o·ni's foramen
Pac·chi·o·ni's fossae
Pac·chi·o·ni's granulations
pac·chi·o·ni·an depressions
pac·chi·o·ni·an foramen
pac·chi·o·ni·an granulations
pace·mak·er
    artificial p.
    asynchronous p.
    cardiac p.
    cardiac p., artificial
    catheter p.
    Chardack-Greatbatch p.
    cilium p.
    Cyberlith p.
    demand p.
    ectopic p.
    external p.
    fixed-rate p.
    gastric p.
    p. of heart
    implanted p.
    internal p.
    Nathan p.
    radio-frequency p.
    shifting p.

pace·mak·er *(continued)*
    Spectrax programmable
      Medtronic p.
    synchronous p.
    transthoracic p.
    transvenous p.
    uterine p.
    ventricular p.
    wandering p.
pa·chom·e·ter
Pa·chon's method
pachy·bleph·a·ron
pachy·bleph·a·ro·sis
pachy·ce·phal·ic
pachy·ceph·a·lous
pachy·ceph·a·ly
pachy·chei·lia
pachy·chro·mat·ic
pachy·dac·tyl·ia
pachy·dac·ty·ly
pachy·der·ma
    p. vesicae
pachy·der·ma·to·cele
pachy·der·ma·tous
pachy·der·mic
pachy·der·mo·peri·os·to·sis
pachy·glos·sia
pa·chyg·na·thous
pachy·gy·ria
pachy·lep·to·men·in·gi·tis
pachy·men·in·ges
pachy·men·in·gi·tis
    cerebral p.
    p. cervicalis hypertrophica
    circumscribed p.
    external p.
    fibrinohemorrhagic p.
    hemorrhagic internal p.
    hypertrophic spinal p.
    internal p.
    p. intralamellaris
    purulent p.
    pyogenic p.
    serous internal p.
    spinal p.
    suppurative p.
    syphilitic p.
pachy·men·in·gop·a·thy

pachy·me·ninx *pl.* pachy·me·
   nin·ges
pachy·ne·ma
pa·chyn·sis
pa·chyn·tic
pachy·onych·ia
   p. congenita
pachy·pel·vi·peri·to·ni·tis
pachy·peri·os·teo·der·ma
pachy·peri·os·ti·tis
pachy·peri·to·ni·tis
pachy·pleu·ri·tis
pachy·rhi·zid
pachy·sal·pin·gi·tis
pachy·sal·pin·go-ova·ri·tis
pachy·tene
pachy·vag·i·nal·itis
pach·y·vag·i·ni·tis
   cystic p.
pac·i·fi·er
pac·ing
   atrial p.
   cardiac p.
   diaphragm p.
   endocardial p.
   epicardial p.
   overdrive p.
   paired p.
   programmed p.
   sequential p.
   ventricular p.
Pa·ci·ni's corpuscles
pa·cin·i·an
pa·cin·i·tis
pack
   cold p.
   dry p.
   full p.
   half p.
   hot p.
   ice p.
   internuclear p.
   Mikulicz p.
   one sheet p.
   partial p.
   periodontal p.
   salt p.
   surgical p.

pack *(continued)*
   three-quarters p.
   throat p.
   wet p.
   wet-sheet p.
pack·er
pack·ing
   denture p.
pad
   abdominal p.
   Bichat's fat p.
   buccal fat p.
   butterfly p.
   dinner p.
   fat p.
   gum p's
   infrapatellar fat p.
   knuckle p's
   occlusal p.
   Passavant's p.
   periarterial p.
   retrodiscal p.
   retromolar p.
   retropatellar fat p.
   sucking p.
   suctorial p.
   synovial fat p.
Pad·gett's dermatome
pad·i·mate A
pad·i·mate O
Pae·cilo·my·ces
   P. variotii
Pae·der·us
PAF — platelet activating
   factor
PAF-ac·e·ther
PAFD — percutaneous
   abscess and fluid drainage
PAGE — polyacrylamide gel
   electrophoresis
Pa·gen·stech·er's ointment
Pa·get's cell
Pa·get's disease
Pa·get's necrosis
Pa·get's tests
Pa·get-von Schroet·ter
   syndrome
pa·get·ic

pag·et·oid
Pag·i·tane
pa·go·pha·gia
pa·go·plex·ia
PAH — para-aminohippuric acid
PAHA — para-aminohippuric acid
Pah·vant Val·ley fever
Pah·vant Val·ley plague
PAI — plasminogen activator inhibitor
pai·don·yx
pain
    atypical facial p.
    bearing-down p.
    boring p.
    Brodie's p.
    central p.
    Charcot's p's
    cross-referred p.
    dilating p's
    eccentric p.
    evoked contralateral p.
    expulsive p's
    false p's
    fulgurant p's
    gas p's
    girdle p.
    griping p.
    growing p's
    heterotopic p.
    homotopic p.
    hunger p.
    intermenstrual p.
    jumping p.
    labor p's
    lancinating p.
    lightning p's
    middle p.
    osteocopic p.
    phantom limb p.
    piercing p.
    postprandial p.
    precordial p.
    premonitory p's
    psychic p.
    psychogenic p.

pain (continued)
    referred p.
    rest p.
    root p.
    shooting p's
    spot p's
    stabbing p.
    starting p's
    terebrant p.
    terebrating p.
    thalamic p.
    vasculosympathetic facial p.
    wandering p.
paint
    antiseptic p.
    Castellani's p.
pair
    base p.
    buffer p.
    ion p.
pair·ing
    base p.
    distributive p.
    exchange p.
    somatic p.
pa·ja·ro·e·llo
Pa·jot's hook
Pa·jot's law
Pa·jot's maneuver
pak·u·rin
Pal's stain
Pal·ade
pal·aeo·cer·e·bel·lum
pal·aeo·cor·tex
pa·la·ta
pal·a·tal
pal·ate
    artificial p.
    bony p.
    bony hard p.
    cleft p.
    gothic p.
    hard p.
    osseous p.
    pendulous p.
    primary p.
    secondary p.

pal·ate *(continued)*
 smoker's p.
 soft p.
 submucous cleft p.
pal·a·tine
pal·a·ti·tis
pal·a·to·glos·sal
pal·a·tog·na·thous
pal·a·to·graph
pal·a·tog·ra·phy
pal·a·to·max·il·lary
pal·a·to·myo·graph
pal·a·to·my·og·ra·phy
pal·a·to·na·sal
pal·a·top·a·gus
pal·a·to·pha·ryn·ge·al
pal·a·to·pha·ryn·go·plas·ty
pal·a·to·plas·ty
 Wardill p.
pal·a·to·ple·gia
pal·a·to·prox·i·mal
pal·a·tor·rha·phy
pal·a·to·sal·pin·ge·us
pal·a·tos·chi·sis
pa·la·tum *pl.* pa·la·ta
 p. durum
 p. durum osseum
 p. fissum
 p. molle
 p. ogivale
 p. osseum
pa·le·en·ceph·a·lon
pa·leo·cer·e·bel·lar
pa·leo·cer·e·bel·lum
pa·leo·cor·tex
pa·leo·gen·e·sis
pa·leo·ge·net·ic
pa·leo·ki·net·ic
pa·leo-olive
pa·leo·pal·li·um
pa·leo·pa·thol·o·gy
pa·leo·ru·brum
pa·leo·sen·sa·tion
pa·leo·stri·a·tal
pa·leo·stri·a·tum
pa·leo·thal·a·mus
pali·ci·ne·sia
pali·gra·phia

pali·ki·ne·sia
pali·la·lia
pal·in·drome
pal·in·dro·mia
pal·in·dro·mic
pal·in·gen·e·sis
pal·in·gra·phia
pal·in·mne·sis
pal·i·no·dia
pal·i·nop·sia
pal·in·phra·sia
pali·phra·sia
pal·i·sade
pal·la·di·um
pall·an·es·the·sia
pall·es·the·sia
pall·es·thet·ic
pall·hyp·es·the·sia
pal·li·al
pal·li·ate
pal·li·a·tive
pal·li·dal
pal·li·dec·to·my
pal·li·do·an·sec·tion
pal·li·do·an·sot·o·my
pal·li·dof·u·gal
pal·li·do·hy·po·tha·lam·ic
pal·li·doi·do·sis
pal·li·dot·o·my
pal·li·dum
 p. I
 p. II
pal·li·dus
 globus p.
pal·li·um
pal·lor
 elevational p.
 temporal p.
palm
 handball p.
pal·ma *pl.* pal·mae
 p. manus
 palmae plicatae
pal·mae
pal·man·es·the·sia
pal·mar
pal·mar·is
pal·mate

pal·ma·ture
pal·mes·the·sia
pal·mes·thet·ic
pal·mi·tal
pal·mi·tate
pal·mit·ic acid
pal·mi·tin
pal·mi·to·le·ic acid
pal·mi·tone
pal·mi·to·yl-CoA
pal·mi·to·yl-CoA hyd·ro·lase
pal·mo·men·tal
pal·mus
palp
palp·a·ble
pal·pate
pal·pa·tion
    bimanual p.
    light touch p.
pal·pa·tom·e·try
pal·pa·to·per·cus·sion
pal·pe·bra *pl.* pal·pe·brae
    p. inferior
    p. superior
    p. tertius
pal·pe·brae
pal·pe·bral
pal·pe·bral·is
pal·pe·brate
pal·pe·bra·tion
pal·pe·bri·tis
pal·pi·form
pal·pi·tate
pal·pi·ta·tion
PALS — periarterial
  lymphoid sheath
pal·sy
    acute thyrotoxic bulbar p.
    atonic cerebral p.
    Bell's p.
    bilateral cord p.
    birth p.
    brachial p.
    bulbar p.
    cerebral p.
    craft p.
    cranial nerve p.
    creeping p.

pal·sy *(continued)*
    crossed leg p.
    diver's p.
    epidemic infantile p.
    Erb's p.
    facial p.
    hammer p.
    hod-carriers' p.
    hypotonic cerebral p.
    infantile cerebral p.
    infantile progressive
      bulbar p.
    inherited bulbar p.
    ischemic p.
    jake p.
    Klumpke's p.
    Landry's p.
    lateral popliteal p.
    lead p.
    minimal cerebral p.
    night p.
    occupational p.
    ocular p.
    painters' p.
    palate p.
    pharyngeal p.
    posticus p.
    pressure p.
    printer's p.
    progressive supranuclear p.
    pseudobulbar p.
    radial p.
    Saturday night p.
    scriveners' p.
    shaking p.
    spastic bulbar p.
    supranuclear p.
    tardy median p.
    tardy ulnar p.
    Todd's p.
    transverse p.
    unilateral cord p.
    wasting p.
Pal·tauf's dwarf
Pal·tauf stain
pal·u·dism
Pal·u·drine
pam·a·brom

pam·a·quine
   p. naphthoate
pam·a·to·lol sul·fate
Pam·ine
Pam·i·syl
pam·o·ate
pam·pin·i·form
pam·pin·ocele
pam·ple·gia
PAN — periodic alternating
  nystagmus
    polyarteritis nodosa
Pan
pan·a·cea
pan·ac·i·nar
pan·ag·glu·tin·a·ble
pan·ag·glu·ti·na·tion
pan·ag·glu·ti·nin
pan·an·gi·itis
   diffuse necrotizing p.
pan·an·xi·e·ty
pan·ar·te·ri·tis
   p. nodosa
pan·ar·thri·tis
pan·at·ro·phy
   p. of Gowers
pan·au·to·no·mic
pan·blas·tic
pan·car·di·tis
   rheumatic p.
pan·cav·er·no·si·tis
pan·chro·mat·ic
pan·chro·mia
Pan·coast's suture
Pan·coast's syndrome
Pan·coast's tumor
pan·co·lec·to·my
pan·cre·al·gia
pan·cre·as *pl.* pan·cre·a·ta
   aberrant p.
   p. accessorium
   accessory p.
   annular p.
   Aselli's p.
   divided p.
   p. divisum
   dorsal p.
   lesser p.

pan·cre·as *(continued)*
   unciform p.
   ventral p.
   Willis' p.
   Winslow's p.
pan·cre·a·ta
pan·cre·a·tal·gia
pan·cre·a·tec·to·my
pan·cre·at·ic
pan·cre·at·i·co·du·o·de·nal
pan·cre·at·i·co·du·o·de·nec·
  to·my
pan·cre·at·i·co·du·o·de·nos·
  to·my
pan·cre·at·i·co·en·ter·os·to·
  my
pan·cre·at·i·co·gas·tros·to·
  my
pan·cre·at·i·co·je·ju·nos·to·
  my
pan·cre·at·i·co·splen·ic
pan·cre·a·tin
pan·cre·a·ti·tis
   acute hemorrhagic p.
   calcereous p.
   centrilobar p.
   chronic relapsing p.
   edematous p.
   interstitial p.
   mumps p.
   perilobar p.
   purulent p.
pan·cre·a·to·du·o·de·nec·to·
  my
pan·cre·a·to·du·o·de·nos·to·
  my
pan·cre·a·to·en·ter·os·to·my
pan·cre·a·to·gen·ic
pan·cre·a·tog·e·nous
pan·cre·a·to·gram
pan·cre·a·tog·ra·phy
   endoscopic retrograde p.
pan·crea·to·lip·ase
pan·cre·ato·lith
pan·cre·a·to·li·thec·to·my
pan·cre·a·to·li·thi·a·sis
pan·cre·a·to·li·thot·o·my
pan·cre·a·tol·y·sis

pan·cre·a·to·lyt·ic
pan·crea·to·meg·a·ly
pan·cre·at·o·my
pan·cre·a·top·a·thy
pan·cre·a·tot·o·my
pan·cre·a·to·trop·ic
pan·cre·a·trop·ic
pan·cre·ec·to·my
pan·cre·li·pase
pan·creo·li·thot·o·my
pan·cre·ol·y·sis
pan·creo·lyt·ic
pan·cre·op·a·thy
pan·creo·priv·ic
pan·creo·ther·a·py
pan·cre·o·trop·ic
pan·creo·zy·min
pan·cul·tured
pan·cu·ro·ni·um bro·mide
pan·cys·ti·tis
pan·cy·tol·y·sis
pan·cy·to·pe·nia
   congenital p.
   Fanconi's p.
   tropical canine p.
pan·cy·to·sis
pan·dem·ic
pan·dem·ic·i·ty
Pan·der's islands
Pan·der's layer
Pan·der's nucleus
pan·dic·u·la·tion
Pán·dy's reaction
Pán·dy's test
pan·dys·auto·no·mia
pan·el
pan·elec·tro·scope
pan·en·ceph·a·li·tis
   Pette-Döring p.
   subacute sclerosing p.
pan·en·dog·ra·phy
pan·en·do·scope
   oral p.
pan·en·dos·co·py
pan·epi·zo·ot·ic
pan·es·the·sia
pan·es·thet·ic
Pa·neth's cells

pang
   breast p.
   brow p.
pan·gen·e·sis
pan·glos·sia
Pan·go·nia
pan·hem·a·to·pe·nia
   primary splenic p.
Pan·hep·rin
pan·hy·drom·e·ter
pan·hy·dro·sis
pan·hy·per·emia
pan·hy·po·gam·ma·glob·u·lin·emia
pan·hy·po·go·nad·ism
pan·hy·po·pi·tu·i·ta·rism
   prepubertal p.
pan·hys·ter·ec·to·my
pan·hys·tero·col·pec·to·my
pan·hys·tero-ooph·o·rec·to·my
pan·hys·tero·sal·pin·gec·to·my
pan·hys·ter·o·sal·pin·go-ooph·o·rec·to·my
pan·ic
   homosexual p.
pan·im·mu·ni·ty
Pan·iz·za's plexus
Panje voice button
pan·leu·ko·pe·nia
pan·lob·u·lar
pan·mix·ia
pan·mix·is
Pan·my·cin
pan·my·eloid
pan·my·elo·pa·thia
pan·my·elop·a·thy
   constitutional infantile p.
pan·my·elo·phthi·sis
pan·my·e·lo·sis
Pan·ner's disease
pan·neu·ri·tis
   p. epidemica
pan·neu·ro·sis
pan·nic·u·lal·gia
pan·nic·u·lec·to·my

pan·nic·u·li
pan·nic·u·li·tis
    LE p.
    lupus p.
    nodular nonsuppurative p.
    relapsing febrile nodular
      nonsuppurative p.
    subacute nodular
      migratory p.
    Weber-Christian p.
pan·nic·u·lus *pl.* pan·nic·u·li
    p. adiposus
    p. carnosus
    hanging p.
pan·nus
    p. carateus
    degenerative p.
    p. degenerativus
    glaucomatous p.
    phlyctenular p.
    p. siccus
    p. trachomatosus
pa·nod·ic
pano·pho·bia
pan·oph·thal·mia
pan·oph·thal·mi·tis
pan·op·tic
pan·os·te·itis
pan·oti·tis
pan·pho·bia
pan·ple·gia
pan·proc·to·co·lec·to·my
pan·ret·i·nal
Pansch's fissure
pan·scle·ro·sis
pan·sen·si·tive
pan·sep·tum
pan·si·nu·itis
pan·si·nus·ec·to·my
pan·si·nus·itis
pan·sper·mia
pan·sper·mic
pan·sper·my
pan·sphyg·mo·graph
pan·sporo·blast
Pan·sporo·blas·ti·na
Pan·stron·gy·lus
    P. geniculatus

Pan·stron·gy·lus (continued)
    P. infestans
    P. megistus
pan·sys·tol·ic
pan·ta·chro·mat·ic
pan·tal·gia
pan·ta·mor·phia
pan·ta·mor·phic
pan·tan·en·ceph·a·ly
pan·tan·ky·lo·bleph·a·ron
pan·ta·tro·phia
pan·tat·ro·phy
Pan·ter·ic
pan·te·the·ine
pan·the·nol
pan·ther·ine
pan·thod·ic
Pan·tho·lin
pant·ing
pan·to·chro·mism
pan·to·graph
pan·to·ic acid
pan·to·mo·gra·phic
pan·to·mog·ra·phy
pan·to·mor·phia
pan·to·mor·phic
Pan·to·paque
pan·to·pho·bia
pan·to·scop·ic
pan·to·then
pan·to·then·ate
pan·to·the·nic acid
pan·to·the·nol
pan·to·trop·ic
pan·to·yl·tau·rine
pan·trop·ic
pan·tur·bi·nate
Pa·num's area
pa·nus
pan·uve·itis
Pan·war·fin
pan·zer·herz
pan·zo·ot·ic
PAP — peroxidase-antiperoxid-
    ase
pa·pa·in
Pap·a·nic·o·laou's stain test
Pa·pav·er

pa·pav·er·ine hy·dro·chlo·
   ride
pa·pav·er·ine sul·fate
pa·paw
pa·pa·ya
pap·a·yo·tin
pa·per
   alkannin p.
   amboceptor p.
   aniline acetate p.
   antigen p.
   articulating p.
   azolitmin p.
   bibulous p.
   biuret p.
   blue litmus p.
   Congo red p.
   filter p.
   indicator p.
   lacmoid p.
   litmus p.
   niter p.
   occluding p.
   potassium nitrate p.
   red litmus p.
   saltpeter p.
   test p.
   turmeric p.
Pa·pez circuit
Pa·pez theory
pa·pil·la *pl.* pa·pil·lae
   acoustic p.
   anal p.
   arcuate papillae of tongue
   Bergmeister's p.
   bile p.
   calciform papillae
   capitate papillae
   circumvallate papillae
   clavate papillae
   papillae conicae
   conical papillae
   conoid papillae of tongue
   p. corii
   p. of corium
   corolliform papillae of
      tongue
   dental p.

pa·pil·la *(continued)*
   dentinal p.
   p. dentis
   dermal p.
   p. dermatis
   duodenal p., major
   duodenal p., minor
   p. duodeni major
   p. duodeni minor
   p. duodeni [Santorini]
   filiform papillae
   papillae filiformes
   papillae foliatae
   foliate papillae
   fungiform papillae
   papillae fungiformes
   gingival p.
   gingivalis
   gustatory papillae
   hair p.
   ileal p.
   p. ilealis
   p. ileocaecalis
   ileocecal p.
   p. ileocecalis
   p. incisiva
   incisive p.
   interdental p.
   p. interdentalis
   interproximal p.
   lacrimal p.
   p. lacrimalis
   lagenar p.
   lenticular papillae
   papillae lenticulares
   papillae lentiformes
   lingual papillae
   papillae linguales
   major duodenal p.
   p. mammae
   mammary p.
   medial papillae of tongue.
   minor duodenal p.
   p. of Morgagni
   nerve p.
   p. nervi optici
   obtuse papillae of tongue
   optic p.

pa·pil·la *(continued)*
　palatine p.
　parotid p.
　p. parotidea
　p. pili
　renal papillae
　papillae renales
　retromolar p.
　p. of Santorini
　simple papillae of tongue
　skin p.
　small papillae of tongue
　p. spiralis
　sublingual p.
　tactile papillae
　urethral p.
　papillae vallatae
　vallate papillae
　vascular p.
　p. of Vater
　villous papillae of tongue
pa·pil·lae
pap·il·lary
pap·il·late
pa·pil·la·tion
pap·il·lec·to·my
pa·pil·le·de·ma
pap·il·lif·er·ous
pa·pil·li·form
pap·il·li·tis
　necrotizing p.
　necrotizing renal p.
pa·pil·lo·ad·e·no·cys·to·ma
pa·pil·lo·car·ci·no·ma
pap·il·lo·ma
　p. canaliculum
　p. choroideum
　cockscomb p.
　cutaneous p.
　ductal p.
　fibroepithelial p.
　hirsutoid p's of penis
　Hopmann's p.
　intracanalicular p.
　intracystic p.
　intraductal p.
　inverted p.
　p. molle

pap·il·lo·ma *(continued)*
　rabbit p.
　rabbit oral p.
　Shope p.
　transitional cell p.
　p. venereum
　villous p.
　warty p.
pap·il·lo·ma·to·sis
　confluent and reticulate p.
　juvenile laryngeal p.
　malignant p. of Degos
　recurrent respiratory p.
pap·il·lom·a·tous
pap·il·lo·ma·vi·rus
　human p.
　rabbit p.
　Shope p.
Pa·pil·lon-Le·fèvre syndrome
pa·pil·lop·a·thy
　ischemic p.
pap·il·lo·ret·i·ni·tis
pa·pil·lose
pap·il·lo·sphinc·ter·ot·o·my
pap·il·lo·tome
pap·il·lot·o·my
pa·pil·lu·la
pa·po·va
Pa·po·va·vi·ri·dae
pa·po·va·vi·rus
Pap·pen·heim's stain
pap·pose
pap·u·lar
pap·u·la·tion
pap·ule
　Gottron's p's
　moist p.
　mucous p.
　painful piezogenic pedal p's
　pearly penile p's
　piezogenic p's
　prurigo p.
　split p's
pap·u·lo·er·y·the·ma·tous
pap·u·loid
pap·u·lo·pus·tu·lar
pap·u·lo·pus·tule

pap·u·lo·sis
    lymphomatoid p.
    malignant atrophic p.
    miliary p.
pap·u·lo·squa·mous
pap·u·lo·ve·sic·u·lar
PAPVR — partial anomalous
  pulmonary venous return
pap·y·ra·ceous
para
para-ac·ti·no·my·co·sis
para-al·bu·min·emia
para-am·i·no·ben·zo·ic acid
para-an·al·ge·sia
para-an·es·the·sia
para-aor·tic
para-ap·pen·di·ci·tis
para·ban·ic acid
para·bi·gem·i·nal
par·ab·i·on
par·ab·i·ont
para·bio·sis
    dialytic p.
    vascular p.
para·bi·ot·ic
para·blast
para·blas·tic
para·blep·sia
para·bu·lia
para·car·di·ac
para·car·mine
para·ca·sein
para·cel·lu·lose
par·a·cel·si·an
Par·a·cel·sus
para·cen·es·the·sia
para·cen·te·sis
    abdominal p.
    p. abdominis
    p. cordis
    p. ovarii
    p. pericardii
    p. pulmonis
    p. thoracis
    p. tunicae vaginalis
    p. tympani
    p. vesicae
para·cen·tet·ic

para·cen·tral
para·ceph·a·lus
para·cer·e·bel·lar
para·cer·vix
par·ac·et·al·de·hyde
par·ac·et·a·mol
para·chlo·ral·ose
para·chlo·ro·meta·xy·le·nol
para·chlo·ro·phe·nol
    camphorated p.
para·chol·era
para·chor·dal
Par·a·chor·do·des
para·chro·ma·tin
para·chro·ma·tism
para·chro·ma·top·sia
para·clin·i·cal
para·clo·nus
para·cnem·is
para·cne·mid·i·on
Para·coc·cid·i·oi·des bra·sil·
   i·en·sis
para·coc·cid·i·oi·do·my·co·sis
para·co·li·tis
para·col·pi·tis
para·col·pi·um
para·cone
para·co·nid
para·cor·tex
par·acou·sis
para·cox·al·gia
para·crine
para·cry·stals
par·acu·sia
    p. acris
    p. duplicata
    p. loci
    p. willisiana
par·acu·sis
    p. of Willis
para·cys·tic
para·cys·ti·tis
para·cys·ti·um
para·cyt·ic
para·den·tal
para·den·ti·tis
para·den·ti·um
para·den·to·sis

para·derm
para·des·mose
para·did·y·mal
para·did·y·mis
para·di·meth·yl·ami·no·
   benz·al·de·hyde
Para·di·one
para·dip·sia
para·don·to·sis
para·dox
    neurotic p.
    Opie p.
    Weber's p.
para·dox·i·cal
paradoxus
    pulsus p.
para·dys·en·tery
para·ec·cri·sis
para·en·do·crine
para·epi·lep·sy
para·equi·lib·ri·um
para·esoph·a·ge·al
para·falx
para·fas·cic·u·lar
Par. aff. — L. pars affecta (the
   part affected)
par·af·fin
    hard p.
    liquid p.
    liquid p., light
    pliable p.
    soft p., white
    soft p., yellow
par·af·fin·o·ma
Para·fi·la·ria mul·ti·pap·il·
   lo·sa
para·fla·gel·late
Par·a·flex
para·floc·cu·lus
para·for·mal·de·hyde
Para·fos·sa·ru·lus
    P. manchouricus
para·fo·ve·al
para·func·tion
para·func·tion·al
para·gam·ma·cism
para·gan·glia

para·gan·gli·o·ma
    medullary p.
    nonchromaffin p.
para·gan·gli·on pl. para·gan·
   glia
    adrenergic p.
    aortic p.
    cardiac p.
    cholinergic p.
para·gen·e·sis
para·ge·net·ic
para·gen·i·ta·lis
para·geu·sia
para·geu·sic
par·ag·glu·ti·na·tion
par·ag·na·thus
par·ag·no·sis
para·gom·pho·sis
par·a·gon·i·mi·a·sis
par·a·gon·i·mo·sis
Para·gon·i·mus
    P. africanus
    P. heterotrema
    P. kellicotti
    P. ringeri
    P. westermani
Para·gor·di·us
para·gram·ma·tism
para·gran·u·lo·ma
para·gra·phia
para·he·mo·phil·ia
para·he·pat·ic
para·hep·a·ti·tis
para·he·red·i·tary
para·hex·yl
para·hor·mone
para·hyp·no·sis
para·hy·po·phy·sis
para·in·flu·en·za
para·in·flu·en·zal
para·ker·a·tin·ized
para·ker·a·to·sis
    p. ostracea
    p. psoriasiformis
    p. scutularis
    p. variegata

para·ki·ne·sia
para·ki·net·ic
Pa·ral
para·la·lia
   p. literalis
para·lamb·da·cism
par·al·bu·min
par·al·de·hyde
par·al·de·hyd·ism
para·lep·sy
para·lex·ia
para·lex·ic
par·al·ge·sia
par·al·ges·ic
par·al·gia
para·li·nin
par·al·lac·tic
par·al·lag·ma
par·al·lax
   binocular p.
   crossed p.
   direct p.
   heteronymous p.
   homonymous p.
   stereoscopic p.
   uncrossed p.
   vertical p.
par·al·lel
par·al·lel·om·e·ter
par·al·ler·gic
par·al·ler·gy
para·lo·gia
   thematic p.
pa·ral·o·gism
pa·ral·o·gy
pa·ral·y·ses
pa·ral·y·sis *pl.* pa·ral·y·ses
   abducens p.
   abducens-facial p.,
     congenital
   p. of accommodation
   acoustic p.
   acute ascending spinal p.
   acute atrophic p.
   acute bulbar p.
   p. agitans
   p. agitans, juvenile (of
     Hunt)

pa·ral·y·sis *(continued)*
   alcoholic p.
   alternate p.
   alternating p.
   ambiguo-accessorius p.
   ambiguo-accessorius-hypogl-
     ossal p.
   ambiguohypoglossal p.
   ambiguospinothalamic p.
   anesthesia p.
   anterior spinal p.
   arsenical p.
   ascending p.
   ascending tick p.
   association p.
   asthenic bulbar p.
   asthenobulbospinal p.
   atrophic muscular p.
   atrophic spinal p.
   Avellis's p.
   axillary nerve p.
   basal-ganglionic p.
   Bell's p.
   bifacial p.
   bilateral p.
   bilateral laryngeal
     abductor p.
   birth p.
   brachial p.
   brachial plexus p.
   brachiofacial p.
   Brown-Séquard's p.
   bulbar p.
   bulbospinal p.
   cage p.
   central p.
   central facial p.
   centrocapsular p.
   cerebral p.
   cerebral spastic infantile p.
   cerebral sympathetic p.
   Chastek p.
   circumflex p.
   common peroneal nerve p.
   complete p.
   compression p.
   congenital abducens-facial
     p.

pa·ral·y·sis *(continued)*
  congenital oculofacial p.
  congenital p. of horizontal
    gaze
  conjugate p.
  cortical p.
  creeping p.
  crossed p.
  cruciate p.
  crossed hypoglossal p.
  crural p.
  crutch p.
  Cruveilhier's p.
  cubital p.
  decubitus p.
  Dejerine-Klumpke p.
  diaphragmatic p.
  diphtheric p.
  diphtheritic p.
  divers'p.
  drunkards' arm p.
  Duchenne's p.
  Duchenne-Erb p.
  epidemic infantile p.
  epidural ascending spinal
    p.
  Erb's p.
  Erb syphilitic spinal p.
  Erb-Duchenne p.
  esophageal p.
  essential p.
  extraocular p.
  facial p.
  false p.
  familial hyperkalemic
    periodic p.
  familial hypokalemic
    periodic p.
  familial infantile bulbar p.
  familial periodic p.
  familial recurrent p.
  familial spastic p.
  faucial p.
  Felton's p.
  femoral nerve p.
  flaccid p.
  fowl p.
  functional p.
  p. of gaze

pa·ral·y·sis *(continued)*
  general p.
  general p. of the insane
  ginger p.
  glossolabial p.
  glossopharyngolabial p.
  Gubler's p.
  Gubler-Millard p.
  hereditary cerebrospinal p.
  histrionic p.
  hyperkalemic periodic p.
  hypoglossal p.
  hypokalemic periodic p.
  hysterical p.
  idiopathic facial p.
  immune p.
  immunologic p.
  incomplete p.
  Indian bow p.
  infantile p.
  infantile, cerebral, ataxic
    p.
  infantile cerebrocerebellar
    diplegic p.
  infantile spastic p.
  infantile spinal p.
  infectious bulbar p.
  inferior alternate p.
  infranuclear p.
  ischemic p.
  Jackson's p.
  jake p.
  Jamaica ginger p.
  juvenile p.
  juvenile distal atrophic p.
  Klumpke's p.
  Klumpke-Dejerine p.
  Kussmaul's p.
  Kussmaul-Landry p.
  labial p.
  labioglossolaryngeal p.
  labioglossopharyngeal p.
  Landry's p.
  laryngeal p.
  laryngeal abductor p.
  lead p.
  lingual p.
  Lissauer's p.

pa·ral·y·sis *(continued)*
Little's p.
local p.
lover's p.
masticatory p.
medial popliteal nerve p.
median p.
medullary tegmental p's
mesencephalic p.
Millard-Gubler p.
mimetic p.
mixed p.
morning p.
motor p.
motor trigeminal p.
musculocutaneous nerve p.
musculospiral p.
myogenic p.
myopathic p.
narcosis p.
neurogenic p.
normokalemic periodic p.
p. notariorum
nuclear p.
obstetric p.
obturator nerve p.
occupational p.
ocular p.
oculofacial p., congenital
oculomotor p.
organic p.
palatal p.
parotitic p.
parturient p.
periodic p., thyrotoxic
peripheral p.
peripheral facial p.
peroneal p.
pharyngeal p.
phonetic p.
phrenic p.
postdiphtheric p.
postdormital p.
postepileptic p.
posthemiplegic p.
posticus p.
Pott's p.
pressure p.

pa·ral·y·sis *(continued)*
progressive bulbar p.
pseudobulbar p.
pseudohypertrophic
  muscular p.
psychic gaze p.
radial p.
Ramsay Hunt p.
range p.
recurrent laryngeal nerve
  p.
reflex p.
Remak's p.
Rieder's p.
rucksack p.
Saturday night p.
sensory p.
serratus anterior p.
serum p.
sleep p.
sodium-responsive periodic
  p.
spastic p.
spastic spinal p.
spinal accessory nerve p.
spinomuscular p.
Sunday morning p.
superior laryngeal nerve p.
supranuclear p.
suxamethonium p.
tegmental mesencephalic
  p.
tick p.
Todd's p.
tourniquet p.
trigeminal p.
trigeminal masticator p.
trochlear p.
ulnar nerve p.
unilateral p.
unilateral vocal cord p.
p. vacillans
vagal p.
vagoaccessory hypoglossal
  p.
vasomotor p.
Vernet's p.
vestibular p.

pa·ral·y·sis *(continued)*
    Volkmann's ischemic p.
    waking p.
    wasting p.
    Weber's p.
    Werdnig-Hoffmann p.
    Winkelman's p.
    writers'p.
    Zenker's p.
par·a·lys·or
par·a·lyt·ic
par·a·lyt·o·gen·ic
par·a·lyz·ant
par·a·lyze
par·a·lyz·er
para·mag·net·ic
para·mag·ne·tism
para·mas·ti·gote
para·mas·ti·tis
para·mas·toid
para·mas·toid·itis
para·me·a·tal
par·a·me·cia
Par·a·me·ci·um
para·me·ci·um *pl.* para·me·cia
para·me·di·al
para·me·di·an
para·med·ic
para·med·i·cal
para·me·nia
para·me·ni·sci·tis
para·me·nis·cus
para·me·si·al
pa·ram·e·ter
    pharmacokinetic p's
para·meth·a·di·one
para·meth·a·sone ac·e·tate
para·me·tri·al
par·a·met·ric
para·me·tris·mus
para·me·trit·ic
para·me·tri·tis
    anterior p.
    posterior p.
para·me·tri·um
para·me·trop·a·thy
par·am·i·do·ac·e·to·phe·none

para·mim·ia
para·mi·tome
par·am·ne·sia
Par·amoe·ba
para·mo·lar
para·morph
para·mor·phia
para·mor·phine
Par·am·phis·to·ma·toi·dea
par·am·phi·sto·mi·a·sis
Par·am·phis·to·mum
para·mu·cin
para·mu·sia
para·mu·ta·ble
para·mu·ta·gen·ic
para·mu·ta·tion
para·my·elin
par·am·y·loi·do·sis
para·my·oc·lo·nus
    p. multiplex
para·myo·sin
par·a·my·o·sin·o·gen
para·myo·tone
para·myo·to·nia
    ataxia p.
    p. congenita
    symptomatic p.
para·myo·to·nus
Para·myxa
Par·a·myx·ea
Par·a·myx·i·da
Para·myxo·vi·ri·dae
para·myxo·vi·rus
par·an·al·ge·sia
para·na·sal
para·neo·pla·sia
para·neo·plas·tic
para·neph·ric
para·ne·phri·tis
    lipomatous p.
para·ne·phro·ma
para·neph·ros *pl.* para·neph·roi
par·an·es·the·sia
para·neu·ral
para·ni·tro·sul·fa·thi·a·zole
par·a·noia
    Sander's p.

par·a·noi·ac
par·a·noid
par·a·no·mia
   visual p.
para·nor·mal
para·nos·ic
para·no·sis
para·nu·cle·ar
para·nu·cle·o·lus
para·nu·cle·us *pl.* para·nu·
   clei
para·om·phal·ic
para·op·er·a·tive
para·oral
para·os·mia
para·pan·cre·at·ic
para·pa·re·sis
   spastic p.
para·pa·ret·ic
para·pe·de·sis
para·peri·to·ne·al
para·per·tus·sis
para·pes·tis
para·pha·ryn·ge·al
para·pha·sia
   central p.
   literal p.
   verbal p.
para·pha·sic
para·pha·sis
para·phe·mia
para·phen·yl·ene·di·amine
pa·ra·phia
para·phil·ia
para·phil·i·ac
para·phi·mo·sis
para·pho·bia
para·pho·nia
   p. puberum
pa·raph·o·ra
para·phra·sia
para·phre·nia
   involutional p.
   late p.
para·phren·ic
para·phre·ni·tis
pa·raph·y·se·al
pa·raph·y·sis

para·pin·e·al
para·plasm
para·plas·mic
para·plas·tic
para·plas·tin
para·plec·tic
para·ple·gia
   alcoholic p.
   ataxic p.
   cerebral p.
   cervical p.
   Erb's spastic p.
   Erb's syphilitic spastic p.
   familial spastic p.
   flaccid p.
   functional p.
   hereditary spastic p.
   hysterical p.
   Jamaican spastic p.
   peripheral p.
   Pott's p.
   reflex p.
   senile p.
   South Indian p.
   spastic p.
   spastic p., congenital
   spastic p., infantile
   spastic p., primary
   p. superior
   syphilitic p.
   toxic p.
para·ple·gia-in-ex·ten·sion
para·ple·gia-in-flex·ion
para·ple·gic
para·ple·gi·form
para·pleu·ri·tis
para·pneu·mo·nia
par·apoph·y·sis
par·apo·plexy
Para·pox·vi·rus
par·a·pox·vi·rus
para·prax·ia
para·prax·is
para·proc·ti·tis
para·proc·ti·um
para·pro·fes·sion·al
para·pros·ta·ti·tis
para·pro·tein

para·pro·tein·emia
par·ap·sia
par·ap·sis
para·pso·ri·a·sis
   p. acuta
   acute p.
   atrophic p.
   chronic p.
   p. guttata
   guttate p.
   large plaque p.
   p. lichenoides
   p. lichenoides chronica
   p. maculata
   p. en plaques
   poikilodermic p.
   poikilodermatous p.
   retiform p.
   small plaque p.
   p. varigata
   p. varioliformis acuta
   p. varioliformis chronica
para·psy·chol·o·gy
para·pyk·no·mor·phous
para·pyle
para·py·ram·id·al
para·quat
para·rec·tal
para·re·du·cine
para·re·flex·ia
para·re·nal
para·rhi·zo·cla·sia
para·rho·ta·cism
para·ro·san·i·line
   p. pamoate
par·ar·rhyth·mia
par·ar·thria
para·sa·cral
para·sag·it·tal
Par·a·sal
para·sal·pin·ge·al
para·sal·pin·gi·tis
para·scap·u·lar
Par·as·car·is
para·scar·la·ti·na
para·scar·let
para·se·cre·tion
para·sel·lar

para·sex·u·al
para·sex·u·al·i·ty
para·sig·ma·tism
para·si·noi·dal
para·si·nu·soi·dal
par·a·site
   accidental p.
   allantoic p.
   animal p.
   autochthonous p.
   celozoic p.
   cytozoic p.
   digenetic p.
   diheteroxenic p.
   ectophytic p.
   ectozoic p.
   endophytic p.
   entozoic p.
   euroxenous p.
   eurytrophic p.
   facultative p.
   false p.
   hematozoic p.
   heterogenetic p.
   incidental p.
   intermittent p.
   intracellular p.
   karyozoic p.
   malarial p.
   obligatory p.
   occasional p.
   optimal p.
   periodic p.
   permanent p.
   plant p.
   specific p.
   spurious p.
   stenotrophic p.
   temporary p.
   teratoid p.
   vegetable p.
par·a·si·te·mia
par·a·sit·ic
par·a·sit·i·ci·dal
par·a·sit·i·cide
par·a·sit·i·cus
par·a·sit·i·fer
par·a·si·tif·er·ous

par·a·sit·ism
   extracellular p.
   intracellular p.
   multiple p.
para·sit·iza·tion
par·a·si·tize
par·a·si·to·gen·e·sis
par·a·si·to·gen·ic
par·a·si·toid
par·a·si·toid·ism
par·a·si·tol·o·gist
par·a·si·tol·o·gy
par·a·si·tome
par·a·si·to·sis
par·a·si·to·trope
par·a·si·to·trop·ic
par·a·si·tot·ro·pism
par·a·si·tot·ro·py
para·small·pox
para·so·ma
para·som·nia
para·spa·di·as
para·spasm
para·spas·mus
   p. faciale
para·spe·cif·ic
para·sple·nic
para·ster·nal
para·stri·ate
para·stru·ma
para·sui·cide
para·sym·pa·thet·ic
para·sym·path·i·co·to·nia
para·sym·pa·thin
para·sym·pa·tho·lyt·ic
para·sym·pa·tho·mi·met·ic
para·sym·pa·tho·para·lyt·ic
para·sym·pa·tho·to·nia
para·syn·an·che
para·syn·ap·sis
para·syn·de·sis
para·syno·vi·tis
para·sys·to·le
para·tae·ni·al
para·tar·si·um
para·ten·e·sis
para·ten·ic
para·ten·on

para·ter·mi·nal
para·thi·on
para·thor·mone
para·thy·mia
para·thy·rin
para·thy·roid
para·thy·roid·al
para·thy·roid·ec·to·mize
para·thy·roid·ec·to·my
para·thy·roid·in
para·thy·roid·o·ma
para·thy·rop·a·thy
para·thy·ro·pri·val
para·thy·ro·pri·via
para·thy·ro·priv·ic
para·thy·rop·ri·vous
para·thy·ro·troph·ic
para·thy·ro·trop·ic
para·to·nia
para·ton·ic
para·ton·sil·lar
para·tope
para·tose
para·tra·cho·ma
para·troph·ic
pa·rat·ro·phy
para·tu·bal
para·tu·ber·cu·lo·sis
para·tu·ber·cu·lous
para·type
para·typh·li·tis
para·ty·phoid
para·typ·ic
para·typ·i·cal
para·um·bil·i·cal
para·un·gual
para·ure·ter·ic
para·ure·thra
para·ure·thral
para·ure·thri·tis
para·uter·ine
para·vac·cin·ia
para·vag·i·nal
para·vag·i·ni·tis
para·val·vu·lar
para·ve·nous
para·ven·tric·u·lar
para·ver·te·bral

para·ves·i·cal
para·vi·ta·min·o·sis
par·ax·i·al
par·ax·on
para·zone
par·ben·da·zole
par·co·na·zole hy·dro·chlo·
  ride
Pa·ré, Ambroise
Pa·ré suture
par·ec·ta·sia
par·ec·ta·sis
par·ec·tro·pia
Par·e·drine
par·e·gor·ic
par·elec·tro·nom·ic
par·elec·tron·o·my
par·el·e·i·din
par·en·ce·pha·lia
par·en·ceph·a·li·tis
par·en·ceph·a·lo·cele
par·en·ceph·a·lon
par·en·ceph·a·lous
par·en·chy·ma
  p. glandulare prostatae
  p. prostatae
  p. testis
  p. of testis
par·en·chy·mal
par·en·chym·a·ti·tis
par·en·chym·a·tous
par·en·chym·u·la
pa·ren·tal
pa·ren·ter·al
pa·ren·ter·ic
par·ent·ing
par·epi·did·y·mal
par·epi·did·y·mis
par·epi·gas·tric
pa·re·sis
  canal p.
  galloping p.
  general p.
  juvenile p.
  vestibular canal p.
par·eso·an·al·ge·sia
par·eso·an·es·the·sia
Par·est

par·es·the·sia
  Berger's p.
  Bernhardt's p.
  visceral p.
par·es·thet·ic
par·es·the·ti·ca
  meralgia p.
pa·ret·ic
pa·reu·nia
par·fo·cal
par·gy·line hy·dro·chlo·ride
Par·ham band
par·i·ca
pa·ric·ine
pa·ri·es *pl.* pa·ri·etes
  p. anterior gastricus
  p. anterior vaginae
  p. anterior ventriculi
  p. caroticus cavitatis
    tympanicae
  p. externus ductus
    cochlearis
  p. inferior orbitae
  p. jugularis cavitatis
    tympanicae
  p. labyrinthicus cavitatis
    tympanicae
  p. lateralis orbitae
  p. mastoideus cavitatis
    tympanicae
  p. medialis orbitae
  p. membranaceus bronchi
  p. membranaceus cavitatis
    tympanicae
  p. membranaceus tracheae
  p. posterior gastricus
  p. posterior vaginae
  p. posterior ventriculi
  p. superior orbitae
  p. tegmentalis cavitatis
    tympanicae
  p. tympanicus ductus
    cochlearis
  p. vestibularis ductus
    cochlearis
pa·ri·e·tal
pa·ri·e·tes

pa·ri·e·ti·tis
pa·ri·e·to·fron·tal
pa·ri·e·tog·ra·phy
   gastric p.
pa·ri·e·to·mas·toid
pa·ri·e·to·oc·cip·i·tal
pa·ri·e·to·sphe·noid
pa·ri·e·to·splanch·nic
pa·ri·e·to·squa·mo·sal
pa·ri·e·to·tem·po·ral
pa·ri·e·to·vis·ce·ral
Pa·ri·naud's oculoglandular
   syndrome
pa·ri pas·su
par·i·ty
Park's aneurysm
Par·ker's fluid
Par·ker-Kerr suture
Par·kin·son's disease
Par·kin·son's facies
Par·kin·son's sign
par·kin·so·ni·an
par·kin·son·ism
   atherosclerotic p.
   drug-induced p.
   hemiplegic p.
   intoxication p.
   juvenile p.
   postencephalitic p.
   symptomatic p.
   traumatic p.
   vascular p.
Par·lo·del
Par·nate
par·oc·cip·i·tal
par·odon·top·a·thy
par·ol·fac·tory
par·ol·i·vary
par·o·mo·my·cin
   p. sulfate
par·om·pha·lo·cele
Pa·ro·na's space
par·oni·ria
par·onych·ia
   herpetic p.
   p. tendinosa
par·o·nych·i·al
pa·ron·y·cho·my·co·sis

par·oöph·o·ric
par·ooph·o·ri·tis
par·oöph·o·ron
par·oph·thal·mia
par·oph·thal·mon·cus
par·op·sis
par·or·chid·i·um
par·or·chis
par·orex·ia
par·os·mia
par·os·phre·sia
par·os·phre·sis
par·os·te·al
par·os·te·itis
par·os·te·o·sis
par·os·ti·tis
par·os·to·sis
pa·rot·ic
pa·rot·id
pa·rot·i·de·an
pa·rot·i·dec·to·my
pa·rot·i·di·tis
pa·rot·i·do·auric·u·lar·is
pa·rot·i·do·scir·rhus
par·o·tin
par·oti·tis
   celiac p.
   epidemic p.
   p. phlegmonosa
   postoperative p.
   staphylococcal p.
   tropical suppurative p.
par·ous
par·ovar·i·an
par·ovar·i·ot·o·my
par·ova·ri·tis
par·ovar·i·um
par·ox·ysm
par·ox·ys·mal
Par·pan·it
Par·rot's atrophy of newborn
Par·rot's disease
Par·rot's pseudoparalysis
Par·ry-Rom·berg syndrome
pars *pl.* par·tes
   p. abdominalis
   p. alaris
   p. alveolaris

pars *(continued)*
p. amorpha
p. analis
p. annularis
p. anterior
p. ascendens
p. atlantica
p. autonomica
p. basilaris
p. basolateralis
p. buccalis
p. buccopharyngea
p. calcaneocuboidea
p. calcaneonavicularis
p. cardiaca
p. cartilaginea
p. caudalis
p. cavernosa
p. centralis
p. ceratopharyngea
p. cerebralis
p. cervicalis
p. chondropharyngea
p. ciliaris
p. clavicularis
p. coccygea
p. cochlearis
p. compacta
p. convoluta
p. corneoscleralis
p. corticalis
p. corticomedialis
p. costalis
p. cranialis
p. cricopharyngea
p. cruciformis
p. cupularis
p. descendens
p. dextra
p. distalis
p. dorsalis
p. endocrina
p. exocrina
p. fetalis
p. fibrillaris
p. fibrosa
p. flaccida
p. frontalis

pars *(continued)*
p. functionalis
partes genitales
p. glabra
p. glossopharyngea
p. granulosa
p. grisea
p. horizontalis
p. iliaca
p. inferior
p. inflexa
p. infraclavicularis
p. infralobaris
p. infrasegmentalis
p. infundibularis
p. insularis
p. interarticularis
p. intercartilaginea
p. intermedia
p. intermembranacea
p. intersegmentalis
p. interstialis
p. intracanicularis
p. intracranialis
p. intralaminaris
p. intraocularis
p. intrasegmentalis
p. iridica
p. labialis
p. lacrimalis
p. laryngea
p. lateralis
p. lenticulothalamicus
p. libera
p. lumbalis
p. magnocellularis
p. mamillaris
p. marginalis
p. mastoidea
p. medialis
p. mediastinalis
p. membranacea
p. mobilis
p. muscularis
p. mylopharyngea
p. nasalis
p. nervosa
p. obliqua

pars *(continued)*
    p. occipitalis
    p. occlusa
    p. olfactoria
    p. opercularis
    p. optica
    p. oralis
    p. orbitalis
    p. ossea
    p. palpebralis
    p. parasympathetica
    p. parasympathica
    p. parietalis
    p. parvocellularis
    p. patens
    p. pelvina
    p. peripherica
    p. perpendicularis
    p. petrosa
    p. pharyngea
    p. pigmentosa
    p. plana
    p. plicata
    p. postcommunicalis
    p. posterior
    p. postlaminaris
    p. postsulcalis
    p. precommunicalis
    p. prelaminaris
    p. presulcalis
    p. prevertebralis
    p. profunda
    p. prostatica
    p. pterygopharyngea
    p. pylorica
    p. quadrata
    p. radiata
    p. recta
    p. reticularis
    p. retrolentiformis
    p. rostralis
    p. sacralis
    p. sphenoidalis
    p. spinalis
    p. spongiosa
    p. squamosa
    p. sternalis
    p. sternocostalis

pars *(continued)*
    p. subcutanea
    p. subfrontalis
    p. sublentiformis
    p. superficialis
    p. superior
    p. supraclavicularis
    p. supraoptica
    p. sympathetica
    p. sympathica
    p. tecta
    p. temporalis
    p. tensa
    p. terminalis
    p. thalamolenticularis
    p. thoracalis
    p. thoracica
    p. thyropharyngea
    p. tibiocalcanea
    p. tibiocalcaneus
    p. tibionavicularis
    p. tibiotalaris
    p. transversa
    p. transversaria
    p. triangularis
    p. tuberalis
    p. tympanica
    p. umbilicalis
    p. uterina
    p. uvealis
    p. vagalis
    p. ventralis
    p. vertebralis
    p. vestibularis
    p. villosa
Par·si·dol
Par·son·age-Tur·ner neuralgia
Par·son·age-Tur·ner
    syndrome
pars pla·ni·tis
part
    abdominal p. of aorta
    abdominal p. of esophagus
    abdominal p. of ureter
    accessory p. of parotid
      gland
    alar p. of nasalis muscle
    alveolar p. of mandible

part *(continued)*

ascending p. of aorta
basilar p. of occipital bone
bony p. of auditory tube
bony p. of nasal septum
broad p. of anterior
annular ligament
cardiac p. of stomach
cartilaginous p. of auditory
tube
cervical p. of trachea
ciliary p. of retina
colic p. of omentum
condylar p. of occipital
bone
convoluted p. of kidney
lobule
costal p. of diaphragm
cranial p. of accessory
nerve
cupular p. of epitympanic
recess
cupulate p. epitympanic
recess
deep p. of parotid gland
descending p. of aorta
descending p. of duodenum
exoccipital p. of occipital
bone
first p. of duodenum
flaccid p. of tympanic
membrane
fourth p. of duodenum
horizontal p. of duodenum
inferior p. of duodenum
infraclavicular p. of
brachial plexus
intercartilaginous p. of
glottis
intermembranous p. of
glottis
interstitial p. of uterine
tube
intervaginal p. of cervix
intramural p. of uterine
tube
iridal p. of retina
jugular p. of occipital bone

part *(continued)*

lambdoidal p. of anterior
annular ligament
laryngeal p. of pharynx
lateral p. of cricothyroid
ligament
lateral p. of occipital bone
lateral p. of sacrum
lumbar p. of autonomic
nervous system
lumbar p. of diaphragm
magnocellular p. of red
nucleus
mamillary p. of temporal
bone
membranous p. of
interventricular septum
membranous p. of male
urethra
membranous p. of nasal
septum
mobile p. of nasal septum
nasal p. of frontal bone
nasal p. of pharynx
occipital p. of occipital
bone
oral p. of pharynx
palpebral p. of lacrimal
gland
parietal p. of pelvic fascia
pectineal p. of inguinal
ligament
pelvic p. of ureter
petrous p. of temporal bone
presenting p.
pyloric p. of stomach
sagittal p. of left portal
vein
second p. of duodenum
spinal p. of accessory nerve
spongiose p. of male
urethra
squamous p. of occipital
bone
squamous p. of temporal
bone
sternal p. of diaphragm

part *(continued)*
  sternocostal p. of
    diaphragm
  subphrenic p. of esophagus
  superficial p. of parotid
    gland
  superior p. of anterior
    annular ligament
  superior p. of duodenum
  tabular p. of occipital bone
  tendinous p. of epicranius
    muscle
  tense p. of tympanic
    membrane
  third p. of duodenum
  third p. of quadriceps
    femoris muscle
  thoracic p. of aorta
  transverse p. of anterior
    annular ligament
  transverse p. of left portal
    vein
  tympanic p. of temporal
    bone
  umbilical p. of left portal
    vein
  vaginal p. of cervix
  vertebral p. of diaphragm
  visceral p. of pelvic fascia
Part. aeq. — L. partes
  aequales (equal parts)
par·tal
par·tes
par·the·no·car·py
par·the·no·gen·e·sis
  artificial p.
par·the·no·pho·bia
par·tho·gen·e·sis
par·ti·ci·pant-ob·serv·er
par·ti·cle
  alpha p.
  attraction p.
  beta p.
  C p.
  chromatin p's
  collodion p's
  colloid p's
  core p.

par·ti·cle *(continued)*
  Dane p.
  disperse p's
  elementary p.
  elementary p's of
    mitochondria
  high-velocity p's
  kappa p's
  lens p.
  nuclear p's
  viral p.
  Zimmermann's elementary
    p's
par·tic·u·late
par·tin·i·um
Par·ti·pi·lo method
par·ti·tion
  oropharyngeal p.
par·ti·tion·ing
  gastric p.
par·tri·cin
Partsch's operation
par·tu·ri·ent
par·tu·ri·fa·cient
par·tu·ri·om·e·ter
par·tu·ri·tion
  double p.
par·tus
  p. maturus
  p. preparator
Part. vic. — L. partitis vicibus
  (in divided doses)
pa·ru·lis
par·um·bil·i·cal
par·u·ria
par·vi·cel·lu·lar
par·vi·loc·u·lar
par·vo·line
Par·vo·vi·ri·dae
par·vo·vi·rus
par·vule
Pa·ry's disease
Pary·phos·to·mum
PAS — para-aminosalicylic
  acid
    periodic acid-Schiff
Pas·cal's law
pas·cal

Pas·cheff's conjunctivitis
Pasch·en's bodies
Pasch·en's corpuscles
Pasch·en's granules
Pa·schu·tin's degeneration
PASG — pneumatic antishock
  garment
Pa·si·ni-Pie·ri·ni syndrome
pas·pal·ism
pas·sage
    adiabatic fast p.
    blind p.
    cloacal p.
    false p.
    serial p.
Pas·sa·vant's bar
Pas·sa·vant's cushion
Pas·sa·vant's pad
Pas·sa·vant's ridge
pass·band
pas·ser
    foil p.
Pas·si·flo·ra
pas·sive
pas·siv·ism
pas·siv·i·ty
Past. — Pasteurella
paste
    aluminum p.
    desensitizing p.
    dextrinated p.
    Ihle's p.
    impression p.
    Lassar's p.
    Lassar's betanaphthol p.
    Lassar's plain zinc p.
    Leunbach's p.
    Nitrol p.
    Piffard's p.
    Teflon p.
    triamcinolone acetonide
      dental p.
    Unna p.
    zinc oxide p.
    zinc oxide and eugenol p.
    zinc oxide and salicylic acid
      p.

paste *(continued)*
    zinc oxide p. with salicylic
      acid
    zipp p.
pas·ter
pas·tern
Pas·teur, Louis
Pas·teur's effect
Pas·teur's method
Pas·teur's reaction
Pas·teur's theory
Pas·teur-Cham·ber·land filter
Pas·teur·el·la
    P. aerogenes
    P. haemolytica
    P. multocida
    P. novicida
    P. pestis
    P. pfaffii
    P. pneumotropica
    P. pseudotuberculosis
    P. septica
    P. septicaemiae
    P. tularensis
    P. ureae
Pas·teur·el·la·ceae
Pas·teur·el·leae
pas·teur·el·lo·sis
pas·teur·ism
pas·teur·iza·tion
pas·teur·iz·er
Pas·tia's lines
Pas·tia's sign
pas·tille
past-point·ing
PAT — paroxysmal atrial
  tachycardia
Pa·tau syndrome
patch
    Bayer p.
    Bitot's p's
    butterfly p.
    Carrel p.
    cotton-wool p's
    herald p.
    Hutchinson's p.
    MacCallum's p.
    mucous p.

patch *(continued)*
    opaline p.
    Peyer's p's
    salmon p.
    sentinel p.
    shagreen p.
    smokers' p.
    soldiers' p's
    white p.
pat·e·fac·tion
Pat·ein's albumin
Pa·tel·la's disease
pa·tel·la
    p. alta
    p. bipartita
    bipartite p.
    p. cubiti
    floating p.
    p. partita
    slipping p.
pa·tel·la·plas·ty
pa·tel·lar
pat·el·lec·to·my
pat·el·li·form
pa·tel·lo·fem·o·ral
pa·tel·lom·e·ter
pat·en·cy
pat·ent
Pat·er·son's syndrome
Pat·er·son-Brown Kel·ly
  syndrome
Pat·er·son-Kel·ly syndrome
Pa·tey's operation
path
    condyle p.
    copulation p.
    incisor p.
    p. of insertion
    ionization p.
    lateral condyle p.
    mean free p.
    milled-in p's
    occlusal p.
    occlusal p., generated
    p. of removal
pa·the·ma *pl.* pa·the·mas, pa·
  them·a·ta
path·er·gia

path·er·gic
path·er·gy
pa·thet·ic
path·find·er
Pa·thi·lon
patho·an·a·tom·i·cal
patho·anat·o·my
patho·bi·ol·o·gy
Path·o·cil
patho·cli·sis
path·odon·tia
patho·for·mic
patho·gen
patho·gen·e·sis
    drug p.
patho·gen·e·sy
patho·ge·net·ic
path·o·gen·ic
patho·ge·nic·i·ty
path·og·e·ny
pa·thog·no·mon·ic
path·og·no·my
path·og·nos·tic
pa·thog·ra·phy
patho·log·ic
patho·log·i·cal
pa·thol·o·gist
    speech p.
pa·thol·o·gy
    anatomic p.
    cellular p.
    chemical p.
    clinical p.
    comparative p.
    dental p.
    experimental p.
    forensic p.
    functional p.
    general p.
    geographical p.
    internal p.
    medical p.
    molecular p.
    oral p.
    special p.
    speech p.
    surgical p.
patho·mi·me·sis

patho·mim·ia
patho·mim·ic·ry
patho·mor·phism
patho·mor·phol·o·gy
patho·neu·ro·sis
patho·no·mia
pa·thon·o·my
patho-oc·clu·sion
patho·pho·bia
patho·phor·e·sis
patho·phys·i·ol·o·gy
patho·poi·e·sis
patho·psy·chol·o·gy
patho·psy·cho·sis
pa·tho·sis
pa·thot·ro·pism
path·way
    afferent p.
    alternative complement p.
    amphibolic p.
    atrio-His p.
    auditory p's
    biosynthetic p.
    classic complement p.
    common p. of coagulation
    distribution p.
    efferent p.
    Embden-Meyerhof p.
    Embden-Meyerhof-Parnas
       p.
    Entner-Doudoroff p.
    extrinsic p. of coagulation
    final common p.
    gustatory p's
    internuncial p.
    intrinsic p. of coagulation
    ketodeoxygluconate p.
    lipoxygenase p.
    metabolic p.
    olfactory p's
    optical p's
    pallidofugal p's
    pentose phosphate p.
    phosphogluconate p.
    properdin p.
    reaction p.
    reentrant p.
    spinocervicothalamic p.

pa·tient
pa·tient-day
Pat·rick's sign
Pat·rick's test
pa·tri·lin·e·al
pat·ro·cli·nous
pa·tro·gen·e·sis
pat·ten
pat·tern
    action p.
    arch p.
    A-V p's
    beam p.
    Christmas tree p.
    cloverleaf p.
    dicing p.
    diffraction p.
    fingerprint p.
    fixed action p.
    honeycomb p.
    interference p.
    juvenile p.
    loop p.
    muscle p.
    occlusal p.
    sedimentation p.
    signet-ring p.
    sine-wave p.
    skeletal p.
    starry-sky p.
    startle p.
    stimulus p.
    wax p.
    wear p.
    whorl p.
pat·tern·ing
pat·ty
    cottonoid p.
pat·u·lin
pat·u·lous
pau·ci·ar·tic·u·lar
pau·ci·syn·ap·tic
Paul's test
Paul's treatment
Paul-Bun·nell test
Paul-Bun·nell-Da·vid·sohn
    test
Paul-Mix·ter tube

Paul·ing-Corey helix
paunch
pause
 cardiac p.
 compensatory p.
 post-extrasystolic p.
 sinus p.
Pau·tri·er's abscess
Pau·tri·er's microabscess
pa·vé
pave·ment·ing
pa·vex
pa·vil·ion
 p. of the ear
 p. of the oviduct
 p. of the pelvis
pav·ing stone de·gen·er·a·tion
Pav·lov, Ivan Petrovich
Pav·lov's pouch
Pav·lov's stomach
pa·vor
 p. diurnus
 p. nocturnus
Pav·u·lon
Pa·vy's disease
Paw·lik's triangle
Paw·lik's trigone
PAWP — pulmonary artery
wedge pressure
Payr's clamp
Payr's disease
pa·zox·ide
PB — Pharmacopoeia
Britannica (British
Pharmacopoeia)
 pressure breathing
PBC — primary biliary
cirrhosis
PBG — porphobilinogen
PBI — protein-bound iodine
PBPI — penile brachial
pressure index
PC — palmitoyl carnitine
 phosphatidyl choline
 phosphocreatine
P.C. — L. pondus civile
(avoirdupois weight)

p.c. — L. post cibum (after
meals)
PCA — passive cutaneous
anaphylaxis
 patient-controlled
 analgesic
PCB — polychlorinated
biphenyl
PcB — near point of
convergence to the
intercentral base line
PCG — phonocardiogram
pCi — picocurie
PCM — protein-calorie
malnutrition
PCNL — percutaneous
nephrostolithotomy
PCO — polycystic ovary
P_{CO_2} — carbon dioxide partial
pressure (tension)
P_{CO_2} — carbon dioxide partial
pressure (tension)
pCO_2 — carbon dioxide partial
pressure (tension)
PCP — phencyclidine
hydrochloride
 Pneumocystis carinii
pneumonia
PCR — polymerase chain
reaction
PCV — packed cell volume
PCW — pulmonary capillary
wedge
PD — interpupillary distance
 prism diopter
PDA — patent ductus
arteriosus
 posterior descending artery
PDGF — platelet-derived
growth factor
PDI — periodontal disease
index
PDLL — poorly differentiated
lymphocytic lymphoma
PE — phosphatidylethanol-
amine
 physical examination
 potential energy

PE — phosphatidylethanol-
  amine *(continued)*
    pulmonary edema
    pulmonary embolism
peak
    biclonal p.
    Bragg p.
    kilovolts p.
    monoclonal p.
peak·om·e·ter
Pé·an's forceps
pearl
    Bohn's p's
    Elschnig's p's
    enamel p.
    epidermic p's
    epithelial p's
    Epstein's p's
    gouty p.
    Laënnec's p's
    parakeratotic p.
Pear·son's product-moment
  correlation coefficient
peau
    p. de chagrin
    p. d'orange
peb·ble
pé·brine
pe·ca·zine
pec·cant
pec·ca·ti·pho·bia
pechy·agra
Pec·quet's cistern
Pec·quet's duct
Pec·quet's reservoir
pec·ten *pl.* pec·ti·nes
    p. of anal canal
    p. analis
    p. ossis pubis
pec·te·nine
pec·te·ni·tis
pec·te·no·sis
pec·te·not·o·my
pec·tic
pec·tic ac·id
pec·tin
pec·ti·nate
Pec·ti·na·tus

pec·tin·e·al
pec·tin·i·form
pec·ti·za·tion
Pec·to·bac·te·ri·um
pec·to·lyt·ic
pec·to·ra
pec·to·ral
pec·to·ral·gia
pec·to·ra·lis
pec·to·ril·o·quy
    aphonic p.
    whispered p.
    whispering p.
pec·to·roph·o·ny
pec·tose
pec·tous
pec·tun·cu·lus
pec·tus *pl.* pec·to·ra
    p. carinatum
    p. excavatum
    p. gallinatum
    p. recurvatum
ped·al
pe·dar·throc·a·ce
ped·atro·phia
ped·er·ast
ped·er·as·ty
ped·er·in
pe·des
Ped·i·a·flor
pedi·al·gia
Pe·di·a·my·cin
pe·di·at·ric
pe·di·a·tri·cian
pe·di·at·rics
pe·di·at·rist
pe·di·at·ry
ped·i·cel
ped·i·cel·late
ped·i·cel·lat·ed
ped·i·cel·la·tion
ped·i·cle
    cone p.
    Filatov-Gillies tubed p.
    p. of lung
    p. of vertebral arch
ped·i·cled
pe·dic·u·lar

pe·dic·u·late
pe·dic·u·lat·ed
pe·dic·u·la·tion
pe·dic·u·li
pe·dic·u·li·cide
Ped·i·cu·li·dae
pe·dic·u·lo·sis
    p. capillitii
    p. capitis
    p. corporis
    p. inguinalis
    p. palpebrarum
    p. pubis
    p. vestimenti
    p. vestimentorum
pe·dic·u·lous
Pe·dic·u·lus
    P. humanus
    P. humanus capitis
    P. humanus corporis
    P. humanus humanus
    P. humanus vestimentorum
    P. inguinalis
    P. pubis
    P. vestimenti
pe·dic·u·lus *pl.* pe·dic·u·li
    p. arcus vertebrae
    p. pulmonis
ped·i·cure
ped·i·gree
ped·i·lu·vi·um
Pe·dio·coc·cus
    P. acidilactici
    P. cerevisiae
    P. halophilus
    P. pentosaceus
    P. urinae-equi
pe·dio·don·tia
pe·dio·nal·gia
pedi·pha·lanx
pedi·stib·u·lum
pe·di·tis
pe·do·baro·ma·crom·e·ter
pe·do·bar·om·e·ter
pe·do·don·tia
pe·do·don·tics
pe·do·don·tist
pe·do·dy·na·mom·e·ter

pe·dog·a·my
pe·do·gen·e·sis
pe·do·graph
pe·dol·o·gist
pe·dol·o·gy
pe·dom·e·ter
pe·do·mor·phic
pe·do·mor·phism
pe·dop·a·thy
pe·do·phil·ia
pe·do·phil·ic
pe·do·pho·bia
pe·dor·thic
pe·dor·thics
pe·dor·thist
pe·dun·cle
    cerebellar p., caudal
    cerebellar p., cranial
    cerebellar p., inferior
    cerebellar p., middle
    cerebellar p., pontine
    cerebellar p., rostral
    cerebellar p., superior
    p's of cerebellum
    cerebral p.
    p. of cerebrum
    p. of flocculus
    frontal thalamic p.
    p. of mamillary body
    olfactory p.
    pineal p.
    p. of pineal body
    p. of thalamus, caudal
    p. of thalamus, inferior
pe·dun·cu·lar
pe·dun·cu·lat·ed
pe·dun·cu·lot·o·my
pe·dun·cu·lus *pl.* pe·dun·cu·li
    p. cerebellaris caudalis
    p. cerebellaris cranialis
    p. cerebellaris inferior
    p. cerebellaris medius
    p. cerebellaris pontinus
    p. cerebellaris rostralis
    p. cerebellaris superior
    pedunculi cerebelli
    p. cerebralis
    p. cerebri

pe·dun·cu·lus *(continued)*
    p. corporis mamillaris
    p. corporis pinealis
    p. flocculi
    p. thalami anterior
    p. thalami caudalis
    p. thalami frontalis
    p. thalami inferior
    p. thalami posterior
    p. thalami superior
    p. vitellinus
peel
    bitter orange p.
    lemon p.
    lip p.
pee·nash
PEEP — positive
  end-expiratory pressure
Peet's operation
PEFR — peak expiratory flow
  rate
PEG — pneumoenceph-
  alography
    polyethylene glycol
peg
    bone p.
    epithelial p's
    rete p's
Peg·a·none
pe·gli·col 5 ole·ate
pe·gol·o·gy
peg·o·ter·ate
peg·ox·ol 7 ste·a·rate
Pel's crises
Pel-Eb·stein disease
Pel-Eb·stein fever
Pel-Eb·stein pyrexia
Pel-Eb·stein symptom
pe·lade
pel·age
Pel·a·mis
    P. bicolor
pel·ar·gon·ic acid
Pel·e·cyp·o·da
Pel·ger's nuclear anomaly
Pel·ger-Hu·ët nuclear anomaly
pel·ger·oid
pel·i·di·si

pel·i·o·sis
    p. hepatis
    p. of liver
Pel·i·zae·us-Merz·bach·er
  disease
pel·lag·ra
    monkey p.
    p. sine pellagra
    typhoid p.
pel·lag·ra·gen·ic
pel·lag·ral
pel·lag·ra·min
pel·lag·rin
pel·la·groid
pel·lag·rol·o·gist
pel·lag·rol·o·gy
pel·lag·rose
pel·la·gro·sis
pel·lag·rous
pel·lant
pel·late
Pel·le·gri·ni's disease
Pel·le·gri·ni-Stie·da disease
pel·let
    foil p.
pel·li·cle
    brown p.
    dental p.
pel·lic·u·lar
pel·lic·u·lous
Pel·liz·zi's syndrome
pel·lote
pel·lu·cid
Pe·lo·bi·on·ti·da
pe·loid
pe·lol·o·gy
Pelo·myxa
pe·lop·a·thy
pe·lo·ther·a·py
pel·ta
pel·tate
pel·ta·tin
pel·ves
pel·vic
pel·vi·cal·i·ce·al
pel·vi·cal·y·ce·al
pel·vi·cel·lu·li·tis

pel·vi·ceph·a·log·ra·phy
pel·vi·ceph·a·lom·e·try
pel·vi·fem·o·ral
pel·vi·fix·a·tion
pel·vi·li·thot·o·my
pel·vim·e·ter
    Budin's p.
    Martin's p.
pel·vim·e·try
    combined p.
    digital p.
    external p.
    instrumental p.
    internal p.
    manual p.
    x-ray p.
pel·vi·og·ra·phy
pel·vio·il·eo·neo·cys·tos·to·my
pel·vio·li·thot·o·my
pel·vio·neo·cys·tos·to·my
pel·vio·ne·os·to·my
pel·vio·peri·to·ni·tis
pel·vio·plas·ty
pel·vio·ra·di·og·ra·phy
pel·vi·os·co·py
pel·vi·os·to·my
pel·vi·ot·o·my
pel·vi·peri·to·ni·tis
pel·vi·ra·di·og·ra·phy
pel·vi·rec·tal
pel·vi·roent·gen·og·ra·phy
pel·vis *pl.* pel·ves, pelvises
    achondroplastic p.
    p. aequabiliter justo minor
    p. aequabiliter justo major
    android p.
    anthropoid p.
    assimilation p.
    asymmetrical p.
    beaked p.
    bifid p.
    blunderbuss p.
    bony p.
    brachypellic p.
    contracted p.
    cordate p.
    cordiform p.

pel·vis *(continued)*
    coxalgic p.
    coxarthrolisthetic p.
    Deventer's p.
    dolichopellic p.
    dwarf p.
    elastic p.
    extrarenal p.
    false p.
    flat p.
    frozen p.
    funnel-shaped p.
    giant p.
    greater p.
    gynecoid p.
    hardened p.
    high-assimilation p.
    infantile p.
    inverted p.
    p. justo major
    p. justo minor
    juvenile p.
    kyphorachitic p.
    kyphoscoliorachitic p.
    kyphoscoliotic p.
    kyphotic p.
    large p.
    lesser p.
    lordotic p.
    low-assimilation p.
    p. major
    mesatipellic p.
    p. minor
    Nägele's p.
    p. nana
    oblique p.
    obliquely contracted p.
    p. obtecta
    p. ossea
    osteomalacic p.
    Otto p.
    p. ovalis
    p. plana
    platypellic p.
    platypelloid p.
    Prague p.
    pseudo-osteomalacic p.
    pseudospider p.

pel·vis *(continued)*
    rachitic p.
    renal p.
    p. renalis
    Robert's p.
    Rokitansky's p.
    p. rotunda
    round p.
    rubber p.
    scoliotic p.
    simple flat p.
    small p.
    spider p.
    p. spinosa
    split p.
    spondylolisthetic p.
    p. spuria
    stove-in p.
    triangular p.
    triradiate p.
    true p.
    p. of ureter
pel·vi·sa·cral
pel·vi·sa·crum
pel·vi·scope
pel·vi·sec·tion
pel·vi·ster·num
pel·vi·therm
pel·vit·o·my
pel·vi·tro·chan·te·ri·an
pel·vi·ure·ter·al
pel·vi·ure·tero·ra·di·og·ra·phy
pel·vo·cal·i·ce·al
pel·vo·cal·i·ec·ta·sis
pel·vos·co·py
pel·vo·spon·dy·li·tis
    p. ossificans
pely·ceph·a·lom·et·ry
pely·col·o·gy
pem·er·id ni·trate
pem·o·line
pem·phi·goid
    benign mucosal p.
    benign mucous membrane p.
    bullous p.
    bullous p., localized

pem·phi·goid *(continued)*
    cicatricial p.
    localized chronic p.
pem·phi·gus
    benign familial p.
    Brazilian p.
    p. contagiosus
    p. erythematosus
    p. foliaceus
    ocular p.
    South American p.
    syphilitic p.
    p. vegetans
    p. vulgaris
    wildfire p.
pem·pi·dine tar·trate
Pen·brit·in
pen·bu·to·lol sul·fate
Pen·de's sign
pen·del·luft
Pendred's syndrome
pen·du·lar
pen·du·lous
pen·du·lum
    Pulfrich's p.
pe·nec·to·my
pen·e·tra·bil·i·ty
pen·e·trance
    complete p.
    genetic p.
pen·e·trant
pen·e·trat·ing
pen·e·tra·tion
pen·e·trom·e·ter
Pen·field epilepsy
Pen·field syndrome
pen·flur·i·dol
pe·ni·al
pen·i·ci·din
pen·i·cil·la·mine
pen·i·cil·lan·ic acid
pen·i·cil·li
pen·i·cil·li·ary
pen·i·cil·lic acid
pen·i·cil·lin
    aluminum p.
    benzathine p. G
    benzyl p. potassium

pen·i·cil·lin *(continued)*
    benzyl p. sodium
    buffered crystalline p. G
    clemizole p.
    depot p.
    p. dihydro F sodium
    dimethoxyphenyl p.
     sodium
    p. F
    p. G
    p. G benzathine
    p. G potassium
    p. G procaine
    p. G sodium
    isoxazolyl p.
    p. K
    p. N
    p. O
    p. O potassium
    p. O sodium
    phenoxymethyl p.
    potassium phenoxymethyl
     p.
    repository p.
    p. V
    p. V benzathine
    p. V hydrabamine
    p. V potassium
    p. X
pen·i·cil·lin·ase
pen·i·cil·lin-fast
pen·i·cil·lin·ic acid
pen·i·cil·li·o·sis
Pen·i·cil·li·um
    P. chrysogenum
    P. citrinum
    P. crustaceum
    P. glaucum
    P. notatum
    P. patulum
    P. uticale
pen·i·cil·lo·ic acid
pen·i·cil·loyl-pol·y·ly·sine
pen·i·cil·lus *pl.* pen·i·cil·li
    penicilli arteriae lienalis
    penicilli arteriae splenicae
    p. splenis
Pe·nic·u·li·na

pe·nic·u·lus *pl.* pe·nic·u·li
pe·nile
pen·il·lam·ine
pen·il·lo·al·de·hyde
pe·nis
    p. captivus
    chordeic p.
    cleft p.
    clubbed p.
    concealed p.
    double p.
    p. palmatus
    p. plastica
    webbed p.
pe·nis·chi·sis
pe·ni·tis
Penn seroflocculation reaction
pen·nate
pen·ni·form
pen·ny·ro·yal
pe·no·scro·tal
Pen·rose drain
pen·ta·ba·sic
pen·ta·chlo·ro·phe·nol
pen·ta·chro·mic
pen·ta·cyc·lic
pen·tad
pen·ta·dac·tyl
pen·ta·ene
pen·ta·eryth·ri·tol
    p. chloral
    p. tetranitrate
pen·ta·eryth·ri·tyl
    p. tetranitrate
pen·ta·gas·trin
pen·tal·o·gy
    p. of Fallot
pen·ta·mer
pen·ta·meth·a·zene
pen·ta·meth·yl·ene·di·amine
pen·ta·meth·yl·ene·tet·ra·zol
pen·ta·meth·yl·mel·amine
pen·tam·i·dine
    aerosolized p.
    p. isethionate
pen·tane
1,5-pen·tane·di·ol
pen·ta·pep·tide

pen·ta·pi·per·ide meth·yl·
  sul·fate
pen·ta·pi·per·i·um meth·yl·
  sul·fate
pen·ta·pyr·ro·li·din·i·um
  bi·tar·trate
pen·ta·so·my
Pen·tas·to·ma
pen·ta·stome
pen·ta·sto·mi·a·sis
pen·ta·sto·mid
Pen·ta·sto·mida
pen·ta·tom·ic
Pen·ta·trich·o·mo·nas
    P. hominis
pen·ta·va·lent
pen·taz·o·cine
    p. hydrochloride
    p. lactate
pent·dyo·pent
pen·tene
2-pen·ten·yl·pen·i·cil·lin
pen·te·tate cal·ci·um tri·so·
  di·um
pen·te·tic acid
pen·thi·e·nate bro·mide
Pen·thrane
pen·thrit
Pen·tids
pen·tiz·i·done so·di·um
pen·to·bar·bi·tal
    p. sodium
pen·to·bar·bi·tone
pen·to·lin·i·um tar·trate
pen·ton
pen·to·san
    methyl p.
pen·to·sa·zon
pen·tose
    p. nucleotide
    p. phosphate
pen·tos·emia
pen·tose·nu·cle·ic acid
pen·to·side
pen·tos·uria
pen·tos·uric
pen·to·syl

pen·to·syl·trans·fer·ase
Pen·to·thal
    P. sodium
pen·tox·ide
pen·tox·i·fyl·line
pen·tri·ni·trol
Pen·tri·tol
Pen·try·ate
pen·tyl
pent·yl·ene·tet·ra·zol
pen·um·bra
Pen-Vee
Pen·zoldt's reagent
Pen·zoldt's test
Pen·zoldt-Fish·er test
peo·til·lo·ma·nia
pe·ot·o·my
PEP — phosphoenol pyruvate
pep·lo·mer
pep·los
pep·per
    cayenne p.
Pep·per's syndrome
Pep·per's type
pep·per·mint
pep·sic
pep·si·gogue
pep·sin
    p. A.
    p. B.
    p. C.
pep·sin·ate
pep·sin·ia
pep·sin·if·er·ous
pep·sin·o·gen
pep·sin·og·e·nous
pep·sin·uria
pep·stat·in
Pep·tav·lon
pep·tic
pep·tid
    N-formylmethionyl p's
pep·ti·dase
pep·tide
    atrial natriuretic p. (ANP)
    C p.

pep·tide *(continued)*
    corticotropin-like
      intermediate lobe p.
      (CLIP)
    N-formylmethionyl p's
    signal p.
    p. T
    vasoactive intestinal p.
      (VIP)
pep·tide hy·dro·lase
pep·ti·der·gic
pep·ti·do·gly·can
pep·ti·do·lyt·ic
pep·ti·dyl
pep·ti·dyl-tRNA
pep·ti·dyl·trans·fer·ase
pep·ti·za·tion
Pep·to·coc·ca·ceae
Pep·to·coc·cus
    P. anaerobius
    P. asaccharolyticus
    P. constellatus
    P. magnus
pep·to·gen·ic
pep·tog·e·nous
pep·tol·y·sis
pep·to·lyt·ic
pep·tone
pep·ton·ic
pep·to·nize
pep·ton·uria
    enterogenous p.
    hepatogenous p.
    nephrogenic p.
    puerperal p.
    pyogenic p.
Pep·to·strep·to·coc·cus
    P. anaerobius
    P. lanceolatus
    P. micros
    P. parvulus
    P. productus
pep·to·tox·in
per·a·ceph·a·lus
per·ac·e·tate
per·ace·tic acid
per·ac·id
per·acid·i·ty

per·acute
Per·an·dren
per anum
per·ar·tic·u·la·tion
per·ax·il·lary
Per·a·zil
per·bor·ax
per·cen·tile
per·cen·tu·al
per·cept
per·cep·tion
    abstract p.
    depth p.
    extrasensory p. (ESP)
    facial p.
    stereognostic p.
    subliminal p.
per·cep·tive
per·cep·tiv·i·ty
per·cep·to·ri·um
per·cep·tuo·mo·tor
per·chlo·rate
per·chlor·ic acid
per·chlo·ride
per·chlor·meth·ane
per·chlor·meth·yl·for·mate
per·chlor·o·eth·y·lene
per·chlo·ro·naph·tha·lene
per·cip·i·ent
per·co·late
per·co·la·tion
per·co·la·tor
Per·coll
per·co·morph
per con·tig·u·um
per con·tin·u·um
Per·cor·ten
per·cuss
per·cus·si·ble
per·cus·sion
    auscultatory p.
    bimanual p.
    chest wall p.
    comparative p.
    deep p.
    direct p.
    drop p.
    drop stroke p.

per·cus·sion *(continued)*
   finger p.
   fist p.
   Goldscheider's p.
   immediate p.
   instrumental p.
   Korányi's p.
   Krönig's p.
   Lerch's p.
   mediate p.
   Murphy's p.
   palpatory p.
   paradoxical p.
   pencil p.
   piano p.
   Plesch's p.
   pleximetric p.
   respiratory p.
   slapping p.
   strip p.
   tangential p.
   threshold p.
   topographic p.
per·cus·sor
per·cu·ta·ne·ous
per cu·tem
per·cu·teur
per·en·ceph·a·ly
per·en·ni·al
Pe·rez's sign
per·fec·tion·ism
per·fil·con A
per·fla·tion
per·fo·rans *pl.* per·fo·ran·tes
   p. manus
per·for·ate
per·fo·rat·ed
per·fo·ra·tion
   Bezold's p.
   mechanical p.
   p. of nasal septum
   pathologic p.
   radicular p.
per·fo·ra·tor
per·fo·ra·to·ri·um
per·fri·ca·tion
per·frig·er·a·tion
per·fu·sate

per·fuse
per·fu·sion
   regional p.
per·fu·sion·ist
per·go·lide mes·y·late
per·hex·i·line mal·e·ate
per·i·ac·i·nal
per·i·ac·i·nous
Per·i·ac·tin
peri·ad·e·ni·tis
   p. mucosa necrotica
   recurrens
peri·ad·ven·ti·tial
peri·ali·en·itis
peri·am·pul·lary
peri·anal
peri·an·gi·itis
peri·an·gio·cho·li·tis
peri·an·gi·o·ma
peri·anth
peri·aor·tic
peri·aor·ti·tis
peri·apex
peri·ap·i·cal
peri·ap·pen·di·ci·tis
   p. decidualis
peri·ap·pen·dic·u·lar
peri·apt
peri·aq·ue·duc·tal
peri·ar·te·ri·al
peri·ar·te·ri·o·lar
peri·ar·te·ri·tis
   disseminated necrotizing p.
   p. gummosa
   p. nodosa
   syphilitic p.
peri·ar·thric
peri·ar·thri·tis
   p. calcarea
   p. of shoulder
peri·ar·tic·u·lar
peri·atri·al
peri·au·ric·u·lar
peri·ax·i·al
peri·ax·il·lary
peri·ax·o·nal
peri·blast
peri·bron·chi·al

peri·bron·chi·o·lar
peri·bron·chio·li·tis
peri·bron·chi·tis
peri·bul·bar
peri·bur·sal
peri·cal·i·ce·al
peri·cal·lo·sal
peri·cal·y·ce·al
peri·can·a·lic·u·lar
peri·cap·il·lary
peri·cap·su·lar
peri·car·dec·to·my
peri·car·di·ac
peri·car·di·al
peri·car·di·cen·te·sis
peri·car·di·ec·to·my
peri·car·dio·cen·te·sis
peri·car·di·ol·y·sis
peri·car·dio·me·di·as·ti·ni·tis
   adhesive p.
peri·car·dio·phren·ic
peri·car·dio·pleu·ral
peri·car·di·or·rha·phy
peri·car·di·os·to·my
peri·car·di·ot·o·my
peri·car·dit·ic
peri·car·di·tis
   acute benign p.
   acute exudative p.
   acute fibrinous p.
   adhesive p.
   amebic p.
   bacterial p.
   bread-and-butter p.
   p. calculosa
   carcinomatous p.
   constrictive p.
   dry p.
   p. with effusion
   p. epistenocardiaca
   p. externa et interna
   external p.
   fibrinous p.
   fibrous p.
   hemorrhagic p.
   idiopathic p.
   leukemic p.
   localized p.

peri·car·di·tis *(continued)*
   malignant p.
   mediastinal p.
   p. obliterans
   obliterating p.
   purulent p.
   rheumatic p.
   septic p.
   serofibrinous p.
   p. sicca
   suppurative p.
   tuberculous p.
   uremic p.
   p. villosa
   viral p.
peri·car·di·um
   adherent p.
   bread-and-butter p.
   calcified p.
   cardiac p.
   p. fibrosum
   fibrous p.
   parietal p.
   p. serosum
   serous p.
   shaggy p.
   visceral p.
peri·car·dot·o·my
peri·ca·val
peri·ce·cal
peri·ce·ci·tis
peri·cel·lu·lar
peri·ce·men·tal
peri·ce·men·ti·tis
   apical p.
   chronic suppurative p.
peri·ce·men·tum
peri·cen·tral
peri·cen·tri·o·lar
peri·ce·phal·ic
peri·cho·lan·gi·tis
peri·cho·le·cys·ti·tis
   gaseous p.
peri·chon·dri·al
peri·chon·dri·tis
peri·chon·dri·um
peri·chon·dro·ma
peri·chord

peri·chor·dal
peri·cho·ri·oi·dal
peri·cho·roi·dal
peri·chrome
peri·ci·sion
Per·i·clor
peri·co·lic
peri·co·li·tis
    p. dextra
    membranous p.
    p. sinistra
peri·co·lon·itis
peri·col·pi·tis
peri·con·chal
peri·con·chi·tis
peri·cor·ne·al
peri·cor·o·nal
peri·cor·o·ni·tis
peri·cox·itis
peri·cra·ni·al
peri·cra·ni·tis
peri·cra·ni·um
peri·cy·cle
peri·cys·tic
peri·cys·ti·tis
peri·cys·ti·um
peri·cyte
peri·cy·ti·al
peri·cy·to·ma
peri·dec·to·my
peri·def·er·en·ti·tis
peri·den·drit·ic
peri·dens
peri·den·tal
peri·den·ti·um
peri·derm
peri·der·mal
peri·des·mic
peri·des·mi·tis
peri·des·mi·um
pe·rid·ia
peri·did·y·mis
peri·did·y·mi·tis
pe·rid·i·um *pl.* pe·rid·ia
per·i·di·ver·tic·u·li·tis
peri·duc·tal
peri·duc·tile
peri·du·o·de·ni·tis

peri·du·ral
peri·du·ro·gram
peri·du·rog·ra·phy
peri·en·ceph·a·li·tis
peri·en·ceph·a·log·ra·phy
peri·en·ceph·a·lo·men·in·gi·
    tis
peri·en·ter·ic
peri·en·ter·itis
peri·en·ter·on
peri·ep·en·dy·mal
peri·epi·the·li·o·ma
peri·esoph·a·ge·al
peri·esoph·a·gi·tis
peri·fas·cic·u·lar
peri·fis·tu·lar
peri·fo·cal
peri·fol·lic·u·lar
peri·fol·lic·u·li·tis
    p. capitis abscedens et
      suffodiens
    superficial pustular p.
peri·gan·gli·itis
peri·gan·gli·on·ic
peri·gas·tric
peri·gas·tri·tis
peri·gem·mal
peri·glan·du·lar
peri·glan·du·li·tis
peri·gli·al
peri·glos·si·tis
peri·glot·tic
peri·glot·tis
peri·graft
peri·he·pat·ic
peri·hep·a·ti·tis
    p. chronica hyperplastica
    gonococcal p.
peri·her·ni·al
peri·hi·lar
peri·hy·poph·y·si·al
peri-in·su·lar
peri-is·let
peri·je·ju·ni·tis
peri·kary·on *pl.* peri·karya
peri·ker·at·ic
peri·ky·ma·ta *sing.* peri·ky·
    ma

peri·lab·y·rinth
peri·lab·y·rin·thi·tis
peri·la·ryn·ge·al
peri·lar·yn·gi·tis
peri·len·tic·u·lar
peri·le·sion·al
peri·lig·a·men·tous
peri·lim·bal
peri·lo·bar
peri·lob·u·li·tis
peri·lymph
peri·lym·pha
peri·lym·phad·e·ni·tis
peri·lym·phan·ge·al
peri·lym·phan·gi·tis
peri·lym·phat·ic
peri·mac·u·lar
peri·mas·ti·tis
peri·med·ul·lary
peri·men·in·gi·tis
pe·rim·e·ter
    arc p.
    dental p.
    projection p.
peri·met·ric
peri·me·trit·ic
peri·me·tri·tis
peri·me·tri·um
peri·met·ro·sal·pin·gi·tis
    encapsulating p.
pe·rim·e·try
    flicker p.
    quantitative p.
peri·mol·y·sis
peri·my·cin
peri·my·elis
peri·my·eli·tis
peri·my·elog·ra·phy
peri·my·lol·y·sis
peri·myo·car·di·tis
peri·myo·en·do·car·di·tis
peri·myo·me·tri·um
peri·myo·si·tis
peri·mys·ia
peri·mys·i·al
peri·mys·i·itis
peri·mys·itis

peri·mys·i·um *pl.* peri·mys·ia
    external p.
    p. externum
    internal p.
    p. internum
peri·na·tal
peri·na·tol·o·gist
peri·na·tol·o·gy
peri·ne·al
peri·neo·cele
peri·ne·om·e·ter
peri·neo·plas·ty
peri·neo·rec·tal
peri·ne·or·rha·phy
    Emmet-Studdiford p.
peri·neo·scro·tal
peri·neo·syn·the·sis
peri·ne·ot·o·my
peri·neo·vag·i·nal
peri·neo·vag·i·no·rec·tal
peri·neo·vul·var
peri·neph·ri·al
peri·neph·ric
peri·ne·phrit·ic
peri·ne·phri·tis
peri·neph·ri·um
peri·ne·um
    anterior p.
    posterior p.
    watering-can p.
peri·neu·ral
peri·neu·ri·al
peri·neu·rit·ic
peri·neu·ri·tis
peri·neu·ri·um
peri·nu·cle·ar
peri·oc·u·lar
pe·ri·od
    absolute refractory p.
    acceleration p.
    antepartum p.
    child-bearing p.
    critical p.
    deceleration p.
    eclipse p.
    ejection p.
    p. of emptying

pe·ri·od *(continued)*
 fertile p.
 p. of filling
 G_1 p.
 G_2 p.
 gestational p.
 half-life p.
 incubation p.
 induction p.
 intrapartum p.
 isoelectric p.
 isometric p.
 p. of isometric contraction
 p. of isometric relaxation
 isovolumic p.
 lag p.
 latency p.
 latent p.
 M p.
 menstrual p.
 monthly p.
 neonatal p.
 patient p.
 perinatal p.
 postneonatal p.
 postpartum p.
 postsphygmic p.
 prefunctional p.
 prenatal p.
 prepatent p.
 presphygmic p.
 prodromal p.
 puerperal p.
 quarantine p.
 reaction p.
 refractory p.
 relative refractory p.
 reproductive p.
 S p.
 safe p.
 silent p.
 sphygmic p.
 steady p.
 Wenckebach p.
per·io·date
pe·ri·od·ic
per·iod·ic acid

pe·ri·o·dic·i·ty
 diurnal p.
 filarial p.
 lunar p.
 malarial p.
 nocturnal p.
 subperiodic p.
peri·odon·tal
peri·odon·tia
peri·odon·tics
peri·odon·tist
peri·odon·ti·tis
 acute local p.
 adult p.
 apical p.
 chronic apical p.
 chronic suppurative p.
 juvenile p.
 marginal p.
 prepubertal p.
 rapidly progressive p.
 simple p.
 p. simplex
 suppurative p.
peri·odon·ti·um *pl.* peri·odon·tia
 p. insertionis
 p. protectoris
peri·odon·tol·o·gy
peri·odon·to·scope
peri·odon·to·sis
peri·om·phal·ic
peri·onych·ia
peri·onych·i·um
peri·onyx
peri·onyx·is
peri·ooph·o·ri·tis
peri·ooph·o·ro·sal·pin·gi·tis
peri·oo·the·ci·tis
peri·op·er·a·tive
peri·oph·thal·mia
peri·oph·thal·mic
peri·oph·thal·mi·tis
peri·op·tom·e·try
peri·oral
peri·or·bit
peri·or·bi·ta

peri·or·bi·tal
peri·or·bi·ti·tis
peri·or·chi·tis
    p. adhaesiva
    p. purulenta
peri·or·chi·um
peri·os·te·al
peri·os·te·itis
peri·os·teo·ede·ma
peri·os·te·o·ma
peri·os·teo·med·ul·li·tis
peri·os·teo·my·eli·tis
peri·os·teo·phyte
peri·os·te·or·rha·phy
peri·os·teo·sis
peri·os·teo·tome
peri·os·te·ot·o·my
peri·os·te·ous
peri·os·te·um
    alveolar p.
    p. alveolare
    p. cranii
peri·os·ti·tis
    p. albuminosa
    albuminous p.
    diffuse p.
    hemorrhagic p.
    p. hyperplastica
    p. interna cranii
    orbital p.
    precocious p.
peri·os·to·sis
    hyperplastic p.
peri·otic
peri·ova·ri·tis
peri·ovu·lar
peri·pachy·men·in·gi·tis
peri·pan·cre·at·ic
peri·pan·cre·a·ti·tis
peri·pap·il·lary
peri·par·tum
peri·pa·tel·lar
peri·pa·tet·ic
peri·pe·ni·al
peri·peri·car·di·tis
peri·pha·ci·tis
peri·phak·us
peri·pha·ryn·ge·al

pe·riph·er·ad
pe·riph·er·al
pe·riph·er·aphose
peri·pher·ic
pe·riph·ero·cen·tral
pe·riph·ero·cep·tor
pe·riph·ero·mit·tor
pe·riph·ero·phose
pe·riph·ery
peri·phle·bit·ic
peri·phle·bi·tis
    sclerosing p.
peri·pho·ria
peri·phre·ni·tis
Peri·pla·ne·ta
    P. americana
    P. australasiae
peri·plasm
peri·plas·mic
peri·pleu·ral
peri·pleu·ri·tis
peri·plo·cin
peri·plo·cy·ma·rin
peri·plog·e·nin
peri·pneu·mo·nia
    p. notha
peri·pneu·mo·ni·tis
peri·po·lar
peri·po·le·sis
peri·po·ri·tis
peri·por·tal
peri·proc·tal
peri·proc·tic
peri·proc·ti·tis
peri·pros·tat·ic
peri·pros·ta·ti·tis
peri·py·eli·tis
peri·py·le·phle·bi·tis
peri·py·lic
peri·py·lo·ric
peri·ra·dic·u·lar
peri·rec·tal
peri·rec·ti·tis
peri·re·nal
peri·rhi·nal
peri·rhi·zo·cla·sia
peri·sal·pin·gi·tis
peri·sal·pin·go·opho·ri·tis

peri·sal·pin·go-ova·ri·tis
peri·sal·pinx
peri·scle·ri·um
peri·scop·ic
peri·sig·moid·itis
peri·si·nu·itis
peri·sin·u·ous
peri·sin·u·si·tis
peri·sper·ma·ti·tis
    p. serosa
peri·splanch·nic
peri·splanch·ni·tis
peri·splen·ic
peri·sple·ni·tis
    p. cartilaginea
peri·spon·dyl·ic
peri·spon·dy·li·tis
    Gibney's p.
Peri·spo·ri·a·ceae
pe·ris·so·dac·ty·lous
peri·stal·sis
    mass p.
    retrograde p.
    reversed p.
peri·stal·tic
peri·stal·tin
peri·staph·y·line
peri·stome
peri·sto·mi·al
peri·stru·mi·tis
peri·stru·mous
peri·sy·no·vi·al
peri·sy·no·vi·tis
peri·syr·in·gi·tis
peri·tec·to·my
peri·ten·din·e·um
peri·ten·di·ni·tis
    adhesive p.
    p. calcarea
    p. crepitans
    p. serosa
peri·ten·di·nous
peri·te·non
peri·ten·o·ne·um
peri·ten·o·ni·tis
peri·ten·on·ti·tis
peri·the·ci·um
peri·the·li·al

peri·the·li·o·ma
peri·the·li·um
    Eberth's p.
peri·tho·rac·ic
peri·thy·re·oid·itis
peri·thy·roi·di·tis
pe·rit·o·mist
peri·tom·ize
pe·rit·o·my
peri·to·ne·al
peri·to·ne·al·gia
peri·to·ne·al·ize
peri·to·neo·cen·te·sis
peri·to·neo·cly·sis
peri·to·ne·og·ra·phy
peri·to·neo·mus·cu·lar
peri·to·ne·op·a·thy
peri·to·neo·peri·car·di·al
peri·to·neo·pexy
peri·to·neo·plas·ty
peri·to·neo·scope
peri·to·ne·os·co·py
peri·to·neo·tome
peri·to·ne·ot·o·my
peri·to·neo·ve·nous
peri·to·ne·um
    abdominal p.
    intestinal p.
    parietal p.
    p. parietale
    urogenital p.
    p. urogenitale
    visceral p.
    p. viscerale
peri·to·nism
peri·to·ni·tis
    acute sterile p.
    adhesive p.
    benign paroxysmal p.
    bile p.
    biliary p.
    chemical p.
    p. chronica fibrosa
      encapsulans
    chyle p.
    circumscribed p.
    p. deformans
    diaphragmatic p.

peri·to·ni·tis *(continued)*
    diffuse p.
    p. encapsulans
    encysted p.
    familial paroxysmal p.
    fibrocaseous p.
    gas p.
    general p.
    hemorrhagic p.
    localized p.
    meconium p.
    pelvic p.
    perforative p.
    periodic p.
    puerperal p.
    purulent p.
    septic p.
    serous p.
    silent p.
    terminal p.
    traumatic p.
    tuberculous p.
peri·to·ni·za·tion
peri·to·nize
peri·ton·sil·lar
peri·ton·sil·li·tis
peri·tra·che·al
Per·i·trate
peri·trich
peri·trich·ia
peri·trich·i·da
pe·rit·ri·chous
peri·tro·chan·ter·ic
peri·tu·ber·cu·lo·sis
peri·typh·lic
peri·typh·li·tis
    p. actinomycotica
peri·um·bil·i·cal
peri·un·gual
peri·ure·ter·al
peri·ure·ter·ic
peri·ure·ter·itis
    p. plastica
peri·ure·thral
peri·ure·thri·tis
peri·uter·ine
peri·vag·i·nal
peri·vag·i·ni·tis

peri·vas·cu·lar
peri·vas·cu·lar·i·ty
peri·vas·cu·li·tis
peri·ve·ni·tus
peri·ve·nous
peri·ven·tric·u·lar
peri·ver·te·bral
peri·ves·i·cal
peri·ve·sic·u·lar
peri·ve·sic·u·li·tis
peri·vis·cer·al
peri·vis·cer·itis
peri·vi·tel·line
peri·vul·var
peri·xe·ni·tis
per·ker·a·to·sis
per·la·pine
per·lèche
Per·lia's nucleus
Perls' stain
Perls' test
perl·sucht
per·man·ga·nate
per·man·gan·ic acid
per·me·a·bil·i·ty
    differential p.
    magnetic p.
per·me·a·ble
per·me·ant
per·me·ase
per·me·at·al
per·me·ate
per·me·a·tion
Per·mi·til
per·na
per·na·sal
per·nic·i·o·si·form
per·ni·cious
per·nio *pl.* per·ni·o·nes
per·ni·o·sis
pe·ro·bra·chi·us
pe·ro·ceph·a·lus
pe·ro·ceph·a·ly
pe·ro·chi·rus
pe·ro·cor·mus
pe·ro·dac·ty·lus
pe·ro·dac·ty·ly
pero·me·lia

pe·rom·e·lus
pe·ro·nar·thro·sis
per·o·ne
per·o·ne·al
pe·ro·neo·cu·boi·de·us
pe·ro·neo·tib·i·al
pe·ro·ne·us
    p. accessorius digiti minimi
    p. accessorius quartus
pe·ro·nia
Per. op. emet. — L. peracta
  operatione emetici (when the
  action of the emetic is over)
pe·ro·pus
per·oral
per os
pe·ro·sis
pe·ro·so·mus
pe·ros·o·my
pe·ro·splanch·nia
per·os·se·ous
pe·rot·ic
pe·rox·i·dase
per·ox·i·da·tic
pe·rox·ide
pe·rox·i·some
per·oxy·ace·tic acid
per·oxy·ac·yl·ni·trate
per·oxy·dol
per·phen·a·zine
per pri·mam
per pri·mam in·ten·ti·o·nem
per rec·tum
Per·rin-Fer·ra·ton disease
Per·ron·ci·to's apparatus
Per·ron·ci·to's spirals
per·salt
per sal·tum
Per·san·tine
per se·cun·dam
per se·cun·dam in·ten·ti·o·
  nem
per·sev·er·ate
per·sev·er·a·tion
per·sist·ence
    hereditary p. of fetal
      hemoglobin (HPFH)
per·sis·ter

per·so·na
per·so·nal·i·ty
    affective p. (disorder)
    alternating p.
    anankastic p.
    antisocial p. (disorder)
    as-if p.
    avoidant p. (disorder)
    borderline p. (disorder)
    compulsive p.
    cycloid p. (disorder)
    cyclothymic p. (disorder)
    dependent p. (disorder)
    dissociative p.
    double p.
    dual p.
    dyssocial p.
    epileptoid p. (disorder)
    explosive p.
    histrionic p. (disorder)
    hysterical p.
    inadequate p.
    multiple p.
    narcissistic p. (disorder)
    obsessive p.
    obsessive-compulsive p.
     (disorder)
    paranoid p. (disorder)
    passive p.
    passive aggressive p.
     (disorder)
    passive-dependent p.
    psychopathic p.
    sadistic p. (disorder)
    schizoid p. (disorder)
    schizothymic p.
    schizotypal p. (disorder)
    seclusive p.
    shut-in p.
    self-defeating p. (disorder)
    split p.
    split-off p.
per·son·o·log·ic
per·so·nol·o·gy
per·spi·ra·tio
    p. insensibilis
per·spi·ra·tion
    insensible p.

per·spi·ra·tion *(continued)*
    sensible p.
per·sua·sion
per·sul·fate
per·sul·fide
per·sul·fur·ic acid
per·tech·ne·tate
Per·thes' disease
Per·thes' test
Per·tik's diverticulum
Per·to·frane
per tu·bam
per·tu·ba·tion
per·tu·cin
per·tus·sal
per·tus·sis
per·tus·soid
per va·gi·nam
per·ve·nous
per·ver·sion
    polymorphous p.
    sexual p.
per·vert
per·vi·gil·i·um
per·vi·ous
pes *pl.* pe·des
    p. abductus
    p. adductus
    p. anserinus
    p. calcaneus
    p. cavus
    p. cerebri
    congenital convex p. valgus
    p. equinovalgus
    equinovarus p.
    p. febricitans
    p. gigas
    p. hippocampi
    p. hippocampi major
    p. hippocampi minor
    p. pedunculi
    p. planovalgus
    p. planus
    p. pronatus
    p. supinatus
    p. valgus
    p. varus

pes·sa·ry
    air-ball p.
    cheek p.
    contraceptive p.
    cup p.
    diaphragm p.
    doughnut p.
    Hodge's p.
    lever p.
    Mayer's p.
    Menge's p.
    prolapsed p.
    retroversion p.
    ring p.
    Smith's p.
    stem p.
    Thomas p.
pes·si·mism
    therapeutic p.
pes·si·mum
pes·su·lum
pes·ti·ce·mia
pes·ti·cide
    hard p.
    nonpersistent p.
    persistent p.
    soft p.
pes·tif·er·ous
pes·ti·lence
pes·ti·len·tial
pes·tis
    p. ambulans
    p. bubonica
    p. equorum
    p. fulminans
    p. major
    p. minor
    p. siderans
    p. varilosa
pes·ti·vi·rus
pes·tle
pes·tol·o·gy
PET — positron emission
  tomography
    preeclamptic toxemia
pet·a·lo·bac·te·ria
pe·te·chia *pl.* pe·tech·iae

pe·te·chia
  calcaneal petechiae
pe·te·chiae
pe·te·chi·al
pe·te·chi·om·e·ter
Pe·ters anomaly
Pe·ters' ovum
Pe·ters syndrome
Pe·ter·sen's bag
peth·i·dine hy·dro·chlo·ride
pet·i·o·late
pet·i·o·lat·ed
pet·i·ole
  epiglottic p.
pet·i·oled
pe·ti·o·lus
  p. epiglottidis
Pe·tit's canal
Pe·tit's hernia
Pe·tit's law
Pe·tit's ligament
Pe·tit's sinus
Pe·tit's triangle
pe·tit mal
  atonic p. m.
  myoclonic p. m.
Pe·trén's diet
Pe·trén's treatment
Pé·tre·quin's ligament
pet·ri·chlo·ral
Pe·tri dish
Pe·tri plate
Pe·tri reaction
Pe·tri test
pet·ri·fac·tion
pé·tris·sage
pe·tro·bas·i·lar
pet·roc·cip·i·tal
pe·trog·e·nous
pet·ro·late
pet·ro·la·tum
  p. album
  hydrophilic p.
  liquid p.
  liquid p., heavy
  liquid p., light
  p. liquidum
  p. liquidum leve

pet·ro·la·tum (continued)
  white p.
pe·tro·le·um
pet·rol·iza·tion
pet·ro·mas·toid
pet·ro-oc·cip·i·tal
pet·ro·pha·ryn·ge·us
pe·tro·sa
pe·tro·sal
pet·ro·sal·pin·go·staph·y·li·
  nus
pet·ro·sec·to·my
pet·ro·si·tis
pe·tro·so·mas·toid
pet·ro·sphe·noid
pet·ro·squa·mo·sal
pet·ro·squa·mous
pet·ro·staph·y·li·nus
pet·rous
pet·rous·itis
Pe·trusch·ky's litmus whey
Pe·trusch·ky's spinalgia
PETT — positron emission
  transaxial tomography
Pet·ten·kof·er's test
Pet·ten·kof·er's theory
pet·ty·mor·rel
Pet·ze·ta·ki's reaction
Pet·ze·ta·ki's test
Petz·val's curvature
Peu·ce·tia
  P. viridans
Peutz-Je·ghers syndrome
pex·ia
pex·ic
pex·in
pex·is
Pey·er's glands
Pey·er's insulae
Pey·er's patches
Pey·er's plaques
pey·o·te
Pey·ro·nie's disease
Pey·rot's thorax
Pfan·nen·stiel's incision
PFC — plaque-forming cell
Pfeif·fer's bacillus
Pfeif·fer's disease

Pfeif·fer's phenomenon
Pfeif·fer's reaction
Pfeif·fer's syndrome
Pfeif·fer-Com·berg method
Pflü·ger's cords
Pflü·ger's law
Pflü·ger's tubes
PFT — parafascicular thalamotomy
Pfuhl's sign
Pfuhl-Jaffé sign
PG — Pharmacopoeia Germanica (German Pharmacopeia)
    prostaglandin
pg — picogram
PGD_2, PGE_2, PGF_2, αPGI_2, etc. — symbols for various prostaglandins
pgm — picogram
Ph — Pharmacopeia
pH — hydrogen ion concentration (potential of hydrogen ion)
PHA — phytohemagglutinin
pha·ci·tis
phaco·ana·phy·lax·is
phaco·cele
phaco·cyst
phaco·cys·tec·to·my
phaco·cys·ti·tis
phaco·emul·si·fi·ca·tion
phaco·er·y·sis
phaco·glau·co·ma
phaco·hy·men·itis
phac·oid
phac·oid·itis
phac·oido·scope
pha·col·y·sin
phac·ol·y·sis
phaco·lyt·ic
pha·co·ma
phaco·ma·la·cia
phac·o·ma·to·sis
phaco·meta·cho·re·sis
phaco·met·e·ce·sis
pha·com·e·ter
phaco·pal·in·gen·e·sis

phaco·pla·ne·sis
phaco·scle·ro·sis
phaco·scope
pha·cos·co·py
phaco·sco·tas·mus
phaco·ther·a·py
phaco·tox·ic
Phaen·i·cia
    P. cuprina
    P. sericata
phaeo·hy·pho·my·co·sis
phage
phag·e·de·na
    p. gangrenosa
    geometric p.
    sloughing p.
    p. tropica
phag·e·den·ic
phage·ly·sis
phage-typ·ing
phago·cyt·a·ble
phago·cyte
    alveolar p's
    endothelial p.
    fixed p.
    free p.
    habitual p's
    mononuclear p.
phago·cyt·ic
phago·cy·tin
phago·cyt·ize
phago·cy·tol·y·sis
phago·cy·to·lyt·ic
phago·cy·tose
phago·cy·to·sis
    induced p.
    spontaneous p.
    surface p.
phago·cy·tot·ic
phago·frag·ma·tome
phago·kary·o·sis
phago·log·i·cal
pha·gol·y·sis
phago·ly·so·some
phago·lyt·ic
phago·ma·nia
phago·pho·bia
phago·plasm

phago·py·ro·sis
phago·some
phago·troph
phago·troph·ic
phago·type
pha·ki·tis
pha·ko·ma
   retinal p.
phak·o·ma·to·sis *pl.* phak·o·
   ma·to·ses
   Bourneville's p.
pha·lan·ge·al
pha·lan·gec·to·my
pha·lan·ges
phal·an·gette
   drop p.
phal·an·gi·tis
phal·an·gi·za·tion
pha·lan·go·pha·lan·ge·al
phal·an·go·sis
pha·lanx *pl.* pha·lan·ges
   Deiters' phalanges
   phalanges digitorum
      manus
   phalanges digitorum pedis
   phalanges of fingers
   p. distalis digitorum manus
   p. distalis digitorum pedis
   p. media digitorum manus
   p. media digitorum pedis
   p. prima digitorum manus
   p. prima digitorum pedis
   p. proximalis digitorum
      manus
   p. proximalis digitorum
      pedis
   p. secunda digitorum
      manus
   p. secunda digitorum pedis
   p. tertia digitorum manus
   p. tertia digitorum pedis
   phalanges of toes
   ungual p. of fingers
   ungual p. of toes
Phal·en's maneuver
Phal·en's sign
Phal·en's test
Phal·la·les

phal·lal·gia
phal·lan·as·tro·phe
phal·lan·eu·rysm
phal·lec·to·my
phal·li
phal·lic
phal·li·form
phal·lin
phal·li·tis
phal·lo·camp·sis
phal·lo·cryp·sis
phal·lo·dyn·ia
phal·loid
phal·loid·in
phal·loid·ine
phal·lon·cus
phal·lo·plas·ty
   reconstructive p.
phal·lor·rha·gia
phal·lor·rhea
phal·lot·o·my
Phal·lus
phal·lus *pl.* phal·li
phan·er·o·gam
phan·ero·ge·net·ic
phan·er·o·gen·ic
phan·ero·plasm
phan·er·o·sis
   fat p.
Phan·o·dorn
phan·ta·sia
phan·tasm
phan·ta·sy
phan·to·geu·sia
phan·tom
   flood p.
   Schultze p.
phan·u·rane
phar — pharmaceutical
   pharmacopeia
   pharmacy
pharm — pharmaceutical
   pharmacopeia
   pharmacy
Phar B — L. Pharmaciae
   Baccalaureus (Bachelor of
   Pharmacy)

Phar C — Pharmaceutical Chemist
phar·ci·dous
Phar D — Pharmaciae Doctor (Doctor of Pharmacy)
Phar G — Graduate in Pharmacy
Phar M — Pharmaciae Magister (Master of Pharmacy)
phar·ma·cal
phar·ma·ceu·tic
phar·ma·ceu·ti·cal
phar·ma·ceu·tics
phar·ma·ceu·tist
phar·ma·cist
phar·ma·co·chem·is·try
phar·ma·co·di·ag·no·sis
phar·ma·co·dy·nam·ic
phar·ma·co·dy·nam·ics
phar·ma·co·en·do·cri·nol·o·gy
phar·ma·co·ep·i·de·mi·ol·o·gy
phar·ma·co·ge·net·ics
phar·ma·cog·nos·tics
phar·ma·cog·no·sy
phar·ma·cog·ra·phy
phar·ma·co·ki·net·ics
phar·ma·co·log·ic
phar·ma·col·o·gist
phar·ma·col·o·gy
    biochemical p.
    marine p.
phar·ma·co·ma·nia
phar·ma·co·met·rics
phar·ma·con
phar·ma·co-or·yc·tol·o·gy
phar·ma·co·pe·dia
phar·ma·co·pe·dics
phar·ma·co·pe·ia
phar·ma·co·pe·ial
phar·ma·co·pho·bia
phar·ma·co·phore
phar·ma·co·poe·ia
phar·ma·co·psy·cho·sis
phar·ma·co·ra·di·og·ra·phy

phar·ma·co·roent·gen·og·ra·phy
phar·ma·co·ther·a·peu·tics
phar·ma·co·ther·a·py
phar·ma·cy
    chemical p.
    clinical p.
    galenic p.
Pharm D — Doctor of Pharmacy
phar·yn·gal·gia
phar·yn·ge·al
phar·yn·gec·ta·sia
phar·yn·gec·to·my
phar·yn·gem·phrax·is
phar·yn·ge·us
phar·yn·gism
phar·yn·gis·mus
phar·yn·git·ic
phar·yn·gi·tid
phar·yn·gi·tis
    acute lymphonodular p.
    atrophic p.
    catarrhal p.
    chronic p.
    croupous p.
    diphtheritic p.
    follicular p.
    gangrenous p.
    glandular p.
    granular p.
    p. herpetica
    hypertrophic p.
    p. keratosa
    membranous p.
    phlegmonous p.
    plague p.
    p. sicca
    ulceromembranous p.
    p. ulcerosa
pha·ryn·go·cele
pha·ryn·go·cer·a·to·sis
pha·ryn·go·con·junc·ti·vi·tis
pha·ryn·go·dyn·ia
pha·ryn·go·epi·glot·tid·e·an
pha·ryn·go·ep·i·glot·tid·e·an
pha·ryn·go·esoph·a·ge·al

pha·ryn·go·esoph·a·go·plas·ty

pha·ryn·go·esoph·a·gus

pha·ryn·go·glos·sal

pha·ryn·go·glos·sus

pha·ryn·go·ker·a·to·sis

pha·ryn·go·la·ryn·ge·al

pha·ryn·go·lar·yn·gec·to·my

pha·ryn·go·lar·yn·gi·tis

pha·ryn·go·lith

pha·ryn·gol·o·gy

pha·ryn·gol·y·sis

pha·ryn·go·max·il·lary

pha·ryn·go·my·co·sis

pha·ryn·go·na·sal

pha·ryn·go-oral

pha·ryn·go·pal·a·tine

pha·ryn·go·pa·ral·y·sis

pha·ryn·gop·a·thy

pha·ryn·go·pe·ris·to·le

pha·ryn·go·plas·ty

   Hynes p.

pha·ryn·go·ple·gia

pha·ryn·go·rhi·ni·tis

pha·ryn·go·rhi·nos·co·py

pha·ryn·gor·rha·gia

pha·ryn·gor·rhea

pha·ryn·go·sal·pin·gi·tis

pha·ryn·go·scle·ro·ma

pha·ryn·go·scope

pha·ryn·gos·co·py

pha·ryn·go·spasm

pha·ryn·go·ste·no·sis

pha·ryn·gos·to·ma

pha·ryn·gos·to·my

pha·ryn·go·tome

pha·ryn·got·o·my

   anterior p.

   external p.

   infrahyoid p.

   internal p.

   lateral p.

   median p.

   subhyoid p.

   transhyoid p.

   translingual p.

   transthyroid p.

   transverse p.

pha·ryn·go·ton·sil·li·tis

pha·ryn·go·ty·phoid

pha·ryn·go·xe·ro·sis

phar·ynx

   laryngeal p.

   oral p.

   primitive p.

phase

   active p.

   alpha p.

   anal p.

   apophylactic p.

   aqueous p.

   beta p.

   cholesteric p.

   continuous p.

   coupling p.

   p. of decline

   diastolic p. of concentration

   diastolic isometric p.

   disperse p.

   effective lethal p.

   erythrocytic p.

   estrin p.

   exponential p.

   external p.

   G_1 p.

   G_2 p.

   genital p.

   hematic p.

   inductive p.

   internal p.

   lag p.

   latency p.

   logarithmic p.

   luteal p.

   m p.

   meiotic p.

   menstrual p.

   motofacient p.

   negative p.

   nephrographic p.

   nonmotofacient p.

   Nonne-Apelt p.

   oedipal p.

   oral p.

   oral-incorporative p.

phase *(continued)*
    oral-sadistic p.
    oral-sucking p.
    phallic p.
    positive p.
    postmeiotic p.
    postmenstrual p.
    preambivalent p.
    pregenital p.
    premeiotic p.
    prereduction p.
    premenstrual p.
    preoedipal p.
    progestational p.
    proliferative p.
    reduction p.
    repulsion p.
    resting p.
    s p.
    secretory p.
    smectic p.
    specific p.
    stance p.
    stationary p.
    supernormal recovery p.
    swing p.
    synaptic p.
    systolic p. of concentration
pha·se·o·la·min
pha·se·o·lin
pha·se·o·lu·na·tin
pha·sic
pha·sin
pha·sein
phas·mid
Phas·mid·ia
PhB — British Pharmacopoeia
PhD — Doctor of Philosophy
Phe — phenylalanine
Phelps' operation
Phe-Mer-Nite
Phe·mer·ol
phem·fil·con A
Phem·is·ter graft
Phem·is·ter oper·ation
phem·i·tone
phen·a·caine hy·dro·chlo·ride
phe·nac·e·mide

phe·nac·e·tin
phen·a·cet·o·lin
phe·nac·e·tu·ric acid
phe·nac·e·tyl·uria
phen·a·gly·co·dol
phe·na·kis·to·scope
phe·nan·threne
phe·nan·thro·lene
phen·an·to·in
phe·nate
phe·naz·o·cine hy·dro·bro·mide
phen·a·zone
phen·a·zo·pyr·i·dine hy·dro·chlo·ride
phen·ben·i·cil·lin
phen·ben·za·mine
phen·bu·ta·zone so·di·um glyc·er·ate
phen·cy·cli·dine hy·dro·chlo·ride
phen·di·met·ra·zine tar·trate
phene
phen·el·zine sul·fate
Phen·er·gan
phen·eth·a·nol
phe·neth·i·cil·lin
    p. potassium
phen·eth·yl
phen·eth·yl·bi·guan·ide
phe·net·i·din
phe·net·i·din·uria
phen·for·min hy·dro·chlo·ride
phen·go·pho·bia
phe·nic acid
phe·nin·da·mine tar·trate
phen·in·di·one
phen·ir·amine mal·e·ate
Phe·nis·tix
phen·met·ra·zine hy·dro·chlo·ride
phe·no·bar·bi·tal
    p. sodium
phe·no·bar·bi·tone
phe·no·copy
phe·no·de·vi·ant
phe·no·ge·net·ics

phe·nol
   camphorated p.
   p. liquefactum
   liquefied p.
   p. red
phe·no·lase
phe·no·late
phe·no·lat·ed
Phe·no·lax
phe·no·le·mia
phe·nol·ic
phe·nol·iza·tion
phe·nol·o·gist
phe·nol·o·gy
phe·nol·phthal·ein
phe·nol sul·fa·tase
phe·nol·sul·fon·ic acid
phe·nol·sul·fon·phthal·ein
phe·nol·tet·ra·chlo·ro·
  phthal·ein
phe·nol·uria
phe·nom
phe·nom·e·nol·o·gy
phe·nom·e·non *pl.* phe·nom·
  e·na
   abstinence p.
   adhesion p.
   anaphylactoid p.
   Anderson's p.
   aqueous-influx p.
   Arias-Stella p.
   arm p.
   p. of Arthus
   Ascher's negative glass-rod
    p.
   Ascher's positive glass-rod
    p.
   Aschner's p.
   Ashman's p.
   Aubert's p.
   Austin Flint p.
   autokinetic visible light p.
   Babinski's p.
   Becker's p.
   Bell's p.
   Berry-Dedrick p.
   blood-influx p.
   Bordet-Gengou p.

phe·nom·e·non *(continued)*
   Bowditch p.
   brake p.
   break-off p.
   Browning's p.
   Chase-Sulzberger p.
   cheek p.
   clasp-knife p.
   cogwheel p.
   cold agglutination p.
   Collie p.
   critical epileptic p.
   crossed phrenic nerve p.
   crus p.
   Cushing's p.
   Dale p.
   Danysz's p.
   Davenport p.
   dawn p.
   Debre's p.
   declamping p.
   Dejerine-Lichtheim p.
   Denys-Leclef p.
   d'Herelle's p.
   diaphragm p.
   diaphragmatic p.
   doll's head p.
   Donath p.
   Doppler p.
   double pain p.
   Duckworth's p.
   Erb's p.
   Erben's p.
   erythrocyte adherence p.
   escape p.
   extinction p.
   face p.
   facialis p.
   fall-and-rise p.
   Felton's p.
   fern p.
   Fick's p.
   finger p.
   first set p.
   flicker p.
   Foix and Thévenard p.
   Frégoli's p.
   Friedreich's p.

phe·nom·e·non *(continued)*
   Galassi's pupillary p.
   Gärtner's p.
   Gengou p.
   Gerhardt's p.
   glass-rod p., positive
   glass-rod p., negative
   Goldblatt p.
   Gowers' p.
   Grasset's p.
   Grasset-Gaussel p.
   great-toe p.
   Gunn's p.
   Gunn's pupillary p.
   halisteresis p.
   Hamburger p.
   Hammerschlag's p.
   Hata p.
   Hayflick's p.
   Hecht p.
   Hektoen p.
   Hering's p.
   Hertwig-Magendie p.
   hip-flexion p.
   Hochsinger's p.
   Hoeppli's p.
   Hoffmann's p.
   Holmes' p.
   Holmes-Stewart p.
   Houssay p.
   Huebener-Thomsen-Frieden-
      reich p.
   Hunt's paradoxical p.
   iceberg p.
   ideomotor p.
   immune-adherence p.
   inattention p.
   intercritical epileptic p.
   interference p.
   interictal epileptic p.
   inverse (inverted) Marcus
      Gunn p.
   irradiation p.
   Isakower p.
   jaw-winking p.
   Jod-Basedow p.
   Kanagawa p.
   Kienböck's p.

phe·nom·e·non *(continued)*
   Kleist's p.
   Koch's p.
   Koebner's p.
   Kohnstamm's p.
   Kühne's muscular p.
   Lavrentiev's p.
   LE (lupus erythematosus)
      cell p.
   Leede-Rumpel p.
   leg p.
   Le Grand-Geblewics p.
   Leichtenstern's p.
   Lewis' p.
   Liacopoulos p.
   Lichtheim's p.
   Liesegang's p.
   lip p.
   Litten's diaphragm p.
   Lucio's p.
   Lust's p.
   Lyon p.
   Marcus Gunn p.
   Marcus Gunn pupillary p.
   Marin Amat p.
   Mayer-Reisch p.
   Meirowsky p.
   Mills-Reincke p.
   multiplication p. of
      Lavrentiev
   muscle p.
   Narsaroff's p.
   neck p.
   Negro's p.
   Neisser-Wechsberg p.
   Neufeld's p.
   Orbeli p.
   orbicularis p.
   Orgel p.
   paradoxical diaphragm p.
   paradoxical p. of dystonia
   paradoxical pupillary p.
   peroneal-nerve p.
   Perroncito's p.
   Pfeiffer's p.
   phi p.
   phrenic p.
   Piltz-Westphal p.

phe·nom·e·non *(continued)*
  Pool's p.
  Porret's p.
  prezone p.
  private cinema p.
  pronation p.
  prozone p.
  psi p.
  Purkinje's p.
  Queckenstedt's p.
  quellung p.
  radial p.
  Raynaud's p.
  rebound p.
  reclotting p.
  red cell adherence p.
  release p.
  Riddoch's p.
  Rieger's p.
  Ritter-Rollet p.
  R-on-T p.
  Rumpel-Leede p.
  Rust's p.
  Sanarelli's p.
  satellite p.
  Schellong-Strisower p.
  Schlesinger's p.
  Schramm's p.
  Schüller's p.
  Schultz-Charlton p.
  second-set p.
  setting sun p.
  Sherrington p.
  shot-silk p.
  Shwartzman p.
  Shwartzman-Sanarelli p.
  Simonsen p.
  Sinkler's p.
  Solovieff's p.
  Somogyi p.
  Soret p.
  Souques' p.
  springlike p.
  staircase p.
  Staub-Traugott p.
  Strassman's p.
  Straus' p.
  Strümpell p.

phe·nom·e·non *(continued)*
  p. of successive contrast
  Sulzberger-Chase p.
  Theobald Smith's p.
  Thomsen p.
  Thomsen-Friedenreich p.
  tibial p.
  tip-of-the-tongue p.
  toe p.
  tongue p.
  treadmill p.
  Trousseau's p.
  Tullio p.
  Twort-d'Herelle p.
  Tyndall p.
  Wartenberg's p.
  Wassermann-Takaki p.
  Wedensky's p.
  Wenckebach p.
  Westphal's p.
  Westphal-Piltz p.
  Wever-Bray p.
  Williams'p.
  zone p.
phe·non
phe·no·pro·pa·zine
phe·no·thi·a·zine
phe·no·type
  Bombay p.
  Cellano p.
  McLeod p.
phe·no·typ·ic
Phe·nox·ene
phen·ox·ide
phe·noxy·benz·amine hy·dro·
  chlo·ride
α-phen·oxy·eth·yl·pen·i·cil·
  lin po·tas·si·um [al·pha-]
phe·no·zy·gous
phen·pro·cou·mon
phen·pro·meth·amine hy·dro·
  chlo·ride
phen·pro·pi·o·nate
phen·sux·i·mide
phen·ter·mine
  p. hydrochloride
phen·tol·amine
  p. hydrochloride

phen·tol·amine *(continued)*
   p. mesylate
Phen·u·rone
phen·yl
   p. aminosalicylate
   p. carbinol
   p. hydrate
   p. hydroxide
   p. mercury acetate
   p. mercury nitrate
   p. salicylate
phen·yl·ace·tic acid
phen·yl·ac·e·tyl·urea
   deficiency
phen·yl·al·a·nine
phen·yl·al·a·nine am·mo·
   nia-ly·ase
phen·yl·al·a·nine 4-hy·drox·
   y·lase
phen·yl·al·a·nine 4-mono·ox·
   y·gen·ase
phen·yl·al·a·nin·emia
phen·yl·al·a·nyl
phen·yl·bu·ta·zone
phen·yl·car·bi·nol
phen·yl·di·meth·yl·py·ra·zo·
   lon
phe·ny·lene
p-phen·yl·ene·di·amine
phen·yl·eph·rine hy·dro·chlo·
   ride
phen·yl·eth·yl·bar·bi·tu·ric
   acid
phen·yl·gly·co·lic acid
phen·yl·hy·dra·zine
phe·nyl·hy·dra·zone
phe·nyl·ic
phe·nyl·ic acid
phen·yl·in·dane·di·one
phen·yl·ke·ton·uria (PKU)
   atypical p.
   classic p.
   Fölling's p.
   maternal p.
   p. II
   p. III
phen·yl·lac·tic acid

phen·yl·mer·cu·ric
   p. acetate
   p. nitrate
phen·yl·meth·a·nol
phen·yl·meth·yl·bar·bi·tu·ric
   acid
phen·yl·osa·mide
phen·yl·pro·pa·nol·amine hy·
   dro·chlo·ride
phen·yl·pro·pi·o·nate
   testosterone p.
phen·yl·pro·pyl·meth·yl·am·
   ine hy·dro·chlo·ride
phen·yl·py·ru·vate
phen·yl·py·ru·vic acid
phen·yl·py·ru·vic·ac·i·du·ria
phe·nyl·quin·o·line
phen·yl·thio·car·ba·mide
phe·nyl·thio·hy·dan·to·in
phen·yl·thio·urea
phen·yl·tol·ox·amine cit·rate
phen·y·ram·i·dol hy·dro·
   chlo·ride
phen·y·to·in
   p. sodium
pheo·chrome
pheo·chro·mo·blast
pheo·chro·mo·blas·to·ma
pheo·chro·mo·cyte
pheo·chro·mo·cy·to·ma
   malignant p.
phe·re·sis
pher·o·mone
pheth·ar·bi·tal
PhG — Graduate in
   Pharmacy
     Pharmacopoeia Germanica
     (German Pharmacopeia)
phi·al
phi·a·lide
Phi·a·loph·o·ra
phi·a·lo·phore
phi·a·lo·spore
phi·li·a·ter
Phil·ip's glands
Phi·lippe-Gom·bault tract
phil·ly·rin

phil·trum
phi·mo·si·ec·to·my
phi·mo·sis
    labial p.
    p. vaginalis
phi·mot·ic
pHi·so·Hex
phle·bal·gia
phleb·an·es·the·sia
phleb·an·gi·o·ma
phleb·ar·te·ri·ec·ta·sia
phleb·as·the·nia
phleb·ec·ta·sia
    p. laryn-gis
phleb·ec·ta·sis
phleb·ec·to·my
phleb·ec·to·pia
phleb·ec·to·py
phleb·em·phrax·is
phleb·ex·air·e·sis
phle·bis·mus
phle·bit·ic
phle·bi·tis
    adhesive p.
    anemic p.
    blue p.
    chlorotic p.
    gouty p.
    p. migrans
    migrating p.
    obliterating p.
    obstructive p.
    plastic p.
    productive p.
    proliferative p.
    puerperal p.
    p. saltans
    septic p.
    sinus p.
    suppurative p.
phle·boc·ly·sis
    drip p.
    slow p.
phlebo·dy·nam·ics
phlebo·dy·na·mom·e·try
phlebo·fi·bro·sis
phle·bog·e·nous
phlebo·gram

phlebo·graph
phle·bog·ra·phy
phleb·oid
phlebo·lith
phlebo·li·thi·a·sis
phle·bol·o·gy
phlebo·ma·nom·e·ter
phlebo·me·tri·tis
phlebo·nar·co·sis
phlebo·phle·bos·to·my
phleb·oph·thal·mot·o·my
phlebo·pi·ezom·e·try
phlebo·plas·ty
phlebo·rhe·og·ra·phy
phleb·or·rha·gia
phle·bor·rha·phy
phleb·or·rhex·is
phlebo·scle·ro·sis
    portal p.
phle·bo·sis
phleb·os·ta·sia
phle·bos·ta·sis
phlebo·ste·no·sis
phlebo·throm·bo·sis
phlebo·tome
phle·bot·o·mist
phle·bot·o·mize
Phle·bot·o·mus
    P. argentipes
    P. chinensis
    P. flaviscutellatus
    P. intermedius
    P. longipes
    P. major
    P. martini
    P. noguchi
    P. orientalis
    P. papatasii
    P. pedifer
    P. perniciosus
    P. pessoai
    P. sergenti
    P. verrucarum
phle·bot·o·my
    bloodless p.
phlegm
phleg·ma·sia
    p. alba dolens

phleg·ma·sia *(continued)*
    p. alba dolens
      puerperarum
    cellulitic p.
    p. cerulea dolens
    thrombotic p.
phleg·mat·ic
phleg·mon
    Holz p.
    pancreatic p.
    periurethral p.
phleg·mo·no·sis
phleg·mon·ous
phlo·em
phlo·gis·tic
phlo·gis·ton
phlo·go·cyte
phlo·go·cy·to·sis
phlo·go·gen
phlo·go·gen·ic
phlo·gog·e·nous
phlo·got·ic
phlo·rhi·zin
phlo·rhi·zi·nize
phlo·rid·zin
phlo·rid·zin·ize
phlo·ri·zin
phlo·ro·glu·cin
phlo·ro·glu·ci·nol
phlor·rhi·zin
phlox·ine
    p. B
phlyc·ten
phlyc·te·na *pl.* phlyc·te·nae
phlyc·te·nar
phlyc·te·noid
phlyc·ten·u·la *pl.* phlyc·ten·u·lae
phlyc·ten·u·lar
phlyc·ten·ule
phlyc·ten·u·lo·sis
    allergic p.
    tuberculous p.
pho·bia
    school p.
    simple p.
    social p.
pho·bic

pho·bo·pho·bia
Pho·cas' disease
pho·co·me·lia
pho·com·e·lus
phol·co·dine tar·trate
phon
pho·naco·scope
pho·na·cos·co·py
pho·nal
phon·an·gi·og·ra·phy
phon·ar·te·rio·gram
phon·ar·te·rio·gra·phic
phon·ar·te·ri·og·ra·phy
phon·as·the·nia
pho·na·tion
    subenergetic p.
    superenergetic p.
pho·na·to·ry
phon·au·to·graph
pho·neme
pho·ne·mic
phon·en·do·scope
phon·en·do·skia·scope
pho·net·ic
pho·net·ics
pho·ni·a·tri·cian
pho·ni·at·rics
phon·ic
phon·ics
pho·nism
pho·no·an·gi·og·ra·phy
pho·no·aus·cul·ta·tion
pho·no·car·dio·gram
pho·no·car·dio·graph
    fetal p.
    logarithmic p.
pho·no·car·dio·gra·phic
pho·no·car·di·og·ra·phy
    intracardiac p.
pho·no·cath·e·ter
pho·no·cath·e·ter·i·za·tion
    intracardiac p.
pho·no·elec·tro·car·dio·scope
pho·no·gram
pho·nol·o·gy
pho·no·my·oc·lo·nus
pho·no·myo·gram
pho·no·my·og·ra·phy

pho·nop·athy
pho·no·pho·bia
pho·nop·sia
phono·re·cep·tor
pho·no·re·no·gram
pho·no·scope
pho·nos·co·py
pho·no·se·lec·to·scope
pho·no·stetho·graph
phor·bin
pho·ria
pho·ria·scope
Phor·mia
    P. regina
pho·ro·blast
pho·ro·cyte
pho·ro·cy·to·sis
pho·rol·o·gy
pho·rom·e·ter
pho·rom·e·try
pho·ront
pho·ro-op·tom·e·ter
Pho·rop·tor
pho·ro·scope
pho·ro·tone
pho·ro·zo·on
phose
phos·gene
phos·gen·ic
pho·sis
phos·pha·gen
phos·pha·gen·ic
phos·pha·tase
    leukocyte alkaline p. (LAP)
phos·phate
    acid p.
    alkaline p.
    ammoniomagnesium p.
    carbamoyl p.
    creatine p.
    cyclic p.
    earthy p.
    ferric p.
    ferric p., soluble
    guanidine p.
    high-energy p.
    low-energy p.
    normal p.

phos·phate *(continued)*
    polyestradiol p.
    stellar p.
    trimagnesium p.
    triorthocresyl p.
    triose p.
    triple p.
phos·phate ace·tyl·trans·fer·ase
phos·phat·ed
phos·pha·te·mia
phos·phat·ic
phos·pha·ti·date
phos·pha·tide
phos·pha·ti·dic acid
phos·pha·ti·do·sis *pl.* phos·pha·ti·do·ses
phos·pha·ti·dyl
phos·pha·ti·dyl·cho·line
phos·pha·ti·dyl·cho·line-cho·les·ter·ol acyl·trans·fer·ase
phos·pha·ti·dyl·cho·line-ster·ol ac·yl·trans·fer·ase
phos·pha·ti·dyl·eth·a·nol·amine
    p. methyltransferase
phos·pha·ti·dyl·glyc·er·ol
phos·pha·ti·dyl·ino·si·tide
phos·pha·ti·dyl·in·o·si·tol
    p. 4,5-bisphosphate (PIP$_2$)
    p. 4-phosphate (PIP)
phos·pha·ti·dyl·ser·ine
phos·pha·ti·dyl·trans·fer·ase
phos·pha·top·to·sis
phos·pha·tu·ria
    renal p.
phos·phene
    accommodation p.
phos·phide
phos·phine
phos·phite
3′-phos·pho·aden·o·sine
5′-phos·pho·sul·fate
phos·pho·cre·a·tine
phos·pho·di·es·ter
phos·pho·di·es·ter·ase
phos·pho·di·hy·drox·y·ac·e·tone

phos·pho·enol·py·ru·vate car·boxy·ki·nase (GTP)
phos·pho·enol·py·ru·vate car·box·yl·ase
phos·pho·enol·py·ru·vic acid
phos·pho·fruct·al·do·lase
6-phos·pho·fruc·to·ki·nase
6-phos·pho·fruc·to-2-ki·nase
phos·pho·fruc·to·mu·tase
phos·pho·ga·lac·tose uri·dyl·yl·trans·fer·ase
phos·pho·glob·u·lin
phos·pho·glu·co·ki·nase
phos·pho·glu·co·mu·tase
phos·pho·glu·co·nate de·hy·dro·gen·ase (de·car·box·yl·at·ing)
6-phos·pho·glu·con·ic acid
phos·pho·glu·co·pro·tein
phos·pho·glu·cose isom·er·ase
phos·pho·glyc·er·ac·e·tal
3-phos·pho·glyc·er·al·de·hyde
phos·pho·glyc·er·ate
2-phos·pho·glyc·er·ate
3-phos·pho·glyc·er·ate
phos·pho·glyc·er·ate ki·nase
phos·pho·glyc·er·ate mu·tase
2-phos·pho·gly·cer·ic acid
3-phos·pho·gly·cer·ic acid
phos·pho·glyc·er·ide
phos·pho·glyc·ero·mu·tase
3-phos·pho·glyc·er·oyl phos·phate
phos·pho·guan·i·dine
phos·pho·hexo·isom·er·ase
phos·pho·hexo·ki·nase
phos·pho·ino·si·tide
phos·pho·ke·to·lase
Phos·pho·line
   P. iodide
phos·pho·lip·ase
   platelet p.
phos·pho·lip·ase A$_1$
phos·pho·lip·ase A$_2$
phos·pho·lip·ase B
phos·pho·lip·ase C
phos·pho·lip·ase D
phos·pho·lip·id

phos·pho·lip·i·de·mia
phos·pho·lip·in
phos·pho·man·nose isom·er·ase
phos·pho·mev·a·lon·ate ki·nase
phos·pho·mo·lyb·dic acid
phos·pho·mono·es·ter·ase
phos·pho·mu·tase
phos·pho·nate
phos·pho·ne·cro·sis
phos·phon·ic acid
phos·pho·ni·um
phos·phono·ace·tic acid
phos·phono·for·mate
   trisodium p.
phos·phono·lip·id
phos·phono·my·cin
phos·pho·nu·cle·ase
4'-phos·pho·pan·te·the·ine
phos·pho·pe·nia
phos·pho·pro·tein
phos·pho·pro·tein phos·pha·tase
phos·pho·pto·maine
phos·pho·py·ru·vate car·boxy·ki·nase
phos·pho·py·ru·vate car·box·yl·ase
phos·pho·py·ru·vic acid
phos·phor
phos·pho·rat·ed
phos·pho·res·cence
phos·pho·res·cent
phos·pho·ri·bo·isom·er·ase
phos·pho·ri·bo·ki·nase
phos·pho·ri·bose
phos·pho·ri·bo·syl·amine
5-phos·pho·ri·bo·syl·gly·cin·amide syn·thase
phos·pho·ri·bo·syl·py·ro·phos·phate
phos·pho·ri·bo·syl·py·ro·phos·phate syn·the·tase
phos·pho·ri·bo·syl·trans·fer·ase
phos·pho·ri·bu·lo·ki·nase
phos·pho·ri·bu·lose

phos·phor·ic acid
phos·phor·ic acid, diluted
phos·phor·ic acid, glacial
phos·pho·rism
phos·pho·rized
phos·pho·rol·y·sis
phos·phoro·scope
phos·pho·rous
phos·pho·rous acid
phos·phor·pe·nia
phos·phor·uria
phos·pho·rus
 p. 32
 amorphous p.
 black p.
 labeled p.
 ordinary p.
 radioactive p.
 red p.
 white p.
 yellow p.
phos·phor·yl
phos·phor·y·lase
 purine nucleoside p.
phos·phor·y·lase ki·nase
phos·phor·y·lase ki·nase
 phos·pha·tase
phos·phor·y·lase phos·pha·tase
phos·phor·y·la·tion
 oxidative p.
 substrate-level p.
phos·pho·ser·ine
phos·pho·sphin·go·side
phos·pho·sug·ar
phos·pho·thre·o·nine
phos·pho·trans·fer·ase
phos·pho·tri·ose
phos·pho·tung·state
phos·pho·tung·stic acid
phos·pho·vi·tel·lin
phos·phu·re·sis
phos·phu·ret·ic
phos·phu·ria
phos·vi·tin
phot
pho·tal·gia
pho·tal·lo·chro·my

pho·tau·gia·pho·bia
pho·te·ryth·rous
pho·tes·the·sis
pho·tic
pho·tism
pho·to·abla·tion
pho·to·ac·tin·ic
pho·to·ac·tive
pho·to·al·ler·gen
pho·to·al·ler·gic
pho·to·al·ler·gy
pho·to·au·to·troph
pho·to·au·to·troph·ic
pho·to·bac·te·ria
pho·to·bi·o·log·ic
pho·to·bi·o·logical
pho·to·bi·ol·o·gy
pho·to·bi·ot·ic
pho·to·ca·tal·y·sis
pho·to·cat·a·lyst
pho·to·cat·a·lyt·ic
pho·to·cat·a·lyz·er
pho·to·cath·ode
pho·to·cau·ter·i·za·tion
pho·to·cep·tor
pho·to·chem·i·cal
pho·to·chem·is·try
pho·to·che·mo·ther·a·py
pho·to·chro·mo·gen
pho·to·chro·mo·gen·ic
pho·to·chro·mo·ge·nic·i·ty
pho·to·co·ag·u·la·tion
pho·to·co·ag·u·la·tor
pho·to·con·duc·tiv·i·ty
pho·to·con·vul·sive
pho·to·cu·ta·ne·ous
pho·to·den·si·tom·e·ter
pho·to·der·ma·ti·tis
 polymorphous p.
pho·to·der·ma·to·sis
pho·to·di·ode
pho·to·dis·in·te·gra·tion
pho·to·dis·rup·tion
pho·tod·ro·my
pho·to·dy·nam·ic
pho·to·dy·nam·ics
pho·to·dyn·ia
pho·to·dys·pho·ria

pho·to·elec·tric
pho·to·elec·tron
pho·to·emis·sion
pho·to·er·y·the·ma
pho·to·es·thet·ic
pho·to·fis·sion
pho·to·flu·o·ro·gram
pho·to·flu·o·rog·ra·phy
pho·to·flu·o·ro·scope
pho·to·fluo·ros·co·py
pho·to·frac·tion
pho·to·gas·tro·scope
pho·to·gene
pho·to·gen·e·sis
pho·to·gen·ic
pho·tog·ra·phy
    fluorescein fundus p.
pho·to·hal·ide
pho·to·hap·ten
pho·to·hem·a·ta·chom·e·ter
pho·to·hen·ric
pho·to·het·ero·troph
pho·to·het·ero·troph·ic
pho·tohm·ic
pho·to·in·ac·ti·va·tion
pho·to·ki·ne·sis
pho·to·ki·net·ic
pho·to·ky·mo·graph
pho·to·la·bile
pho·tol·o·gy
pho·to·lu·min·es·cence
pho·tol·y·sis
pho·to·lyte
pho·to·lyt·ic
pho·to·ma
pho·to·mag·ne·tism
pho·tom·e·ter
    flame p.
    flicker p.
    Förster's p.
pho·to·met·he·mo·glo·bin
pho·tom·e·try
    flicker p.
    internal standard flame p.
pho·to·mi·cro·graph
pho·to·mi·crog·ra·phy
pho·to·mi·cro·scope
pho·to·mi·cros·co·py

pho·to·mor·pho·gen·e·sis
pho·to·mo·tor
pho·to·myo·clon·ic
pho·to·myo·clo·nus
    hereditary p.
pho·to·my·o·gen·ic
pho·ton
pho·ton·cia
pho·to-onych·ol·y·sis
pho·to-ox·i·da·tion
pho·to·par·ox·ys·mal
pho·to·patho·log·ic
pho·top·a·thy
pho·to·peak
pho·to·per·cep·tive
pho·to·pe·ri·od
pho·to·pe·ri·od·ic
pho·to·pe·ri·o·dic·i·ty
pho·to·pe·ri·od·ism
pho·to·phar·ma·col·o·gy
pho·to·phil·ic
pho·to·pho·bia
pho·to·pho·bic
pho·to·phos·phor·y·la·tion
    cyclic p.
pho·toph·thal·mia
    flash p.
pho·to·pia
pho·top·ic
pho·to·pig·ment
pho·to·ple·thys·mog·ra·phy
pho·to·prod·uct
pho·to·pro·tec·tion
pho·to·pro·ton
pho·top·sia
pho·top·sin
pho·top·sy
pho·to·ptar·mo·sis
pho·top·tom·e·ter
pho·top·tom·e·try
pho·to·ra·di·a·tion
pho·to·ra·di·om·e·ter
pho·to·re·ac·tion
pho·to·re·ac·ti·va·tion
pho·to·re·cep·tion
pho·to·re·cep·tive
pho·to·re·cep·tor
pho·to·res·pi·ra·tion

pho·to·ret·i·ni·tis
pho·to·ret·i·nop·a·thy
pho·to·re·ver·sal
pho·to·scan
pho·to·scan·ner
pho·to·scin·ti·gram
pho·to·scope
pho·tos·co·py
pho·to·sen·si·tive
pho·to·sen·si·tiv·i·ty
pho·to·sen·si·ti·za·tion
    contact p.
pho·to·sen·si·tize
pho·to·sta·ble
pho·to·stetho·scope
pho·to·syn·the·sis
pho·to·tax·is
pho·to·ther·a·py
    ultraviolet p.
pho·to·ther·mal
pho·to·ther·my
pho·to·tim·er
pho·tot·o·nus
pho·to·to·pia
pho·to·tox·ic
pho·to·tox·ic·i·ty
pho·to·tox·is
pho·to·troph·ic
pho·to·trop·ic
pho·tot·ro·pism
pho·to·tur·bido·met·ric
pho·to·va·por·iza·tion
pho·tox·y·lin
pho·tron·re·flec·tom·e·ter
pho·tu·ria
phren·i·co·cos·tal
PHPPA — *p*-hydroxyphenylpyr-
    uvic acid
phrag·mo·plast
phren
phre·nal·gia
phre·nec·to·my
phren·em·phrax·is
phre·net·ic
phren·ic
phren·i·cec·to·my
phren·i·cla·sia
phren·i·cla·sis

phren·i·co·ex·air·e·sis
phren·i·co·ex·er·e·sis
phren·i·co·neu·rec·to·my
phren·i·cot·o·my
phren·i·co·trip·sy
phre·ni·tis
phreno·car·dia
phreno·col·ic
phreno·colo·pexy
phreno·cos·tal
phreno·dyn·ia
phreno·gas·tric
phreno·glot·tic
phreno·graph
phreno·he·pat·ic
phre·nol·o·gist
phre·nol·o·gy
phreno·peri·car·di·tis
phreno·ple·gia
phren·op·to·sis
phreno·sin
phreno·sin·ic acid
phreno·spasm
phreno·splen·ic
phreno·ster·ol
phren·o·trop·ic
phric·to·path·ic
phro·ne·ma
phry·nin
phryno·der·ma
phry·nol·y·sin
phthal·ate
phthal·e·in
    alpha-naphthol p.
    orthocresol p.
phthal·e·in·om·e·ter
phthal·ic acid
phthal·in
phthalo·cy·a·nine
phthal·yl·sul·fa·cet·amide
phthal·yl·sul·fa·thi·a·zole
phthal·yl·sul·fon·a·zole
phthin·oid
phthi·o·col
phthi·o·ic acid
phthir·i·a·sis
    p. capitis
    p. corporis

phthir·i·a·sis *(continued)*
    p. inguinalis
    pubic p.
Phthi·rus
    P. pubis
phthis·ic
phthi·sis
    aneurysmal p.
    p. bulbi
    p. corneae
    dorsal p.
    essential p.
    Mediterranean p.
    p. nodosa
    nonbacillary p.
    ocular p.
    p. pancreatica
phy·co·chrome
phy·co·chro·mo·pro·tein
phy·co·er·y·thrin
Phy·co·my·ce·tae
phy·co·my·cete
Phy·co·my·ce·tes
phy·co·my·ce·to·sis
    subcutaneous p.
phy·co·my·ce·tous
phy·co·my·co·sis
    cerebral p.
    p. entomophthorae
    subcutaneous p.
phy·go·ga·lac·tic
phy·la
phy·lac·tic
phy·lac·to·trans·fu·sion
phy·lax·is
phy·let·ic
Phyl·lan·thus
    P. engleri
phyl·lid·ea
phyl·lode
phyl·lo·des
phyl·lo·er·y·thrin
phyl·loid
phyl·lo·lith
phyl·lo·pyr·role
phyl·lo·quin·one
phy·lo·gen·e·sis
phy·lo·ge·net·ic

phy·lo·gen·ic
phy·log·e·ny
phy·lum *pl.* phy·la
phy·ma *pl.* phy·ma·ta
phy·ma·ta
phy·ma·to·rhu·sin
phy·ma·tor·rhys·in
Phy·sa·lia
phy·sal·i·des
phys·a·lif·er·ous
phy·sal·i·form
phy·sal·i·phore
phys·a·liph·o·rous
phys·a·lis *pl.* phys·al·i·des
phys·al·li·za·tion
Phys·a·lop·tera
    P. caucasica
    P. mordens
    P. rara
    P. truncata
phys·a·lop·ter·i·a·sis
phys·e·al
phys·ia·tri·cian
phys·iat·rics
phys·iat·rist
phys·iat·ry
phys·ic
phys·i·cal
phy·si·cian
    admitting p.
    p. assistant
    attending p.
    emergency p.
    family p.
    forensic p.
    resident p.
Phy·sick's oper·ation
Phy·sick's pouches
phys·i·co·chem·i·cal
phys·i·co·gen·ic
phys·i·co·ther·a·peu·tics
phys·i·co·ther·a·py
phys·ics
phys·io·chem·i·cal
phys·io·chem·is·try
phys·io·gen·e·sis
phys·i·og·no·my
phys·i·og·no·sis

phys·i·o·log·ic
phys·i·o·log·i·cal
phys·i·o·log·i·co·an·a·tom·i·
  cal
phys·i·ol·o·gist
phys·i·ol·o·gy
  antenatal p.
  applied p.
  aviation p.
  cellular p.
  comparative p.
  dental p.
  developmental p.
  general p.
  hominal p.
  human p.
  morbid p.
  pathologic p.
  special p.
  vegetable p.
phys·i·ol·y·sis
phys·io·med·i·cal·ism
phys·i·om·e·try
phys·io·neu·ro·sis
phys·i·on·o·my
phys·io·patho·log·ic
phys·io·pa·thol·o·gy
phys·i·oph·y·ly
phys·io·ther·a·peu·tic
phys·io·ther·a·peu·tist
phys·io·ther·a·pist
phys·io·ther·a·py
phy·sique
phy·sis
phy·so·cele
Phy·so·ceph·a·lus
phy·so·ceph·a·ly
phy·so·hem·a·to·me·tra
phy·so·hy·dro·me·tra
phy·so·me·tra
Phy·sop·sis
phy·so·pyo·sal·pinx
Phy·so·stig·ma
phy·so·stig·mine
  p. salicylate
  p. sulfate
phy·so·stig·min·ism
phyt·ag·glu·ti·nin

phyt·al·bu·min
phyt·al·bu·mose
phy·tan·ic acid
phy·tan·ic acid α-hy·droxy·
  lase
6-phy·tase
phy·tate
phy·tic acid
phy·tid
phy·tin
phy·to·a·lex·in
phy·to·an·a·phy·lac·to·gen
phy·to·be·zoar
phy·to·chem·is·try
phy·to·chin·in
phy·to·dem·ic
phy·to·der·ma
phy·to·de·tri·tus
phy·to·flag·el·late
phy·to·gen·e·sis
phy·to·ge·net·ic
phy·to·gen·ic
phy·tog·e·nous
phy·to·hem·ag·glu·ti·nin
phy·to·hor·mone
phy·toid
phy·tol
Phy·to·mas·ti·goph·o·ra
Phy·to·mas·ti·goph·o·rea
phy·to·mas·ti·goph·o·re·an
phy·to·mel·in
phy·to·men·a·di·one
phy·to·mi·to·gen
phy·to·na·di·one
phy·ton·o·sis
phy·to·par·a·site
phy·to·path·o·gen·ic
phy·to·pa·thol·o·gy
phy·top·a·thy
phy·toph·a·gous
phy·to·pho·to·der·ma·ti·tis
phy·to·plank·ton
phy·to·plasm
phy·to·pre·cip·i·tin
phy·to·sen·si·tin·o·gen
phy·to·sis
phy·to·ste·rol·in
phy·to·ther·a·py

phy·to·tox·ic
phy·to·tox·in
phy·to·tri·cho·be·zoar
phy·to·vi·tel·lin
phy·tox·y·lin
phy·tyl·men·a·qui·none
PI — periodontal index
    protamine insulin
pia
    p. mater
pia-ar·ach·ni·tis
pia-arach·noid
pia-glia
pi·al
pia ma·ter
    p. m. encephali
    p. m. spinalis
pia·ma·tral
pi·an
    p. bois
    hemorrhagic p.
pi·ar·ach·ni·tis
pi·ar·ach·noid
pi·ar·he·mia
pi·as·tri·ne·mia
pi·blok·to
PIC — polymorphism
    information content
PICA — posterior inferior
    communicating artery
pi·ca
Pic·chi·ni syndrome
Pic·co·lo·mi·ni's striae
pick
    apical p.
    crane p.
    root p.
Pick's bodies
Pick's cell
Pick's disease
pick·ling
pick·wick·i·an syndrome
pi·co·am·pere (pA)
pi·co·cu·rie
pi·cod·na·vi·rus
pi·co·gram
pi·co·li·ter (pl)
pi·co·mole (pmol)

pi·co·pi·co·gram
Pi·cor·na·vi·ri·dae
pi·cor·na·vi·rus
pi·co·unit
pic·ram·ic acid
pic·rate
pic·ric acid
pic·ro·car·mine
pic·ro·geu·sia
pic·rol
pic·ro·ni·gro·sin
pic·ro·podo·phyl·lin
Pic·ror·rhi·za
pic·ro·sac·cha·rom·e·ter
pic·ro·scle·ro·tine
pic·ro·tox·in
pic·ro·tox·in·ism
PID — pelvic inflammatory
    disease
PIE — pulmonary infiltration
    with eosinophilia
pie·bald
pie·bald·ism
piece
    chief p.
    connecting p.
    end p.
    Fd p.
    middle p.
    principal p.
    secretory p.
pie crust·ing
pi·e·dra
    black p.
    white p.
Pi·e·draia
Pi·e·drai·a·ceae
pier
Pi·erre Ro·bin syndrome
Pier·sol's point
pi·es·es·the·sia
pi·esim·e·ter
    Hales'p.
pi·ezal·lo·chro·my
pi·ez·es·the·sia
pi·ezo·car·dio·gram
pi·ezo·chem·is·try
pi·ezo·elec·tric

pi·ezo·elec·tric·i·ty
pi·ezom·e·ter
PIF — prolactin inhibiting
  factor
    proliferation inhibitory
      factor
pi·far·nine
pig·bel
pig·ment
    bile p.
    blood p.
    cone p.
    endogenous p.
    exogenous p.
    fatty p.
    hematogenous p.
    hepatogenous p.
    lipid p.
    lipochrome p.
    malarial p.
    melanotic p.
    respiratory p's
    visual p.
    wear and tear p's
pig·men·tary
pig·men·ta·tion
    addisonian dermal p.
    arsenic p.
    exogenous p.
    gingival p.
    hematogenous p.
    vagabond's p.
pig·ment·ed
pig·men·to·der·mia
pig·men·to·gen·e·sis
pig·men·to·gen·ic
pig·men·tol·y·sis
pig·men·to·phage
pig·men·to·phore
Pig·net's formula
Pig·net's index
Pig·net's standard
pig·skin
pig·tail
PIH — prolactin-inhibiting
  hormone
pi·itis
pik·ro·my·cin

Pil. — L. pilula (pill)
    L. pilulae (pills)
Pi·la
    P. conica
pi·la *pl.* pi·lae
pi·lae
pi·lar
pil·a·ry
pi·las·ter
    p. of Broca
pi·la·tion
Pil·cher bag
pile
    muscular p.
    prostatic p.
    sentinel p.
    thermoelectric p.
    thrombosed p.
    voltaic p.
piles
pi·le·us
pi·li
pi·li·al
pi·li·ate
pi·li·a·tion
Pil·i·dae
pi·li·form
pi·li·mic·tio
pi·li·mic·tion
pi·lin
pill
    birth control p. (BCP)
    chalybeate p's
    combined oral
      contraceptive p.
    enteric p.
    ferrous carbonate p's
    ferruginous p's
    hexylresorcinol p's
    morning-after p.
    oral contraceptive p's
      (OCP)
    radio p.
    sequential oral p.
pil·lar
    p. of Corti's organ
    p's of diaphragm

pil·lar *(continued)*
    p. of fauces, anterior
    p. of fauces, posterior
    p. of fornix, anterior
    p. of fornix, posterior
    p's of soft palate
    Uskow's p's
pil·let
pil·lion
pil·low
    Frejka p.
pill-roll·ing
pi·lo·be·zoar
pi·lo·car·pine
    p. hydrochloride
    p. nitrate
Pi·lo·car·pus
pi·lo·cys·tic
pi·lo·cyt·ic
pi·lo·erec·tion
pi·lo·jec·tion
pi·lol·o·gy
pi·lo·ma·tri·co·ma
pi·lo·ma·trix·o·ma
pi·lo·mo·tor
pi·lo·ni·dal
pi·lose
pi·lo·se·ba·ceous
Piltz's reflex
Piltz's sign
Piltz-West·phal phenomenon
pil·u·la *pl.* pil·u·lae
pil·u·lar
pil·ule
pi·lus *pl.* pi·li
    p. annulatus
    p. cuniculatus
    F p.
    p. incarnatus
    p. incarnatus recurvus
    pili multigemini
    sex p.
    p. tortus
Pima
pi·mel·ic acid
pim·e·li·tis
pim·e·lo·ma
pim·e·lop·ter·yg·i·um

pim·el·or·thop·nea
pim·e·lo·sis
pim·el·uria
pi·me·tine hy·dro·chlo·ride
pi·min·o·dine es·y·late
pi·mo·zide
Pim·pi·nel·la
pim·ple
pin
    Ender p.
    friction-retained p.
    Hagie p.
    incisal guide p.
    Kuntscher p.
    retention p.
    self-threading p.
    sprue p.
    Steinmann p.
pin·a·cy·a·nole
Pi·nard's maneuver
pince-ci·seaux
pince·ment
pin·cers
    key p.
    pulp p.
Pind·borg tumor
pin·do·lol
pine
    white p.
pin·e·al
pin·e·al·ec·to·my
pin·e·al·ism
pin·e·a·lo·blas·to·ma
pin·e·a·lo·cyte
pin·e·a·lo·cy·to·ma
pin·e·a·lo·ma
    ectopic p.
pin·e·a·lop·a·thy
pi·nene
pin·eo·blas·to·ma
pin·eo·cy·to·ma
pin·gue·cu·la *pl.* pin·gue·cu·lae
pin·i·form
pink·eye
pin·lay
pin·ledge
pin·na

pin·nal
pino·cyte
pino·cyt·ic
pino·cy·to·sis
    reverse p.
pino·cy·tot·ic
pino·some
Pi·no·yel·la
    P. simii
Pins' sign
pint
pin·ta
pin·tid
pi·nus
pin·worm
pio·epi·the·li·um
pi·on
pi·o·ne·mia
Pi·oph·i·la
    P. casei
pi·or·thop·nea
Pi·o·trow·ski's sign
PIP — phosphatidylinositol
    4-phosphate
PIP$_2$ — phosphatidylinositol
    4,5-biphosphate
pi·pam·a·zine
pi·pam·pe·rone
Pip·a·nol
pip·aze·thate
pi·pen·zo·late bro·mide
pip·er·a·cet·a·zine
pi·per·a·cil·lin so·di·um
pi·per·az·i·dine
pi·per·a·zine
    p. citrate
    p. edetate calcium
    p. phosphate
    p. tartrate
pi·per·id·o·late hy·dro·chlo·
    ride
pi·per·ine
pi·per·ism
pi·per·o·caine hy·dro·chlo·
    ride
pi·per·ox·an hy·dro·chlo·ride
pi·pet
pi·pette

pi·pette
    Pasteur p.
Pi·pi·zan
pi·po·bro·man
pi·po·sul·fan
pip·o·ti·a·zine pal·mi·tate
pip·ox·o·lan hy·dro·chlo·ride
γ-pip·ra·dol [gam·ma-]
pi·pra·drol hy·dro·chlo·ride
pip·ro·zo·lin
Pip·to·ceph·a·lus
piq·ui·zil hy·dro·chlo·ride
pi·qûre
Pi·ra·caps
pir·an·da·mine hy·dro·chlo·
    ride
pir·ben·i·cil·lin so·di·um
pir·bu·ter·ol hy·dro·chlo·ride
Pi·re·nel·la
    P. conica
pir·fen·i·done
Pi·rie bone
pir·i·form
Pir·o·goff's amputation
Pir·o·goff's angle
pir·o·late
pir·o·la·za·mide
piro·men
pi·ro·plasm
Pi·ro·plas·ma
Pi·ro·plas·mia
pi·ro·plas·mid
Pi·ro·plas·mi·da
pi·ro·plas·mo·sis
    tropical p.
pir·ox·i·cam
pir·pro·fen
Pir·quet's cutireaction
Pir·quet's reaction
Pir·quet's test
pis·ci·cide
Pis·cid·ia
pis·ci·din
pi·si·an·nu·lar·is
pi·si·form
pi·si·for·mis
pi·si·meta·car·pus
Pis·ka·cek's sign

pi·so·tri·que·tral
pis·til
pis·ton
    McGee p.
    Shea p.
    stapedectomy p.
PIT — plasma iron turnover
pit
    anal p.
    arm p.
    auditory p.
    basilar p.
    coated p's
    costal p.
    ear p.
    gastric p's
    Gaul's p's
    Herbert's p's
    lens p.
    nasal p.
    oblong p. of arytenoid
      cartilage
    olfactory p.
    otic p.
    postanal p.
    primitive p.
    pterygoid p.
    p. of the stomach
    suprameatal p.
    triangular p. of arytenoid
      cartilage
pitch
    absolute p.
    black p.
    Burgundy p.
    Canada p.
    naval p.
pitch·blende
pith
pith·e·coid
pith·ing
Pit·kin's menstruum
Pi·to·cin
Pi·tres' sections
Pi·tres' sign
Pi·tres·sin
pit·ting
pi·tu·i·cyte

pi·tu·i·ta
pi·tu·i·tar·i·gen·ic
pi·tu·i·ta·rism
pi·tu·i·tar·i·um
pi·tu·i·tary
    anterior p.
    pharyngeal p.
    posterior p.
    whole p.
pi·tu·i·tec·to·my
pi·tu·i·tous
Pi·tu·i·trin
pit·y·ri·a·sis
    p. alba
    p. amiantacea
    p. capitis
    p. circinata
    p. furfuracea
    Gilbert's p.
    lichenoid p. acute
    lichenoid p. chronic
    p. lichenoides acuta
    p. lichenoides chronica
    p. lichenoides et
      varioliformis acuta
    p. linguae
    p. maculata
    p. rosea
    p. rotunda
    p. rubra
    p. rubra pilaris
    p. sicca
    p. simplex
    p. steatoides
    p. versicolor
    p. vulgaris
pit·y·roid
Pit·y·ros·po·rum
    P. orbiculare
    P. ovale
piv·a·late
piv·am·pi·cil·lin hy·dro·chlo·
  ride
piv·ot
    occlusal p.
pix·el
pi·zo·ty·line
PK — pyruvate kinase

PKU — phenylketonuria
PLA-car·bon
pla·ce·bo
    active p.
    impure p.
place·ment
    lingual p.
pla·cen·ta *pl.* pla·cen·tae, pla·
    cen·tas
    accessory p.
    p. accreta
    adherent p.
    allantoic p.
    annular p.
    battledore p.
    bidiscoidal p.
    bilobate p.
    bilobed p.
    p. bipartita
    bipartite p.
    chorioallantoic p.
    choriovitelline p.
    p. circumvallata
    circumvallate p.
    cirsoid p.
    p. cirsoides
    deciduate p.
    deciduous p.
    p. diffusa
    p. dimidiata
    dimidiate p.
    discoid p.
    p. discoidea
    Duncan p.
    duplex p.
    endotheliochorial p.
    epitheliochorial p.
    p. fenestrata
    fenestrated p.
    fetal p.
    p. foetalis
    fundal p.
    furcate p.
    hemochorial p.
    hemodichorial p.
    hemoendothelial p.
    hemomonochorial p.
    hemotrichorial p.

pla·cen·ta *(continued)*
    horseshoe p.
    incarcerated p.
    p. increta
    labyrinthine p.
    lobed p.
    p. marginalis
    p. marginata
    maternal p.
    p. membranacea
    multilobate p.
    multilobed p.
    p. multipartita
    p. nappiformis
    nondeciduate p.
    nondeciduous p.
    panduriform p.
    p. panduriformis
    p. percreta
    p. previa
    p. previa centralis
    p. previa marginalis
    p. previa partialis
    p. reflexa
    reniform p.
    p. reniformis
    retained p.
    Schultze's p.
    p. spuria
    p. succenturiata
    succenturiate p.
    syndesmochorial p.
    trapped p.
    p. triloba
    trilobate p.
    p. tripartita
    tripartite p.
    p. triplex
    tubal-cornual p.
    p. uterina
    uterine p.
    varicose p.
    velamentous p.
    villous p.
    yolk-sac p.
    zonary p.
    zonular p.

pla·cen·tal
Pla·cen·ta·lia
pla·cen·ta·tion
pla·cen·ti·form
pla·cen·ti·tis
pla·cen·to·gen·e·sis
pla·cen·to·gram
pla·cen·tog·ra·phy
   indirect p.
pla·cen·toid
pla·cen·tol·o·gist
pla·cen·tol·o·gy
   comparative p.
pla·cen·to·ma
pla·cen·top·a·thy
pla·cen·to·sis
pla·cen·tu·la
Pla·ci·do's disk
Plac·i·dyl
plac·ode
   auditory p.
   dorsolateral p's
   epibranchial p's
   lens p.
   olfactory p.
   optic p.
   otic p.
plac·oid
pla·fond
pla·gio·ce·phal·ic
pla·gio·ceph·a·lism
pla·gio·ceph·a·ly
plague
   ambulatory p.
   black p.
   bubonic p.
   domestic p.
   glandular p.
   hemorrhagic p.
   lung p.
   meningeal p.
   murine p.
   Pahvant Valley p.
   pharyngeal p.
   pneumonic p.
   pulmonic p.
   septicemic p.
   siderating p.

plague *(continued)*
   sylvatic p.
   tarbagan p.
   urban p.
   white p.
pla·kins
pla·na
pla·nar
pla·nar·i·an
plan·chet
Planck's constant
Planck's theory
plane
   Addison's p's
   Aeby's p.
   auricular p. of sacral bone
   auriculoinfraorbital p.
   axial p.
   axial p. of tooth
   axial wall p.
   axiolabiolingual p.
   axiomesiodistal p.
   Baer's p.
   base p.
   bite p.
   Blumenbach's p.
   Bolton's p.
   Bolton-nasion p.
   Broadbent-Bolton p.
   Broca's p.
   buccolingual p.
   Camper's p.
   coronal p.
   cove p.
   cusp p.
   datum p.
   Daubenton's p.
   eye-ear p.
   facial p.
   first parallel pelvic p.
   Frankfort horizontal p.
   frontal p.
   frontoparallel p.
   guide p.
   guiding p.
   Hensen's p.
   Hodge's p's
   horizontal p.

plane *(continued)*
  p. of inlet of pelvis
  intercristal p.
  interparietal p. of occipital bone
  interspinal p.
  intertubercular p.
  labiolingual p.
  Listing's p.
  Ludwig's p.
  mandibular p.
  mean foundation p.
  Meckel's p.
  median p.
  median-raphe p.
  mesiodistal p.
  midpelvic p.
  midsagittal p.
  Morton's p.
  nasion-postcondylare p.
  nuchal p.
  occipital p.
  occlusal p.
  p. of occlusion
  orbital p.
  orbital p. of frontal bone
  parasagittal p.
  pelvic p.
  pelvic p., narrow
  pelvic p. of greatest dimension
  pelvic p. of inlet
  pelvic p. of least dimension
  pelvic p., wide
  pelvic p. of outlet
  popliteal p. of femur
  principal p.
  p's of reference
  p. of regard
  sagittal p.
  semicircular p. of frontal bone
  semicircular p. of parietal bone
  semicircular p. of squama temporalis
  SN (sella-nasion) p.
  spinous p.

plane *(continued)*
  sternal p.
  sternoxiphoid p.
  subcostal p.
  supracrestal p.
  suprasternal p.
  temporal p.
  thoracic p.
  tooth p.
  transpyloric p.
  transtubercular p.
  transverse p.
  umbilical p.
  vertical p.
  visual p.
pla·ni·gram
pla·nig·ra·phy
pla·nim·e·ter
plan·ing
  root p.
plani·tho·rax
plank·ton
plan·ning
  family p.
pla·no·cel·lu·lar
pla·no·con·cave
pla·no·con·vex
pla·no·cyte
pla·no·gram
pla·nog·ra·phy
pla·nor·bid
Pla·nor·bi·dae
Pla·nor·bis
pla·no·topo·ki·ne·sia
pla·no·val·gus
plan·ta pe·dis
plan·tag·i·nis se·men
Plan·ta·go
plan·tal·gia
plan·tar
plan·ta·ris
plan·ta·tion
plan·ti·flex·ion
plan·ti·grade
plan·u·la
  invaginate p.
pla·num *pl.* pla·na
  p. interspinale

pla·num *(continued)*
    p. intertuberculare
    p. nuchale
    p. occipitale
    p. orbitale
    p. popliteum femoris
    p. semilunatum
    p. sphenoidale
    p. sternale
    p. subcostale
    p. supracristale
    p. temporale
    p. transpyloricum
pla·nu·ria
plaque
    argyrophil p's
    atheromatous p.
    attachment p's
    bacterial p.
    bacteriophage p.
    dental p.
    fibromyelinic p's
    fibrous p.
    gelatinoid p.
    Hollenhorst p's
    Hutchinson's p's
    Lichtheim p's
    mucin p.
    mucous p.
    opaline p.
    Peyer's p's
    Randall's p's
    Redlich-Fisher miliary p's
    senile p's
    shagreen p.
    talc p's
Pla·que·nil
plasm
    germ p.
plas·ma
    antihemophilic human p.
    blood p.
    citrated p.
    dried human p.
    fresh frozen p.
    hyperimmune p.
    normal human p.
    oxalate p.

plas·ma *(continued)*
    pooled p.
    salt p.
    seminal p.
    true p.
plas·ma·blast
plas·ma·crit
plas·ma·cyte
plas·ma·cyt·ic
plas·ma·cy·toid
plas·ma·cy·to·ma
    cutaneous p.
    extramedullary p.
    multiple p. of bone
    peripheral p.
    solitary p.
plas·ma·cy·to·sis
plas·ma·gel
plas·ma·gene
plas·ma·haut
plas·mal
plas·ma·lem·ma
plas·mal·o·gen
Plas·ma·nate
plas·man·ic acid
plas·ma·phe·re·sis
plas·mar·rhex·is
plas·ma·ther·a·py
plas·mat·ic
plas·ma·tog·a·my
plas·ma·tor·rhex·is
plas·ma·to·sis
plas·men·ic acid
plas·mic
plas·mid
    conjugative p.
    F p.
    F′ p.
    oligomeric p.
    R p.
    resistance p.
    self-transmissible p.
plas·min
plas·min·o·gen
plas·mo·cyte
plas·mo·cy·to·ma
plas·mo·dia
plas·mo·di·al

plate 1021

plas·mo·di·blast
plas·mo·di·ci·dal
plas·mo·di·cide
Plas·mo·di·i·dae
plas·mo·di·tropho·blast
Plas·mo·di·um
    P. falciparum
    P. malariae
    P. ovale
    P. perniciosum
    P. tenue
    P. vivax
plas·mo·di·um *pl.* plas·mo·dia
    exoerythrocytic p.
plas·mog·a·my
plas·mo·gen
plas·moid
plas·mol·o·gy
plas·mol·y·sis
plas·mo·lyt·ic
plas·mo·lyz·a·bil·i·ty
plas·mo·lyz·a·ble
plas·mo·lyze
plas·mo·ma
plas·mon
plas·mo·nu·cle·ic acid
plas·mop·ty·sis
plas·mor·rhex·is
plas·mos·chi·sis
plas·mo·sin
plas·mot·o·my
plas·mo·tropho·blast
plas·son
plas·te·in
plas·ter
    adhesive p.
    dental p.
    impression p.
    model p.
    mustard p.
    p. of Paris
    salicylic acid p.
    sterile adhesive p.
plas·tic
    modeling p.
plas·tic·i·ty
plas·ti·ci·zer
plas·tid

plas·tin
plas·tin·a·tion
plas·to·chon·dria
plas·to·chro·ma·nol
plas·to·cy·te·mia
plas·to·cy·to·pe·nia
plas·to·cy·to·sis
plas·to·dy·na·mia
plas·tog·a·my
plas·to·gel
plas·to·quin·one
plas·to·some
plas·tron
plate
    alar p.
    anal p.
    auditory p.
    axial p.
    basal p.
    basal p. of cranium
    basal p. of Winckler
    base p.
    bite p.
    bone p.
    cardiogenic p.
    cell p.
    cerebellar p.
    chorionic p.
    clinoid p.
    collecting p.
    cortical p.
    cough p.
    counting p.
    p. of cranial bone, inner
    p. of cranial bone, outer
    cribriform p.
    cribriform p. of ethmoid
      bone
    cuticular p.
    cutis p.
    decidual p.
    deck p.
    dental p.
    dermomyotome p.
    die p.
    dorsal p.
    dorsal thalamic p.
    dorsolateral p.

plate *(continued)*
    Eggers' p.
    end p.
    epiphyseal p.
    equatorial p.
    ethmovomerine p.
    facial p.
    floor p.
    foot p.
    frontal p.
    frontonasal p.
    growth p.
    horizontal p. of palatine bone
    Ishihara p's
    jumping the bite p.
    Kingsley p.
    Kühne's terminal p's
    Lane p's
    lateral mesoblastic p.
    lawn p.
    lingual p.
    location p.
    Mancini p's
    meatal p.
    medullary p.
    mesial p.
    metaphase p.
    middle p.
    Moe p.
    motor end p.
    muscle p.
    nail p.
    nephrotome p.
    neural p.
    notochordal p.
    nuclear p.
    optic p.
    oral p.
    orbital p. of ethmoid bone
    orbital p. of frontal bone
    palatal p.
    palate p.
    paper p.
    parachordal p.
    parietal p.
    perpendicular p. of ethmoid bone

plate *(continued)*
    perpendicular p. of palatine bone
    Petri p.
    pharyngeal p.
    polar p's
    pole p's
    pour p.
    prechordal p.
    prochordal p.
    primitive joint p.
    pterygoid p., external
    pterygoid p., internal
    pterygoid p., lateral
    pterygoid p., medial
    quadrigeminal p.
    reticular p.
    roof p.
    segmental p.
    Sherman p.
    sole p.
    spiral p.
    spread p.
    spring p.
    Strasburger's cell p.
    streak p.
    subgerminal p.
    tantalum p.
    Tarin's p.
    tarsal p's
    terminal p.
    tympanic p.
    urethral p.
    vascular foot p.
    ventral p.
    ventrolateral p.
    vertical p. of palatine bone
    visceral p.
    wing p.
pla·teau
    Geiger p.
    tibial p.
    ventricular p.
plate·let
    Bizzozero p's
    blood p.
    giant p.
plate·let·phe·re·sis

pla·ti·nec·to·my
plat·ing
    replica p.
pla·tin·ic
plat·i·node
Pla·ti·nol
plat·i·no·sis
plat·i·nous
plat·i·num
    p. chloride
    chordal p.
    p. diamminodichloride
cis–plat·i·num II
platy·ba·sia
platy·ce·lous
platy·ce·phal·ic
plat·y·ceph·a·ly
platy·cne·mia
platy·cne·mic
platy·co·ria
platy·cra·nia
platy·glos·sal
platy·hel·minth
Platy·hel·min·thes
platy·hi·er·ic
platy·kne·mia
platy·kur·tic
platy·me·ria
platy·me·ric
platy·mor·phia
platy·mor·phic
platy·my·a·ri·al
platy·my·a·ri·an
platy·my·oid
platy·onych·ia
platy·opia
platy·pel·lic
platy·pel·loid
platy·phyl·line
pla·typ·nea
platy·po·dia
Plat·yr·rhi·na
plat·yr·rhine
pla·tys·ma
pla·tys·mal
platy·spon·dyl·ia
platy·spon·dyl·i·sis
platy·spo·ri·na

platy·staph·y·line
plat·y·sten·ce·phal·ic
plat·y·sten·ceph·a·lism
platy·sten·ceph·a·ly
platy·trope
plau·ra·cin
Plaut's angina
Play·fair's treatment
plea·sure
    function p.
    organ p.
Plec·to·my·ce·tes
plec·tron
plec·trum
PLED — periodic lateralized
  epileptiform discharge
pledge
    Nightingale p.
pled·get
pleg·a·pho·nia
plei·a·des
pleio·chlo·ru·ria
pleio·tro·pia
plei·o·trop·ic
plei·ot·ro·pism
plei·ot·ro·py
Pleis·toph·o·ra
plek·tron
pleo·caryo·cyte
pleo·chro·ic
pleo·chro·ism
pleo·chro·mat·ic
pleo·chro·ma·tism
pleo·chro·mo·cy·to·ma
pleo·co·ni·al
pleo·cy·to·sis
pleo·karyo·cyte
pleo·mas·tia
pleo·mas·tic
pleo·ma·zia
pleo·mor·phic
pleo·mor·phism
pleo·mor·phous
pleo·nasm
pleo·nex·ia
ple·on·os·te·o·sis
    Leri's p.
pleo·no·tia

ple·op·tics
ple·op·to·phor
ple·ro·cer·coid
ple·ro·sis
Plesch's percussion
Plesch's test
ple·si·og·na·thus
Ple·si·o·mo·nas
    P. shigelloides
ple·sio·mor·phism
ple·sio·mor·phous
ple·si·opia
ples·ses·the·sia
ples·si·graph
ples·sim·e·ter
ples·si·met·ric
ples·sor
pleth·o·ra
ple·thor·ic
ple·thys·mo·gram
ple·thys·mo·graph
    body p.
    digital p.
    finger p.
    jerkin p.
ple·thys·mog·ra·phy
    air-cuff p.
    dynamic venous p.
    impedance p.
    strain-gauge p.
    thermistor p.
    tympanic p.
    venous occlusion p.
ple·thys·mom·e·ter
pleu·ra *pl.* pleu·rae
    cervical p.
    costal p.
    p. costalis
    diaphragmatic p.
    p. diaphragmatica
    mediastinal p.
    p. mediastinalis
    parietal p.
    p. parietalis
    pericardiac p.
    p. pericardiaca
    p. pulmonalis
    pulmonary p.

pleu·ra *(continued)*
    visceral p.
    p. visceralis
pleu·ra·cen·te·sis
pleu·ra·cot·o·my
pleu·rae
pleu·ral
pleu·ral·gia
pleu·ral·gic
pleu·ram·ni·on
pleu·ra·poph·y·sis
pleu·rec·to·my
pleu·ri·sy
    acute p.
    adhesive p.
    basal p.
    benign dry p.
    blocked p.
    cholesterol p.
    chronic p.
    chyliform p.
    chyloid p.
    chylous p.
    circumscribed p.
    costal p.
    diaphragmatic p.
    diffuse p.
    double p.
    dry p.
    p. with effusion
    encysted p.
    epidemic p.
    exudative p.
    fibrinous p.
    hemorrhagic p.
    ichorous p.
    indurative p.
    interlobular p.
    latent p.
    mediastinal p.
    metapneumonic p.
    plastic p.
    primary p.
    proliferating p.
    pulmonary p.
    pulsating p.
    purulent p.
    sacculated p.

pleu·ri·sy *(continued)*
  secondary p.
  serofibrinous p.
  serous p.
  single p.
  suppurative p.
  typhoid p.
  visceral p.
  wet p.
pleu·rit·ic
pleu·ri·tis
pleu·ri·tog·e·nous
pleu·ro·bron·chi·tis
pleu·ro·cele
pleu·ro·cen·te·sis
pleu·ro·cen·trum
Pleu·ro·cer·i·dae
pleu·ro·cho·le·cys·ti·tis
pleu·ro·cu·ta·ne·ous
pleu·rod·e·sis
pleu·ro·dont
pleu·ro·dyn·ia
  epidemic p.
pleu·ro·gen·ic
pleu·rog·e·nous
pleu·rog·ra·phy
pleu·ro·hep·a·ti·tis
pleu·ro·lith
pleu·rol·y·sis
pleu·ro·me·lus
pleu·ro·pa·ri·e·to·pexy
pleu·ro·peri·car·di·al
pleu·ro·peri·car·di·tis
pleu·ro·peri·to·ne·al
pleu·ro·per·i·to·ne·um
pleu·ro·pneu·mo·nia
pleu·ro·pneu·mo·nol·y·sis
pleu·ro·pul·mo·nary
pleur·or·rhea
pleu·ros·co·py
pleu·ro·so·ma
pleu·ro·so·mus
pleu·ro·thot·o·nos
pleu·ro·thot·o·nus
pleu·ro·tin
pleu·ro·tome
pleu·rot·o·my
pleu·ro·ty·phoid

pleu·ro·vis·cer·al
plex·al
plex·ec·to·my
plex·i·form
plex·im·e·ter
plex·i·met·ric
plex·im·e·try
plex·i·tis
  acute p.
plex·o·gen·ic
plex·om·e·ter
plex·op·a·thy
  lumbar p.
plex·or
plex·us *pl.* plex·us, plex·us·es
  annular p.
  anococcygeal p.
  anserine p.
  p. anserinus
  anterior bronchial p.
  anterior esophageal p.
  anterolateral p. of
   Santorini
  aortic p., abdominal
  aortic p., thoracic
  p. aorticus
  p. aorticus abdominalis
  p. aorticus thoracalis
  p. aorticus thoracicus
  areolar p.
  p. arteriae chorioideae
  p. arteriae ovaricae
  Auerbach's p.
  p. auricularis posterior
  autonomic p's
  p. autonomici
  basilar p.
  p. basilaris
  Batson's p.
  biliary p.
  brachial p.
  p. brachialis
  bulbar p.
  cardiac p.
  p. cardiacus
  p. caroticus communis
  p. caroticus externus
  p. caroticus internus

plex·us *(continued)*
    carotid p.
    carotid p., common
    carotid p., external
    carotid p., internal
    p. cavernosus
    cavernous p.
    celiac p.
    p. celiacus
    cephalic ganglionated p.
    cervical p.
    p. cervicalis
    p. cervicobrachialis
    choroid p.
    p. choroideus
    coccygeal p.
    p. coccygeus
    coccygeal vascular p.
    p. coeliacus
    colic p., left
    colic p., middle
    colic p., right
    corneal p.
    p. coronarius cordis anterior
    p. coronarius cordis posterior
    coronary p's, gastric
    coronary p. of heart, anterior
    coronary p. of heart, posterior
    coronary p's of stomach, superior
    crural p.
    Cruveilhier's p.
    cystic p.
    deep cervical p.
    deep stroma p.
    deferential p.
    p. deferentialis
    dental p., inferior
    dental p., superior
    p. dentalis inferior
    p. dentalis superior
    diaphragmatic p.
    enteric p.
    p. entericus

plex·us *(continued)*
    epigastric p.
    esophageal p.
    p. esophageus
    Exner's p.
    external iliac p.
    external maxillary p.
    facial p.
    p. of facial artery
    p. facialis
    femoral p.
    p. femoralis
    fundamental p.
    p. gangliosus ciliaris
    gastric p's
    p. gastrici
    p. gastricus anterior
    p. gastricus inferior
    p. gastricus posterior
    p. gastricus superior
    gastroepiploic p., left
    p. haemorrhoidalis
    Heller's p.
    hemorrhoidal p.
    hepatic p.
    p. hepaticus
    Hovius' p.
    hypogastric p.
    p. hypogastricus
    ileocolic p.
    iliac p's
    p. iliaci
    p. iliacus externus
    inferior vesical p.
    infraorbital p.
    inguinal p.
    p. inguinalis
    p. intercavernosus
    intercavernous p.
    intermediate p.
    intermesenteric p.
    p. intermesentericus
    internal carotid venous p.
    internal maxillary p.
    interradial p.
    intestinal p., submucous
    intramural p.
    p. intraparotideus

plex·us *(continued)*
  intrascleral p.
  ischiadic p.
  Jacobson's p.
  Jacques p.
  jugular p.
  p. jugularis
  laryngeal p.
  lateral p.
  Leber's p.
  lienal p.
  p. lienalis
  lingual p.
  p. lingualis
  p. lumbalis
  lumbar p.
  p. lumbaris
  lumboaortic
    intermesenteric p.
  lumbosacral p.
  p. lumbosacralis
  lymphatic p.
  p. lymphaticus
  p. lymphaticus axillaris
  axillary lymphatic p.
  p. mammarius
  p. mammarius internus
  mammary venous p.
  p. maxillaris externus
  p. maxillaris internus
  maxillary p.
  Meissner's p.
  meningeal p.
  p. meningeus
  mesenteric p., inferior
  mesenteric p., superior
  p. mesentericus inferior
  p. mesentericus superior
  molecular p.
  myenteric p.
  p. myentericus
  nasopalatine p.
  nerve p.
  p. nervorum spinalium
  nervous p.
  obturator p.
  occipital p.
  p. occipitalis

plex·us *(continued)*
  p. oesophageus
  ophthalmic p.
  p. ophthalmicus
  ovarian p.
  p. ovaricus
  pampiniform p.
  p. pampiniformis
  pancreatic p.
  p. pancreaticus
  pancreaticoduodenal p.
  Panizza's p's
  parotid p. of facial nerve
  p. parotideus nervi facialis
  p. patellae
  patellar p.
  pelvic p.
  periarterial p.
  p. periarterialis
  pericorneal p.
  periesophageal p. of veins
  perivascular p.
  p. perivascularis
  pharyngeal p.
  p. pharyngealis
  p. pharyngeus
  p. pharyngeus ascendens
  phrenic p.
  p. phrenicus
  popliteal p.
  p. popliteus
  preaortic p's
  presacral p.
  prevertebral p's
  primary p.
  prostatic p.
  prostaticovesical p.
  p. prostaticus
  pterygoid p.
  p. pterygoideus
  pudendal p.
  p. pudendalis
  p. pulmonalis anterior
  p. pulmonalis posterior
  pulmonary p.
  pulmonary p., anterior
  pulmonary p., posterior
  pyloric p.

plex·us *(continued)*
    Quénu p.
    Ranvier's p.
    p. of Raschkow
    rectal p's, inferior
    rectal p's, middle
    rectal p., superior
    p. rectales inferiores
    p. rectales medii
    p. rectalis superior
    Remak's p.
    renal p.
    p. renalis
    sacral p.
    sacral lymphatic p.
    p. sacralis
    Santorini's p.
    Sappey's subareolar p.
    sciatic p.
    sinocarotid p.
    solar p.
    spermatic p.
    p. spermaticus
    p. of spinal nerves
    splenic p.
    p. splenicus
    Stensen's p.
    stroma p.
    sub-basal p.
    subclavian p.
    p. subclavius
    subendocardiac p.
    subendocardial terminal p.
    subepithelial p.
    submolecular p.
    submucosal p.
    p. submucosus
    submucous p.
    subpapillary p.
    subpapillary venous p.
    subpericardial p.
    subsartorial p.
    p. subsartorialis
    subserosal p.
    p. subserosus
    subtrapezius p.
    supraradial p.
    suprarenal p.

plex·us *(continued)*
    p. suprarenalis
    p. sympathici
    p. temporalis superficialis
    testicular p.
    p. testicularis
    thoracic aortic p.
    p. thyreoideus impar
    p. thyreoideus inferior
    p. thyreoideus superior
    thyroid p., inferior
    thyroid p., superior
    thyroid p., unpaired
    thyroid venous p.
    tonsillar p.
    Trolard's p.
    tympanic p.
    p. tympanicus
    p. tympanicus [Jacobsoni]
    ureteric p.
    p. uretericus
    urorectal p.
    uterine p.
    p. uterinus
    uterovaginal p.
    p. uterovaginalis
    uterovaginal venous p.
    vaginal p.
    p. vaginalis
    vascular p.
    p. vasculosus
    p. venosus
    p. venosus areolaris
    p. venosus pterygoideus
    p. venosus rectalis
    p. venosus sacralis
    p. venosus suboccipitalis
    p. venosus uterinus
    p. venosus vaginalis
    p. venosus vertebralis
      externus anterior
    p. venosus vertebralis
      externus posterior
    p. venosus vertebralis
      internus anterior
    p. venosus vertebralis
      internus posterior
    p. venosus vesicalis

plex·us *(continued)*
venous p.
venous p., areolar
venous p., hemorrhoidal
venous p., prostatic
venous p., rectal
venous p., sacral
venous p., suboccipital
venous p., uterine
venous p., vaginal
venous p., vesical
venous p. of foot, dorsal
venous p. of foramen ovale
venous p. of hand, dorsal
venous p. of hypoglossal
  canal
vertebral p.
vertebral p's, internal
vertebral p's, external
p. vertebralis
vertebral venous p.
vesical p.
p. vesicale
p. vesicalis
vesicoprostatic p.
vidian p.
p. villosae gastricae
visceral p's
p. viscerales
pli·ca *pl.* pli·cae
plicae alares
plicae ampullares tubae
  uterinae
p. aryepiglottica
p. axillaris anterior
p. axillaris posterior
plicae caecales
p. caecalis vascularis
plicae cecales
p. cecalis vascularis
p. chordae tympani
p. choroidea
plicae ciliares
plicae circulares
plicae circulares
  [Kerkringi]
plicae conniventes
p. cordae utero-inguinalis

pli·ca *(continued)*
p. duodenalis inferior
p. duodenalis superior
p. duodenojejunalis
p. duodenomesocolica
p. epigastrica
p. epigastrica peritonaei
epiglottic p.
p. fimbriata
plicae gastricae
p. gastropancreatica
p. glossoepiglottica
  lateralis
p. glossoepiglottica
  mediana
p. hepatopancreatica
p. hypogastrica
p. ileocaecalis
p. incudis
p. interarytenoidea
p. interureterica
plicae iridis
p. lacrimalis
p. lacrimalis [Hasneri]
p. longitudinalis duodeni
p. lunata
p. mallearis anterior
p. mallearis posterior
p. membranae tympani
  externa anterior
p. membranae tympani
  externa posterior
p. nervi laryngei
plicae palatinae
  transversae
plicae palmatae
p. palpebronasalis
p. paraduodenalis
p. pubovesicalis
p. recti
p. rectouterina
p. rectouterina [Douglasi]
p. salpingopalatina
p. salpingopharyngea
p. semilunaris
plicae semilunares coli
p. semilunaris conjunctivae
p. sigmoidea coli

pli·ca *(continued)*
    p. spiralis
    p. stapedis
    p. sublingualis
    p. synovialis
    p. synovialis infrapatellaris
    p. synovialis patellaris
    plicae transversales recti
    p. triangularis
    plicae tubales tubae
      uterinae
    plicae tubariae tubae
      uterinae
    plicae tunicae mucosae
    p. umbilicalis lateralis
    p. umbilicalis media
    p. umbilicalis medialis
    p. umbilicalis mediana
    p. urachi
    p. ureterica
    plicae vaginae
    p. venae cavae sinistrae
    p. ventricularis
    p. vesicalis transversa
    p. vestibularis
    plicae villosae
    p. vocalis
pli·cae
pli·cate
pli·ca·tion
    caval p.
pli·cec·to·my
pli·cot·o·my
pli·ers
Plim·mer's bodies
plint
plinth
ploi·dy
plom·bage
plop
plot
    Kurie p.
    Lineweaver-Burk p.
plo·to·ly·sin
plo·to·spas·min
plo·to·tox·in
PLT — primed lymphocyte
  typing

PLT — primed lymphocyte
  typing
    psittacosis-lymphogranu-
      loma venereum-trachoma
plug
    cervical p.
    copulation p.
    Corner's p.
    Dittrich's p's
    Ecker's p.
    epithelial p.
    Imlach's fat p.
    kite-tailed p.
    meconium p.
    mucous p.
    Traube's p's
    vaginal p.
    yolk p.
Plugge's test
plug·ger
    amalgam p.
    gold p.
    root canal p.
plum·bage
plum·ba·go
plum·bic
plum·bism
plum·bo·ther·a·py
plu·mer·i·cin
Plum·mer's disease
Plum·mer's sign
Plum·mer-Vin·son syndrome
plu·mose
plump·er
plum·u·la
plu·ri·de·fi·cient
plu·ri·fo·cal
plu·ri·glan·du·lar
plu·ri·grav·i·da
plu·ri·loc·u·lar
plu·ri·men·or·rhea
plu·ri·nu·cle·ar
plu·ri·or·i·fi·cial
plu·rip·a·ra
plu·ri·par·i·ty
plu·ri·par·tite
plu·ri·po·lar
plu·ri·po·tent

plu·ri·po·ten·tial
plu·ri·po·ten·ti·al·i·ty
plu·ri·re·sis·tant
plu·ri·tis·su·lar
plu·ri·vis·cer·al
plu·to·nism
plu·to·ni·um
PMB — polymorphonuclear
 basophil leukocytes
  postmenopausal bleeding
PME — polymorphonuclear
 eosinophil leukocytes
PMI — point of maximal
 impulse
PML — progressive multifocal
 leukoencephalopathy
PMM — pentamethylmelamine-
PMMA — polymethyl
 methacrylate
PMN — polymorphonuclear
 neutrophil leukocytes
PMR — proportionate
 mortality ratio
PMS — postmenstrual stress
 premenstrual syndrome
PMSG — pregnant mare
 serum gonadotropin
PMT — premenstrual tension
PN — peripheral nerve
 peripheral neuropathy
 polyneuritis
PND — paroxysmal nocturnal
 dyspnea
pneo·gas·ter
pneo·gram
pneo·graph
pne·om·e·ter
pneo·scope
PNET — peripheral
 neuroectodermal tumor
pneu·mal
pneu·mar·thro·gram
pneu·mar·throg·ra·phy
pneu·mar·thro·sis
pneu·ma·scope
pneu·ma·the·mia
pneu·mat·ic
pneu·mat·ics

pneu·ma·tin·u·ria
pneu·ma·tism
pneu·ma·ti·za·tion
 mastoid p.
pneu·ma·tized
pneu·ma·to·car·dia
pneu·ma·to·cele
 p. cranii, extracranial p.
 intracranial p.
 parotid p.
 scrotal p.
pneu·ma·to·ceph·a·lus
pneu·ma·to·dysp·nea
pneu·ma·to·gram
pneu·ma·to·graph
pneu·ma·tom·e·ter
pneu·ma·tom·e·try
pneu·ma·to·phore
pneu·ma·tor·rha·chis
pneu·ma·to·sis
 p. cystoides intestinalis
 p. cystoides intestinorum
 intestinal p.
 p. intestinalis
 p. pulmonum
pneu·ma·to·ther·a·py
pneu·ma·tu·ria
pneu·ma·type
pneu·mec·to·my
pneum·en·ceph·a·log·ra·phy
pneu·mo·al·veo·log·ra·phy
pneu·mo·am·ni·os
pneu·mo·an·gio·gram
pneu·mo·an·gi·og·ra·phy
pneu·mo·arc·tia
pneu·mo·ar·throg·ra·phy
pneu·mo·ba·cil·lus
 Friedländer's p.
pneu·mo·bac·ter·ine
pneu·mo·bil·ia
pneu·mo·blas·to·ma
pneu·mo·bul·bar
pneu·mo·bul·bous
pneu·mo·car·di·al
pneu·mo·car·dio·graph
pneu·mo·car·di·og·ra·phy
pneu·mo·cele
pneu·mo·cen·te·sis

pneu·mo·ceph·a·lus
pneu·mo·cho·le·cys·ti·tis
pneu·mo·chy·sis
pneu·mo·coc·cal
pneu·mo·coc·ce·mia
pneu·mo·coc·ci
pneu·mo·coc·cic
pneu·mo·coc·ci·dal
pneu·mo·coc·col·y·sis
pneu·mo·coc·co·sis
pneu·mo·coc·co·su·ria
pneu·mo·coc·cus *pl.* pneu·mo·
　coc·ci
pneu·mo·co·lon
pneu·mo·co·ni·o·sis
　asbestos p.
　bauxite p.
　p. of coal workers
　collagenous p.
　complicated p.
　diatomaceous earth p.
　fractional p.
　noncollagenous p.
　rheumatoid p.
　p. siderotica
　talc p.
pneu·mo·cra·nia
pneu·mo·cra·ni·um
pneu·mo·cys·tic
Pneu·mo·cys·tis
　P. carinii
pneu·mo·cys·tog·ra·phy
pneu·mo·cys·to·sis
pneu·mo·cys·to·to·mog·ra·
　phy
pneu·mo·cyte
　granular p.
　membranous p.
pneu·mo·der·ma
pneu·modo·graph
pneu·mo·dy·nam·ics
pneu·mo·em·py·e·ma
pneu·mo·en·ceph·a·li·tis
pneu·mo·en·ceph·a·lo·gram
pneu·mo·en·ceph·a·lo·gra·
　phy
pneu·mo·en·ceph·a·lo·my·
　elo·gram

pneu·mo·en·ceph·a·lo·my·
　elog·ra·phy
pneu·mo·en·ceph·a·los
pneu·mo·en·ter·itis
　p. of calves
pneu·mo·fas·cio·gram
pneu·mo·ga·lac·to·cele
pneu·mo·gas·tric
pneu·mo·gas·trog·ra·phy
pneu·mo·gas·tros·co·py
pneu·mo·gram
pneu·mo·graph
pneu·mog·ra·phy
　cerebral p.
　retroperitoneal p.
pneu·mo·gy·no·gram
pneu·mo·he·mia
pneu·mo·he·mo·peri·car·di·
　um
pneu·mo·he·mo·tho·rax
pneu·mo·hy·dro·me·tra
pneu·mo·hy·dro·peri·car·di·
　um
pneu·mo·hy·dro·tho·rax
pneu·mo·kid·ney
pneu·mo·lith
pneu·mo·li·thi·a·sis
pneu·mol·o·gy
pneu·mol·y·sin
pneu·mol·y·sis
pneu·mo·ma·la·cia
pneu·mo·mas·sage
pneu·mo·me·di·as·ti·no·gram
pneu·mo·me·di·as·ti·nog·ra·
　phy
pneu·mo·me·di·as·ti·num
pneu·mo·mel·a·no·sis
pneu·mom·e·ter
pneu·mo·mon·i·li·a·sis
pneu·mo·my·co·sis
pneu·mo·my·elog·ra·phy
pneu·mo·nec·ta·sia
pneu·mo·nec·ta·sis
pneu·mo·nec·to·my
pneu·mo·ne·de·ma
pneu·mo·ne·mia
pneu·mo·nere

pneu·mo·nia
    abortive p.
    acute p.
    p. alba
    alcoholic p.
    amebic p.
    anthrax p.
    apex p.
    apical p.
    p. apostematosa
    aspiration p.
    atypical p.
    atypical bronchial p.
    bacterial p.
    bilious p.
    bronchial p.
    brooder p.
    Buhl's desquamative p.
    caseous p.
    cat p.
    catarrhal p.
    central p.
    cerebral p.
    cheesy p.
    chronic p.
    chronic eosinophilic p.
    chronic fibrous p.
    cold agglutinin p.
    congenital aspiration p.
    contagious p. of horses
    contusion p.
    core p.
    Corrigan's p.
    creeping p.
    croupous p.
    deglutition p.
    dermal p.
    desquamative p.
    desquamative interstitial
      p.
    p. dissecans
    double p.
    Eaton agent p.
    embolic p.
    ephemeral p.
    ether p.
    fibrinous p.
    fibrous p.

pneu·mo·nia *(continued)*
    fibrous p., chronic
    Friedländer's p.
    Friedländer's bacillus p.
    gangrenous p.
    giant cell p.
    Hecht's p.
    hypostatic p.
    indurative p.
    infective p. of goats
    influenzal p.
    influenza virus p.
    inhalation p.
    p. interlobularis purulenta
    interstitial p.
    interstitial plasma cell p.
    intrauterine p.
    Kaufman's p.
    Klebsiella p.
    lipid p.
    lipoid p.
    lobar p.
    lobular p.
    Löffler's p.
    Louisiana p.
    lymphoid interstitial p.
    p. malleosa
    massive p.
    metastatic p.
    migratory p.
    mycoplasmal p.
    obstructive p.
    oil-aspiration p.
    organizing p.
    parenchymatous p.
    Pittsburgh p.
    plague p.
    plasma cell p.
    pleuritic p.
    pleurogenetic p.
    pleurogenic p.
    pneumococcal p.
    pneumocystis p.
    Pneumocystis carinii p.
    primary atypical p.
    purulent p.
    rheumatic p.
    secondary p.

pneu·mo·nia *(continued)*
  septic p.
  staphylococcal p.
  streptococcal p.
  superficial p.
  suppurative p.
  terminal p.
  toxemic p.
  transplantation p.
  traumatic p.
  tuberculous p.
  tularemic p.
  typhoid p.
  unresolved p.
  vagus p.
  varicella p.
  viral p.
  wandering p.
  white p.
  woolsorter's p.
pneu·mon·ic
pneu·mo·ni·tis
  acute interstitial p.
  aspiration p.
  chemical p.
  cholesterol p.
  eosinophilic p.
  granulomatous p.
  hypersensitivity p.
  interstitial p.
  lymphocytic interstitial p.
  malarial p.
  pneumocystis p.
  rheumatic p.
  uremic p.
pneu·mo·no·cele
pneu·mo·no·cen·te·sis
pneu·mo·no·cir·rho·sis
pneu·mo·no·coc·cus
pneu·mo·no·cyte
  granular p.
  membranous p.
pneu·mo·no·en·ter·itis
pneu·mo·no·graph
pneu·mo·nog·ra·phy
pneu·mo·nol·y·sis
pneu·mo·no·mel·a·no·sis
pneu·mo·nom·e·ter

pneu·mo·no·mo·ni·li·a·sis
pneu·mo·no·my·co·sis
pneu·mo·no·pal·u·dism
pneu·mo·nop·a·thy
  eosinophilic p.
pneu·mo·no·pexy
pneu·mo·noph·thi·sis
pneu·mo·no·pleu·ri·tis
pneu·mo·no·re·sec·tion
pneu·mo·nor·rha·gia
pneu·mo·nor·rha·phy
pneu·mo·no·sis
pneu·mo·no·ther·a·py
pneu·mo·not·o·my
pneu·mo-or·bi·tog·ra·phy
pneu·mo·pal·u·dism
pneu·mop·a·thy
pneu·mo·peri·car·di·tis
pneu·mo·peri·car·di·um
pneu·mo·peri·to·ne·al
pneu·mo·peri·to·ne·um
  transabdominal p.
pneu·mo·peri·to·ni·tis
pneu·mo·pexy
pneu·mo·pha·gia
pneu·mo·pho·nia
pneu·mo·ple·thys·mog·ra·phy
pneu·mo·pleu·ri·tis
pneu·mo·pleu·ro·pa·ri·e·to·
  pexy
pneu·mo·pre·cor·di·um
pneu·mo·pre·peri·to·ne·um
pneu·mo·py·elog·ra·phy
pneu·mo·pyo·peri·car·di·um
pneu·mo·pyo·tho·rax
pneu·mo·ra·chi·cen·te·sis
pneu·mo·ra·chis
pneu·mo·ra·di·og·ra·phy
pneu·mo·re·sec·tion
pneu·mo·re·tro·peri·to·ne·
  um
pneu·mo·roent·geno·gram
pneu·mo·roent·gen·og·ra·phy
pneu·mor·rha·gia
pneu·mo·sep·ti·ce·mia
pneu·mo·se·ro·sa
pneu·mo·se·ro·tho·rax
pneu·mo·sil·i·co·sis

pneu·mo·tacho·graph
pneu·mo·ta·chom·e·ter
pneu·mo·tach·y·graph
pneu·mo·tax·ic
pneu·mo·ther·a·py
pneu·mo·ther·mo·mas·sage
pneu·mo·tho·rax
    artificial p.
    clicking p.
    closed p.
    diagnostic p.
    extrapleural p.
    induced p.
    open p.
    pressure p.
    spontaneous p.
    sucking p.
    tension p.
    therapeutic p.
    traumatic p.
    valvular p.
pneu·mo·to·mog·ra·phy
pneu·mot·o·my
pneu·mo·trop·ic
pneu·mot·ro·pism
pneu·mo·tym·pa·num
pneu·mo·uria
Pneu·mo·vax
    P. 23
pneu·mo·ven·tri·cle
pneu·mo·ven·tric·u·li
pneu·mo·ven·tric·u·log·ra·phy
pneu·mo·vi·rus
pneu·sis
PNH — paroxysmal nocturnal hemoglobinuria
PNPB — positive-negative pressure breathing
PO — L. per os (by mouth, orally)
POA — pancreatic oncofetal antigen
Po_2 — oxygen partial pressure (tension)
pO_2 — oxygen partial pressure (tension)

Pocill. — L. pocillum (a small cup)
pock
pock·et
    absolute p.
    complex p.
    compound p.
    endocardial p's
    gingival p.
    infrabony p.
    intra-alveolar p.
    intrabony p.
    periodontal p.
    pyorrhea p.
    Rathke's p.
    regurgitant p's
    relative p.
    retraction p.
    Seessel's p.
    simple p.
    subcrestal p.
    suprabony p.
    supracrestal p.
    supragingival p.
    true p.
    p's of Zahn
pock·mark
Pocul. — L. poculum (cup)
poc·u·li·form
poc·u·lum
    p. Diogenis
po·dag·ra
pod·a·gral
po·dag·ric
pod·a·grous
po·dal·gia
po·dal·ic
pod·ar·thri·tis
pod·ede·ma
pod·en·ceph·a·lus
po·dia
po·di·at·ric
po·di·a·trist
po·di·a·try
po·di·tis
po·di·um *pl.* po·dia

podo·cyte
podo·derm
podo·dy·na·mom·e·ter
podo·dyn·ia
podo·gram
podo·graph
po·dol·o·gy
podo·phyl·lin
podo·phyl·lo·tox·in
po·doph·yl·lous
Podo·phyl·lum
podo·phyl·lum
podo·pom·pho·lyx
podo·tro·chi·li·tis
Poe·cil·ia
    P. reticulata
po·go·ni·a·sis
po·go·ni·on
Po·go·no·myr·mex
pOH — hydroxide ion
  concentration (potential of
  hydroxide ion)
Pohl's test
poi·e·tin
poi·ki·lo·blast
poi·ki·lo·car·y·no·sis
poi·ki·lo·cyte
poi·ki·lo·cy·the·mia
poi·ki·lo·cy·to·sis
poi·ki·lo·der·ma
    p. atrophicans vasculare
    p. of Civatte
    congenital p.
    p. congenitale
    p. congenitale of Thomson
    p. vasculare atrophicans
poi·ki·lo·der·ma·to·myo·si·
  tis
poi·ki·lo·ploid
poi·ki·lo·ploidy
poi·ki·los·mo·sis
poi·ki·los·mot·ic
poi·ki·lo·sta·sis
poi·ki·lo·therm
poi·ki·lo·ther·mal
poi·ki·lo·ther·mic
poi·ki·lo·ther·mism
poi·ki·lo·ther·my

poi·ki·lo·throm·bo·cyte
poi·ki·lo·thy·mia
poin
point
    p. A
    absolute near p.
    absorbent p.
    Addison's p.
    alveolar p.
    apophysiary p.
    p. Ar
    p. of Arrhigi
    auricular p.
    p. B
    p. Ba
    Barker's p.
    p. of Béclard
    p. Bo
    Boas' p.
    boiling p.
    boiling p., normal
    Bolton p.
    Bolton registration p.
    Brewer's p.
    Broadbent registration p.
    Broca's p.
    Cannon's p.
    cardinal p's
    p. of centricity
    Chauffard's p.
    cold rigor p.
    condenser p.
    conjugate p.
    contact p.
    convenience p.
    p. of convergence
    convergence near p.
    corresponding p's
    Cova's p.
    craniometric p.
    critical p.
    crossover p.
    p. D
    deaf p.
    de Mussy's p.
    Desjardins' p.
    p. of direction
    disparate p's

point *(continued)*
 p. of dispersion
 p. of divergence
 dorsal p.
 p's douloureux
 E p.
 p. of election
 Erb's p.
 eye p.
 far p.
 p. of fixation
 focal p.
 freezing p.
 fusion p.
 Galliot's p.
 glenoid p.
 Guéneau de Mussy's p.
 gutta-percha p.
 Hallé's p.
 Hartmann's critical p.
 heat-rigor p.
 hinge-axis p.
 Hirschfeld's silver p.
 homologous p.
 hysteroepileptogenous p.
 hysterogenic p.
 ice p.
 identical p's
 image p.
 p. of incidence
 incisal p.
 isobestic p.
 isoelectric p.
 isoionic p.
 J p.
 jugal p.
 jugomaxillary p.
 Keen's p.
 Kienböck-Adamson p's
 Kocher's p.
 Krafft p.
 lacrimal p.
 Lanz's p.
 leak p.
 McBurney's p.
 McEwen's p.
 Mackenzie's p.
 malar p.

point *(continued)*
 p. of maximal impulse
 maximum occipital p.
 median mandibular p.
 Méglin's p.
 melting p.
 mental p.
 metopic p.
 midinguinal p.
 motor p.
 Munro's p.
 Mussy's p.
 nasal p.
 near p.
 near p., absolute
 near p., relative
 neutral p.
 nodal p's
 object p.
 occipital p.
 ossification p.
 ossification p., primary
 ossification p., secondary
 painful p's
 paper p.
 Pauly's p.
 phrenic-pressure p.
 Piersol's p.
 p. Po.
 pour p.
 preauricular p.
 pressure p.
 pressure-arresting p.
 pressure-exciting p.
 principal p's
 p. of proximal contact
 p. R
 Ramond's p.
 reflection p.
 refraction p.
 p. of regard
 registration p.
 retromandibular tender p.
 Robson's p.
 root canal p.
 p. SE
 set p.
 silver p.

point *(continued)*
  p. SO
  spinal p.
  stereoidentical p's
  p. of Sudeck
  subnasal p.
  subtemporal p.
  supra-auricular p.
  supraclavicular p.
  supranasal p.
  supraorbital p.
  sylvian p.
  thermal death p.
  trigger p.
  triple p.
  Trousseau's apophysiary
    p's
  Valleix's p's
  vital p.
  Vogt's p.
  Vogt-Hueter p.
  Voillemier's p.
  Weber's p.
  p. Z
  Ziemssen's motor p's
point·er
  back p.
  hip p.
poin·til·lage
Poi·ri·er's glands
Poi·ri·er's line
poise
Poi·seuille's law
Poi·seuille's space
poi·son
  acrid p.
  acronarcotic p.
  acrosedative p.
  arrow p.
  catalyst p.
  contact p.
  corrosive p.
  fatigue p.
  fugu p.
  gonyaulax p.
  hemotropic p.
  irritant p.
  mitotic p.

poi·son *(continued)*
  muscle p.
  narcotic p's
  paralytic shellfish p.
  puffer p.
  sedative p's
  shellfish p.
  toot p.
  vascular p.
  whelk p.
poi·son ivy
poi·son oak
poi·son su·mac
poi·son·ing
  acetaminophen p.
  acetanilid p.
  acetylsalicylic acid p.
  akee p.
  alcohol p.
  aminopyrine p.
  amphetamine p.
  aniline p.
  antimony p.
  arsenic p.
  aspirin p.
  barbiturate p.
  benzene p.
  beryllium p.
  blood p.
  bongkrek p.
  bromide p.
  broom p.
  callistin shellfish p.
  carbon disulfide p.
  carbon monoxide p.
  cheese p.
  chemical fume p.
  chloral hydrate p.
  corncockle p.
  coyotillo p.
  cyanide p.
  dural p.
  elasmobranch p.
  ergot p.
  esowasure-gai p.
  fish p.
  fluoride p., chronic
  fluorine p., chronic

poi·son·ing *(continued)*
    food p.
    forage p.
    fugu p.
    gossypol p.
    gymnothorax p.
    heavy metal p.
    iron p.
    larkspur p.
    lead p.
    loco p.
    manganese p.
    meat p.
    mercury p.
    milk p.
    molybdenum p.
    mushroom p.
    mussel p.
    naphthol p.
    nitroaniline p.
    nutmeg p.
    O_2 p.
    paraldehyde p.
    parathyroid p.
    phenol p.
    phenytoin p.
    phosphorus p.
    pitch p.
    potato p.
    puffer p.
    salmon p.
    salmonellal food p.
    salt p.
    saturnine p.
    sausage p.
    scombroid p.
    selenium p.
    shellfish p.
    silver p.
    spider p.
    staphylococcal food p.
    tempeh p.
    tetrachlorethane p.
    tetraodon p.
    thallium p.
    thorn apple p.
    TNT p.
    tobacco p.

poi·son·ing *(continued)*
    trinitrotoluene p.
    whelk p.
    zinc p.
poi·son·ous
Pois·son distribution
Pois·son-Pear·son formula
poi·tri·naire
poke·root
poke·weed
pol·a·cril·in
    p. potassium
Po·land's anomaly
Po·land's syndrome
po·lar
Po·lar·amine
po·la·rim·e·ter
po·la·rim·e·try
po·lar·i·scope
po·lar·i·scop·ic
po·lar·is·co·py
po·lar·is·tro·bom·e·ter
po·lar·i·ty
    dynamic p.
    operon p.
po·lar·iza·tion
    circular p.
    elliptical p.
    plane p.
    rotatory p.
po·lar·ize
po·lar·iz·er
po·laro·gram
po·laro·gra·phic
po·lar·og·ra·phy
Po·lar·oid
po·laro·plast
pol·dine meth·yl·sul·fate
pole
    animal p.
    anterior p. of eyeball
    anterior p. of lens
    antigerminal p.
    apical p.
    caudal p.
    cephalic p.
    cranial p.
    frontal p.

pole *(continued)*
    germinal p.
    inferior p. of kidney
    inferior p. of testis
    negative p.
    nutritive p.
    occipital p.
    pelvic p.
    placental p.
    positive p.
    posterior p. of eyeball
    posterior p. of lens
    temporal p.
    twin p.
    upper p. of kidney
    upper p. of testis
    vegetal p.
    vegetative p.
    vitelline p.
po·li
pol·i·ca·pram
po·lice·man
poli·clin·ic
pol·i·en·ceph·a·li·tis
pol·i·en·ceph·a·lo·my·eli·tis
po·lio
po·lio·ci·dal
po·lio·clas·tic
po·lio·dys·tro·phia
    p. cerebri
    p. cerebri progressiva
      infantalis
po·lio·dys·tro·phy
    p. cerebri
    progressive cerebral p.
po·lio·en·ceph·a·li·tis
    p. acuta hemorrhagica
    p. acuta infantum
    acute bulbar p.
    p. infectiva
    inferior p.
    p. of Marie-Strümpell
    posterior p.
    superior hemorrhagic p.
    Wernicke's acute
      hemorrhagic upper p.
po·lio·en·ceph·a·lo·me·nin·
  go·my·eli·tis

po·lio·en·ceph·a·lo·my·eli·tis
po·lio·en·ceph·a·lo·my·elop·
  a·thy
    carcinomatous p.
po·lio·en·ceph·a·lop·a·thy
    Alpers p.
po·lio·en·ceph·a·lo·trop·ic
po·lio·my·el·en·ceph·a·li·tis
po·lio·my·elit·ic
po·lio·my·eli·ti·ci·dal
po·lio·my·eli·tis
    abortive p.
    acute anterior p.
    acute lateral p.
    anterior p.
    ascending p.
    bulbar p.
    bulbospinal p.
    cerebral p.
    chronic anterior p.
    encephalitic p.
    endemic p.
    epidemic p.
    nonparalytic p.
    paralytic p.
    postinoculation p.
    post-tonsillectomy p.
    postvaccinal p.
    spinal paralytic p.
    spinobulbar p.
po·lio·my·elo·en·ceph·a·li·tis
po·lio·my·elop·a·thy
po·lio·neu·ro·mere
po·li·o·sis
    p. circumscripta
po·lio·vi·rus
poli·pro·pene
pol·ish·ing
poli·sog·ra·phy
Pol·it·zer's bag
Pol·it·zer's cone
Pol·it·zer's speculum
Pol·it·zer's test
pol·it·zer·iza·tion
    negative p.
pol·kis·sen
pol·la·ki·dip·sia
pol·la·ki·su·ria

pol·la·ki·uria
pol·len
pol·le·no·gen·ic
pol·le·no·sis
pol·lex *pl.* pol·li·ces
   p. extensus
   p. flexus
   p. valgus
   p. varus
pol·lic·i·za·tion
pol·li·na·tion
pol·lin·ic
pol·li·ni·um
pol·li·no·sis
pol·lo·dic
pol·lu·tion
   noise p.
po·lo·cyte
po·lo·ni·um
pol·ox·a·lene
pol·ox·al·kol
pol·ox·a·mer
   p. 182L
   p. 188
   p. 331
pol·ster
pol·toph·a·gy
po·lus *pl.* po·li
   p. anterior bulbi oculi
   p. anterior lentis
   p. frontalis hemispherii
     cerebri
   p. occipitalis hemispherii
     cerebri
   p. posterior bulbi oculi
   p. posterior lentis
   p. temporalis hemispherii
     cerebri
poly
poly A — polyadenylate
   polyadenylic acid
Pol·ya's oper·ation
poly·ac·id
poly·ac·ryl·am·ide gel
poly·ac·rylo·ni·trile
poly·ad·e·ni·tis
   malignant p.
poly·ad·e·no·ma

poly·ad·e·no·ma·to·sis
poly·ad·e·nop·a·thy
poly·ad·e·no·sis
poly·ad·e·nous
pol·y·a·den·y·late
poly·ad·e·nyl·a·tion
poly·ag·glu·tin·abil·i·ty
poly·al·co·hol·ism
poly·al·ge·sia
poly·am·ide
poly·amine
poly·an·dry
poly·an·gi·itis
poly·ar·ter·itis
   p. nodosa
poly·ar·thric
poly·ar·thri·tis
   benign p.
   chronic osteolytic p.
   chronic secondary p.
   chronic villous p.
   p. destruens
   infectious p.
   peripheral p.
   p. rheumatica acuta
   rheumatoid p.
   tuberculous p.
   vertebral p.
   xanthomatous p.
poly·ar·throp·a·thy
poly·ar·thro·sis
   progressive p.
pol·y·ar·tic·u·lar
poly·atom·ic
poly·auxo·troph
poly·auxo·troph·ic
poly·avi·ta·min·o·sis
poly·ax·on
poly·ax·on·ic
poly·az·iz
poly·ba·sic
poly·blast
poly·blen·nia
poly·bu·ti·late
poly·car·bo·phil
poly·cel·lu·lar
poly·cen·tric
poly·cen·tric·i·ty

poly·chei·ria
poly·che·mo·ther·a·py
poly·chlo·rin·at·ed bi·phen·yl
  (PCB)
poly·chlo·ru·ria
poly·cho·lia
poly·chon·dri·tis
    chronic atrophic p.
    p. chronica atrophicans
    relapsing p.
poly·chon·dro·path·ia
poly·chon·drop·a·thy
poly·chrest
poly·chro·ma·sia
poly·chro·ma·tia
poly·chro·mat·ic
poly·chro·mato·cyte
poly·chro·ma·to·cy·to·sis
poly·chro·mato·phil
poly·chro·ma·to·phil·ia
poly·chro·ma·to·phil·ic
poly·chro·ma·to·sis
poly·chro·me·mia
poly·chro·mic
poly·chro·mo·phil
poly·chro·mo·phil·ia
poly·chy·lia
poly·cil·lin
poly·clin·ic
poly·clin·i·cal
poly·clo·nal
poly·clo·nia
poly·co·ria
    p. spuria
    p. vera
poly·crot·ic
pol·yc·ro·tism
poly·cy·clic
poly·cy·cline
poly·cy·e·sis
poly·cys·tic
poly·cys·to·ma
poly·cyte
poly·cy·the·mia
    absolute p.
    appropriate p.
    benign p.
    chronic splenomegalic p.

poly·cy·the·mia *(continued)*
    compensatory p.
    familial p.
    p. hypertonica
    inappropriate p.
    myelopathic p.
    primary p.
    relative p.
    p. rubra
    p. rubra vera
    secondary p.
    splenomegalic p.
    spurious p.
    stress p.
    p. vera
poly·dac·tyl·ia
poly·dac·tyl·ism
poly·dac·ty·ly
poly·de·fi·cient
poly·de·oxy·ri·bo·nu·cleo·tide
poly·de·oxy·ri·bo·nu·cle·o·
    tide syn·thase (ATP)
poly·dip·sia
poly·dis·per·soid
poly·don·tia
poly·dys·pla·sia
    hereditary ectodermal p.
poly·dys·spon·dy·lism
poly·dys·troph·ic
poly·dys·tro·phy
    pseudo-Hurler p.
poly·elec·tro·lyte
poly·em·bry·o·ma
poly·em·bry·o·ny
poly·emia
    p. hyperalbuminosa
    p. polycythaemica
poly·en·do·crine
poly·en·do·cri·no·ma
poly·en·do·cri·nop·a·thy
poly·ene
poly·er·gic
poly·es·the·sia
poly·es·thet·ic
poly·es·tra·di·ol phos·phate
poly·es·trous
poly·eth·a·dene

poly·eth·y·lene
    p. terephthalate
poly·eth·y·lene gly·col
poly·fer·ose
Po·lyg·a·la
poly·ga·lac·tia
po·lyg·a·lin
po·lyg·a·mous
po·lyg·a·my
poly·gan·gli·on·ic
poly·gene
pol·y·gen·ic
poly·glac·tin 910
poly·glan·du·lar
poly·glob·u·lism
poly·gly·col·ic acid
po·lyg·na·thus
Poly·go·na·tum
poly·gram
poly·graph
    Keeler's p.
po·lyg·y·ny
poly·gy·ria
poly·he·dral
poly·het·er·ox·en·ous
poly·hex·ose
poly·hi·dro·sis
poly·hy·brid
poly·hy·dram·ni·os
poly·hy·dric
poly·hy·dru·ria
poly·hy·per·men·or·rhea
poly·hy·po·men·or·rhea
poly·id·ro·sis
poly·in·fec·tion
poly·ion·ic
poly·karyo·cyte
poly·ke·tide
poly·ki·ne·ty
poly·kol
poly·lec·i·thal
poly·lep·tic
poly·lob·u·lar
poly·ly·sine
poly·ma·con
poly·mas·tia
poly·mas·ti·gi·da
poly·mas·ti·gote

poly·ma·zia
poly·me·lia
po·lym·e·lus
poly·me·nia
poly·men·or·rhea
poly·mer
    addition p.
    condensation p.
po·lym·er·ase
poly·me·ria
poly·mer·ic
poly·mer·iza·tion
poly·mer·ize
poly·meta·car·pia
poly·meta·phos·phate
poly·meta·tar·sia
poly·meth·yl
    p. methacrylate
poly·mi·cro·bi·al
poly·mi·cro·bic
poly·mi·cro·gy·ria
poly·mi·cro·lipo·ma·to·sis
poly·mi·cro·tome
Po·lym·nia
poly·morph
poly·mor·pha
poly·mor·phic
poly·mor·phism
    balanced p.
    chromosome p.
    genetic p.
    restriction fragment length
      p. (RFLP)
    transient p.
poly·mor·pho·cel·lu·lar
poly·mor·pho·cyte
poly·mor·pho·nu·cle·ar
    filament p.
    nonfilament p.
poly·mor·phous
poly·mox
poly·my·al·gia
    p. arteritica
    p. rheumatica
poly·my·a·ri·an
poly·my·oc·lo·nus
poly·my·op·a·thy

poly·myo·si·tis
   hemorrhagic p.
   trichinous p.
poly·myx·in
   p. B sulfate
poly·ne·sic
poly·neu·ral
poly·neu·ral·gia
poly·neu·ric
poly·neu·rit·ic
poly·neu·ri·tis
   acute febrile p.
   acute idiopathic p.
   acute infective p.
   acute postinfectious p.
   anemic p.
   ascending p.
   p. cerebralis menieriformis
   endemic p.
   p. endemica
   cranial p.
   diabetic p.
   Guillain-Barré p.
   infectious p.
   Jamaica ginger p.
   postinfectious p.
   p. potatorum
   progressive hypertrophic p.
   triorthocresyl phosphate p.
poly·neu·ro·myo·si·tis
poly·neu·ro·ni·tis
poly·neu·rop·a·thy
   acromegalic p.
   acute febrile p.
   acute postinfectious p.
   alcoholic p.
   amyloid p.
   buckthorn p.
   carcinomatous p.
   cranial p.
   diabetic p.
   erythredema p.
   familial recurrent p.
   isoniazid p.
   paraneoplastic p.
   recurrent p.
   relapsing p.
   uremic p.

poly·neu·ro·ra·dic·u·li·tis
poly·nu·cle·ar
poly·nu·cle·ate
poly·nu·cle·at·ed
poly·nu·cle·o·lar
poly·nu·cle·o·lus
poly·nu·cleo·ti·dase
poly·nu·cleo·tide
poly·nu·cleo·tide ad·e·nyl·yl·
   trans·fer·ase
poly·nu·cleo·tide li·gase
poly·nu·cleo·tide phos·pha·
   tase
pol·y·nu·cle·o·tide phos·
   phor·y·lase
poly·odon·tia
poly·ol de·hy·dro·gen·ase
poly·o·ma
poly·o·ma·vi·rus
poly·onych·ia
poly·opia
   binocular p.
   p. monophthalmica
poly·op·sia
poly·or·chi·dism
poly·or·chis
poly·or·chism
poly·orex·ia
poly·os·tot·ic
poly·otia
poly·ov·u·lar
poly·ov·u·la·to·ry
pol·y·ox·y·eth·y·lene 50 ste·
   a·rate
poly·ox·yl
   p. 5 oleate
   p. 10 oleyl ether
   p. 20 celostearyl ether
   p. 50 stearate
pol·yp
   adenomatous p.
   antrochoanal p.
   aural p.
   cardiac p.
   cervical p.
   choanal p's
   cutaneous fibrous p.
   endometrial p's

pol·yp *(continued)*
    fibrinous p.
    fibrous p.
    fleshy p.
    gelatinous p.
    gum p.
    Hopmann's p.
    hydatid p.
    inflammatory p.
    juvenile p's
    lipomatous p.
    lymphoid p's
    myomatous p.
    nasal p's
    osseous p.
    pedunculated p.
    retention p's
    sessile p.
    tooth p.
poly·pap·il·lo·ma trop·i·cum
poly·para·si·tism
poly·path·ia
poly·pec·to·my
poly·pep·ti·dase
poly·pep·tide
    gastric inhibitory p. (GIP)
    pancreatic p.
    vasoactive intestinal p.
     (VIP)
poly·pep·ti·de·mia
poly·pep·ti·dor·rha·chia
poly·peri·os·ti·tis
    p. hyperesthetica
poly·pha·gia
poly·pha·lan·gia
poly·pha·lan·gism
poly·phar·ma·ceu·tic
poly·phar·ma·cy
poly·phase
poly·pha·sic
poly·phen·ic
poly·phe·nol·ox·i·dase
po·lyph·e·ny
poly·pho·bia
poly·phos·phate
poly·phos·pho·ino·si·tide
poly·phy·let·ic
poly·phy·le·tism

poly·phy·le·tist
poly·phy·odont
poly·pi
pol·yp·if·er·ous
po·lyp·i·form
poly·pi·o·nia
poly·plas·tic
poly·plax
poly·ple·gia
poly·pleu·ro·dia·phrag·mot·o·my
poly·ploid
poly·ploi·dy
pol·yp·nea
pol·yp·ne·ic
poly·po·dia
poly·poid
poly·poi·do·sis
pol·yp·o·rin
pol·yp·o·rous
Pol·yp·o·rus
poly·po·sia
poly·po·sis
    acquired multiple p.
    adenomatous p. coli
    p. coli
    familial p.
    familial p. coli
    familial intestinal p.
    gastric p.
    p. gastrica
    intestinal p.
    p. intestinalis
    multiple familial p.
    nasal p.
    p. ventriculi
po·lyp·o·tome
po·lyp·o·trite
poly·pous
poly·prag·ma·sy
poly·pty·chi·al
pol·y·pus *pl.* pol·y·pi
    p. angiomatodes
    p. cysticus
    p. hydatidosus
    p. telangiectodes
poly·ra·dic·u·li·tis
poly·ra·dic·u·lo·neu·ri·tis

poly·ra·dic·u·lo·neu·ri·tis
    acute idiopathic p.
pol·y·ra·dic·u·lo·neu·rop·a·
  thy
    acute postinfective p.
    inflammatory acute p.
poly·ri·bo·nu·cleo·tide
poly·ri·bo·nu·cleo·tide nu·
  cleo·ti·dyl·trans·fer·ase
poly·ri·bo·some
pol·yr·rhea
poly·sac·cha·rid·ase
poly·sac·cha·ride
    p. A
    p. B
    bacterial p's
    core p.
    gastric p.
    immune p's
    O-specific p.
    pneumococcus p.
    specific p's
poly·sac·cha·rose
poly·sar·cia
poly·sar·cous
poly·sce·lia
po·lys·ce·lus
poly·scle·ro·sis
poly·scope
poly·sen·si·tiv·i·ty
poly·sen·so·ry
poly·se·ro·si·tis
    familial recurrent p.
    periodic p.
    recurrent p.
    tuberculous p.
poly·si·al·ia
poly·si·nu·sec·to·my
poly·si·nu·si·tis
poly·so·mat·ic
poly·so·ma·ty
poly·some
poly·so·mia
poly·so·mic
poly·so·mus
poly·so·my
poly·sor·bate
poly·sper·mia

poly·sper·mism
poly·sper·my
    pathological p.
    physiological p.
poly·spike-wave
poly·sple·nia
poly·stich·ia
poly·sty·rene
poly·sus·pen·soid
poly·sy·nap·tic
poly·syn·brachy·dac·ty·ly
poly·syn·dac·ty·ly
poly·syn·o·vi·tis
poly·syph·i·lide
poly·tef
poly·ten·di·ni·tis
poly·ten·di·no·bur·si·tis
poly·tene
poly·te·ni·za·tion
poly·teno·syn·o·vi·tis
poly·te·ny
poly·tet·ra·flu·o·ro·eth·y·
  lene
poly·the·lia
poly·the·lism
poly·thene
poly·thet·ic
poly·thi·a·zide
po·lyt·o·cous
poly·to·mo·gram
poly·to·mo·graph·ic
poly·to·mog·ra·phy
poly·trich·ia
poly·tri·cho·sis
Po·lyt·ri·chum
poly·tro·phia
poly·troph·ic
po·lyt·ro·phy
pol·y·trop·ic
poly·typ·ic
poly·un·guia
poly·un·sat·u·rat·ed
poly·uria
poly·uri·dyl·ic acid
poly·va·lent
poly·vi·nyl
    p. acetate
    p. chloride

poly·vi·nyl·ac·e·tate
poly·vi·nyl·ben·zene
poly·vi·nyl·chlo·ride
poly·vi·nyl·pyr·rol·i·done
po·made
Po·mat·i·op·sis
po·ma·tum
Pom·e·roy's operation
pom·pho·ly·he·mia
pom·pho·lyx
po·mum
    p. adami
pon·ceau B
    p. 3 B
Pon·cet's disease
Pon·cet's operation
Pon·cet's rheumatism
Pond. — L. pondere (by
  weight)
pon·der·al
Pon·di·min
pon·do·stat·u·ral
po·ne·si·a·trics
Pon·fick's shadow
Pon·gi·dae
po·no·graph
po·nos
pons *pl.* pon·tes
    p. cerebelli
    p. hepatis
    p. tarini
    p. varolii
pons-ob·lon·ga·ta
Pon·stel
pon·tes
Pon·ti·ac fever
pon·ti·bra·chi·um
pon·tic
pon·tic·u·lar
pon·tic·u·lus
    p. auriculae
    p. hepatis
    p. promontorii
pon·tile
pon·tine
pon·tis
    basis p.
pon·to·bul·bar

pon·to·bul·bia
Pon·to·caine
pon·to·cer·e·bel·lar
pon·to·med·ul·lary
pon·to·mes·en·ce·phal·ic
pon·toon
pon·to·pe·dun·cu·lar
pool
    abdominal p.
    gene p.
    metabolic p.
    recirculating lymphocyte p.
Pool's phenomenon
Pool-Schles·in·ger sign
POP — plaster of Paris
pop·les
pop·lit·e·al
pop·lit·e·us
    p. minor
pop·py
pop·u·la·tion
    closed p.
    Segi's p.
    standard p.
POR — problem-oriented
  record
por·ade·nia
por·ad·e·ni·tis
    p. nostras
    subacute inguinal p.
    p. venerea
por·ad·e·no·lym·phi·tis
por·al
por·ce·lain
    aluminous p.
    dental p.
    high fusing p.
    metal-bonding p.
    synthetic p.
por·ce·la·ne·ous
por·cine
    p. xenograft
pore
    acoustic p., osseous,
      external
    acoustic p., osseous,
      internal
    alveolar p's

pore *(continued)*
  biliary p.
  birth p.
  Galen's p.
  genital p.
  gustatory p.
  interalveolar p's
  p's of Kohn
  mammary p.
  nuclear p's
  slit p's
  sweat p.
  taste p.
  urinary p.
  p's of Vieussens
por·en·ce·phal·ic
por·en·ceph·a·li·tis
por·en·ceph·a·lous
por·en·ceph·a·ly
  schizocephalic p.
  traumatic p.
por·fi·ro·my·cin
Por·ges-Her·mann-Pe·rutz
  reaction
Por·ges-Mei·er reaction
Por·ges-Mei·er test
po·ri
Po·rif·e·ra
po·rin
po·rio·ma·nia
po·ri·on
po·ro·cele
po·ro·ceph·a·li·a·sis
Poro·ce·phal·i·da
Poro·ce·phal·i·dae
po·ro·ceph·a·lo·sis
Po·ro·ceph·a·lus
  P. armillatus
  P. constrictus
  P. denticulatus
poro·fo·con
po·ro·ker·a·to·sis
  disseminated superficial
    actinic p.
  p. excentrica
  p. of Mantoux
  p. of Mibelli

po·ro·ker·a·to·sis *(continued)*
  p. palmaris et plantaris
    disseminata
po·ro·ker·a·tot·ic
po·ro·ma
  eccrine p.
po·ro·plas·tic
po·ro·sis
  cerebral p.
po·ros·i·ty
po·rot·ic
po·rot·o·my
por·ous
por·phin
por·pho·bi·lin
por·pho·bi·lin·o·gen
por·pho·bi·lin·o·gen de·am·
  in·ase
por·pho·bi·lin·o·gen syn·
  thase
por·pho·bi·lin·o·gen·uria
por·phy·ran
por·phy·ria
  acquired p.
  acute p.
  acute intermittent p.
  congenital erythropoietic p.
  congenital photosensitive
    p.
  p. cutanea tarda
    hereditaria
  p. cutanea tarda
    symptomatica
  cutaneous p.
  erythropoietic p.
  p. erythropoietica
  hepatic p.
  p. hepatica
  mixed p.
  ovulocyclic p.
  photosensitive p.
  South African genetic p.
  Swedish genetic p.
  p. variegata
  variegate p.
por·phy·rin
por·phy·rin·emia
por·phy·rin·o·gen

por·phyr·in·op·a·thy
por·phy·rin·uria
por·phy·ris·mus
por·phy·ri·za·tion
por·phy·rox·ine
por·phyr·uria
por·phy·ryl
Por·ro's cesarean section
por·ta *pl.* por·tae
    p. hepatis
    p. labyrinthi
    p. lienis
    p. of lung
    p. omenti
    p. of omentum
    p. pulmonis
    p. renis
    p. of spleen
por·ta·ca·val
por·tal
    p. of entry
    hepatic p.
    intestinal p., anterior
    intestinal p., posterior
    velopharyngeal p.
porte-ai·guille
porte·pol·ish·er
porte-pol·ish·er
Por·ter, Rodney Robert
Por·ter's sign
Por·ter's test
Por·ter-Sil·ber chromogens
  test
Por·te·us maze test
por·tio *pl.* por·ti·o·nes
    p. dura paris septimi
    p. intermedia nervi acustici
    p. major nervi trigemini
    p. minor nervi trigemini
    p. mollis paris septimi
    p. supravaginalis cervicis
    p. vaginalis cervicis
por·ti·o·nes
por·ti·plex·us
port·lig·a·ture
por·to·en·ter·os·to·my
por·to·gram

por·tog·ra·phy
    percutaneous transhepatic
      p.
    portal p.
    splenic p.
    umbilical p.
por·to·sys·tem·ic
por·to·ve·no·gram
por·to·ve·nog·ra·phy
po·rus *pl.* po·ri
    p. acusticus externus
    p. acusticus externus
      osseus
    p. acusticus internus
    p. acusticus internus osseus
    p. galeni
    p. gustatorius
    p. opticus
    p. sudoriferus
Po·sa·da's mycosis
Po·sa·da-Wer·ni·cke disease
po·si·tion
    Albert's p.
    anatomical p.
    batrachian p.
    Bertel's p.
    Bonner's p.
    Bozeman's p.
    Brickner p.
    bronchoscopic p.
    cadaveric p.
    Caldwell p.
    Casselberry's p.
    centric p.
    cis p.
    coiled p.
    decerebrate p.
    decorticate p.
    decubitus p.
    Depage's p.
    depressive p.
    dorsal p.
    dorsal elevated p.
    dorsal lithotomy p.
    dorsal recumbent p.
    dorsal rigid p.
    dorsosacral p.

po·si·tion *(continued)*
    Duncan's p.
    eccentric p.
    Edebohls' p.
    electrical heart p.
    Elliot's p.
    emprosthotonos p.
    English p.
    flipper p.
    Fowler's p.
    froglike p.
    frontal anterior p.
    frontal posterior p.
    frontal transverse p.
    frontoanterior p.
    frontoposterior p.
    frontotransverse p.
    Fuchs p.
    p. of function
    Gaynor-Hart p.
    genucubital p.
    genufacial p.
    genupectoral p.
    heart p.
    high pelvic p.
    hinge p.
    hinge p., condylar
    hinge p., mandibular
    hinge p., terminal
    horizontal p.
    intercuspal p.
    jackknife p.
    Jones' p.
    knee-chest p.
    knee-elbow p.
    kneeling-squatting p.
    Kraske p.
    lateral recumbent p.
    lateroabdominal p.
    leapfrog p.
    ligamentous p.
    lithotomy p.
    Mayer p.
    Mayo-Robson p.
    mentoanterior p.
    mentoposterior p.
    mentotransverse p.
    mentum anterior p.

po·si·tion *(continued)*
    mentum posterior p.
    mentum transverse p.
    Noble's p.
    nuchal hitch p.
    obstetrical p.
    occipitoanterior p.
    occipitoposterior p.
    occipitosacral p.
    occipitotransverse p.
    occiput anterior p.
    occiput posterior p.
    occiput sacral p.
    occiput transverse p.
    occlusal p.
    opisthotonos p.
    orthopnea p.
    orthopneic p.
    orthotonos p.
    physiologic rest p.
    posterior border p.
    primary p. of gaze
    prone p.
    protrusive p.
    rest p.
    Robson's p.
    Rose's p.
    sacroanterior p.
    sacroposterior p.
    sacrotransverse p.
    sacrum anterior p.
    sacrum posterior p.
    sacrum transverse p.
    scapula anterior p.
    scapula posterior p.
    scapuloanterior p.
    scapuloposterior p.
    scorbutic p.
    semi-Fowler p.
    semiaxial p.
    semiprone p.
    semireclining p.
    Simon's p.
    Sims' p.
    Stern's p.
    submentovertex p.
    supine p.
    terminal hinge p.

po·si·tion *(continued)*
  Titterington p.
  trans p.
  Trendelenburg's p.
  tripod p.
  Valentine's p.
  verticosubmental p.
  Waters p.
  Waters p., reverse
po·si·tion·er
  tooth p.
pos·i·tive
  biologic false p.
pos·i·tro·ceph·a·lo·gram
pos·i·tron
Pos·ner's reaction
Pos·ner's test
po·so·log·ic
po·sol·o·gy
Pos·sum
post
  abutment p.
  implant p.
  status p.
post·abor·tal
post·ac·i·dot·ic
post·al·bu·min
post·an·es·thet·ic
post·apo·plec·tic
post·au·di·to·ry
post·au·ra·le
post·au·ric·u·lar
post·ax·i·al
post·bra·chi·al
post·bra·chi·um
post·bul·bar
post·cap·il·lary
post·car·di·nal
post·car·di·ot·o·my
post·ca·va
post·ca·val
post·ce·cal
post·cen·tral
post·cen·tra·lis
post·ci·bal
post ci·bum
post·cis·ter·na
post·co·i·tal

post·con·cep·tu·al
post·con·dy·la·re
post·con·vul·sive
post·cor·nu
post·cra·ni·al
post·cu·bi·tal
post·dam·ming
post·di·as·tol·ic
post·di·crot·ic
post·diph·ther·ic
post·dor·mi·tal
post·dor·mi·tum
post·duc·tal
post·ec·dy·sis
post·em·bry·on·ic
post·en·ceph·a·lic
post·ep·i·lep·tic
pos·te·ri·ad
pos·ter·i·or
pos·tero·an·te·ri·or
pos·tero·clu·sion
pos·tero·ex·ter·nal
pos·tero·in·fe·ri·or
pos·tero·in·ter·nal
pos·tero·lat·er·al
pos·tero·me·di·al
pos·tero·me·di·an
pos·tero·pa·ri·e·tal
pos·tero·su·pe·ri·or
pos·tero·tem·po·ral
pos·ter·u·la
post·esoph·a·ge·al
post·ex·po·sure
post·fe·brile
post·gan·gli·on·ic
post·gle·noid
post·glo·mer·u·lar
post·hemi·ple·gic
post·he·pat·ic
post·hep·a·tit·ic
post·her·pet·ic
pos·thet·o·my
pos·thio·plas·ty
post·hip·po·cam·pal
pos·thi·tis
pos·tho·lith
post·hu·mous
post·hy·oid

post·hyp·not·ic
post·hy·po·gly·ce·mic
post·hy·poph·y·sis
post·hy·pox·ic
post·ic·tal
pos·ti·cus
post·in·fec·tive
post·is·chi·al
post·ma·lar·i·al
post·mas·tec·to·my
post·mas·toid
post·ma·ture
post·ma·tur·i·ty
post·max·il·lary
post·me·di·as·ti·nal
post·me·di·as·ti·num
post·mei·ot·ic
post·meno·pau·sal
post·men·strua
post·mes·en·ter·ic
post·min·i·mus *pl.* post·min·i·mi
post·mi·ot·ic
post·mi·tot·ic
post·mor·tal
post mor·tem
post·mor·tem
post·na·res
post·na·ri·al
post·nar·is
post·na·sal
post·na·tal
post·neu·rit·ic
post·op·er·a·tive
post·ov·u·la·tory
post·pal·a·tine
post·pa·lu·tal
post·para·lyt·ic
post par·tum
post·par·tum
post·phle·bit·ic
post·pi·tu·i·tary
post·pleu·rit·ic
post·pneu·mon·ic
post·po·lio
post·pon·tile
post·pran·di·al
post·pu·ber·al

post·pu·ber·tal
post·pu·ber·ty
post·pu·bes·cence
post·pu·bes·cent
post·py·ram·i·dal
post·re·nal
post·ro·lan·dic
post·scar·la·ti·nal
Post sing. sed. liq. — L. post singulas sedes liquidas (after every loose stool)
post·si·nu·soi·dal
post·sphe·noid
post·sphyg·mic
post·splen·ic
post·ste·not·ic
post·syl·vi·an
post·sy·nap·tic
post·sys·tol·ic
post-tec·ta
post-throm·bot·ic
post-trau·mat·ic
post-tre·mat·ic
post-tus·sis
pos·tu·late
    Ehrlich's p.
    Koch's p's
pos·tur·al
pos·ture
    decerebrate p.
    decorticate p.
    Drosin's p's
post·vac·ci·nal
post·vac·cin·i·al
post·vi·tal
post·zone
post·zos·ter
post·zy·got·ic
pot·a·ble
pot AGT — potential abnormality of glucose tolerance
Po·tain's sign
Pot·a·mon
pot·ash
    caustic p.
    sulfurated p.
pot·as·se·mia

po·tas·sic
po·tas·si·um
    p. acetate
    p. alum
    p. aspartate and
      magnesium aspartate
    p. bicarbonate
    p. bichromate
    p. bitartrate
    p. bromide
    p. carbonate
    p. chlorate
    p. chloride
    p. citrate
    p. cyanide
    p. dichromate
    p. dihydrogen phosphate
    p. ferricyanide
    p. glucaldrate
    p. gluconate
    p. glycerophosphate
    p. guaiacolsulfonate
    p. hydroxide
    p. iodate
    p. iodide
    p. mercuric iodide
    p. metaphosphate
    p. nitrate
    p. penicillin G
    p. perchlorate
    p. permanganate
    p. phenoxymethyl
      penicillin
    p. phosphate
    p. phosphate, dibasic
    p. phosphate, monobasic
    propicillin p.
    radioactive p.
    p. sodium tartrate
    p. sorbate
    p. sulfate
    p. tartrate
    p. thiocyanate
Po·tas·si·um Tri·plex
po·ten·cy
    prospective p.
    reactive p.
po·ten·tia

po·ten·tial
    action p.
    after-p.
    after-p., negative
    after-p., positive
    average evoked p.
    bioelectric p.
    biotic p.
    chemical p.
    cochlear p.
    cochlear microphonic p.
    compound action p.
    demarcation p.
    early vertex p.
    electrocortical p.
    electrode p.
    electrotonic p.
    endocochlear p.
    evoked p.
    evoked cortical p's
    excitatory postsynaptic p.
    fasciculation p.
    fibrillation p's
    generator p.
    giant p.
    ground p.
    hyperpolarizing p.
    inhibitory postequilibrium
      p.
    inhibitory postsynaptic p.
    injury p.
    late vertex p.
    life p.
    membrane p.
    miniature end-plate p's
    morphogenetic p.
    motor unit p.
    myopathic p.
    negative summating p.
    Nernst p.
    nerve p.
    oxidation-reduction p.
    pacemaker p.
    polyphasic p.
    polyspike p.
    postsynaptic p's
    receptor p.

po·ten·tial *(continued)*
  redox p.
  reinnervation p.
  reproductive p.
  resting p.
  ripple p.
  somatosensory evoked p.
    (SEP)
  spike p.
  spinal evoked p.
  standard electrode p.
  standard reduction p.
  streaming p.
  summating p.
  transmembrane p.
  utricular DC p.
  vertex p.
  visual evoked p.
  zeta p.
po·ten·ti·al·iza·tion
po·ten·ti·a·tion
  paradoxical p.
  post-tetanic p.
po·ten·ti·a·tor
po·ten·ti·om·e·ter
po·ten·tize
po·ti·fi·ca·tion
po·tion
po·to·ma·nia
Pott's abscess
Pott's aneurysm
Pott's curvature
Pott's disease
Pott's dwarfism
Pott's fracture
Pott's paraplegia
Pott's puffy tumor
Pott's tumor
Pot·ten·ger's sign
Pot·ter's facies
Pot·ter treatment
Pot·ter version
Pot·ter-Bucky diaphragm
Pot·ter-Bucky grid
Potts oper·ation
Potts-Smith-Gib·son operation
Pö·tzel syndrome

pouch
  abdominovesical p.
  allantochorionic p's
  anal p.
  anterior p. of Tröltsch
  branchial p.
  Broca's p.
  craniobuccal p.
  craniopharyngeal p.
  Dennis-Brown p.
  p. of Douglas
  enterocoelic p.
  gill p.
  guttural p's
  Hartmann's p.
  Heidenhain p.
  hepatorenal p.
  hyomandibular p.
  ileocecal p.
  laryngeal p.
  Morison's p.
  neurobuccal p.
  obturator p.
  paracystic p.
  pararectal p.
  paravesical p.
  Pavlov p.
  perineal p., deep
  perineal p., superficial
  pharyngeal p.
  Physick's p's
  posterior p. of Tröltsch
  Prussak's p.
  Rathke's p.
  rectouterine p.
  rectovaginal p.
  rectovesical p.
  Seessel's p.
  superficial perineal p.
  uteroabdominal p.
  uterovesical p.
  vesicouterine p.
  visceral p.
  Willis' p.
  Zenker's p.
pou·drage
  pleural p.

poul·tice
pound
Pou·part's ligament
Pou·part's line
Po·van
pov·er·ty
    p. of movement
po·vi·done
po·vi·done-io·dine
pow·der
    aluminum hydroxide p.
    bleaching p.
    blood-plasma p.
    p. of chalk, aromatic
    p. of chalk, aromatic, with
      opium
    chalk p., compound
    Dalmatian insect p.
    Dover's p.
    dusting p.
    dusting p., absorbable
    effervescent p's, compound
    furazolidone and
      nifuroxime p.
    glycyrrhiza p., compound
    Goa p.
    impalpable p.
    iodochlorhydroxyquin p.,
      compound
    licorice p., compound
    methylbenzethonium
      chloride p.
    nystatin topical p.
    Persian insect p.
    Seidlitz p's
    senna p., compound
    sodium bicarbonate and
      calcium carbonate p.
    sodium bicarbonate and
      magnesium oxide p.
    talcum p.
    tissue p.
    tolnaftate p.
    triacetin p.
    zinc sulfate p., compound
pow·er
    acoustic p.
    candle p.

pow·er *(continued)*
    carbon dioxide-combining
      p.
    CO_2-combining p.
    defining p.
    dioptric p.
    resolving p.
pox
    Kaffir p.
    wart p.
Pox·vi·ri·dae
pox·vi·rus
PP — postpartum
    L. punctum proximum
      (near point of
      accommodation)
PP_i — pyrophosphate
p.p. — L. post prandium (after
    meals)
PPCA — proserum
    prothrombin conversion
    accelerator
PPCF — plasmin prothrombin
    converting factor
PPD — purified protein
    derivative (tuberculin)
ppg — picopicogram
PPLO — pleuropneumonia-like-
    organisms
ppm — parts per million
PPO — preferred provider
    organization
Ppt — precipitate
    prepared
P-pul·mo·na·le syndrome
PQ — permeability quotient
    plastoquinone
PR — prosthion
    L. punctum remotum (far
      point of accommodation)
PRA — plasma renin activity
Pr — presbyopia
    prism
prac·tice
    contract p.
    family p.
    general p.
    group p.

prac·tice *(continued)*
    individual p.
    panel p.
    prepaid group p.
    private p.
    solo p.
prac·ti·tion·er
    general p.
    indigenous p.
    nurse p.
prac·to·lol
Pra·der-Lab·hart-Wil·li
    syndrome
prae·cox
    dementia p.
prae·pu·ti·um
prag·mat·ag·no·sia
prag·mat·am·ne·sia
pral·i·dox·ime
    p. chloride
    p. iodide
    p. mesylate
pra·mox·ine hy·dro·chlo·ride
pran·di·al
pra·no·li·um chlo·ride
Pran·tal
pra·seo·dym·i·um
P. rat. aetat. — L. pro ratione
    aetatis (in proportion to age)
pra·tique
Praus·nitz-Küst·ner reaction
Praus·nitz-Küst·ner test
Prax·ag·o·ras of Cos
prax·i·ol·o·gy
prax·is
pra·ze·pam
pra·zi·quan·tel
pra·zo·sin hy·dro·chlo·ride
pre·adap·ta·tion
pre·ad·i·po·cyte
pre-AIDS
pre·al·bu·min
    thyroxine-binding p.
      (TBPA)
pre·am·pli·fi·er
pre·an·es·the·sia
pre·an·es·thet·ic

pre·aor·tic
pre·atax·ic
pre·au·ra·le
pre·au·ric·u·lar
pre·ax·i·al
pre·bac·il·lary
pre·base
pre·be·ta-lipo·pro·tein
    sinking p.
pre·be·ta·lipo·pro·tein·emia
pre·bi·ot·ic
pre·blad·der
pre·bra·chi·al
pre·bra·chi·um
pre·can·cer
pre·can·cer·o·sis
pre·can·cer·ous
pre·cap·il·lary
pre·car·cin·o·gen
pre·car·ci·nom·a·tous
pre·car·di·nal
pre·car·di·um
pre·car·ti·lage
pre·ca·va
pre·ce·men·tum
pre·cen·tral
pre·chor·dal
pre·cip·i·ta·ble
pre·cip·i·tant
pre·cip·i·tate
    alum p.
    immune p.
    keratic p's
    keratic p's, mutton-fat
    pigmented keratic p's
    white p.
pre·cip·i·ta·tion
    electrostatic p. of dust
    group p.
    isoelectric p.
    salt p.
    tuberculin p. (TP)
pre·cip·i·tin
pre·cip·i·tin·o·gen
pre·cip·i·to·gen
pre·ci·sion
pre·clin·i·cal
pre·cli·val

pre·clot·ting
pre·co·cious
pre·coc·i·ty
   heterosexual p.
   isosexual p.
   sexual p.
   skeletal p.
pre·cog·ni·tion
pre·col·lag·e·nous
pre·co·ma
pre·com·mis·su·ral
pre·com·mis·sure
pre·con·scious
pre·cor·dia
pre·cor·di·al
pre·cor·di·al·gia
pre·cor·di·um
pre·cor·nu
pre·cos·tal
pre·crit·i·cal
pre·cu·ne·al
pre·cu·ne·ate
pre·cu·ne·us
pre·cur·sor
   mast-cell p.
pre·da·tion
pre·da·tor
pre·den·tin
pre·di·a·be·tes
pre·di·as·to·le
pre·di·a·stol·ic
pre·di·crot·ic
pre·di·ges·tion
pre·dis·pose
pre·dis·pos·ing
pre·dis·po·si·tion
   convulsive p.
   epileptic p.
pre·di·ver·tic·u·lar
pred·ni·mus·tine
pred·nis·o·lone
   p. acetate
   p. butylacetate
   p. sodium phosphate
   p. sodium succinate for
    injection
   p.-21-stearoylglycolate
   p. succinate

pred·nis·o·lone *(continued)*
   p. tebutate
pred·ni·sone
pre·dor·mi·tal
pre·dor·mi·tum
pre·duc·tal
pre·eclamp·sia
pre·eclamp·tic
pre·el·a·cin
pre·epi·glot·tic
pre·erup·tive
pre·ex·ci·ta·tion
   ventricular p.
pre-ex·po·sure
pre·fi·brot·ic
pre·for·ma·tion
pre·for·ma·tion·ist
pre·fron·tal
pre·func·tion·al
pre·gan·gli·on·ic
pre·gen·i·tal
Pregl's test
pre·glo·mer·u·lar
preg·nan·cy
   abdominal p.
   ampullar p.
   angular p.
   bigeminal p.
   broad ligament p.
   cervical p.
   combined p.
   compound p.
   cornual p.
   ectopic p.
   exochorial p.
   extra-amniotic p.
   extrauterine p.
   fallopian p.
   false p.
   gemellary p.
   heterotopic p.
   hydatid p.
   hysteric p.
   incomplete p.
   interstitial p.
   intraligamentary p.
   intraligamentous p.
   intramural p.

preg·nan·cy *(continued)*
  intraperitoneal p.
  intrauterine p.
  isthmic p.
  membranous p.
  mesenteric p.
  molar p.
  multiple p.
  mural p.
  nervous p.
  ovarian p.
  ovario-abdominal p.
  oviductal p.
  parietal p.
  phantom p.
  plural p.
  primary ovarian p.
  prolonged p.
  pseudointraligamentary p.
  sarcofetal p.
  sarcohysteric p.
  spurious p.
  stump p.
  tubal p.
  tuboabdominal p.
  tuboligamentary p.
  tubo-ovarian p.
  tubouterine p.
  twin p.
  uteroabdominal p.
  utero-ovarian p.
  uterotubal p.
preg·nane
preg·nane·di·ol
preg·nane·tri·ol
preg·nant
preg·nene
preg·nen·in·o·lone
preg·nen·o·lone
preg·nen·o·lone suc·ci·nate
pre·go·ni·um
pre·hal·lux
pre·hen·sile
pre·hen·sion
pre·he·pat·ic
pre·he·pat·i·cus
pre·hor·mone
pre·hy·oid

pre·hy·po·phys·e·al
pre·hy·po·phys·i·al
pre·hy·poph·y·sis
pre·ic·tal
pre·in·duc·tion
pre·in·su·la
pre·in·va·sive
pre·io·ta·tion
Prei·ser's disease
Preisz-No·card bacillus
pre·kal·li·kre·in
pre·lac·te·al
pre·lep·to·tene
pre·leu·ke·mia
pre·leu·ke·mic
pre·lim·bic
pre·lo·cal·iza·tion
pre·lo·co·mo·tion
pre·ma·lig·nant
Prem·a·rin
pre·ma·ture
pre·ma·tur·i·ty
pre·max·il·la
pre·max·il·lary
pre·med·i·cal
pre·med·i·cant
pre·med·i·ca·tion
pre·mei·ot·ic
pre·mel·a·no·some
pre·me·nar·chal
pre·me·nar·che
pre·me·nar·che·al
pre·meno·pau·sal
pre·men·strua
pre·men·stru·al
pre·men·stru·um *pl.* pre·men·
  strua
pre·mi·tot·ic
pre·mo·lar
pre·mon·i·to·ry
pre·mono·cyte
pre·mor·bid
pre·mor·tal
pre·mu·ni·tion
pre·mu·ni·tive
pre·my·elo·blast
pre·my·elo·cyte
pre·nar·co·sis

pre·nar·cot·ic
pre·na·res
pre·na·sa·le
pre·na·tal
pre·neo·plas·tic
pre·oc·cip·i·tal
pre·oed·i·pal
pre·op·er·a·tive
pre·oper·cu·lum
pre·op·tic
pre·ov·u·la·tory
pre·ox·y·gen·a·tion
pre·para·lyt·ic
prep·a·ra·tion
    allergenic protein p's
    biomechanical p.
    cavity p.
    corrosion p.
    cover-glass p.
    cytologic filter p.
    hanging-drop p.
    Hata p.
    heart-lung p.
    impression p.
    surgical p.
pre·pa·ret·ic
pre·par·tal
pre·pa·tel·lar
pre·pa·ten·cy
pre·pa·tent
pre·per·cep·tion
pre·peri·to·ne·al
pre·pla·cen·tal
pre·pol·lex
pre·pon·der·ance
    ventricular p.
pre·po·ten·tial
pre·pran·di·al
pre·pro·cess·ing
pre·pro·hor·mone
pre·pro·in·su·lin
pre·pro·phage
pre·pro·pro·tein
pre·pros·thet·ic
pre·pro·tein
pre·pu·ber·al
pre·pu·ber·tal
pre·pu·ber·ty

pre·pu·bes·cence
pre·pu·bes·cent
pre·puce
    p. of clitoris
    p. of penis
    redundant p.
pre·pu·tial
pre·pu·ti·ot·o·my
pre·pu·ti·um
    p. clitoridis
    p. penis
pre·py·lor·ic
pre·rec·tal
pre·re·nal
pre·ren·nin
pre·re·pro·duc·tive
pre·ret·i·nal
Pres·a·mine
pres·by·acu·sia
pres·by·at·rics
pres·by·car·dia
pres·by·cu·sis
pres·by·esoph·a·gus
pres·by·ope
pres·byo·phre·nia
pres·by·opia
pres·by·op·ic
pre·scap·u·la
pre·scap·u·lar
pre·scle·rot·ic
pre·scribe
pre·scrip·tion
    shotgun p.
pre·se·cre·tin
pre·se·cre·to·ry
pre·seg·men·ter
pre·se·nile
pre·se·nil·i·ty
pre·se·ni·um
pre·sent
pre·sen·ta·tion
    acromion p.
    antigen p.
    arm p.
    breech p.
    breech p., complete
    breech p., double
    breech p., frank

pre·sen·ta·tion *(continued)*
    breech p., incomplete
    breech p., single
    brow p.
    cephalic p.
    compound p.
    double footling p.
    face p.
    footling p.
    funis p.
    hand and head p.
    longitudinal p.
    oblique p.
    parietal p.
    pelvic p.
    placental p.
    polar p.
    shoulder p.
    single footling p.
    torso p.
    transverse p.
    trunk p.
    vertex p.
pre·ser·va·tive
pre·si·nu·soi·dal
pre·so·mite
pre·sper·ma·tid
pre·sphe·noid
pre·sphyg·mic
pre·spon·dy·lo·lis·the·sis
press
    French p.
pres·som·e·ter
    Jarcho p.
pres·sor
pres·so·re·cep·tive
pres·so·re·cep·tor
pres·so·sen·si·tive
pres·so·sen·si·tiv·i·ty
    reflexogenic p.
pres·sure
    absolute p.
    after p.
    airway p.
    alveolar p.
    ambulatory venous p.
    amniotic p.
    arterial p.

pres·sure *(continued)*
    atmospheric p.
    back p.
    barometric p.
    biting p.
    blood p.
    brain p.
    capillary p.
    central venous p. (CVP)
    cerebrospinal p.
    colloid osmotic p.
    continuous positive airway
      p. (CPAP)
    critical closing p.
    diastolic p.
    Donders' p.
    endocardial p.
    expiratory p.
    filtration p.
    hydrostatic p.
    hyperbaric p.
    p. of ideas
    imbibition p.
    inspiratory p.
    inspiratory triggering p.
    interstitial p.
    intra-abdominal p.
    intracranial p.
    intramyometrial p.
    intraocular p.
    intrapulmonary p.
    intraspinal p.
    intrathecal p.
    intrathoracic p.
    intratympanic p.
    intraventricular p.
    jugular venous p.
    mean circulatory filling p.
    mutation p.
    nasal continuous positive
      airway p. (CPAP)
    negative p.
    negative end-expiratory p.
    occlusal p.
    oncotic p.
    osmotic p.
    osmotic p., effective
    partial p.

pres·sure *(continued)*
   perfusion p.
   portal venous p.
   positive p.
   positive end-expiratory p.
    (PEEP)
   pulmonary p.
   pulmonary artery wedge p.
   pulmonary capillary wedge
    p.
   pulse p.
   radiation p.
   selection p.
   solution p.
   p. of speech
   splenic pulp p.
   standard p.
   subambient p.
   subatmospheric p.
   surface p.
   systolic p.
   thought p.
   tissue p.
   transairway p.
   transmural p.
   transpulmonary p.
   transthoracic p.
   vapor p.
   venous p.
   ventilator p.
   posterior p.
   water vapor p.
   wedge p.
   wedged hepatic vein p.
   zero end-expiratory p.
pre·ster·num
pre·stri·ate
pre·su·bic·u·lum
pre·sump·tive
pre·sup·pu·ra·tive
pre·syl·vi·an
pre·symp·tom
pre·symp·to·mat·ic
pre·syn·ap·tic
pre·sys·to·le
pre·sys·tol·ic
pre·tar·sal
pre·tec·tal

pre·tec·tum
pre·term
pre·ter·mi·nal
preth·ca·mide
pre·thy·roi·de·al
pre·thy·roi·de·an
pre·tu·ber·cu·lo·sis
pre·tu·ber·cu·lous
pre·ure·thri·tis
prev AGT — previous
   abnormality of glucose
   tolerance
prev·a·lence
   period p.
   point p.
pre·ven·tion
pre·ven·tive
pre·ven·to·ri·um
pre·ven·tric·u·lo·sis
pre·ven·tric·u·lus
pre·ver·mis
pre·ver·te·bral
pre·ver·tig·i·nous
pre·ves·i·cal
pre·vi·a·ble
pre·vi·ta·min
Pré·vost's law
Pré·vost's sign
Prey·er's reflex
Prey·er's test
pre·zone
pre·zo·nu·lar
pre·zy·ga·poph·y·sis
pre·zy·got·ic
PRF — prolactin releasing
   factor
PRH — prolactin-releasing
   hormone
pri·a·pism
pri·a·pi·tis
pri·a·pus
Price-Jones curve
Price-Jones method
Priess·nitz bandage
Priess·nitz compress
pril·o·caine hy·dro·chlo·ride
pri·ma·cy
   genital p.

pri·ma·cy *(continued)*
    phallic p.
pri·mal
pri·ma·my·cin
prim·a·quine phos·phate
pri·mary
pri·mate
Pri·ma·tes
primed
prime mov·er
prim·er
    cavity p.
prim·i·done
pri·mi·grav·id
pri·mi·grav·i·da
    elderly p.
pri·mip·a·ra *pl.* pri·mip·a·rae
pri·mi·par·i·ty
pri·mip·a·rous
pri·mit·iae
prim·i·ti·va·tion
prim·i·tive
pri·mor·di·al
pri·mor·di·um *pl.* pri·mor·dia
    genital p.
    lens p.
prim·ver·ose
Prin·a·dol
prin·ceps
Prin·ci·pen
prin·ci·ple
    active p.
    Bragg-Gray p.
    Doppler p.
    Fick p.
    Huygens (Huyghens) p.
    immediate p.
    Le Chatelier p.
    luteinizing p.
    mass action p.
    melanophore dilating p.
    organic p.
    pleasure p.
    pleasure-pain p.
    proximate p.
    reality p.
    repetition-compulsion p.
    Venturi p.

Prin·gle's disease
Pri·nos ver·ti·cel·la·tus
Prinz·met·al's angina
pri·on
Pri·on·urus
Pris·co·line
prism
    adamantine p's
    enamel p's
    Maddox p.
    Nicol p.
    Risley's p.
pris·ma *pl.* pris·ma·ta
    prismata adamantina
pris·ma·ta
pris·mat·ic
pris·moid
pris·mop·tom·e·ter
pris·mo·sphere
pris·op·tom·e·ter
priv·i·lege
    admitting p's
    conversion p.
    staff p's
Pri·vine
PRL — prolactin
Prl — prolactin
p.r.n. — L. pro re nata
    (according as circumstances
    may require)
Pro — proline
pro·ac·cel·er·in
pro·ac·ti·no·my·cin
pro·ac·ti·va·tor
    C3 p. (C3PA)
pro·ad·i·fen hy·dro·chlo·ride
pro·al
pro·am·ni·on
pro·an·gio·ten·sin
pro·at·las
pro·az·amine
prob·a·bil·i·ty
    birth order p.
    conditional p.
    prior p.
    reproduction p.
    significance p.
pro·bac·te·rio·phage

pro·band
pro·bang
Pro-Ban·thine
pro·bar·bi·tal
probe
    Anel's p.
    blood flow p.
    blunt p.
    Bowman's p.
    Brackett's p's
    bullet p.
    calibrated p.
    drum p.
    electric p.
    eyed p.
    fiberoptic p.
    Girdner's p.
    Girdner's electric p.
    heat p.
    lacrimal p.
    memory p.
    oligonucleotide p.
    periodontal p.
    pocket p.
    root canal p.
    scintillation p.
    scissors p.
    telephonic p.
    ultrasound p.
    uterine p.
    vertebrated p.
    WHO (World Health
    Organization) periodontal
    p.
pro·ben·e·cid
pro·bit
pro·bos·cis
pro·bu·col
pro·cain·amide hy·dro·chlo·ride
pro·caine
    p. amide hydrochloride
    p. hydrochloride
    p. penicillin G
pro·cal·lus
pro·car·ba·zine hy·dro·chlo·ride
pro·car·boxy·pep·ti·dase

pro·car·cin·o·gen
Pro·caryo·tae
pro·ca·tarc·tic
pro·ca·tarx·is
pro·ce·dure
    Anderson p.
    Aries-Pitanguy p.
    Bosworth p.
    Bristow p.
    Brock's p.
    Cockett p.
    Dale p.
    Darrach p.
    DuVal p.
    Ewart's p.
    exteriorization p.
    Feulgen p.
    Glenn p.
    Gomori-Takamatsu p.
    Hartmann's p.
    Hassab p.
    Husni p.
    Ilizarov leg-lengthening p.
    Jannetta p.
    Kazanjian's p.
    Kestenbach-Anderson p.
    Kuhnt-Szymanowski p.
    Ladd's p.
    Lester Martin p.
    Linton p.
    May p.
    Merindino p.
    Mikulicz's p.
    Mustard p.
    Nichol p.
    Ober-Barr p.
    Palma p.
    Potts p.
    Puestow p.
    push-back p.
    Rashkind p.
    second-look p.
    Senning p.
    shelf p.
    Shirodkar p.
    Soave p.
    Stamey's p.
    stereotaxic p.

pro·ce·dure *(continued)*
    Sugiura p.
    Swenson pull-through p.
    Tanner's p.
    V-Y p.
    Valsalva's p.
    Womack p.
    Zancolli p.
pro·ce·lous
pro·cen·tri·ole
pro·ce·phal·ic
pro·cer·coid
pro·ce·rus
pro·cess
    ABC p.
    accessory p. of lumbar
      vertebrae
    accessory p. of sacrum,
      spurious
    acromial p.
    acromion p.
    acute p. of helix
    alar p.
    aliform p.
    alveolar p.
    ameloblastic p.
    anconeal p.
    angular p. of frontal bone,
      external
    articular p.
    ascending p's of vertebrae
    auditory p.
    axillary p.
    axis-cylinder p.
    basilar p.
    Beccari p.
    p. of Blumenbach
    calcaneal p.
    calcanean p.
    capitular p.
    caudate p.
    ciliary p's
    Civinini's p.
    clinoid p.
    cochleariform p.
    condylar p.
    condyloid p.
    conoid p.

pro·cess *(continued)*
    coracoid p.
    coronoid p.
    costal p.
    cubital p.
    deep p. of submandibular
      gland
    Deiters' p.
    dendritic p.
    dental p.
    dentoid p.
    ensiform p.
    epiphyseal p.
    ethmoidal p.
    ethmoidal p. of Macalister
    facial p.
    falciform p.
    floccular p.
    folian p.
    p. of Folius
    foot p.
    frontal p.
    frontal p., external
    frontonasal p.
    frontosphenoidal p.
    funicular p.
    globular p.
    Gottstein's basal p.
    hamate p.
    hamular p.
    head p.
    incisive p.
    inferior articular p.
    inframalleolar p.
    infraorbital p.
    infundibular p.
    Ingrassia's p.
    intercondylar p.
    intrajugular p.
    jugular p.
    lacrimal p.
    lateral p.
    lenticular p.
    lentiform p.
    long p. of malleus
    lumbocostal p.
    malar p.
    mamillary p.

pro·cess *(continued)*
 mandibular p.
 marginal p.
 mastoid p.
 maxillary p.
 medial angular p.
 medial p.
 mental p.
 middle clinoid p.
 muscular p.
 nasal p.
 notochordal p.
 oblique p.
 occipital p.
 p. of odontoblast
 odontoblastic p.
 odontoid p.
 olecranon p.
 orbital p.
 palatal p.
 palatine p.
 papillary p.
 paracondyloid p.
 paroccipital p.
 paramastoid p.
 petrosal p.
 postauditory p.
 posterior clinoid p.
 posterior p. of talus
 postglenoid p.
 postmeatal p.
 primary p.
 pterygoid p.
 pterygopalatine p.
 pterygoquadrate p.
 pterygospinous p.
 pyramidal p.
 random p.
 Rau's p.
 ravian p.
 restiform p. of Henle
 retromandibular p.
 schizophrenic p.
 secondary p.
 small p. of Soemmering
 sphenoidal p.
 spinous p.

pro·cess *(continued)*
 spinous p. of sacrum,
  spurious
 Stieda's p.
 stochastic p.
 styloid p.
 sucker p.
 superior articular p.
 supracondylar p.
 synovial p.
 temporal p.
 Todd's p.
 Tomes p.
 transverse p.
 trochlear p.
 unciform p.
 uncinate p.
 ungual p.
 vaginal p.
 vermiform p.
 vertebral p.
 vocal p.
 xiphoid p.
 zygomatic p.
 zygomatico-orbital p.
pro·cess·ing
 signal p.
pro·ces·sor
pro·ces·sus *pl.* pro·ces·sus
 p. accessorii spurii
 p. accessorius
 p. alaris ossis ethmoidalis
 p. alveolaris maxillae
 p. anterior mallei
 p. anterior mallei [Folii]
 p. articularis
 p. axillaris
 p. brevis incudis
 p. brevis mallei
 p. calcaneus
 p. caudatus hepatis
 p. ciliares
 p. clinoideus anterior
 p. clinoideus medius
 p. clinoideus posterior
 p. cochleariformis
 p. condylaris
 p. condyloideus

pro·ces·sus *(continued)*
- p. coracoideus
- p. coronoideus
- p. costalis
- p. costarius
- p. ethmoidalis
- p. falciformis
- p. Ferreini lobuli corticalis renis
- p. frontalis
- p. frontosphenoidalis
- p. gracilis
- p. of Ingrassia
- p. intrajugularis
- p. jugularis
- p. lacrimalis
- p. lateralis
- p. lenticularis incudis
- p. mamillaris
- p. marginalis
- p. mastoideus
- p. maxillaris
- p. medialis
- p. muscularis
- p. orbitalis
- p. palatinus maxillae
- p. papillaris hepatis
- p. paramastoideus
- p. phalangeus
- p. posterior sphenoidalis
- p. posterior tali
- p. pterygoideus
- p. pterygospinosus
- p. pterygospinosus [Civinini]
- p. pyramidalis
- p. retromandibularis
- p. sphenoidalis
- p. spinosus
- p. styloideus
- p. supracondylaris humeri
- p. supracondyloideus humeri
- p. supraepicondylaris humeri
- p. temporalis
- p. transversus
- p. trochlearis calcanei

pro·ces·sus *(continued)*
- p. uncinatus
- p. vaginalis
- p. vermiformis
- p. vocalis
- p. xiphoideus
- p. zygomaticus

pro·chei·lon
Pro·chlo·ro·phy·ta
pro·chlor·pem·a·zine
pro·chlor·per·a·zine
- p. edisylate
- p. maleate

pro·chon·dral
pro·chor·dal
pro·cho·ri·on
pro·chro·mo·some
pro·ci·den·tia
- p. uteri

pro·cin·o·nide
pro·clin·a·tion
pro·co·ag·u·lant
pro·col·la·gen
pro·col·lag·e·nase
pro·col·la·gen-ly·sine, 2-oxo·glu·ta·rate 5-di·oxy·gen·ase
pro·col·la·gen pep·ti·dase
pro·col·la·gen-pro·line, 2-oxo·glu·ta·rate 4-di·oxy·gen·ase
pro·col·la·gen *N*-pro·tein·ase
pro·con·cep·tive
pro·con·dyl·ism
pro·con·ver·tin
pro·cre·a·tion
pro·cre·a·tive
proc·tal·gia
- p. fugax

proc·ta·tre·sia
proc·tec·ta·sia
proc·tec·to·my
proc·ten·clei·sis
proc·teu·ryn·ter
proc·teu·ry·sis
proc·ti·tis
- epidemic gangrenous p.
- factitial p.
- radiation p.
- ulcerative p.

proc·to·cele
proc·to·cly·sis
proc·to·coc·cy·pexy
proc·to·co·lec·to·my
proc·to·co·li·tis
proc·to·co·lon·os·co·py
proc·to·col·po·plas·ty
proc·to·cys·to·cele
proc·to·cys·to·plas·ty
proc·to·cys·to·tome
proc·to·cys·tot·o·my
proc·to·dae·um
proc·to·de·um
proc·to·dyn·ia
Proc·to·foam-HC
proc·to·gen·ic
proc·to·log·ic
proc·tol·o·gist
proc·tol·o·gy
proc·to·pa·ral·y·sis
proc·to·peri·neo·plas·ty
proc·to·peri·ne·or·rha·phy
proc·to·pexy
proc·to·plas·ty
proc·to·ple·gia
proc·to·poly·pus
proc·top·to·sis
proc·tor·rha·gia
proc·tor·rha·phy
proc·tor·rhea
proc·to·scope
    Tuttle's p.
proc·tos·co·py
proc·to·sig·moid
proc·to·sig·moi·dec·to·my
proc·to·sig·moi·di·tis
proc·to·sig·moi·do·pexy
proc·to·sig·moi·do·scope
proc·to·sig·moi·dos·co·py
proc·to·spasm
proc·tos·ta·sis
proc·to·stat
proc·to·ste·no·sis
proc·tos·to·my
proc·to·tome
proc·tot·o·my
    external p.
    internal p.

proc·tot·o·my *(continued)*
    linear p.
proc·to·val·vot·o·my
pro·cum·bent
pro·cur·sive
pro·cur·va·tion
pro·cu·ti·cle
pro·cy·cli·dine hy·dro·chlo·ride
pro·cy·cli·dine metho·chlo·ride
pro·do·lic acid
pro·dro·ma *pl.* pro·dro·ma·ta
pro·dro·mal
pro·dro·ma·ta
pro·drome
    epileptic p.
pro·dro·mic
pro-drug
prod·uct
    cleavage p.
    contact activation p.
    decay p.
    end p.
    fibrinolytic split p's
    fission p.
    gene p., primary
    spallation p's
    substitution p.
pro·duc·tive
pro·ec·dy·sis
pro·elas·tase
pro·emi·al
pro·en·ceph·a·lus
pro·en·ceph·a·ly
pro·en·zyme
pro·eryth·ro·blast
pro·eryth·ro·cyte
pro·es·tro·gen
pro·es·trum
pro·fa·dol hy·dro·chlo·ride
pro·fen·amine
pro·fes·sion·al
    allied health p.
Pro·fes·sion·al Stan·dards Re·view Or·gan·i·za·tion
Pro·feta's law
pro·fi·bri·nol·y·sin

Pro·fi·chet's disease
Pro·fi·chet's syndrome
pro·fil·ac·tin
pro·file
    antigenic p.
    biochemical p.
    blood p.
    facial p.
    health p.
    histochemical p.
    personality p.
    urethral pressure p.
pro·fil·er
    beam p.
pro·fil·in
pro·fil·om·e·try
    urethral pressure p.
pro·fla·vine
pro·flu·vi·um
    p. seminis
pro·fon·dom·e·ter
pro·fun·da·plas·ty
pro·fun·do·plas·ty
pro·fun·dus
prog·a·mous
pro·gas·ter
pro·gas·trin
pro·ge·nia
pro·gen·i·tal
pro·gen·i·tor
prog·e·ny
pro·ge·ria
pro·ges·ta·tion·al
pro·ges·te·roid
pro·ges·te·rone
pro·ges·tin
pro·ges·to·gen
pro·ges·to·mi·met·ic
pro·glos·sis
pro·glot·tid
pro·glot·tis *pl.* pro·glot·ti·des
pro·glu·mide
Pro·gly·cem
prog·na·thia
prog·na·thic
prog·na·thism
    mandibular p.
prog·na·thom·e·ter

prog·na·thous
prog·nose
prog·no·sis
prog·nos·tic
prog·nos·ti·cate
prog·nos·ti·cian
pro·go·no·ma
    melanotic p.
pro·gran·u·lo·cyte
    early p.
pro·grav·id
pro·gres·sion
    backward p.
    cross-legged p.
    metadromic p.
pro·gres·sive
pro·guan·il hy·dro·chlo·ride
Pro·gyn·on
pro·his·tio·cyte
pro·hor·mone
pro·in·su·lin
pro·jec·tion
    Caldwell's p.
    eccentric p.
    erroneous p.
    essential p.
    geniculostriate p.
    impersonal p.
    left anterior oblique p.
    left posterior oblique p.
    Low-Beers p.
    neuronal p.
    pontocerebellar p.
    right anterior oblique p.
    right posterior oblique p.
    thalamocortical p's
    Towne p.
    Waters p.
pro·kal·li·kre·in
pro·karyo·blast
pro·kary·on
pro·karyo·sis
pro·kary·ote
pro·kary·ot·ic
Pro·ke·ta·zine
pro·la·bi·um
pro·lac·tin
pro·lac·ti·no·ma

pro·lam·in
pro·lan
pro·lapse
    acute cervical disk p.
    anal p.
    p. of anterior lip of cervix
    p. of anus
    p. of the cord
    p. of female urethra
    frank p.
    p. of intervertebral disk
    p. of the iris
    lumbar disk p.
    Morgagni's p.
    occult p. of cord
    rectal p.
    p. of rectum
    p. of uterus
pro·lap·sus
    p. ani
    p. recti
    p. uteri
Pro·lene
pro·lep·sis
pro·lep·tic
pro·leu·ko·cyte
pro·li·dase
pro·li·dase deficiency
pro·lif·er·ate
pro·lif·er·a·tion
    bile duct p.
    fibroplastic p.
    mesangial p.
pro·lif·er·a·tive
pro·lif·er·ous
pro·lif·ic
pro·lig·er·ous
pro·lin·ase
pro·line
    p. hydroxyproline
      glycinuria
pro·line de·hy·dro·gen·ase
pro·line di·pep·ti·dase
pro·line hy·drox·y·lase
pro·lin·emia
pro·line-5-ox·i·dase
pro·lin·tane hy·dro·chlo·ride
Pro·lix·in

Pro·loid
prolo·ther·a·py
Pro·lu·ton
pro·lyl
pro·lyl di·pep·ti·dase
pro·lyl hy·drox·y·lase
pro·lym·pho·blast
pro·lym·pho·cyte
PROM — premature rupture
    of membranes
pro·man·ide
pro·mas·ti·gote
pro·ma·zine hy·dro·chlo·ride
pro·mega·karyo·cyte
pro·meg·a·lo·blast
pro·meta·phase
pro·meth·a·zine hy·dro·chlo·
    ride
pro·meth·es·trol di·pro·pi·o·
    nate
pro·me·thi·um
pro·mine
prom·i·nence
    Ammon's scleral p.
    cephalic p.
    p. of facial canal
    laryngeal p.
    p. of lateral semicircular
      canal
    mallear p. of tympanic
      membrane
    spiral p.
    styloid p.
    tubal p.
prom·i·nen·tia *pl.* prom·i·
nen·tiae
    p. canalis facialis
    p. canalis semicircularis
      lateralis
    p. foraminalis
    p. frontonasalis
    p. laryngea
    p. mallearis membranae
      tympani
    p. malleolaris membranae
      tympani
    p. mandibularis
    p. spiralis

prom·i·nen·tia *(continued)*
    p. styloidea
prom·i·nen·tiae
pro·mi·to·sis
pro·mono·cyte
prom·on·to·ri·um *pl.* prom·
  on·to·ria
    p. cavitatis tympanicae
    p. faciei
    p. ossis sacri
    p. tympani
prom·on·to·ry
    p. of the middle ear
    pelvic p.
    p. of sacrum
    tympanic p.
    p. of tympanic cavity
pro·mo·ter
    eosinophil stimulator p.
pro·mo·tion
pro·mox·o·lane
pro·my·elo·blast
pro·my·elo·cyte
pro·nase
pro·nate
pro·na·tion
pro·na·to·flex·or
pro·na·tor
pro·na·tor-su·pi·na·tor
prone
pro·neph·ron
pro·neph·ros *pl.* pro·neph·roi
Pro·nes·tyl
pro·net·a·lol
pro·neth·a·lol
prong
pro·no·grade
pro·nom·e·ter
pro·nor·mo·blast
    Sabin's p.
Pron·to·sil
pro·nu·cle·us
    female p.
    male p.
pro·opio·mel·a·no·cor·tin
pro-ot·ic
proö·var·i·um
    dental p.

Pro·pa·drine
prop·a·gate
pro·pa·ga·tion
prop·a·ga·tive
pro·pal·i·nal
pro·pane
pro·pan·i·did
pro·pa·nol
pro·pan·o·lide
pro·pan·the·line bro·mide
pro·par·a·caine hy·dro·chlo·
  ride
pro·par·gyl
pro·pa·tyl ni·trate
pro·pene
pro·pe·nyl
pro·pep·sin
pro·pep·tone
pro·pep·ton·uria
pro·per·din
pro·peri·to·ne·al
prop·er·ty
    colligative p.
pro·phage
pro·phase
pro·phen·py·rid·amine
pro·phy·lac·tic
pro·phy·lax·is
    causal p.
    chemical p.
    clinical p.
    collective p.
    dental p.
    drug p.
    gametocidal p.
    individual p.
    mechanical p.
    oral p.
    serum p.
    suppressive p.
pro·phyr·ism
pro·pi·cil·lin
pro·pio·lac·tone
pro·pi·o·ma·zine hy·dro·chlo·
  ride
pro·pi·o·nate
pro·pi·o·nate car·box·y·lase
pro·pi·on·i·bac·ter

Pro·pi·on·i·bac·te·ri·a·ceae
Pro·pi·on·i·bac·te·ri·um
    P. acnes
    P. freudenreichii
    P. granulosum
    P. jensenii
pro·pi·on·ic acid
pro·pi·on·ic·ac·i·de·mia
pro·pio·ni·trile
pro·pi·o·nyl
pro·pi·o·nyl-CoA car·boxy·lase
pro·pi·o·nyl-cho·line
pro·pi·ram fu·mar·ate
pro·plas·ma·cyte
pro·plas·min
Proplast
pro·plas·tid
pro·pons
pro·por·phy·rin·o·gen ox·i·dase
pro·por·tion
    femininity p.
    masculinity p.
    mutant p.
    optimal p.
pro·pos·i·ta pro·pos·i·tae
pro·pos·i·tus *pl.* pro·pos·i·ti
pro·poxy·caine hy·dro·chlo·ride
pro·poxy·phene
    p. hydrochloride
    p. napsylate
pro·pran·o·lol
    p. hydrochloride
pro·pri·e·tary
pro·prio·cep·tion
pro·prio·cep·tive
pro·prio·cep·tor
pro·prio·spi·nal
pro·pro·tein
prop·tom·e·ter
prop·to·sis
pro·pul·sion
pro·pyl
    p. gallate
prop·y·lene
    p. glycol

prop·y·lene *(continued)*
    p. oxide
pro·pyl·hex·e·drine
pro·pyl·io·done
pro·pyl·par·a·ben
pro·pyl·thio·ura·cil
pro·qua·zone
pro re na·ta
pro·ren·nin
pro·ren·o·ate po·tas·si·um
Pro·ro·cen·trum
pro·rox·an hy·dro·chlo·ride
pror·sad
pro·ru·bri·cyte
pro·scil·lar·i·din
pro·se·cre·tin
pro·sect
pro·sec·tion
pro·sec·tor
pros·en·ceph·a·lon
proso·coele
proso·de·mic
pros·o·dy
proso·gas·ter
proso·pag·no·sia
proso·pal·gia
proso·pal·gic
proso·pan·tri·tis
proso·pec·ta·sia
proso·phe·no·sia
proso·pla·sia
pros·o·po·an·os·chi·sis
pros·o·po·di·ple·gia
pros·o·po·dys·mor·phia
pros·o·po·neu·ral·gia
pros·o·pop·a·gus
pros·o·po·ple·gia
pros·o·po·ple·gic
pros·o·pos·chi·sis
pros·o·po·spasm
proso·po·ster·no·dym·ia
pros·o·po·ster·no·dy·mus
proso·po·ster·no·pa·gus
pros·o·po·tho·ra·cop·a·gus
pros·ta·cy·clin
pros·ta·glan·din
pros·ta·glan·din en·do·per·ox·ide syn·thase

Δ13-pros·ta·glan·din re·duc·tase

pros·ta·glan·din syn·the·tase

pros·ta·lene

pros·ta·no·ic acid

pros·ta·noid

Pros·taph·lin

pros·ta·ta

pros·ta·tal·gia

pros·ta·tauxe

pros·tate
    funnel-neck p.

pros·ta·tec·to·my
    perineal p.
    retropubic p.
    retropubic prevesical p.
    suprapubic transvesical p.
    transurethral p.

pros·ta·tel·co·sis

pros·tat·ic

pros·tat·i·co·ves·i·cal

pros·tat·i·co·ve·sic·u·lec·to·my

pros·ta·tism
    vesical p.

pros·ta·tisme
    p. sans prostate

pros·ta·ti·tic

pros·ta·ti·tis
    allergic p.
    bacterial p.
    eosinophilic p.
    fungal p.
    nonspecific granulomatous
        p.

pros·ta·to·cys·ti·tis

pros·ta·to·cys·tot·o·my

pros·ta·to·dyn·ia

pros·ta·tog·ra·phy

pros·ta·to·lith

pros·ta·to·li·thot·o·my

pros·ta·to·meg·a·ly

pros·ta·tom·e·ter

pros·tat·o·my

pros·ta·to·myo·mec·to·my

pros·ta·tor·rhea

pros·ta·tot·o·my

pros·ta·to·tox·in

pros·ta·to·ve·sic·u·lec·to·my

pros·ta·to·ve·sic·u·li·tis

pros·tax·ia

pro·ster·na·tion

pros·the·ca *pl.* pros·the·cae

pros·the·sis *pl.* pros·the·ses
    Angelchick p.
    antireflux p.
    Aufranc-Turner p.
    Austin Moore p.
    Bechtol hip p.
    Björk-Shiley aortic valve p.
    Blom-Singer voice p.
    caged-ball p.
    Charnley's p.
    Charnley total hip p.
    Charnley-Mueller hip p.
    cleft palate p.
    Cronin p.
    Cutter SCDK p.
    dental p.
    disk valve p.
    endoskeletal p.
    exoskeletal p.
    feeding p.
    heart valve p.
    knitted vascular p.
    maxillofacial p.
    McKee-Farrar p.
    modular p.
    Munster p.
    myoelectric p.
    Neville p.
    Niebauer p.
    ocular p.
    Panje voice p.
    penile p.
    pneumatic p.
    speech-aid p.
    Starr-Edwards p.
    Syme p.
    Thompson p.
    tracheoesophageal fistula
        voice button p.
    woven vascular p.

pros·thet·ic

pros·thet·ics
    dental p.

pros·thet·ics *(continued)*
  denture p.
  facial p.
  maxillofacial p.
pros·the·tist
pros·thi·on
pros·tho·don·tia
pros·tho·don·tics
pros·tho·don·tist
Pros·tho·gon·i·mus
pros·tho·ker·a·to·plas·ty
Pro·stig·min
Pros·tin E2
Pros·tin F2 Alpha
pros·tra·tion
  heat p.
  nervous p.
pro·tac·tin·i·um
pro·ta·gon
pro·tal
Pro·tal·ba
pro·tal·bu·mose
pro·tam·in·ase
pro·ta·mine
  p. sulfate
pro·tan
pro·tan·drous
prot·an·dry
pro·ta·nom·al
pro·ta·nom·a·lous
pro·ta·nom·a·ly
pro·ta·nope
pro·ta·no·pia
pro·ta·nop·ic
pro·ta·nop·sia
Pro·ta·phane NPH
Pro·tea
pro·te·an
pro·te·ase
pro·tec·tant
pro·tec·tion
  Caldwell's p.
  passive p.
pro·tec·tive
pro·tec·tor
  hearing p.
  LATS p.

pro·tec·tor *(continued)*
  LATS (long-acting thyroid
    stimulator) p.
  nipple p.
Pro·te·eae
pro·tein
  p. A
  alcohol-soluble p.
  allosteric p.
  α-chain p. [alpha-]
  amyloid A (AA) p.
  amyloid light chain (AL) p.
  autologous p.
  bacterial p.
  bacterial cellular p.
  Bence Jones p.
  binding p.
  bone morphogenetic p.
  p. C
  C4 binding p.
  calcium-binding p.
  carrier p.
  cationic p's
  coagulated p.
  coat p.
  complete p.
  compound p.
  conjugated p.
  constitutive p's
  control p's
  cord p's
  corticosteroid-binding p.
  C-reactive p.
  denatured p.
  derived p.
  encephalitogenic p.
  eosinophil major basic p.
  fibrillar p.
  fibrous p.
  floating p.
  G p.
  Gc p.
  globular p.
  guanyl-nucleotide-binding
    p.
  Hektoen, Kretschmer, and
    Welker p.
  heme-thiolate p.

pro·tein *(continued)*
    heterologous p.
    p. hydrolysate
    immune p's
    incomplete p.
    insoluble p.
    iodized p.
    iron-sulfur p.
    p. kinase
    liquid p.
    M p.
    maintenance p.
    matrix p.
    mild silver p.
    myelin basic p. (MBP)
    myeloma p.
    native p.
    nonhistone chromosomal p.
    nonstructural p.
    partial p.
    periplasmic binding p's
    plasma p's
    plasma p. fraction
    R p.
    racemized p.
    retinol binding p. (RBP)
    ribonuclear p.
    p. S
    S p.
    serum p's
    serum amyloid A (SAA) p.
    silver p., mild
    silver p., strong
    simple p.
    staphylococcal p. A
    synthetic p.
    Tamm-Horsfall p.
    thyroid binding p.
    thyroxine-binding p.
    transport p.
    whole p.
    p. Z
pro·tein·a·ceous
pro·tein·ase
pro·tein·emia
    Bence Jones p.
    broad-beta p.
    floating-beta p.

pro·tein-glu·ta·mine γ-glu·ta·myl·trans·fer·ase
pro·tein ly·sine 6-ox·i·dase
pro·tein·ic
pro·tein ki·nase
pro·tein·o·chrome
pro·tein·og·e·nous
pro·tein·ol·o·gy
pro·tein·o·sis
    lipoid p.
    pulmonary alveolar p.
    tissue p.
pro·tein·pho·bia
pro·tein·uria
    accidental p.
    adventitious p.
    anoxemic p.
    asymptomatic p.
    athletic p.
    Bence Jones p.
    benign p.
    cardiac p.
    colliquative p.
    dietetic p.
    digestive p.
    effort p.
    emulsion p.
    enterogenic p.
    essential p.
    exercise p.
    false p.
    febrile p.
    functional p.
    gestational p.
    globular p.
    gouty p.
    hematogenous p.
    hemic p.
    intermittent p.
    intrinsic p.
    isolated p.
    light-chain p.
    lordotic p.
    march p.
    mixed p.
    nephrogenous p.
    nonselective p.
    orthostatic p.

pro·tein·uria *(continued)*
    overflow p.
    palpatory p.
    paroxysmal p.
    persistent p.
    physiologic p.
    postrenal p.
    postural p.
    p. prae-tuberculosa
    prerenal p.
    pseudo-p.
    pyogenic p.
    regulatory p.
    renal p.
    residual p.
    selective p.
    serous p.
    transient p.
    true p.
pro·tein·uric
pro·teo·clas·tic
pro·teo·gly·can
pro·teo·lip·id
pro·teo·lip·in
pro·te·ol·y·sis
pro·teo·lyt·ic
pro·teo·meta·bol·ic
pro·teo·me·tab·o·lism
pro·teo·pec·tic
pro·teo·pep·sis
pro·teo·pep·tic
pro·teo·pex·ic
pro·teo·pexy
pro·te·ose
pro·teo·se·mia
pro·te·os·uria
pro·ter
Pro·tero·glypha
pro·tero·gly·phic
pro·te·uria
pro·te·uric
Pro·te·us
    P. inconstans
    P. mirabilis
    P. myxofaciens
    P. penneri
    P. vulgaris
pro·te·us *pl.* pro·tei

pro·thal·lus
pro·thi·pen·dyl hy·dro·chlo·ride
pro·throm·bin
pro·throm·bin·ase
    extrinsic p.
    intrinsic p.
pro·throm·bin·o·gen
pro·throm·bi·no·gen·ic
pro·throm·bi·no·pe·nia
pro·thy·mo·cyte
pro·tio·dide
pro·ti·re·lin
pro·tist
    eukaryotic p.
    higher p.
    lower p.
    prokaryotic p.
Pro·tis·ta
pro·ti·um
pro·to·al·bu·mose
pro·to·anem·o·nin
pro·to·bi·ol·o·gy
pro·to·blast
pro·to·blas·tic
pro·to·bro·chal
pro·to·cary·on
pro·to·cat·e·chu·ic acid
pro·to·chlo·ride
pro·to·chlo·ro·phyll
pro·to·chon·dral
pro·to·chon·dri·um
pro·to·chor·date
Pro·to·coc·ci·di·i·da
pro·to·col
    Balke p.
    Bruce p.
    citrovorum rescue p.
    leucovorin rescue p.
    Memorial Sloan-Kettering p.
    neon particle p.
    test p.
pro·to·cone
pro·to·co·nid
pro·to·co·op·er·a·tion
pro·to·cop·ro·por·phyr·ia
pro·to·di·as·to·le

pro·to·di·a·stol·ic
pro·to·du·o·de·num
pro·to·elas·tin
pro·to·elas·tose
pro·to·fi·bril
pro·to·fil·a·ment
pro·to·gas·ter
pro·to·glob·u·lose
pro·to·go·no·cyte
pro·tog·y·nous
pro·tog·y·ny
pro·to·heme
pro·to·he·min
pro·to·io·dide
pro·to·ky·lol hy·dro·chlo·ride
Pro·to·mas·tig·i·da
pro·tom·e·ter
Pro·to·mo·na·di·na
pro·ton
pro·to·nate
pro·to·neph·ron
pro·to·neph·ros
pro·to·neu·ron
pro·to·ni·trate
pro·to-on·co·gene
Pro·to·pam
pro·to·path·ic
pro·to·pec·ten
pro·to·phyl·lin
Pro·to·phy·ta
pro·to·pia·no·ma
pro·to·pine
pro·to·pla·sia
pro·to·plasm
    functional p.
    granular p.
    superior p.
pro·to·plas·mat·ic
pro·to·plas·mic
pro·to·plas·mol·y·sis
pro·to·plast
pro·to·por·phyr·ia
    erythrohepatic p.
    erythropoietic p.
pro·to·por·phy·rin
pro·to·por·phy·rin·o·gen ox·i·dase
pro·to·por·phy·rin·uria

pro·to·pro·te·ose
pro·top·sis
pro·to·salt
pro·to·spasm
Pro·to·spi·ru·ra
pro·to·spore
pro·to·sto·ma
pro·to·stome
Pro·to·sto·mia
Pro·to·stron·gy·lus
pro·to·sul·fate
pro·to·syph·i·lis
Pro·to·the·ca
    P. wickerhamii
    P. zopfii
pro·to·the·co·sis
pro·to·troph
pro·to·troph·ic
pro·tot·ro·phy
pro·tot·ro·py
pro·to·type
pro·to·ver·a·trine
pro·to·ver·ine
pro·to·ver·te·bra
pro·tox·ide
Pro·to·zoa
pro·to·zoa
pro·to·zo·a·cide
pro·to·zo·ag·glu·ti·nin
pro·to·zo·al
pro·to·zo·an
pro·to·zo·ia·sis
pro·to·zo·ol·o·gy
    clinical p.
pro·to·zo·on *pl.* pro·to·zoa
pro·to·zo·o·phage
pro·to·zo·o·sis
pro·to·zoo·ther·a·py
pro·tract
pro·trac·tion
    mandibular p.
    maxillary p.
pro·trac·tor
pro·trans·glu·tam·i·nase
pro·trip·ty·line hy·dro·chlo·ride
pro·tru·sio
    p. acetabuli

pro·tru·sion
    acetabular p.
    bimaxillary p.
    bimaxillary dentoalveolar
      p.
    intervertebral disk p.
    intrapelvic p.
    lateral p.
pro·tryp·sin
pro·tu·ber·ance
    Bichat's p.
    p. of chin
    frontal p.
    laryngeal p.
    mental p.
    natiform p.
    occipital p., transverse
    palatine p.
    parietal p.
    tubal p.
pro·tu·ber·an·tia
    p. laryngea
    p. mentalis
    p. occipitalis externa
    p. occipitalis interna
Proust-Lich·theim maneuver
pro-UK — prourokinase
Pro·vell
pro·ven·tric·u·lus
Pro·vera
pro·ver·te·bra
Pro·vi·den·cia
    P. alcalifaciens
    P. rettgeri
    P. stuartii
pro·vid·er
    preferred p. organization
      (PPO)
pro·vi·ral
pro·vi·rus
pro·vi·sion·al
pro·vi·ta·min
    p. D
pro·voc·a·tive
Pro·wa·zek's bodies
Pro·wa·zek-Greeff bodies
prox·a·zole
    p. citrate

prox·e·mics
prox·i·mad
prox·i·mal
prox·i·ma·lis
prox·i·mate
prox·i·mo·atax·ia
prox·i·mo·buc·cal
prox·i·mo·cep·tor
prox·i·mo·la·bi·al
prox·i·mo·lin·gual
proxy
pro·zo·nal
pro·zone
PRPP — phosphoribosylpyro-
    phosphate
PRU — peripheral resistance
    unit
pru·al
pru·i·nate
Pru·let
Pru·nel·la
Pru·nus
    P. amygdalu
    P. communi
    P. serotin
    P. virginiana
pru·rig·i·nous
pru·ri·go
    p. agria
    Besnier's p.
    p. of Besnier
    Besnier p. of pregnancy
    p. chronica multiformis
    dermographic p.
    p. estivalis
    p. ferox
    flexural p.
    p. gestationis of Besnier
    p. of Hebra
    Hutchinson summer p.
    leukodermic p.
    melanotic p.
    p. mitis
    nodular p.
    p. simplex
    summer p. of Hutchinson
    p. infantilis
    p. vulgaris

pru·ri·go *(continued)*
    winter p.
pru·rit·ic
pru·rit·o·gen·ic
pru·ri·tus
    p. ani
    aquagenic p.
    autotoxic p.
    p. hiemalis
    p. scroti
    senile p.
    p. senilis
    symptomatic p.
    uremic p.
    p. vulvae
Prus·sak's fibers
Prus·sak's pouch
Prus·sak's space
prus·si·ate
prus·sic acid
PS — phosphatidylserine
ps — per second
psa·lis
psal·te·ri·al
psal·te·ri·um
Psal·y·do·lyt·ta
psam·mo·car·ci·no·ma
psam·mo·ma
psam·mom·a·tous
psam·mo·sar·co·ma
psam·mo·ther·a·py
psam·mous
psau·os·co·py
psel·a·phe·sia
psel·lism
pseud·acou·sis
pseud·acous·ma
pseud·ac·ti·no·my·co·sis
pseud·agraph·ia
pseud·al·bu·mi·nu·ria
Pseu·dal·les·che·ria boy·dii
pseud·am·ne·sia
Pseud·am·phis·to·mum
    P. truncatum
pseud·an·gi·na
pseud·an·ky·lo·sis
pseud·aphia
pseud·ar·thri·tis

pseud·ar·thro·sis
Pseud·ech·is
pseud·en·ceph·a·lus
pseud·es·the·sia
pseu·di·no·ma
pseu·do·ab·scess
pseu·do·ac·an·tho·sis
    p. nigricans
pseu·do·aceph·a·lus
pseu·do·ac·ro·meg·a·ly
pseu·do·ac·ti·no·my·co·sis
pseu·do·ag·glu·ti·na·tion
pseu·do·ag·gres·sion
pseu·do·agram·ma·tism
pseu·do·agraph·ia
pseu·do·al·bu·mi·nu·ria
pseu·do·al·leles
pseu·do·al·lel·ic
pseu·do·al·le·lism
pseu·do·al·ve·o·lar
pseu·do·amen·or·rhea
pseu·do·ana·phy·lac·tic
pseu·do·ana·phy·lax·is
pseu·do·ane·mia
    p. angiospastica
pseu·do·an·eu·rysm
pseu·do·an·gi·na
pseu·do·an·ky·lo·sis
pseu·do·an·odon·tia
pseu·do·an·tag·o·nist
pseu·do·apha·sia
pseu·do·ap·o·plexy
pseu·do·ap·pen·di·ci·tis
    p. zooparasitica
pseu·do-Ar·gyll Rob·ert·son
    pupil
pseu·do-Ar·gyll Rob·ert·son
    syndrome
pseu·do·ar·thro·sis
pseu·do·aster·e·og·no·sis
pseu·do·asth·ma
pseu·do·ath·e·to·sis
pseu·do·at·ro·pho·der·ma
    col·li
pseu·do-Ba·bin·ski sign
pseu·do·bac·il·lus
pseu·do·bac·te·ri·um
pseu·do·bas·e·dow

pseu·do·bron·chi·ec·ta·sis
pseu·do·bul·bar
pseu·do·car·ti·lage
pseu·do·car·ti·lag·i·nous
pseu·do·cast
pseu·do·cele
pseu·do·ceph·a·lo·cele
pseu·do·chan·cre
    p. redux
pseu·do·cho·le·cys·ti·tis
pseu·do·cho·les·te·a·to·ma
pseu·do·cho·lin·es·ter·ase
pseu·do·cho·rea
pseu·do·chrom·es·the·sia
pseu·do·chro·mid·ro·sis
pseu·do·chro·mo·some
pseu·do·chy·lous
pseu·do·cir·rho·sis
pseu·do·clau·di·ca·tion
pseu·do·clo·nus
pseu·do·co·arc·ta·tion
    p. of the aorta
pseu·do·coele
pseu·do·coe·lom
pseu·do·coel·o·mate
pseu·do·col·loid
pseu·do·col·o·bo·ma
pseu·do·cop·u·la·tion
pseu·do·cor·pus lu·te·um
pseu·do·cow·pox
pseu·do·cox·al·gia
pseu·do·cri·sis
pseu·do·croup
pseu·do·cryp·tor·chid·ism
pseu·do·cy·a·nin
pseu·do·cy·e·sis
pseu·do·cy·lin·droid
pseu·do·cyst
    p's of lung
    pancreatic p.
    pararenal p.
    pulmonary p's
pseu·do·de·cid·ua
pseu·do·de·men·tia
    hysterical p.
pseu·do·dex·tro·car·dia
pseu·do·di·a·be·tes
    stress p.

pseu·do·di·a·stol·ic
pseu·do·diph·the·ria
pseu·do·dom·i·nance
pseu·do·dom·i·nant
pseu·do·dys·en·tery
pseu·do·ede·ma
pseu·do·elas·tin
pseu·do·em·bry·on·ic
pseu·do·em·phy·se·ma
pseu·do·en·ceph·a·lo·ma·la·
  cia
pseu·do·en·do·me·tri·tis
pseu·do·eo·sin·o·phil
pseu·do·ephed·rine
    p. hydrochloride
pseu·do·ep·i·lep·sy
pseu·do·epiph·y·sis
pseu·do·ero·sion
pseu·do·er·y·sip·e·las
pseu·do·es·the·sia
pseu·do·ex·fo·li·a·tion
pseu·do·exo·pho·ria
pseu·do·ex·oph·thal·mos
pseu·do·ex·tro·phy
pseu·do·far·cy
pseu·do·fluc·tu·a·tion
pseu·do·fol·lic·u·li·tis
pseu·do·frac·ture
pseu·do·fruc·tose
pseu·do·gan·gli·on
    Bochdalek's p.
    Cloquet's p.
    Valentin's p.
pseu·do·gene
    dispersed p.
    processed p.
pseu·do·ges·ta·tion
pseu·do·geus·es·the·sia
pseu·do·geu·sia
pseu·do·glan·ders
pseu·do·gli·o·ma
pseu·do·glob·u·lin
pseu·do·glot·tic
pseu·do·glot·tis
pseu·do·glu·co·sa·zone
pseu·do·gon·or·rhea
pseu·do·gout
pseu·do·graph·ia

pseu·do·gyn·e·co·mas·tia
pseu·do·hal·lu·ci·na·tion
pseu·do·hau·stra·tion
pseu·do·hel·minth
pseu·do·hem·ag·glu·ti·na·
   tion
pseu·do·he·ma·tu·ria
pseu·do·hemi·a·car·di·us
pseu·do·he·mo·phil·ia
   p. hepatica
pseu·do·he·mop·ty·sis
pseu·do·he·red·i·tary
pseu·do·her·maph·ro·dism
pseu·do·her·maph·ro·dite
   female p.
   male p.
pseu·do·her·maph·ro·dit·ism
   female p.
   male p.
pseu·do·her·nia
pseu·do·het·ero·to·pia
pseu·do-Hur·ler's disease
pseu·do-Hur·ler's
   polydystrophy
pseu·do·hy·dro·ceph·a·lus
   traumatic internal p.
pseu·do·hy·dro·ceph·a·ly
pseu·do·hy·dro·ne·phro·sis
pseu·do·hy·os·cy·amine
pseu·do·hy·per·ka·le·mia
pseu·do·hy·per·tri·cho·sis
pseu·do·hy·per·troph·ic
pseu·do·hy·per·tro·phy
   muscular p.
pseu·do·hy·po·al·dos·ter·on·
   ism
pseu·do·hy·po·na·tre·mia
pseu·do·hy·po·para·thy·roi·
   dism
pseu·do·hy·po·phos·pha·ta·
   sia
pseu·do·hy·po·thy·roi·dism
pseu·do·ic·ter·us
pseu·do·in·farc·tion
pseu·do·in·flu·en·za
pseu·do·in·ti·ma
pseu·do·ion
pseu·do·iso·chro·mat·ic

pseu·do·iso·cy·a·nin
pseu·do·jaun·dice
pseu·do·ker·a·tin
pseu·do·la·mel·lar
pseu·do·leu·ke·mia
pseu·do·li·po·ma
pseu·do·li·thi·a·sis
pseu·do·lo·gia
   p. fantastica
pseu·do·lux·a·tion
pseu·do·lym·pho·ma
   p. of Spiegler-Fendt
Pseu·do·lynch·ia
   P. canariensis
   P. maurah
pseu·do·ma·lig·nan·cy
pseu·do·mam·ma
pseu·do·ma·nia
pseu·do·mas·tur·ba·tion
pseu·do·mega·co·lon
pseu·do·mel·a·no·ma
pseu·do·mel·a·no·sis
pseu·do·me·lia
   p. paraesthetica
pseu·do·mem·brane
pseu·do·mem·bra·nelle
pseu·do·mem·bra·nous
pseu·do·me·nin·gi·tis
pseu·do·men·stru·a·tion
pseu·do·met·he·mo·glo·bin
pseu·do·mi·cro·ceph·a·lus
pseu·do·mi·cro·ceph·a·ly
pseu·do·mil·i·um
pseu·do·mo·nad
Pseu·do·mo·na·da·ceae
Pseu·do·mo·na·da·les
Pseu·do·mo·na·di·neae
Pseu·do·mo·nas
   P. acidovorans
   P. aeruginosa
   P. alcaligenes
   P. cepacia
   P. diminuta
   P. eisenbergii
   P. fluorescens
   P. mallei
   P. maltophilia
   P. multivorans

Pseu·do·mo·nas (continued)
   P. paucimobilis
   P. pertucinogena
   P. pickettii
   P. pseudoalcaligenes
   P. pseudomallei
   P. putida
   P. putrefaciens
   P. stanieri
   P. stutzeri
   P. syncyanea
   P. testosteroni
   P. thomasii
   P. vesicularis
Pseu·do·mo·nil·ia
pseu·do·mor·phine
pseu·do·mo·tor
pseu·do·mu·cin
pseu·do·mu·ci·nous
pseu·do·my·as·the·nia
pseu·do·my·ce·li·um
pseu·do·my·ia·sis
pseu·do·my·o·pia
pseu·do·myo·to·nia
pseu·do·myx·o·ma
   p. peritonei
pseu·do·myxo·vi·rus
pseu·do·nar·cot·ic
pseu·do·nar·co·tism
pseu·do·neo·plasm
pseu·do·neu·ri·tis
pseu·do·neu·ro·ma
pseu·do·neu·ro·no·pha·gia
pseu·do·nu·cle·o·lus
pseu·do·nys·tag·mus
pseu·do-ob·struc·tion
   intestinal p.
pseu·do-ochro·no·sis
pseu·do-op·to·gram
pseu·do-os·teo·ma·la·cia
pseu·do-ovum
pseu·do·pap·il·le·de·ma
pseu·do·pa·ral·y·sis
   p. agitans
   arthritic general p.
   congenital atonic p.
   generalized alcoholic p.
   Parrot's p.

pseu·do·pa·ral·y·sis
  (continued)
   syphilitic p.
pseu·do·para·ple·gia
pseu·do·par·a·site
pseu·do·pa·re·sis
pseu·do·par·kin·son·ism
pseu·do·pe·lade
   Brocq's p.
pseu·do·pel·lag·ra
pseu·do·pep·tone
pseu·do·peri·car·di·al
pseu·do·peri·to·ni·tis
pseu·do·pha·kia
   p. adiposa
   p. fibrosa
pseu·do·phleg·mon
   Hamilton p.
pseu·do·pho·tes·the·sia
pseu·do·phyl·lid
Pseu·do·phyl·lid·ea
pseu·do·phyl·lid·e·an
pseu·do·plasm
pseu·do·plas·mo·di·um
pseu·do·ple·gia
pseu·do·pneu·mo·nia
pseu·do·pock·et
pseu·do·pod
pseu·do·po·dia
pseu·do·po·di·o·spore
pseu·do·po·di·um *pl.* pseu·do·
   po·dia
pseu·do·po·lio·my·eli·tis
pseu·do·poly·cy·the·mia
pseu·do·poly·me·lia
   p. paraesthetica
pseu·do·pol·yp
pseu·do·pol·y·po·sis
pseu·do·por·en·ceph·a·ly
pseu·do-Pott's disease
pseu·do·preg·nan·cy
pseu·do·prog·na·thism
pseu·do·pro·tein·uria
pseu·do·pseu·do·hy·po·para·
   thy·roid·ism
pseud·op·sia
pseu·do·psy·cho·sis
pseu·do·pter·yg·i·um

pseu·do·pto·sis
pseu·do·pty·al·ism
pseu·do·pu·ber·ty
  heterosexual p.
  isosexual p.
  precocious p.
pseu·do·ra·bies
  bovine p.
pseu·do·re·ac·tion
pseu·do·re·duc·tion
pseu·do·rem·i·nis·cence
pseu·do·ret·in·i·tis pig·men·to·sa
pseu·do·rheu·ma·tism
pseu·do·rick·ets
pseu·do·ro·sette
pseu·do·sar·co·ma
pseu·do·scar·la·ti·na
pseu·do·scle·re·ma
pseu·do·scle·ro·der·ma
pseu·do·scle·ro·sis
  Jakob spastic p.
  Neumayer's amyotrophic
    lateral p.
  spastic p.
  p. spastica
  Strümpell-Westphal p.
  Westphal-Strümpell p.
pseu·do·scro·tum
pseu·do·se·nil·i·ty
pseu·do·sign
  Babinski p.
pseu·do·small·pox
pseud·os·mia
pseu·do·so·lu·tion
pseu·do·sto·ma
pseu·do·stra·bis·mus
pseu·do·stra·ti·fied
pseu·do·stro·phan·thin
pseu·do·struc·ture
pseu·do·ta·bes
  diabetic p.
  pupillotonic p.
pseu·do·tet·a·nus
pseu·do·tho·rax
pseu·do·thrill
pseu·do·tox·in
pseu·do·tra·cho·ma

pseu·do·tris·mus
pseu·dot·ro·pine
pseu·do·trun·cus ar·te·ri·o·sus
pseu·do·tu·ber·cle
pseu·do·tu·ber·cu·lo·ma
  silicotic p.
  p. silicoticum
pseu·do·tu·ber·cu·lo·sis
  p. hominis streptothrica
pseu·do·tu·bule
pseu·do·tu·mor
  p. cerebri
  orbital p.
pseu·do·tym·pa·ni·tes
pseu·do·ty·phus
pseu·do·ure·mia
pseu·do·uri·dine
pseu·do·uri·dyl·ate
pseu·do·uri·dyl·ic acid
pseu·do·vac·u·ole
pseu·do·valve
pseu·do·ven·tri·cle
pseu·do·ver·mi·cule
pseu·do·ver·mic·u·lus
pseu·do·ver·ti·go
pseu·do·vil·lus
pseu·do·vi·ron
pseu·do·vi·ta·min B$_{12}$
pseu·do·voice
pseu·do·vom·it·ing
pseu·do·xan·tho·ma elas·ti·cum
psi
psi — pounds per square inch
psi·co·fur·a·nine
psi·lo·cin
psi·lo·cy·bin
psi·lo·sis pig·men·to·sa
psit·ta·cine
psit·ta·co·sis
pso·as
pso·dy·mus
pso·itis
pso·pho·gen·ic
psor·a·len
psor·en·ter·itis
pso·ri·as·i·form

pso·ri·a·sis
  annular p.
  p. annularis
  p. annulata
  arthritic p.
  p. arthropathica
  p. arthopica
  Barber's p.
  p. buccalis
  circinate p.
  p. circinata
  p. diffusa
  discoid p.
  p. discoidea
  erythrodermic p.
  exfoliative p.
  p. figurata
  figurate p.
  flexural p.
  follicular p.
  p. follicularis
  p. geographica
  p. guttata
  guttate p.
  p. gyrata
  gyrate p.
  inverse p.
  p. inveterata
  p. linguae
  napkin p.
  nummular p.
  p. nummularis
  p. orbicularis
  p. ostracea
  ostraceous p.
  palmar p.
  p. of palms and soles
  provoked p.
  p. punctata
  pustular p., generalized
  pustular p., localized
  rupioid p.
  p. rupioides
  seborrheic p.
  ungual p.
  p. universalis
  unstable p.
  volar p.

pso·ri·a·sis *(continued)*
  von Zumbusch's p.
  p. vulgaris
  Zumbusch's p.
pso·ri·at·ic
Pso·roph·o·ra
psor·oph·thal·mia
Pso·rop·tes
pso·ro·sper·mi·o·sis
PSP — phenolsulfonphthalein
PSRO — professional
  standards review
  organization
psy·chal·ga·lia
psy·chal·gia
psy·chal·gic
psy·cha·nop·sia
psy·chas·the·nia
psy·cha·tax·ia
psy·che
psy·che·del·ic
psy·cher·go·graph
psy·chi·at·ric
psy·chi·at·rics
psy·chi·a·trist
psy·chi·a·try
  biological p.
  community p.
  comparative p.
  consultation liaison p.
  cross-cultural p.
  cultural p.
  descriptive p.
  dynamic p.
  existential p.
  experimental p.
  forensic p.
  geriatric p.
  industrial p.
  liaison p.
  occupational p.
  organic p.
  orthomolecular p.
  phenomenological p.
  preventive p.
  political p.
  social p.
  transcultural p.

psy·chic
psy·cho·acous·tics
psy·cho·ac·ti·va·tor
psy·cho·ac·tive
psy·cho·an·a·lep·tic
psy·cho·anal·y·sis
  adlerian p.
  classic p.
  jungian p.
psy·cho·an·a·lyst
psy·cho·an·a·lyt·ic
psy·cho·au·di·to·ry
psy·cho·bi·o·log·i·cal
psy·cho·bi·ol·o·gist
psy·cho·bi·ol·o·gy
psy·cho·ca·thar·sis
psy·cho·chem·is·try
psy·cho·chrome
psy·cho·chrom·es·the·sia
psy·cho·cor·ti·cal
psy·cho·cu·ta·ne·ous
psy·cho·di·ag·no·sis
psy·cho·di·ag·nos·tics
Psy·cho·di·dae
psy·cho·dom·e·ter
psy·cho·dom·e·try
Psy·cho·do·py·gus
psy·cho·dra·ma
psy·cho·dy·nam·ics
  adaptational p.
psy·cho·dys·lep·tic
psy·cho·gal·van·ic
psy·cho·gal·va·nom·e·ter
psy·cho·gen·der
psy·cho·gen·e·sis
psy·cho·gen·ic
psy·cho·ger·i·at·ric
psy·cho·ger·i·a·tri·cian
psy·cho·ger·i·at·rics
psy·cho·gog·ic
psy·cho·gram
psy·cho·graph
psy·cho·his·tory
psy·cho·in·fan·til·ism
psy·cho·ki·ne·sis
psy·cho·lag·ny
psy·cho·lep·sy
psy·cho·lep·tic

psy·cho·lin·guis·tics
psy·cho·log·ic
psy·cho·log·i·cal
psy·chol·o·gist
psy·chol·o·gy
  abnormal p.
  adlerian p.
  analytic p.
  animal p.
  applied p.
  behavioristic p.
  child p.
  clinical p.
  cognitive p.
  community p.
  comparative p.
  counseling p.
  criminal p.
  depth p.
  developmental p.
  dynamic p.
  environmental p.
  experimental p.
  gestalt p.
  humanistic p.
  individual p.
  industrial p.
  infant p.
  Janet's p.
  jungian p.
  physiologic p.
  social p.
psy·chom·e·ter
psy·cho·me·tri·cian
psy·cho·met·rics
psy·chom·e·try
psy·cho·mo·tor
psy·cho·neu·ral
psy·cho·neu·ro·sis *pl.* psy·cho·neu·ro·ses
  defense p.
  obsessive-compulsive p.
psy·cho·no·mics
psy·chon·o·my
psy·cho·path
  sexual p.
psy·cho·path·ia
  p. sexualis

psy·cho·path·ic
psy·cho·pa·thol·o·gy
psy·chop·a·thy
psy·cho·phar·ma·col·o·gy
psy·cho·phys·i·cal
psy·cho·phys·ics
psy·cho·phys·io·log·ic
psy·cho·phys·i·ol·o·gy
psy·cho·ple·gia
psy·cho·ple·gic
psy·cho·pol·i·tics
psy·cho·pro·phy·lax·is
psy·cho·se·da·tion
psy·cho·sed·a·tive
psy·cho·sen·so·ri·al
psy·cho·sen·so·ry
psy·cho·ses
psy·cho·sex·u·al
psy·cho·sex·u·al·i·ty
psy·cho·sin
psy·cho·sis *pl.* psy·cho·ses
  affective p.
  alcoholic p's
  alcoholic polyneuritic p.
  alternating p.
  p. of association
  atypical p.
  bipolar p.
  bipolar affective p.
  brief reactive p.
  bromide p.
  buffoonery p.
  chronic epileptic p.
  circular p.
  climacteric p.
  depressive p.
  drug p.
  functional p.
  housewife's p.
  hysterical p.
  induced p.
  involutional p.
  Korsakoff's p.
  manic p.
  manic-depressive p.
  organic p.
  paranoiac p.
  paranoid p.

psy·cho·sis *(continued)*
  periodic p.
  polyneuritic p.
  p. polyneuritica
  postpartum p.
  prison p.
  puerperal p.
  reactive p.
  reactive depressive p.
  schizoaffective p.
  schizophrenic p.
  schizophreniform p.
  senile p.
  situational p.
  symbiogenic p.
  symbiotic p.
  symbiotic infantile p.
  tardive p.
  toxic p.
  unipolar p.
  Wernicke-Korsakoff p.
psy·cho·so·cial
psy·cho·so·mat·ic
psy·cho·so·mi·met·ic
psy·cho·stim·u·lant
psy·cho·sur·gery
psy·cho·syn·drome
  focal brain p.
psy·cho·syn·the·sis
psy·cho·tech·nics
psy·cho·ther·a·peu·tics
psy·cho·ther·a·pist
psy·cho·ther·a·py
  brief p.
  contractual p.
  directive p.
  dynamic p.
  existential p.
  family p.
  group p.
  hypnotic p.
  personologic p.
  psychoanalytic p.
  suggestive p.
  supportive p.
  transactional p.
psy·chot·ic
psy·chot·o·gen

psy·chot·o·gen·ic
psy·choto·mi·met·ic
psy·cho·trop·ic
psy·chro·al·gia
psy·chro·es·the·sia
psy·chro·lu·sia
psy·chrom·e·ter
    sling p.
psy·chro·phile
psy·chro·phil·ic
psy·chro·phore
psy·chro·ther·a·py
psyl·li·um
    p. hydrophilic mucilloid
PT — physical therapist
    physical therapy
    prothrombin time
PTA — plasma
  thromboplastin antecedent
  (blood coagulation Factor XI)
ptar·mic
ptar·mus
PTC — phenylthiocarbamide
    plasma thromboplastin
    component (blood
    coagulation Factor IX)
PTCA — percutaneous
  transluminal coronary
  angioplasty
PTEN — pentaerythritol
  tetranitrate
pter·i·dine
pter·in
    p. deaminase
pte·ri·on
pter·nal·gia
pte·ro·ic acid
pter·op·ter·in
pter·o·yl
pter·o·yl·glu·ta·mate
pter·o·yl·glu·tam·ic acid
pter·o·yl·tri·glu·tam·ic acid
pte·ryg·i·um *pl.* pte·ryg·ia
    congenital p.
    p. unguis
pter·y·goid
pter·y·go·man·dib·u·lar
pter·y·go·max·il·lary

pter·y·go·pal·a·tine
PTF — plasma
  thromboplastin factor
PTFE — polytetrafluroethylene-
PTH — parathyroid hormone
pthi·ri·a·sis
    p. pubis
pti·lo·sis
pto·maine
pto·main·emia
pto·maino·tox·ism
pto·ma·tine
pto·ma·top·sia
pto·ma·top·sy
pto·mat·ro·pine
pto·ma·trop·ism
ptosed
pto·sis
    p. adiposa
    false p.
    Horner's p.
    p. lipomatosis
    morning p.
    p. sympathetica
    traumatic p.
    waking p.
ptot·ic
PTT — activated partial
  thromboplastin time
    partial thromboplastin
    time
pty·al·a·gogue
pty·a·lec·ta·sis
pty·a·lin
pty·a·lism
pty·a·lize
pty·alo·cele
    sublingual p.
pty·al·o·gen·ic
pty·a·log·ra·phy
pty·a·lo·li·thi·a·sis
pty·a·lo·li·thot·o·my
pty·a·lo·re·ac·tion
pty·a·lor·rhea
pty·a·lose
pty·oc·ri·nous
pu·bar·che
pu·ber·al

pu·ber·pho·nia
pu·ber·tal
pu·ber·tas
   p. praecox
pu·ber·ty
   delayed p.
   precocious p.
pu·bes
pu·bes·cence
pu·bes·cent
pu·bic
pu·bio·plas·ty
pu·bi·ot·o·my
pu·bis *pl.* pu·bes
pu·bo·ca·ver·no·sus
pu·bo·coc·cyg·e·al
pu·bo·coc·cy·ge·us
pu·bo·fem·o·ral
pu·bo·per·i·to·ne·al·is
pu·bo·pros·tat·ic
pu·bo·rec·tal
pu·bo·tib·i·al
pu·bo·trans·ver·sal·is
pu·bo·ves·i·cal
pu·bo·ves·i·cal·is
PUD — peptic ulcer disease
pu·den·da
pu·den·dag·ra
pu·den·dal
pu·den·dum *pl.* pu·den·da
   female p.
   p. femininum
   p. muliebre
Pu·denz-Hey·er valve
pu·dic
pu·er·i·cul·ture
pu·er·ile
pu·er·pera
pu·er·per·al
pu·er·per·al·ism
pu·er·per·ant
pu·er·pe·ri·um
Pue·stow procedure
puff
   chromosome p's
   veiled p.
puff·er
   pink p.

puff·ing
pu·gil
pu·gil·lus
puits de De·ver·gie
Pu·lex
   P. irritans
pu·lex *pl.* pu·li·ces
Pul·frich's pendulum
Pul·heems
pu·lic·i·cide
Pu·lic·i·dae
pu·li·co·sis
pull
pul·lu·late
pul·lu·la·tion
pul·mo *pl.* pul·mo·nes
   p. dexter
   p. sinister
pul·mo·aor·tic
pul·mo·gram
pul·mo·lith
pul·mom·e·ter
pul·mom·e·try
pul·mo·nal
pul·mo·nary
pul·mo·nate
pul·mo·nec·to·my
pul·mo·nes
pul·mon·ic
pul·mon·is
pul·mo·ni·tis
pul·mo·no·he·pat·ic
pul·mo·nol·o·gist
pul·mo·nol·o·gy
pul·mo·no·per·i·to·ne·al
pul·mo·tor
pulp
   coronal p.
   dead p.
   dental p.
   devitalized p.
   digital p.
   enamel p.
   exposed p.
   hair p.
   mummified p.
   necrotic p.
   nonvital p.

pulp *(continued)*
    putrescent p.
    radicular p.
    red p.
    p. of spleen
    splenic p.
    tooth p.
    vertebral p.
    vital p.
    white p.
pul·pa *pl.* pul·pae
    p. coronale
    p. dentis
    p. lienis
    p. radicularis
    p. splenica
pul·pal
pul·pal·gia
pul·pec·to·my
    partial p.
pul·pi·form
pul·pit·i·des
pul·pi·tis *pl.* pul·pit·i·des
    anachoretic p.
    closed p.
    hyperplastic p.
    open p.
pulp·less
pul·pot·o·my
pul·py
pul·sate
pul·sa·tile
pul·sa·tion
    expansile p.
    suprasternal p.
pul·sa·tor
    Bragg-Paul p.
pulse
    abdominal p.
    abrupt p.
    allorhythmic p.
    alternating p.
    anacrotic p.
    anadicrotic p.
    anatricrotic p.
    apical p.
    arachnoid p.
    atrial liver p.

pulse *(continued)*
    atrial venous p.
    atriovenous p.
    biferious p.
    bisferious p.
    bigeminal p.
    cannon ball p.
    capillary p.
    carotid p.
    catadicrotic p.
    catatricrotic p.
    centripetal venous p.
    collapsing p.
    Corrigan's p.
    coupled p.
    dicrotic p.
    digitalate p.
    dropped-beat p.
    elastic p.
    entoptic p.
    epigastric p.
    equal p.
    febrile p.
    filiform p.
    formicant p.
    frequent p.
    full p.
    funic p.
    gate p.
    hard p.
    hepatic p.
    high-tension p.
    infrequent p.
    intermittent p.
    irregular p.
    jerky p.
    jugular p.
    Kussmaul's p.
    labile p.
    low-tension p.
    Monneret's p.
    monocrotic p.
    nail p.
    paradoxical p.
    parvus et tardus p.
    pistol-shot p.
    plateau p.
    polycrotic p.

pulse *(continued)*
    quadrigeminal p.
    quick p.
    Quincke's p.
    radial p.
    respiratory p.
    retrosternal p.
    Riegel's p.
    running p.
    sharp p.
    short p.
    slow p.
    soft p.
    strong p.
    tense p.
    thready p.
    tricrotic p.
    trigeminal p.
    trip-hammer p.
    undulating p.
    unequal p.
    vagus p.
    venous p.
    vermicular p.
    vibrating p.
    water-hammer p.
    wiry p.
pulse·less
pul·sel·lum *pl.* pul·sel·la
pul·sion
pul·sus *pl.* pul·sus
    p. abdominalis
    p. aequalis
    p. alternans
    p. biferiens
    p. bisferiens
    p. bigeminus
    p. celer
    p. cordis
    p. differens
    p. filiformis
    p. formicans
    p. fortis
    p. frequens
    p. heterochronicus
    p. irregularis perpetuus
    p. magnus
    p. magnus et celer

pul·sus *(continued)*
    p. mollis
    p. monocrotus
    p. oppressus
    p. paradoxus
    p. parvus
    p. parvus et tardus
    p. plenus
    p. tardus
    p. trigeminus
    p. undulosus
    p. vacuus
    p. venosus
pul·ta·ceous
pulv. — L. pulvis (powder)
pul·ver·iza·tion
pul·ver·u·lent
pul·vi·nar
    p. thalami
    p. tunicae internae
      segmenti arterialis
      anastomosis arteriovenae
      glomeriformis
pul·vi·nate
pul·vis
pu·mex
pum·ice
pump
    air p.
    Alvegniat's p.
    blood p.
    breast p.
    calcium p.
    cardiac balloon p.
    Carrel-Lindberg p.
    dental p.
    infusion p.
    infusion-withdrawal p.
    intra-aortic balloon p.
    Lindbergh p.
    McGaw p.
    muscle p.
    Na^+-K^+ p.
    peristaltic p.
    rotary p.
    saliva p.
    sodium p.
    sodium-potassium p.

pump *(continued)*
  stomach p.
pump-oxy·gen·a·tor
pu·na
punch
  Acufex p.
  Gass scleral p.
  kidney p.
  Murphy's kidney p.
  pin p.
  plate p.
  rubber dam p.
  sphenoidal p.
punch·drunk
punched-out
punc·ta
punc·tate
punc·ti·form
punc·to·graph
punctuation
  Schüffner's p.
punc·tum *pl.* punc·ta
  p. caecum
  puncta dolorosa
  p. lacrimale
  puncta lacrimalia
  p. luteum
  p. nasale inferius
  p. ossificationis
  p. ossificationis primarium
  p. ossificationis
    secundarium
  p. proximum
  p. remotum
  puncta vasculosa
punc·tum·e·ter
punc·ture
  Bernard's p.
  cisternal p.
  cranial p.
  diabetic p.
  epigastric p.
  exploratory p.
  heat p.
  intracisternal p.
  Kronecker's p.
  lumbar p.
  Marfan's epigastric p.

punc·ture *(continued)*
  Quincke's p.
  spinal p.
  splenic p.
  sternal p.
  subdural p.
  suboccipital p.
  suprapubic p.
  thecal p.
  tibial p.
  tracheoesophageal p.
  transethmoidal p.
  ventricular p.
pun·gent
Pun·nett square
Pun·ti·us
  P. javanicus
PUO — pyrexia of unknown
  origin
pu·pa
pu·pal
pu·pil
  Adie's p.
  Argyll Robertson p.
  artificial p.
  Behr's p.
  bounding p.
  Bumke's p.
  cat's-eye p.
  cornpicker's p's
  double p.
  fixed p.
  Horner's p.
  Hutchinson's p.
  keyhole p.
  Marcus Gunn p.
  multiple p.
  myotonic p.
  pinhole p.
  pseudo-Argyll Robertson p.
  Robertson's p.
  skew p's
  stiff p.
  tonic p.
pu·pil·la
pu·pil·lary
pu·pil·la·to·nia
Pu·pil·li·dae

pu·pil·lo·con·stric·tion
pu·pil·lo·graph
pu·pil·log·ra·phy
pu·pil·lom·e·ter
pu·pil·lom·e·try
pu·pil·lo·mo·tor
pu·pil·lo·ple·gia
pu·pil·lo·scope
pu·pil·los·co·py
pu·pil·lo·sta·tom·e·ter
pu·pil·lo·to·nia
pu·pip·a·rous
pu·piv·o·rous
Pur·dy's method
Pur·dy's test
pur·ga·tion
pur·ga·tive
    saline p.
purge
pu·ric
pu·ri·form
pu·rine
    amino p.
    methyl p's
pu·rin·emia
pu·rin·emic
pu·rine-nu·cleo·side phos·phor·y·lase
pu·rine-5′-nu·cleo·ti·dase
Pu·rine·thol
pu·rino·lyt·ic
pu·rin·om·e·ter
Pur·kin·je's cells
Pur·kin·je's fibers
Pur·kin·je's image
Pur·kin·je's layer
Pur·kin·je's network
Pur·kin·je's phenomenon
Pur·kin·je's shift
Pur·kin·je's vesicle
Pur·kin·je-San·son mirror images
Pur·mann's method
Pu·ro·di·gin
pu·ro·hep·a·ti·tis
pu·ro·mu·cous
pu·ro·my·cin
    p. hydrochloride

pur·ple
    bromcresol p.
    visual p.
Pur·pu·ra
pur·pu·ra
    acute vascular p.
    allergic p.
    anaphylactoid p.
    p. angioneurotica
    p. annularis telangiectodes
    p. arthritica
    athrombocytopenic p.
    autoimmune thrombocytopenic p.
    benign hyperglobulinemic p.
    brain p.
    p. bullosa
    cachectic p.
    drug p.
    dysproteinemic p.
    essential p.
    factitious p.
    fibrinolytic p.
    p. fibrinolytica
    p. fulminans
    hemogenic p.
    p. hemorrhagica
    Henoch's p.
    Henoch-Schönlein p.
    p. hyperglobulinemica
    idiopathic p.
    idiopathic thrombocytopenic p.
    itching p.
    lung p. with nephritis
    Majocchi's p.
    malignant p.
    mechanical p.
    p. nervosa
    p. of newborn
    nonthrombocytopenic p.
    orthostatic p.
    palpable p.
    p. pigmentosa chronica
    psychogenic p.
    p. pulicans

pur·pu·ra *(continued)*
   p. rheumatica
   Schönlein p.
   Schönlein-Henoch p.
   p. scorbutica
   senile p.
   p. senilis
   p. simplex
   steroid p.
   symptomatic p.
   thrombocytopenic p.
   thrombocytopenic p.,
      idiopathic
   thrombocytopenic p.,
      secondary
   thrombocytopenic p.,
      thrombotic
   p. thrombolytica
   thrombopenic p.
   thrombotic
      thrombohemolytic p.
   p. urticans
   p. variolosa
   Waldenström's
      hyperglobulinemic p.
pur·pu·rea·gly·co·side
   p. C.
pur·pu·ric
pur·pu·ric acid
pur·pu·rif·e·rous
pur·pu·rin
pur·pu·rine
pur·pu·rin·uria
pur·pu·rog·e·nous
pur·shi·a·nin
Purt·scher's angiopathic
   retinopathy
Purt·scher's disease
pu·ru·lence
pu·ru·len·cy
pu·ru·lent
pu·ru·loid
pus *pl.* pu·ra
   anchovy sauce p.
   blue p.
   burrowing p.
   cheesy p.

pus *(continued)*
   curdy p.
   green p.
   ichorous p.
   laudable p.
   p. laudandum
   sanious p.
Pu·sey's emulsion
push·back
   palatal p.
pus·tu·la *pl.* pus·tu·lae
pus·tu·lar
pus·tu·la·tion
pus·tule
   amniotic p's
   compound p.
   malignant p.
   multilocular p.
   postmortem p.
   primary p.
   secondary p.
   simple p.
   spongiform p.
   spongiform p. of Kogoj
   unilocular p.
pus·tu·lo·sis
   acral p.
   p. palmaris et plantaris
   palmoplantar p.
   p. vacciniformis acuta
   p. varioliformis acuta
pu·ta·men
Put·nam type
Put·nam-Da·na syndrome
pu·tre·fac·tion
pu·tre·fac·tive
pu·tre·fy
pu·tres·cence
pu·tres·cent
pu·tres·cen·tia uteri
pu·tres·cine
pu·trid
Put·ti syndrome
put·ty
   Horsley's p.
Pu·us·epp's reflex
PUVA — psoralen plus
   ultraviolet A

PV — peripheral vascular
    plasma volume
    polycythemia vera
    portal vein
PVC — polyvinyl chloride
PVD — peripheral vascular
    disease
PVP — polyvinylpyrrolidone
PVP-I — povidone-iodine
PWM — pokeweed mitogen
py·ar·thro·sis
Pyc·nan·the·mum
py·ec·chy·sis
py·elec·ta·sia
py·elec·ta·sis
py·el·ic
py·elit·ic
py·eli·tis
    calculous p.
    cystic p.
    p. cystica
    defloration p.
    encrusted p.
    p. glandularis
    p. granulosa
    p. gravidarum
    hematogenous p.
    hemorrhagic p.
    suppurative p.
    urogenous p.
py·elo·cal·i·ce·al
py·elo·cali·ec·ta·sis
py·elo·cys·ti·tis
py·elo·cys·to·sto·mo·sis
py·elo·flu·o·ros·co·py
py·elo·gram
    dragon p.
py·elo·graph
py·elog·ra·phy
    air p.
    antegrade p.
    ascending p.
    p. by elimination
    excretion p.
    intravenous p.
    lateral p.
    respiration p.
    retrograde p.

py·elog·ra·phy *(continued)*
    wash-out p.
py·elo·il·eo·cu·ta·ne·ous
py·elo·in·ter·sti·tial
py·elo·li·thot·o·my
py·elom·e·try
py·elo·ne·phri·tis
    acute p.
    ascending p.
    calculous p.
    chronic bacterial p.
    chronic p.
    hematogenous p.
    p. of pregnancy
    xanthogranulomatous p.
py·elo·ne·phro·sis
py·elop·a·thy
py·elo·phle·bi·tis
py·elo·plas·ty
py·elos·co·py
py·elos·to·my
py·elot·o·my
py·elo·ure·ter·al
py·elo·ure·ter·ec·ta·sis
py·elo·ure·ter·og·ra·phy
py·elo·ure·ter·ol·y·sis
py·elo·ure·tero·plas·ty
py·elo·ve·nous
py·em·e·sis
py·e·mia
    arterial p.
    cryptogenic p.
    otogenous p.
    portal p.
py·e·mic
Py·e·mo·tes
    P. ventricosus
py·en·ceph·a·lus
py·e·sis
py·gal
py·gal·gia
pyg·ma·li·on·ism
pyg·my
py·go·amor·phus
py·go·did·y·mus
py·gom·e·lus
py·gop·a·gus
    p. parasiticus

py·gop·a·gy
py·ic
pyk·nic
pyk·no·cyte
pyk·no·cy·to·ma
pyk·no·cy·to·sis
pyk·no·dys·os·to·sis
pyk·no·ep·i·lep·sy
pyk·no·lep·sy
pyk·nom·e·ter
pyk·nom·e·try
pyk·no·mor·phic
pyk·no·mor·phous
pyk·no·phra·sia
pyk·no·plas·son
pyk·no·sis
pyk·no·so·ma·tic
pyk·not·ic
py·la
py·lar
Pyle's disease
py·le·phle·bec·ta·sis
py·le·phle·bi·tis
   adhesive p.
py·le·throm·bo·phle·bi·tis
py·le·throm·bo·sis
py·lic
PYLL — potential years of life
   lost
py·lon
py·lo·ral·gia
py·lo·rec·to·my
py·lo·ric
py·lo·ri·ste·no·sis
py·lo·ri·tis
py·lo·ro·di·la·tor
py·lo·ro·di·o·sis
py·lo·ro·du·o·de·ni·tis
py·lo·ro·gas·trec·to·my
py·lo·ro·my·ot·o·my
py·lo·ro·plas·ty
   double p.
   Finney p.
   Heineke-Mikulicz p.
py·lo·ros·co·py
py·lo·ro·spasm
   congenital p.
   reflex p.

py·lo·ro·ste·no·sis
py·lo·ros·to·my
py·lo·rot·o·my
py·lo·rus
pyo·ar·thro·sis
pyo·blen·nor·rhea
pyo·ca·lix
pyo·cele
   frontal sinus p.
pyo·ce·lia
pyo·ceph·a·lus
pyo·che·zia
pyo·cin
pyo·coc·cic
pyo·coc·cus
pyo·col·po·cele
pyo·col·pos
pyo·cy·an·ic
pyo·cy·a·nin
pyo·cy·a·no·gen·ic
pyo·cy·a·no·sis
pyo·cyst
pyo·cys·tis
pyo·cyte
pyo·der·ma
   chancriform p.
   p. chancriforme faciei
   p. faciale
   p. gangrenosum
   malignant p.
   oral p.
   p. vegetans
   verrucous p.
pyo·der·ma·ti·tis
   p. vegetans
pyo·der·ma·to·sis
pyo·der·mia
pyo·fe·cia
pyo·gen·e·sis
pyo·gen·ic
py·og·e·nous
pyo·he·mia
pyo·he·mo·tho·rax
pyo·hy·dro·ne·phro·sis
py·oid
pyo·lab·y·rin·thi·tis
pyo·me·tra
pyo·me·tri·tis

pyo·me·tri·um
pyo·my·o·ma
pyo·myo·si·tis
    tropical p.
pyo·ne·phri·tis
pyo·neph·ro·li·thi·a·sis
pyo·neph·ro·sis
    calculous p.
pyo·ne·phrot·ic
pyo-ovar·i·um
pyo·pen
pyo·peri·car·di·tis
pyo·peri·car·di·um
pyo·peri·to·ne·um
pyo·peri·to·ni·tis
pyo·pha·gia
py·oph·thal·mia
py·oph·thal·mi·tis
pyo·phy·lac·tic
pyo·phy·so·me·tra
pyo·pla·nia
pyo·pneu·mo·cho·le·cys·ti·tis
pyo·pneu·mo·cyst
pyo·pneu·mo·hep·a·ti·tis
pyo·pneu·mo·peri·car·di·tis
pyo·pneu·mo·peri·car·di·um
pyo·pneu·mo·peri·to·ne·um
pyo·pneu·mo·peri·to·ni·tis
pyo·pneu·mo·tho·rax
pyo·poi·e·sis
pyo·poi·et·ic
py·op·ty·sis
pyo·py·elec·ta·sis
py·or·rhea
    p. alveolaris
    Schmutz p.
py·or·rhe·al
pyo·ru·bin
pyo·sal·pin·gi·tis
pyo·sal·pin·go-ooph·o·ri·tis
pyo·sal·pin·go-oo·the·ci·tis
pyo·sal·pinx
pyo·sap·re·mia
pyo·scle·ro·sis
pyo·sep·ti·ce·mia
py·o·sis
    p. of Corlett
    p. of Manson

pyo·sper·mia
pyo·stat·ic
pyo·sto·ma·ti·tis
    p. vegetans
pyo·tho·rax
    subphrenic p.
pyo·tox·in·emia
pyo·um·bil·i·cus
pyo·ura·chus
pyo·ure·ter
pyo·ve·sic·u·lo·sis
pyo·xan·thine
pyo·xan·those
pyr·a·brom
py·ra·cin
py·ra·hex·yl
Pyr·a·lis
    P. farinalis
pyr·a·mid
    age-sex p.
    p. of cerebellum
    p. of Ferrein
    p's of kidney
    Lalouette's p.
    p. of light
    Malacarne's p.
    p's of Malpighi
    p. of medulla oblongata
    medullary p.
    olfactory p.
    petrous p.
    population p.
    renal p's
    star p.
    p. of temporal bone
    p. of temporal bone, of
      Arnold
    p. of thyroid
    p. of tympanum
    p. of vermis
    p. of vestibule
    Wistar's p's
py·ram·i·dal
py·ram·i·da·le
py·ram·i·da·lis
py·ram·i·des
Py·ram·i·don
py·ram·i·dot·o·my

py·ram·i·dot·o·my
   spinal p.
pyr·a·mis *pl.* py·ram·i·des
   p. cerebelli
   pyramides Malpighii
   p. medullae oblongatae
   p. ossis temporalis
   pyramides renales
   pyramides renales
      [Malpighii]
   p. vermis
   p. vestibuli
py·ran
py·ra·nis·a·mine mal·e·ate
py·ra·nose
py·ran·o·side
py·ran·tel
   p. pamoate
   p. tartrate
py·ran·yl
py·ra·thi·a·zine hy·dro·chlo·
   ride
py·ra·zin·amide
py·ra·zine
py·ra·zo·fur·in
pyr·az·o·lone
py·rec·tic
py·rene
py·re·noid
py·re·nol·y·sis
Py·re·no·my·ce·tes
py·re·ther·a·py
py·re·thrin
py·re·thron
py·re·thrum
py·ret·ic
py·ret·o·gen
py·re·to·gen·e·sis
py·re·to·ge·net·ic
py·re·to·gen·ic
py·re·tog·e·nous
py·re·tog·ra·phy
py·re·tol·o·gy
py·re·tol·y·sis
py·re·to·ther·a·py
py·re·to·ty·pho·sis
py·rex·ia *pl.* py·rex·iae
   heat p.

py·rex·ia *(continued)*
   Pel-Ebstein p.
py·rex·i·al
py·rex·in
py·rex·i·o·gen·ic
Pyr·i·ben·za·mine
pyr·i·dine
Py·rid·i·um
pyr·i·do·stig·mine bro·mide
pyr·i·dox·al
   p. kinase
   p. phosphate
pyr·i·dox·amine
   p. phosphate
pyr·i·dox·ic acid
pyr·i·dox·i·lat·ed
pyr·i·dox·ine
   p. dehydrogenase
   p. hydrochloride
pyr·i·dox·ol
   p. phosphate
pyr·i·form
pyr·il·amine mal·e·ate
pyr·i·meth·amine
py·rim·i·dine
pyr·in·o·line
pyr·i·thi·amine
pyr·i·thi·one zinc
py·ro·bo·rate
py·ro·bo·ric acid
py·ro·cat·e·chin
py·ro·cat·e·chol
py·ro·dex·trin
py·ro·gal·lol
py·ro·gen
   bacterial p.
   endogenous p.
   exogenous p's
   leukocytic p.
py·ro·ge·net·ic
py·ro·gen·ic
py·rog·e·nous
py·ro·glob·u·lin
py·ro·glob·u·lin·emia
py·ro·glu·ta·mase
py·ro·glu·ta·mate
py·ro·glu·ta·mate hy·dro·lase
py·ro·glu·tam·ic acid

py·ro·lag·nia
py·ro·lig·ne·ous
py·rol·y·sis
py·ro·ma·nia
    erotic p.
py·rom·e·ter
py·rone
Py·ro·nil
py·ro·nin
    p. B
    p. G
    p. Y
py·ro·nine
py·ro·nin·o·phil·ia
py·ro·nino·phil·ic
py·ro·pho·bia
py·ro·phos
py·ro·phos·pha·tase
    inorganic p.
py·ro·phos·phate
    ferric p.
    stannous p.
py·ro·phos·phate ri·
  bose-P-syn·the·tase
py·ro·phos·pho·ki·nase
py·ro·phos·pho·mev·a·lon·
    ate
py·ro·phos·pho·ric acid
py·ro·phos·phor·ol·y·sis
py·ro·phos·pho·ryl·ase
py·ro·phos·pho·trans·fer·ase
py·ro·sis

py·rot·ic
pyro·val·er·one hy·dro·chlo·
    ride
pyr·ox·amine mal·e·ate
py·roxy·lin
pyr·ro·bu·ta·mine phos·phate
pyr·ro·caine
    p. hydrochloride
pyr·role
pyr·rol·i·dine
pyr·ro·line
Δ^1-pyr·ro·line-5-car·box·y·
    late de·hy·dro·gen·ase
pyr·ro·line-5-car·box·y·late
    re·duc·tase
pyr·rol·ni·trin
pyr·ro·lo·por·phyr·ia
py·ru·vate
py·ru·vate car·box·y·lase
py·ru·vate de·car·box·y·lase
py·ru·vate de·hy·dro·gen·ase
py·ru·ve·mia
py·ru·vic acid
pyr·vin·i·um pam·o·ate
pyth·i·o·sis
py·tho·gen·e·sis
py·tho·gen·ic
py·thog·e·nous
py·u·ria
    abacterial p.
    miliary p.
PZI — protamine zinc insulin

Q

Q — ubiquinone
Q — electric charge
    heat
    reaction quotient
Q_{10} — temperature coefficient
    ubiquinone
$\dot{Q}$ — rate of blood flow

q — long arm of a
    chromosome
q. — L. quaque (each, every)
q — electric charge
    probability of an
        alternative event
    ubiquinone

q.d. — L. quaque die (every day)

Q fever

q.h. — L. quaque hora (every hour)

q.i.d. — L. quater in die (four times a day)

q.l. — L. quantum libet (as much as desired)

qns — quantity not sufficient

q.o.d. — every other day

q.p. — L. quantum placeat (as much as desired)

q.q.h. — L. quaque quarta hora (every four hours)

Qq. hor. — L. quaque hora (every hour)

q.s. — L. quantum satis (sufficient quantity)

q-sort

q.suff. — L. quantum sufficit (as much as suffices)

Quaa·lude

quack·ery

quack·sal·ver

quad·er

Quad·ra·moid

quad·ran·gle

quad·ran·gu·lar

quad·rant
dental q.

quad·ran·tal

quad·rant·an·o·pia

quad·rant·an·op·sia

quad·ran·tec·to·my

quad·rate

quad·ra·ti·pro·na·tor

quad·ra·tus

qua·dri·ba·sic

qua·dri·ceps

qua·dri·ceps·plas·ty

qua·dri·cus·pid

qua·dri·den·tate

qua·dri·dig·i·tate

quad·ri·gem·i·nal

quad·ri·ge·mi·num *pl.* quad·ri·ge·mi·na

quad·ri·gem·i·nus

quad·ri·lat·er·al
Celsus' q.

quad·ri·loc·u·lar

quad·rip·a·ra

quad·ri·pa·re·sis

quad·ri·par·tite

quad·ri·ple·gia

quad·ri·ple·gic

quad·ri·po·lar

quad·ri·sect

quad·ri·sec·tion

quad·ri·tu·ber·cu·lar

quad·ri·va·lent

quad·ru·ped

quadrupl. — L. quadruplicato (four times as much)

quad·rup·let

Quain's degeneration

Quain's fatty heart

qua·le

qua·lim·e·ter

qual·i·ta·tive

qual·i·tive

qual·i·ty

quan·ta

quan·tal

quan·tile

quan·tim·e·ter

quan·ti·tate

quan·ti·ta·tive

quan·ti·ty
vectorial q.

quan·ti·za·tion

quan·tized

quan·tum *pl.* quan·ta
q. of light

quan·tum li·bet

quan·tum pla·cet

quan·tum sat·is

quan·tum suf·fi·cit

quan·tum vis

quar·an·tine

quart

quar·tan
double q.
triple q.

quar·ta·na
   q. duplex
   q. triplex
quar·ter
   false q.
quar·tet
quar·tile
quar·tip·a·ra
quar·ti·sect
quar·ti·ster·nal
quartz
Quar·zan
qua·si·dip·loid
qua·si·dom·i·nance
qua·si·dom·i·nant
quas·sa·tion
Quas·sia
quas·sia
quas·sin
Quat. — L. quattuor (four)
qua·ter in die
qua·ter·nary
Qua·tre·fages' angle
qua·ze·pam
qua·zo·dine
Queck·en·stedt's phenomenon
Queck·en·stedt's sign
Queck·en·stedt's test
Queck·en·stedt-Stoo·key test
Quel·i·cin
quel·lung
quench·ing
   color q.
   fluorescence q.
   thermal q.
Qué·nu-Mu·ret sign
Qué·nu plex·us
quer·ce·tin
   q.-3-rutinoside
Quer·cus
Quer·vain's disease
Ques·tran
Quet·e·let's rule
Que·venne's iron
Quey·rat's erythroplasia
Quick test
quick·lime
quick·en·ing

Quide
quil·la·ia
quil·lain
Quil·la·ja
quin·a·crine hy·dro·chlo·ride
quin·al·bar·bi·tone
quin·al·dic acid
quin·al·din·ic acid
quin·a·quina
Quincke's disease
Quincke's edema
Quincke's meningitis
Quincke's pulse
Quincke's puncture
Quincke's sign
quin·es·trol
quin·eth·a·zone
quin·fa·mide
quin·ges·ta·nol ac·e·tate
quin·ges·trone
quin·hy·drone
quin·ic acid
Quin·i·dex
quin·i·dine
   q. gluconate
   q. polygalacturonate
   q. sulfate
qui·nine
   β-q.
   q. and urea hydrochloride
   q. dihydrochloride
   q. ethylcarbonate
   q. hydrochloride
   q. sulfate
qui·nin·ism
qui·nin·ize
quin·o·cide hy·dro·chlo·ride
quin·oid
quin·ol
quin·o·line
quin·o·lone
qui·none
quin·o·noid
Quin·o·ra
quin·o·vin
Quinq. — L. quinque (five)
quin·que·cus·pid
quin·que·tu·ber·cu·lar

quin·que·va·lent
quin·qui·na
quin·sy
    lingual q.
Quint. — L. quintus (fifth)
quin·tan
quin·tes·sence
quin·tile
quin·tip·a·ra
quin·ti·ster·nal
quin·tup·let
quit·tor
    simple q.
    skin q.
    subhorny q.
    tendinous q.
quo·ad vi·tam
Quo·tane
Quotid. — L. quotidie (daily)
quo·tid·i·an

quo·tient
    achievement q.
    albumin q.
    Ayala's q.
    blood q.
    caloric q.
    D q.
    D/N (dextrose/nitrogen) q.
    developmental q.
    growth q.
    intelligence q.
    phonation q.
    protein q.
    rachidian q.
    reaction q.
    respiratory q.
    spinal q.
q.v. — L. quantum vis (as much as you please)
    quod vide (which see)

R

R — Behnkin's unit
    radical
    Rankine scale
    rate
    Réaumur scale
    rectal
    resistance
    respiration
    respiratory exchange ratio
    rhythm
    right
    roentgen
    rough (colony)
    rub
R. — L. remotum (far)
R — gas constant
    resistance
℞ — L. recipe (take)
R_A — airway resistance

R_{AW} — airway resistance
R_e — Reynold's number
r — drug resistance
    ring chromosome
r — correlation coefficient
    distance radius
    drug resistance
r_s — Spearman's rank correlation coefficient
ρ — correlation coefficient
    electric charge density
    mass density
Raa·be's test
rab·bet·ting
rab·bit·pox
rab·e·la·i·sin
ra·bi·ci·dal
rab·id

ra·bies
    dumb r.
    furious r.
    paralytic r.
    sullen r.
ra·bi·form
ra·ce·mase
ra·ce·mate
ra·ce·me·thi·o·nine
ra·ce·mic
ra·ce·mi·za·tion
rac·e·mose
ra·ceph·e·drine hy·dro·chlo·ride
rac·e·phen·i·col
ra·chi·al
ra·chi·al·bu·mi·nim·e·ter
ra·chi·al·bu·mi·nim·e·try
ra·chi·al·gia
ra·chi·an·al·ge·sia
ra·chi·an·es·the·sia
ra·chi·cen·te·sis
ra·chid·i·al
ra·chid·i·an
ra·chi·graph
ra·chil·y·sis
ra·chio·camp·sis
ra·chio·cen·te·sis
ra·chio·chy·sis
ra·chi·odyn·ia
ra·chio·ky·pho·sis
ra·chi·om·e·ter
ra·chio·my·eli·tis
ra·chi·op·a·gus
ra·chi·op·a·thy
ra·chio·sco·li·o·sis
ra·chio·tome
ra·chi·ot·o·my
ra·chip·a·gus
ra·chi·re·sis·tance
ra·chi·re·sis·tant
ra·chis
ra·chis·ag·ra
ra·chis·chi·sis
    r. partialis
    r. posterior
    r. totalis
ra·chi·sen·si·bil·i·ty

ra·chi·sen·si·ble
ra·chit·ic
ra·chi·tis
    r. fetalis annularis
    r. fetalis micromelica
    r. tarda
rach·i·tism
ra·chit·o·gen·ic
rach·i·tome
ra·chit·o·my
ra·cial
Ra·cine syndrome
rad — absorbed dose of ionizing radiation
    radian
rad. — L. radix (root)
ra·dar·ky·mo·gram
ra·dar·ky·mog·ra·phy
ra·dec·to·my
ra·di·a·bil·i·ty
ra·di·a·ble
ra·di·ad
ra·di·al
ra·di·a·lis
ra·di·an
ra·di·ant
ra·di·ate
ra·di·a·ther·my
ra·di·a·tio *pl.* ra·di·a·ti·o·nes
    r. acustica
    r. corporis callosi
    r. corporis striati
    r. optica
    r. pyramidalis
    radiationes thalamicae anteriores
    radiationes thalamicae centrales
    radiationes thalamicae posteriores
ra·di·a·tion
    α-r.
    acoustic r.
    adaptive r.
    alpha r.
    annihilation r.
    auditory r.
    β-r.

ra·di·a·tion *(continued)*
  background r.
  backscattered r.
  beta r.
  braking r.
  Cerenkov r.
  characteristic r.
  r. of corpus callosum
  corpuscular r's
  electromagnetic r.
  fractionated r.
  γ-r.
  gamma r.
  geniculocalcarine r.
  geniculotemporal r.
  r. of Gratiolet
  hard r.
  heterogeneous r.
  homogeneous r.
  Huldshinsky's r.
  infrared r.
  interstitial r.
  ionizing r.
  irritative r.
  mitogenetic r.
  mitogenic r.
  monochromatic r.
  monoenergetic r.
  nuclear r.
  occipitothalamic r.
  optic r.
  photochemical r.
  protracted r.
  pyramidal r.
  Rollier's r.
  striatothalamic r.
  supervoltage r.
  tegmental r.
  thalamic r.
  thalamic r's, anterior
  thalamic r's, central
  thalamic r's, posterior
  thalamic r's, superior
  thalamotemporal r.
  useful-beam r.
  visual r.
  Wernicke's r.
  white r.

ra·di·a·ti·o·nes
rad·i·cal
  acid r.
  alcohol r.
  color r.
  free r.
rad·i·cal-ion
rad·i·ces
ra·dic·i·form
rad·i·cle
rad·i·cot·o·my
ra·dic·u·la
ra·dic·u·lal·gia
ra·dic·u·lar
ra·dic·u·lec·to·my
ra·dic·u·li·tis
  spinal r.
ra·dic·u·lo·gan·gli·o·ni·tis
ra·dic·u·lo·med·ul·lary
ra·dic·u·lo·me·nin·go·my·eli·tis
ra·dic·u·lo·my·elop·a·thy
ra·dic·u·lo·neu·ri·tis
ra·dic·u·lo·neu·rop·a·thy
  hypertrophic interstitial r.
ra·dic·u·lop·a·thy
  brachial r.
  cervical r.
  spinal r.
  spondylotic caudal r.
ra·di·ec·to·my
ra·dii
ra·dio·ab·la·tion
ra·dio·ac·tive
ra·dio·ac·tiv·i·ty
  artificial r.
  induced r.
  natural r.
ra·dio·al·ler·go·sor·bent
ra·dio·au·to·gram
ra·dio·au·to·graph
ra·dio·au·tog·ra·phy
ra·dio·bi·cip·i·tal
ra·dio·bi·o·log·i·cal
ra·dio·bi·ol·o·gist
ra·dio·bi·ol·o·gy
ra·dio·cal·ci·um
ra·dio·car·bon

ra·dio·car·ci·no·gen·e·sis
ra·dio·car·dio·gram
ra·dio·car·di·og·ra·phy
ra·dio·car·pal
ra·dio·car·pus
ra·dio·chem·is·try
ra·dio·chro·ism
ra·dio·cin·e·mato·graph
ra·dio·co·balt
ra·dio·col·loids
ra·dio·cur·a·ble
ra·dio·cys·ti·tis
ra·di·ode
ra·dio·dense
ra·dio·den·si·ty
ra·dio·der·ma·ti·tis
ra·dio·di·ag·no·sis
ra·dio·di·ag·nos·tics
ra·dio·dig·i·tal
ra·dio·don·tics
ra·di·odon·tist
ra·dio·do·sim·e·try
ra·dio·ecol·o·gy
ra·dio·elec·tro·car·dio·gram
ra·dio·elec·tro·car·di·o·graph
ra·dio·elec·tro·car·di·og·ra·
  phy
ra·dio·el·e·ment
ra·dio·en·ceph·a·lo·gram
ra·dio·en·ceph·a·log·ra·phy
ra·dio·epi·der·mi·tis
ra·dio·ep·i·the·li·o·ma
ra·dio·epi·the·li·tis
ra·dio·fre·quen·cy
ra·dio·gal·li·um
ra·dio·gen·e·sis
ra·di·o·gen·ic
ra·dio·gold
ra·dio·gram
ra·dio·graph
    bite-wing r.
    cephalometric r.
    extraoral r.
    intraoral r.
    lateral oblique jaw r.
    lateral ramus r.
    lateral skull r.
    maxillary sinus r.

ra·dio·graph *(continued)*
    occlusal r.
    panoramic r.
    periapical r.
    submental vertex r.
    survey r.
    Towne projection r.
    Waters view r.
ra·dio·graph·ic
ra·di·og·ra·phy
    body section r.
    digital r.
    double contrast r.
    electron r.
    mass r.
    miniature r., mass
    mucosal relief r.
    neutron r.
    panoramic r.
    sectional r.
    selective r.
    serial r.
    spot-film r.
ra·dio·hu·mer·al
ra·dio·im·mu·ni·ty
ra·dio·im·mu·no·as·say
ra·dio·im·mu·no·de·tec·tion
ra·dio·im·mu·no·dif·fu·sion
ra·dio·im·mu·no·elec·tro·
  pho·re·sis
ra·dio·im·mu·no·im·ag·ing
ra·dio·im·mu·no·pre·cip·i·
  ta·tion
ra·dio·im·mu·no·scin·tig·ra·
  phy
ra·dio·im·mu·no·sor·bent
ra·dio·in·di·ca·tor
ra·dio·io·din·at·ed
ra·dio·io·dine
ra·dio·iron
ra·dio·iso·tope
    carrier-free r.
ra·dio·ky·mog·ra·phy
ra·dio·lead
ra·dio·le·sion
ra·dio·li·gand
ra·di·o·log·ic
ra·di·o·log·i·cal

ra·di·ol·o·gist
  dental r.
ra·di·ol·o·gy
  dental r.
  nuclear r.
  oral r.
ra·dio·lu·cen·cy
ra·dio·lu·cent
ra·di·o·lus
ra·di·ol·y·sis
ra·di·om·e·ter
ra·dio·mi·crom·e·ter
ra·dio·mi·met·ic
ra·dio·mus·cu·lar
ra·dio·mu·ta·tion
ra·dio·ne·cro·sis
ra·dio·neph·rog·ra·phy
ra·dio·neu·ri·tis
ra·di·o·ni·tro·gen
ra·dio·nu·clide
  metastable r.
  parent r.
ra·dio-opac·i·ty
ra·di·opac·i·ty
ra·dio·pal·mar
ra·di·opaque
ra·dio·par·en·cy
ra·dio·par·ent
ra·dio·pa·thol·o·gy
ra·dio·pel·vim·e·try
ra·dio·phar·ma·ceu·ti·cal
ra·dio·phar·ma·col·o·gy
ra·dio·phar·ma·cy
ra·dio·pho·bia
ra·dio·phos·pho·rus
ra·dio·pho·tog·ra·phy
ra·dio·phy·lax·is
ra·dio·phys·ics
ra·dio·plas·tic
ra·dio·po·tas·si·um
ra·dio·po·ten·ti·a·tion
ra·dio·prax·is
ra·dio·pul·mo·nog·ra·phy
ra·dio·re·ac·tion
ra·dio·re·cep·tor
ra·dio·re·nog·ra·phy
ra·dio·re·sis·tance
ra·dio·re·sis·tant

ra·dio·re·spon·sive
ra·di·os·co·py
ra·dio·sen·si·bil·i·ty
ra·dio·sen·si·tive
ra·dio·sen·si·tive·ness
ra·dio·sen·si·tiv·i·ty
ra·dio·sen·si·ti·zer
ra·dio·so·di·um
ra·dio·spi·rom·e·try
ra·dio·ster·eo·as·say
ra·dio·ste·re·os·co·py
ra·dio·stron·ti·um
ra·dio·sul·fur
ra·dio·tel·em·e·try
ra·dio·tel·lu·ri·um
ra·dio·than·a·tol·o·gy
ra·dio·ther·a·peu·tics
ra·dio·ther·a·pist
ra·dio·ther·a·py
  arc r.
  contact r.
  fast neutron r.
  interstitial r.
  intracavitary r.
  supervoltage r.
  whole-body r.
ra·dio·ther·my
ra·dio·thy·rox·ine
ra·di·ot·o·my
ra·dio·tox·emia
ra·dio·tra·cer
ra·dio·trans·par·en·cy
ra·dio·trans·par·ent
ra·di·o·trop·ic
ra·di·ot·ro·pism
ra·dio·ul·nar
ra·di·sec·to·my
ra·di·um
ra·di·us *pl.* ra·dii
  r. curvus
  r. fixus
  radii of lens
  radii lentis
  Van der Waals r.
ra·dix *pl.* ra·di·ces
  r. arcus vertebrae
  r. clinica
  r. dentis

ra·dix *(continued)*
  r. facialis
  r. linguae
  r. mesenterii
  r. nasi
  r. penis
  r. pili
  r. pulmonis
  r. unguis
ra·don
Ra·do·vi·ci reflex
Ra·do·vi·ci sign
Rae·der syndrome
raf·fi·nose
ra·fox·a·nide
rage
  sham r.
rag·o·cyte
Rah·nel·la
RAI — radioactive iodine
ra·i·gan
Rail·li·e·ti·na
rail·li·e·ti·ni·a·sis
Raim·iste's sign
Rai·ney's tube
Rai·ney's tubule
rale
  amphoric r.
  atelectatic r.
  border r.
  bronchial r.
  bubbling r.
  cavernous r.
  cellophane r.
  clicking r.
  collapse r.
  consonating r.
  crackling r.
  crepitant r.
  dry r.
  extrathoracic r.
  gurgling r.
  guttural r.
  r. indux
  laryngeal r.
  marginal r.
  metallic r.
  moist r.

rale *(continued)*
  mucous r.
  r. muqueux
  pleural r.
  r. redux
  r. de retour
  sibilant r.
  sonorous r.
  subcrepitant r.
  tracheal r.
  Velcro r.
  vesicular r.
  whistling r.
Ralfe's test
ra·mal
Ram·an effect
RAMC — Royal Army
  Medical Corps
ramex
ra·mi
ram·i·cot·o·my
ram·i·fi·ca·tion
rami·form
ram·i·fy
rami·sec·tion
ram·i·sec·to·my
ram·itis
ra·mol·lisse·ment
Ra·mon's flocculation test
Ra·món y Ca·jal, Santiago
Ram·ond's sign
ra·mose
ram·part
  maxillary r.
Ram·say Hunt disease
Ram·say Hunt syndrome
Rams·den's eyepiece
Ram·stedt operation
ram·u·lus *pl.* ram·u·li
ra·mus *pl.* ra·mi
  r. acetabularis
  r. acromialis
  rami alveolares
  r. anastomoticus
  r. anterior
  rami arteriosi
  rami articulares
  r. ascendens

ra·mus *(continued)*
r. atrialis
rami atrioventriculares
r. auricularis
rami bronchiales
rami buccales
rami calcanei
r. calcarinus
rami capsulae internae
rami capsulares
rami cardiaci
rami caroticotympanici
r. carpalis dorsalis
r. carpalis palmaris
r. carpeus dorsalis
r. carpeus palmaris
rami caudati
rami celiaci
rami centrales
 anteromediales
r. chiasmaticus
rami choroidei mediales
rami choroidei posteriores
rami choroidei ventriculi
 lateralis
rami choroidei ventriculi
 tertii
r. choroideus ventriculi
 quarti
r. cingularis
r. circumflexus
r. clavicularis
r. clivi
r. cochlearis
rami coeliaci
r. colicus
r. collateralis
r. colli
r. communicans
r. communicans albus
r. communicans cochlearis
r. communicans griseus
rami corporis amygdaloidei
r. corporis callosi dorsalis
rami corporis geniculati
 lateralis
r. costalis lateralis
r. cricothyroideus

ra·mus *(continued)*
r. cutaneus
r. deltoideus
rami dentales
r. descendens
r. dexter
r. digastricus
r. dorsalis
rami duodenales
rami epididymales
rami epiploici
rami esophagei
r. externus
rami fauciales
r. femoralis
r. frontalis
rami ganglionares
r. ganglionis trigemini
rami gastrici
r. genitalis
rami gingivales
r. glandularis
rami globi pallidi
rami helicini
rami hepatici
r. hyoideus
r. hypothalamicus
r. ilealis
r. iliacus
r. inferior
r. infrahyoideus
r. infrapatellaris
rami inguinales
rami intercostales
rami interganglionares
r. internus
r. interventricularis
 anterior
r. interventricularis
 posterior
rami interventriculares
 septales
r. of ischium
rami isthmi faucium
r. of jaw
rami labiales anteriores
rami labiales inferiores
rami labiales posteriores

ra·mus *(continued)*
  rami labiales superiores
  rami laryngopharyngei
  r. lateralis
  rami lienales
  r. lingualis
  r. lumbalis
  rami malleolares
  rami mammarii
  rami mammarii externi
  rami mammarii laterales
  rami mammarii mediales
  r. of mandible
  r. mandibulae
  r. marginalis dexter
  r. marginalis mandibulae
  r. marginalis sinister
  r. marginalis tentorii
  r. mastoideus
  r. meatus acustici interni
  r. medialis
  rami mediastinales
  rami ad medullam
    oblongatam
  rami medullares
  r. membranae tympani
  r. meningeus
  r. meningeus accessorius
  r. meningeus anterior
  r. meningeus medius
  r. meningeus posterior
  r. meningeus recurrens
  r. mentalis
  rami musculares
  r. mylohyoideus
  rami nasales anteriores
  rami nasales externi
  rami nasales interni
  rami nasales laterales
  rami nasales mediales
  rami nasales posteriores
    inferiores
  rami nasales posteriores
    superiores
  r. nasociliaris
  r. nervi oculomotorii
  r. nodi atrioventricularis
  r. nodi sinuatrialis

ra·mus *(continued)*
  rami nuclei rubris
  rami nucleorum
    hypothalamicorum
  r. obturatorius
  r. occipitalis
  r. occipitotemporalis
  rami oesophagei
  rami omentales
  r. orbitalis
  r. orbitofrontalis
  r. ossis ischii
  r. ossis pubis
  r. ovaricus
  r. ovarii
  r. palmaris
  r. palmaris profundus
  r. palmaris superficialis
  rami palpebrales
  rami palpebrales inferiores
  r. palpebralis
  rami pancreatici
  rami parietales
  r. parieto-occipitalis
  r. parotideus
  rami pectorales
  rami pedunculares
  r. perforans
  rami perforantes
  rami pericardiaci
  rami peridentales
  rami perineales
  r. petrosus
  r. petrosus superficialis
  rami pharyngeales
  r. pharyngeus
  rami phrenicoabdominales
  r. plantaris profundus
  rami ad pontem
  r. posterior
  r. posterolateralis dexter
  r. profundus
  rami prostatici
  rami pterygoidei
  r. pubicus
  r. of pubis
  r. of pubis, ascending
  r. of pubis, descending

ra·mus *(continued)*
  rami pulmonales
  rami radiculares
  r. renalis
  rami sacrales laterales
  r. saphenus
  rami scrotales anteriores
  rami scrotales posteriores
  rami septales anteriores
  rami septales posteriores
  r. septi nasi
  r. sinister
  r. sinus carotici
  r. sinus cavernosi
  rami spinales
  rami splenici
  r. stapedius
  rami sternales
  r. sternocleidomastoideus
  r. stylohyoideus
  r. stylopharyngeus
  rami subendocardiales
  rami submaxillares
  rami subscapulares
  rami substantiae nigrae
  rami substantiae
   perforatae anterioris
  r. superficialis
  r. superior
  r. suprahyoideus
  rami suprarenales
  r. sympatheticus
  r. sympathicus
  rami temporales
  rami temporales anteriores
  rami temporales
   intermedii
  r. temporales posteriores
  r. tentorii basalis
  r. tentorii marginalis
  rami thalamici
  rami thymici
  r. thyrohyoideus
  r. tonsillae
  r. tonsillaris
  r. tentorii
  rami tracheales
  rami tractus optici

ra·mus *(continued)*
  r. transversus
  rami trigeminales et
   trochleares
  r. tubalis
  r. tubarius
  rami tuberis cinerei
  r. ulnaris
  rami ureterici
  rami vaginales
  rami ventrales
  r. ventriculi sinistri
   posterior
  rami vestibulares
  rami viscerales
  r. volaris
  r. volaris profundus
  r. volaris superficialis
  rami zygomatici
  r. zygomaticofacialis
  r. zygomaticotemporalis
ran·cid
ran·cid·i·fy
ran·cid·i·ty
Ran·dall's plaques
Ran·dolph's test
ran·dom
ran·dom·iza·tion
ran·dom·ize
range
  r. of accommodation
  r. of audibility
  audiofrequency r.
  dynamic r.
  interquartile r.
  r. of motion
  normal r.
  r. of normal
  reference r.
  thermal comfort r.
ran·i·my·cin
ra·nine
ra·ni·ti·dine
rank
Ranke's angle
Ranke's complex
Ranke's formula
Ranke's stages

Ran·so·hoff sign
ran·u·la
   pancreatic r.
ran·u·lar
Ra·nun·cu·lus
Ran·vier's crosses
Ran·vier's disk
Ran·vier's node
Ran·vier's segment
Ra·oult's law
rape
   statutory r.
ra·pha·nia
ra·phe *pl.* ra·phae
   abdominal r.
   amniotic r.
   r. of ampulla
   r. anococcygea
   anococcygeal r.
   anogenital r.
   buccal r.
   r. corporis callosi
   horizontal r. of eye
   longitudinal r. of tongue
   median r. of medulla
     oblongata
   r. mediana medullae
     oblongatae
   median r. of neck, posterior
   median r. of perineum
   median r. of pons
   r. mediana pontina
   r. of medulla oblongata
   r. medullae oblongatae
   r. mesencephali
   r. palati
   palatine r.
   palpebral r., lateral
   r. palpebralis lateralis
   r. penis
   perineal r.
   r. perinealis
   r. perinei
   r. of perineum
   r. pharyngis
   r. of pharynx
   r. of pons
   r. pontis

ra·phe *(continued)*
   pterygomandibular r.
   r. pterygomandibularis
   r. scroti
   r. of scrotum
rap·port
rap·tus
rar·e·fac·tion
   bone r.
RAS — reticular activating
   system
ras·ce·ta
rash
   ammonia r.
   antitoxin r.
   astacoid r.
   brown-tail r.
   butterfly r.
   canker r.
   caterpillar r.
   diaper r.
   drug r.
   enema r.
   heat r.
   heliotrope r.
   hydatid r.
   lobster r.
   medicinal r.
   mulberry r.
   nettle r.
   rose r.
   scarlet r.
   serum r.
   summer r.
   vaccination r.
   wandering r.
Rash·kind procedure
ra·sion
Ras·mus·sen's aneurysm
ras·pa·to·ry
RAST — radioallergosorbent
   test
Ras·tel·li's operation
rast·er
ra·su·ra
rat
   albino r.
   BBr.

rat *(continued)*
- black r.
- brown r.
- Egyptian r.
- fa/fa r.
- Fischer 344 r.
- Holtzman r.
- Long-Evans r.
- Norwegian gray r.
- roof r.
- Sprague-Dawley r.
- white r.
- Wistar r.
- wood r.
- Zucker r.

rate
- abortion r.
- absorption r.
- adjusted r.
- adjusted death r.
- admission r.
- age-specific r.
- attack r.
- background counting r.
- basal metabolic r.
- birth r.
- Boeckh's r.
- Boeckh-Kuczynski r.
- carrier r.
- case r.
- case fatality r.
- cause-specific death r.
- circulation r.
- conduction r.
- corrected survival r.
- counting r.
- crude r.
- crude annual general death r.
- crude annual live birth r.
- crude survival r.
- death r.
- DEF r.
- discharge r.
- DMF r.
- dose r.
- early neonatal death r.
- effective fertility r.

rate *(continued)*
- equivalent average death r.
- erythrocyte sedimentation r. (ESR)
- false-negative r.
- false-positive r.
- fatality r.
- female reproduction r.
- fertility r.
- fetal death r.
- five-year survival r.
- frame r.
- glomerular filtration r. (GFR)
- general fertility r.
- gross female reproduction r.
- growth r.
- heart r.
- incidence r.
- infant mortality r.
- instantaneous growth r.
- instantaneous r.
- Kuczynski's r.
- lethality r.
- marital fertility r.
- marriage r.
- maternal mortality r.
- mendelian r.
- morbidity r.
- mortality r.
- mutation r.
- natality r.
- neonatal mortality r.
- net female reproductive r.
- nupitality r.
- oocyst r.
- output exposure r.
- parasite r.
- parity-specific birth r.
- peak expiratory flow r. (PEFR)
- perinatal mortality r.
- population growth r.
- postneonatal death r.
- prevalence r.
- puerperal mortality r.
- pulse r.

rate *(continued)*

    real-time r.
    relative survival r.
    replacement r.
    reproduction r.
    respiration r.
    response r.
    secondary attack r.
    sedimentation r.
    sex-specific death r.
    sickness r.
    single nephron glomerular
      filtration r.
    specific r.
    specific birth r.
    specific death r.
    sporozoite r.
    standardized r.
    standardized death r.
    steroid metabolic clearance
      r.
    steroid production r.
    steroid secretory r.
    survival r.
    stillbirth r.
    total fertility r.
    true r. of natural increase
    Westergren sedimentation
      r.

Rath·ke's column
Rath·ke's cyst
Rath·ke's fold
Rath·ke's pouch
Rath·ke's trabecula
Rath·ke's tumor
rat·i·cide
rat·ing
    behavior r.
ra·tio
    absolute terminal
      innervation r.
    AC/A r.
    A/G r. (albumin/globulin)
    age dependency r.
    ALT/AST r.
    arm r.
    assimilation efficiency r.
    base r.

ra·tio *(continued)*

    base pair r.
    beam uniformity r.
    birth-death r.
    body-weight r.
    cardiothoracic r.
    case fatality r.
    cell color r.
    channels r.
    clinical crown–clinical root
      r.
    concentration r.
    cross-products r.
    cup-to-disk r.
    curative r.
    death-to-case r.
    dependency r.
    D/N r. (dextrose/nitrogen)
    economic dependency r.
    expiratory exchange r.
    extraction r.
    F r.
    fetal death r.
    F:P r.
    galvanic tetanus r.
    general fertility r.
    G/N r. (glucose/nitrogen)
    grid r.
    gyromagnetic r.
    hand r.
    holdaway r.
    human blood r.
    ^{131}I conversion r.
    innervation r.
    inspiratory-expiratory
      phase time r.
    isophane r.
    K:A r.
    karyoplasmic r.
    ketogenic-antiketogenic r.
    L/S (lecithin/sphingo-
      myelin) r.
    M/E (myeloid/erythroid) r.
    masculinity r.
    mendelian r.
    middle-ear areal r.
    myeloid/erythroid r.
    nuclear magnetogyric r.

ra·tio *(continued)*
    nucleocytoplasmic r.
    nucleoplasmic r.
    nutritive r.
    ocular micrometer r.
    odds r.
    ossicular lever r.
    P/O r.
    parity progression r.
    peak-to-total r.
    polymorphonuclear-lympho-
        cyte r.
    potency r.
    primary sex r.
    proportionate mortality r.
        (PMR)
    protein efficiency r.
    radioactive iodide
        conversion r.
    respiratory exchange r.
    risk/benefit r.
    saliva-to-plasma
        radioiodine r.
    sampling r.
    secondary sex r.
    sex r.
    signal-to-noise r.
    standardized morbidity r.
        (SMR)
    standardized mortality r.
        (SMR)
    stimulation r. (SR)
    therapeutic r.
    urea excretion r.
    variance r.
    ventilation-perfusion r.
    zeta sedimentation r. (ZSR)
ra·tion
    basal r.
ra·tion·al
ra·tio·nale
ra·tion·al·iza·tion
rat-tails
rat·tle·snake
Rat·tus
    R. norvegicus
    R. rattus
    R. rattus alexandrinus

Rau's apophysis
Rau's process
Rau·ber's layer
Rauch·fuss' triangle
rausch·brand
Rau·scher's leukemia virus
Rau-Sed
Rau·ser·pa
Rau·wi·loid
Rau·wol·fia
    R. serpentina
rau·wol·fia
    r. serpentina
    r. serpentina, powdered
Rau·zide
Ra·vi·us
ray
    α-r's
    actinic r.
    alpha r's
    anode r's
    antirachitic r's
    astral r.
    β-r's
    beta r's
    Bucky's r's
    caloric r.
    canal r's
    cathode r's
    central r.
    characteristic r's
    characteristic fluorescent
        r's
    chemical r.
    convergent r.
    cortical r.
    cosmic r's
    δ-r's
    delta r's
    digital r.
    direct r.
    divergent r's
    Dorno's r's
    dynamic r's
    erythema-producing r's
    Finsen r's
    fluorescent r's
    γ-r's

ray *(continued)*
    gamma r's
    glass r's
    Goldstein's r's
    grenz r's
    hard r's
    heat r's
    incident r.
    indirect r's
    infrared r's
    infra roentgen r's
    intermediate r's
    Lenard r's
    luminous r's
    Lyman r's
    medullary r.
    necrobiotic r's
    parallel r's
    pigment-producing r's
    polar r.
    positive r's
    primary r's
    reflected r.
    refracted r.
    roentgen r's
    s r's
    Sagnac r's
    scattered r's
    Schumann r's
    secondary r.
    soft r's
    ultraviolet r's
    ultra x-r.
    vital r's
    W r's
    x-r's
Ray·leigh scattering law
Ray·mond's apoplexy
Ray·mond-Ces·tan
Ray·naud's disease
Ray·naud's gangrene
Ray·naud's phenomenon
razor
    Occam's r.
RBBB — right bundle branch
  block
RBC — red blood cell
    red blood (cell) count

RBC IT — red blood cell iron turnover
RBE — relative biological effectiveness
RBF — renal blood flow
RBP — retinol binding protein
RCM — Royal College of Midwives
RCN — Royal College of Nursing
RCOG — Royal College of Obstetricians and Gynaecologists
RCP — Royal College of Physicians
rcp — reciprocal translocation
RCS — Royal College of Surgeons
RCU — red cell utilization
RCVS — Royal College of Veterinary Surgeons
RD — reaction of degeneration
    retinal detachment
rd — rutherford
RDA — recommended daily allowance
RDE — receptor-destroying enzyme
RDS — respiratory distress syndrome
RE — retinol equivalent
    right eye
re·a·ble·ment
re·ab·sorb
re·ab·sorp·tion
    facultative water r.
    intestinal r.
    obligatory water r.
    tubular r.
re·act
re·ac·tance
re·ac·tant
    acute phase r.
re·ac·tion
    accelerated r.
    acetic acid r.
    acid r.

re·ac·tion *(continued)*
   acrosome r.
   acute situational r.
   acute stress r.
   adjustment r.
   alarm r.
   alkaline r.
   allergic r.
   allograft r.
   alphanaphthol r.
   anamnestic r.
   anaphylactic r.
   anaphylactoid r.
   anaplerotic r.
   anergastic r.
   annihilation r.
   anniversary r.
   anthrone r.
   antigen-antibody r.
   antiglobulin r.
   anxiety r.
   argentaffin r.
   Arias-Stella r.
   arousal r.
   Arthus r.
   Arthus-type r.
   Ascoli's r.
   associative r.
   axon r.
   axonal r.
   Bachman's r.
   Bareggi's r.
   Bekhterev's r.
   Bence Jones r.
   bi-bi r.
   biphasic r.
   Bittorf's r.
   biuret r.
   blocking r.
   bombardment r.
   Bordet and Gengou r.
   Brieger's r.
   Brieger's cachexia r.
   browning r's
   Burchard-Liebermann r.
   cadaveric r.
   Calmette's r.
   Cannizzaro's r.

re·ac·tion *(continued)*
   capsular r.
   capsule swelling r.
   capture r.
   carbamino r.
   cascade r.
   Casoni's r.
   chain r.
   Chopra antimony r.
   chromaffin r.
   cockade r.
   colloidal gold r.
   complement fixation r.
   conglutination r.
   consensual r.
   consensual light r.
   conversion r.
   Coombs and Gell r.
   crisis r.
   cross r.
   cutaneous r.
   cytotoxic r.
   Dale r.
   decidual r.
   defense r.
   r. of degeneration
   delayed hypersensitivity r.
   delayed-type
     hypersensitivity r.
   depot r.
   depressive r.
   dermotuberculin r.
   desmoplastic r.
   diazo r.
   Dick r.
   digitonin r.
   displacement r.
   dissociative r.
   dopa r.
   downgrading r.
   duplicative r.
   dysergastic r.
   Ebbecke's r.
   eczematoid r.
   egg yellow r.
   Ehrlich's diazo r.
   electric r.
   eosinopenic r.

re·ac·tion *(continued)*
  Erb's r.
  equilibrium r.
  erythrocyte sedimentation
    r.
  r. of exhaustion
  Fahraeus r.
  Felix-Weil r.
  Fernandez r.
  Feulgen r.
  fight-or-flight r.
  first-order r.
  focal r.
  foreign body r.
  Forssman antigen-antibody
    r.
  fuchsinophil r.
  Gangi's r.
  gemistocytic r.
  Gerhardt's r.
  Ghilarducci's r.
  Gmelin's r.
  Goetsch skin r.
  gold r.
  graft-vs.-host r.
  Grignard's r.
  gross stress r.
  group r.
  Gruber's r.
  Gruber-Widal r.
  Gubler's r.
  Gunning r.
  hemagglutination-inhibition-
    r.
  hemianopic pupillary r.
  hemiopic pupillary r.
  hemoclastic r.
  Henle's r.
  Herxheimer's r.
  heteroclytic r.
  Hill's r.
  heterophil antibody r.
  homograft r.
  hunting r.
  hyperkinetic r. of
    childhood
  hypersensitivity r.
  id r.

re·ac·tion *(continued)*
  r. of identity
  immediate hypersensitivity
    r.
  immune r.
  indirect light r.
  indirect pupillary r.
  indophenol r.
  infusion r.
  intracutaneous r.
  intradermal r.
  involutional psychotic r.
  isomorphous provocative r.
  Ito-Reenstierna r.
  Jaffé r.
  Jarisch-Herxheimer r.
  johnin r.
  Jolly's r.
  Jones-Mote r.
  Keller-Killian r.
  Knaus r.
  Koch's r.
  Kveim's r.
  Lange's r.
  late r.
  lengthening r.
  lepra r.
  lepromin r.
  leukemic r.
  leukemoid r.
  Lewis'r.
  Lieben's r.
  Liebermann-Burchard r.
  local anesthetic r.
  Loeb's decidual r.
  Loewi's r.
  Lohmann r.
  lymphocyte transfer r.
  Machado r.
  Machado-Guerreiro r.
  macrophage disappearance
    r.
  manic-depressive r.
  Mantoux r.
  Marañón's r.
  Marchi's r.
  Mátéfy's r.
  Millon's r.

re·ac·tion *(continued)*
- Mitsuda r.
- mixed agglutination r.
- mixed antiglobulin r.
- mixed leukocyte r.
- mixed lymphocyte r.
- Molisch's r.
- Moloney r.
- Montenegro r.
- Morelli's r.
- Moritz r.
- mouse tail r.
- myasthenic r.
- myotonic r.
- myotonic pupillary r.
- myotonoid r.
- Nadi r.
- Nagler's r.
- near-point r.
- negative supporting r.
- negative therapeutic r.
- Neill-Mooser r.
- Neisser's r.
- Neufeld's r.
- neurotonic r.
- neutral r.
- Nile blue r.
- ninhydrin r.
- r. of nonidentity
- Nonne-Apelt r.
- normal lymphocytic transfer r.
- nucleal r.
- obsessive-compulsive r.
- Oestreicher's r.
- ophthalmic r.
- orbicularis r.
- oxidase r.
- pain r.
- Pándy's r.
- paradoxical pupillary r.
- parallergic r.
- Parish r.
- r. of partial identity
- PAS r.
- passive Arthus r.
- passive cutaneous anaphylaxis r.

re·ac·tion *(continued)*
- Pasteur's r.
- Paul-Bunnell r.
- periodic acid–Schiff r.
- peroxidase r.
- Petri r.
- Petzetaki's r.
- Pfeiffer's r.
- phobic r.
- photochemical r.
- Pinkerton-Mooser r.
- Pirquet r.
- Porges-Pollatschek r.
- pneumococcus capsule swelling r.
- Porter-Silber r.
- positive supporting r.
- Posner's r.
- Prausnitz-Küstner r.
- precipitin r.
- primary r. of Nissl
- prozone r.
- pseudoallergic r.
- pseudomyotonic r.
- psychosomatic r.
- psychotic depressive r.
- puncture r.
- quellung r.
- rage r.
- retrobulbar pupil r.
- reversal r.
- reverse passive Arthus r.
- reversible r.
- Rivalta's r.
- Roger's r.
- Rubino's r.
- Russo r.
- Sanarelli-Schwartzman r.
- sarcoid tissue r.
- Schardinger's r.
- Schick r.
- Schultz-Charlton r.
- Schultz-Dale r.
- scrotal r.
- second-order r.
- second-set r.
- sedimentation r.
- Selivanoff r.

re·ac·tion *(continued)*
  serological r.
  serum r.
  serum sickness–like r.
  Sgambati's r.
  shortening r.
  Shwartzman r., generalized
  Shwartzman r., localized
  skin r.
  soluble immune complex r.
  spring r.
  startle r.
  statokinetic r.
  stemming r.
  Straus' r.
  stress r.
  supporting r's
  sympathetic stress r.
  Szent-Györgyi r.
  Tanret's r.
  tendon r.
  thread r.
  thyroid function r.
  tilt r.
  toxin-antitoxin r.
  Trambusti's r.
  trigger r.
  tuberculin r.
  tuberculin-type r.
  Turnbull's blue r.
  upgrading r.
  vaccinoid r.
  vestibular pupillary r.
  vital r.
  Voges-Proskauer r.
  von Pirquet's r.
  Waaler-Rose r.
  Wassermann r.
  Watson-Schwartz r.
  Weil-Felix r.
  Wernicke's r.
  wheal and erythema r.
  wheal and flare r.
  white-graft r.
  Widal's r.
  Wolff-Calmette r.
  Wolff-Eisner r.
  xanthoproteic r.

re·ac·tion *(continued)*
  xanthydrol r.
  zed r.
  zero-order r.
  Zimmermann r.
re·ac·tion-for·ma·tion
re·ac·ti·vate
re·ac·ti·va·tion
  r. of serum
re·ac·ti·va·tor
  cholinesterase r.
re·ac·tive
re·ac·tiv·i·ty
  vascular r.
Re·ac·trol
Read's formula
read·i·ness
  explosion r.
  reading r.
read·ing
  lip r.
  speech r.
  wet r.
read·through
re·a·gent
  amino-acid r.
  arsenic–sulfuric acid r.
  benzidine r.
  Bial's r.
  biuret r.
  Black's r.
  Bogg's r.
  Bohme's r.
  Bonchardat's r.
  Brücke's r.
  Cleland's r.
  Cramer's 2.5 r.
  Cross and Bevan's r.
  diazo r.
  dinitrosalicylic acid r.
  Ehrlich's aldehyde r.
  Ehrlich's diazo r.
  formalin–sulfuric acid r.
  Frohn's r.
  general r.
  Gies' biuret r.
  Grignard's r.
  Hager's r.

re·a·gent *(continued)*
    Hahn oxine r.
    Haines' r.
    Ilosvay's r.
    Izar's r.
    Lloyd's r.
    Mandelin's r.
    Marme's r.
    Marquis' r.
    Mayer's r.
    Mecke's r.
    Meyer's r.
    Millon's r.
    Mörner's r.
    Moro's r.
    Nadi r.
    Nakayama r.
    Nessler's r.
    Ninhydrin r.
    Noguchi's r.
    Obermayer's r.
    Pappenheim's r.
    Penzoldt's r.
    Rosenthaler's r.
    Schaer's r.
    Scheibler's r.
    Schiff's r.
    Schweitzer's r.
    Scott-Wilson r.
    selenious–sulfuric acid r.
    Soldaini's r.
    Spiegler's r.
    splenic r.
    Sulkowitch's r.
    Sumner's r.
    Tanret's r.
    Triboulet's r.
    Tsuchiya r.
    Uffelmann's r.
    vanadic–sulfuric acid r.
    Wolff's r.
re·a·gin
    atopic r.
re·a·gin·ic
re·al·gar
rea·mer
    chamfer r.
re·am·pu·ta·tion

re·an·i·mate
re·ar·range·ment
    Amadori r.
re·at·tach·ment
Ré·au·mur's scale
Ré·au·mur's thermometer
re·base
re·bound
    REM r.
re·breath·ing
re·cal·ci·fi·ca·tion
re·call
    free r.
re·can·al·iza·tion
re·ca·pit·u·la·tion
re·cei·ver
re·cep·tac·u·lum *pl.* re·cep·tac·u·la
    r. chyli
    r. ganglii petrosi
    r. Pecqueti
re·cep·to·ma
re·cep·tor
    adrenergic r's
    α-adrenergic r's
    β-adrenergic r.
    B cell antigen r's
    central r's
    cholinergic r's
    complement r's.
    contact r.
    contiguous r.
    cutaneous r.
    distance r.
    equilibratory r's
    estrogen r.
    Fc r's
    genital r's
    gravity r's
    gustatory r.
    H_1, H_2 r's
    IgE r's
    immune adherence r.
    insulin r's
    length r.
    low-density lipoprotein (LDL) r's
    muscarinic r's

re·cep·tor *(continued)*
    muscle r.
    N_1-r's
    N_2-r's
    nicotinic r's
    olfactory r.
    pain r.
    Pinkus-Iggo r.
    pressure r.
    progesterone r.
    static r's
    stretch r.
    T cell antigen r's
    tactile r.
    taste r.
    tension r.
    tissue r.
    touch r.
    visual r.
    volume r's
re·cep·tor·ol·o·gy
re·cess
    accessory r. of elbow
    acetabular r.
    Arlt's r.
    attic r.
    cerebellopontile r.
    chiasmatic r.
    cochlear r. of vestibule
    conarial r.
    costodiaphragmatic r. of
      pleura
    costomediastinal r. of
      pleura
    duodenojejunal r.
    elliptical r. of vestibule
    epitympanic r.
    r. of fourth ventricle,
      lateral
    hepatoenteric r.
    hepatorenal r.
    Hyrtl's r.
    incisive r.
    inferior duodenal r.
    inferior ileocecal r.
    inferior omental r.
    infundibular r.
    infundibuliform r.

re·cess *(continued)*
    r. of infundibulum
    interpeduncular r.
    intersigmoidal r.
    labyrinthine r.
    laryngopharyngeal r.
    lateral r. of rhomboid fossa
    r. of lesser omental cavity
    lienal r.
    mesenteric r.
    mesocolic r.
    nasopalatine r.
    r. of nasopharynx, lateral
    neuroporic r.
    optic r.
    paracolic r's
    paraduodenal r.
    r. of pelvic mesocolon
    peritoneal r's
    pharyngeal r., middle
    phrenicohepatic r's
    pineal r.
    piriform r.
    pleural r's
    pneumatoenteric r.
    pontocerebellar r.
    posterior r. of
      interpeduncular fossa
    posterior r. of tympanic
      membrane
    Reichert's r.
    retroannular r.
    retrocecal r.
    retroduodenal r.
    right subhepatic r.
    r. of Rosenmüller
    sacciform r. of articulation
      of elbow
    sacciform r. of distal
      radioulnar articulation
    sphenoethmoidal r.
    spherical r. of vestibule
    splenic r.
    subhepatic r's
    subphrenic r's
    subpopliteal r.
    superior duodenal r.
    superior ileocecal r.

re·cess *(continued)*
    superior omental r.
    superior r. of tympanic
        membrane
    suprapineal r.
    supratonsillar r.
    Tarini's r.
    r's of Tröltsch
    tubotympanic r.
    utricular r.
    r. of vestibule
re·ces·sion
    angle r.
    bone r.
    clitoral r.
    gingival r.
    r. of ocular muscle
    tendon r.
re·ces·sive
re·ces·sive·ness
re·ces·sus *pl.* re·ces·sus
    r. cerebellopontis
    r. chiasmatis
    r. cochlearis vestibuli
    r. costodiaphragmaticus
        pleurae
    r. costomediastinalis
        pleurae
    r. duodenalis inferior
    r. duodenalis superior
    r. duodenojejunalis
    r. ellipticus vestibuli
    r. epitympanicus
    r. hepatorenalis
    r. ileocaecalis inferior
    r. ileocaecalis superior
    r. ileocecalis inferior
    r. ileocecalis superior
    r. inferior omentalis
    r. infundibuli
    r. intersigmoideus
    r. lateralis fossae
        rhomboidei
    r. lateralis ventriculi
        quarti
    r. lienalis
    r. membranae tympani
        anterior

re·ces·sus *(continued)*
    r. membranae tympani
        posterior
    r. membranae tympani
        superior
    r. opticus
    r. paracolici
    r. paraduodenalis
    r. pharyngealis
    r. pharyngeus
    r. pharyngeus
        [Rosenmülleri]
    r. phrenicohepatici
    r. phrenicomediastinalis
    r. phrenicomediastinalis
        pleurae
    r. pinealis
    r. piriformis
    r. pleurales
    r. pneumatoentericus
    r. posterior fossae
        interpeduncularis [Tarini]
    r. pro utriculo
    r. retrocaecalis
    r. retrocecalis
    r. retroduodenalis
    r. sacciformis articulationis
        cubiti
    r. sacciformis articulationis
        radioulnaris distalis
    r. sphenoethmoidalis
    r. sphericus vestibuli
    r. splenicus
    r. subhepatici
    r. subphrenici
    r. subpopliteus
    r. superior omentalis
    r. suprapinealis
    r. triangularis
    r. tubotympanicus
re·cid·i·va·tion
re·cid·i·vism
re·cid·i·vist
rec·i·pe
re·cip·i·ent
    universal r.
re·cip·io·mo·tor

re·cip·ro·ca·tion
  active r.
  passive r.
re·ci·proc·i·ty
Reck·ling·hau·sen's canals
Reck·ling·hau·sen's disease
Reck·ling·hau·sen-Ap·pel·
  baum disease
Rec·lus' disease
re·cog·nin
re·cog·ni·tion
  cell r.
  immunologic r.
  multiple codon r.
  pattern r.
re·coil
  passive r.
re·com·bi·nant
  r. DNA
  hGH-r.
re·com·bi·na·tion
  bacterial r.
  intrachromosomal r.
  mitotic r.
  molecular r.
re·com·pres·sion
re·con·di·tion·ing
re·con·sti·tu·tion
re·con·struc·tion
  Bucknall's r. of urethra
  image r. from projections
re·con·struc·tor
  dynamic spatial r. (DSR)
re·con·tour
rec·ord
  chew-in r., functional
  dental identification r.
  face-bow r.
  interocclusal r.
  interocclusal r., centric
  interocclusal r., eccentric
  interocclusal r., lateral
  interocclusal r., protrusive
  jaw relation r.
  maxillomandibular r.
  medical r.
  occluding centric relation
    r.

rec·ord *(continued)*
  patient r.
  problem-oriented r. (POR)
  profile r.
  protrusive r.
  terminal jaw relation r.
  unit r.
re·cord·er
  pulse volume r.
  strip-chart r.
re·cord·ing
  depth r.
re·cov·ery
  spontaneous r.
rec·re·ment
rec·re·men·ti·tious
re·cru·des·cence
re·cru·des·cent
re·cruit·ment
  loudness r.
Rect. — L. rectificatus
  (rectified)
rec·tal
rec·tal·gia
rec·tec·to·my
rec·ti·fi·ca·tion
  full-wave r.
  half-wave r.
  spontaneous r.
rec·ti·fied
rec·ti·fi·er
  thermionic r.
rec·tis·chi·ac
rec·ti·tis
rec·to·ab·dom·i·nal
rec·to·anal
rec·to·cele
rec·to·cly·sis
rec·to·coc·cy·ge·al
rec·to·coc·cy·pexy
rec·to·co·li·tis
rec·to·cu·ta·ne·ous
rec·to·cys·tot·o·my
rec·to·la·bi·al
rec·to·peri·ne·or·rha·phy
rec·to·pexy
rec·to·plas·ty
rec·to·ro·mano·scope

rec·to·ro·ma·nos·co·py
rec·tor·rha·phy
rec·to·scope
rec·tos·co·py
rec·to·sig·moid
rec·to·sig·moi·dec·to·my
rec·to·sig·moid·itis
rec·to·ste·no·sis
rec·tos·to·my
rec·to·tome
rec·tot·o·my
rec·to·ure·thral
rec·to·uter·ine
rec·to·vag·i·nal
rec·to·ves·i·cal
rec·to·ves·tib·u·lar
rec·to·vul·var
Rec·tules
rec·tum
rec·tus
    r. accessorius
re·cum·bent
re·cu·per·ate
re·cu·per·a·tion
re·cu·per·a·tive
re·cur·rence
re·cur·rent
re·cur·va·tion
re·cur·va·tum
red
    alizarin r.
    alizarin r. S
    alizarin water-soluble r.
    aniline r.
    basic r. 2
    basic r. 9
    bordeaux r.
    bromphenol r.
    carmine r.
    cerasine r.
    chlorophenol r.
    Congo r.
    cotton r.
    cotton r. B
    cotton r. C
    cotton r. 4 B
    cresol r.
    dianil r. 4 C

red *(continued)*
    dianin r. 4 B
    direct r.
    direct r. 4 B
    fast r. B or P
    fast r. P
    indigo r.
    indoxyl r.
    magdala r.
    methyl r.
    naphthaline r.
    neutral r.
    oil r.
    oil r. IV
    oil r. O
    phenol r.
    provisional r.
    scarlet r.
    scarlet r. sulfonate
    senitol r.
    sudan r.
    toluylene r.
    tony r.
    trypan r.
    vital r.
re·de·cus·sate
red·foot
re·dia *pl.* re·diae
re·dif·fer·en·ti·a·tion
Redig. in pulv. — L. redigatur
    in pulverem (let it be reduced
    to powder)
Red. in pulv. — L. reductus in
    pulverem (reduced to powder)
red·in·te·gra·tion
re·dis·lo·ca·tion
Red·i·sol
Red·lich-Ober·stei·ner area
re·dox
re·dresse·ment
red tide
re·duce
re·duced
re·du·ci·ble
re·duc·tant
re·duc·tase
    5α-r.
    lipoamide r.

re·duc·tion
  delayed r.
  r. of chromosomes
  closed r.
  r. en bloc
  r. en masse
  hydrostatic r.
  immediate r.
  meiotic r.
  mitotic r.
  open r.
  somatic r.
  weight r.
redun·dan·cy
re·dun·dant
re·du·pli·cat·ed
re·du·pli·ca·tion
re·du·vi·id
Re·du·vi·i·dae
Re·du·vi·us
  R. personatus
red·wa·ter
Reed's cells
Reed-Hodg·kin disease
Reed-Stern·berg cells
reef
reef·ing
  stomach r.
re·en·trant
re·en·try
re·epi·the·li·al·iza·tion
Rees's test
Rees-Eck·er fluid
Rees-Eck·er solution
Reese-Ells·worth retino-
  blastoma classification (I–V)
re·ex·ci·ta·tion
re·ex·pand
re·fect
re·fec·tion
re·fec·tious
re·fer·able
re·fer·ral
re·ferred
re·fine
re·flect
re·flect·ed
re·flec·tion

re·flec·tion
  specular r.
re·flec·tor
  dental r.
  specular r.
re·flex
  abdominal r's
  abdominal cutaneous r.
  abdominocardiac r.
  Abrams' r.
  Abrams' heart r.
  acceleratory r.
  accommodation r.
  Achilles tendon r.
  acoustic r.
  acoustic stapedial r.
  acousticopalpebral r.
  acousticospinal r.
  acquired r.
  acromial r.
  adductor r.
  adductor r. of foot
  adductor r. of thigh
  allied r's
  anal r.
  anal wink r.
  ankle r.
  antagonistic r's
  antagonistic anterior tibial
    r. of Piotrowski
  anticus r.
  antigravity r.
  aortic r.
  aponeurotic r.
  Aschner's r.
  atriopressor r.
  attention r. of pupil
  attitudinal r's
  audito-oculogyric r.
  auditory r.
  auditory-palpebral r.
  aural r.
  auricle r.
  auriculocervical nerve r.
  auriculopalpebral r.
  auriculopressor r.
  autonomic r.
  axon r.

re·flex *(continued)*
- Babinski's r.
- Babkin r.
- Bainbridge r.
- Balduzzi's r.
- Barkman's r.
- basal joint r.
- behavior r.
- Bekhterev's r.
- Bekhterev's deep r.
- Bekhterev-Mendel r.
- bending r.
- Benedeck's r.
- biceps r.
- Bing's r.
- bladder r.
- blink r.
- body-righting r.
- bowing r.
- brachioradialis r.
- Brain's r.
- Brain's quadrupedal r.
- bregmocardiac r.
- Brissaud's r.
- Brudzinski's r.
- bulbocavernous r.
- bulbomimic r.
- bulbospongiosus r.
- Capps r.
- cardiac r.
- cardiac depressor r.
- carotid body r.
- carotidosympathoatrial r.
- carotidovagoatrial r.
- carotidoventricular r.
- carotid sinus r.
- carpophalangeal r.
- cat's eye r.
- celiac plexus r.
- cephalopalpebral r.
- cerebral cortex r.
- cerebropupillary r.
- Chaddock r.
- chain r.
- chin r.
- chin-jerk r.
- chocked r.
- Chodzko's r.

re·flex *(continued)*
- ciliary r.
- ciliospinal r.
- clasping r.
- clasp-knife r.
- cochleo-orbicular r.
- cochleopalpebral r.
- cochleopupillary r.
- cochleostapedial r.
- coitus r.
- concealed r.
- conditioned r.
- conjunctival r.
- consensual r.
- consensual light r.
- contralateral r.
- convergence r.
- convergency r.
- convulsive r.
- coordinated r.
- corneal r.
- corneomandibular r.
- corneopterygoid r.
- corneomental r.
- coronary r.
- corticopupillary r.
- costal arch r.
- costal periosteal r.
- costopectoral r.
- cough r.
- cranial r.
- cremasteric r.
- crossed r.
- cuboidodigital r.
- cutaneous r.
- cutaneous pupillary r.
- dartos r.
- Darwin's r.
- darwinian r.
- dazzle r.
- deep r.
- deep tendon r. (DTR)
- deep abdominal r's
- defecation r.
- defense r.
- deglutition r.
- delayed r.
- deltoid r.

re·flex *(continued)*
 depressor r.
 digital r.
 direct r.
 direct light r.
 disynaptic r.
 diving r.
 doll's eye r.
 dorsal r.
 dorsocuboidal r.
 dorsum pedis r.
 ejaculation r.
 elbow r.
 embrace r.
 emergency light r.
 enterogastric r.
 epigastric r.
 Erben's r.
 erector spinae r.
 Escherich's r.
 esophagosalivary r.
 extensor r.
 extensor thrust r.
 external auditory meatus
  r.
 external hamstring r.
 external oblique r.
 eyeball compression r.
 eyeball-heart r.
 eyelid closure r.
 facial r.
 faucial r.
 femoral r.
 femoroabdominal r.
 finger flexor r.
 finger-thumb r.
 flexion r. of leg
 flexor r., paradoxical
 flexor withdrawal r.
 flight r.
 fontanel r.
 foveal r.
 foveolar r.
 front-tap r.
 fundus r.
 fusion r.
 gag r.
 Galant's r.

re·flex *(continued)*
 galvanic skin r.
 Gamper's r.
 gastrocnemius r.
 gastrocolic r.
 gastroileal r.
 gastropancreatic r.
 gastrosalivary r.
 Gault's cochleopalpebral r.
 Geigel's r.
 genital r.
 Gifford's r.
 Gifford-Galassi r.
 glabellar tap r.
 glossary r.
 gluteal r.
 Gordon's r.
 Gower-Henry r.
 grasp r.
 grasping r.
 great toe r.
 gripping r.
 Grünfelder's r.
 Guillain-Barré r.
 gustolacrimal r.
 H-r.
 Haab's r.
 hamstring r.
 heart r.
 heel-tap r.
 heel r. of Weingrow
 Hering-Breuer r.
 Hirschberg's r.
 Hoffmann's r.
 Hughes's r.
 hyperactive myotactic r.
 hypochondrial r.
 hypogastric r.
 hypothenar r.
 ileogastric r.
 inborn r.
 indirect r.
 infraspinatus r.
 inguinal r.
 intercoronary r.
 internal hamstring r.
 interscapular r.
 intersegmental r.

re·flex *(continued)*
- intestinal r.
- intestinointestinal r.
- inverted radial r.
- investigatory r.
- iris contraction r.
- ischemic r.
- jaw r.
- jaw jerk r.
- Joffroy's r.
- Juster r.
- juvenile r.
- Kehrer's r.
- Kisch's r.
- knee flexion r.
- knee jerk r.
- Kocher's r.
- labyrinthine righting r.
- lacrimal r.
- Laehr-Henneberg hard palate r.
- Landau r.
- laryngeal r.
- latent r.
- laughter r.
- let-down r.
- lid r.
- Liddell and Sherrington r.
- light r.
- lip r.
- little toe r.
- Livierato's r.
- lordosis r.
- Lovén r.
- lower abdominal r.
- lower abdominal periosteal r.
- lumbar r.
- lung r.
- Lust's r.
- McCarthy's r.
- McCormac's r.
- McDowall r.
- macular r.
- Magnus and de Kleijn neck r's
- mandibular r.
- Marey's r.

re·flex *(continued)*
- Marinesco-Radovici r.
- mark-time r.
- mass r.
- Mayer's r.
- medioplantar r.
- mediopubic r.
- menace r.
- Mendel's r.
- Mendel-Bekhterev r.
- Mendel's dorsal r. of foot
- metacarpohypothenar r.
- metacarpothenar r.
- metatarsal r.
- micturition r.
- middle ear r.
- milk ejection r.
- milk let-down r.
- Mondonesi's r.
- monosynaptic r. (MSR)
- Morley's peritoneocutaneous r.
- Moro's r.
- Moro embrace r.
- motor r.
- muscular r.
- myenteric r.
- myopic r.
- myotatic r.
- nasal r.
- nasofacial r.
- nasolabial r.
- nasomental r.
- naso-ocular r.
- nasopulmonary r.
- near r.
- neck r's
- neck righting r.
- nociceptive r's
- nociceptive r. of Riddoch and Buzzard
- nose-bridge-lid r.
- nose-eye r.
- nostril r.
- obliquus r.
- ocular counter-rolling r.
- ocular fixation r.
- ocular righting r.

re·flex *(continued)*
  oculoauditory r.
  oculocardiac r.
  oculocephalic r.
  oculocephalogyric r.
  oculogastric r.
  oculopharyngeal r.
  oculopupillary r.
  oculosensory cell r.
  oculovagal r.
  oculovestibular r.
  olecranon r.
  Oppenheim's r.
  optical righting r.
  opticofacial winking r.
  opticopalpebral r.
  orbicularis r.
  orbicularis oculi r.
  orbicularis oris r.
  orbicularis pupillary r.
  orbiculopupillary r.
  orienting r.
  pain r.
  palatal r.
  palatine r.
  palm-chin r.
  palmar r.
  palmomental r.
  palpebral r.
  panting r.
  paradoxical pupillary r.
  patellar r.
  patelloadductor r.
  pathologic r.
  Pavlov's r.
  pectoral r.
  Peiper's r.
  pendular r.
  penile r.
  penis r.
  perception r.
  perianal r.
  pericardial r.
  periosteal r.
  periosteoradial r.
  peritoneointestinal r.
  pharyngeal r.
  phasic r.

re·flex *(continued)*
  Philippson's r.
  pilomotor r.
  Piltz's r.
  Piotrowski r.
  placing r.
  plantar r.
  plantar flexor r.
  platysmal r.
  polysynaptic r.
  positive supporting r.
  postural r.
  pressor r.
  pressoreceptor r.
  Preyer's r.
  primitive r.
  pronator r.
  proprioceptive r.
  protective r.
  protective laryngeal r.
  psychic r.
  psychocardiac r.
  psychogalvanic r.
  puboadductor r.
  pulmonocoronary r.
  pupillary r.
  pupillary skin r.
  Puusepp's r.
  pyelovesical r.
  quadriceps r.
  quadrupedal extensor r.
  radial r.
  radiobicipital r.
  radioperiosteal r.
  radiopronator r.
  Radovici r.
  rectal r.
  rectus abdominis r.
  red r.
  regional r.
  Reimer's r.
  Remak's r.
  renal r.
  renointestinal r.
  renorenal r.
  renoureteral r.
  resistance r.
  retrobulbar pupillary r.

re·flex *(continued)*
  retromalleolar r.
  reversed pupillary r.
  Riddoch's mass r.
  righting r.
  Roger's r.
  Romberg r.
  rooting r.
  Rossolimo's r.
  Ruggeri's r.
  Saenger's r.
  scapular r.
  scapulohumeral r.
  Schäffer's r.
  Schunkel r.
  scratch r.
  scrotal r.
  segmental r.
  semimembranosus r.
  semitendinosus r.
  senile r.
  sensory blinking r.
  sexual r.
  shot-silk r.
  simple r.
  sinus r.
  skin r.
  skin pupillary r.
  sneezing r.
  Snellen's r.
  snout r.
  sole r.
  sole-tap r.
  Somagyi's r.
  somatointestinal r.
  spinal r.
  spino-adductor r.
  stapedial r.
  stapedius r.
  startle r.
  static r.
  static adaptation r.
  static attitudinal r.
  statokinetic r.
  statotomic r's
  stepping r.
  sternobrachial r.
  Stookey r.

re·flex *(continued)*
  stretch r.
  Strümpell's r.
  styloradial r.
  sucking r.
  superficial r.
  superficial abdominal r.
  supinator r.
  supinator longus r.
  supporting r's
  supraorbital r.
  suprapatellar r.
  suprapubic r.
  supraumbilical r.
  swallowing r.
  tactile r.
  tapetal light r.
  tarsophalangeal r.
  tendon r.
  tensor fasciae latae r.
  testicular compression r.
  thigh crossed lengthening
    r.
  threat r.
  Throckmorton's r.
  thumb r.
  tibialis posterior r.
  tibioadductor r.
  toe r.
  tonic r.
  tonic neck r.
  tonic plantar r.
  tonic vibration r.
  trained r.
  triceps r.
  triceps surae r.
  trigeminocervical r.
  trigeminofacial r.
  trigeminus r.
  Trömner's r.
  tympanic r.
  trochanter r.
  ulnar r.
  unconditioned r.
  unloading r.
  upper abdominal periosteal
    r.
  upper deep abdominal r.

re·flex *(continued)*
  urinary r's
  utricular r.
  vagal pupillary r.
  vagovagal r.
  vagus r.
  vascular r.
  vasomotor r.
  vasopressor r's
  vasovagal r.
  venorespiratory r.
  vertebra prominens r.
  vesical r.
  vesicointestinal r.
  vestibular r's
  vestibulo-ocular r.
  vestibulospinal r.
  virile r.
  visceral r.
  visceral traction r.
  viscerocardiac r.
  visceromotor r.
  viscerosensory r.
  viscerotrophic r.
  visual orbicularis r.
  visuocortical r.
  vomiting r.
  von Mering r.
  walking r.
  Wartenberg r.
  water-silk r.
  Weingrow's r.
  Weiss's r.
  Westphal's pupillary r.
  Westphal-Piltz r.
  wink r.
  withdrawal r.
  wrist clonus r.
  wrist flexion r.
  zygomatic r.
re·flex·o·gen·ic
re·flex·og·e·nous
re·flexo·graph
re·flex·ol·o·gy
re·flex·om·e·ter
re·flex·om·e·try
re·flexo·phil
re·flexo·ther·a·py

re·flux
  abdominojugular r.
  duodenogastric r.
  esophageal r.
  gastroesophageal r.
  hepatojugular r.
  intrarenal r.
  pyelolymphatic r.
  pyelorenal r.
  pyelosinus r.
  pyelotubular r.
  pyelovenous r.
  urethrovesiculo-differ-
    ential r.
  vesicoureteral r.
  vesicoureteric r.
re·fract
re·frac·ta do·si
re·frac·tile
re·frac·tion
  double r.
  dynamic r.
  manifest r.
  ocular r.
  static r.
re·frac·tion·ist
re·frac·tive
re·frac·tiv·i·ty
re·frac·tom·e·ter
re·frac·tom·e·try
re·frac·tor
re·frac·to·ry
re·frac·ture
re·fran·gi·bil·i·ty
re·fran·gi·ble
re·fresh
re·frig·er·a·tion
re·frin·gent
Ref·sum's disease
Ref·sum's syndrome
re·fuin
re·fu·sion
REG — radioencephalogram
re·gain·er
  space r.
re·gain·er-main·tain·er
Re·gaud's (Re·gaut's) method

Re·gaud and La·cas·sagne
  technique
re·gen·er·a·tion
    epimorphic r.
    morphallactic r.
reg·i·men
    chemotherapeutic r.
    sanitary r.
re·gio *pl.* re·gi·o·nes
    r. abdominalis
    regiones abdominales
    r. acromialis
    r. analis
    r. antebrachialis anterior
    r. antebrachialis posterior
    r. antibrachii radialis
    r. antibrachii ulnaris
    r. antibrachii volaris
    r. auricularis
    r. axillaris
    r. brachialis anterior
    r. brachialis posterior
    r. buccalis
    r. calcanea
    regiones capitis
    r. carpalis anterior
    r. carpalis posterior
    regiones cervicales
    r. cervicalis anterior
    r. cervicalis lateralis
    r. cervicalis posterior
    r. clavicularis
    regiones colli
    r. colli anterior
    r. colli lateralis
    r. colli posterior
    r. costalis lateralis
    r. coxae
    r. cruralis anterior
    r. cruralis posterior
    r. cubitalis anterior
    r. cubitalis posterior
    r. deltoidea
    r. dorsalis manus
    r. dorsalis pedis
    regiones dorsales
    r. epigastrica
    regiones faciales

re·gio *(continued)*
    r. femoralis anterior
    r. femoralis posterior
    r. frontalis
    r. genualis anterior
    r. genualis posterior
    r. genus anterior
    r. genus posterior
    r. glutealis
    r. hyoidea
    r. hypochondriaca [dextra
      et sinistra]
    r. hypogastrica
    r. hypothalamica anterior
    r. hypothalamica dorsalis
    r. hypothalamica
      intermedia
    r. hypothalamica posterior
    r. infraclavicularis
    r. inframammaria
    r. infraorbitalis
    r. infrascapularis
    r. infratemporalis
    r. inguinalis [dextra et
      sinistra]
    r. interscapularis
    r. labialis inferior
    r. labialis superior
    r. laryngea
    r. lateralis [dextra/sinistra]
    r. lumbalis
    r. malleolaris lateralis
    r. malleolaris medialis
    r. mammaria
    r. mastoidea
    r. mediana dorsi
    r. mentalis
    r. nasalis
    r. nuchalis
    r. occipitalis
    r. olecrani
    r. olfactoria
    r. oralis
    r. orbitalis
    r. palpebralis inferior
    r. palpebralis superior
    r. parietalis
    r. parotideomasseterica

re·gio *(continued)*
 r. patellaris
 r. pectoralis
 regiones pectorales
 r. perinealis
 regiones plantares
  digitorum pedis
 r. plantaris pedis
 regiones pleuropulmonales
 r. presternalis
 r. pubica
 r. pudendalis
 r. respiratoria
 r. retromalleolaris lateralis
 r. retromalleolaris medialis
 r. sacralis
 r. scapularis
 r. sternalis
 r. sternocleidomastoidea
 r. subhyoidea
 r. submaxillaris
 r. supraorbitalis
 r. suprascapularis
 r. suprasternalis
 r. suralis
 regiones talocrurales
  anterior et posterior
 r. temporalis
 r. thyreoidea
 r. trochanterica
 r. umbilicalis
 regiones unguiculares
  digitorum manus
 regiones unguiculares
  digitorum pedis
 r. urogenitalis
 r. vertebralis
 regiones volares digitorum
  manus
 r. volaris manus
 r. zygomatica
re·gion
 abdominal r.
 r. of accommodation
 antebrachial r., radial
 antebrachial r., ulnar
 antebrachial r., volar
 anterior r. of neck

re·gion *(continued)*
 axillary r.
 basilar r.
 Broca's r.
 buccal r.
 calcaneal r.
 cervical r.
 ciliary r.
 cingulate r.
 constant (C) r.
 dorsal lip r.
 encephalic r.
 epigastric r.
 external r.
 extrapolar r.
 facial r's
 femoral r.
 focal r.
 frontal r.
 Geiger r.
 genitourinary r.
 gluteal r.
 gustatory r.
 hinge r.
 homology r's
 hypencephalic r.
 hypervariable r's
 hypochondriac r.
 hypogastric r.
 I r.
 iliac r.
 infraclavicular r.
 infrahyoid r.
 inframammary r.
 infraorbital r.
 infrascapular r.
 infraspinous r.
 infratemporal r.
 inguinal r.
 intermediate hypothalamic
  r.
 ischiorectal r.
 lateral abdominal r.
 lateral r. of neck
 r's of leg, anterior and
  posterior
 limbic r.
 lumbar r.

re·gion *(continued)*
    mammary r.
    mental r.
    motor r.
    mylohyoid r.
    r. of nape
    nasal r.
    nuchal r.
    occipital r.
    ocular r.
    olfactory r.
    opticostriate r.
    oral r.
    orbital r.
    parietal r.
    parietotemporal r.
    parotideomasseteric r.
    patellar r.
    pectoral r's
    pelvic r.
    perineal r.
    plantar r's of toes
    popliteal r.
    posterior r. of neck
    precordial r.
    prefrontal r.
    preoptic r.
    presumptive r.
    pretectal r.
    proportional r.
    pterygomaxillary r.
    pubic r.
    respiratory r.
    retromaxillary r.
    rolandic r.
    sacral r.
    sacrococcygeal r.
    scapular r.
    sensory r.
    sternocleidomastoid r.
    subauricular r.
    submandibular r.
    submaxillary r.
    submental r.
    subphrenic r.
    subscapular r.
    subthalamic r.
    supraclavicular r.

re·gion *(continued)*
    suprainguinal r.
    supraomental r.
    suprapubic r.
    supraspinous r.
    tegmental r.
    temporal r.
    trabecular r.
    umbilical r.
    urogenital r.
    variable (V) r.
    V_H r.
    vertebral r.
    vestibular r.
    V_L r.
    vestibular r.
    volar r's of fingers
    volar r. of hand
    zygomatic r.
re·gion·al
re·gi·o·nes
reg·is·ter
    immunization r.
reg·is·trant
reg·is·trar
reg·is·tra·tion
    r. of functional form
    maxillomandibular r.
    occlusal r.
reg·is·try
    cancer r.
Reg·i·tine
Reg·o·nol
re·gres·sion
    curvilinear r.
    linear r.
    multiple r.
    nonlinear r.
re·gres·sive
Reg·ro·ton
reg·u·lar
reg·u·la·tion
    down r.
    fertility r.
    menstrual r.
    ontogenetic r.
reg·u·la·tor
reg·u·lon

re·gur·gi·tant
re·gur·gi·tate
re·gur·gi·ta·tion
    aortic r.
    duodenal r.
    functional r.
    mitral r.
    pulmonic r.
    tricuspid r.
    valvular r.
    vesicoureteral r.
re·ha·bil·i·tate
re·ha·bil·i·ta·tion
    alaryngeal voice r.
    functional r.
    mouth r.
    occlusal r.
    oral r.
re·ha·bil·i·tee
re·ha·la·tion
Reh·fuss' method
Reh·fuss' test
Reh·fuss' tube
re·hy·dra·tion
Rei·chel's cloacal duct
Rei·chert's canal
Rei·chert's cartilage
Rei·chert's membrane
Rei·chert's method
Rei·chert's recess
Rei·chert's scar
Rei·chert's substance
Reich·mann's disease
Reich·mann's syndrome
Reich·stein, Tadeus
Reid's base line
Rei·fen·stein syndrome
Reil's insula
Reil's ribbon
Reil's sulcus
Reil's trigone
Reil·ly bodies
re·im·plan·ta·tion
re·in·fec·tion
re·in·force·ment
    delayed r.
    differential r.
    fixed interval r.

re·in·force·ment *(continued)*
    fixed ratio r.
    negative r.
    positive r.
    primary r.
    r. of reflex
    secondary r.
    variable interval r.
    variable ratio r.
re·in·forc·er
re·in·fu·sate
re·in·fu·sion
Rein·ke's crystalloids
Rein·ke's crystals
re·in·ner·va·tion
re·in·oc·u·la·tion
re·in·te·gra·tion
re·in·tu·ba·tion
re·in·ver·sion
re·in·vo·ca·tion
Reis·sei·sen's muscles
Reiss·ner's fiber
Reiss·ner's membrane
Rei·ter's disease
Rei·ter's syndrome
re·it·er·a·ture
re·jec·tion
    acute r.
    acute cellular r.
    allograft r.
    cellular r.
    chronic r.
    first-set r.
    graft r.
    hyperacute r.
    immunologic r.
    second-set r.
re·ju·ve·nes·cence
re·lapse
    intercurrent r.
    mucocutaneous r.
    rebound r.
re·laps·ing
re·la·tion
    acentric r.
    buccolingual r.
    centric r.
    centric jaw r.

re·la·tion *(continued)*
    convenience r. of teeth
    cusp-fossa r.
    dynamic r's
    eccentric r.
    eccentric jaw r.
    intermaxillary r.
    jaw r.
    jaw-to-jaw r.
    lateral occlusal r.
    mass-energy r.
    maxillomandibular r.
    median jaw r.
    median retruded jaw r.
    object r.
    occlusal r.
    occlusal jaw r.
    posterior border jaw r.
    protrusive jaw r.
    range-energy r.
    rest jaw r.
    ridge r.
    static r's
    unstrained jaw r.
    vertical r.
re·la·tion·ship
    blood r.
    confidential r.
    dose-response r.
    linear r.
re·lax·ant
    muscle r.
    smooth muscle r.
re·lax·a·tion
    isometric r.
    isovolumetric r.
    longitudinal r.
    mecystatic r.
re·lax·in
re·learn·ing
re·lease
    contracture r.
    laryngeal r.
re·li·a·bil·i·ty
re·lief
    gingival r.
re·lieve
re·line

re·lu·cence
re·lux·a·tion
REM — rapid eye movements
  (sleep)
rem
Re·mak's axon
Re·mak's band
Re·mak's fibers
Re·mak's ganglion
Re·mak's paralysis
Re·mak's plexus
Re·mak's reflex
Re·mak's sign
Re·mak's symptom
Re·mak's type
re·me·di·al
rem·e·dy
    concordant r's
    inimic r's
    specific r.
    tissue r's
Re·mij·ia
re·min·er·al·i·za·tion
re·mis·sion
re·mit·tence
re·mit·tent
rem·nant
    acroblastic r.
    allantoic r.
    dermal r.
remodeling
    bone r.
re·mo·ti·va·tion
re·mo·val
    pulp r.
re·my·eli·na·tion
ren *pl.* re·nes
    r. mobilis
    r. unguliformis
Re·nac·i·din
re·nal
re·na·tu·ra·tion
Ren·aut's bodies
ren·cu·lus *pl.* ren·cu·li
Ren·du-Os·ler-Web·er disease
Ren·du-Os·ler-Web·er
  syndrome
re·nes

Ren·ese
reni·cap·sule
re·nic·u·lus *pl.* re·nic·u·li
ren·i·form
re·nin
    big r.
re·nin·ism
    primary r.
re·nin·o·ma
reni·pel·vic
reni·por·tal
ren·net
ren·nin
re·no·cor·ti·cal
re·no·cu·ta·ne·ous
re·no·cys·to·gram
re·no·gas·tric
re·no·gen·ic
Re·no·graf·in
re·no·gram
    isotope r.
    radionuclide r.
re·nog·ra·phy
    emission r.
re·no·in·tes·ti·nal
re·nop·a·thy
re·no·pri·val
Re·no·quid
re·no·troph·ic
re·no·trop·ic
re·no·vas·cu·lar
Re·no·vist
Ren·shaw inhibition
ren·ule .
re·nun·cu·lus
Reo·vir·i·dae
reo·vi·rus
re·ox·i·da·tion
re·ox·y·gen·a·tion
Rep. — L. repetatur (let it be
    repeated)
rep
re·pair
    Brown-McDowell r.
    Cecil-Culp r.
    DuVries hammer toe r.
    excision r.
    Lich-Gregoire r.

re·pair *(continued)*
    Lichtenstein hernia r.
    pants-over-vest r.
re·par·a·tive
re·pa·ten·cy
re·pel·lent
re·pel·ler
re·per·co·la·tion
re·per·cus·sion
re·per·cus·sive
re·per·fu·sion
re·pe·ta·tur
re·place·ment
    isomorphous r.
    reciprocal r.
re·plant
re·plan·ta·tion
    intentional r.
re·plen·ish·er
re·ple·tion
rep·li·case
rep·li·cate
rep·li·ca·tion
    conservative r.
    DNA r.
    nonconservative r.
    semiconservative r.
rep·li·con
Re·poise
re·po·lar·iza·tion
re·po·si·tion·ing
    jaw r.
    muscle r.
re·pos·i·tor
re·pos·i·to·ry
rep·re·sen·ta·tion
    sensorimotor r.
re·pres·sion
    catabolite r.
    coordinate r.
    endproduct r.
    enzyme r.
    gene r.
re·pres·sor
    active r.
    inactive r.
re·pro·duc·tion
    asexual r.

re·pro·duc·tion *(continued)*
  bisexual r.
  cytogenic r.
  sexual r.
  somatic r.
  unisexual r.
re·pro·duc·tive
rep·ro·mi·cin
re·pro·ter·ol hy·dro·chlo·ride
rep·til·ase
rep·tile
Rep·til·ia
  capillary r.
re·pul·lu·la·tion
re·pul·sion
re·quire·ment
  minimum daily r. (MDR)
RES — reticuloendothelial
  system
re·sa·zu·rin
re·scin·na·mine
res·cue
  citrovorum r.
  folinic acid r.
  leucovorin r.
re·search
  clinical r.
re·sect
re·sec·ta·ble
re·sec·tion
  levator r.
  gastric r.
  Girdlestone r.
  mandibular r.
  maxillary r.
  Mikulicz r.
  pulmonary r.
  root r.
  submucosal r.
  submucous r.
  transurethral r.
  transurethral prostatic r.
    (TURP)
  wedge r.
re·sec·to·scope
re·sec·tos·co·py
res·ene
res·er·pine

Res·er·poid
re·serve
  alkali r.
  alkaline r.
  breathing r.
  cardiac r.
  lifetime r.
  respiratory r.
re·ser·voir
  chromatin r.
  r. of infection
  Koch r.
  Mainz pouch urinary r.
  Ommaya r.
  Pecquet's r.
  Rickham r.
re·set·tle·ment
  occupational r.
re·shap·ing
res·i·den·cy
res·i·dent
re·sid·ua
re·sid·u·al
  postvoiding r.
res·i·due
  day r.
re·sid·u·um *pl.* re·sid·ua
  gastric r.
re·sil·i·ence
re·sil·i·en·cy
re·sil·i·ent
res·in
  acrylic r's
  activated r.
  anion-exchange r.
  autopolymer r.
  azure A carbacrylic r.
  carbacrylamine r's
  cation-exchange r.
  cholestyramine r.
  cold-curing r.
  composite r.
  copolymer r.
  direct filling r.
  epoxy r.
  guaiacum r.
  heat-curing r.
  ion exchange r.

res·in *(continued)*
    phentermine r.
    podophyllum r.
    polyamine-methylene r.
    polyester r.
    quick-cure r.
    quinine carbacrylic r.
    self-curing r.
    styrene r.
    sulfonated polystyrene r.
    synthetic r.
    vinyl r.
Res·i·nat
res·i·noid
res·i·nous
res ip·sa lo·qui·tur
re·sis·tance
    acquired radiation r.
    airway r.
    basilar membrane r.
    capillary r.
    cogwheel r.
    drug r.
    ego r.
    electrical r.
    environmental r.
    expiratory r.
    hybrid r.
    id r.
    input r.
    insulin r.
    internal r.
    natural r.
    peripheral r.
    phenotypic r.
    pulmonary r.
    pulmonary vascular r.
    superego r.
    total peripheral r.
    total pulmonary r.
    vascular r.
re·sis·tant
re·sis·tiv·i·ty
re·sis·tor
res·ite
res·ole
res·o·lu·tion
    angular r.

res·o·lu·tion *(continued)*
    axial r.
    azimuthal r.
    depth r.
    energy r.
    lateral r.
    longitudinal r.
    range r.
    spatial r.
    transverse r.
re·solve
re·sol·vent
res·o·nance
    amphoric r.
    bandbox r.
    bell-metal r.
    cavernous r.
    cough r.
    cracked-pot r.
    electron paramagnetic r.
      (e.p.r.)
    electron spin r.
    hydatid r.
    nasal r.
    nuclear magnetic r.
    osteal r.
    proton magnetic r. (p.m.r.)
    shoulder-strap r.
    skodaic r.
    tympanic r.
    tympanitic r.
    vesicular r.
    vesiculotympanic r.
    vocal r.
    whispering r.
    wooden r.
res·o·nant
res·o·na·tor
    Oudin r.
re·sorb
re·sor·bent
re·sor·cin
re·sor·ci·nism
re·sor·ci·nol
    r. monoacetate
re·sor·ci·nol·phthal·e·in
re·sorp·tion
    apical root r.

re·sorp·tion *(continued)*
  bone r.
  external root r.
  gingival r.
  horizontal r.
  idiopathic r.
  internal r.
  physiologic r.
  rear r.
  root r.
  surface root r.
  tooth r., external
  tooth r., internal
  tubular r.
  undermining r.
  vertical r.
res·pir·a·ble
res·pi·ra·tion
  abdominal r.
  absent r.
  accelerated r.
  aerobic r.
  amphoric r.
  anaerobic r.
  artificial r.
  asthmoid r.
  ataxic r.
  Austin Flint r.
  Biot's r.
  Bouchut's r.
  bronchial r.
  bronchocavernous r.
  bronchovesicular r.
  cavernous r.
  cell r.
  cerebral r.
  Cheyne-Stokes r.
  cogwheel r.
  collateral r.
  controlled diaphragmatic r.
  Corrigan's r.
  costal r.
  diaphragmatic r.
  diffusion r.
  direct r.
  divided r.
  electrophrenic r.
  external r.

res·pi·ra·tion *(continued)*
  fetal r.
  forced r.
  granular r.
  harsh r.
  indefinite r.
  intermittent positive
    pressure r. (IPPR)
  internal r.
  interrupted r.
  jerky r.
  Kussmaul's r.
  Kussmaul-Kien r.
  labored r.
  meningitic r.
  metamorphosing r.
  mouth-to-mouth r.
  nervous r.
  paradoxical r.
  pendelluft r.
  periodic r.
  placental r.
  puerile r.
  rude r.
  Seitz's metamorphosing r.
  slow r.
  spontaneous r's
  stertorous r.
  supplementary r.
  suppressed r.
  thoracic r.
  tidal r.
  tissue r.
  transitional r.
  tubular r.
  vesicular r.
  vesiculocavernous r.
  vicarious r.
  wavy r.
res·pi·ra·tor
  cabinet r.
  cuirass r.
  demand r.
  Drinker r.
  Engström r.
  protective r.
res·pi·ra·to·ry
res·pi·ra·to·ry sys·tem

res·pi·rom·e·ter
res·pi·rom·e·try
re·spon·de·at su·pe·ri·or
re·sponse
   allergic r.
   anal r.
   anamnestic r.
   anticipatory r.
   autoimmune r.
   average evoked r.
   Babinski r.
   booster r.
   brain stem evoked r.
   conditioned r.
   corneal r.
   Cornell r.
   delayed r.
   delayed conditioned r.
   disinhibition r.
   dose r.
   dynamic r.
   evoked r.
   extensor plantar r.
   flare r.
   frequency r.
   fright r.
   galvanic skin r.
   ice water r.
   immediate r.
   immune r.
   lysogenic r.
   lytic r.
   memory r.
   middle latency r.
   orienting r.
   placing r.
   postauricular r.
   primary immune r.
   psychogalvanic r. (PGR)
   quantal r.
   rage r.
   recall r.
   reticulocyte r.
   Rinne's r.
   secondary immune r.
   second-set r.
   somatosensory evoked r.
    (SER)

re·sponse *(continued)*
   startle r.
   stretch r.
   thalamic r.
   triple r. (of Lewis)
   unconditioned r.
   vestibular placing r.
   visual evoked r.
   wink r.
rest
   aberrant r.
   adrenal r.
   bed r.
   carbon r.
   caudal medullary r.
   cingulum r.
   embryonic r.
   epithelial r.
   fetal r.
   incisal r.
   lingual r.
   Malassez r.
   mesonephric r.
   occlusal r.
   precision r.
   recessed r.
   semiprecision r.
   suprarenal r.
   surface r.
   Walthard's cell r's
rest·bite
re·ste·no·sis
   false r.
   true r.
res·ti·bra·chi·um
res·ti·form
res·tis
res·ti·tu·tio
   r. ad integrum
res·ti·tu·tion
res·to·ra·tion
   buccal r.
   cusp r.
   facial r.
   pin-ledge r.
   prosthetic r.
re·stor·a·tive

re·straint
  chemical r.
  mechanical r.
  medicinal r.
re·stric·tion
  MHC r.
re·sub·limed
re·sul·tant
re·su·pi·na·tion
re·sus·ci·ta·tion
  cardiac r.
  cardiopulmonary r. (CPR)
  colloid r.
  crystalloid r.
  fluid r.
  r. of the heart
  hypertonic r.
  mouth-to-mouth r.
  mouth-to-nose r.
  oral r.
re·sus·ci·ta·tor
  cardiopulmonary r.
re·su·ture
re·tain·er
  continuous bar r.
  direct r.
  Hawley r.
  indirect r.
  intracoronal r.
  matrix r.
  space r.
re·tard
  expiratory r.
re·tar·date
  ineducable r.
re·tar·da·tion
  cultural-familial mental r.
  intrauterine growth r.
    (IUGR)
  mental r.
  psychomotor r.
  psychosocial r.
retch·ing
re·te pl. re·tia
  acromial r.
  r. acromiale
  r. arteriosum
  r. arteriosum dermidis

re·te (continued)
  r. arteriosum subpapillare
  articular r.
  articular cubital r.
  articular r. of elbow
  articular r. of knee
  r. articulare cubiti
  r. articulare genus
  calcaneal r.
  r. calcaneum
  r. canalis hypoglossi
  carpal r., dorsal
  r. carpale dorsale
  r. carpi dorsale
  r. cutaneum
  dorsal venous r. of foot
  dorsal venous r. of hand
  r. dorsale pedis
  r. foraminis ovalis
  r. of Haller
  r. Halleri
  r. lymphocapillare
  malleolar r., lateral
  malleolar r., medial
  r. malleolare laterale
  r. malleolare mediale
  malpighian r.
  r. mirabile
  r. mirabile of kidney
  r. mucosum
  r. nasi
  r. olecrani
  r. ovarii
  r. of patella
  r. patellae
  r. patellare
  r. patellaris
  plantar r.
  plantar venous r.
  r. subpapillare
  r. testis
  r. testis [Halleri]
  r. vasculosum articulare
  r. venosum
  r. venosum dorsale manus
  r. venosum dorsale pedis
  r. venosum plantare
  retia venosa vertebrarum

re·ten·tion
    bladder r.
    denture r.
    direct r.
    indirect r.
    surgical r.
    urinary r.
    r. of urine
re·te·the·li·o·ma
re·tia
re·ti·al
re·tic·u·la
re·tic·u·lar
re·tic·u·late
re·tic·u·lat·ed
re·tic·u·la·tion
    dust r.
re·tic·u·lin
    r. M
re·tic·u·li·tis
re·tic·u·lo·cyte
re·tic·u·lo·cy·to·gen·ic
re·tic·u·lo·cy·to·pe·nia
re·tic·u·lo·cy·to·sis
re·tic·u·lo·en·do·the·li·al
re·tic·u·lo·en·do·the·li·o·ma
re·tic·u·lo·en·do·the·li·o·sis
    leukemic r.
re·tic·u·lo·en·do·the·li·um
re·tic·u·lo·his·tio·cy·tary
re·tic·u·lo·his·ti·o·cy·to·ma
    r. of Crosti
re·tic·u·lo·his·ti·o·cy·to·sis
    multicentric r.
re·tic·u·loid
    actinic r.
re·ti·cu·lo·lym·pho·sar·co·ma
re·tic·u·lo·ma
re·tic·u·lo·pe·nia
re·tic·u·lo·peri·the·li·um
re·tic·u·lo·pi·tu·i·cyte
re·tic·u·lo·plas·mo·cy·to·ma
re·tic·u·lo·po·dia
re·tic·u·lo·po·di·um
re·tic·u·lo·sis
    benign r.
    bony r.

re·tic·u·lo·sis *(continued)*
    familial hemophagocytic r.
    familial histiocytic r.
    histiocytic medullary r.
    lipomelanic r.
    pagetoid r.
    primary r. of brain
re·tic·u·lo·spi·nal
re·tic·u·lo·the·li·um
    agranular r.
re·tic·u·lot·o·my
re·tic·u·lum *pl.* re·tic·u·la
    agranular r.
    agranular endoplasmic r.
    arachnoid r.
    Chiari's r.
    Ebner's r.
    endoplasmic r.
    granular r.
    nuclear r.
    reticula lienis
    rough endoplasmic r.
    sarcoplasmic r.
    smooth endoplasmic r.
    splenic r.
    stellate r.
    r. trabeculare sclerae
    r. trabeculare anguli
      iridocornealis
re·ti·form
ret·i·na
    cilial r.
    cilioiridial r.
    coarctate r.
    detached r.
    detachment of r.
    iridial r.
    Kandori's fleck r.
    leopard r.
    nasal r.
    shot-silk r.
    temporal r.
    tigroid r.
    watered-silk r.
Ret·in-A
ret·i·nac·u·lum *pl.* ret·i·nac·u·la
    r. of arcuate ligament

ret·i·nac·u·lum *(continued)*
    r. capsulae articularis
        coxae
    caudal r.
    r. caudale
    r. costae ultimae
    retinacula cutis
    extensor r. of foot, inferior
    extensor r. of foot, superior
    extensor r. of hand
    r. extensorum manus
    flexor r. of ankle
    flexor r. of foot
    flexor r. of hand
    r. flexorum manus
    r. of hip joint
    r. ligamenti arcuati
    r. patellae laterale
    r. patellae mediale
    patellar r., lateral
    patellar r., medial
    peroneal r., inferior
    peroneal r., superior
    r. tendinum
    retinacula unguis
    Weitbrecht's r.
ret·i·nae com·mo·tio
ret·i·nal
    11-*cis r.*
    all-*trans r.*
ret·i·nal
    r. pigment epithelium
ret·i·nal·de·hyde
ret·i·nal isom·er·ase
ret·ine
ret·i·nene
ret·i·ni·tis
    actinic r.
    albuminuric r.
    r. albuminurica
    apoplectic r.
    azotemic r.
    central angiospastic r.
    r. centralis serosa
    r. circinata
    circinate r.
    Coats' r.
    diabetic r.

ret·i·ni·tis *(continued)*
    disciform r.
    exudative r.
    gravidic r.
    hypertensive r.
    Jacobson's r.
    Jensen's r.
    leukemic r.
    metastatic r.
    nephritic r.
    r. pigmentosa
    r. pigmentosa sine
        pigmento
    r. proliferans
    proliferating r.
    r. punctata albescens
    punctate r.
    renal r.
    r. sclopetaria
    serous r.
    solar r.
    splenic r.
    r. stellata
    striate r.
    suppurative r.
    syphilitic r.
    r. syphilitica
    uremic r.
ret·i·no·blas·to·ma
ret·i·no·cer·e·bel·lo·an·gio·
    ma·to·sis
ret·i·no·cho·roid
ret·i·no·cho·roi·di·tis
    r. juxtapapillaris
    toxoplasmic r.
ret·i·no·di·al·y·sis
ret·i·no·graph
ret·i·nog·ra·phy
ret·i·no·ic ac·id
13-*cis*-ret·i·no·ic acid
ret·i·noid
ret·i·nol
ret·i·no·ma·la·cia
ret·i·no·pap·il·li·tis
ret·i·nop·a·thy
    actinic r.
    apoplectic r.
    arteriosclerotic r.

ret·i·nop·a·thy *(continued)*
    central angiospastic r.
    central disk-shaped r.
    central serous r.
    chloroquine r.
    circinate r.
    diabetic r.
    eclamptic r.
    exudative r.
    hemorrhagic r.
    hypertensive r.
    leukemic r.
    macular r.
    r. of prematurity
    pigmentary r.
    proliferative r.
    Purtscher's angiopathic r.
    purulent r.
    renal r.
    rubella r.
    septic r.
    sickle cell r.
    splenic r.
    stellate r.
    suppurative r.
    thioridazine r.
    toxemic r. of pregnancy
ret·i·no·pexy
ret·i·no·pho·tos·co·py
ret·i·no·pi·e·sis
ret·i·nos·chi·sis
ret·i·no·scope
ret·i·nos·co·py
ret·i·no·sis
ret·i·no·top·ic
ret·i·no·tox·ic
reti·so·lu·tion
reti·sper·sion
re·to·peri·the·li·um
Re·tor·ta·mo·nad·i·da
Re·tor·tam·o·nas
re·to·thel
re·to·the·li·al
re·to·the·li·um
re·tract
re·trac·tile
re·trac·tion
    clot r.

re·trac·tion *(continued)*
    gingival r.
    head r.
    lid r.
    mandibular r.
    massive vitreous r.
    systolic r.
    uterine r.
re·trac·tor
    abdominal r.
    Army-Navy r.
    Aufricht r.
    Emmet's r.
    Moorehead's r.
    palate r.
    periosteal r.
    rake r.
    rib r.
    self-retaining r.
    tonsil pillar r.
    vein r.
re·trad
re·treat
    vegetative r.
re·triev·al
    information r.
ret·ro·ac·tion
ret·ro·au·ric·u·lar
ret·ro·buc·cal
ret·ro·bul·bar
ret·ro·cal·ca·neo·bur·si·tis
ret·ro·cath·e·ter·ism
ret·ro·ce·cal
ret·ro·ce·dent
ret·ro·cer·vi·cal
ret·ro·ces·sion
    r. of uterus
ret·ro·cli·na·tion
ret·ro·coch·le·ar
ret·ro·col·lic
ret·ro·col·ic
ret·ro·col·lis
ret·ro·con·duc·tion
ret·ro·cru·ral
ret·ro·cur·sive
ret·ro·de·vi·a·tion
ret·ro·dis·place·ment
ret·ro·du·o·de·nal

ret·ro·du·ral
ret·ro·fill·ing
ret·ro·flexed
ret·ro·flex·ion
    r. of uterus
ret·ro·gas·se·ri·an
ret·ro·gna·thia
ret·ro·gnath·ic
ret·ro·gnath·ism
ret·ro·grade
ret·rog·ra·phy
ret·ro·gres·sion
ret·ro·il·lu·mi·na·tion
ret·ro·in·fec·tion
ret·ro·in·su·lar
ret·ro·irid·i·an
ret·ro·jec·tion
ret·ro·len·tic·u·lar
ret·ro·lis·the·sis
ret·ro·mas·toid
ret·ro·mo·lar
ret·ro·mor·pho·sis
ret·ro·peri·to·ne·al
ret·ro·peri·to·ne·um
ret·ro·peri·to·ni·tis
ret·ro·phar·yn·gi·tis
ret·ro·phar·ynx
ret·ro·pla·cen·tal
ret·ro·pla·sia
ret·ro·posed
ret·ro·po·si·tion
ret·ro·pul·sion
ret·ror·sine
ret·ro·si·nus
ret·ro·sple·ni·al
ret·ro·spon·dy·lo·lis·the·sis
ret·ro·stal·sis
ret·ro·ster·nal
ret·ro·sym·phys·i·al
ret·ro·tar·sal
ret·ro·uter·ine
ret·ro·ver·sio·flex·ion
ret·ro·ver·sion
    r. of uterus
ret·ro·vert·ed
ret·ro·ves·i·cal
Ret·ro·vir·i·dae
ret·ro·vi·rus

ret·ro·vi·rus
    human lymphotrophic r.
re·tru·sion
    mandibular r.
Rett syndrome
re·turn
    venous r.
Ret·zi·us' cavity
Ret·zi·us' fibers
Ret·zi·us' foramen
Ret·zi·us' lines
Ret·zi·us' space
Ret·zi·us' striae
Ret·zi·us' stripes
Ret·zi·us' veins
Reuss' color charts
Reuss' tables
re·vac·ci·na·tion
re·vas·cu·lar·iza·tion
re·ve·hent
Re·ver·din's graft
Re·ver·din's needle
re·ver·sal
    epinephrine r.
    r. of gradient
    sex r.
re·ver·sal-for·ma·tion
re·verse tran·scrip·tase
re·ver·si·ble
re·ver·sion
    antigenic r.
    genotypic r.
    Mantoux r.
    phenotypic r.
re·ver·tant
Re·vil·liod's sign
re·vi·ves·cence
re·viv·i·fi·ca·tion
rev·o·lute
rev·o·lu·tion
    demographic r.
re·vul·sant
re·vul·sion
re·vul·sive
re·ward
    token r.
re·warm·ing
Reye syndrome

Rey·nals permeability factor
Rey·nold's test
Rez·i·pas
RF — releasing factor
  rheumatoid factor
RFA — right frontoanterior
RFLP — restriction fragment
  length polymorphism
RFP — right frontoposterior
RFPS(Glasgow) — Royal
  Faculty of Physicians and
  Surgeons of Glasgow
RFT — right frontotransverse
RGN — Registered General
  Nurse (Scotland)
RH — releasing hormone
Rh — rhesus factor
  rhodium
Rhab·di·a·soi·dea
rhab·dit·ic
rhab·dit·i·form
Rhab·di·tis
rhab·di·toid
Rhab·di·toi·dea
rhab·do·cyte
rhab·doid
rhab·do·myo·blast
rhab·do·myo·blas·to·ma
rhab·do·myo·chon·dro·ma
rhab·do·my·ol·y·sis
  familial paroxysmal r.
  exertional r.
  idiopathic r.
rhab·do·my·o·ma
rhab·do·myo·myx·o·ma
rhab·do·myo·sar·co·ma
Rhab·do·ne·ma
rhab·dos
rhab·do·sar·co·ma
rhab·do·sphinc·ter
Rhab·do·vir·i·dae
rhab·do·vi·rus
rha·co·ma
rhae·bo·cra·nia
rhae·bo·sce·lia
rhae·bo·sis
rhag·a·des
rha·gad·i·form

rhag·io·crine
rhag·i·on·id
Rhag·i·on·i·dae
rham·ni·nose
rham·nose
rham·no·side
Rham·nus
Rh an·ti·body
rha·pha·nia
rha·phe
Rha·zes
Rh blood group
rhe
rheg·ma
rheg·ma·tog·e·nous
rhe·ni·um
rheo·base
rheo·en·ceph·a·log·ra·phy
rhe·ol·o·gy
Rheo·mac·ro·dex
rhe·om·e·ter
rhe·om·e·try
rheo·nome
rheo·scope
rheo·stat
rhe·os·to·sis
rheo·ta·chyg·ra·phy
rheo·tax·is
  negative r.
  positive r.
rheo·tome
rheo·trope
rhe·ot·ro·pism
rhe·sus (Rh)
Rhe·um
rheum
rheu·ma
rheu·mar·thri·tis
rheu·ma·tal·gia
rheu·mat·ic
  r. heart disease
rheu·ma·tid
rheu·ma·tism
  apoplectic r.
  articular r., acute
  articular r., chronic
  Besnier's r.
  cerebral r.

rheu·ma·tism *(continued)*
   desert r.
   gonorrheal r.
   r. of the heart
   Heberden's r.
   inflammatory r.
   lumbar r.
   MacLeod's capsular r.
   muscular r.
   nodose r.
   nonarticular r.
   osseous r.
   palindromic r.
   Poncet's r.
   subacute r.
   synovial r.
   tuberculous r.
   visceral r.
rheu·ma·tis·mal
rheu·ma·to·gen·ic
rheu·ma·toid
rheu·ma·to·log·ic
rheu·ma·tol·o·gist
rheu·ma·tol·o·gy
rheu·ma·to·sis
rheu·mic
rhex·is
Rh fac·tor
rhi·go·sis
rhi·got·ic
rhi·nal
rhi·nal·gia
rhin·al·ler·go·sis
rhi·nec·to·my
   total r.
rhin·ede·ma
rhin·en·ce·pha·lia
rhin·en·ce·phal·ic
rhin·en·ceph·a·lon
rhin·en·ceph·a·lus
rhin·en·chy·sis
rhin·es·the·sia
rhin·eu·ryn·ter
rhin·i·on
rhi·nism
rhi·ni·tis
   acute catarrhal r.
   allergic r.

rhi·ni·tis *(continued)*
   anaphylactic r.
   atopic r.
   atrophic r.
   atrophic r. of swine
   r. caseosa
   chronic catarrhal r.
   croupous r.
   dyscrinic r.
   fibrinous r.
   gangrenous r.
   granulomatous r.
   hypertrophic r.
   inclusion-body r.
   infective r.
   intrinsic r.
   r. medicamentosa
   membranous r.
   nonseasonal allergic r.
   perennial r.
   perennial allergic r.
   periodic r.
   polypoid r.
   porcine inclusion body r.
   pseudomembranous r.
   purulent r.
   scrofulous r.
   r. sicca
   syphilitic r.
   tuberculous r.
   vasomotor r.
rhi·no·an·e·mom·e·ter
rhi·no·an·tri·tis
rhi·no·by·on
rhi·no·can·thec·to·my
rhi·no·cele
rhi·no·ceph·a·lus
Rhi·no·ceph·a·lus an·nu·la·
   tus
rhi·no·ceph·a·ly
rhi·no·chei·lo·plas·ty
rhi·no·clei·sis
rhi·no·coele
rhi·no·dac·ryo·lith
rhi·no·dym·ia
rhi·no·dyn·ia
rhi·no·en·to·moph·tho·ro·
   my·co·sis

Rhi·no·es·trus
rhi·nog·e·nous
rhi·no·hy·per·pla·sia
rhi·no·ky·pho·sis
rhi·no·la·lia
    r. aperta
    r. clausa
    open r.
rhi·no·lar·yn·gi·tis
rhi·no·lar·yn·gol·o·gy
rhi·no·lith
rhi·no·li·thi·a·sis
rhi·nol·o·gist
rhi·nol·o·gy
rhi·no·ma·nom·e·ter
rhi·no·ma·nom·e·try
rhi·nom·e·ter
rhi·nom·mec·to·my
rhi·no·my·co·sis
rhi·no·ne·cro·sis
rhi·no·nem·me·ter
rhi·no·neu·ro·sis
rhi·no·path·ia
    r. vasomotoria
rhi·nop·a·thy
    vasomotor r.
rhi·no·pha·ryn·ge·al
rhi·no·phar·yn·gi·tis
    r. mutilans
rhi·no·pha·ryn·go·cele
rhi·no·pha·ryn·go·lith
rhi·no·phar·ynx
rhi·no·pho·nia
rhi·no·phy·co·my·co·sis
rhi·no·phy·ma
rhi·no·plas·tic
rhi·no·plas·ty
    augmentation r.
    Carpue's r.
    English r.
    Indian r.
    Joseph r.
    Italian r.
    reconstructive r.
    tagliacotian r.
    Tagliacozzi r.
rhi·no·pneu·mo·ni·tis
    equine viral r.

rhi·no·poly·pus
rhi·nor·rha·gia
rhi·nor·rha·phy
rhi·nor·rhea
    cerebrospinal r.
rhi·no·sal·pin·gi·tis
rhi·no·scle·ro·ma
rhi·no·scope
rhi·no·scop·ic
rhi·nos·co·py
    anterior r.
    median r.
    posterior r.
rhi·no·spo·rid·i·o·sis
Rhi·no·spo·rid·i·um see·beri
rhi·no·steg·no·sis
rhi·no·ste·no·sis
rhi·not·o·my
    lateral r.
rhi·no·tra·che·itis
rhi·no·vac·ci·na·tion
rhi·no·vi·ral
rhi·no·vi·rus
Rhi·pi·cen·tor
Rhi·pi·ceph·a·lus
    R. appendiculatus
    R. bursa
    R. capensis
    R. decoloratus
    R. evertsi
    R. sanguineus
    R. simus
rhi·zan·es·the·sia
rhi·zo·blast
rhi·zo·don·tro·py
rhi·zo·don·try·py
Rhi·zog·ly·phus
    R. parasiticus
rhi·zoid
rhi·zoi·dal
rhi·zol·y·sis
rhi·zome
rhi·zo·me·lia
rhi·zo·mel·ic
rhi·zo·me·nin·go·my·eli·tis
rhi·zo·mere
rhi·zo·neure
rhi·zo·plast

rhi·zo·pod
Rhi·zop·o·da
rhi·zo·po·di·um *pl.* rhi·zo·po·
  dia
Rhi·zo·pus
  R. nigricans
rhi·zot·o·my
  anterior r.
  dorsal r.
  posterior r.
  retrogasserian r.
  trigeminal r.
rho
  Spearman's r.
rho·da·mine
  r. B
rho·da·nate
rho·da·nese
rho·dan·ic acid
rho·da·nine
Rho·din's fixative
rho·di·um
Rhod·ni·us pro·lix·us
rho·do·gen·e·sis
rho·do·my·cin
rho·do·phy·lac·tic
rho·do·phy·lax·is
rho·dop·sin
Rho·do·tor·u·la
  R. glutinis
  R. rubra
rho·do·tor·u·lo·sis
rho·do·tox·in
RhoGAM
rhom·ben·ce·phal·ic
rhom·ben·ceph·a·li·tis
rhom·ben·ceph·a·lon
rhom·bo·coele
rhom·boid
  Michaelis's r.
rhom·bo·mere
rhon·chal
rhon·chi·al
rhon·chus *pl.* rhon·chi
  sibilant r.
Rho·pa·lo·psyl·lus ca·vic·o·la
rhop·try
rho·ta·cism

r-HuEPO — recombinant
  human erythropoietin
Rhus
rhythm
  accelerated idioventricular
    r.
  agonal r.
  alpha r.
  atrioventricular r.
  Berger r.
  beta r.
  bigeminal r.
  biological r.
  cantering r.
  cardiac r.
  circadian r.
  circus r.
  coronary sinus r.
  coupled r.
  delta r.
  ectopic r.
  escape r.
  fetal r.
  gallop r.
  gamma r.
  idionodal r.
  idioventricular r.
  infradian r.
  isochronal r.
  junctional r.
  metachronal r.
  nodal r.
  nyctohemeral r.
  parasystolic r.
  pendulum r.
  quadrigeminal r.
  quadruple r.
  reciprocal r.
  reciprocating r.
  sinus r.
  sinusoidal r.
  theta r.
  train-wheel r.
  triple r.
  ultradian r.
  ventricular r.
rhyth·meur
rhyth·mic

rhyth·mi·cal
rhyth·mic·i·ty
rhyt·i·dec·to·my
rhyt·i·do·plas·ty
rhyt·i·do·sis
RI — recession index
RIA — radioimmunoassay
rib
    abdominal r's
    asternal r's
    bicipital r.
    bifid r.
    branched r.
    cervical r.
    false r's
    floating r's
    fused r.
    slipping r.
    spurious r's
    sternal r's
    sternebral r.
    Stiller's r.
    true r's
    vertebral r's
    vertebrochondral r's
    vertebrocostal r's
    vertebrosternal r's
    Zahn's r's
ri·bam·i·nol
ri·ba·vi·rin
Rib·bert's theory
ri·bo·fu·ra·nose
rib·bon
    r. of Reil
    synaptic r.
Ribes' ganglion
ri·bi·tol
ri·bo·des·ose
ri·bo·fla·vin
    r. 5′-phosphate
ri·bo·fla·vin ki·nase
ri·bo·fu·ra·no·syl·ad·e·nine
ri·bo·fu·ra·no·syl·cy·to·sine
ri·bo·fu·ra·no·syl·gua·nine
ri·bo·nu·cle·ase
    r. I
    r. II
    pancreatic r.

ri·bo·nu·cle·ic acid
    heterogenous nuclear RNA
      (hnRNA)
    messenger RNA (mRNA)
    ribosomal RNA (rRNA)
    transfer RNA (tRNA)
ri·bo·nu·cleo·pro·tein
ri·bo·nu·cleo·side
ri·bo·nu·cleo·side di·phos·
    phate re·duc·tase
ri·bo·nu·cleo·tide
ri·bo·nu·cleo·tide re·duc·tase
ri·bo·prine
ri·bo·py·ra·nose
ri·bose
ri·bose nu·cle·ic acid
ri·bose-5-phos·phate isom·er·
    ase
ri·bose-phos·phate py·ro·
    phos·pho·ki·nase
ri·bo·side
ri·bo·so·mal
ri·bo·some
ri·bos·uria
ri·bo·syl
ri·bo·syl·thy·mine
5-ri·bo·syl·uri·dine
ri·bo·thy·mi·dine
ri·bo·vi·rus
ri·bu·lose
    r. 1,5-diphosphate
    r. 5-phosphate
ri·bu·lose-bi·phos·phate car·
    boxy·lase
ri·bu·lose-phos·phate 3-epim·
    er·ase
RIC — Royal Institute of
    Chemistry
rice
    r. polishings
    white r.
Rich·ards, Dickinson Woodruff,
    Jr.
Rich·ard·son's sign
Ri·chet, Charles Robert
Ri·chet's aneurysm
Ri·chet's fascia

Rich·ter's hernia
Rich·ter's syndrome
Rich·ter-Mon·ro line
ri·cin
ri·cin·ism
ri·cin·ole·ic acid
Ric·i·nus
rick·ets
    acute r.
    adult r.
    anticonvulsant r.
    beryllium r.
    celiac r.
    familial hypophosphatemic
      r.
    familial vitamin
      D–resistant r.
    fat r.
    fetal r.
    hemorrhagic r.
    hepatic r.
    late r.
    lean r.
    pancreatic r.
    pseudodeficiency r.
    refractory r.
    renal r.
    resistant r.
    scurvy r.
    tardy r.
    vitamin D–dependent r.
    vitamin D–refractory r.
    vitamin D–resistant r.
rick·ett·se·mia
Rick·ett·sia
    R. akamushi
    R. akari
    R. australis
    R. burnetii
    R. canis
    R. conorii
    R. diaporica
    R. mooseri
    R. muricola
    R. nipponic
    R. orientalis
    R. pediculi
    R. prowazekii

Rick·ett·sia (continued)
    R. quintana
    R. rickettsii
    R. sennetsu
    R. sibirica
    R. tsutsugamushi
    R. typhi
rick·ett·sia *pl.* rick·ett·siae
Rick·ett·si·a·ceae
rick·ett·si·al
Rick·ett·si·a·les
rick·ett·si·al·pox
rick·ett·si·ci·dal
Rick·ett·si·eae
rick·ett·si·ol·o·gy
rick·ett·si·o·sis
    north Asian tick-borne r.
    canine r.
rick·ett·sio·stat·ic
Ri·co·le·sia
ric·tal
ric·tus
RID — radial
  immunodiffusion
Rid·doch's reflex
Rid·e·al-Walk·er coefficient
ridge
    alveolar r.
    alveolar r., residual
    anal r.
    apical ectodermal r.
    basal r.
    bicipital r., anterior
    bicipital r., external
    bicipital r., internal
    bicipital r., outer
    bicipital r., posterior
    buccocervical r.
    buccogingival r.
    bulbar r's
    carotid r.
    cerebral r's of cranial
      bones
    deltoid r.
    dental r.
    dermal r's
    digital r's
    edentulous r.

ridge *(continued)*
- epicondylic r., lateral
- epicondylic r., medial
- epipericardial r.
- ganglion r.
- gastrocnemial r.
- genital r.
- germ r.
- gluteal r. of femur
- gonadal r.
- healing r.
- r. of humerus
- incisal r.
- interarticular r. of head of rib
- interosseous r.
- intertrochanteric r.
- interureteric r.
- linguocervical r.
- linguogingival r.
- longitudinal r. of hard palate
- Mall's r.
- mammary r.
- r. of mandibular neck
- marginal r.
- medullary r.
- mesonephric r.
- middle r. of femur
- milk r.
- mylohyoid r.
- r. of neck of rib
- nephrogenic r.
- neural r.
- r. of nose
- oblique r.
- oblique r's of scapula
- Outerbridge's r.
- palatine r's, transverse
- papillary r's
- Passavant's r.
- pectoral r.
- pharyngeal r.
- pterygoid r.
- pulmonary r.
- radial r. of wrist
- residual r.
- residual alveolar r.

ridge *(continued)*
- rete r's
- rough r. of femur
- semicircular r.
- skin r's
- sublingual r.
- superciliary r.
- supinator r.
- supplemental r.
- supracondylar r., lateral
- supracondylar r., medial
- supraorbital r.
- suprarenal r.
- synaptic r.
- taste r's
- temporal r.
- tentorial r.
- transverse r.
- trapezoid r.
- triangular r.
- tubercular r. of sacrum
- ulnar r. of wrist
- urethral r.
- urogenital r.
- wolffian r.

rid·gel
ridg·ing
ridg·ling
Rid·ley's sinus
Rie·del's lobe
Rie·del's disease
Rie·del's struma
Rie·del's thyroiditis
Rie·der's cell
Rie·der's cell leukemia
Rie·der's lymphocyte
Rie·gel's pulse
Rie·ger's anomaly
Rie·ger's syndrome
Rieg·ler's test
Riehl's melanosis
Ries·man's pneumonia
Ries·man's sign
Ri·et·ti, Grep·pi, and Mi·che·li's anemia
Rieux's hernia
RIF — right iliac fossa
Rif·a·din

rif·a·mide
rif·am·pi·cin
rif·am·pin
rif·a·my·cin
Rift Val·ley fever
Riga-Fede disease
Riggs' disease
right-hand·ed
ri·gid·i·ty
    α-r.
    anatomical r.
    cadaveric r.
    clasp-knife r.
    cogwheel r.
    decerebrate r.
    extrapyramidal r.
    γ-r.
    hemiplegic r.
    hysterical r.
    lead-pipe r.
    muscular r.
    mydriatic r.
    nuchal r.
    pallidal r.
    paratonic r.
    parkinsonian r.
    pathologic r.
    postmortem r.
    spasmodic r.
    spastic r.
rig·or
    acid r.
    calcium r.
    heat r.
    instantaneous r. mortis
    r. mortis
    r. tremens
    water r.
Ri·ley's virus
Ri·ley-Day syndrome
Ri·ley-Smith syndrome
rim
    r. of abrasion
    bite r.
    occlusion r.
    record r.
ri·ma *pl.* ri·mae
    r. glottidis

ri·ma *(continued)*
    r. glottidis cartilaginea
    r. glottidis membranacea
    intercartilaginous r.
    intermembranous r.
    r. oris
    r. palpebrarum
    r. pudendi
    r. respiratoria
    r. vestibuli
    r. vocalis
    r. vulvae
Rim·ac·tane
r··mae
ri·mal
ri·man·ta·dine hy·dro·chlo·ride
Rim·i·fon
rim·i·ter·ol hy·dro·bro·mide
rim·ose
rim·u·la *pl.* rim·u·lae
rin·der·pest
Rind·fleisch's cells
Rind·fleisch's folds
ring
    abdominal r., deep
    abdominal r., external
    abdominal inguinal r.
    abdominal r., internal
    abdominal r., superficial
    Albl's r.
    amnion r.
    anal r.
    annular r's
    annular r. of Gerlach
    apical r.
    atrial r.
    Balbiani's r's
    Bandl's r.
    benzene r.
    Bickel's r.
    Braun's r.
    Cabot's r's
    Cannon's r.
    carbocyclic r.
    cardiac lymphatic r.
    casting r.
    ciliary r.

ring *(continued)*
    ciliary r. of iris
    closing r. of
      Winkler-Waldeyer
    common tendinous r.
    conjunctival r.
    constriction r.
    contact r.
    contractile r.
    contraction r.
    coronary r.
    crural r.
    Döllinger's tendinous r.
    Donder's r.
    esophageal r.
    Falope r.
    femoral r.
    fibrocartilaginous r. of
      tympanic membrane
    fibrous r., interpubic
    fibrous r's of heart
    fibrous r. of intervertebral
      disk
    Fleischer r.
    Fleischer-Strümpell r.
    Fleischer keratoconus r.
    furan r.
    germ r.
    glaucomatous r.
    Graefenberg r.
    hymenal r.
    infancy r.
    r. of iris, greater
    heterocyclic r.
    homocyclic r.
    inguinal r., deep
    inguinal r., external
    inguinal r., internal
    inguinal r., superficial
    isocyclic r.
    Kayser-Fleischer r.
    r. of iris, lesser
    Landolt's r's
    Liesegang r's
    Löwe's r.
    Lower's r's
    lower esophageal
      contraction r.

ring *(continued)*
    lymphoid r.
    Maxwell's r.
    neonatal r.
    Newton's r's
    Ochsner's r.
    olive r.
    pathologic retraction r.
    pericorneal lymphatic r.
    periosteal bone r.
    physiologic retraction r.
    pleural r's
    polar r.
    posterior limiting r.
    pyran r.
    retraction r.
    Schatzki's r.
    Schwalbe's r.
    Schwalbe's anterior border
      r.
    scleral r.
    signet r.
    Soemmering's r.
    subchorial closing r.
    tantalum r.
    tendinous r., common
    terminal r.
    tonsillar r.
    tracheal r's
    tympanic r.
    umbilical r.
    vascular r.
    venous r. of Haller
    r. of Vieussens
    Vossius' r.
    Waldeyer's tonsillar r.
    Wimberger's r.
    Zinn's r.
ring·bin·den
Ring·er's injection
Ring·er's irrigation
Ring·er's mixture
Ring·er's solution
ring·worm
    anthropophilic r.
    r. of the beard
    black-dot r.
    r. of the body

Ritchie-Black III

ring·worm *(continued)*
    crusted r.
    ectothrix r.
    endothrix r.
    r. of the face
    r. of the feet
    geophilic r.
    gray-patch r.
    r. of the groin
    r. of the hand
    honeycomb r.
    hypertrophic r.
    r. of the nails
    r. of the scalp
Rinne's response
Rinne's test
Ri·o·lan's anastomosis
Ri·o·lan's arch
Ri·o·lan's bone
Ri·o·lan's muscle
Ri·o·lan's nosegay
Ri·o·lan's ossicle
rio·mit·sin
Ri·o·pan
ri·pa
ri·pa·ri·an
Ri·pault's sign
ri·pa·ze·pam
RIPHH — Royal Institute of Public Health and Hygiene
RISA — radioactive iodinated serum albumin
risk
    absolute r.
    assumption of r.
    attributable r.
    competing r.
    empiric r.
    genetic r.
    insurable r.
    population-attributable r.
    relative r.
Ris·ley's prism
ris·o·caine
Ris·ser jacket
RIST — radioimmunosorbent test

Ris·tel·la mel·a·nin·o·gen·i·ca
ris·to·ce·tin
ri·sus
    r. caninus
    r. sardonicus
Rit·a·lin
Rit·gen maneuver
Rit·gen method
rit·o·drine
Rit·ter's disease
Rit·ter's fiber
Rit·ter-Rol·let phenomenon
Rit·ter-Rol·let sign
Rit·ter-Val·li law
rit·u·al
ri·val·ry
    binocular r.
    retinal r.
    sibling r.
Ri·val·ta's reaction
Ri·val·ta's test
Ri·va-Roc·ci sphygmomanometer
Riv·ers cocktail
Riv·iere's sign
ri·vi·ni·an
Ri·vi·nus' canals
Ri·vi·nus' ducts
Ri·vi·nus' foramen
Ri·vi·nus' gland
Ri·vi·nus' incisure
Ri·vi·nus' notch
Ri·vi·nus' segment
ri·vus *pl.* ri·vi
    r. lacrimalis
riz·i·form
RKY — roentgenkymography
RLF — retrolental fibroplasia
RLL — right lower lobe (of lungs)
RLQ — right lower quadrant
RMA — right mentoanterior
RML — right middle lobe (of lungs)
RMP — right mentoposterior
RMT — right mentotransverse

RN — Registered Nurse
RNA — ribonucleic acid
    heterogenous nuclear RNA
        (hnRNA)
    informational RNA
    isoacceptor transfer RNA
    messenger RNA
    nuclear RNA (nRNA)
    polycystic messenger RNA
    ribosomal RNA
    soluble RNA
    template RNA
    transfer RNA
RNase
RNA-di·rect·ed DNA po·lym·
    er·ase
RNA di·rect·ed RNA po·lym·
    er·ase
RNA nu·cleo·tid·yl·trans·fer·
    ase
RNA po·lym·er·ase
RNP — ribonucleoprotein
ROA — right occipitoanterior
Ro·ba·late
Ro·bax·in
Rob·bins, Frederick Chapman
ro·ben·i·dine hy·dro·chlo·ride
Rob·ert's ligament
Rob·ert's pelvis
Rob·erts' test
Rob·ert·shaw tube
Rob·ert·son's pupil
Rob·ert·son's sign
rob·in
Rob·in's anomalad
Rob·in's syndrome
Rob·in·son's circle
Ro·bi·nul
Ro·bi·son ester
Ro·bi·son es·ter de·hy·dro·
    gen·ase
Ro·bi·tus·sin
Rob·les disease
Rob·son's line
Rob·son's point
Rob·son's position
ro·bust
ro·bust·ness

ROC — receiver operating
    characteristics
Ro·ceph·in
Ro·cha·li·maea
    R. quintana
Ro·cher's drawer test
Ro·cher's sign
Ro·chon-Du·vig·neaud
    syndrome
rod
    analyzing r.
    Auer r's
    basal r.
    Corti's r's
    enamel r's
    germinal r.
    Harrington r.
    r's of Heidenhain
    König's r's
    Luque r.
    Maddox r's
    Meckel's r.
    muscle r.
    olfactory r.
    Reichmann's r.
    retinal r.
ro·den·ti·cide
ro·den·tine
rod-mono·chro·mat
ro·do·caine
Roe·der·er's ecchymosis
Roe·der·er's obliquity
roent·gen
roent·gen·ky·mo·graph
roent·gen·ky·mog·ra·phy
roent·geno·car·dio·gram
roent·geno·cin·e·ma·tog·ra·
    phy
roent·geno·gram
roent·geno·graph
roent·geno·graph·ic
roent·gen·og·ra·phy
    body section r.
    double contrast r.
    magnification r.
    mass r.
    mucosal relief r.
    sectional r.

roent·gen·og·ra·phy
  (continued)
    selective r.
    spot film r.
roent·geno·ky·mo·graph
roent·gen·ol·o·gist
roent·gen·ol·o·gy
roent·geno·lu·cent
roent·gen·om·e·ter
roent·gen·om·e·try
roent·gen·opaque
roent·geno·par·ent
roent·geno·scope
roent·gen·os·co·py
roent·geno·ther·a·py
    intraoral r.
roent·gen rays
roe·teln
    intravaginal r.
ro·flu·rane
Ro·ger's bruit
Ro·ger's disease
Ro·ger's murmur
Ro·ger's reaction
Ro·ger's symptom
Ro·ger-Jo·sué test
Ro·gers' sphygmomanometer
Röhl's marginal corpuscles
Ro·ki·tan·sky's disease
Ro·ki·tan·sky's diverticulum
Ro·ki·tan·sky's pelvis
Ro·kin·tan·sky-Asch·off sinus
Ro·kin·tan·sky-Cush·ing ulcer
ro·lan·dic
Ro·lan·do, Luigi
Ro·lan·do's angle
Ro·lan·do's cells
Ro·lan·do's line
ro·lan·dom·e·ter
role
    gender r.
role-play·ing
ro·let·a·mide
rolf·ing
ro·li·tet·ra·cy·cline
    r. nitrate
roll
    cotton r.

roll (continued)
    iliac r.
    jelly r.
    scleral r.
roll·er
Rol·ler's nucleus
Rol·le·ston's rule
Rol·let's stroma
Rol·lier's radiation
Rol·lier's treatment
ROM — range of motion
    rupture of membranes
Ro·maña's sign
ro·mano·pexy
ro·mano·scope
Ro·ma·nov·sky's (Ro·ma·now·
    sky's) stain
Ro·ma·nov·sky's (Ro·ma·now·
    sky's) method
Rom·berg's disease
Rom·berg's sign
Rom·berg's spasm
Rom·berg's station
Rom·berg's trophoneurosis
Rom·berg-How·ship syndrome
rom·berg·ism
Ro·mil·ar
Rom·mel·aere's sign
Ron·do·my·cin
ron·geur
    Adson r.
Ro·ni·a·col
ro·nid·a·zole
Rönne's nasal step
ron·nel
rönt·gen·og·ra·phy
Rood method
roof
    r. of orbit
    r. of skull
    r. of tympanum
room
    anechoic r.
    birthing r.
    consulting r.
    delivery r.
    intensive therapy r.
    labor r.

room *(continued)*
    operating r.
    postdelivery r.
    predelivery r.
    recovery r.
room·ing-in
root
    anatomical r.
    aortic
    r. of arch of vertebra
    belladonna r.
    bitter r.
    clinical r.
    r. of clitoris
    deadly nightshade r.
    dorsal r.
    facial r.
    r. of hair
    internal olfactory r.
    licorice r.
    lingual r.
    r. of lung
    mandrake r.
    r. of mesentery
    motor r.
    r. of nail
    r. of nose
    orizaba jalap r.
    orris r.
    palatine r.
    parasympathetic r. of
      ciliary ganglion
    r. of penis
    penile r.
    physiological r.
    puccoon r.
    red r.
    retained r.
    spinal r's
    spinal vestibular r.
    sweet r.
    r. of tongue
    r. of tooth
    ventral r.
root·let
    flagellar r.
ROP — right occipitoposterior
ro·pi·zine

Ror·schach test
ro·sa·cea
    granulomatous r.
    lupoid r.
    ocular r.
    papular r.
ro·sac·ic acid
ro·sa·mi·cin
ro·san·i·line
ro·sa·ry
    rachitic r.
rose
    r. bengal
Rose's position
Rose's test
Rose-Waa·ler test
ro·se·in
Ro·sen·bach's erysipeloid
Ro·sen·bach's sign
Ro·sen·bach's syndrome
Ro·sen·mül·ler's body
Ro·sen·mül·ler's gland
Ro·sen·mül·ler's node
Ro·sen·mül·ler's organ
Ro·sen·thal's canal
Ro·sen·thal syndrome
Ro·sen·thal's test
Ro·sen·thal's vein
Ro·sen·zweig's test
ro·se·o·la
    r. infantilis
    r. infantum
    syphilitic r.
    r. typhosa
    r. urticata
Ro·ser's sign
Ro·ser-Braun sign
ro·sette
    E r.
    EAC r.
    Homer Wright r.
    malarial r.
    Wintersteiner's r.
ro·sin
Ro·sin's test
Ros·ma·ri·nus
ro·so·lic acid
ro·sox·a·cin

Ross, Sir Ronald
Ross' black spores
Ross' bodies
Ross·bach's disease
Ros·so·li·mo's reflex
Ros·so·li·mo's sign
Ros·tan's asthma
ros·tel·lum *pl.* ros·tel·la
ros·trad
ros·tral
ros·tra·lis
ros·trate
ros·tri·form
ros·trum *pl.* ros·tra, ros·trums
    r. corporis callosi
    r. of corpus callosum
    sphenoidal r.
    r. sphenoidale
ROT — right
  occipitotransverse
ro·tam·e·ter
ro·ta·ry
ro·tate
ro·ta·tion
    external r.
    internal r.
    lateral r.
    manual r.
    medial r.
    molecular r.
    optical r.
    renal r.
    specific r.
    van Ness r.
    wheel r.
ro·ta·tor
ro·ta·to·ry
ro·ta·vi·rus
Rotch's sign
ro·te·none
ro·texed
ro·tex·ion
Roth's (Rot's) disease
Roth's (Rot's) syndrome
Roth's spots
Roth's vas aberrans
Roth-Bern·hardt disease
Roth-Bern·hardt syndrome

Ro·the·ra's test
Roth·ia
    R. dentocariosus
Roth·man-Ma·kai syndrome
Roth·mund syndrome
Roth·mund-Thom·son
  syndrome
Roths·child's sign
rot·lauf
Ro·tor syndrome
ro·to·sco·li·o·sis
ro·tox·amine
    r. tartrate
Rot·ter's nodes
Rot·ter's test
rott·le·ra
rott·ler·in
rouge
Rou·get's bulb
Rou·get's cells
Rou·get's muscle
rough·age
Rough·ton-Scho·lan·der
  method
Roug·non-Heb·er·den disease
rou·leau *pl.* rou·leaux
round·worm
Rous, Francis Peyton
Rous sarcoma
Rous test
Rous·sy-De·je·rine syndrome
Rous·sy-Lé·vy disease
Rous·sy-Lé·vy hereditary
  ataxic dystasia
Rous·sy-Lé·vy syndrome
Rou·vi·ère's node
Roux's anastomosis
Roux-en-Y
Ro·vi·ghi's sign
Rov·sing's sign
Rown·tree-Ger·agh·ty test
RPF — renal plasma flow
R Ph — Registered
  Pharmacist
rpm — revolutions per minute
RPR — rapid plasma reagin
  (test)

RPS — renal pressor substance

RQ — recovery quotient
respiratory quotient

RRA — radioreceptor assay
Registered Record Administrator

RRL — Registered Record Librarian

rRNA — ribosomal RNA

RS — respiratory syncytial (virus)

RScA — right scapuloanterior

RSCN — Registered Sick Children's Nurse

RScP — right scapuloposterior

RSM — Royal Society of Medicine

RSNA — Radiological Society of North America

RSP — right sacroposterior

RST — right sacrotransverse

RSTMH — Royal Society of Tropical Medicine and Hygiene

RSV — respiratory syncytial virus
Rous sarcoma virus

RTA — renal tubular acidosis

RTF — resistance transfer factor

RU — rat unit

rub
  friction r.
  pericardial r.
  pleural r.
  pleuritic r.
  pleuropericardial r.

rub·ber dam
ru·be·fa·cient
ru·bel·la
ru·bel·li·form
ru·be·o·la
ru·be·o·sis
  r. iridis
  r. retinae
ru·ber
ru·ber·ous

ru·bes·cent
ru·bid·i·um
  r. and ammonium bromide
ru·bid·o·my·cin
ru·big·i·nous, ru·big·i·nose
ru·bin
Ru·bin's test
Ru·bin·stein syndrome
Ru·bin·stein-Tay·bi syndrome
ru·bi·vi·rus
Rub·ner's law
Rub·ner's test
ru·bor
  dependent r.
ru·bor·ous
ru·bre·ser·ine
ru·bri·blast
ru·bric
ru·bri·cyte
ru·bro·bul·bar
ru·bro·cer·e·bel·lar
ru·bro·glio·cla·din
ru·bro·ol·i·vary
ru·bro·re·tic·u·lar
ru·bro·spi·nal
ru·bro·tha·lam·ic
ru·brous
Ru·bus
ruc·tus
ru·di·ment
  hair r.
  hepatic r.
  hippocampal r.
  lens r.
  r. of vaginal process
ru·di·men·ta·ry
ru·di·men·tum pl. ru·di·men·ta
  r. processus vaginalis
Ru·di·mi·cro·spo·rea
rue
Ru·fen
Ruf·fi·ni's brushes
Ruf·fi·ni's corpuscles
Ruf·fi·ni's cylinder
Ruf·fi·ni's organ
ru·fo·chro·mo·my·cin
ru·fous

ru·ga *pl.* ru·gae
    rugae gastricae
    rugae palatinae
    palatine rugae
    r. of scrotum
    rugae of stomach
    r. of urinary bladder
    rugae of vagina
    rugae vaginales
ru·gae
Rug·ge·ri's reflex
Rug·ge·ri's sign
ru·gine
    Lempert r.
ru·gi·tus
ru·gose
ru·gous
ru·gos·i·ty
RUL — right upper lobe (of a lung)
rule
    Allen's r.
    American Law Institute r.
    analytic r.
    Anstie's r.
    Aston's r.
    Arey's r.
    Bartholomews'r. of fourths
    Bastedo's r.
    Bergmann's r.
    Budin's r.
    Clark's r.
    Clark's body area r.
    Cowling's r.
    delivery date r.
    dermatomal r.
    Dilling's r.
    discovery r.
    Durham r.
    Eichler's r.
    Fahrenholtz r.
    Fried's r.
    Fuhrman's r.
    Gibson's r.
    Goodsall's r.
    Haase's r.
    Hamburger's r.
    Hardy-Weinberg r.

rule *(continued)*
    His r.
    Hudson's lactone r.
    Jackson's r.
    Knaus r.
    Liebermeister's r.
    Lossen's r.
    McDonald's r.
    M'Naghten r.
    Nägele's r.
    r. of nines
    octet r.
    r. of outlet
    phase r.
    Quetelet's r.
    Rolleston's r.
    Szidat r.
    van't Hoff's r.
    Weinberg's r.
    Young's r.
rum·ble
    diastolic r.
Rum·pel-Leede phenomenon
Rum·pel-Leede sign
Rum·pel-Leede test
Run·dles-Falls anemia
Run·dles-Falls syndrome
Rune·berg's anemia
Rune·berg's disease
Rune·berg's type
Rune·berg's formula
ru·pia
ru·pi·al
ru·pi·oid
rup·ture
    artifical r. of membranes
    defense r.
    extracapsular r.
    incidental r.
    intracapsular r.
    r. of membranes (ROM)
    premature r. of membranes (PROM)
    prolonged r. of membranes
    spontaneous r.
    traumatic r.
RUQ — right upper quadrant
Rus·co·ni's anus

Rush, Benjamin
Rus·sell's bodies
Rus·sell's double sugar agar
Rus·sell effect
Rus·sell syndrome
Russell traction
Rus·sell's viper
Rus·sell's viper venom
Rus·so's reaction
Rus·so's test
Rust's disease
Rust's phenomenon
Rust's sign
Rust's syndrome
ru·the·ni·um
ruth·er·ford
ruth·er·ford·i·um
ru·ti·do·sis
ru·tin

ru·ti·nose
ru·to·side
Ruysch's glomeruli
Ruysch's membrane
Ruysch's muscle
Ruysch's tube
Ruysch's tunic
Ruysch's veins
ruysch·ian membrane
RV — residual volume
RVA — rabies vaccine
    absorbed
RVH — right ventricular
    hypertrophy
℞ — L. recipe, take
rye
    spurred r.
Ryle tube

S

S — sacral vertebrae (S1–S5)
    serum
    siemens
    smooth (colony)
    sone
    spherical lens
    substrate
    sulfur
    Svedberg unit
S. — L. signa (mark)
S — entropy
S_1 — first heart sound
S_2 — second heart sound
S_3 — third heart sound
S_4 — fourth heart sound
S_f — Svedberg flotation unit
s — second
s. — L. semis (half)
    L. sinister (left)
$\bar{s}$ — L. sine (without)

s — sample standard deviation
s^{-1} — reciprocal second
σ — standard deviation
S.A. — L. secundum artem
    (according to art)
SAA — severe aplastic anemia
Saath·off's test
sa·ber-legged
Sa·bethes
Sa·bin's megaloblast
Sa·bin's pronormoblast
Sa·bin's vaccine
Sa·bin-Feld·man dye test
sab·i·nism
sab·i·nol
Sab·ou·raud's dextrose agar
Sab·ou·rau·dia
Sab·ou·rau·di·tes
sab·u·lous
sa·bur·ra

sa·bur·ral
sab·u·lum
sac
    abdominal s.
    air s's
    allantoic s.
    alveolar s's
    amniotic s.
    aneurysmal s.
    aortic s.
    chorionic s.
    conjunctival s.
    dental s.
    dural s.
    embryonic s.
    enamel s.
    endolymphatic s.
    epiploic s.
    gestation s.
    greater s. of peritoneum
    s. of Gruber
    heart s.
    hernial s.
    Hilton's s.
    lacrimal s.
    laryngeal s.
    lesser s. of peritoneal
      cavity
    Lower's s's
    lymphatic s's
    omental s.
    pericardial s.
    peritoneal s.
    pleural s.
    posterior lymph s's
    preputial s.
    pudendal s.
    retroperitoneal lymph s.
    serous s.
    splenic s.
    synovial s.
    tear s.
    tubotympanic s.
    vaginal s.
    vitelline s.
    yolk s.
sac·brood
sac·cade

sac·cad·ic
sac·cate
sac·cha·ra·scope
sac·cha·rate
sac·cha·rat·ed
sac·char·eph·i·dro·sis
sac·char·ic acid
sac·cha·ride
sac·cha·rif·er·ous
sac·char·i·fi·ca·tion
sac·cha·rim·e·ter
    Einhorn's s.
    fermentation s.
    Lohnstein's s.
sac·cha·rin
    s. calcium
    s. sodium
sac·cha·rine
sac·char·i·nol
sac·cha·ri·num
sac·cha·ro·bi·ose
sac·cha·ro·co·ria
sac·cha·ro·ga·lac·tor·rhea
sac·cha·ro·lyt·ic
sac·cha·ro·me·ta·bol·ic
sac·cha·ro·me·tab·o·lism
sac·cha·rom·e·ter
Sac·cha·ro·my·ces
    S. albicans
    S. anginae
    S. bayanus
    S. cantliei
    S. capillitii
    S. carlsbergensis
    S. cerevisiae
    S. dairensis
    S. ellipsoideus
    S. exiguus
    S. galacticolus
    S. glutinis
    S. granulomatosus
    S. guttulatus
    S. hansenii
    S. hominis
    S. lemonnieri
    S. lithogenes
    S. mesentericus
    S. mycoderma

Sac·cha·ro·my·ces (continued)
S. *neoformans*
S. *pastorianus*
S. *rubrum*
S. *subcutaneus tumefaciens*
S. *tumefaciens albus*
sac·cha·ro·my·ces *pl.* sac·cha·ro·my·cetes
Busse's s.
Sac·cha·ro·my·ce·ta·cea
sac·cha·ro·my·ce·tes
sac·cha·ro·my·cet·ic
sac·cha·ro·my·ce·tol·y·sis
Sac·cha·ro·my·cop·sis
S. *guttulatus*
sac·cha·ro·pine
sac·cha·ro·pine de·hy·dro·gen·ase
sac·cha·ror·rhea
sac·cha·ro·san
sac·cha·rose
sac·cha·ros·uria
Sac·cha·rum
sac·cha·rum lac·tis
sac·cha·ru·ria
sac·ci·form
sac·cu·lar
sac·cu·lat·ed
sac·cu·la·tion
cecal s's
s's of colon
uterine s.
sac·cule
air s's
alveolar s's
laryngeal s.
s. of larynx
sac·cu·li
sac·cu·lot·o·my
sac·cu·lo·coch·le·ar
sac·cu·lus *pl.* sac·cu·li
sacculi alveolares
s. communis
s. dentis
s. endolymphaticus
s. lacrimalis
s. laryngis
s. Morgagnii

sac·cu·lus *(continued)*
s. proprius
s. rotundus
s. sphaericus
s. ventricularis
s. vestibularis
sac·cus *pl.* sac·ci
s. conjunctivalis
s. endolymphaticus
s. lacrimalis
s. vaginalis
SACH — single axis cushion heel (foot)
Sachs' disease
Sachsse's test
sa·crad
sa·cral
sa·cral·gia
sa·cral·iza·tion
lumbar s.
sa·crar·thro·gen·ic
sa·crec·to·my
sac·ri·fice
sa·cro·an·te·ri·or
sa·cro·coc·cy·ge·al
sa·cro·coc·cyx
sa·cro·cox·al·gia
sa·cro·cox·itis
sa·cro·dyn·ia
sa·cro·il·i·ac
sa·cro·il·i·itis
sa·cro·lis·the·sis
sa·cro·lum·bar
sa·cro·peri·ne·al
sa·cro·pos·te·ri·or
sa·cro·prom·on·to·ry
sa·cro·sci·at·ic
sa·cro·spi·nal
sa·crot·o·my
sa·cro·trans·verse
sa·cro·uter·ine
sa·cro·ver·te·bral
sa·crum
assimilation s.
tilted s.
sac·to·sal·pinx
sad·dle
bounded s.

sad·dle *(continued)*
    denture base s.
    free-end s.
sad·dle·nose
sa·dism
    anal s.
    oral s.
sa·dist
sa·dis·tic
sa·do·ma·so·chism
sa·do·ma·so·chis·tic
Sae·misch's operation
Sae·misch's section
Sae·misch's ulcer
Saeng·er's macula
Saeng·er's reflex
Saeng·er's sign
Sae·thre-Chot·zen syndrome
Saff
Saf·flor
safranin O
saf·ra·nine
saf·ra·no·phil·ic
saf·rene
saf·rol
saf·ro·sin
sag·it·tal
sag·it·ta·lis
sa·go
Sah·li's method
Sah·li's reaction
Sah·li's test
St. Aig·non's disease
St. An·tho·ny's disease
St. Clair Thom·son's curet
St. Vi·tus' dance
S.A.L. — L. secundum artis
  leges (according to the rules
  of art)
sal
    s. ammoniac
    s. diureticum
    s. soda
    s. volatile
Sala's cells
sal·abra·sion
sal·acet·amide
sal·a·man·der

sal·a·man·der·in
sal·an·tel
sal·a·zo·sul·fa·pyr·i·dine
sal·bu·ta·mol
sal·ca·to·nin
sal·co·lex
sal·eth·amide mal·e·ate
sal·i·cyl·al·de·hyde
sal·i·cyl·amide
sal·i·cyl·an·i·lide
sal·i·cyl·ate
    s. meglumine
    theophylline calcium s.
sal·i·cyl·at·ed
sal·i·cyl·a·zo·sul·fa·pyr·i·
  dine
sal·i·cyl·emia
sal·i·cyl·ic
sal·i·cyl·ic acid
sal·i·cyl·ism
sal·i·cyl·sal·i·cyl·ic acid
sal·i·cyl·sul·fon·ic acid
sal·i·cyl·ur·ic acid
sa·li·ent
sal·i·fi·a·ble
sal·i·fy
sa·lim·e·ter
sa·line
    hypertonic s.
    hypotonic s.
    normal s. (NS)
    physiological s.
sa·lin·i·ty
sal·i·nom·e·ter
sal·it
sa·li·va
    chorda s.
    ganglionic s.
    lingual s.
    parotid s.
    ropy s.
    sublingual s.
    submaxillary s.
    sympathetic s.
sal·i·vant
sal·i·var·ia
sal·i·var·i·an
sal·i·vary

sal·i·vate
sal·i·va·tion
sal·i·va·tor
sal·i·va·to·ry
sal·i·vo·li·thi·a·sis
Salk vaccine
Sal·kow·ski's method
Sal·kow·ski's test
sal·mi·ac
sal·min
Sal·mo·nel·la
   S. agona
   S. arizonae
   S. bongor
   S. choleraesuis
   S. choleraesuis var.
    kuzendorf
   S. choleraesuis var.
    typhisuis
   S. enteritidis
   S. enteritidis serotype
    agona
   S. enteritidis serotype
    heidelberg
   S. enteritidis serotype
    hirschfeldii
   S. enteritidis serotype
    infantis
   S. enteritidis serotype
    newport
   S. enteritidis serotype
    paratyphi A
   S. enteritidis serotype
    schottmuelleri
   S. enteritidis serotype
    sendai
   S. enteritidis serotype
    typhimurium
   S. heidelberg
   S. hirschfeldii
   S. houtenae
   S. infantis
   S. morgani
   S. newport
   S. paratyphi
   S. paratyphi A
   S. paratyphi B
   S. paratyphi C

Sal·mo·nel·la (continued)
   S. salamae
   S. schottmuelleri
   S. sendai
   S. suipestifer
   S. typhi
   S. typhimurium
   S. typhisuis
   S. typhosa
sal·mo·nel·la *pl.* sal·mo·nel·
  lae
sal·mo·nel·lal
Sal·mo·nel·leae
sal·mo·nel·lo·sis
sal·mon-patch
sal·o·coll
sa·lol
Sal·o·mon's test
sal·pin·gec·to·my
sal·pin·gem·phrax·is
sal·pin·gi·an
sal·pin·gi·on
sal·pin·git·ic
sal·pin·gi·tis
  chronic interstitial s.
  chronic vegetating s.
  eustachian s.
  follicular s.
  gonococcal s.
  hemorrhagic s.
  hypertrophic s.
  s. isthmica nodosa
  mural s.
  nodular s.
  parenchymatous s.
  s. profluens
  pseudofollicular s.
  purulent s.
  tuberculous s.
sal·pin·go·cele
sal·pin·gog·ra·phy
sal·pin·go·li·thi·a·sis
sal·pin·gol·y·sis
sal·pin·go·pal·a·tine
sal·pin·go-ooph·o·rec·to·my
sal·pin·go-ooph·o·ri·tis
sal·pin·go-ooph·oro·cele
sal·pin·go-oo·the·ci·tis

sal·pin·go-oo·the·co·cele
sal·pin·go-ovar·i·ec·to·my
sal·pin·go-ovar·i·ot·o·my
sal·pin·go·peri·to·ni·tis
sal·pin·go·pexy
sal·pin·go·pha·ryn·ge·al
sal·pin·go·plas·ty
sal·pin·gor·rha·phy
sal·pin·go·sal·pin·gos·to·my
sal·pin·gos·co·py
sal·pin·go·staph·y·line
sal·pin·go·sto·mat·o·my
sal·pin·go·sto·mato·plas·ty
sal·pin·gos·to·my
sal·pin·go·the·cal
sal·pin·got·o·my
sal·pinx
    s. auditiva
    s. uterina
sal·sa·late
salt
    acid s.
    artificial s.
    artificial Carlsbad s.
    artificial Kissingen s.
    basic s.
    bile s's
    bone s's
    buffer s.
    Carlsbad s.
    common s.
    complex s.
    diuretic s.
    double s.
    effervescent s's
    effervescent artificial
     Vichy s.
    Epsom s.
    Glauber's s.
    halide s.
    haloid s.
    iodized s.
    neutral s.
    normal s.
    Plimmer's s.
    Preston's s.
    Rochelle s.
    Seignette's s.

salt *(continued)*
    smelling s's
    Wurster's s's
sal·ta·tion
sal·ta·to·ri·al
sal·ta·to·ric
sal·ta·to·ry
Sal·ter fracture (I through VI)
Sal·ter's line
salt·ing in
salt·ing out
salt·pe·ter
    Chile s.
sa·lu·bri·ous
sal·ure·sis
sal·uret·ic
Sal·u·ron
sal·u·tary
sa·lute
    allergic s.
Sal·u·ten·sin
Sal·u·ten·sin-Demi
sa·lut·ing
sal·var·san
    silver s.
    sulfoxylate s.
salve
Sal·via
Sal·yr·gan
sa·ly·sal
Salz·mann's nodular corneal
  dystrophy
SAM — systolic anterior
  motion
sam·an·dar·i·dine
sam·an·da·rine
sa·mar·i·um
sam·ple
    biased s.
    matched s.
    paired s's
    random s.
    representative s.
    stratified s.
    systematic s.
samp·ling
    chorionic villus s. (CVS)
    cluster s.

samp·ling *(continued)*
    duplicate portion s.
    Haldane-Priestley s.
    multistage s.
    quota s.
    random s.
    sequential s.
Samp·son's cyst
San·a·rel·li's phenomenon
san·a·tive
san·a·to·ri·um
san·a·to·ry
Sanc·to·ri·us
san·cy·cline
sand
    brain s.
    hydatid s.
    intestinal s.
san·dal·wood
san·da·rac
sand crack
San·der's disease
San·der's paranoia
San·ders bed
San·ders' disease
San·ders forceps
San·ders incision
San·ders laryngoscope
sand·fly
San·di·son-Clark chamber
San·dril
Sand·ström's bodies
Sand·ström'glands
Sand·with's bald tongue
sand·worm
sane
San·fi·lip·po's disease
San·fi·lip·po's syndrome
San·ger Brown ataxia
san·guic·o·lous
san·gui·fa·cient
san·guif·er·ous
san·gui·fi·ca·tion
san·gui·mo·tor
san·gui·mo·to·ry
san·gui·nar·ia
san·gui·na·rine
san·guine

san·guin·e·ous
san·gui·ni·fi·ca·tion
san·guin·o·lent
san·gui·no·poi·et·ic
san·gui·no·pu·ru·lent
san·gui·nous
san·gui·re·nal
san·guis
san·gui·su·ga
san·guiv·o·rous
sa·ni·es
sa·nio·pu·ru·lent
sa·nio·se·rous
sa·ni·ous
san·i·tar·i·an
san·i·tar·i·um
san·i·tary
san·i·ta·tion
san·i·ti·za·tion
san·i·tize
san·i·ty
San·o·rex
San·sert
San·som's sign
San·son's images
san·ta·lum
    s. rubrum
san·ton·i·ca
san·to·nin
San·to·ri·ni's cartilages
San·to·ri·ni's duct
San·to·ri·ni's fissure
San·to·ri·ni's ligament
San·to·ri·ni's muscle
San·to·ri·ni's papilla
San·to·ri·ni's plexus
San·to·ri·ni's tubercle
sap
    cell s.
    nuclear s.
sa·phe·na
saph·e·nec·to·my
sa·phe·nous
sap·id
sa·pin
sa·po
    s. domesticus
    s. mollis

sa·po *(continued)*
    s. mollis medicinalis
    s. viridis
sa·pog·e·nin
sa·po·na·ceous
Sa·po·nar·ia
sa·po·na·tus
sa·pon·i·fi·a·ble
sa·pon·i·fi·ca·tion
sa·pon·i·fy
sap·o·nin
    cholan s's
    triterpenoid s's
sap·o·phore
sa·po·ros·i·ty
sap·o·tal·ene
sa·po·tox·in
Sap·pey's fibers
Sap·pey's ligament
Sap·pey's nucleus
Sap·pey's veins
sap·phism
Sap·pin·ia di·ploi·dea
sa·prin
sa·probe
sa·pro·bic
Sap·ro·leg·nia
Sap·ro·leg·ni·a·les
sap·ro·no·sis
sa·proph·a·gous
sa·proph·i·lous
sap·ro·phyte
sap·ro·phyt·ic
sap·ro·troph
sap·ro·zo·ic
sap·ro·zo·ite
sap·ro·zoo·no·sis
sar·al·a·sin ac·e·tate
Sar·bó's sign
Sar·ci·na
sar·ci·na *pl.* sar·ci·nae
sar·co·blast
sar·co·car·ci·no·ma
sar·co·cele
sar·co·cyst
Sar·co·cys·ti·dae
sar·co·cys·tin

Sar·co·cys·tis
    S. bovihominis
    S. hominis
    S. lindemanni
    S. suihominis
sar·co·cys·to·sis
sar·co·cyte
Sar·co·di·na
sar·co·dine
sar·co·din·i·an
sar·co·en·chon·dro·ma
sar·co·gen·ic
sar·cog·lia
sar·co·hy·dro·cele
sar·coid
    Boeck's s.
    s. of Boeck
    Darier-Roussy s.
    multiple benign s.
    Salem s.
    Schaumann's s.
    Spiegler-Fendt s.
sar·coi·do·sis
    beryllium s.
    cerebral s.
    s. cordis
    Danielssen-Boeck s.
    hypercalcemic s.
    intrathoracic s.
    muscular s.
    myocardial s.
sar·co·lac·tic acid
sar·co·lem·ma
sar·co·lem·mic
sar·co·lem·mous
sar·co·ly·sis
sar·co·lyte
L-sar·co·ly·sin
sar·co·ma *pl.* sar·co·mas, sar·
  co·ma·ta
    Abernethy's s.
    adipose s.
    alveolar soft part s.
    ameloblastic s.
    botryoid s.
    s. botryoides
    cerebral reticulum cell s.

sar·co·ma *(continued)*
  chloromatous s.
  chondroblastic s.
  circumscribed cerebellar
    arachnoid s.
  s. colli uteri hydropicum
    papillare
  s. cutaneum
    telangiectaticum
    multiplex
  deciduocellular s.
  embryonal s.
  endometrial stromal s.
  Ewing's s.
  fascial s.
  fibroblastic s.
  fowl s.
  giant cell s.
  glandular s.
  granulocytic s.
  histiocytic s.
  Hodgkin's s.
  idiopathic multiple
    pigmented hemorrhagic s.
  immunoblastic s. of B cells
  immunoblastic s. of T cells
  intracanalicular s.
  Jensen's s.
  Kaposi's s.
  Kupffer cell s.
  leukocytic s.
  lymphangioendothelial s.
  lymphatic s.
  melanotic s.
  mixed cell s.
  monstrocellular s.
  multiple idiopathic
    hemorrhagic s.
  myeloid s.
  neurogenic s.
  osteoblastic s.
  osteogenic s.
  osteoid s.
  osteolytic s.
  parosteal s.
  periductal s.
  periosteal s.
  s. of peripheral nerve

sar·co·ma *(continued)*
  polymorphous s.
  pseudo–Kaposi s.
  reticulum cell s.
  Rous s.
  serocystic s.
  spindle-cell s.
  synovial s.
  telangiectatic s.
  s. of testis
  Walker s.
sar·co·ma·gen·ic
Sar·co·mas·ti·goph·o·ra
sar·co·ma·ta
sar·co·ma·toid
sar·co·ma·to·sis
  s. cutis
  general s.
  meningeal s.
sar·co·ma·tous
sar·co·mere
sar·co·meso·the·li·o·ma
sar·co·neme
Sar·coph·a·ga
Sar·co·phag·i·dae
sar·co·plasm
sar·co·plas·mic
sar·co·plast
sar·co·poi·et·ic
Sar·cop·syl·la
  S. penetrans
Sar·cop·tes
  S. scabiei
sar·cop·tic
Sar·cop·ti·dae
sar·cop·ti·do·sis
sar·cop·toid
sar·co·sine
sar·co·sine de·hy·dro·gen·ase
sar·co·si·ne·mia
sar·co·sis
sar·co·some
Sar·co·spo·rid·ia
sar·co·spo·rid·i·a·sis
sar·co·spo·rid·i·o·sis
sar·cos·to·sis
sar·co·style
sar·cot·ic

sar·co·tu·bules
sar·cous
sar·don·ic
sa·rin
sar·men·tog·e·nin
Sa·ro·tham·nus
sar·pi·cil·lin
Sar·ra·ce·nia
sar·sa·pa·ril·la
sar·sa·sapo·gen·in
Sas·sa·fras
SATA — spatial average
  temporal average
sat·el·lite
    bacterial s.
    centriolar s.
    chromosomal s.
    nucleolar s.
    pericentriolar s.
    perineuronal s.
    perivascular s.
sat·el·li·tism
sat·el·li·to·sis
sa·ti·a·tion
sa·ti·e·ty
Sat·ter·thwaite's method
Sat·tler's layer
sat·u·rat·ed
sat·u·ra·tion
    arterial oxygen s. (SaO_2)
    blood oxygen s.
    oxygen s.
sat·ur·nine
sat·ur·nism
sat·y·ri·a·sis
sat·y·ro·ma·nia
sau·cer
    auditory s.
sau·cer·iza·tion
sau·cer·ize
Sau·er's vaccine
Sau·er·bruch's cabinet
Sau·er·bruch's prosthesis
sau·na
Saund·by's test
Saun·ders' disease
Saun·ders' sign
Saus·sure's hygrometer

Sau·vi·neau's ophthalmoplegia
Sav·age's perineal body
sav·in
saw
    Adams' s.
    Albee s.
    amputating s.
    bayonet s.
    Butcher's s.
    crown s.
    Farabeuf's s.
    Gigli's wire s.
    Hey's s.
    hole s.
    separating s.
    Shrady's s.
    subcutaneous s.
    Stryker s.
saxi·fra·gant
saxi·tox·in
Sax·torph's maneuver
Sayre's apparatus
SBE — subacute bacterial
  endocarditis
SC — closure of the semilunar
  valves
    secretory component
scab
    foot s.
    head s.
    sheep s.
sca·bet·ic
sca·bi·cide
sca·bies
    cat s.
    crusted s.
    Norwegian s.
    sarcoptic s.
sca·bi·et·ic
sca·la *pl.* sca·lae
    s. media
    s. of Löwenberg
    s. tympani
    s. vestibuli
sca·lar
sca·lar·i·form
scald

scale
  absolute s.
  absolute temperature s.
  adhesive s.
  Apgar s.
  Baumé's s.
  Bayley s. of infant
    development
  Berkow s.
  Brazelton behavioral s.
  Cattell Infant Intelligence
    S.
  Celsius s.
  centigrade s.
  Charrière s.
  Clark's s.
  Columbia Mental Maturity
    S.
  developmental s.
  dichotomous s.
  Dubowitz s.
  Dubowitz infant maturity
    s.
  Dunfermline s.
  Esterman s.
  Fahrenheit s.
  French s.
  Gaffky s.
  Gesell developmental s's
  Glasgow coma s.
  Global Assessment S.
  gray s.
  homigrade s.
  hydrometer s.
  interval s.
  Karnofsky s.
  Karnofsky rating s.
  Kelvin s.
  Minnesota preschool s.
  nominal s.
  nonlinear s.
  ordinal s.
  Outerbridge s.
  pH s.
  Rankine s.
  rating s.
  ratio s.
  Réaumur s.

scale *(continued)*
  Sörensen s.
  Stanford-Binet intelligence
    s.
  Tanner developmental s.
  temperature s.
  Vineland social maturity s.
  Wechsler Adult
    Intelligence s. (WAIS)
  Wechsler Intelligence S.
    for Children (WISC)
  Zung depression s.
sca·lene
sca·le·nec·to·my
sca·le·not·o·my
sca·le·nus
sca·ler
  chisel s.
  deep s.
  double-ended s.
  hoe s.
  sickle s.
  superficial s.
  ultrasonic s.
  watch-spring s.
scal·ing
  deep s.
  root s.
  subgingival s.
  ultrasonic s.
scal·lop·ing
  vertebral s.
scalp
  gyrate s.
scal·pel
  plasma s.
scal·pri·form
scal·prum
sca·ly
scam·mo·nia
scam·mo·ny
  Mexican s.
scan
  B s.
  bone s.
  bone-marrow s.
  brain s.
  C s.

scan *(continued)*
   CAT s.
   C-mode s.
   compound s.
   CT s.
   gallium s.
   gamma s.
   HIDA (hepato-
     iminodiacetic acid) s.
   liver s.
   mechanical compound s.
   Meckel s.
   medronate s.
   MUGA (multiple gaited
     acquisition) s.
   perfusion s.
   PIPIDA s.
   Positron s.
   PYP (pyrophosphate) s.
   radioactive s.
   sector s.
   single sweep s.
   technetium s.
   thallium myocardial s.
   ventilation-perfusion s.
   V/Q s.
scan·di·um
scan·ner
   duplex s.
   EMI s.
   gated s. CT
   mechanical real-time s.
   multicrystal whole-body s.
   PET (Positron emission
     tomography) s.
   rectilinear s.
   scintillation s.
   small parts s.
   tomographic s.
scan·ning
   line s.
   linear s.
   radioisotope s.
   ventilation-perfusion s.
sca·nog·ra·phy
scan·sion
scan·so·ri·us
Scan·zo·ni's maneuver

Scan·zo·ni's operation
scape·goat·ing
sca·pha
sca·phi·on
scapho·ce·pha·lia
scapho·ce·phal·ic
scapho·ceph·a·lism
scapho·ceph·a·lous
scapho·ceph·a·ly
scapho·hy·dro·ceph·a·lus
scapho·hy·dro·ceph·a·ly
scaph·oid
scaph·oid·itis
   tarsal s.
scapho·lu·nate
Scap·to·co·sa
   S. raptoria
scap·u·la *pl.* scap·u·lae
   alar s.
   s. alata
   elevated s.
   Graves' s.
   scaphoid s.
   winged s.
scap·u·lal·gia
scap·u·lar
scap·u·lary
scap·u·lec·to·my
scap·u·lo·an·te·ri·or
scap·u·lo·cla·vic·u·lar
scap·u·lo·dyn·ia
scap·u·lo·hu·mer·al
scap·u·lo·pexy
scap·u·lo·pos·te·ri·or
sca·pus *pl.* sca·pi
   s. penis
   s. pili
scar
   bridle s.
   cortical s.
   hesitation s's
   hypertrophic s.
   icepick s's
   mature s.
   Reichert's s.
   shilling s's
   tissue paper s.
   ulceration s.

scar *(continued)*
    white s. of ovary
scar·a·bi·a·sis
Scar·di·no's uteropelvioplasty
scarf
    Mayor's s.
scar·i·fi·ca·tion
scar·i·fi·ca·tor
scar·i·fi·er
scar·i·fy
scar·la·ti·na
    s. anginosa
    s. haemorrhagica
    malignant s.
    s. papulosa
    s. pruriginosa
    puerperal s.
    s. pustulosa
    s. rheumatica
scar·lat·i·nal
scar·lat·i·nel·la
scar·la·tin·i·form
scar·lat·i·noid
scar·let
    Biebrich s., water-soluble
    s. G
    s. R
Scar·pa's fascia
Scar·pa's fluid
Scar·pa's foramen
Scar·pa's ganglion
Scar·pa's ligament
Scar·pa's membrane
Scar·pa's nerve
Scar·pa's sheath
Scar·pa's staphyloma
Scar·pa's triangle
scar·ring
    web s.
SCAT — sheep cell
  agglutination test
    sickle cell anemia test
sca·te·mia
sca·tol
scato·lo·gia
scato·log·ic
sca·tol·o·gy
sca·to·ma

sca·toph·a·gy
scato·phil·ia
sca·tos·co·py
scat·ter
    coherent s.
    forward s.
    light s.
scat·ter·gram
scat·ter·ing
    coherent s.
    Compton s.
    Rayleigh s.
    Thomson s.
scat·ter·plot
scat·u·la
scav·en·ger
ScD — Doctor of Science
ScDA — L. scapulodextra
  anterior (right
  scapuloanterior)
ScDP — L. scapulodextra
  posterior (right
  scapuloposterior)
Sce·do·spo·ri·um
sce·lal·gia
scel·o·tyr·be
Scha·cher's ganglion
Scha·cho·wa's spiral tubes
Schae·fer sign
Scha·fer's method
Scha·fer syndrome
Schäf·fer's reflex
Scham·berg's dermatosis
Scham·berg's disease
Schanz's disease
Schanz's syndrome
Schar·din·ger's enzyme
Schar·din·ger's reaction
schar·lach R
Schat·zki's ring
Schau·dinn's fluid
Schau·mann's bodies
Schau·mann's disease
Schau·mann's sarcoid
Schau·mann's syndrome
Schau·ta's operation
Schau·ta-Wert·heim operation
Sche·de's clot

sched·ule
   fixed interval s.
   fixed ratio s.
   Gesell developmental s.
   s. of reinforcement
   variable interval s.
   variable ratio s.
Scheie's syndrome
Schei·ner's experiment
sche·ma
   Hamberger's s.
sche·mat·ic
sche·mato·gram
sche·mato·graph
Scher·er's test
sche·ro·ma
Scheu·er·mann's disease
Scheu·er·mann's kyphosis
Schick's reaction
Schick's sign
Schick's test
Schief·fer·deck·er's disk
Schief·fer·deck·er's theory
Schiff's biliary cycle
Schiff's reagent
Schiff's test
Schil·der's disease
Schil·der's encephalitis
Schil·der-Ad·di·son complex
Schil·ler's test
Schil·ling blood count
Schil·ling test
Schim·mel·busch's disease
schin·dy·le·sis
Schi·otz's tonometer
Schir·mer's test
schis·ta·sis
schis·to·ce·lia
schis·to·ceph·a·lus
schis·to·coe·lia
schis·to·cor·mia
schis·to·cor·mus
schis·to·cys·tis
schis·to·cyte
schis·to·cy·to·sis
schis·to·glos·sia
schis·to·me·lia
schis·tom·e·lus

schis·to·pro·so·pia
schis·to·pros·o·pus
schis·tor·a·chis
schis·to·sis
Schis·to·so·ma
   S. *haematobium*
   S. *intercalatum*
   S. *japonicum*
   S. *mansoni*
   S. *mekongi*
schis·to·so·ma·ci·dal
schis·to·so·ma·cide
schis·to·so·mal
Schis·to·so·ma·toi·dea
schis·to·some
schis·to·so·mia
schis·to·so·mi·a·sis
   Asiatic s.
   bladder s.
   cerebral s.
   cutaneous s.
   eastern s.
   genitourinary s.
   s. haematobia
   hepatic s.
   s. intercalatum
   intestinal s.
   s. japonica
   Manson's s.
   s. mansoni
   Oriental s.
   pulmonary s.
   rectal s.
   urinary s.
   vesical s.
   visceral s.
schis·to·so·mi·ci·dal
schis·to·so·mi·cide
Schis·to·so·mum
schis·to·so·mus
schis·to·ster·nia
schis·to·tho·rax
schis·to·tra·che·lus
schiz·am·ni·on
schiz·ax·on
schiz·en·ce·phal·ic
schiz·en·ceph·a·ly
schizo·af·fec·tive

Schizo·blas·to·spo·ri·on
schizo·ce·pha·lia
schizo·coe·lic
schizo·cor·tex
schizo·cyte
schizo·cy·to·sis
schizo·gen·e·sis
schi·zog·e·nous
schi·zog·o·ny
schizo·gy·ria
schiz·oid
schizo·ki·ne·sis
schizo·my·cete
Schizo·my·ce·tes
schizo·my·co·sis
schiz·ont
schi·zon·ti·cide
schizo·nych·ia
schizo·pha·sia
schizo·phre·nia
   acute s.
   ambulatory s.
   atypical s.
   borderline s.
   catatonic s.
   childhood s.
   disorganized s.
   hebephrenic s.
   iatrogenic s.
   latent s.
   nuclear s.
   paranoid s.
   paraphrenic s.
   prepsychotic s.
   process s.
   prodromal s.
   pseudoneurotic s.
   pseudopsychopathic s.
   reactive s.
   residual s.
   schizo-affective s.
   simple s.
   undifferentiated s.
schizo·phren·ic
schizo·phren·i·form
Schizo·phy·ceae
schizo·pro·so·pia
Schizo·py·ren·i·da

schizo·tho·rax
schizo·to·nia
schizo·trich·ia
schizo·trop·ic
schizo·try·pa·no·sis
schiz·o·tryp·a·no·so·mi·a·sis
Schiz·o·tryp·a·num
   S. cruzi
schizo·zo·ite
schlaf·krank·heit
schlaf·sucht
Schlat·ter's disease
Schlat·ter's sprain
Schlat·ter-Os·good disease
Schlemm's canal
Schlemm's ligaments
Schlep·per
Schle·sin·ger's phenomenon
Schle·sin·ger's sign
Schlich·ter test
Schlich·ting dystrophy
Schlös·ser's treatment
Schluss·ko·ag·u·lum
Schmi·del's anastomosis
Schmi·del's ganglion
Schmidt's diet
Schmidt's syndrome
Schmidt's test
Schmidt-Lan·ter·man clefts
Schmidt-Lan·ter·man
   incisures
Schmidt-Lan·ter·man segment
Schmin·cke tumor
Schmitz bacillus
Schmorl's body
Schmorl's disease
Schmorl's nodule
Schna·bel's caverns
schnauz·krampf
Schnei·der's carmine
schnei·de·ri·an membrane
Scho·ber test
Schoe·ma·ker's line
Schoen·gas·tia
Scho·lan·der's apparatus
Scholz's disease
Scholz-Biel·schow·sky-
   Hen·ne·berg sclerosis

Scholz-Green·field disease
Schön's theory
Schön·bein's reaction
Schön·bein's test
Schön·lein's disease
Schön·lein's purpura
Schön·lein-Hen·och disease
Schön·lein-Hen·och purpura
Schön·lein-Hen·och syndrome
Schott's bath
Schott's treatment
Schott·mül·ler's disease
schra·dan
Schre·ger's band
Schre·ger's lines
Schre·ger's striae
Schre·ger's zones
Schrei·ber's maneuver
Schroe·der's disease
Schroe·der's fibers
Schroe·der's test
Schroe·der van der Kolk's law
Schrön's granule
Schrön-Much granules
Schroth's treatment
Schröt·ter's chorea
Schu·chardt's incision
Schüff·ner's dots
Schüff·ner's granules
Schüff·ner's punctuation
Schüff·ner's stippling
Schül·ler's disease
Schül·ler's method
Schül·ler's phenomenon
Schül·ler's syndrome
Schül·ler-Chris·tian disease
Schül·ler-Chris·tian syndrome
Schultz's angina
Schultz's disease
Schultz's syndrome
Schultz-Charl·ton reaction
Schultz-Charl·ton phenomenon
Schultz-Charl·ton test
Schultz-Dale reaction
Schult·ze's bundle
Schult·ze's cells
Schult·ze's fold
Schult·ze's sign

Schult·ze's test
Schult·ze's tract
Schult·ze's type
Schult·ze-Chvos·tek sign
Schumm's test
Schütz's micrococcus
Schwa·bach's test
Schwach·man syndrome
Schwal·be's corpuscles
Schwal·be's fissure
Schwal·be's foramen
Schwal·be's nucleus
Schwal·be's ring
Schwal·be's sheath
Schwal·be's space
Schwann's cell
Schwann's membrane
Schwann's nucleus
Schwann's sheath
Schwann's substance
schwan·ni·tis
schwan·no·gli·o·ma
schwan·no·ma
    granular cell s.
    malignant s.
schwan·no·sis
Schwartz-Bart·ter syndrome
Schwartz-Jam·pel myotonia
Schwartz-Jam·pel syndrome
Schwart·ze's mastoidectomy
Schwart·ze's operation
Schwart·ze's sign
Schwarz activator
Schwarz appliance
Schweig·ger-Sei·del sheath
schwei·ne·rot·lauf
schwei·ne·seuche
Schweit·zer's reagent
schwelle
Schwen·in·ger's method
Schwen·in·ger-Buz·zi
    anetoderma
sci·age
sci·aly·scope
sci·at·ic
sci·at·i·ca
SCID — severe combined
    immunodeficiency

sci·ence
    applied s.
    behavioral s.
    food s.
    forensic s.
    life s's
    natural s.
    pure s.
sci·en·tist
sci·er·opia
scil·la
scil·la·bi·ose
scil·la·ren
scil·lir·o·side
scil·lism
scil·lit·ic
Scin·tad·ren
scin·ti·an·gi·og·ra·phy
scin·ti·gram
scin·ti·graph
scin·ti·graph·ic
scin·tig·ra·phy
    thyroidal lymph node s.
scin·til·lat·ing sco·to·ma
scin·til·la·tion
scin·til·la·tor
scin·ti·pho·to·graph
scin·ti·pho·tog·ra·phy
scin·tis·can
scin·ti·scan·ner
sci·on
sci·op·o·dy
scir·rhoid
scir·rho·ma
    s. caminianorum
scir·rhoph·thal·mia
scir·rhous
scir·rhus
scis·sile
scis·sion
scis·si·par·i·ty
scis·sor·ing
scis·sors
    canalicular s.
    cannula s.
    craniotomy s.
    Dandy s.
    Fox s.

scis·sors *(continued)*
    Liston's s.
    Smellie's s.
    stitch s.
scis·su·ra
scis·su·ral
scis·sors-bite
ScLA — L. scapulolaeva
  anterior (left scapuloanterior)
scle·ra *pl.* scle·rae
    blue s.
scle·rad·e·ni·tis
scle·ral
scle·ra·ti·tis
scle·ra·tog·e·nous
scle·rec·ta·sia
scle·rec·ta·sis
scle·rec·to·iri·dec·to·my
scle·rec·to·iri·do·di·al·y·sis
scle·rec·tome
scle·rec·to·my
scle·re·de·ma
    s. adultorum
    Buschke's s.
    s. neonatorum
scle·re·ma
    s. adiposum
    s. adultorum
    s. cutis
    s. neonatorum
scle·ren·ce·pha·lia
scle·ren·ceph·a·ly
scle·ri·a·sis
scle·ri·rit·o·my
scle·ri·tis
    annular s.
    anterior s.
    brawny s.
    s. necroticans
    necrotizing s.
    nodular s.
    posterior s.
scle·ro·ad·i·pose
scle·ro·blas·te·ma
scle·ro·blas·tem·ic
scle·ro·cho·roi·di·tis
    s. anterior
    s. posterior

scle·ro·con·junc·ti·val
scle·ro·con·junc·ti·vi·tis
scle·ro·cor·nea
scle·ro·cor·ne·al
scle·ro·dac·tyl·ia
scle·ro·dac·ty·ly
scle·ro·der·ma
  annular s.
  circumscribed s.
  diffuse s.
  generalized s.
  linear s.
  localized s.
  s. neonatorum
  paramedian s.
  progressive s.
  pulmonary s.
  systemic s.
scle·ro·der·ma·to·myo·si·tis
scle·ro·der·ma·tous
scle·ro·der·mi·tis
scle·ro·des·mia
scle·ro·gen·ic
scle·rog·e·nous
scle·ro·gum·ma·tous
scle·ro·gy·ria
scle·roid
scle·ro·iri·tis
scle·ro·ker·a·ti·tis
scle·ro·ker·a·to·iri·tis
scle·ro·ker·a·to·sis
scle·ro·ma
  s. respiratorium
scle·ro·ma·la·cia
scle·ro·me·ninx
scle·ro·mere
scle·rom·e·ter
scle·ro·mu·cin
scle·ro·myx·ede·ma
scle·ro·nych·ia
scle·ro·nyx·is
scle·ro-ooph·o·ri·tis
scle·ro-oo·the·ci·tis
scle·roph·thal·mia
scle·ro·pro·tein
scle·ro·sal
scle·ro·sant
scle·ro·sar·co·ma

scle·ro·scope
scle·rose
scle·rosed
sclé·rose en plaques
scle·ros·ing
scle·ro·sis
  acute diffuse familial
    infantile cerebral s.
  Alzheimer s.
  amyotrophic lateral s.
  annular s.
  anterolateral s.
  arterial s.
  arteriocapillary s.
  arteriolar s.
  atrophic s.
  Baló's concentric s.
  bone s.
  bulbar multiple s.
  Canavan's diffuse s.
  central areolar choroidal s.
  cerebral centrolobar s.
  cerebral diffuse s.
  cerebrospinal s.
  choroidal s.
  combined s.
  s. of corpora cavernosa
  dentinal s.
  s. dermatis
  diaphyseal s.
  diffuse s.
  diffuse cerebral s.
  diffuse cortical s.
  diffuse mesangial s.
  diffuse systemic s.
  disseminated s.
  dorsolateral s.
  endocardial s.
  Erb's s.
  familial centrolobar s.
  familial centrolobular s.
  focal s.
  focal glomerular s.
  gastric s.
  glomerular s.
  hereditary spinal s.
  hyperplastic s.
  insular s.

scle·ro·sis *(continued)*
 Krabbe-type diffuse s.
 laminar cortical s.
 lateral s.
 lateral spinal s.
 lenticular nuclear s.
 lobar s.
 mantle s.
 Marie's s.
 mesial temporal s.
 miliary s.
 Mönckeberg's s.
 multiple s.
 nodular s.
 nuclear s.
 Pelizaeus-Merzbacher s.
 posterior s.
 posterior spinal s.
 posterolateral s.
 presenile s.
 primary lateral s.
 primary systemic s.
 progressive lateral s.
 progressive systemic s.
 renal arteriolar s.
 Scholz cerebral s.
 Scholz-Bielschowsky-
  Henneberg s.
 subendocardial s.
 sudanophilic diffuse s.
 systemic s.
 systemic duodenal s.
 systemic s. of kidney
 s. tuberosa
 tuberous s.
 unicellular s.
 vascular s.
 valvular s.
 venous s.
 ventrolateral s.
scle·ro·skel·e·ton
scle·ro·ste·no·sis
scle·ros·te·o·sis
scle·ros·to·my
scle·ro·ther·a·py
 endoscopic s.
 injection s.
scle·ro·tia

scle·rot·ic
scle·rot·i·ca
scle·rot·ic acid
scle·rot·i·cec·to·my
scle·rot·i·co·cho·roid·itis
Scle·ro·tin·ia
Scle·ro·tin·i·a·ceae
scle·ro·tin·ic acid
scle·ro·ti·tis
scle·ro·ti·um
scle·ro·tized
scle·ro·tome
scle·rot·o·my
 anterior s.
 posterior s.
scle·rous
scle·ro·zone
ScLP — L. scapulolaeva
 posterior (left
 scapuloposterior)
SCM — State Certified
 Midwife
scob·i·nate
sco·le·ces
sco·le·ci·a·sis
sco·lec·i·form
sco·le·coid
sco·le·col·o·gy
sco·lex *pl.* sco·le·ces
sco·lio·ky·pho·sis
sco·lio·lor·do·sis
sco·lio·me·ter
sco·lio·ra·chit·ic
sco·li·o·si·om·e·try
sco·li·o·sis
 Brissaud's s.
 cicatricial s.
 congenital s.
 coxitic s.
 empyematic s.
 fixed s.
 functional s.
 habit s.
 inflammatory s.
 ischiatic s.
 mobile s.
 myopathic s.
 ocular s.

sco·li·o·sis *(continued)*
    ophthalmic s.
    organic s.
    osteopathic s.
    paralytic s.
    rachitic s.
    rheumatic s.
    sciatic s.
    static s.
    structural s.
sco·li·o·som·e·ter
sco·li·ot·ic
sco·lio·tone
Sco·lo·pen·dra
sco·lop·sia
scom·broid
Scom·broi·dea
scom·bro·tox·ic
scom·bro·tox·in
scoop
    Mules's s.
sco·pa·fun·gin
sco·pa·rin
sco·pa·ri·us
scope
    Olympus s's
sco·po·la
sco·po·lag·nia
sco·pol·a·mine
    s. hydrobromide
    s. methylbromide
Sco·po·lia
sco·pom·e·ter
sco·pom·e·try
sco·po·mor·phin·ism
sco·po·phil·ia
sco·po·pho·bia
scop·to·lag·nia
scop·to·phil·ia
scop·to·pho·bia
scop·u·la
Scop·u·lar·i·op·sis
scop·u·lar·i·op·so·sis
scor·bu·tic
scor·bu·ti·gen·ic
scor·bu·tus
scor·di·ne·ma

score
    Apgar s.
    Bishop s.
    Donaldson s.
    Eastman visual function s.
    Gleason s.
    Kurtzke disability status s.
    LAP (leukocyte alkaline
      phosphatase) s.
    lod s.
    recovery s.
    standardized s.
scor·ings
scor·pi·on
    devil s.
    hairy s.
scor·pi·on·ism
Sco·to·bac·te·ria
sco·to·bac·te·ri·um
sco·to·chro·mo·gen
sco·to·chro·mo·gen·ic
sco·to·chro·mo·ge·nic·i·ty
sco·to·din·ia
sco·to·ma *pl.* sco·to·ma·ta
    absolute s.
    annular s.
    arcuate s.
    aural s.
    s. auris
    Bjerrum's s.
    cecocentral s.
    central s.
    centrocecal s.
    color s.
    cuneate s.
    flittering s.
    hemianopic s.
    insular s.
    mental s.
    motile s's
    negative s.
    paracecal s.
    paracentral s.
    pericecal s.
    peripapillary s.
    peripheral s.
    physiologic s.

sco·to·ma *(continued)*
    positive s.
    relative s.
    ring s.
    scintillating s.
    Seidel's s.
    suppression s.
    zonular s.
sco·to·ma·graph
sco·to·ma·ta
sco·tom·a·tous
sco·tom·e·ter
    Bjer-rum's s.
sco·tom·e·try
sco·to·mi·za·tion
sco·to·phil·ia
sco·to·pho·bia
sco·to·pho·bin
sco·to·pia
sco·top·ic
sco·top·sin
sco·tos·co·py
sco·to·ther·a·py
scr — scruple
scra·pie
scratch·er
    Kratz s.
screen
    Bjerrum s.
    dream s.
    fluorescent s.
    intensifying s.
    oral s.
    tangent s.
    vestibular s.
screen·ing
    chest s.
    genetic s.
    mass s.
    multiphasic s.
    multiple s.
    neonatal s.
    prenatal s.
    prescriptive s.
screw
    dentin s.
    expansion s.
screw·worm

Scrib·ner shunt
scrib·o·ma·nia
scro·bic·u·late
scro·bic·u·lus
    s. cordis
scrof·u·la
scrof·u·lo·der·ma
    s. gummosa
    papular s.
    tuberculous s.
    ulcerative s.
    verrucous s.
scrof·u·lous
scro·tal
scro·tec·to·my
scro·ti·tis
scro·to·cele
scro·to·plasty
scro·tum
    s. lapillosum
    lymph s.
    watering-can s.
scru·ple
scru·pu·los·i·ty
scul·te·tus
scu-PA — single chain
    urokinase-type plasminogen
    activator
scur·vy
    alpine s.
    biochemical s.
    hemorrhagic s.
    infantile s.
    land s.
    sea s.
    subclinical s.
scu·tate
scute
    tympanic s.
scu·ti·form
scu·tu·lar
scu·tu·lum *pl.* scu·tu·la
scu·tum
    s. pectoris
scyb·a·la
scyb·a·lous
scyb·a·lum *pl.* scyb·a·la
scy·phoid

Scy·ta·lid·i·um hy·a·lin·um
scy·thro·pas·mus
scy·to·blas·te·ma
SD — skin dose
　　standard deviation
　　sudden death
SDA — L. sacrodextra
　anterior (right sacroanterior)
　　specific dynamic action
SDE — specific dynamic effect
SDP — L. sacrodextra
　posterior (right
　sacroposterior)
SDS — sodium dodecyl sulfate
SDS-PAGE — SDS–polyacrylam-
　ide gel electrophoresis
SDT — L. sacrodextra
　transversa (right
　sacrotransverse)
SE — standard error
　　sphenoethmoidal suture
seal
　　border s.
　　double s.
　　peripheral s.
　　posterior palatal s.
　　velopharyngeal s.
seal·ant
　　dental s.
　　fissure s.
　　pit and fissure s.
seal·er
　　endodontic s.
　　root canal s.
seal·ing
　　fissure s.
seam
　　osteoid s.
　　pigment s.
search·er
Sea·shore test
sea·sick·ness
seat
　　basal s.
　　rest s.
seat·worm
se·ba·ceous
se·bia·gog·ic

se·bif·er·ous
Seb·i·leau's bands
Seb·i·leau's hollow
se·bip·a·rous
sebo·lith
sebo·poi·e·sis
seb·or·rhea
　　s. adiposa
　　eczematoid s.
　　nasolabial s.
　　s. oleosa
　　s. sicca
seb·or·rhe·al
seb·or·rhe·ic
seb·or·rhe·id
seb·or·rhi·a·sis
sebo·trop·ic
se·bum
　　cutaneous s.
　　s. cutaneum
　　s. palpebrale
　　s. preputiale
sec — second
Se·ca·le
sec·a·lose
Se·cer·nen·tea
Sech·en·off's center
Seck·el dwarf
Seck·el syndrome
sec·la·zone
se·clu·sio pu·pil·lae
se·co·bar·bi·tal
　　s. sodium
se·co·dont
Sec·o·nal
se·cond
　　gray per s.
　　inverse s.
　　milliampere s's
　　reciprocal s.
se·con·dary
se·cond in·ten·tion
seco·ste·roid
se·cre·ta
se·cret·a·gogue
se·crete
se·cre·tin
　　gastric s.

se·cre·tion
  antilytic s.
  external s.
  gastric s.
  internal s.
  neurohumoral s.
  paralytic s.
se·cre·to·gogue
se·cre·to·in·hib·i·to·ry
se·cre·to·mo·tor
se·cre·to·mo·tory
se·cre·tor
se·cre·to·ry
sec·tile
sec·tio *pl.* sec·tio·nes
  s. cadaveris
  sectiones cerebelli
  sectiones corporum
    quadrigeminorum
  sectiones hypothalami
  sectiones isthmi
  s. mediana
  sectiones medullae
    oblongatae
  sectiones medullae spinalis
  sectiones mesencephalicae
  sectiones mesencephali
  sectiones pedunculi cerebri
  sectiones pontis
  sectiones telencephali
  sectiones thalamencephali
  sectiones thalami et
    metathalami
sec·tion
  abdominal s.
  celloidin s.
  cesarean s.
  cesarean s., cervical
  cesarean s., classic
  cesarean s., corporeal
  cesarean s., extraperitoneal
  cesarean s., Latzko's
  cesarean s., lower segment
  cesarean s., Munro Kerr
  cesarean s., Porro
  cesarean s., transperitoneal
  coronal s.
  cross s.

sec·tion *(continued)*
  frontal s.
  frozen s.
  ground s.
  low cervical cesarean s.
  paraffin s.
  perineal s.
  Pitres's's
  pituitary stalk s.
  postmortem cesarean s.
  radical cesarean s.
  root s.
  Saemisch's s.
  sagittal s.
  semithin s.
  serial s.
  step s.
  transverse s.
  trigeminal root s.
  ultrathin s.
sec·ti·o·nes
sec·tion·ing
  surgical s.
sec·tor
  Sommer s.
sec·to·ri·al
se·cun·di·grav·i·da
se·cun·di·na *pl.* se·cun·di·nae
  s. uteri
se·cun·di·nes
se·cun·dip·a·ra
se·cun·di·par·i·ty
se·cun·dip·a·rous
se·cun·dum ar·tem
SED — skin erythema dose
se·date
se·da·tion
  conscious s.
sed·a·tive
  Battley s.
  cardiac s.
  cerebral s.
  gastric s.
  general s.
  intestinal s.
  nerve trunk s.
  nervous s.
  respiratory s.

sed·a·tive *(continued)*
   spinal s.
   vascular s.
sed·en·tary
se·di·gi·tate
Sé·dil·lot's operation
sed·i·ment
   urinary s.
sed·i·ment·a·ble
sed·i·men·ta·tion
   erythrocyte s.
   formalin-ether s. (Ritchie)
   Westergren s. rate
sed·i·men·ta·tor
sed·i·men·tom·e·ter
seed
   cardamom s.
   celery s.
   larkspur s.
   plantago s.
   psyllium s.
   radiogold (^{198}Au) s.
   radon s.
See·lig·mül·ler's sign
Sees·sel's pocket
Sees·sel's pouch
Sé·glas type
seg·ment
   arterial s. of glomeriform
     arteriovenous anasto-
     mosis
   arterial s's of kidney
   body s.
   bronchopulmonary s.
   ceratobranchial s.
   connecting s.
   cranial s's
   differential s.
   epibranchial s.
   Fc s.
   frontal s.
   hepatic s's
   hypobranchial s.
   interannular s.
   internodal s.
   s's of kidney
   s's of liver
   lower uterine s.

seg·ment *(continued)*
   medullary s.
   mesoblastic s.
   mesodermal s.
   muscle s.
   neural s.
   occipital s.
   pairing s's
   parietal s.
   pharyngobranchial s.
   postcommunical s.
   PR s.
   primitive s.
   protovertebral s.
   pubic s. of the pelvis
   Ranvier's s's
   renal s's
   rivinian s.
   s. of Rivinus
   rod s.
   RS-T s.
   sacral s.
   Schmidt-Lanterman s.
   spinal s.
   s's of spinal cord
   ST s.
   ST-T s.
   thin s.
   upper uterine s.
   uterine s.
   venous s's of kidney
   venous s's of liver
seg·men·ta
seg·men·tal
seg·men·ta·tion
   complete s.
   haustral s.
   metameric s.
   partial s.
   regular s.
   rhythmic s.
   unequal s.
seg·men·ter
Seg·men·ti·na
seg·men·tum *pl.* seg·men·ta
   s. arteriale anastomosis
     arteriovenae glomeri-
     formis

seg·men·tum *(continued)*
   segmenta
     bronchopulmonalia
   segmenta hepatis
   s. internodale
   segmenta medullae
     spinalis
   segmenta renalia
   s. venosum anastomosis
     arteriovenae glomeri-
     formis
seg·re·ga·tion
   nuclear s.
seg·re·ga·tor
seg·re·some
Sé·guin's sign
Sé·guin's signal symptom
Sehrt's clamp
Sehrt's compressor
Sei·del's scotoma
Sei·del's sign
Sei·de·lin bodies
Seid·litz powder
Seid·litz powder test
Seig·nette's salt
Seip-Law·rence syndrome
seis·es·the·sia
seis·mes·the·sia
seis·mo·car·dio·gram
seis·mo·car·di·og·ra·phy
seis·mo·ther·a·py
Sei·tel·ber·ger's disease
Sei·tel·ber·ger's dystrophy
Seitz's sign
sei·zure
   absence s.
   audiogenic s.
   cerebral s.
   complex partial s.
   cough s.
   drop s.
   erotic s.
   febrile s.
   generalized s.
   jackknife s.
   major motor s.
   minor motor s.
   myoclonic s.

sei·zure *(continued)*
   paralytic s.
   photogenic s.
   psychomotor s.
   reflex anoxic s.
   tonic-clonic s.
   traumatic s.
   uncinate s.
se·junc·tion
sek·is·a·nine
se·la·chi·an
se·lec·tion
   artificial s.
   complete s.
   darwinian s.
   directional s.
   disruptive s.
   diversifying s.
   germinal s.
   incomplete s.
   multiple s.
   natural s.
   normalizing s.
   progeny s.
   sexual s.
   single s.
   stabilizing s.
   truncate s.
se·lec·tive
se·lec·tiv·i·ty
se·lene
   s. unguium
sel·e·nide
se·le·ni·um
   s. sulfide
se·le·no·cys·teine
se·le·no·dont
se·le·no·me·thi·o·nine
se·le·no·meth·yl·nor·cho·les·
  te·rol
Se·le·no·mo·nas
se·le·no·sis
self
   idealized s.
   true s.
self-ab·sorp·tion
self-an·ti·gen
self-ar·tic·u·lat·ing

self-con·scious·ness
self-dif·fer·en·ti·a·tion
self-di·ges·tion
self-es·teem
self-ex·tinc·tion
self-fer·men·ta·tion
self-fer·ti·li·za·tion
self-hyp·no·sis
self-im·age
self-in·duc·tance
self-in·fec·tion
self·ing
self-lim·it·ed
self-lim·it·ing
self-re·cog·ni·tion
self-sug·ges·tion
self-sus·pen·sion
self-tol·er·ance
self·wise
Sel·i·va·noff's (Sel·i·wa·
   now's) test
Sel·i·va·noff's reaction
sel·la pl. sel·lae
   empty s.
   empty s. syndrome
   s. turcica
sel·lar
Sel·lick maneuver
Sel·sun
   S. Blue
Sel·ter's disease
Sel·ye syndrome
se·man·tic
se·man·tics
se·ma·si·ol·o·gy
se·mei·og·ra·phy
se·mei·ol·o·gy
se·mei·ot·ic
se·mei·ot·ics
sem·el·in·ci·dent
semel in d. — L. semel in die
   (once a day)
sem·el·par·i·ty
sem·el·pa·rous
se·men
se·me·nol·o·gist
se·me·nol·o·gy
se·me·nu·ria

semi·al·de·hyde
semi·apo·chro·mat
semi·apo·chro·mat·ic
semi·ca·nal
   s. of auditory tube
   s. of humerus
   s. of tensor tympani muscle
semi·ca·na·lis pl. semi·ca·na·
   les
   s. musculi tensoris tympani
   s. tubae auditivae
semi·car·ba·zide
semi·car·ba·zone
semi·car·ti·lag·i·nous
semi·co·ma
semi·co·ma·tose
semi·con·duc·tor
semi·con·scious
semi·cris·ta pl. semi·cris·tae
   s. incisiva
semi·de·cus·sa·tion
semi·dia·gram·mat·ic
semi·dom·i·nance
semi·flex·ion
semi·fluc·tu·at·ing
Semih. — L. semihora (half an
   hour)
Sem·i·kon
semi·lu·nar
semi·lu·na·re
semi·lux·a·tion
semi·mem·bra·nous
sem·i·nal
semi·nar·co·sis
sem·i·na·tion
sem·i·nif·er·ous
sem·i·nis
sem·i·nol·o·gist
sem·i·nol·o·gy
sem·i·no·ma
   ovarian s.
   spermatocytic s.
semi·nor·mal
sem·i·nose
sem·i·nu·ria
se·mi·og·ra·phy
se·mi·ol·o·gy
semi·or·bic·u·lar

se·mi·ot·ic
semi·para·site
semi·pen·ni·form
semi·per·me·a·ble
semi·ple·gia
semi·pri·vate
semi·pro·na·tion
semi·prone
semi·quan·ti·ta·tive
semi·quin·one
semi·re·cum·bent
se·mis
semi·sid·er·a·tio
semi·som·nus
semi·so·por
semi·spi·na·lis
semi·star·va·tion
semi·sul·cus *pl.* semi·sul·ci
semi·su·pi·na·tion
semi·su·pine
semi·syn·thet·ic
Sem·i·tard
semi·ten·di·nous
semi·ter·tian
Sem·li·ki For·est encephalitis
Sem·li·ki For·est virus
Sem·mel·weis, Ignaz Philipp
Se·mon's law
Se·mon's sign
Se·mon-Her·ing hypothesis
Se·mon-Her·ing theory
Se·mon-Ro·sen·bach law
Sem·oxy·drine
Sem·ple's vaccine
se·mus·tine
Se·near-Ush·er syndrome
Se·ne·cio
     S. jacobae L. (Compositae)
sen·e·ga
sen·e·gen·in
se·nes·cence
     dental s.
se·nes·cent
Sengs·tak·en-Blake·more tube
se·nile
se·nil·ism
se·nil·i·ty
se·ni·um

se·ni·um
     s. praecox
sen·na
sen·no·side
se·no·graph
se·nog·ra·phy
Sen·o·kot
se·no·pia
sen·sa·tion
     articular s.
     chromatic s.
     cincture s.
     common s.
     concomitant s.
     cutaneous s.
     delayed s.
     dermal s.
     eccentric s.
     epigastric s.
     external s.
     general s.
     generalized epileptic
        somatic s.
     girdle s.
     gnostic s's
     internal s.
     joint s.
     kinesthetic s.
     light s.
     objective s.
     palmesthetic s.
     primary s.
     proprioceptive s.
     protopathic s.
     radiating s.
     referred s.
     reflex s.
     secondary s.
     skin s.
     strain s.
     subjective s.
     tactile s.
     transferred s.
     vascular s.
     visceral s.
     s. of warmth
sense
     body s.

sense *(continued)*
    chemical s.
    color s.
    dermal s.
    equilibrium s.
    form s.
    internal s.
    interoceptive s's
    joint s.
    joint position s.
    kinesthetic s.
    labyrinthine s.
    light s.
    muscle s.
    muscular s.
    obstacle s.
    pain s.
    s. of pitch
    posture s.
    pressure s.
    proprioceptive s.
    seventh s.
    sixth s.
    space s.
    special s.
    static s.
    stereognostic s.
    tactile s.
    temperature s.
    time s.
    tone s.
    vestibular s.
    visceral s.
Sen·sib·amine
sen·si·bil·i·ty
    articular s.
    binaural s.
    bone s.
    common s.
    cortical s.
    cutaneous s.
    deep s.
    dissociation s.
    electromuscular s.
    epicritic s.
    gnostic s.
    interoceptive s.
    joint s.

sen·si·bil·i·ty *(continued)*
    kinesthetic s.
    mesoblastic s.
    muscular s.
    myotatic s.
    nervous s.
    pallesthetic s.
    palmesthetic s.
    proprioceptive s.
    protopathic s.
    recurrent s.
    somesthetic s.
    splanchnesthetic s.
    touch s.
    two-point s.
    uterine s.
    vibratory s.
sen·si·bil·i·za·tion
sen·si·ble
sen·sif·er·ous
sen·sig·e·nous
sen·sim·e·ter
sen·si·tive
sen·si·tiv·i·ty
    antibiotic s.
    autoerythrocyte s.
    deep s.
    delayed s.
    diagnostic s.
    differential s.
    primaquine s.
    proportional s.
    suxamethonium s.
    thermal s.
    trophic s.
    vibratory s.
sen·si·ti·za·tion
    active s.
    autoerythrocyte s.
    passive s.
    photodynamic s.
    Rh s.
sen·si·tized
sen·si·tiz·er
sen·so·mo·bile
sen·so·mo·bil·i·ty
sen·so·mo·tor
sen·so·pa·ral·y·sis

sen·sor
sen·so·ri·al
sen·so·ri·glan·du·lar
sen·so·ri·me·tab·o·lism
sen·so·rim·e·try
sen·so·ri·mo·tor
sen·so·ri·mus·cu·lar
sen·so·ri·neu·ral
sen·so·ri·um
    general s.
sen·so·ri·vas·cu·lar
sen·so·ri·vaso·mo·tor
sen·so·ry
sen·su·al·ism
sen·tence
    Babcock s.
sen·ti·ent
sen·ti·nel
SEP — somatosensory evoked
  potential
sep·a·loid
sep·a·ra·tion
    AC (acromioclavicular)
      joint s.
    eschar s.
    s. of placenta
    shoulder s.
sep·a·ra·tor
sep·a·zo·ni·um chlo·ride
sep·e·don
sep·e·do·no·gen·e·sis
se·per·i·dol hy·dro·chlo·ride
Seph·a·dex
se·pia
se·pi·um
sep·sin
sep·sis
    s. agranulocytica
    burn wound s.
    catheter s.
    gas s.
    incarcerated s.
    s. intestinalis
    s. lenta
    oral s.
    postabortal s.
    puerperal s.
Sep·sis vi·o·la·cea

Sept. — L. septem (seven)
sep·ta
sep·tal
sep·tan
sep·ta·nose
sep·tate
sep·ta·tion
sep·ta·tome
sep·tec·to·my
sep·te·mia
sep·tic
sep·ti·ce·mia
    acute fulminating
      meningococcal s.
    bronchopulmonary s.
    Bruce's s.
    cryptogenic s.
    fowl s.
    hemorrhagic s.
    s. hemorrhagica
    lymphovenous s.
    metastasizing s.
    morphine injector's s.
    phlebitic s.
    plague s.
    puerperal s.
    sputum s.
sep·ti·ce·mic
sep·ti·cine
sep·ti·co·py·emia
    cryptogenic s.
    metastatic s.
    spontaneous s.
sep·ti·co·py·emic
sep·ti·form
sep·ti·grav·i·da
sep·tile
sep·ti·me·tri·tis
sep·ti·neu·ri·tis
    Nicolau's s.
sep·tip·a·ra
sep·ti·va·lent
sep·to·mar·gi·nal
sep·to·na·sal
sep·to·plas·ty
sep·to·rhi·no·plas·ty
sep·tos·to·my
    balloon atrial s.

sep·to·tome
sep·tot·o·my
sep·tu·la
sep·tu·lum *pl.* sep·tu·la
  septula testis
sep·tum *pl.* sep·ta
  s. alveoli
  aorticopulmonary s.
  s. atriorum cordis
  atrioventricular s. of heart
  s. atrioventriculare cordis
  s. of auditory tube
  s. auricularum
  Bigelow's s.
  bony s. of eustachian canal
  bony s. of nose
  bronchial s.
  s. bronchiale
  bucconasal s.
  bulbar s.
  s. bulbi urethrae
  s. canalis musculotubarii
  s. cartilagineum nasi
  cervical s., intermediate
  s. cervicale intermedium
  cloacal s.
  s. of Cloquet
  s. corporum cavernosorum
    clitoridis
  crural s.
  dorsal median s.
  Douglas' s.
  enamel s.
  femoral s.
  s. femorale
  s. femorale [Cloqueti]
  s. of frontal sinuses
  gingival s.
  s. glandis penis
  s. of glans penis
  gum s.
  hemal s.
  iliopectineal s.
  s. inferius
  interalveolar s.
  septa interalveolaria
  interatrial s. of heart
  s. interatriale cordis

sep·tum *(continued)*
  interauricular s.
  interdental s.
  s. intermedium
  intermuscular s.
  interplacental s.
  interradicular s.
  s. interradiculare
  intersegmental s.
  interventricular s. of heart
  s. interventriculare cordis
  s. intra-alveolarium
  Körner s.
  s. linguae
  lingual s.
  s. lucidum
  median s., dorsal
  median s., posterior
  s. medianum dorsale
  s. medianum posterius
  mediastinal s.
  s. mediastinale
  s. membranaceum nasi
  s. membranaceum
    ventriculorum cordis
  membranous s. of nose
  s. mobile nasi
  mobile s. of nose
  s. musculare
    ventriculorum cordis
  s. of musculotubal canal
  nasal s.
  s. nasi
  s. nasi osseum
  neural s.
  orbital s.
  s. orbitale
  osseous s. of nose
  parietal s.
  s. pectiniforme
  pellucid s.
  s. pellucidum
  s. penis
  pericardioperitoneal s.
  pericardiopleural s.
  pharyngeal s.
  placental s.
  pleuroperitoneal s.

sep·tum *(continued)*
s. pontis
posterior s.
s. posticum
precommissural s.
s. precommissurale
s. primum
rectovaginal s.
s. rectovaginale
rectovesical s.
s. rectovesicale
s. renis
s. scroti
s. of scrotum
s. secundum
s. sinuum frontalium
s. sinuum sphenoidalium
sphenoidal s.
s. of sphenoidal sinuses
spiral s.
spurious s.
s. spurium
subarachnoidal s.
septa of testis
s. of tongue
tracheoesophageal s.
transverse s. of ampulla
s. transversum
true s.
s. tubae
urorectal s.
s. of ventricles of heart
ventricular s.
s. ventriculorum cordis
s. verum
sep·tup·let
seq. luce — L. sequenti luce
(the following day)
se·quel
se·que·la *pl.* se·que·lae
postpolio sequelae
postpoliomyelitis sequelae
se·quence
amino acid s.
amniotic band s.
base s.
canonical s.

se·quence *(continued)*
Carr-Purcell-Meiboom-Gill s.
coding s.
complementary base s.
consensus s.
deformation s.
disruption s.
flanking s.
intervening s.
leader s.
malformation s.
nearest neighbor s.
regulatory s.
Robin s.
termination s.
se·quen·tial
se·ques·ter
se·ques·tra
se·ques·tral
se·ques·trant
se·ques·tra·tion
biochemical s.
bronchopulmonary s.
pulmonary s.
se·ques·trec·to·my
se·ques·trot·o·my
se·ques·trum *pl.* se·ques·tra
primary s.
secondary s.
tertiary s.
se·quoi·o·sis
SER — smooth endoplasmic reticulum
somatosensory evoked reponse
Ser — serine
se·ra
ser·ac·tide ac·e·tate
ser·al
se·ral·bu·min
se·ran·gi·tis
Ser-Ap-Es
se·ra·phe·re·sis
Se·ra·pi·on
Ser·ax
sere
se·rem·pi·on

Se·re·ni·um
Se·ren·til
Ser·fin
Ser·gent's white adrenal line
se·ri·al
se·ri·al·o·graph
ser·i·cin
se·ri·cite
Ser·i·co·pel·ma
    S. communis
se·ries
    basophil s.
    basophilic s.
    electrochemical s.
    eosinophil s.
    eosinophilic s.
    erythrocyte s.
    erythrocytic s.
    gastrointestinal s.
    granulocyte s.
    granulocytic s.
    Hofmeister s.
    homologous s.
    leukocytic s.
    lymphocyte s.
    lymphocytic s.
    lyotropic s.
    monocyte s.
    monocytic s.
    myelocytic s.
    myelogenous s.
    myeloid s.
    natural radioactive s.
    neptunium s.
    neutrophil s.
    neutrophilic s.
    plasmacyte s.
    plasmacytic s.
    radioactive s.
    thorium s.
    thrombocyte s.
    thrombocytic s.
ser·i·flux
ser·ine
ser·ine car·boxy·pep·ti·dase
ser·ine hy·droxy·meth·yl·
  trans·fer·ase
ser·ine pro·tein·ase

se·ri·os·co·py
seri·scis·sion
se·ro·al·bu·min·ous
se·ro·al·bu·min·uria
se·ro·co·li·tis
se·ro·con·ver·sion
se·ro·con·vert
se·ro·cul·ture
se·ro·cys·tic
se·ro·di·ag·no·sis
se·ro·di·ag·nos·tic
se·ro·en·te·ri·tis
se·ro·epi·de·mi·ol·o·gy
se·ro-fast
se·ro·fib·rin·ous
se·ro·fi·brous
se·ro·floc·cu·la·tion
se·ro·flu·id
se·ro·glob·u·lin
se·ro·group
se·ro·hem·or·rhag·ic
se·ro·li·pase
se·ro·log·ic
se·ro·log·i·cal
se·rol·o·gist
se·rol·o·gy
    diagnostic s.
    forensic s.
se·rol·y·sin
se·ro·ma
se·ro·mem·bra·nous
se·ro·mu·coid
se·ro·mu·cous
se·ro·mu·cus
se·ro·mus·cu·lar
Sero·my·cin
se·ro·neg·a·tive
se·ro·neg·a·tiv·i·ty
se·ro·peri·to·ne·um
se·ro·phil·ic
se·ro·plas·tic
se·ro·pneu·mo·tho·rax
se·ro·pos·i·tive
se·ro·pos·i·tiv·i·ty
se·ro·prog·no·sis
se·ro·pu·ru·lent
se·ro·pus
se·ro·re·ac·tion

se·ro·re·lapse
se·ro·re·sis·tant
se·ro·re·sis·tance
se·ro·re·ver·sal
se·ro·sa
se·ro·sal
se·ro·sa·mu·cin
se·ro·san·guin·e·ous
se·rose
se·ro·se·rous
se·ro·si·tis *pl.* se·ro·sit·i·des
   adhesive s.
   infectious avian s.
   multiple s.
se·ros·i·ty
se·ro·sur·vey
se·ro·sy·no·vi·al
se·ro·syn·o·vi·tis
se·ro·ther·a·py
se·ro·tho·rax
se·ro·ton·er·gic
sero·to·nin
sero·to·nin·er·gic
se·ro·type
   heterologous s.
   homologous s.
se·rous
se·ro·vac·ci·na·tion
se·ro·var
se·ro·zyme
Ser·pa·sil
ser·pent
ser·pen·ta·ria
Ser·pen·tes
ser·pen·tine
ser·pig·i·nous
ser·rat·ed
Ser·ra·tia
   S. liquefaciens
   S. marcescens
   S. odorifera
   S. plymuthica
   S. proteamaculans
   S. rubidaea
ser·ra·tion
ser·ra·tus
   s. anterior
serre·fine

Ser·res' angle
Ser·res' glands
ser·ru·late
Ser·to·li's cell
Ser·to·li's column
Ser·to·li's tumor
Ser·to·li-cell-on·ly syndrome
se·rum *pl.* se·rums, se·ra
   active s.
   alkaline blood s.
   anti-gas-gangrene s.
   anti-Rh s.
   antianthrax s.
   antibotulinus s.
   anticholera s.
   anticomplementary s.
   anticrotalus s.
   antidiphtheria s.
   antiglobulin s.
   antilymphocyte s. (ALS)
   antimeningococcus s.
   antiophidic s.
   antiplague s.
   antiplatelet s.
   antipneumococcus s.
   antirabies s.
   antireticular cytotoxic s.
   antisnakebite s.
   antitetanic s. (A.T.S.)
   antitoxic s.
   antitubercle s.
   antitularenase s.
   articular s.
   bacteriolytic s.
   Behring s.
   blister s.
   blood s.
   blood grouping s's
   Bogomolets s.
   Calmette s.
   Cattani s.
   Cheron s.
   convalescence s.
   convalescent s.
   Coombs s.
   despeciated s.
   Felix Vi s.
   Felton s.

Sestamibi Persantine thallium scan

se·rum *(continued)*
    Flexner s.
    foreign s.
    Foshay s.
    glycerin s.
    heterologous s.
    homologous s.
    hyperimmune s.
    immune s.
    inactivated s.
    s. lactis
    Löffler's s.
    Lorrain Smith blood s.
    lymphatolytic s.
    monospecific s.
    monovalent s.
    multipartial s.
    muscle s.
    normal s.
    normal human s.
    North American
      antisnakebite s.
    pericardial s.
    polyvalent s.
    pooled s.
    pregnancy s.
    pregnant mare's s.
    prophylactic s.
    quality control s.
    Roux s.
    Sclavo's s.
    specific s.
    truth s.
    Yersin s.
se·ru·mal
se·rum·ci·dal
se·rum-fast
se·rum·uria
Serv. — L. serva (keep,
  preserve)
ser·vo·mech·a·nism
ser·yl
ses·a·me
ses·a·moid
ses·a·moi·di·tis
sesquih. — L. sesquihora (an
  hour and a half)
ses·qui·ho·ra

ses·qui·ox·ide
ses·qui·sul·fate
ses·qui·sul·fide
ses·sile
Ses·sin·ia
set
    Barraquer-Krumeich-Swing-
      er refractive s.
    mental s.
    phalangeal s.
    preparatory s.
se·ta *pl.* se·tae
se·ta·ceous
Se·tar·ia
    S. cervi
    S. cervina
    S. equina
    S. labiatopapillosa
Setch·e·now's centers
Setch·e·now's nuclei
se·tif·er·ous
se·tig·er·ous
se·ton
set-point
set·up
    diagnostic s.
Seu·tin's bandage
Se·ver's disease
se·vo·flu·rane
se·vum
sew·age
    activated s.
    domestic s.
    septic s.
sex
    chromosomal s.
    endocrinologic s.
    genetic s.
    gonadal s.
    morphological s.
    nuclear s.
    psychological s.
    social s.
sex-con·di·tioned
sex·dig·i·tate
sex·duc·tion
sex-in·flu·enced
sex·iv·a·lent

sex-lim·it·ed
sex-linked
sex·ol·o·gy
sex·op·a·thy
sex-spe·cif·ic
sex·tan
sex·ti·grav·i·da
sex·tip·a·ra
sex·tup·let
sex·u·al
sex·u·al·i·ty
   infantile s.
   pregenital s.
sex·u·al·iza·tion
Sey·der·helm's solution
Sé·za·ry cell
Sé·za·ry erythroderma
Sé·za·ry syndrome
SF — spinal fluid, synovial
  fluid
SFEMG — single fiber
  electromyography
Sgam·ba·ti's reaction
Sgam·ba·ti's test
SGOT — serum
  glutamic-oxaloacetic
  transaminase
SGPT — serum glutamate
  pyruvate transaminase
SH — serum hepatitis
shad·ow
   acoustic s.
   bat's wing s.
   heart s.
   Purkinje's s's
   snowstorm s.
   sound s.
shad·ow-cast·ing
Shaf·fer's method
shaft
   s. of femur
   s. of fibula
   hair s.
   s. of humerus
   s. of metacarpal bone
   s. of metatarsal bone
   s. of penis
   s. of phalanx of fingers

shaft *(continued)*
   s. of phalanx of toes
   s. of radius
   s. of rib
   s. of tibia
   s. of ulna
sha·green
shakes
   hatter's s.
   helium s.
   kwaski s.
   spelter s.
   Teflon s.
sham-feed·ing
shank
shap·ing
Shar·pey's fibers
Sha·ver's disease
Shear's test
shear
shears
   bandage s.
   Liston s.
   malleus s.
sheath
   arachnoid s.
   axillary s.
   bulbar s.
   carotid s.
   caudal s.
   chordal s.
   common synovial flexor s.
   common s. of tendons of
     peroneal muscles
   common s. of testis and
     spermatic cord
   connective tissue s. of Key
     and Retzius
   crural s.
   dentinal s.
   dural s.
   enamel prism s.
   enamel rod s.
   endoneurial s.
   epithelial s.
   s. of eyeball
   fascial s. of prostate
   female s.

sheath *(continued)*
- femoral s.
- fibrous s's of fingers
- fibrous s. of kidney
- fibrous s. of liver
- fibrous s. of optic nerve
- fibrous s. of spermatozoon
- fibrous s. of tendon
- fibrous s's of toes
- s. of Henle
- Hertwig s.
- s. of Hertwig
- Huxley s.
- intermeningeal s. of optic nerve
- s. of Key and Retzius
- lamellar s.
- masculine s.
- Mauthner's s.
- medullary s.
- meningeal s's of optic nerve
- microfilarial s.
- mitochondrial s.
- mucous s's
- mucous s., intertubercular
- mucous s. of tendon
- mucous s's of tendons of fingers
- mucous s's of tendons of toes
- myelin s.
- Neumann s.
- s. of Neumann
- neurilemmal s.
- notochordal s.
- nucleated s.
- s's of optic nerve
- s. of optic nerve, external
- s. of optic nerve, internal
- s. of optic nerve, outer meningeal
- peel-away s.
- periarterial lymphatic s.
- periarterial lymphoid s. (PALS)
- periesophageal s.
- perinephric s.

sheath *(continued)*
- perivascular s.
- pial s.
- pipestem s.
- s. of plantar tendon of long peroneal muscle
- primitive s.
- prism s.
- s. of prostate
- rectus s.
- s. of rectus abdominis muscle
- rod s.
- root s.
- Scarpa's s.
- Schwalbe's s.
- s. of Schwann
- Schweigger-Seidel s.
- spiral s.
- s. of styloid process
- synovial s.
- tendinous s.
- s. of thymus
- thyroid s.

Sheehan's syndrome
Shee·hy syndrome
sheep-pox
sheet
- β-s.
- beta s.
- β-pleated s.
- beta pleated s.
- draw s.
- drip s.
- pleated s.
- secretory s.

shelf
- Blumer s.
- buccal s.
- dental s.
- mesocolic s.
- palatine s.
- rectal s.

shel·lac
Shen·ton's arch
Shen·ton's line
Shep·herd's fracture

Sher·man plate
Sher·man unit
Sher·man-Bour·quin unit
Sher·man-Mun·sell unit
Sher·ren's triangle
Sher·ring·ton's law
shi·at·su
shield
    amputation s.
    Buller's s.
    circumcision s.
    Dalkon s.
    embryonic s.
    eye s.
    Faraday s.
    Fuller s.
    heat s.
    lead s.
    nipple s.
    oral s.
    phallic s.
    skull s.
shield·ing
shift
    antigenic s.
    axis s.
    chemical s.
    chloride s.
    Doppler s.
    s. down
    frame s.
    s. of Hamburger
    isohydric s.
    s. to the left
    midline s.
    permanent threshold s.
    phase s.
    Purkinje s.
    regenerative blood s.
    s. to the right
    temporary threshold s.
Shi·ga's bacillus
Shi·ga's toxin
Shi·gel·la
    S. ambigua
    S. arabinotarda type A
    S. arabinotarda type B
    S. boydii

Shi·gel·la (continued)
    S. ceylonensis
    S. dysenteriae
    S. etousae
    S. flexneri
    S. newcastle
    S. paradysenteriae
    S. parashigae
    S. schmitzii
    S. shigae
    S. sonnei
shi·gel·la *pl.* shi·gel·lae
shi·gel·lo·sis
shik·i·mene
shin
    bucked s's
    cucumber s.
    saber s.
    sore s's
shin·bone
shin·gles
Shi·rod·kar's procedure
shiv·er
shiv·er·ing
shock
    acoustic s.
    anaphylactic s.
    anaphylactoid s.
    anesthesia s.
    apoplectic s.
    asthmatic s.
    burn s.
    cardiac s.
    cardiogenic s.
    cerebral s.
    culture s.
    declamping s.
    deferred s.
    delayed s.
    diastolic s.
    electric s.
    electrotherapeutic s.
    endotoxic s.
    endotoxin s.
    Forssman s.
    heart s.
    hematogenic s.
    hemoclastic s.

shock *(continued)*
    hemorrhagic s.
    histamine s.
    hypoglycemic s.
    hypovolemic s.
    insulin s.
    irreversible s.
    neural s.
    neurogenic s.
    obstetric s.
    oligemic s.
    osmotic s.
    paralytic s.
    peptone s.
    pleural s.
    postoperative s.
    primary s.
    protein s.
    secondary s.
    septic s.
    serum s.
    shell s.
    spinal s.
    surgical s.
    testicular s.
    traumatic s.
    vasogenic s.
shoe
    Charlier's s.
    Scarpa's s.
Shope papilloma
short·sight·ed
short·sight·ed·ness
short-wind·ed·ness
shot-com·pres·sor
shot·ty
shoul·der
    bull's-eye s.
    drop s.
    frozen s.
    knocked-down s.
    linguogingival s.
    loose s.
    round s's
    stubbed s.
shoul·der-blade
shoul·der slip
Shoul·dice herniorrhaphy

show
show·er
    uric acid s.
Shra·dy's saw
Shrap·nell's membrane
shrink·age
shrink·er
    stump s.
shud·der
shuf·fle
    exon s.
shunt
    arteriovenous (A-V) s.
    Buselmeier s.
    cardiovascular s.
    cavomesenteric s.
    Denver s.
    dialysis s.
    Drapanas s.
    endolymphatic-mastoid s.
    endolymphatic s.
    end-to-side s.
    Glenn s.
    hexose monophosphate s.
    internal s.
    Javid s.
    left-to-right s.
    LeVeen peritoneovenous s.
    Linton s.
    lymphaticovenous s.
    mesoatrial s.
    mesocaval s.
    otic-periotic s.
    pentose s.
    peritoneosubarachnoid s.
    peritoneothecal s.
    peritoneovenous s.
    PFTE (polyfluoro-
        tetraethylene) s.
    portacaval s.
    portorenal s.
    portosystemic s.
    postcaval s.
    pulmonary s.
    Quinton-Scribner s.
    renal-splenic venous s.
    reversed s.
    right-to-left s.

shunt *(continued)*
   salpingothecal s.
   Scribner s.
   side-to-side s.
   splenorenal s.
   splenorenal s., distal
   Stookey-Scarff s.
   subduroperitoneal s.
   subduropleural s.
   Thomas s.
   Thomas appliqué s.
   Torkildsen s.
   total s.
   ureterothecal s.
   ventriculoatrial s.
   ventriculojugular s.
   ventriculoperitoneal s.
   ventriculopleural s.
   ventriculovenous s.
   Warren s.
shut·tle
   glycerol phosphate s.
   malate-aspartate s.
Shwach·man syndrome
Shwach·man-Di·a·mond
   syndrome
Shwartz·man phenomenon
Shwartz·man reaction
Shwartz·man-San·a·rel·li
   phenomenon
Shy-Drager syndrome
SI — soluble insulin
   stimulation index
   Système International
     d'Unites (International
     System of Units)
SIADH — syndrome of
   inappropriate antidiuretic
   hormone
si·al·a·den
si·al·ad·e·nec·to·my
si·al·ad·e·ni·tis
   chronic nonspecific s.
si·al·ad·e·nog·ra·phy
si·al·ad·e·nop·athy
   benign lymphoepithelial s.
si·al·ad·e·no·sis
si·al·ad·e·not·o·my

si·a·la·gog·ic
si·al·a·gogue
si·a·late
si·al·ec·ta·sia
sia·lec·ta·sis
si·al·em·e·sis
si·al·ic
si·al·ic acid
si·al·i·dase
si·a·line
si·al·ism
si·al·is·mus
si·a·li·tis
si·a·lo·ad·e·nec·to·my
si·a·lo·ad·e·ni·tis
si·a·lo·ad·e·not·o·my
si·alo·aero·pha·gia
si·alo·aer·oph·a·gy
si·alo·an·gi·ec·ta·sis
si·alo·an·gi·itis
si·alo·an·gi·og·ra·phy
si·alo·an·gi·tis
si·alo·cele
si·alo·do·chi·tis
si·alo·do·cho·plas·ty
si·alo·duc·ti·tis
si·alo·gas·trone
si·a·log·e·nous
si·alo·gog·ic
si·alo·gogue
si·alo·gram
si·alo·graph
si·a·log·ra·phy
si·alo·lith
si·alo·li·thi·a·sis
si·alo·li·thot·o·my
si·al·o·ma
si·alo·meta·pla·sia
   necrotizing s.
si·a·lom·e·ter
si·a·lom·e·try
si·alo·mu·cin
si·a·lon
si·alo·pha·gia
si·alo·pro·tein
si·a·lor·rhea
si·a·los·che·sis
si·a·lo·se·mei·ol·o·gy

si·alo·sis
si·alo·ste·no·sis
si·alo·sy·rinx
sib
sib·i·lant
sib·i·lus
Sib·ley-Leh·nin·ger test
sib·ling
sib·ship
Sib·son's aponeurosis
Sib·son's fascia
Sib·son's furrow
Sib·son's groove
Sib·son's notch
Si·card's syndrome
sic·cant
sic·co·la·bile
sic·co·sta·bile
sic·cus
sick
sick bay
sick·le
sick·le·mia
sick·le·mic
sick·ler
sick·ling
sick·ness
    acute serum s.
    acute sleeping s.
    aerial s.
    African sleeping s.
    air s.
    altitude s.
    athletes's.
    aviation s.
    balloon s.
    bay s.
    black s.
    Borna s.
    bush s.
    caisson s.
    car s.
    Ceylon s.
    chronic serum s.
    chronic sleeping s.
    compressed-air s.
    decompression s.
    drug-induced serum s.

sick·ness *(continued)*
    East African sleeping s.
    falling s.
    Gambian sleeping s.
    grass s.
    green s.
    green tobacco s.
    high-altitude s.
    Indian s.
    Jamaican vomiting s.
    laughing s.
    microwave s.
    mid-African sleeping s.
    morning s.
    motion s.
    mountain s.
    ozone s.
    painted s.
    radiation s.
    railroad s.
    Rhodesian sleeping s.
    sea s.
    secondary radiation s.
    serum s.
    sleeping s.
    space s.
    spotted s.
    talking s.
    vomiting s.
    West African sleeping s.
    x-ray s.
    Zambezi sleeping s.
Sid·bury syndrome
s.i.d. — L. semel in die (once a
  day)
side
    balancing s.
    functioning s.
    nonfunctioning s.
    working s.
side-bone
side-cut·ting
side ef·fect
sid·er·amine
sid·er·in·uria
sid·er·ism
sid·ero·blast
    ringed s.

sid·ero·chrome
sid·ero·cyte
sid·ero·cy·to·sis
sid·ero·der·ma
sid·ero·fi·bro·sis
sid·er·og·e·nous
sid·ero·my·cin
sid·ero·pe·nia
sid·ero·pe·nic
sid·ero·phage
sid·ero·phil
sid·ero·phil·in
sid·er·oph·i·lous
sid·ero·phone
sid·ero·phore
sid·ero·scope
sid·er·o·sil·i·co·sis
sid·er·o·sis
    s. bulbi
    s. conjunctivae
    hematogenous s.
    hepatic s.
    nutritional s.
    pulmonary s.
    urinary s.
sid·er·ot·ic
sid·er·ous
SIDS — sudden infant death syndrome
Sieg·bahn unit
Sie·gert's sign
Sie·gle's otoscope
sie·mens
Sie·mer·ling's nucleus
Sieur's sign
Sieur's test
sieve
    molecular s.
sie·vert
SIg — surface immunoglobulin
Sig. — L. signetur (let it be labeled)
sigh
    Hefke-Turner s.
sight
    day s.
    far s.

sight (continued)
    long s.
    near s.
    night s.
    old s.
    second s.
    short s.
Sig·ma method
sig·ma
sig·ma·sism
sig·ma·tism
sig·moid
sig·moid·ec·to·my
sig·moid·itis
sig·moido·pexy
sig·moido·proc·tos·to·my
sig·moido·rec·tos·to·my
sig·moido·scope
sig·moid·os·co·py
sig·moido·sig·moi·dos·to·my
sig·moid·os·to·my
sig·moid·ot·o·my
sig·moido·ves·i·cal
Sig·mund's glands
sign
    Aaron's s.
    Abadie's s.
    Abrahams's.
    accessory s.
    Achilles tendon s.
    Ahlfeld s.
    air bronchogram s.
    air-cushion s.
    Allis' s.
    Alri s.
    Amoss's.
    anatomical snuffbox s.
    Andral's s.
    André-Thomas s.
    Anghelescu's s.
    antecedent s.
    anterior tibial s.
    anticus s.
    Apley s.
    Argyll Robertson pupil s.
    Arroyo's s.
    Aschner's s.
    assident s.

sign *(continued)*
    associated abduction s.
    Auenbrugger's s.
    Aufrecht's s.
    auscultatory s.
    Babinski's s's
    Babinski's toe s.
    Baccelli's s.
    Baillarger's s.
    Balduzzi s.
    Ballance's s.
    Ballet's s.
    Bamberger's s.
    bandage s.
    Bárány's s.
    Bard's s.
    Barré's s.
    Barré's pyramidal s.
    Bastian-Bruns' s.
    Battle's s.
    Beccaria s.
    Becker's s.
    Béclard's s.
    Beevor's s.
    Behier-Hardy s.
    Bekhterev's s.
    Bell's s.
    Bergara-Wartenberg s.
    Berger's s.
    Bergman's s.
    Bespaloff s.
    Bethea's s.
    Bezold's s.
    Biederman's s.
    Biermer's s.
    Biernacki's s.
    Bikele s.
    Binda's s.
    Bing s.
    Bing's entotic s.
    Biot's s.
    Bird's s.
    Bjerrum's s.
    Blatin's s.
    Blumberg's s.
    Boas s.
    Bonnet's s.
    Bordier-Fränkel s.

sign *(continued)*
    Borsieri's s.
    Boston's s.
    Bouchard's s.
    Bouillaud's s.
    Bouveret s.
    Boyce's s.
    Bozzolo's s.
    Bragard's s.
    Branham's s.
    Braun von Fernwald s.
    Braunwald s.
    Braxton Hicks' s.
    Brenner s.
    Brickner's s.
    Broadbent's s.
    Broadbent's inverted s.
    Brockenbrough's s.
    Brodie's s.
    Brown Kelly s.
    Brown-Séquard's s.
    Brudzinski's s.
    Brunati's s.
    Bruns' s.
    Bryant's s.
    Burger's s.
    Burghart's s.
    Burton's s.
    Calkins s.
    camelot s.
    candlewax s.
    Cantelli's s.
    Capps s.
    Carabelli's s.
    Cardarelli's s.
    cardinal s's
    cardiorespiratory s.
    Carman's s.
    Carnett's s.
    Carvallo s.
    Case's pad s.
    Castellino's s.
    caviar s.
    Cegka's s.
    Cestan s.
    Chaddock's s.
    Chadwick s.
    chandelier s.

sign *(continued)*
    Charcot's s.
    Chaussier s.
    Cheyne-Stokes s.
    Chilaiditi s.
    chin-retraction s.
    Chvostek's s.
    Chvostek-Weiss s.
    Clark s.
    Claude s.
    Claude's hyperkinesis s.
    clavicular s.
    claw hand s.
    Cleeman's s.
    clenched fist s.
    closed fist s.
    cobra head s.
    Codman's s.
    cogwheel s.
    coin s.
    Cole's s.
    Collier s.
    Comby s.
    commemorative s.
    Comolli's s.
    complementary opposition
      s.
    compressed tissue s.
    Conillaud s.
    contralateral s.
    Coopernail s.
    Cope's s.
    Corrigan's s.
    coughing s.
    Courtois s.
    Courvoisier's s.
    Cowen's s.
    crescent s.
    Crichton-Browne's s.
    Cruveilhier's s.
    Cullen's s.
    Cumbo s.
    curtain s.
    cushingoid s's
    Dalrymple's s.
    D'Amato's s.
    Damoiseau's s.
    dance s.

sign *(continued)*
    Danforth s.
    Darier's s.
    Davidsohn's s.
    Dawbarn's s.
    Dejerine's s.
    de la Camp's s.
    Delbet's s.
    Delmege's s.
    Demarquay's s.
    Demianoff's s.
    de Musset's s.
    de Mussy's s.
    Dennie's s.
    Desault's s.
    d'Espine's s.
    Dew's s.
    Diakiogiannis s.
    diaphragm s.
    Dixon Mann's s.
    doll's eye s.
    Dorendorf's s.
    dorsocuboidal s.
    double contour s.
    doublet s.
    drawer s.
    Drummond's s.
    DTP s.
    Du Bois' s.
    Duchenne's s.
    Duckworth's s.
    Dugas' s.
    Duncan-Bird s.
    Dupuy-Dutemps s.
    Dupuy-Dutemps and
      Cestan s.
    Dupuytren's s.
    Duroziez's s.
    Dutemps-Cestan s.
    echo s.
    Elliot's s.
    Ellis' s.
    Ely's s.
    Enroth's s.
    Erb's s.
    Erben's s.
    Erichsen's s.
    Erni's s.

sign *(continued)*
- Escherich's s.
- Eustace Smith's s.
- Ewart's s.
- Ewing s.
- external malleolar s.
- extinction s.
- eyelash s.
- fabere s.
- facial s.
- fadir s.
- Faget's s.
- Fajersztajn s.
- Fajersztajn's crossed sciatic s.
- fan s.
- Federici's s.
- femoral s.
- Filipovitch's s.
- finger spread s.
- Finkelstein s.
- Fischer's s.
- fistula s.
- flag s.
- flush-tank s.
- Foerster s.
- fontanelle s.
- forearm s.
- formication s.
- Fournier s.
- Fränkel's s.
- Friedreich's s.
- Froment's paper s.
- front tap s.
- frontal release s.
- Fuchs s.
- Fürbringer's s.
- Gaenslen's s.
- Galeazzi s.
- Gangolphe s.
- Garel's s.
- Gerhardt's s.
- Gianelli's s.
- Gifford's s.
- Gilbert's s.
- glabellar-tap s.
- Glasgow's s.
- Gobiet s.

sign *(continued)*
- Goggia's s.
- Golden s.
- Goldstein's s.
- Goldthwait's s.
- Gonda s.
- Goodell's s.
- Gordon's s.
- Gorissenne s.
- Gottron's s.
- Gowers' s.
- Graefe's s.
- Grancher's s.
- Granger's s.
- Grasset's s.
- Grasset-Bychowski s.
- Grasset-Gaussel-Hoover s.
- Greene's s.
- Grey Turner's s.
- Griesinger's s.
- Griffith's s.
- grip s.
- Grisolle's s.
- Grocco's s.
- Grossman's s.
- Gubler's s.
- Guilland's s.
- Gunn's s.
- Gunn's crossing s.
- Gunn's pupillary s.
- Günzberg s.
- Guye s.
- Guyon's s.
- Hahn's s.
- Halban s.
- Hall's s.
- halo s.
- Hamilton s.
- Hamman's s.
- harlequin s.
- Harris s.
- Hatchcock's s.
- Haudek's s.
- Heberden's s's
- Hefke-Turner s.
- Hegar's s.
- Heilbronner's s.
- Heim-Kreysig s.

sign *(continued)*
  Helbing's s.
  Hellendall's s.
  Hennebert's s.
  Henning's s.
  Hertwig-Magendie s.
  Heryng's s.
  Hicks' s.
  Higouménakis' s.
  Hill's s.
  Hirschberg's s.
  Hochsinger's s.
  Hoehne's s.
  Hoffmann's s.
  Holmes' s.
  Homans' s.
  Hoover's s.
  Hope's s.
  Horn's s.
  Horner's s.
  Horsley's s.
  Howship-Romberg s.
  Hoyne's s.
  Huchard's s.
  Hueter's s.
  Human's s.
  Huntington's s.
  Hutchinson's s.
  hyperkinesis s.
  interossei s.
  Itard-Cholewa s.
  Jaccoud's s.
  Jackson's s.
  Jacquemier's s.
  Jellinek's s.
  Jendrassik's s.
  Joffroy's s.
  Jolly s.
  jugular s.
  Jürgensen's s.
  Kanavel's s.
  Kanter s.
  Kantor's s.
  Karplus' s.
  Kashida's s.
  Keen's s.
  Kehr's s.
  Kellock's s.

sign *(continued)*
  Kelly's s.
  Kerandel's s.
  Kergaradec's s.
  Kernig's s.
  Kerr's s.
  Kestenbaum's s.
  Kleist's s.
  Klemm's s.
  Klippel-Feil s.
  Kluge s.
  Knie's s.
  Kocher's s.
  Koplik's s.
  Korányi's s.
  Kreysig's s.
  Krisovski's (Krisowski's) s.
  Kussmaul's s.
  Küstner's s.
  Ladin's s.
  Laënnec's s.
  Lafora's s.
  Langoria's s.
  Lasègue's s.
  Laugier's s.
  leg s.
  Le Gendre (Legendre) s.
  leg flexion s.
  Leichtenstern's s.
  Lennhoff's s.
  Leri's s.
  Leser-Trélat s.
  levator s.
  Levine's clenched-fist s.
  Lhermitte's s.
  Libman's s.
  Lichtheim's s.
  ligature s.
  Liget s.
  Linder's s.
  Litten's s.
  Livierato's s.
  Lloyd's s.
  Lockwood s.
  Loenen s.
  Lombardi's s.
  long tract s's
  Lorenz s.

sign *(continued)*
- Lucas' s.
- Ludloff's s.
- Lust's s.
- McBurney's s.
- McCarthy s.
- McClintock s.
- McCort s.
- Macewen's s.
- McGinn-White s.
- McMurray s.
- Magendie's s.
- Magendie-Hertwig s.
- Magnan's s.
- Mahler's s.
- Maisonneuve's s.
- Mann's s.
- Mannkopf's s.
- Marañón s.
- Marcus Gunn's pupillary s.
- Marfan's s.
- Marie's s.
- Marie-Foix s.
- Marinesco's s.
- Mayo's s.
- Means's.
- Meltzer's s.
- Mendel-Bekhterev s.
- meniscus s.
- Mennell's s.
- Meunier s.
- Mingazzini s.
- Minor's s.
- Mirchamp's s.
- Möbius' (Moebius') s.
- Moniz s.
- Morquio's s.
- Moschcowitz's s.
- Mosler's s.
- moulage s.
- Moutard-Martin s.
- Müller's s.
- Munson's s.
- Murat's s.
- Murphy's s.
- Musset's s.
- Myerson's s.
- neck s.

sign *(continued)*
- Negro s.
- Neri's s.
- newspaper s.
- niche s.
- Nicoladoni's s.
- Nikolsky's s.
- nostril s.
- Nothnagel s.
- nuchal s.
- Ober's s.
- objective s.
- obturator s.
- oil-drop s.
- Oliver's s.
- Oppenheim's s.
- orange-peel s.
- orbicularis s.
- Ortolani's s.
- Osiander s.
- Osler's s.
- palmoplantar s.
- Parkinson's s.
- Parrot's s.
- Pastia's s.
- patent bronchus s.
- Patrick's s.
- Pende's s.
- Perez's s.
- peroneal s.
- Petruschky s.
- Pfuhl's s.
- Pfuhl-Jaffé s.
- Phalen's s.
- physical s.
- Piltz's s.
- Pinard s.
- Pins's.
- Piotrowski's s.
- Piskacek's s.
- Pitres' s.
- pivot-shift s.
- placental s.
- platysma s.
- plumb-line s.
- Plummer's s.
- pneumatic s.
- Pool-Schlesinger s.

sign *(continued)*
- Porter's s.
- Potain's s.
- Pottenger's s.
- Prehn's s.
- Prévost's s.
- pronation s.
- pseudo-Babinski's s.
- pseudo-Graefe's s.
- psoas s.
- puddle s.
- pyloric string s.
- pyramid s.
- pyramidal s.
- pyramidal tract s. of lower extremities
- Quant's s.
- Queckenstedt's s.
- Quénu-Muret s.
- Quincke's s.
- radialis s.
- Radovici's s.
- railroad track s.
- Raimiste's s.
- Ramond's s.
- Ransohoff s.
- Rasch s.
- Rasin's s.
- Raynaud's s.
- rebound s.
- Remak's s.
- reservoir s.
- Revilliod's s.
- Riesman's s.
- rising sun s.
- Ritter-Rollet s.
- Riviere's s.
- Robertson's s.
- Roche's s.
- Rocher's s.
- Roger's counter s.
- Romaña's s.
- Romberg's s.
- Rommelaere's s.
- root s.
- rope s.
- Rosenbach's s.
- Roser's s.

sign *(continued)*
- Roser-Braun s.
- Rossolimo's s.
- Rotch's s.
- Rothschild's s.
- Rovighi's s.
- Rovsing's s.
- Rucker s.
- Ruggeri's s.
- Rumpel-Leede s.
- Rust's s.
- Saenger's s.
- Sansom's s.
- Sarbó's s.
- Saunders' s.
- scarf s.
- Schaefer s.
- Schepelmann's s.
- Schick's s.
- Schlesinger's s.
- Schultze's s.
- Schultze-Chvostek s.
- Schwartze's s.
- scimitar s.
- Seeligmüller's s.
- Séguin's s.
- Seidel's s.
- Seitz's s.
- Semon's s.
- setting-sun s.
- Shibley's s.
- Siegert's s.
- Signorelli's s.
- Silex's s.
- Simon's s.
- Sisto's s.
- Skoda's s.
- Smith's s.
- Snellen's s.
- soft s's
- Somagyi s.
- Soto-Hall s.
- Souques's.
- Spalding's s.
- spinal s.
- spine s.
- Spurling s.
- Squire's s.

sign *(continued)*
  stairs s.
  steeple s.
  Stellwag's s.
  Sterles' s.
  Sternberg's s.
  Stewart-Holmes s.
  Stierlin's s.
  Stimson s.
  Strauss' s.
  string s.
  Strümpell's s.
  Strunsky's s.
  subjective s.
  Suker's s.
  Sumner's s.
  swinging flashlight s.
  tapir snout s.
  Tarnier s.
  Tay's s.
  Theimich's lip s.
  thermic s.
  thigh s.
  Thomas' s.
  Thomson's s.
  Thornton's s.
  Throckmorton s.
  thumb s.
  thumb print s.
  tibialis s.
  Tinel's s.
  toe s.
  toe spread s.
  Tournay's s.
  Traube's s.
  Trendelenburg's s.
  trepidation s.
  Tresilian's s.
  Trimadeau's s.
  Troisier's s.
  Trömner's s.
  Trousseau's s.
  Turner's s.
  Turyn's s.
  Uhthoff's s.
  Unschuld's s.
  Uriolla s.
  Vanzetti's s.

sign *(continued)*
  Vedder's s's
  vein s.
  Vermel s.
  Vipond s.
  vital s's
  vitropressin s.
  Voltolini's s.
  von Graefe's s.
  von Monakow s.
  von Strümpell s.
  Wartenberg's s.
  Warthin s.
  water lily s.
  Weber's s.
  Wegner's s.
  Weill's s.
  Weiss's s.
  Wernicke's s.
  Westermark's s.
  Westphal's s.
  Widowitz's s.
  Wilder's s.
  Williams's.
  Williamson's s.
  Wilson's .
  Wilson's pronator s.
  Winterbottom's s.
  Wintrich's s.
  Wood's s.
  Zaufal's s.
sig·na
sig·nal
  Doppler velocity s.
  magnetic resonance s.
  nuclear s.
  sensory s.
  s.-to-noise ratio (S/N)
sig·na·ture
signe
  s. de la bandera
  s. de journal
  s. de peau d'orange
sig·net-ring pat·tern
sig·nif·i·cance
  statistical s.
sig·nif·i·cant
Sig·nor·el·li's sign

Sig. n. pro. — L. signa nomine
  proprio (label with the proper
  name)
sig·ua·te·ra
sik·i·mi
sik·i·min
sik·im·i·tox·in
sil·a·fil·con A
sil·a·fo·con A
Si·lain
si·lan·drone
Si·las·tic
si·lence
    electrical s.
si·lent
si·lex
Si·lex's sign
sil·hou·ette
sil·i·ca
sil·i·cate
sil·i·ca·to·sis
si·lic·ea
si·li·ceous
si·lic·ic acid
si·li·cious
sil·i·co·an·thra·co·sis
sil·i·co·flu·o·ride
sil·i·con
    s. carbide
    s. dioxide
    s. dioxide, colloidal
    s. fluoride
sil·i·cone
sil·i·con·o·ma
sil·i·co·pro·tein·o·sis
sil·i·co·sid·er·o·sis
sil·i·co·sis
    infective s.
Sil·i·cote
sil·i·cot·ic
sil·i·co·tu·ber·cu·lo·sis
sil·i·qua
    s. olivae
sil·i·quose
    floss s.
    surgical s.
Sil·va·dene
sil·vat·ic

sil·ver
    s. chloride
    colloidal s.
    Howe's s. nitrate
    s. iodide, colloidal
    methenamine s.
    s. nitrate
    s. nitrate, toughened
    s. picrate
    s. protein, mild
    s. protein, strong
    s. sulfadiazine
Sil·ver-Rus·sell syndrome
Sil·ver·man's needle
sil·ver·skin
Sil·ver·skiöld syndrome
sil·ver wire ef·fect
Sil·ves·ter's method
sil·ves·trene
Sil·vi·us
Sim·a·ru·ba
sim·a·ru·bi·din
sim·es·the·sia
si·meth·i·cone
si·mil·ia si·mil·i·bus cu·ran·
  tur
si·mil·li·mum
Sim·monds' disease
Sim·monds' syndrome
Si·mon's position
Si·mon's septic factor
Si·mon's sign
Si·mo·nart's band
Si·mo·nart's thread
Si·mo·nel·li's test
Si·mons' disease
sim·ple
Simp·son's forceps
Simp·son lamp
Simp·son light
Sims' depressor
Sims' position
Sims' speculum
sim·ul
sim·u·la·tion
sim·u·la·tor
    electrocardiographic s.

sim·u·la·tor *(continued)*
   space s.
Si·mu·li·i·dae
Si·mu·li·um
   S. *damnosum*
   S. *neavei*
   S. *ochraceum*
si·mul·tag·no·sia
si·mul·tan·ag·no·sia
SIMV — synchronized
  intermittent mandatory
  ventilation
si·nal
Sin·ax·ar
sin·ca·lide
sin·cip·i·tal
sin·ci·put
sin·e·fun·gin
Sin·e·quan
sin·ew
   back s.
   weeping s.
sing. — L. singulorum (of
  each)
sin·gle blind
sing·ly
Sin·go·serp
sin·gul·ta·tion
sin·gul·tous
sin·gul·tus
sin·i·grin
sin·is·ter
sin·is·trad
sin·is·tral
sin·is·tral·i·ty
sin·is·trau·ral
sin·is·tro·car·dia
sin·is·tro·cer·e·bral
sin·is·troc·u·lar
sin·is·troc·u·lar·i·ty
sin·is·tro·gy·ra·tion
sin·is·tro·man·u·al
sin·is·trop·e·dal
sin·is·tro·tor·sion
Sin·kler's phenomenon
si·no·atri·al
si·no·au·ric·u·lar
si·no·bron·chi·tis

Si·no·graf·in
si·nog·ra·phy
si·nom·e·nine
Si non val. — L. si non valeat
  (if it is not enough)
si·no·pul·mo·nary
si·no·spi·ral
si·no·ven·tric·u·lar
sin·ter
Sin·trom
sin·u·ate
sinu·at·ri·al
sinu·au·ric·u·lar
sinu·os·i·ty
sin·u·ous
si·nus *pl.* si·nus, si·nus·es
   accessory s's of the nose
   air s.
   alveolar s.
   anal s's
   s. anales
   anterior s's
   s. of anterior chamber
   s. anteriores
   s. aortae
   s. aortae [Valsalvae]
   aortic s.
   Arlt's s.
   s. arteriae pulmonalis
   articular s. of atlas
   articular s. of atlas,
     superior
   articular s. of axis, anterior
   articular s. of vertebrae,
     inferior
   s. of atlas, anterior
   barbers' hair s.
   basilar s.
   s. of Bochdalek
   branchial s.
   Breschet's s.
   s. caroticus
   carotid s.
   s. cavernosus
   cavernous s.
   cerebral s.
   cervical s.
   circular s.

si·nus *(continued)*
s. circularis
s. circularis iridis
coccygeal s.
s. cochleae
s. condylorum femoris
congenital lip s's
s. coronarius
coronary s.
s. of corpus callosum
cortical s's
costal s's of sternum
costodiaphragmatic s.
costomediastinal s. of
  pleura
s. costomediastinalis
  pleurae
costophrenic s.
cranial s's
Cuvier's s's
dental s.
dermal s.
draining s.
s's of dura mater
s. durae matris
s. epididymidis
s. of epididymis
Eternod's s.
ethmoidal s.
s. ethmoidalis
external branchial s.
Forssell's s.
frontal s.
frontal s., bony
s. frontalis
s. frontalis osseus
Guérin's s.
Huguier's s.
s. interarcualis
s. intercavernosi
s. intercavernosus anterior
s. intercavernosus
  posterior
intercavernous s's
intermediate s's
internal branchial s.
s. of internal jugular vein,
  inferior

si·nus *(continued)*
s. of internal jugular vein,
  superior
s. of kidney
lacteal s's
s. lacteus
s. lactiferi
lactiferous s's
laryngeal s.
s. of larynx
lateral s.
s. lienis
longitudinal s., inferior
longitudinal s., superior
lunate s. of radius
lunate s. of ulna
Luschka s.
lymph s's
lymphatic s's
s. of Maier
marginal s's
mastoid s.
s. maxillaris
s. maxillaris [Highmori]
s. maxillaris osseus
maxillary s.
maxillary s., bony
s. mediae
s. medii
medullary s's
Meyer's s.
s. Meyeri
middle s's
middle s. of atlas
s. of Morgagni
mucous s's of male urethra
nasal s's
oblique s. of pericardium
s. obliquus pericardii
occipital s.
s. occipitalis
omphalomesenteric s.
oral s.
Palfyn s.
paranasal s's
s. paranasales
parasinoidal s.
pericardial s.

si·nus *(continued)*
    s. pericardii
    s. pericranii
    peroneal s. of tibia
    Petit's s.
    petro-occipital s.
    petrosal s., inferior
    petrosal s., superior
    s. petrosquamosus
    s. petrosus inferior
    s. petrosus superior
    phrenicocostal s.
    s. phrenicocostalis
    pilonidal s.
    piriform s.
    s. pleurae
    pleural s.
    pleuroperitoneal s.
    s. pocularis
    posterior s's
    s. posterior cavi tympani
    s. posteriores
    preauricular s.
    s. precervicalis
    prostatic s.
    s. prostaticus
    s's of pulmonary trunk
    pyriform s.
    rectal s's
    s. rectales
    s. rectus
    renal s.
    s. renalis
    s. reuniens
    rhomboid s.
    rhomboid s. of Henle
    Ridley's s.
    Rokitansky-Aschoff s's
    sacrococcygeal s.
    sagittal s., inferior
    sagittal s., superior
    s. sagittalis inferior
    s. sagittalis superior
    semilunar s. of tibia
    sigmoid s.
    s. sigmoideus
    soleal s's
    sphenoidal s.

si·nus *(continued)*
    sphenoidal s., bony
    s. sphenoidalis
    s. sphenoidalis osseus
    sphenoparietal s.
    s. sphenoparietalis
    s. of spleen
    splenic s.
    s. splenicus
    straight s.
    subarachnoidal s's
    subcapsular s's
    subpetrosal s.
    superpetrosal s.
    tarsal s.
    s. tarsi
    tentorial s.
    terminal s.
    tonsillar s.
    s. tonsillaris
    transverse s. of dura mater
    transverse s. of
      pericardium
    s. transversus durae matris
    s. transversus pericardii
    traumatic s.
    s. trunci pulmonalis
    s. tympani
    tympanic s.
    s. of tympanic cavity,
      posterior
    s. unguis
    urogenital s.
    s. urogenitalis
    uterine s's
    uteroplacental s.
    s. of Valsalva
    s. of venae cavae
    s. venarum cavarum
    s. venosi durales
    s. venosus
    s. venosus sclerae
    venous s.
    venous s's of dura mater
    venous s. of sclera
    s. ventriculi
si·nus·al

si·nu·si·tis
  barotraumatic s.
  chronic caseous s.
  ethmoidal s.
  frontal s.
  infectious s. of turkeys
  maxillary s.
  papillary s.
  paranasal s.
  sphenoidal s.
si·nu·soid
  hepatic s.
  myocardial s's
  soleal s's
si·nu·soi·dal
si·nu·soi·dal·iza·tion
si·nu·sot·o·my
si·nu·ven·tric·u·lar
sio·my·cin
Si op. sit — L. si opus sit (if it
  is necessary)
si·phon
  carotid s.
si·phon·age
Si·pho·nap·tera
Si·phun·cu·la·ta
Si·phun·cu·li·na
    S. funicola
Sip·ple syndrome
Sip·py diet
Sip·py method
Sip·py treatment
si·qua
si·reno·form
si·reno·me·lia
si·ren·om·e·lus
sir·i·a·sis
SIRS — soluble immune
  response suppressor
sir·up
SISI — short increment
  sensitivity index
sis·mo·ther·a·py
siso·mi·cin
  s. sulfate
sis·so·rex·ia
sis·ter
Sis·ter Mary Jo·seph node

Sis·to's sign
Sis·trunk operation
Sis·tru·rus
site
  active s.
  allosteric s.
  antibody-combining s.
  antigen-binding s.
  antigen-combining s.
  binding s's
  catalytic s.
  combining s.
  donor s.
  fragile s.
  graft donor s.
  hypersensitive s.
  immunologically privileged
    s's
  marker s.
  mutable s.
  nucleotide replacement s.
  operator s.
  peptidyl s.
  privileged s's
  receptor s.
  recipient s.
  restriction s.
sit·fast
si·tol·o·gy
si·to·ma·nia
si·to·pho·bia
si·tos·ter·ol
β-si·tos·ter·ol·emia
si·to·tax·is
si·to·ther·a·py
si·to·tox·in
si·to·tox·ism
si·tot·ro·pism
sit·u·a·tion
si·tus pl. si·tus
  s. inversus
  s. inversus abdominalis
  s. inversus thoracis
  s. inversus viscerum
  s. perversus
  s. solitus
  s. transversus

Si vir. perm. — L. si vires
    permittant (if the strength
    will permit)
size
        achieved family s.
        completed family s.
        sample s.
Sjö·gren's disease
Sjö·gren's syndrome
Sjö·gren-Lars·son syndrome
Sjö·qvist's method
skat·ole
ska·tox·yl
skein
        Holmgren's s's
        test s's
ske·lal·gia
ske·las·the·nia
Ske·lax·in
skel·e·tal
skel·e·tin
skel·e·ti·za·tion
skel·e·to·fusi·mo·tor
skel·e·tog·e·nous
skel·e·tog·e·ny
skel·e·tog·ra·phy
skel·e·tol·o·gy
skel·e·to·mo·tor
skel·e·ton
        appendicular s.
        s. appendiculare
        articulated s.
        axial s.
        s. axiale
        cardiac s.
        fibrous s. of heart
        s. of heart
        thoracic s.
        s. of thorax
        visceral s.
skel·e·to·pia
skel·e·to·py
Skene's ducts
Skene's glands
Skene's tubules
ske·ni·tis
ske·no·scope
skew

skew·foot
skew·ness
ski·am·e·try
skia·po·res·co·py
skia·scope
skia·scope-op·tom·e·ter
ski·as·co·py
Skil·lern's fracture
skim·ming
        plasma s.
skin
        alligator s.
        bronzed s.
        citrine s.
        collodion s.
        crocodile s.
        elastic s.
        farmers' s.
        fish s.
        freeze-dried s.
        glabrous s.
        glossy s.
        India rubber s.
        lax s.
        loose s.
        lyophilized s.
        marble s.
        nail s.
        parchment s.
        piebald s.
        pig s.
        porcupine s.
        sailors' s.
        shagreen s.
Skin·ner box
Skin·ner classification
Ski·o·dan
skip·per
        cheese s.
Sklow·sky's symptom
Sko·da's sign
Sko·da's tympany
sko·da·ic
sko·pom·e·ter
SKSD — streptokinase-
    streptodornase
skull
        Alpert s.

skull *(continued)*
    cloverleaf s.
    hot cross bun s.
    lacuna s.
    maplike s.
    membranous s.
    natiform s.
    steeple s.
    stenobregmatic s.
    tower s.
    West's lacuna s.
    West-Engstler's s.
skull·cap
sl — slyke
SLA — L. sacrolaeva anterior
    (left sacroanterior)
slant
    s. of occlusal plane
SLE — systemic lupus
    erythematosus
sleep
    active s.
    crescendo s.
    D s.
    deep s.
    delta-wave s.
    desynchronized s.
    dreaming s.
    dreamless s.
    electric s.
    electrotherapeutic s.
    fast wave s.
    hypnotic s.
    non–rapid eye movement s.
    NREM s.
    orthodox s.
    paradoxical s.
    paroxysmal s.
    pontine s.
    prolonged s.
    quiet s.
    rapid eye movement s.
    REM s.
    rhomboencephalic s.
    rolandic s.
    S s.
    slow wave s.
    synchronized s.

sleep *(continued)*
    twilight s.
sleep·less·ness
sleep·talk·ing
sleep·walk·ing
slide
    histology s.
    microscope s.
sling
    Glisson's s.
    levator s.
    mandibular s.
    pterygomasseteric s.
    suburethral s.
    s. and swathe
slit
    Cheatle s.
    filtration s's
    gill s.
    pharyngeal s.
    stenopeic s.
    vulvar s.
slit-lamp
    s. biomicroscopy
    s. examination
slope
    lower ridge s.
    mandibular
        anteroposterior ridge s.
slough
    graft s.
slow·ing
    saccadic s.
SLP — L. sacrolaeva posterior
    (left sacroposterior)
SLRT — straight leg raising
    test
SLT — L. sacrolaeva
    transversa (left
    sacrotransverse)
Slu·der's method
Slu·der's neuralgia
Slu·der's syndrome
sludge
    activated s.
    biliary s.
sludg·ing
    s. of blood

slug
slur·ry
slyke
SMA — Sequential Multiple
  Analyzer
    superior mesenteric artery
SMAF — specific macrophage
  arming factor
small·pox
    inoculation s.
SMC — selenomethylnorcholes-
  terol
smear
    bronchoscopic s.
    buccal s.
    buffy coat s.
    cervical s.
    cul-de-sac s.
    cytologic s.
    FGT (female genital tract)
      cytologic s.
    Pap s.
    Papanicolaou s.
    Tzanck s.
    VCE (vagina, ectocervix,
      and endocervix) s.
smeg·ma
    s. embryonum
smeg·ma·lith
smeg·mat·ic
smell-brain
Smel·lie's method
Smel·lie's scissors
Smel·lie-Veit maneuver
smi·la·cin
smi·la·gen·in
Smi·lax
smile (smil·ing) incision
Smith, Hamilton Othanel
Smith's disease
Smith's dislocation
Smith's fracture
Smith's operation
Smith's sign
Smith's test
Smith-Gib·son operation
Smith-Lem·li-Opitz syndrome
Smith-Pe·ter·sen nail

Smith-Rob·in·son operation
Smith·wick's operation
smog
smoke
    mainstream s.
    sidestream s.
smok·ing
    passive s.
SMON — subacute
  myelo-opticoneuropathy
SMR — standard morbidity
  ratio
    standard mortality ratio
    submucous resection
smudg·ing
S.N. — L. secundum naturam
  (according to nature)
snail
snake
    brown s.
    cabbage s.
    colubrid s.
    coral s.
    crotalid s.
    elapid s.
    hair s.
    harlequin s.
    lyre s.
    poisonous s.
    sea s.
    tiger s.
    venomous s.
    viperine s.
snake·root
    Seneca s.
    senega s.
snap
    opening s.
snare
    basket s.
    nasal s.
    tonsil s.
Sned·don-Wil·kin·son disease
sneeze
Snell, George Davis
Snell's law
Snel·len's chart
Snel·len's eye

Snel·len's tests
Snel·len's test type
SNF — skilled nursing facility
Sni·der match test
SNM — Society of Nuclear Medicine
snore
snow
 carbon dioxide s.
snow·ball opa·ci·ties
snow·banks
snow·blind·ness
SNS — sympathetic nervous system
snuff
 anatomical s.-box
Sny·der test
SO — spheno-occipital synchondrosis
SOAP — Subjective, Objective, Assessment, Plan (record)
soap
 carbolic s.
 curd s.
 green s.
 hexachlorophene liquid s.
 medicinal soft s.
 potash s.
 soft s.
 superfatted s.
 zinc s.
soap·stone
SOB — shortness of breath
so·cia
 s. parotidis
so·cial·iza·tion
so·cio·acu·sis
so·ci·o·bi·o·log·ic
so·ci·o·bi·o·log·i·cal
so·cio·bi·ol·o·gist
so·cio·bi·ol·o·gy
so·cio·dra·ma
so·ci·o·gen·ic
so·ci·ol·o·gist
so·ci·ol·o·gy
so·ci·om·e·try
so·cio·path

so·cio·path·ic
so·ci·op·a·thy
so·cio·ther·a·py
sock·et
 adjustable s.
 dry s.
 Dundee s.
 eye s.
 infected s.
 partial-contact s.
 plug-fit s.
 septic s.
 suction s.
 tooth s's
 total-contact s.
so·da
 baking s.
 bicarbonate of s.
 caustic s.
 chlorinated s.
 s. lime
 washing s.
so·dio·cit·rate
so·dio·tar·trate
so·di·um
 s. acetate
 s. acid citrate
 s. acid phosphate
 s. alginate
 s. alizarinsulfonate
 s. arsenate
 s. ascorbate
 s. aurothiomalate
 s. aurothiosulfate
 s. benzoate
 s. bicarbonate
 s. biphosphate
 s. bisulfite
 s. borate
 s. bromide
 s. calcium edetate
 s. caprylate
 s. carbonate
 s. caseinate
 s. cellulose phosphate
 s. chloride
 s. chromate
 s. chromate Cr 51

so·di·um *(continued)*
  s. citrate
  s. fluoride
  s. fluosilicate
  s. folate
  s. glutamate
  s. glycocholate
  s. gold thiosulfate
  s. hydrate
  s. hydroxide
  s. hypochlorite
  s. hyposulfite
  s. iodide
  s. ipodate
  s. lactate
  s. lauryl sulfate
  s. metabisulfite
  s. monofluorophosphate
  s. nitrate
  s. nitrite
  s. nitroferricyanide
  s. nitroprusside
  s. oxybate
  s. para-aminosalicylate
  s. perborate
  s. phosphate
  s. phosphate, dried
  s. phosphate, effervescent
  s. phosphate, exsiccated
  s. phytate
  s. polyphosphate
  s. polystyrene sulfonate
  potassium s. tartrate
  s. propionate
  s. pyroborate
  s. pyrophosphate
  radioactive s.
  s. salicylate
  s. silicofluoride
  s. stearate
  s. stibocaptate
  s. succinate
  s. sulfate
  s. sulfite
  s. sulfite, anhydrous
  s. sulfite, exsiccated
  s. tetraborate
  s. tetradecyl sulfate

so·di·um *(continued)*
  s. thiamylal
  s. thiosulfate
  s. trimetaphosphate
so·di·um-po·tas·si·um aden·o·sine·tri·phos·pha·tase
so·do·ko·sis
so·do·ku
sod·o·mist
sod·o·my
Soem·mer·ing's foramen
Soem·mer·ing's gray substance
Soem·mer·ing's ring
Soem·mer·ing's spot
sof·ten·ing
  anemic s.
  s. of the brain
  colliquative s.
  gray s.
  green s.
  hemorrhagic s.
  inflammatory s.
  mucoid s.
  pyriform s.
  red s.
  s. of the stomach
  white s.
  yellow s.
so·ja bean
so·ko·sho
Sol. — solution
sol
  metal s.
  solid s.
Sol·a·na·ceae
sol·a·na·ceous
so·lan·drine
so·la·ni·dine
so·la·nine
so·la·nism
so·la·noid
So·la·num
  S. carolinense
so·lap·sone
so·lar
so·lar·i·um
so·la·so·dine
so·la·sul·fone

sol·a·tion
Sol·da·i·ni's reagent
Sol·da·i·ni's test
sold·er
sole
so·le·al
So·le·nog·ly·pha
so·le·no·glyph·ic
so·le·noid
so·le·no·nych·ia
So·le·no·po·tes
   S. capillatus
so·le·nop·sin A
So·le·nop·sis
sole plate
sol·fer·i·no
Sol·ga·nal
sol·id
   color s.
Sol·i·da·go
sol·i·dism
sol·ip·sism
sol·ip·sis·tic
sol-lu·nar
sol·pu·gid
Sol·pu·gida
sol·u·bil·i·ty
sol·u·ble
Solu-Cor·tef
so·lum *pl.* so·la
   s. tympani
so·lute
so·lu·tio
so·lu·tion
   acetylcysteine s.
   Albright's s.
   alcoholic s.
   alkaline sodium
     hypochlorite s.
   Alsever s.
   aluminum acetate topical
     s.
   aluminum subacetate
     topical s.
   amaranth s.
   amaranth s., compound
   aminoacetic acid sterile s.
   aminobenzoic acid s.

so·lu·tion *(continued)*
   ammonia s., diluted
   ammonia s., strong
   ammonium acetate s.
   ammonium citrate s.,
     alkaline
   ammonium hydroxide s.,
     diluted
   ammonium hydroxide s.,
     stronger
   anisotonic s.
   antazoline phosphate
     ophthalmic s.
   anticoagulant citrate
     dextrose s.
   anticoagulant citrate
     phosphate dextrose s.
   anticoagulant heparin s.
   antipyrine and benzocaine
     s.
   antiseptic s.
   aqueous s.
   arsenical s.
   arsenious acid s.
   atropine sulfate
     ophthalmic s.
   auxiliary s.
   balanced electrolyte s.
   balanced salt s.
   Basham's s.
   Benedict's s.
   benzalkonium chloride s.
   benzethonium chloride
     topical s.
   Bonain's s.
   borax-carmine s.
   boric acid s.
   Bouin's s.
   Brompton s.
   buffer s.
   Burnett s.
   Burow's s.
   butacaine sulfate s.
   calciferol s.
   calcium cyclamate and
     calcium saccharin s.
   calcium hydroxide topical
     s.

so·lu·tion *(continued)*
   carbachol ophthalmic s.
   carbol-fuchsin topical s.
   cardioplegic s.
   carmine s.
   Carnoy's s.
   carphenazine maleate s.
   centinormal s.
   cetylpyridinium chloride s.
   chloramphenicol
     ophthalmic s.
   chloramphenicol for
     ophthalmic s.
   chymotrypsin for
     ophthalmic s.
   clindamycin palmitate
     hydrochloride for oral s.
   cloxacillin sodium for oral
     s.
   coal tar topical s.
   cochineal s.
   Cohn's s.
   colloid s.
   colloidal s.
   comprehensive s.
   contrast s.
   cresol s., compound
   cresol s., saponated
   crystal violet s.
   cyanocobalamin Co 57 s.
   cyanocobalamin Co 60 s.
   cyclopentamine
     hydrochloride s.
   cyclopentolate hydro-
     chloride ophthalmic s.
   Czapek-Dox s.
   Dakin's s.
   Dakin's s., modified
   Darrow s.
   decimolar s.
   decinormal s.
   demecarium bromide
     ophthalmic s.
   dexamethasone sodium
     phosphate ophthalmic s.
   diatrizoate sodium s.
   diethyltoluamide topical s.

so·lu·tion *(continued)*
   dioctyl calcium
     sulfosuccinate s.
   dioctyl sodium
     sulfosuccinate s.
   diphenoxylate
     hydrochloride and
     atropine sulfate oral s.
   disclosing s.
   docusate sodium s.
   double-normal s.
   Drabkin's s.
   dyclonine hydrochloride
     topical s.
   echothiophate iodide for
     ophthalmic s.
   dl-ephedrine hydrochloride
     s.
   ephedrine sulfate nasal s.
   epinephrine s.
   epinephrine bitartrate
     ophthalmic s.
   epinephrine nasal s.
   epinephryl borate
     ophthalmic s.
   ergocalciferol oral s.
   erythrosine sodium topical
     s.
   Farrant's s.
   Fehling's s.
   ferric subsulfate s.
   ferrous sulfate oral s.
   fiftieth-normal s.
   fixative s.
   Flemming's s.
   fluocinolone acetonide
     topical s.
   fluorouracil topical s.
   Fonio's s.
   formaldehyde s.
   formol-Zenker s.
   Fowler's s.
   gelatin s., special
     intravenous
   gentian violet topical s.
   Gilson's s.
   glycerin oral s.
   gold s.

so·lu·tion *(continued)*
    gold [198]Au s.
    Gowers's.
    Gram's s.
    gram molecular s.
    half-normal s.
    haloperidol oral s.
    Hamdi's s.
    Hanks s.
    hardening s.
    Hartman s.
    Hayem's s.
    hexylcaine hydrochloride
        topical s.
    homatropine hydrobromide
        ophthalmic s.
    hundredth-normal s.
    hydrogen dioxide s.
    hydrogen peroxide topical
        s.
    hydroxyamphetamine
        hydrobromide ophthalmic
        s.
    hydroxypropyl methyl-
        cellulose ophthalmic s.
    hyperbaric s.
    hypertonic s.
    hypobaric s.
    hypotonic s.
    idoxuridine ophthalmic s.
    iodine s., compound
    iodine s., strong
    iodine topical s.
    isobaric s.
    isoflurophate ophthalmic s.
    isotonic s.
    Kaiserling s.
    Krebs-Ringer s.
    Labarraque's s.
    Lang's s.
    Lange's s.
    lead subacetate s.
    lead subacetate s., diluted
    lime s., sulfurated
    liver s.
    Locke's s.
    Locke's s., citrated
    Locke-Ringer's s.

so·lu·tion *(continued)*
    Lugol's s.
    Magendie's s.
    magnesium citrate oral s.
    major s.
    Mayer s.
    merbromin s.
    merbromin s., surgical
    methoxsalen topical s.
    methylcellulose
        ophthalmic s.
    methylrosaniline chloride
        s.
    molal s.
    molar s.
    molecular disperse s.
    Monsel's s.
    nafcillin sodium for oral s.
    naphazoline hydrochloride
        nasal s.
    naphazoline hydrochloride
        ophthalmic s.
    neomycin and polymyxin B
        sulfates and gramicidin
        ophthalmic s.
    neomycin and polymyxin B
        sulfates and
        hydrocortisone otic s.
    neomycin sulfate oral s.
    Nessler's s.
    nitrofurazone topical s.
    nitromersol topical s.
    normal s.
    normal saline s.
    normal salt s.
    normobaric s.
    nortriptyline s.
    Ohlmacher s.
    ophthalmic s.
    Orth's s.
    oxacillin sodium for oral s.
    oxymetazoline
        hydrochloride nasal s.
    paramethadione oral s.
    parathyroid s.
    Perenyi's s.
    phenylephrine
        hydrochloride nasal s.

so·lu·tion *(continued)*

phenylephrine hydro-
chloride ophthalmic s.

physiological salt s.

physiological sodium
chloride s.

physostigmine salicylate
ophthalmic s.

pilocarpine hydrochloride
ophthalmic s.

pilocarpine nitrate
ophthalmic s.

Pitkin's s.

pituitary s.

pituitary s., posterior

potassium arsenite s.

potassium iodide oral s.

potassium phenethicillin
for oral s.

povidone-iodine topical s.

prednisolone sodium
phosphate ophthalmic s.

prochlorperazine edisylate
oral s.

promazine hydrochloride
oral s.

proparacaine hydro-
chloride ophthalmic s.

racemic ephedrine
hydrochloride s.

racephedrine
hydrochloride s.

radiocyanocobalamin s.

radiogold s.

Randall's s.

Rees-Ecker s.

Ringer's s.

Ruge's s.

saline s.

salt s.

saponated cresol s.

saturated s.

Schällibaum's s.

sclerosing s.

scopolamine hydrobromide
ophthalmic s.

seminormal s.

Seyderhelm's s.

so·lu·tion *(continued)*

Shohl's s.

silver nitrate s.,
ammoniacal

silver nitrate ophthalmic s.

sodium chloride s.

sodium chromate Cr 51
sterile s.

sodium citrate and citric
acid s.

sodium cyclamate and
sodium saccharin s.

sodium fluorescein
ophthalmic s.

sodium fluoride oral s.

sodium fluoride and
orthophosphoric acid s.

sodium hypochlorite s.

sodium hypochlorite s.,
diluted

sodium iodide I 125 s.

sodium iodide I 131 s.

sodium pertechnetate
Tc 99m s.

sodium phosphate s.

sodium phosphate and
biphosphate oral s.

sodium phosphate P 32 s.

sodium radioiodide s.

sodium radiophosphate s.

sorbitol s.

standard s.

Suby's G s.

sulfacetamide sodium
ophthalmic s.

sulfisoxazole diolamine
ophthalmic s.

supersaturated s.

surgical s. of chlorinated
soda

susa s.

tenth-normal s.

test s's

tetracaine hydrochloride
ophthalmic s.

tetracaine hydrochloride
topical s.

so·lu·tion *(continued)*
    tetrahydrozoline hydro-
      chloride nasal s.
    tetrahydrozoline hydro-
      chloride ophthalmic s.
    thimerosal topical s.
    thioridazine hydrochloride
      oral s.
    thousandth-normal s.
    Toison's s.
    tolnaftate topical s.
    tribromethyl alcohol s.
    tribromoethanol s.
    tribromoethyl alcohol s.
    trimethadione s.
    triple antibiotic s.
    tropicamide ophthalmic s.
    tuaminoheptane sulfate
      nasal s.
    Tyrode's s.
    Vleminckx's s.
    volumetric s.
    Weigert s.
    xylometazoline
      hydrochloride nasal s.
    Zenker's s.
    Ziehl's s.
    zinc sulfate ophthalmic s.
solv. — L. solve (dissolve)
sol·va·ble
sol·vate
sol·va·tion
sol·ven·cy
sol·vent
    lipid s.
    polar s.
sol·vol·y·sis
So·ma
so·ma
so·mal
som·a·lin
so·ma·plasm
som·as·the·nia
so·ma·tag·no·sia
so·ma·tal·gia
so·mat·as·the·nia
so·mat·es·the·sia
so·mat·es·thet·ic

so·mat·ic
so·mat·i·co·splanch·nic
so·mat·i·co·visc·er·al
so·ma·tist
so·ma·ti·za·tion
so·mato·blast
so·mato·cep·tor
so·mato·chrome
so·mato·cyte
so·mato·derm
so·ma·to·did·y·mus
so·ma·to·dym·ia
so·mato·form
so·ma·to·gen·e·sis
so·ma·to·ge·net·ic
so·ma·to·gen·ic
so·mato·gram
so·ma·tol·o·gy
so·ma·to·mam·mo·tro·pin
    chorionic s.
so·ma·to·me·din
    s. C
so·ma·to·meg·a·ly
so·ma·tom·e·try
so·ma·top·a·gus
so·ma·to·path·ic
so·ma·top·a·thy
so·ma·to·phre·nia
so·mato·plasm
so·ma·to·pleu·ral
so·ma·to·pleure
so·ma·to·psy·chic
so·ma·to·psy·cho·sis
so·ma·tos·chi·sis
so·ma·tos·co·py
so·ma·to·sen·sory
so·ma·to·sex·u·al
so·ma·to·splanch·no·pleur·ic
so·ma·to·stat·in
so·ma·to·stat·i·no·ma
so·ma·to·ther·a·py
so·ma·to·to·nia
so·ma·to·top·ag·no·sia
so·ma·to·top·ic
so·ma·to·trid·y·mus
so·mato·trope
so·mato·troph
so·ma·to·troph·ic

so·ma·to·trop·ic
so·ma·to·tro·pin
so·mato·type
so·mato·typ·ing
so·mato·ty·py
so·mat·ro·pin
Som·bu·lex
so·mes·the·sia
so·mes·thet·ic
SOMI — sternal-occipital-mand-
  ibular immobilizer
so·mite
    cranial s.
    occipital s's
so·mit·ic
som·nam·bu·lance
som·nam·bu·la·tion
som·nam·bu·lism
som·nam·bu·list
som·ni·al
som·ni·fa·cient
som·nif·er·ous
som·nif·ic
som·nil·o·quence
som·nil·o·quism
som·nil·o·quist
som·nil·o·quy
som·no·cin·e·ma·to·graph
som·no·lence
som·no·lent
som·no·len·tia
Som·nos
som·nus
So·mo·gyi effect
So·mo·gyi phenomenon
So·mo·gyi unit
so·nar
so·nar·og·ra·phy
sonde
    s. coudé
Son·der·gaard's cleft
Son·der·mann's canals
sone
son·ic
son·i·cate
son·i·ca·tion
son·i·tus
Sonne dysentery

sono·chem·is·try
so·no·gram
so·nog·ra·pher
so·no·graph·ic
so·nog·ra·phy
    Acuson computed s.
sono·in·ver·sion
so·nol·o·gist
so·nol·o·gy
so·no·lu·cen·cy
so·no·lu·cent
so·no·rous
so·no·scope
so·no·to·mo·gram
so·no·to·mog·ra·phy
so·phis·ti·cate
so·phis·ti·ca·tion
sopho·ma·nia
So·pho·ra
soph·o·re·tin
soph·o·rin
soph·o·rine
so·por
so·po·rif·er·ous
sop·o·rif·ic
so·por·ous
S. op. s. — L. si opus sit (if it is
  necessary)
sorb
sor·be·fa·cient
sor·bent
sor·bic acid
sor·bin
sor·bi·nose
sor·bi·tan
sor·bite
sor·bi·tol
sor·bi·tol de·hy·dro·gen·ase
Sor·bi·trate
sor·bose
Sor·da·ri·a·ciae
sor·des
    s. gastricae
sore
    bed s.
    canker s.
    chrome s.
    Cochin s.

sore *(continued)*
    cold s.
    Delhi s.
    denture s.
    desert s.
    Gallipoli s.
    hard s.
    mixed s.
    Naga s.
    oriental s.
    pressure s.
    primary s.
    soft s.
    umballa s.
    veldt s.
    venereal s.
Sör·en·sen's reagent
So·ret band
So·ret effect
So·ret phenomenon
sore throat
    clergyman's s. t.
    epidemic streptococcal s. t.
    hospital s. t.
    putrid s. t.
    septic s. t.
    spotted s. t.
    streptococcal s. t.
    ulcerated s. t.
so·ri
so·roche
sorp·tion
sort·er
    fluorescence-activated cell
       s. (FACS)
so·rus *pl.* so·ri
S.O.S. — L. si opus sit (if it is
  necessary)
so·ta·lol hy·dro·chlo·ride
so·ter·e·nol hy·dro·chlo·ride
So·to-Hall sign
So·tos syndrome
Sot·tas disease
souf·fle
    cardiac s.
    fetal s.
    funic s.
    funicular s.

souf·fle *(continued)*
    placental s.
    splenic s.
    umbilical s.
    uterine s.
sound
    adventitious s's
    atrial s.
    auscultatory s.
    bandbox s.
    Beatty-Bright friction s.
    bell s.
    Bellocq's s.
    bellows s.
    Benique s.
    bottle s.
    bronchial breath s.
    cardiac s's
    cavernous voice s.
    coin s.
    cracked-pot s.
    cracked-pot s., cranial
    diastolic s.
    diver-bomber s.
    eddy s's
    ejection s's
    entotic s's
    esophageal s.
    first s.
    flapping s.
    fourth s.
    friction s.
    gallop s.
    heart s's
    hippocratic s.
    Korotkoff s's
    lacrimal s.
    LeFort s.
    metallic s.
    muscle s.
    peacock s.
    percussion s.
    pericardial friction s.
    physiological s's
    pistol-shot s.
    post-tussis suction s.
    pulmonic second s.
    respiratory s.

sound *(continued)*
    Santini's booming s.
    second s.
    second s., pulmonic
    shaking s.
    subjective s.
    succussion s's
    third s.
    tick-tack s's
    to-and-fro s.
    urethral s.
    uterine s.
    vesicular breath s's
    water-wheel s.
    white s.
    Winternitz's s.
    xiphisternal crunching s.
Souques' phenomenon
Souques' sign
source
    point s.
south·ern·wood
Sout·tar's tube
sow·dah
Soxh·let's apparatus
soya
soy·bean
sp. — L. spiritus (spirit)
space
    alveolar dead s.
    anatomical dead s.
    antecubital s.
    apical s.
    arachnoid s.
    axillary s.
    Blessig's s's
    Bogros's s.
    Böttcher s.
    Bowman's s.
    bregmatic s.
    Burns' s.
    capsular s.
    cartilage s's
    cathodal dark s.
    cell s's
    chloride s.
    chyle s's
    circumlental s.

space *(continued)*
    Colles' s.
    complemental s.
    corneal s's
    Cotunnius' s.
    Crookes s.
    cupular s.
    Czermak's s's
    dead s.
    s's in dentin
    Disse's s's
    s. of Donders
    Douglas' s.
    epicerebral s.
    epidural s.
    episcleral s.
    epispinal s.
    epitympanic s.
    escapement s's
    extradural s.
    extraperitoneal s.
    filtration s.
    follicular s.
    s's of Fontana
    s. of Forel
    freeway s.
    globular s's of Czermak
    H. s.
    haversian s.
    Henke's s.
    His-Held s.
    His' perivascular s.
    Holzknecht's s.
    iliocostal s.
    interarytenoid s.
    intercostal s.
    intercristal s.
    intercrural s.
    interdental s.
    interfascial s.
    interglobular s's (of Owen)
    interlamellar s's
    intermesoblastic s.
    intermetacarpal s's
    intermetatarsal s's
    interocclusal s.
    interosseous s's
    interpeduncular s.

space *(continued)*
- interpleural s.
- interproximal s.
- interproximate s.
- interradicular s.
- interseptal s.
- interstitial s.
- intervaginal s.
- intervaginal s's of optic nerve
- intervillous s.
- intra-adventitial s.
- intracapsular s.
- intracristal s.
- intrapial s.
- s's of iridocorneal angle
- Kiernan's s's
- Kiesselbach's s.
- Kretschmann's s.
- Kuhnt s's
- Larrey's s's
- leeway s.
- Lesgaft's s.
- s. of Littre
- lymph s.
- lymphatic s.
- Magendie's s's
- Malacarne's s.
- Marie's quadrilateral s.
- marrow s.
- mechanical dead s.
- Meckel's s.
- mediastinal s.
- medullary s.
- meningeal s.
- midpalmar s.
- mitochondrial membrane s.
- Mohrenheim's s.
- Nance's leeway s.
- Nuel's s's
- Obersteiner-Redlich s.
- palmar s.
- parapharyngeal s.
- pararenal s.
- parasinoidal s's
- paraxial s.
- Parona's s.

space *(continued)*
- pelvocrural s.
- perforated s., anterior
- perforated s., posterior
- periaxial s.
- perichorioidal s.
- perichoroidal s.
- perilymphatic s.
- perineal s., deep
- perineal s., superficial
- perineural s.
- pleural s.
- pleuroperitoneal s.
- perineuronal s.
- perinodal s.
- perinuclear s.
- periotic s.
- peripharyngeal s.
- periplasmic s.
- periportal s. of Mall
- perisinusoidal s's
- peritoneal s.
- perivascular s.
- perivitelline s.
- personal s.
- pharyngomaxillary s.
- phrenocostal s.
- physiologic dead s.
- pia-arachnoid s.
- placental blood s.
- plantar s.
- pneumatic s.
- Poiseuille's s.
- popliteal s.
- postnasal s.
- postperforated s.
- preperitoneal s.
- preputial s.
- prevertebral s.
- prevesical s.
- prezonular s.
- proximal s.
- proximate s.
- Prussak's s.
- pterygomandibular s.
- pulp s.
- quadrangular s.
- quadrilateral s. of Marie

space (*continued*)
    relief s.
    respiratory dead s.
    retrobulbar s.
    retrocardiac s.
    retroinguinal s.
    retromylohyoid s.
    retro-ocular s.
    retroperitoneal s.
    retropharyngeal s.
    retropubic s.
    Retzius s.
    Robin's s's
    Schwalbe's s's
    semilunar s.
    septal s.
    subarachnoid s.
    subchorial s.
    subdural s.
    subepicranial s.
    subgingival s.
    submaxillary s.
    subphrenic s.
    subumbilical s.
    suprahepatic s's
    suprapubic s.
    suprasternal s.
    Tarin's s.
    Tenon's s.
    thenar s.
    thiocyanate s.
    third s.
    thyrohyal s.
    Traube's semilunar s.
    Tröltsch's s's
    urogenital s.
    Verga s.
    Virchow-Robin s's
    vitelline s.
    web s.
    Westberg's s.
    yolk s.
    Zang's s.
    zonular s's
spac·er
Spal·ding's sign
Spal·lan·za·ni's law
spal·la·tion

span
    attention s.
    auditory s.
    liver s.
Span·i·op·sis
Span·ish wind·lass
spar
    Iceland s.
spar·ga·no·sis
    ocular s.
spar·ga·num *pl.* spar·ga·na
Spar·ine
spar·ing
    macular s.
    protein s.
    sacral s.
spark
    direct s.
spar·so·my·cin
spar·te·ine
    s. sulfate
spar·tism
spar·ti·um
spasm
    s. of accommodation
    arterial s.
    athetoid s.
    Bell's s.
    blacksmiths' s.
    bowing s.
    bronchial s.
    cadaveric s.
    canine s.
    carpopedal s.
    cerebral s.
    clonic s.
    clonic facial s.
    cynic s.
    dancing s.
    diffuse esophageal s.
    epidemic transient
      diaphragmatic s.
    esophageal s.
    facial s.
    fatigue s.
    fixed s.
    flexion s.

spasm *(continued)*
    flexor s.
    functional s.
    glottic s.
    habit s.
    histrionic s.
    infantile massive s's
    inspiratory s.
    intention s.
    lock s.
    malleatory s.
    massive s.
    masticatory s.
    mimic s.
    mixed s.
    mobile s.
    muscle s.
    myopathic s.
    nictitating s.
    nodding s.
    occupation s.
    oculogyric s.
    pantomimic s.
    pedal s.
    perineal s.
    phonatory s.
    postparalytic facial s.
    professional s.
    progressive torsion s.
    recruitment s.
    respiratory s.
    retrocollic s.
    Romberg's s.
    rotatory s.
    salaam s.
    saltatory s.
    sewing s.
    spinal accessory s.
    stutter s.
    synclonic s.
    tailors' s.
    tetanic s.
    tonic s.
    tonoclonic s.
    torsion s.
    toxic s.
    vascular s.
    West s.

spasm *(continued)*
    winking s.
    writers's.
spas·mod·ic
spas·mo·gen
spas·mo·gen·ic
spas·mol·o·gy
spas·mo·lyg·mus
spas·mol·y·sant
spas·mol·y·sis
spas·mo·lyt·ic
spas·mo·phile
spas·mo·phil·ia
spas·mo·phil·ic
spas·mus
    s. agitans
    s. caninus
    s. coordinatus
    s. muscularis
    s. nictitans
    s. nutans
spas·tic
spas·tic·i·ty
    cerebral s.
    clasp-knife s.
spa·tia
spa·tial
spa·tic
spa·ti·um *pl.* spa·tia
    spatia anguli iridis
      [Fontanae]
    spatia anguli iridocornealis
    s. episclerale
    s. extraperitoneale
    s. intercostale
    s. interfasciale [Tenoni]
    spatia interglobularia
    spatia interossea metacarpi
    spatia interossea metatarsi
    s. intervaginale
    spatia intervaginalia nervi
      optici
    s. perichorioideale
    s. perichoroideale
    s. perilymphaticum
    s. perinei profundum
    s. perinei superficiale
    s. peripharyngeum

spa·ti·um *(continued)*
    s. retroperitoneale
    s. retropharyngeum
    s. retro-pubicum
    s. subdurale
    spatia zonularia
spat·u·la
    s. mallei
    tongue s.
spat·u·lar
spat·u·late
spat·u·la·tion
SPCA — serum prothrombin
    conversion accelerator (blood
    coagulation factor VII)
Spear·man's rank correlation
    coefficient (rho)
spear·mint
spe·cial·ism
spe·cial·ist
    clinical nurse s.
    nurse s.
spe·cial·iza·tion
spe·cial·ize
spe·cial·ty
spe·ci·a·tion
spe·cies
    diovulatory s.
    fugative s.
    monovulatory s.
    morphological s.
    polyovulatory s.
    polytypic s.
    type s.
spe·cies-spe·cif·ic
spe·cif·ic
spec·i·fic·i·ty
    carrier s.
    diagnostic s.
    neuronal s.
spe·cil·lum
spec·i·men
    corrosion s.
    cytologic s.
speck·le
    laser s.

SPECT — single photon
    emission computed
    tomography
spec·ta·cles
    compound s.
    decentered s.
    divided s.
    half-glass s.
    industrial s.
    Masselon's s.
    mica s.
    pantoscopic s.
    periscopic s.
    prismatic s.
    protective s.
    pulpit s.
    safety s.
    stenopeic s.
    tinted s.
    wire frame s.
spec·ti·no·my·cin
    s. hydrochloride
spec·tra
spec·tral
spec·trin
spec·tro·chrome
spec·tro·col·or·im·e·ter
spec·tro·flu·o·rom·e·ter
spec·tro·gram
    olfactory s.
spec·tro·graph
    mass s.
    x-ray s.
spec·trom·e·ter
    mass s.
    Mossbauer s.
    pulse-height s.
    x-ray s.
spec·trom·e·try
    x-ray emission s.
spec·tro·pho·to·flu·o·rom·e·
    ter
spec·tro·pho·tom·e·ter
    absorption s.
spec·tro·pho·tom·e·try
    atomic absorption s.
    flame emission s.
spec·tro·po·lar·im·e·ter

spec·tro·scope
    direct vision s.
spec·tro·scop·ic
spec·tros·co·py
    infrared s.
    microabsorption s.
spec·trum *pl.* spec·tra
    absorption s.
    action s.
    antibiotic s.
    broad-s.
    chemical s.
    chromatic s.
    color s.
    continuous s.
    continuous x-ray s.
    diffraction s.
    electromagnetic s.
    excitation s.
    fluorescence s.
    fortification s.
    gaseous s.
    grafting s.
    invisible s.
    normal s.
    ocular s.
    prismatic s.
    pure s.
    solar s.
    thermal s.
    visible s.
    x-ray s.
spec·u·lum *pl.* spec·u·la
    anal s.
    Aufricht's s.
    aural s.
    bivalve (or bivalved) s.
    Bozeman's s.
    Brinkerhoff's s.
    Cook's s.
    duck-billed s.
    esophageal s.
    eye s.
    Fergusson's s.
    Fränkel's s.
    Gruber's s.
    Hartmann's s.
    s. Helmontii

spec·u·lum *(continued)*
    Kelly's s.
    Killian nasal s.
    Martin's s.
    Martin and Davy s.
    Mathews's.
    nasal s.
    nasopharyngeal s.
    Pedersen s.
    Politzer's s.
    rectal s.
    Siegle's pneumatic ear s.
    Sims's.
    stop s.
    Thudichum s.
    urethral s.
    vaginal s.
    wire bivalve s.
    Yankauer s.
Spee's curvature
Spee's curve
speech
    alaryngeal s.
    ataxic s.
    clipped s.
    echo s.
    esophageal s.
    explosive s.
    incoherent s.
    interjectional s.
    jumbled s.
    mirror s.
    plateau s.
    pressured s.
    scamping s.
    scanning s.
    scattered s.
    slurred s.
    spastic s.
    staccato s.
    tangential s.
    telegraphic s.
spel·en·ce·pha·lia
    breath-holding s.
Spe·mann, Hans
Spe·mann's induction
Spen·cer-Par·ker vaccine
Spen·cer Wells facies

Speng·ler's fragments
Spens' syndrome
sperm
 muzzled s.
sper·ma
sper·ma·ceti
 synthetic s.
sper·ma·cra·sia
sper·mag·glu·ti·na·tion
sper·ma·te·li·o·sis
sper·mat·em·phrax·is
sper·mat·ic
sper·mat·i·cide
sper·ma·tid
sper·ma·tin
sper·ma·tism
sper·ma·ti·tis
sper·ma·to·blast
sper·ma·to·cele
sper·ma·to·ce·lec·to·my
sper·ma·to·ci·dal
sper·ma·to·cyst
sper·ma·to·cys·tec·to·my
sper·ma·to·cys·ti·tis
sper·ma·to·cys·tot·o·my
sper·ma·to·cy·tal
sper·ma·to·cyte
 primary s.
 secondary s.
sper·ma·to·cy·to·gen·e·sis
sper·ma·to·cy·to·ma
sper·ma·to·gen·e·sis
sper·ma·to·gen·ic
sper·ma·tog·e·nous
sper·ma·tog·e·ny
sper·ma·to·gone
sper·ma·to·go·nia
sper·ma·to·go·ni·um *pl.* sper·
 ma·to·go·nia
sper·ma·toid
sper·ma·tol·o·gy
sper·ma·tol·y·sin
sper·ma·tol·y·sis
sper·ma·to·lyt·ic
sper·ma·to·me·rite
sper·ma·to·path·ia
sper·ma·top·a·thy
sper·ma·to·phore

sper·ma·to·poi·et·ic
sper·ma·tor·rhea
 s. dormientum
 false s.
sper·ma·tos·che·sis
sper·ma·to·spore
sper·ma·to·tox·in
sper·mat·ovum
sper·ma·tox·in
sper·ma·to·zoa
sper·ma·to·zo·al
sper·ma·to·zo·i·cide
sper·ma·to·zoid
sper·ma·to·zo·on *pl.* sper·ma·
 to·zoa
sper·ma·tu·ria
sper·mec·to·my
sper·mi·a·tion
sper·mi·ci·dal
sper·mi·cide
sper·mid
sper·mi·dine
sper·mi·duct
sper·mine
 s. phosphate
sper·mio·cyte
sper·mio·gen·e·sis
sper·mio·go·ni·um
sper·mio·gram
sper·mio·te·le·o·sis
sper·mio·te·le·ot·ic
sper·mo·blast
sper·mo·cy·to·ma
sper·mo·lith
sper·mol·oro·pexy
sper·mol·y·sin
sper·mol·y·sis
sper·mo·lyt·ic
sper·mo·neu·ral·gia
Sper·moph·i·lus
sper·mo·phle·bec·ta·sia
sper·mo·plasm
sper·mo·sphere
sper·mo·spore
sper·mo·tox·ic
sper·mo·tox·in
Sper·ry, Roger Wolcott
spes phthi·si·ca

SPF — specific-pathogen free
sp gr — specific gravity
sph — spherical lens
sphac·e·late
sphac·e·la·tion
sphac·e·lin·ic acid
sphac·e·lism
sphac·e·lo·der·ma
sphac·e·loid
sphac·e·lous
sphac·e·lus
Sphae·ria
   S. sinensis
Sphae·ri·a·les
Sphae·roi·des mac·u·la·tus
Sphae·ro·pho·rus
   S. necrophorus
Sphae·ro·ti·lus
spha·gi·as·mus
spha·gi·tis
sphen·eth·moid
sphe·ni·on *pl.* sphe·nia
sphe·no·bas·i·lar
sphe·noc·cip·i·tal
sphe·no·ceph·a·lus
sphe·no·ceph·a·ly
sphe·no·eth·moid
sphe·no·fron·tal
sphe·noid
   Koffler s.
sphe·noi·dal
sphe·noi·dale
   planum s.
sphe·noi·di·tis
sphe·noi·dos·to·my
sphe·noi·dot·o·my
sphe·no·ma·lar
sphe·no·max·il·lary
sphe·no-oc·cip·i·tal
sphe·nop·a·gus
sphe·no·pal·a·tine
sphe·no·pa·ri·e·tal
sphe·no·pe·tro·sal
sphe·nor·bi·tal
sphe·no·sis
sphe·no·squa·mo·sal
sphe·no·tem·po·ral
sphe·not·ic

sphe·no·tribe
sphe·no·trip·sy
sphe·no·tur·bi·nal
sphe·no·vo·mer·ine
sphe·no·zy·go·mat·ic
sphere
   attraction s.
   conflict-free ego s.
   embryotic s.
   Morgagni's s.
   Mule vitreous s.
   neurosecretory s.
   segmentation s.
   vitelline s.
   yolk s.
sphe·res·the·sia
spher·i·cal
sphe·ro·cyl·in·der
sphe·ro·cyte
sphe·ro·cyt·ic
sphe·ro·cy·to·sis
   hereditary s.
sphe·roid
sphe·roi·dal
sphe·roi·din
sphe·ro·lith
sphe·ro·ma
sphe·rom·e·ter
sphe·ro·pha·kia
Spher·oph·o·rous
sphe·ro·plast
sphe·ro·sper·mia
spher·ule
   s's of Fulci
   rod s.
spher·u·lin
sphinc·ter
   anatomic s.
   s. angularis
   s. ani
   artificial s.
   s. of bile duct
   s. of Boyden
   cardiac s.
   cardioesophageal s.
   choledochal s.
   s. of common bile duct
   cornual s.

sphinc·ter *(continued)*
    cricopharyngeal s.
    s. of duct of Wirsung
    duodenal s.
    external s. of anus
    s. of eye
    gastroesophageal s.
    Giordano's s.
    Glisson s.
    Henle's s.
    hepatic s.
    s. of hepatopancreatic
      ampulla
    Hyrtl's s.
    ileal s.
    inguinal s.
    internal s. of anus
    s. iridis
    laryngeal s.
    Lütkens' s.
    Nélaton's s.
    O'Beirne's s.
    s. oculi
    Oddi's s.
    s. oris
    ostial s.
    palatopharyngeal s.
    pancreatic s.
    pharyngoesophageal s.
    physiologic s.
    precapillary s.
    prepyloric s.
    s. pupillae
    pyloric s.
    rectal s.
    segmental s.
    smooth muscle s.
    striated muscle s.
    tubal s.
    s. urethrae
    s. vaginae
    s. vesicae
sphinc·ter·al
sphinc·ter·al·gia
sphinc·ter·ec·to·my
sphinc·ter·ic
sphinc·ter·is·mus
sphinc·ter·itis

sphinc·ter·ol·y·sis
sphinc·tero·plas·ty
sphinc·tero·scope
    Kelly's s.
sphinc·ter·os·co·py
sphinc·tero·tome
sphinc·ter·ot·o·my
    internal s.
sphin·ga·nine
sphin·go·ga·lac·to·side
sphin·go·gly·co·lip·id
sphin·goid
sphin·go·in
sphin·gol
sphin·go·lip·id
sphin·go·lip·i·do·ses
sphin·go·lip·i·do·sis
    cerebral s.
    late onset cerebral s.
sphin·go·lipo·dys·tro·phy
sphin·go·my·e·lin
sphin·go·my·e·lin·ase
sphin·go·my·eli·no·sis
sphin·go·my·e·lin phos·pho·
    di·es·ter·ase
sphin·go·phos·pho·lip·id
sphin·go·sine
sphyg·mic
sphyg·mo·bo·lo·gram
sphyg·mo·bo·lom·e·ter
sphyg·mo·bo·lom·e·try
sphyg·mo·car·dio·gram
sphyg·mo·car·dio·graph
sphyg·mo·car·dio·scope
sphyg·mo·chro·no·graph
sphyg·mo·chro·nog·ra·phy
sphyg·mo·dy·na·mom·e·ter
sphyg·mo·gen·in
sphyg·mo·gram
sphyg·mo·graph
sphyg·mo·graph·ic
sphyg·mog·ra·phy
    jugular pulse s.
sphyg·moid
sphyg·mol·o·gy
sphyg·mo·ma·nom·e·ter
sphyg·mo·ma·nom·e·try
sphyg·mom·e·ter

sphyg·mo·met·ro·graph
sphyg·mo·met·ro·scope
sphyg·mo-os·cil·lom·e·ter
sphyg·mo·pal·pa·tion
sphyg·mo·phone
sphyg·mo·ple·thys·mo·graph
sphyg·mo·scope
    Bishop's s.
sphyg·mos·co·py
sphyg·mo·sys·to·le
sphyg·mo·to·nom·e·ter
sphyg·mo·vis·co·sim·e·try
sphyg·mus
sphy·rec·to·my
sphy·rot·o·my
spi·ca
spic·u·lar
spic·ule
    cemental s.
spic·u·lum *pl.* spic·u·la
spi·der
    arterial s.
    banana s.
    black widow s.
    brown recluse s.
    cat-headed s.
    comb-footed s.
    European wolf s.
    funnel-web s.
    jointed s.
    lynx s.
    tree funnel-web s.
    vascular s.
    wandering s.
    wolf s.
spi·der burst
Spie·gel·berg's criterion
Spie·ghel's line
Spie·gler's reagent
Spie·gler's test
Spie·gler-Fendt sarcoid
Spiel·mey·er-Vogt disease
spi·ge·li·an
Spi·ge·li·us line
spike
    cemental s.
    fever s.
    focal s's

spike *(continued)*
    M s.
    multiple s's
    physiologic occipital s's
    slow s.
spike·nard
    American s.
spik·ing
Spi·lan·thes
    cellular s.
Spil·ler syndrome
spill·way
    occlusal s.
spi·lus
spi·na *pl.* spi·nae
    s. angularis
    s. bifida
    s. bifida anterior
    s. bifida aperta
    s. bifida cystica
    s. bifida manifesta
    s. bifida occulta
    s. bifida posterior
    s. frontalis
    s. helicis
    s. iliaca anterior inferior
    s. iliaca anterior superior
    s. iliaca posterior inferior
    s. iliaca posterior superior
    s. intercondyloidea
    s. ischiadica
    s. ischialis
    s. meatus
    s. mentalis
    s. nasalis anterior maxillae
    s. nasalis ossis frontalis
    s. nasalis ossis palatini
    s. nasalis posterior ossis
     palatini
    s. ossis sphenoidalis
    spinae palatinae
    s. scapulae
    s. suprameatalis
    s. suprameatica
    s. tibiae
    s. trochlearis
    s. tympanica major

spi·na *(continued)*
    s. tympanica minor
    s. ventosa
spi·nal
spi·nal·gia
    Petruschky's s.
spi·na·lis
spi·nant
spi·nate
spin·dle
    aortic s.
    Axenfeld-Krukenberg s.
    Bütschli's nuclear s.
    central s.
    cleavage s.
    complex muscle s.
    enamel s's
    His' s.
    intermediate muscle s.
    Krukenberg's s.
    Kühne's s.
    mitotic s.
    monofibral s.
    muscle s.
    neuromuscular s.
    neurotendinal s.
    nuclear s.
    simple muscle s.
    sleep s's
    tandem s.
    tendon s.
    tigroid s's
    urine s's
spine
    alar s.
    angular s.
    anterior inferior iliac s.
    anterior superior iliac s.
    bamboo s.
    basilar s.
    cervical s.
    Civinini's s.
    cleft s.
    dendritic s.
    dorsal s.
    ethmoidal s. of Macalister
    frontal s., external

spine *(continued)*
    s. of greater tubercle of
      humerus
    s. of helix
    hemal s.
    s. of Henle
    hysterical s.
    iliopectineal s.
    intercondyloid s.
    ischial s.
    s. of ischium
    jugular s.
    kissing s's
    s. of lesser tubercle of
      humerus
    lumbar s.
    lumbosacral s.
    s. of maxilla
    meatal s.
    mental s., external
    nasal s., anterior
    nasal s. of frontal bone
    nasal s. of palatine bone
    nasal s., posterior
    neural s.
    obturator s.
    occipital s., external
    occipital s., internal
    palatine s's
    peroneal s. of os calcis
    pharyngeal s.
    poker s.
    posterior inferior iliac s.
    posterior palatine s.
    posterior superior iliac s.
    s. of pubic bone
    s. of pubis
    railway s.
    rigid s.
    sacral s.
    s. of scapula
    sciatic s.
    s. of sphenoid bone
    sphenoidal s.
    s. of Spix
    suprameatal s.
    thoracic s.
    s. of tibia

spine *(continued)*
    tibial s.
    tibial s. of Macewen
    trochanteric s., greater
    trochanteric s., lesser
    trochlear s.
    tympanic s., anterior
    tympanic s., greater
    tympanic s., lesser
    tympanic s., posterior
    typhoid s.
    s. of vertebra
    vertebral s.
Spi·nel·li's operation
spini·form
spi·nif·u·gal
spi·nip·e·tal
spinn·bar·keit
spi·no·bul·bar
spi·no·cel·lu·lar
spi·no·cer·e·bel·lar
spi·no·cer·e·bel·lum
spi·no·col·lic·u·lar
spi·no·cor·ti·cal
spi·no·cos·tal·is
spi·no·gal·van·iza·tion
spi·no·gle·noid
spi·no·gram
spi·no·mus·cu·lar
spi·no·neu·ral
spi·nop·e·tal
spi·no·sal
spi·nose
spi·no·tec·tal
spi·no·trans·ver·sar·i·us
spi·nous
spin·thar·i·con
spin·thar·i·scope
spin·ther·ism
spin·ther·om·e·ter
spin·ther·o·pia
spin·tom·e·ter
spip·e·rone
spir. — L. spiritus (spirit)
spir·a·cle
spi·rad·e·no·ma
    cylindromatous s.
    eccrine s.

spi·ral
    Curschmann's s's
    Golgi-Rezzonico s.
    Herxheimer's s's
    Perroncito's s's
spir·a·my·cin
spi·reme
spi·ril·la
Spi·ril·la·ceae
spi·ril·le·mia
spi·ril·li·ci·dal
spi·ril·li·cide
spi·ril·lol·y·sis
spi·ril·lo·sis
spi·ril·lo·trop·ic
spi·ril·lot·ro·pism
Spi·ril·lum
    S. *minus*
spi·ril·lum *pl.* spi·ril·la
    s. of Finkler and Prior
    s. of Vincent
spir·it
    ammonia s., aromatic
    s. of ammonia, aromatic
    benzaldehyde s.
    camphor s.
    ether s.
    ether s., compound
    industrial mentholated s.
    mentholated s.
    s. of Mindererus
    s. of nitre
    orange s., compound
    peppermint s.
    proof s.
    rectified s.
    s. of sal volatile
    s. of turpentine
spir·i·tus
Spi·ro's test
Spi·ro·chae·ta
Spi·ro·chae·ta·ceae
Spi·ro·chae·ta·les
spi·ro·che·tal
spi·ro·chete
    Dutton's s.
spi·ro·che·te·mia

spi·ro·che·ti·ci·dal
spi·ro·che·ti·cide
spi·ro·che·tog·e·nous
spi·ro·che·to·ic
spi·ro·che·tol·y·sin
spi·ro·che·tol·y·sis
spi·ro·che·to·lyt·ic
spi·ro·che·to·sis
    s. arthritica
    bronchopulmonary s.
    s. icterohemorrhagica
    s. riverensis
spi·ro·che·tu·ria
spi·ro·gram
spi·ro·graph
spi·rog·ra·phy
spi·roid
spi·ro-in·dex
spi·ro·lac·tone
spi·ro·ma
spi·rom·e·ter
Spi·ro·met·ra
    S. erinaceieuropaei
    S. mansonoides
spi·ro·met·ric
spi·rom·e·try
    bronchoscopic s.
    incentive s.
spir·o·no·lac·tone
spi·ro·phore
spi·ro·scope
spi·ros·co·py
Spi·ru·roi·dea
spis·sat·ed
spis·si·tude
Spit·zer's theory
Spitz·ka's nucleus
Spitz·ka's tract
Spitz·ka-Lis·sau·er column
Spitz·ka-Lis·sau·er tract
splanch·nap·o·phys·e·al
splanch·na·poph·y·sis
splanch·nec·to·pia
splanch·nes·the·sia
splanch·nes·thet·ic
splanch·nic
splanch·ni·cec·to·my
    lumbodorsal s.

splanch·ni·cot·o·my
splanch·no·blast
splanch·no·cele
splanch·no·coele
splanch·no·cra·ni·um
splanch·no·derm
splanch·no·di·as·ta·sis
splanch·nog·ra·phy
splanch·no·lith
splanch·no·lo·gia
splanch·nol·o·gy
splanch·no·meg·a·lia
splanch·no·meg·a·ly
splanch·no·mic·ria
splanch·nop·a·thy
splanch·no·pleu·ral
splanch·no·pleure
splanch·nop·to·sis
splanch·no·scle·ro·sis
splanch·nos·co·py
splanch·no·skel·e·ton
splanch·no·so·mat·ic
splanch·not·o·my
splanch·no·tribe
splash
    gastric s.
    succussion s.
S-plasty
splay·foot
spleen
    accessory s.
    aguecake s.
    bacon s.
    cyanotic s.
    diffuse waxy s.
    enlarged s.
    flecked s. of Feitis
    floating s.
    Gandy-Gamna s.
    hard-baked s.
    lardaceous s.
    movable s.
    porphyry s.
    sago s.
    speckled s.
    wandering s.
    waxy s.
splen

splen
  s. accessorius
sple·nad·e·no·ma
sple·nal·gia
splen·at·ro·phy
sple·nauxe
splen·cer·a·to·sis
splen·cu·lus
sple·nec·ta·sis
sple·nec·to·mize
sple·nec·to·my
  subcapsular s.
sple·nec·to·pia
sple·nec·to·py
sple·nel·co·sis
sple·ne·mia
sple·nem·phrax·is
sple·ne·o·lus
sple·net·ic
sple·ni·al
splen·ic
splen·ic·ter·us
sple·nic·u·lus
splen·i·fi·ca·tion
splen·i·form
splen·in
splen·i·ser·rate
sple·ni·tis
  spodogenous s.
sple·ni·um
  s. corporis callosi
splen·iza·tion
  hypostatic s.
sple·no·blast
sple·no·cele
sple·no·cer·a·to·sis
sple·no·clei·sis
sple·no·col·ic
sple·no·cyte
sple·no·dyn·ia
sple·nog·e·nous
sple·no·gram
sple·no·gran·u·lo·ma·to·sis
  sid·er·ot·i·ca
sple·nog·ra·phy
sple·no·hep·a·to·me·ga·lia
sple·no·hep·a·to·meg·a·ly
sple·noid

sple·no·ker·a·to·sis
sple·no·lap·a·rot·o·my
sple·nol·o·gy
sple·no·lym·phat·ic
sple·nol·y·sin
sple·nol·y·sis
sple·no·ma *pl.* sple·no·mas,
  sple·no·mata
sple·no·ma·la·cia
sple·no·med·ul·lary
sple·no·me·ga·lia
sple·no·meg·a·ly
  chronic malarial s.
  congestive s.
  Egyptian s.
  febrile tropical s.
  Gaucher's s.
  hemolytic s.
  hypercholesterolemic s.
  infectious s.
  infective s.
  myelophthisic s.
  siderotic s.
  spodogenous s.
  thrombophlebitic s.
  tropical s.
sple·nom·e·try
sple·no·my·elog·e·nous
sple·no·my·elo·ma·la·cia
sple·non·cus
sple·no·neph·ric
sple·no·neph·rop·to·sis
sple·no·pan·cre·at·ic
sple·no·pa·rec·ta·sis
sple·nop·a·thy
sple·no·pexy
sple·no·phren·ic
sple·no·pneu·mo·nia
sple·no·por·tog·ra·phy
sple·nop·to·sia
sple·nop·to·sis
sple·no·re·nal
sple·no·re·no·pexy
sple·nor·rha·gia
sple·nor·rha·phy
sple·no·sis
sple·not·o·my
sple·no·tox·in

splen·ule
splen·u·lus *pl.* splen·u·li
sple·nun·cu·lus
splic·ing
    alternative s.
    gene-s.
    RNA s.
splint
    abutment s.
    acrylic resin bite-guard s.
    air s.
    airplane s.
    anchor s.
    Anderson s.
    Angle's s.
    Asch s.
    Balkan s.
    banjo traction s.
    bridge s.
    buddy s.
    Bunnell s's
    caliper s.
    cap s.
    cast bar s.
    cast cap s.
    Chandler felt collar s.
    Chatfield-Girdleston s.
    coaptation s's
    cockup s.
    continuous clasp s.
    Cramer's s.
    crib s.
    Denis Browne s.
    diodontic s.
    drop foot s.
    dynamic s.
    Essig-type s.
    fixed s.
    fixed partial denture s.
    fracture s.
    Frejka pillow s.
    Friedman s.
    functional s.
    Gilmer's s.
    Gunning's s.
    hayrake s.
    Hodgen s.
    interdental s.

splint *(continued)*
    Kanavel's cockup s.
    Keller-Blake s.
    Kingsley s.
    Kirschner wire s.
    labial s.
    ladder s.
    lingual s.
    Liston's s.
    live s.
    Morris external fixation s.
    nasal s.
    open cap s.
    opponens s.
    pillow s.
    plaster s.
    plastic s.
    poroplastic s.
    Porzett s.
    Roger Anderson s.
    shin s's
    Stader s.
    sugar-tong s.
    surgical s.
    talipes hobble s.
    Taylor s.
    therapeutic s.
    Thomas s.
    Thomas knee s.
    Tobruk s.
    Toronto s.
    traction s.
splin·ter
splint·ing
splints
    shin s.
split·ting
    fee s.
    s. of heart sounds
    sagittal s. of mandible
spo·dio·my·eli·tis
spo·dog·e·nous
spo·dog·ra·phy
spok·ing
    cortical s.
spon·dee
spon·dy·lal·gia
spon·dyl·ar·thri·tis

spon·dyl·ar·thri·tis
   s. ankylopoietica
spon·dyl·ar·throc·a·ce
spon·dyl·ex·ar·thro·sis
spon·dy·lit·ic
spon·dy·li·tis
   s. ankylopoietica
   s. ankylosans
   ankylosing s.
   Bekhterev's s.
   s. deformans
   hypertrophic s.
   s. infectiosa
   Kümmell's s.
   Marie-Strümpell s.
   muscular s.
   post-traumatic s.
   rheumatoid s.
   rhizomelic s.
   s. rhizomelica
   s. rhizomélique
   traumatic s.
   s. tuberculosa
   tuberculous s.
   s. typhosa
spon·dy·li·ze·ma
spon·dy·lo·ar·throp·a·thy
spon·dy·loc·a·ce
spon·dy·lod·e·sis
spon·dy·lo·di·dym·ia
spon·dy·lod·y·mus
spon·dy·lo·dyn·ia
spon·dy·lo·lis·the·sis
   congenital s.
   degenerative s.
   dysplastic s.
   isthmic s.
   pathological s.
   traumatic s.
spon·dy·lo·lis·thet·ic
spon·dy·lol·y·sis
spon·dy·lo·ma·la·cia
   s. traumatica
spon·dy·lop·a·thy
   traumatic s.
spon·dy·lop·to·sis
spon·dy·lo·py·o·sis
spon·dy·los·chi·sis

spon·dy·lo·sis
   cervical s.
   s. chronica ankylopoietica
   degenerative s.
   hyperostotic s.
   lumbar s.
   rhizomelic s.
   s. uncovertebralis
spon·dy·lo·syn·de·sis
spon·dy·lo·ther·a·py
spon·dy·lot·ic
spon·dy·lot·o·my
spon·dy·lous
spon·dy·lus
sponge
   Bernays's.
   Bunge s.
   fibrin s.
   gauze s.
   gelatin s.
   gelatin s., absorbable
   peanut s.
   sodium s.
   spermicidal s.
spon·gia
   s. gelatina absorbenda
spon·gi·form
spon·gi·itis
spon·gio·blast
spon·gio·blas·to·ma
   s. multiforme
   polar s.
   s. unipolare
spon·gio·cyte
spon·gio·cy·to·ma
spon·gi·oid
spon·gio·plasm
spon·gio·sa
spon·gio·sa·plas·ty
spon·gi·ose
spon·gi·o·sis
spon·gio·si·tis
spon·gi·ot·ic
spon·gy
spon·ta·ne·ous
Spon·tin
spool

spoon
    Daviel's s.
    sharp s.
    Volkmann's s.
spo·rad·ic
spor·a·din
spo·rad·o·neure
spo·ran·gia
spo·ran·gi·al
spo·ran·gio·phore
spo·ran·gio·spore
spo·ran·gi·um *pl.* spo·ran·gia
spo·ra·tion
spore
    asexual s.
    bacterial s.
    black s's of Ross
    swarm s.
spo·ri·ci·dal
spo·ri·cide
spo·ri·des·min
spo·rif·er·ous
spo·rip·a·rous
spo·ro·ag·glu·ti·na·tion
spo·ro·blast
spo·ro·cyst
spo·ro·duct
spo·ro·gen·e·sis
spo·ro·gen·ic
spo·rog·e·nous
spo·rog·e·ny
spo·rog·o·ny
spo·ront
spo·ro·phore
spo·ro·phyte
spo·ro·plasm
spo·ro·plas·mic
spo·ro·the·ca
Spo·ro·thrix
spo·rot·ri·chin
spo·ro·tri·cho·sis
spo·ro·tri·chot·ic
Spo·rot·ri·chum
Spo·ro·zoa
spo·ro·zoa
spo·ro·zo·an
Spo·ro·zo·ea
spo·ro·zo·ite

spo·ro·zo·oid
spo·ro·zo·on *pl.* spo·ro·zoa
spo·ro·zo·o·sis
sport
spor·u·lar
spor·u·la·tion
    endogenous s.
    exogenous s.
spor·ule
spot
    acoustic s's
    ash leaf s.
    Bitot's s's
    blind s.
    blind s., mental
    blue s.
    Brushfield's s's
    café au lait s's
    Campbell de Morgan s.
    Carleton's s's
    Cayenne pepper s's
    cherry-red s.
    Christopher's s's
    chromatin s.
    cold s.
    conjunctival s's
    cotton-wool s's
    cribriform s's
    deaf s.
    De Morgan's s's
    embryonic s.
    epigastric s.
    eye s.
    flame s's
    focal s.
    Fordyce's s's
    Forschheimer s's
    genital s.
    germinal s.
    gift s's
    hot s.
    hypnogenetic s.
    ink s's
    interpalpebral s.
    Koplik's s's
    lenticular s's
    light s.
    liver s.

spot *(continued)*
- Mariotte's s.
- Maurer's s's
- Maxwell's s.
- milk s's
- milky s's
- mongolian s.
- Mueller s's
- mulberry s.
- orange s.
- pain s's
- pelvic s's
- pink s.
- plague s's
- rose s's
- Roth's s's
- saccular s.
- sacral s.
- shin s's
- Smith-McGuckin s.
- Soemmering's s.
- soldier's s's
- spongy s.
- Stephen's s's
- Tardieu's s's
- Tay's s.
- temperature s's
- tendinous s's
- touch s.
- trigger s.
- Trousseau's s.
- typhoid s's
- Wagner's s.
- warm s's
- Willner s's
- yellow s.

spot·ting

sprain
- acromioclavicular s.
- deltoid s.
- rider's s.
- Schlatter's s.
- tibiofibular s.
- vertebral cervical s.

spray
- ether s.
- lysine pitressin s.
- needle s.

spray *(continued)*
- tyrothricin s.

spread
- electrotonic s.
- gene s.
- secondary s.

spread·er
- gutta-percha s.
- root canal filling s.

Spren·gel's deformity

spring
- auxiliary s.
- bow s.
- closed s.
- coil s.
- finger s.
- Kesling s.
- loop s.
- open s.
- paddle s.
- separating s.
- uprighting s.
- Weiss s's
- Z s.

sprout
- nodal s.
- syncytial s's

sprout·ing

sprue
- celiac s.
- collagenous s.
- non-tropical s.
- refractory s.
- tropical s.
- unclassified s.

sprue-form·er

Spt. — L. spiritus (spirit)

SPTA — spatial peak temporal average

Spu·ma·vi·ri·nae

spu·ma·vi·rus

spur
- calcaneal s.
- cementum s.
- enamel s.
- heel s.
- Morand's s.
- occipital s.

spur (continued)
    olecranon s.
    scleral s.
spu·ri·ous
Spur·ling sign
spur·ring
Spur·way syndrome
spu·tum
    s. aeroginosum
    albuminoid s.
    s. coctum
    s. crudum
    s. cruentum
    globular s.
    green s.
    icteric s.
    moss-agate s.
    mucoid s.
    nummular s.
    prune juice s.
    rusty s.
SQ — subcutaneous
squal·ene
squal·ene mono·oxy·gen·ase
squa·ma pl. squa·mae
    s. alveolaris
    frontal s.
    s. of frontal bone
    s. frontalis
    mental s., external
    occipital s.
    occipital s., superior
    s. occipitalis
    perpendicular s.
    temporal s.
    s. of temporal bone
    s. temporalis
squa·mate
squa·ma·ti·za·tion
squame
    s. of occipital bone
squa·mo·cel·lu·lar
squa·mo·fron·tal
squam·oid
squa·mo·man·dib·u·lar
squa·mo·mas·toid
squa·mo·oc·cip·i·tal
squa·mo·pa·ri·e·tal

squa·mo·pe·tro·sal
squa·mo·sa
squa·mo·sal
squa·mo·so·pa·ri·e·tal
squa·mo·sphe·noid
squa·mo·tem·po·ral
squa·mo·tym·pan·ic
squa·mous
squa·mo·zy·go·mat·ic
square
    Punnett s.
squat·ting
squeeze
    tussive s.
squill
    red s.
    white s.
squil·lit·ic
squint
    accommodative s.
    comitant s.
    concomitant s.
    convergent s.
    divergent s.
    upward and downward s.
Squire's sign
SR — stimulation ratio
sr — steradian
SRBC — sheep red blood cell
SRF — skin reactive factor
    somatotropin releasing
      factor
SRH — somatotropin-releasing-
hormone
SRIF — somatostatin
SRN — State Registered
Nurse (England and Wales)
sRNA — soluble ribonucleic
acid
SRS-A — slow reacting
substance of anaphylaxis
SRT — sedimentation rate
test
    speech reception threshold
SS — somatostatin
ss. — L. semis (one half)
Ssa·ban·e·jew-Frank
operation

SSD — source-skin distance
ssDNA — single-stranded
  DNA
ssRNA — single-stranded
  RNA
SSS — specific soluble
  substance
    sick sinus syndrome
s.s.s. — L. stratum super
  stratum (layer upon layer)
S.S.V. — L. sub signo veneni
  (under a poison label)
ST — stable toxin
    skin test
    standardized test
    survival time
St. — L. stent (let them stand)
    L. stet (let it stand)
sta·bi·late
sta·bile
    heat s.
sta·bi·lim·e·ter
sta·bil·i·ty
    denture s.
    dimensional s.
sta·bil·iza·tion
sta·bi·li·zer
    endodontic s.
sta·bilo·graph
sta·ble
stac·ca·to
sta·chy·drine
stach·y·ose
Stacke's operation
stac·tom·e·ter
Sta·der splint
Sta·de·ri·ni's nucleus
sta·di·um *pl.* sta·dia
    s. acmes
    s. augmenti
    s. caloris
    s. decrementi
    s. defervescentiae
    s. fluorescentiae
    s. frigoris
    s. incrementi
    s. invasionis
    s. sudoris

staff
    s. of Aesculapius
    attending s.
    closed s.
    consulting s.
    house s.
    s. of Wrisberg
Staf·ne's cavity
stage
    algid s.
    amphibolic s.
    anal s.
    bell s.
    cap s.
    cold s.
    defervescent s.
    developmental s.
    dictyotene s.
    emergent s. I
    eruptive s.
    exoerythrocytic s.
    expulsive s.
    s. of fervescence
    first s.
    first s. of labor
    fourth s.
    genital s.
    Gillespie s's of anesthesia
    Guedel s.
    hot s.
    imperfect s.
    incubative s.
    s. of invasion
    knäuel s.
    s's of labor
    latency s.
    mechanical s.
    microscope s.
    oral s.
    oral-sadistic s.
    perfect s.
    phallic s.
    placental s.
    preeruptive s.
    preerythrocytic s.
    premenstrual s.
    prodromal s.

stage *(continued)*
    prodromal s. of labor
    progestational s.
    proliferative s.
    pyretogenic s.
    pyrogenetic s.
    Ranke's s's
    rest s.
    resting s.
    ring s.
    rotation s. of labor
    second s.
    second s. of labor
    seral s.
    stepladder s.
    sweating s.
    Tanner s's
    Tanner developmental s's
      (I–V)
    third s.
    third s. of labor
    tissue s.
    transitional pulp s.
    trypanosome s.
    ugly duckling s.
    vegetative s.
stag·ing
    Greulich and Pyle bone age
      s.
    Marshall and Tanner
      pubertal s.
    pathological s. of
      lymphomas
    Rai s.
    TNM s.
Stäh·li's pigment line
Stahr's gland
stain
    Achucárro's s.
    acid s.
    acid-fast s.
    acid fuchsin s.
    acid phosphatase s.
    Albert's diphtheria s.
    alkaline phosphatase s.
    alum-carmine s.
    Alzheimer s.
    amido black B s.

stain *(continued)*
    amido schwartz s.
    aniline blue black s.
    Anthony capsule s.
    auramine-rhodamine s.
    azan s.
    basic s.
    basic fuchsin s.
    Benda's s.
    Bensley's neutral gentian
      orange G s.
    benzidine and nitro-
      prusside peroxidase s.
    Best's carmine s.
    Bielschowsky's s.
    Biondi-Heidenhain s.
    Bowie s.
    Bunge-Trantenroth s.
    carbol-aniline fuchsin s.
    carbolfuchsin s.
    carbol-gentian violet s.
    Castaneda's s.
    certified s.
    chloracetate esterase s.
    Ciaccio's s.
    Commission Certified s.
    Congo red s.
    contrast s.
    Coomassie blue s.
    counter s.
    cytochemical s.
    Davenport's s.
    Dieterle's s.
    differential s.
    double s.
    Ehrlich's neutral s.
    Ehrlich's triacid s.
    elastica-van Gieson s.
    elastic fibers s.
    electron s's
    electron dense s.
    fluorescent s.
    fluorochrome s.
    Fontana's s.
    Fontana-Masson s.
    Giemsa s.
    Giemsa-Wright s.
    Gimenez s.

stain *(continued)*

gold chloride s.
Gomori's s's
Gomori-Takamatsu s's
Gomori-Wheatley s.
Gomori methenamine
  silver nitrate s.
Goodpasture's s.
Gram's s.
green s.
Gridley s.
Grocott-Gomori
  methenamine-silver
  nitrate s.
Grübler s.
Guenther s.
Gutstein s.
Hale's iron s.
heavy-metal s.
Heidenhain's iron
  hematoxylin s.
hemalum s.
hematoxylin-eosin s.
Hiss capsule s.
histochemical s.
immunofluorescent s.
immunoperoxidase s.
India ink s.
India ink capsule s.
intravital s.
iron s.
Kinyoun s.
Kinyoun carbolfuchsin s.
Kleihauer-Betke s.
lactophenol cotton blue s.
Laidlaw s.
Leder s.
Leifson flagella s.
Leishman's s.
Lendrum's inclusion body
  s.
leukocyte alkaline
  phosphatase s.
lipoid s.
lithium-carmine s.
Löffler's alkaline
  methylene blue s.
Lorrain Smith s.

stain *(continued)*

Luxol fast blue s.
Macchiavellos s.
Mallory's acid fuchsin,
  orange G, and aniline
  blue s.
Mallory's phloxine–
  methylene blue s.
Mallory's phosphotungstic
  acid–hematoxylin s.
Mallory's triple s.
Mallory-Azan s.
Mann's s.
Masson s.
Masson's trichrome s.
Maximow's s.
May-Grünwald s.
May's spore s.
Mayer mucicarmine s.
meconium s.
metachromatic s.
methyl green-pyronine s.
methyl violet s.
Michaelis's.
Milligan's trichrome s.
MSB (Martius yellow,
  scarlet and blue) s.
multiple s.
naphthol blue black s.
negative s.
neutral s.
Nissl s.
nonspecific esterase s.
nuclear s.
Orth s.
Pal's modification of
  Weigert's myelin sheath
  s.
Paltauf s.
Papanicolaou's s.
Pappenheim's s.
PAS s.
periodic acid–Schiff (PAS)
  s.
Perls' s.
peroxidase s.
phloxine-methylene blue s.

stain *(continued)*
    phosphotungstic
        acid–hematoxylin s.
    plasmatic s.
    plasmic s.
    Ponceau S s.
    Ponder-Kinyoun s.
    port-wine s.
    potassium hydroxide s.
    progressive s.
    protoplasmic s.
    Prussian blue s.
    PTAH (phosphotungstic
        acid-hematoxylin s.
    Ranson's pyridine silver s.
    resorcin-fuchsin s.
    Rinehart and Abul-Haj s.
    Romanovsky's
        (Romanowsky's) s.
    Schiff's s.
    selective s.
    Seller's s.
    simple s.
    Smith s.
    Sternheimer-Malbin s.
    substantive s.
    successive s.
    Sudan black B fat s.
    supravital s.
    tartrate-resistant acid
        phosphatase s.
    tetrachrome s.
    toluidine blue s.
    trichrome s.
    triple s.
    Truant auramine-
        rhodamine s.
    tumor s.
    Unna s.
    Unna-Pappenheim s.
    Unna's alkaline methylene
        blue
    van Gieson s.
    Verhoeff's s.
    Verhoeff-van Gieson s.
    vital s.
    von Kossa's s.
    Warthin-Starry silver s.

stain *(continued)*
    Wayson s.
    Weigert's fibrin s.
    Weigert's iron hematoxylin
        s.
    Weigert's neuroglia fiber s.
    Weigert's resorcin-fuchsin
        s.
    Weil's s.
    Wirtz-Conklin spore s.
    Wright's s.
    Ziehl-Neelsen s.
stain·ing
    bipolar s.
    differential s.
    double s.
    fluorescent s.
    intravital s.
    multiple s.
    negative s.
    polar s.
    postvital s.
    preagonal s.
    relief s.
    simple s.
    substantive s.
    supravital s.
    telomeric s.
    terminal s.
    triple s.
    vital s.
stair·case phe·nom·e·non
stal·ag·mom·e·ter
sta·lag·mon
stal·ing
stalk
    allantoic s.
    body s.
    cerebellar s.
    connecting s.
    embryonic s.
    s. of the epiglottis
    hypophysial s.
    infundibular s.
    mesangial s.
    neural s.
    optic s.
    pineal s.

stalk *(continued)*
    pituitary s.
    s. of Rathke's pouch
    s's of thalamus
    yolk s.
stal·li·my·cin hy·dro·chlo·ride
stal·tic
sta·men
Sta·mey's procedure
Sta·mey's test
stam·i·na
stam·mer
stam·mer·ing
Stam·no·so·ma
stan·dard
    Aub-Dubois s's
    Dubois s.
    Harris and Benedict s.
    international biological s.
    nylic s.
    Pignet's s.
    radioactive s.
    reference s.
stan·dard·iza·tion
    biologic s.
    direct s.
    indirect s.
    physiologic s.
stan·dard·ize
stand·by
stand·ing
    reflex s.
stand·still
    atrial s.
    auricular s.
    cardiac s.
    respiratory s.
    sinus s.
    ventricular s.
Stan·ford-Bi·net test
Stan·ley bacillus
Stan·ley Kent
stan·nate
stan·nic
    s. chloride
stan·nif·er·ous
Stan·ni·us ligature

stan·no·sis
stan·nous
stan·num
stan·o·lone
stan·o·zo·lol
Stan·ton's disease
sta·pe·dec·to·my
    partial s.
sta·pe·di·al
sta·pe·di·ol·y·sis
sta·pe·dio·plas·ty
sta·pe·dio·te·not·o·my
sta·pe·dio·ves·tib·u·lar
sta·pes
Staph·cil·lin
staph·i·sa·gria
staph·i·sa·grine
staph·y·la·gra
staph·y·lec·to·my
staph·yl·ede·ma
staph·y·line
staph·y·lin·id
Staph·y·lin·i·dae
staph·y·li·nus
sta·phyl·i·on
staph·y·li·tis
staph·y·lo·an·gi·na
staph·y·lo·co·ag·u·lase
staph·y·lo·coc·cal
staph·y·lo·coc·ce·mia
staph·y·lo·coc·ci
staph·y·lo·coc·cic
staph·y·lo·coc·cin
staph·y·lo·coc·col·y·sin
staph·y·lo·coc·co·sis
Staph·y·lo·coc·cus
    S. albus
    S. aureus
    S. epidermidis
    S. haemolyticus
    S. hominis
    S. pyogenes
    S. saprophyticus
    S. simulans
staph·y·lo·coc·cus *pl.* staph·y·lo·coc·ci
staph·y·lo·der·ma
staph·y·lo·di·al·y·sis

staph·y·lo·ede·ma
staph·y·lo·he·mia
staph·y·lo·he·mol·y·sin
staph·y·lo·ki·nase
staph·y·lo·leu·ko·ci·din
staph·y·lol·y·sin
    α s.
    alpha s.
    β s.
    beta s.
    δ s.
    delta s.
    ε s.
    epsilon s.
    γ s.
    gamma s.
staph·y·lo·ma
    annular s.
    anterior s.
    ciliary s.
    s. corneae
    s. corneae racemosum
    corneal s.
    equatorial s.
    intercalary s.
    posterior s.
    s. posticum
    projecting s.
    retinal s.
    Scarpa's s.
    scleral s.
    uveal s.
staph·y·lom·a·tous
staph·y·lon·cus
staph·y·lo·phar·yn·gor·rha·phy
staph·y·lo·plas·ty
staph·y·lop·to·sia
staph·y·lop·to·sis
staph·y·lor·rha·phy
staph·y·los·chi·sis
staph·y·lo·tome
staph·y·lot·o·my
staph·y·lo·tox·in
stap·ling
    gastric s.
star
    daughter s.

star *(continued)*
    dental s.
    lens s's
    macular s.
    mother s.
    polar s's
    s's of Verheyen
    Winslow's s's
starch
    cassava s.
    corn s.
    s. glycerite
    pregelatinized s.
    sago s.
    soluble s.
stare
    postbasic s.
Star·ling's hypothesis
Star·ling's law
Starr-Ed·wards value
star·ry-sky pat·tern
start·er
star·va·tion
    salt s.
stas·i·mor·phia
stas·i·mor·phy
sta·sis
    ileal s.
    intestinal s.
    papillary s.
    pressure s.
    urinary s.
    venous s.
Stas-Ot·to method
stat. — L. statim
  (immediately)
state
    absent s.
    acute confusional s.
    alcoholic paranoid s.
    alpha s.
    altered s's of consciousness
    anelectrotonic s.
    aneuploid s.
    anxiety s.
    anxiety tension s. (A.T.S.)
    borderline s.
    carrier s.

state *(continued)*
  catelectrotonic s.
  central excitatory s.
  central inhibitory s.
  compulsive s.
  convulsive s.
  correlated s.
  D s.
  delta s.
  dreamy s.
  entatic s.
  epileptic s.
  epileptic clouded s.
  epileptic twilight s.
  euploid s.
  excited s.
  Ganser s.
  ground s.
  haploid s.
  hypnagogic s.
  hypnoid s.
  hypnopompic s.
  lacunar s.
  local excitatory s.
  marble s.
  metastable s.
  obsessive-ruminative s.
  oxidation s.
  persistent vegetative s.
  plastic s.
  pluripotent s.
  postepileptic s.
  refractory s.
  resting s.
  singlet s.
  split-brain s.
  steady s.
  subscurvy s.
  triplet s.
  twilight s.
  vegetative s.
state·ment
  antemortem s.
  uncertainty s.
stath·mo·ki·ne·sis
stat·ic
stat·ics
sta·tim

sta·tion
  anterior s.
  s. of fetus
  olfactory s. of Broca
  posterior s.
  Romberg s.
sta·tion·ary
sta·tis·tic
  kappa s.
sta·tis·tics
  bayesian s.
  Bose-Einstein s.
  distribution-free s.
  Fermi-Dirac s.
  health s.
  medical s.
  nonparametric s.
  vital s.
stato·acous·tic
stato·co·nia
stato·co·ni·um *pl.* stato·co·nia
stato·cyst
stato·ki·net·ic
stato·ki·net·ics
stato·lith
stat·o·lon
sta·tom·e·ter
stato·re·cep·tor
stat·u·ral
sta·ture
sta·tus
  absence s.
  s. anginosus
  s. arthriticus
  s. asthmaticus
  s. calcifames
  s. choreicus
  s. convulsivus
  s. cribalis
  s. cribrosus
  s. criticus
  s. degenerativus
  s. dysgraphicus
  s. dysmyelinatus
  s. dysmyelinisatus
  s. dysraphicus
  s. epilepticus

sta·tus *(continued)*
  s. fibrosus
  focal s.
  s. hemicranicus
  Karnofsky s.
  s. lacunaris
  s. lacunosus
  s. lymphaticus
  s. macrobioticus
    multiparus
  s. marmoratus
  mental s.
  myoclonic s.
  nutrition s.
  petit mal s.
  s. praesens
  psychomotor s.
  s. raptus
  s. spongiosus
  s. thymicolymphaticus
  s. thymicus
  s. verrucosus
  s. vertiginosus
Staub-Trau·gott effect
Staub-Trau·gott test
stau·ri·on
stau·ro·co·nid·i·um *pl.* stau·
  ro·co·nid·ia
stau·ro·ple·gia
stau·ro·spore
staves·acre
stax·is
stay
  s. of white line
STD — sexually transmitted
  disease
    skin test dose
    standard test dose
steal
    extracranial s.
    intracerebral s.
    subclavian s.
    vascular s.
ste·a·ral·de·hyde
ste·a·rate
ste·a·ric acid
ste·ar·i·form
ste·a·rin

ste·a·rop·ten
stearo·yl-CoA de·sat·u·rase
ste·ar·rhea
ste·a·tad·e·no·ma
ste·a·tite
ste·a·ti·tis
ste·ato·cele
ste·a·to·cys·to·ma
  s. multiplex
ste·a·tog·e·nous
ste·a·tol·y·sis
ste·a·to·lyt·ic
ste·a·to·ma *pl.* ste·a·to·ma·
  ta, ste·a·to·mas
ste·a·to·ma·to·sis
ste·a·tom·a·tous
ste·a·tom·ery
ste·a·to·ne·cro·sis
ste·a·to·pyg·ia
ste·a·top·y·gous
ste·a·tor·rhea
  congenital pancreatic s.
  familial s.
  idiopathic s.
ste·a·to·sis
  s. cardiaca
  s. cordis
stech·i·ol·o·gy
stech·i·om·e·try
Stec·lin
Steele-Ri·chard·son-Ols·zew·
  ski syndrome
Steell's murmur
Steen·bock unit
stee·ple sign
stef·fi·my·cin
steg·no·sis
steg·not·ic
Steg·o·my·ia
Stei·dele's complex
Stein's test
Stein-Lev·en·thal syndrome
Stein·brinck's anomaly
Steindler operation
Stei·ner's tumors
Stein·mann's pin
stein·strasse
Stel·a·zine

stel·la *pl.* stel·lae
    s. lentis hyaloidea
    s. lentis iridica
stel·late
stel·lec·to·my
Stel·lite
stel·lu·la *pl.* stel·lu·lae
    stellulae vasculosae
      winslowii
    stellulae of Verheyen
    stellulae verheyenii
Stell·wag's sign
Stell·wag's symptom
stem
    brain s.
    infundibular s.
Sten·der dish
Stene·di·ol
sten·i·on *pl.* sten·ia
Ste·no
steno·breg·mat·ic
steno·car·dia
steno·ce·pha·lia
steno·ceph·a·lous
steno·ceph·a·ly
steno·cho·ria
steno·co·ri·a·sis
steno·cro·ta·phia
steno·crot·a·phy
steno·pe·ic
ste·no·sal
ste·nose
ste·nosed
ste·no·sis
    adult pyloric s.
    aortic s.
    aortic valve s.
    aqueduct s.
    arterial s.
    bronchial s.
    buttonhole mitral s.
    calcified aortic s.
    caroticovertebral s.
    carotid s.
    choanal s.
    cicatricial s.
    congenital aortic s.

ste·no·sis *(continued)*
    congenital hypertrophic
      pyloric s.
    coronary s.
    coronary ostial s.
    critical s.
    cystic duct s.
    fishmouth mitral s.
    granulation s.
    hypertrophic pyloric s.
    idiopathic hypertrophic
      subaortic s.
    infundibular s.
    infundibular pulmonary s.
    laryngeal s.
    lumbar canal s.
    mitral s.
    muscular subaortic s.
    muscular subvalvular s.
    myocardial infundibular s.
    nasal s.
    postdiphtheritic s.
    posterior s. of urethra
    post-tracheostomy s.
    pulmonary s.
    pulmonary artery s.
    pulmonary valve s.
    pyloric s.
    renal artery s.
    spinal s.
    subaortic s.
    subvalvular aortic s.
    supravalvular s.
    tracheal s.
    tricuspid s.
    valvular s.
    vertebral s.
steno·sto·mia
steno·ther·mal
steno·ther·mic
steno·tho·rax
ste·not·ic
ste·nox·e·nous
Sten·sen's canal
Sten·sen's duct
Sten·sen's experiment
Sten·sen's foramen
Sten·sen's plexus

stent
step
    rate-controlling s.
    rate-determining s.
    rate-limiting s.
    Rönne's nasal s.
ste·pha·ni·al
ste·pha·ni·on
Steph·a·no·fi·lar·ia
    S. stilesi
steph·a·no·fi·la·ri·a·sis
Steph·a·nu·rus
    S. dentatus
Ste·phen·son's wave
step·ping
    air s.
ste·ra·di·an
Ster·ane
ster·co·bi·lin
ster·co·bi·lin·o·gen
ster·co·lith
ster·co·ra·ceous
ster·co·ral
ster·co·rar·ia
ster·co·rar·i·an
ster·co·rin
ster·co·ro·lith
ster·co·ro·ma
ster·co·rous
Ster·cu·lia
ster·cus *pl.* ster·co·ra
stere
ster·eo·ag·no·sis
ster·eo·an·es·the·sia
ster·eo·ar·throl·y·sis
ster·eo·aus·cul·ta·tion
ster·eo·blas·tu·la
ster·eo·cam·pim·e·ter
ster·eo·chem·i·cal
ster·eo·chem·is·try
ster·eo·cil·i·um *pl.* ster·eo·
    cil·ia
ster·eo·cine·flu·o·rog·ra·phy
ster·eo·cog·no·sy
ster·eo·col·po·gram
ster·eo·col·po·scope
ster·eo·en·ceph·a·lo·tome
ster·éo·en·ceph·a·lot·o·my

ster·eo·flu·o·ros·co·py
ster·e·og·no·sis
ster·e·og·nos·tic
ster·eo·gram
ster·eo·graph
ster·eo·iso·mer
ster·eo·iso·mer·ic
ster·eo·isom·er·ism
ster·e·ol·o·gy
ster·e·om·e·ter
ster·e·om·e·try
ster·eo·mono·scope
ster·eo·phan·to·scope
ster·eo-oph·thal·mo·scope
Ster·eo-or·thop·ter
ster·eo·pho·rom·e·ter
ster·eo·phoro·scope
ster·eo·pho·to·mi·cro·graph
ster·eo·plasm
ster·e·op·sis
ster·eo·ra·di·og·ra·phy
ster·eo·roent·gen·og·ra·phy
ster·eo·roent·gen·om·e·try
ster·eo·sal·pin·gog·ra·phy
ster·eo·scope
ster·eo·scop·ic
ster·e·os·co·py
ster·eo·ski·ag·ra·phy
ster·eo·spe·cif·ic
ster·eo·spe·ci·fic·i·ty
ster·eo·stro·bo·scope
ster·eo·tac·tic
ster·eo·tax·ic
ster·eo·tax·is
ster·eo·taxy
ster·eo·trop·ic
ster·e·ot·ro·pism
ster·eo·ty·py
ste·ric
ste·rig·ma *pl.* ste·rig·ma·ta
ster·i·lant
ster·ile
ster·ile·ly
ste·ril·i·ty
    absolute s.
    aspermatogenic s.
    dyspermatogenic s.
    female s.

ste·ril·i·ty *(continued)*
    male s.
    normospermatogenic s.
    one-child s.
    partial s.
    primary s.
    relative s.
    secondary s.
    two-child s.
ster·i·li·za·tion
    eugenic s.
    fractional s.
    intermittent s.
    tubal s.
ster·i·lize
ster·i·liz·er
    steam s.
Ster·i·sil
Stern's position
ster·nad
ster·nal
ster·nal·gia
ster·na·lis
Stern·berg's disease
Stern·berg's giant cells
Stern·berg-Reed cells
ster·ne·bra *pl.* ster·ne·brae
Ster·nee·dle
ster·nen
ster·no·cla·vic·u·lar
ster·no·cla·vic·u·la·ris
ster·no·clei·dal
ster·no·clei·do·mas·toid
ster·no·cor·a·coid
ster·no·cos·tal
ster·no·cos·ta·lis
ster·no·dym·ia
ster·nod·y·mus
ster·no·dyn·ia
ster·no·go·ni·om·e·ter
ster·no·hy·oid
ster·no·hy·oi·de·us azy·gos
ster·noid
ster·no·mas·toid
ster·no-om·pha·lop·a·gus
ster·no·pa·gia
ster·nop·a·gus
ster·no·peri·car·di·al

ster·no·scap·u·lar
ster·nos·chi·sis
ster·no·thy·re·oi·de·us
ster·no·thy·roid
ster·not·o·my
    median s.
ster·no·tra·che·al
ster·no·try·pe·sis
ster·no·ver·te·bral
ster·no·xi·phoid
ster·no·xi·phop·a·gus
ster·num
    s. bifidum
    cleft s.
ster·nu·ta·tion
ster·nu·ta·tor
ster·nu·ta·to·ry
stern·zel·len
ste·roid
    adrenocortical s.
    anabolic s.
    s. monooxygenase
ste·roid 11β-mono·oxy·gen·ase
ste·roid 17α-mono·oxy·gen·ase
ste·roid 21-mono·oxy·gen·ase
ste·roi·do·gen·e·sis
ste·roi·do·gen·ic
ste·roid 5α-re·duc·tase
ste·roid sul·fa·tase
ste·rol
ster·tor
    hen-cluck s.
ster·to·rous
ster·yl sul·fa·tase
steth·acous·tic
steth·al·gia
steth·emia
steth·en·do·scope
stetho·cyr·to·graph
steth·odyn·ia
stetho·go·ni·om·e·ter
stetho·graph
steth·og·ra·phy
stetho·kyr·to·graph
steth·om·e·ter
Stetho·my·ia

stetho·my·itis
stetho·my·o·si·tis
stetho·pa·ral·y·sis
stetho·phone
stetho·pho·nom·e·ter
stetho·poly·scope
stetho·scope
    binaural s.
    Cammann's s.
    DeLee-Hillis obstetric s.
    differential s.
    electronic s.
    esophageal s.
    Leff s.
stetho·scop·ic
steth·os·co·py
stetho·spasm
Ste·vens-John·son syndrome
Ste·wart-Holmes sign
Ste·wart-Mo·rel syndrome
Ste·wart-Treves syndrome
STH — somatotropic (growth)
  hormone
sthe·nia
sthen·ic
sthen·om·e·ter
sthen·om·e·try
stib·amine glu·co·side
stib·en·yl
stib·i·al·ism
stib·i·at·ed
stib·ine
stib·in·ic acids
stib·i·um
stib·o·cap·tate
stib·o·phen
sticho·chrome
stick
    sponge s.
Stick·er's disease
Stie·da's disease
Stie·da's fracture
Stie·da's process
Stier·lin's sign
Stier·lin's symptom
stiff·ness
    congenital spasmodic limb
    s.

stiff·ness (continued)
    neck s.
stig·ma pl. stig·mas, stig·ma·
ta
    s. of degeneracy
    follicular s.
    Giuffrida-Ruggieri s.
    Koplik s. of degeneration
    malpighian s's
    professional s's
    syphilitic s's
stig·mal
stig·mas·te·rol
stig·ma·ta
stig·mat·ic
stig·ma·tism
stig·ma·ti·za·tion
stig·ma·tom·e·ter
stil·al·gin
Stil·ba·ceae
stil·baz·i·um io·dide
stil·bene
stil·bes·trol
Stiles-Craw·ford effect
sti·let
sti·lette
Still's disease
Still-Chauf·fard syndrome
still·birth
still·born
Stil·ler's rib
stil·li·cid·i·um
    s. narium
    s. urinae
Stil·ling's canal
Stil·ling's column
Stil·ling's fibers
Stil·ling's fleece
Stil·ling's nucleus
Stil·ling syndrome
Stil·ling-Turk-Du·ane
    syndrome
stil·lin·gia
Stil·phos·trol
sti·lus pl. sti·li
stim·u·lant
    alcoholic s.
    central s.

stim·u·lant *(continued)*
   cerebral s.
   diffusable s.
   general s.
   local s.
   nervous s.
   respiratory s.
   spinal s.
   topical s.
   uterine s.
   vascular s.
   vasomotor s.
stim·u·late
stim·u·la·tion
   areal s.
   audio-visual-tactile s.
   biocular s.
   cerebellar s.
   direct s.
   faradic s.
   indirect s.
   intermittent photic s.
   magnetic s.
   nonspecific s.
   paradoxical s.
   paraspecific s.
   photic s.
   punctual s.
   transcutaneous electrical
      nerve s. (TENS)
stim·u·la·tor
   Bimler s.
   cerebellar s.
   dorsal column s.
   electronic s.
   human thyroid adenylate
      cyclase s's (HTACS)
   interdental s.
   long-acting thyroid s.
      (LATS)
   nerve s.
stim·u·li
stim·u·lon
stim·u·lus *pl.* stim·u·li
   adequate s.
   aversive s.
   chemical s.
   conditioned s.

stim·u·lus *(continued)*
   conditioning s.
   discriminative s.
   electric s.
   eliciting s.
   heterologous s.
   heterotopic s.
   homologous s.
   inadequate s.
   latent s.
   liminal s.
   manifest s.
   maximal s.
   mechanical s.
   minimal s.
   morphogenetic s.
   nomotopic s.
   reinforcing s.
   square wave s.
   subliminal s.
   subthreshold s.
   supraliminal s.
   supramaximal s.
   thermal s.
   threshold s.
   unconditioned s.
stim·u·lus-re·sponse (S-R)
sting
   Irukandji s.
Stint·zing's tables
stip·pling
   basophilic s. of
      erythrocytes
   epiphyseal s.
   gingival s.
   malarial s.
   Maurer's s.
   Schüffner's s.
Stir·ling's modification of
  Gram stain
sti·ro·fos
stir·pi·cul·tur·al
stir·pi·cul·ture
stir·rup
   Finochietto's s.
   swivel s.
stitch
   glover s.

sto·chas·tic
stock·i·net
stock·i·nette
stock·ings
    compression s.
    Jobst s.
    TED (thromboembolic
      disease) s.
stoe·chi·ol·o·gy
Stoerk's blennorrhea
stoi·chi·ol·o·gy
stoi·chio·met·ric
stoi·chi·om·e·try
stoke
Stokes' amputation
Stokes' collar
Stokes' expectorant
Stokes' law
Stokes' operation
Stokes' syndrome
Stokes-Ad·ams disease
Stokes-Ad·ams syndrome
Stok·vis' disease
Stok·vis' test
Stok·vis-Tal·ma syndrome
sto·ma pl. sto·mas, sto·ma·ta
sto·mac·a·ce
stom·ach
    aberrant umbilical s.
    bilocular s.
    cardiac s.
    cascade s.
    cup-and-spill s.
    dumping s.
    honeycomb s.
    hourglass s.
    leather bottle s.
    miniature s.
    Pavlov's s.
    physiologic hourglass s.
    powdered s.
    primitive s.
    sclerotic s.
    thoracic s.
    trifid s.
    upside-down s.
    waterfall s.
    water-trap s.

stom·ach·ache
stom·a·chal
stom·a·chal·gia
sto·mach·ic
stom·a·cho·dyn·ia
sto·ma·de·um
sto·mal
sto·mal·gia
sto·ma·ta
sto·ma·tal
sto·ma·tal·gia
sto·mat·ic
sto·ma·tit·i·des
sto·ma·ti·tis pl. sto·ma·tit·i·des
    acute necrotizing s.
    allergic s.
    angular s.
    aphthobullous s.
    s. aphthosa
    aphthous s.
    s. arsenicalis
    bismuth s.
    catarrhal s.
    contact s.
    denture s.
    epidemic s.
    epizootic s.
    erythematopultaceous s.
    s. exanthematica
    fusospirochetal s.
    gangrenous s.
    gonococcal s.
    gonorrheal s.
    herpetic s.
    infectious s.
    s. intertropica
    lead s.
    s. medicamentosa
    membranous s.
    mercurial s.
    mycotic s.
    s. nicotina
    nonspecific s.
    s. prosthetica
    recurrent aphthous s.
    s. scarlatina
    s. scorbutica

sto·ma·ti·tis *(continued)*
  syphilitic s.
  traumatic s.
  tropical s.
  ulcerative s.
  ulcerative s. of sheep
  uremic s.
  s. venenata
  vesicular s.
  Vincent's s.
sto·ma·toc·a·ce
sto·ma·to·cyte
sto·ma·to·cy·to·sis
sto·ma·to·dyn·ia
sto·ma·to·dys·o·dia
sto·ma·to·gen·e·sis
sto·ma·to·glos·si·tis
sto·ma·tog·nath·ic
sto·ma·tog·ra·phy
sto·ma·to·la·lia
sto·ma·to·log·i·cal
sto·ma·tol·o·gist
sto·ma·tol·o·gy
sto·ma·to·ma·la·cia
sto·ma·to·me·nia
sto·mat·o·my
sto·ma·to·my·co·sis
sto·ma·to·ne·cro·sis
sto·ma·to·no·ma
sto·ma·top·a·thy
sto·ma·to·plas·tic
sto·ma·to·plas·ty
sto·ma·tor·rha·gia
  s. gingivarum
sto·ma·tos·chi·sis
sto·ma·to·scope
sto·ma·tot·o·my
sto·ma·to·ty·phus
sto·men·ceph·a·lus
sto·mi·on
sto·mo·ceph·a·lus
sto·mo·de·al
sto·mo·de·um
sto·mos·chi·sis
Sto·mox·ys
stone
  artificial s.
  bladder s.

stone *(continued)*
  blue s.
  chalk s.
  dental s.
  diamond s.
  kidney s.
  lathe s.
  lung s.
  metabolic s.
  pulp s.
  salivary s.
  s.-searcher
  skin s's
  staghorn s.
  struvite s.
  tear s.
  urate s.
  ureteral s.
  vein s.
  wheel s.
  womb s.
Stook·ey's reflex
Stook·ey-Scarff operation
Stook·ey-Scarff shunt
stool
  bilious s.
  caddy s.
  fatty s.
  lienteric s.
  mucous s.
  pea soup s.
  pipe-stem s.
  rabbit s's
  ribbon s.
  rice-water s's
  sago-grain s.
  silver s.
  spinach s.
stool·ing
stop
  centric s.
  glottal s.
  occlusal s.
  short s.
sto·rax
sto·res·in·ol
stor·i·form

storm
  thyroid s.
  thyrotoxic s.
Storm van Leeu·wen chamber
Stox·il
STP — standard temperature
  and pressure
STPD — standard
  temperature and pressure,
  dry
stra·bis·mal
stra·bis·mic
stra·bis·mol·o·gy
stra·bis·mom·e·ter
stra·bis·mom·e·try
stra·bis·mus
  A s.
  absolute s.
  accommodative s.
  alternating s.
  bilateral s.
  binocular s.
  comitant s.
  concomitant s.
  constant s.
  convergent s.
  cyclic s.
  s. deorsum vergens
  divergent s.
  dynamic s.
  external s.
  incomitant s.
  intermittent s.
  internal s.
  kinetic s.
  latent s.
  manifest s.
  mechanical s.
  monocular s.
  monolateral s.
  muscular s.
  noncomitant s.
  nonconcomitant s.
  nonparalytic s.
  paralytic s.
  relative s.
  seesaw s.
  spasmodic s.

stra·bis·mus (continued)
  suppressed s.
  s. sursum vergens
  unilateral s.
  uniocular s.
  V s.
  vertical s.
stra·bom·e·ter
stra·bom·e·try
strabo·tome
stra·bot·o·my
Stra·chen's disease
Stra·chen's syndrome
Stra·chen-Scott syndrome
strah·len
strain
  cell s.
  congenic s.
  F^+ s.
  F^- s.
  heterologous s.
  Hfr s.
  high-jumper's s.
  homologous s.
  inbred s.
  isogenic s.
  left ventricular s.
  male s.
  neotype s.
  prime s.
  prototrophic s's
  recombinant inbred s.
  reference s.
  resistant s.
  right ventricular s.
  rough s.
  S s.
  smooth s.
  T-s.
  type s.
  vertebral cervical s.
  Vi s.
  wild-type s.
strain·er
strait
  pelvic s., inferior
  pelvic s., superior
strait·jack·et

stra·mo·ni·um
strand
  Billroth's s's
  lateral enamel s.
  plus s.
stran·gal·es·the·sia
stran·gle
stran·gu·lat·ed
stran·gu·la·tion
stran·gu·ria
stran·gu·ry
strap
  crib s.
  Montgomery s's
strap·ping
  Gibney's s.
Stras·bur·ger's cell plate
Strass·burg's test
Strass·man's phenomenon
stra·ta
strat·i·fi·ca·tion
strat·i·fied
strat·i·form
strat·i·gram
stra·tig·ra·phy
stra·tum *pl.* stra·ta
  s. adamantinum
  s. album
  s. basale
  s. cerebrale retinae
  cerebral s. of retina
  s. cinereum
  s. circulare
  s. compactum
  s. corneum unguis
  s. cutaneum
  s. cylindricum
  s. eboris
  s. fibrosum
  s. functionale
  s. ganglionare
  ganglionic s.
  s. gangliosum
  s. germinativum
  s. granulosum
  s. griseum
  s. intermedium
  s. interolivare lemnisci

stra·tum *(continued)*
  s. lacunosum
  s. lemnisci
  s. longitudinale externum
  s. longitudinale gastris
  s. longitudinale internum
  s. longitudinale ventriculi
  s. lucidum
  s. malpighii
  s. medium
  s. moleculare
  s. mucosum
  s. nervosum retinae
  s. neuroepitheliale retinae
  s. neuronorum piriformium
  s. nucleare externum
  s. nucleare internum
  s. nucleare medullae
    oblongatae
  s. opticum
  s. oriens
  s. osteogeneticum
  s. papillare
  pigmented s.
  s. pigmenti
  s. pigmentosum
  s. plexiforme cerebelli
  s. plexiforme externum
  s. plexiforme internum
  s. Purkinje
  s. pyramidale
  s. radiatum
  s. reticulare
  s. spinosum
  s. spongiosum
  s. subendotheliale
  s. submucosum
  submucous s.
  s. subserosum
  s. subvasculare
  s. supravasculare
  s. supravasculosum
  s. synoviale
  s. vasculare
  s. vasculosum
  s. zonale
Straus' phenomenon
Straus' reaction

Straus' test
Strauss' sign
streak
    angioid s's
    fatty s.
    germinal s.
    Knapp's s's
    medullary s.
    meningeal s.
    primitive s.
streak·ing
stream
    axial s.
    blood s.
    s. of consciousness
    electron s.
    hair s's
stream·ing
    cytoplasmic s.
    protoplasmic s.
streb·lo·mi·cro·dac·ty·ly
strength
    biting s.
    dioptric s.
    ego s.
    ionic s.
streph·eno·po·dia
streph·exo·po·dia
strepho·po·dia
strepho·sym·bo·lia
strep·i·tus
strepo·gen·in
strep·tam·ine
strep·ti·ce·mia
strep·ti·dine
strep·to·an·gi·na
strep·to·bac·il·li
Strep·to·bac·il·lus
    S. moniliformis
strep·to·bac·il·lus *pl.* strep·to·ba·cil·li
strep·to·bio·sa·mine
strep·to·cer·ci·a·sis
Strep·to·coc·ca·ceae
strep·to·coc·cal
strep·to·coc·ce·mia
strep·to·coc·ci
strep·to·coc·cic

strep·to·coc·ci·cide
strep·to·coc·col·y·sin
strep·to·coc·co·sis
Strep·to·coc·cus
    S. acidominimus
    S. agalactiae
    S. anaerobius
    S. anginosus
    S. avium
    S. bovis
    S. cremoris
    S. durans
    S. epidemicus
    S. equinus
    S. equisimilis
    S. erysipelatis
    S. faecalis
    S. faecium
    S. foetidus
    S. hemolyticus
    S. lacticus
    S. lactis
    S. lanceolatus
    S. liquefaciens
    S. mastitidis
    S. micros
    S. milleri
    S. mitis
    S. mutans
    S. pneumoniae
    S. pyogenes
    S. salivarius
    S. sanguis
    S. scarlatinae
    S. thermophilus
    S. uberis
    S. viridans
    S. zooepidemicus
strep·to·coc·cus *pl.* strep·to·coc·ci
    alpha s.
    anaerobic s.
    anhemolytic s.
    beta s.
    Fehleisen s.
    gamma s.
    green s.

strep·to·coc·cus *(continued)*
  group A, B, C (etc.)
    streptococci
  hemolytic s.
  indifferent s.
  s. MG
  viridans s.
strep·to·der·ma·ti·tis
strep·to·dor·nase
  streptokinase-s.
strep·to·du·o·cin
strep·to·gen·in
strep·to·he·mol·y·sin
strep·to·ki·nase
  s.-streptodornase
strep·to·leu·ko·cid·in
strep·to·ly·di·gin
strep·tol·y·sin
  s. O
  s. S
strep·to·mi·cro·dac·ty·ly
Strep·to·my·ces
  S. ambofaciens
  S. antibioticus
  S. aureofaciens
  S. griseolus
  S. hygroscopicus
  S. niveus
  S. nogalater
  S. noursei
  S. orientalis
  S. orchidaceus
  S. paraguayensis
  S. rimosus
  S. somaliensis
  S. spectabilis
  S. vinaceus
Strep·to·my·ce·ta·ceae
strep·to·my·cete
strep·to·my·cin
  s. hydrochloride
  s. sulfate
strep·to·my·co·sis
strep·to·ni·grin
strep·to·ni·vi·cin
strep·tose
strep·to·sep·ti·ce·mia
strep·to·thri·cin

Strep·to·thrix
strep·to·zo·cin
strep·to·zo·to·cin
stress
  g s.
  occlusal s.
  post-traumatic s.
stress-break·er
stretch·er
stretch·ing
  pulse s.
stria *pl.* striae
  acoustic striae
  striae albicantes
  s. albicantes gravidarum
  striae of Amici
  s. arcuate olivarum
  striae atrophicae
  auditory striae
  striae of Baillarger
  brown s.
  striae ciliares
  s. diagonalis (Broca)
  striae distensae
  s. fornicis
  s. of Gennari
  striae gravidarum
  habenular s.
  s. of Held
  s. intermedia trigoni
    olfactorii
  s. kaesbekhterevi
  Knapp's striae
  s. lancisii
  Langhans' s.
  lateral olfactory s.
  s. lateralis trigoni olfactorii
  Liesegang's striae
  mallear s. of tympanic
    membrane
  s. mallearis membranae
    tympani
  s. malleolaris membranae
    tympani
  medial olfactory s.
  s. medialis trigoni olfactorii
  striae medullares
  meningitic s.

stria *(continued)*
    s. of Monakow
    Nitabuch's s.
    striae olfactoriae
    olfactory striae
    olfactory s., intermediate
    s. parallelae
    s. of Piccolomini
    Retzius' parallel striae
    Rohr's s.
    Schreger's striae
    s. semicircularis
    s. spinosa
    s. tecta
    s. terminalis
    s. ventriculi tertii
    Wickham's striae
striae
stria·scope
stri·a·tal
stri·ate
stri·at·ed
stri·a·tion
    Baillarger s's
    basal s's
    s's of Frommann
    tabby cat s.
    tigroid s.
stri·a·to·ni·gral
stri·a·to·pal·li·dal
Stri·a·tran
stri·a·tum
stric·ture
    anal s.
    annular s.
    bridle s.
    cicatricial s.
    contractile s.
    esophageal s.
    false s.
    functional s.
    Hunner's s.
    hysterical s.
    impassable s.
    impermeable s.
    irritable s.
    linear s.
    organic s.

stric·ture *(continued)*
    permanent s.
    rectal s.
    recurrent s.
    ring s.
    spasmodic s.
    spastic s.
    string s.
    temporary s.
stric·tur·iza·tion
stric·turo·tome
stric·tur·ot·o·my
stri·dent
stri·dor
    congenital laryngeal s.
    expiratory s.
    inspiratory s.
    laryngeal s.
    s. serraticus
strid·u·lous
string-halt
strio·cel·lu·lar
strio·cer·e·bel·lar
strio·mo·tor
strio·mus·cu·lar
strio·ni·gral
strip
    abrasive s.
    amalgam s.
    lightning s.
    linen s.
    moving s.
    polishing s.
    separating s.
stripe
    s's of Baillarger
    s. of Gennari
    Hensen's s.
    s. of Kaes-Bekhterev
    Mees's s's
    s's of Retzius
    Vicq d'Azyr's s.
strip·per
    external s.
    internal s.
    thrombus s.
    vein s.

strip·ping
    s. of membranes
    s. of pleura
stro·bi·la *pl.* stro·bi·lae
strob·i·la·tion
stro·bile
strob·i·lo·cer·cus
stro·bi·loid
stro·bi·lus
stro·bo·scope
stro·bo·scop·ic
stro·bo·ster·eo·scope
Stro·gan·off's (Stro·gan·ov's) treatment
stroke
    apoplectic s.
    back s.
    cerebral s.
    completed s.
    effective s.
    heat s.
    lacunar s.
    light s.
    lightning s.
    paralytic s.
    progressive s.
    recovery s.
    sun s.
stroke-in-ev·o·lu·tion
stro·ma *pl.* stro·ma·ta
    s. of cornea
    erythrocyte s.
    s. ganglii
    s. glandulae thyroideae
    s. iridis
    s. of iris
    lymphatic s.
    s. ovarii
    s. of ovary
    Rollet's s.
    s. of thyroid gland
    vitreous s.
    s. vitreum
stro·mal
stro·mat·ic
stro·ma·tin
stro·ma·tog·e·nous
stro·ma·tol·y·sis

stro·ma·to·sis
Stro·mey·er's cephalhematocele
strom·uhr
Strong's bacillus
stron·gyle
stron·gy·li
stron·gy·li·a·sis
stron·gy·lid
Stron·gyl·i·dae
stron·gy·li·form
Stron·gy·loi·dea
Stron·gy·loi·des
    S. intestinalis
    S. papillosus
    S. stercoralis
stron·gy·loi·di·a·sis
stron·gy·loi·do·sis
stron·gy·lo·sis
Stron·gy·lus
stron·gy·lus *pl.* stron·gy·li
stron·ti·um
    s. 90
    radioactive s.
stron·ti·ure·sis
stron·ti·uret·ic
stro·phan·thi·din
stro·phan·thin
    G-s.
    s.-G
Stro·phan·thus
stropho·ceph·a·lus
stropho·ceph·a·ly
stropho·so·mia
stropho·so·mus
stroph·u·lus
    s. albidus
struc·tur·al
struc·ture
    antigenic s.
    β-s.
    covalent s.
    denture-supporting s's
    fine s.
    primary s.
    quaternary s.
    secondary s.
    tertiary s.

struc·ture *(continued)*
   toroid s.
strug·gle
   death s.
stru·ma
   s. aberranta
   s. baseos linguae
   s. calculosa
   cast iron s.
   s. colloides
   s. colloides cystica
   s. endothoracica
   s. fibrosa
   s. follicularis
   s. gelatinosa
   Hashimoto's s.
   s. hyperplastica
   ligneous s.
   s. lingualis
   s. lipomatodes aberrata
      renis
   s. lymphatica
   s. lymphomatosa
   s. maligna
   s. nodosa
   s. ovarii
   s. parenchymatosa
   retrosternal s.
   Riedel's s.
   substernal s.
   thymus s.
   s. vasculosa
stru·mec·to·my
   median s.
stru·mi·form
stru·mi·tis
stru·mous
Strüm·pell's disease
Strüm·pell's sign
Strüm·pell's type
Strüm·pell-Leich·ten·stern
   disease
Strüm·pell-Ma·rie disease
Strüm·pell-West·phal
   pseudosclerosis
Strun·sky's sign
Struth·ers' ligament
Struve's test

stru·vite
strych·nine
strych·nin·ism
strych·nin·iza·tion
strych·nino·ma·nia
strych·nism
Strych·nos
STS — serologic test syphilis
   Society of Thoracic
      Surgeons
STU — skin test unit
Stu·art-Bras syndrome
Stu·dent's t-test
study
   case-control s.
   cohort s.
   cross-sectional s.
   descriptive s.
   dynamic s's
   experimental s.
   gastrointestinal s.
   H reflex s.
   intervention s.
   longitudinal s.
   prospective s.
   retrospective s.
   technetium albumin
      (TECA) s.
stump
   conical s.
   ischial-bearing s.
stun
stunt
stupe
stu·pe·fa·cient
stu·pe·fac·tive
stu·por
   anergic s.
   benign s.
   Cairns s.
   catatonic s.
   depressive s.
   epileptic s.
   Kahlbaum's catatonic s.
   melancholic s.
   postconvulsive s.
   spike-wave s.
   s. vigilans

stu·por·ous
stupp
Sturge's disease
Sturge's syndrome
Sturge-Web·er syndrome
Sturge-Web·er-Di·mi·tri
  disease
Sturm's conoid
Sturm's interval
Sturm·dorf operation
stut·ter
stut·ter·ing
  labiochoreic s.
  urinary s.
sty·co·sis
stye *pl.* styes
  meibomian s.
  zeisian s.
sty·let
  endotracheal s.
  lacrimal s.
sty·li·form
sty·lis·cus
sty·lo·glos·sal
sty·lo·glos·sus
sty·lo·hy·al
sty·lo·hy·oid
sty·loid
sty·loid·itis
sty·lo·man·dib·u·lar
sty·lo·mas·toid
sty·lo·max·il·lary
sty·lo·my·loid
sty·lo·po·di·um
sty·lo·staph·y·line
sty·los·teo·phyte
sty·lo·stix·is
sty·lus
sty·ma·to·sis
sty·page
stype
styp·sis
styp·tic
  Binelli s.
  chemical s.
  mechanical s.
  vascular s.
Styp·ven

styr·a·mate
Sty·rax
sty·rax
sty·rene
sty·rol
sty·ro·lene
su. — L. sumat (let him take)
sub·ab·dom·i·nal
sub·ab·dom·i·no·peri·to·ne·
  al
sub·ac·e·tab·u·lar
sub·ac·e·tate
sub·ac·id
sub·a·cid·i·ty
sub·acro·mi·al
sub·acute
sub·al·i·men·ta·tion
sub·anal
sub·an·co·ne·us
sub·ap·i·cal
sub·apo·neu·rot·ic
sub·arach·noid
sub·arach·noid·itis
  acute curable juvenile s.
sub·ar·cu·ate
sub·are·o·lar
sub·as·trag·a·lar
sub·astrin·gent
sub·at·loi·de·an
sub·atom·ic
sub·au·ral
sub·au·ra·le
sub·au·ric·u·lar
sub·ax·i·al
sub·ax·il·lary
sub·ba·sal
sub·bra·chi·al
sub·bra·chy·ce·phal·ic
sub·cal·ca·re·ous
sub·cal·car·ine
sub·cal·lo·sal
sub·cap·su·lar
sub·cap·su·lo·peri·os·te·al
sub·car·bo·nate
sub·car·ti·lag·i·nous
sub·cen·tral
sub·cep·tion
sub·cer·e·bel·lar

sub·cer·e·bral
sub·chlo·ride
sub·chon·dral
sub·chor·dal
sub·cho·ri·on·ic
sub·cho·roi·dal
sub·chron·ic
sub·class
sub·cla·vi·an
sub·cla·vic·u·lar
sub·clin·i·cal
sub·clone
sub·col·lat·er·al
sub·con·junc·ti·val
sub·con·scious
sub·con·scious·ness
sub·cor·a·coid
sub·cor·tex
sub·cor·ti·cal
sub·cos·tal
sub·cos·ta·lis *pl.* sub·cos·ta·
les
sub·cra·ni·al
sub·crep·i·tant
sub·crep·i·ta·tion
sub·cul·ture
sub·cur·a·tive
sub·cu·ta·ne·ous
sub·cu·tic·u·lar
sub·cu·tis
sub·de·lir·i·um
sub·del·toid
sub·den·tal
sub·der·mal
sub·di·a·phrag·mat·ic
sub·dor·sal
sub·duct
sub·duc·tion
sub·du·ral
sub·en·do·car·di·al
sub·en·do·the·li·al
sub·en·do·the·li·um
sub·en·dy·mal
sub·ep·en·dy·mal
sub·ep·en·dy·mo·ma
sub·ep·i·der·mal
sub·ep·i·der·mic
sub·epi·glot·tic

sub·epi·the·li·al
su·ber·i·tin
su·ber·o·sis
sub·ex·ten·si·bil·i·ty
sub·fal·ci·al
sub·fam·i·ly
sub·fas·cial
sub·fe·cun·di·ty
sub·fer·tile
sub·fer·til·i·ty
Sub fin. coct. — L. sub finem
coctionis (toward the end of
boiling)
sub·fis·sure
sub·fla·vous
sub·fo·li·ar
sub·fo·li·um
sub·for·ni·cal
sub·fron·tal
sub·ga·le·al
sub·gal·late
sub·gem·mal
sub·ge·nus
sub·ger·mi·nal
sub·gin·gi·val
sub·gle·noid
sub·glos·sal
sub·glos·si·tis
sub·glot·tic
sub·gran·u·lar
sub·gron·da·tion
sub·gy·rus
sub·he·pat·ic
sub·hu·mer·al
sub·hy·a·loid
sub·hy·oid
sub·hy·oi·de·an
sub·ic·ter·ic
su·bic·u·lar
su·bic·u·lum
    s. cornu ammonis
    s. hippocampi
    s. promontorii cavi
    tympani
    s. of promontory of
    tympanic cavity
sub·il·i·ac
sub·il·i·um

sub·in·flam·ma·tion
sub·in·flam·ma·to·ry
sub·in·tern
sub·in·ti·mal
sub·in·trance
sub·in·trant
sub·in·vo·lu·tion
   chronic s. of uterus
sub·io·dide
sub·ja·cent
sub·ject
sub·jec·tive
sub·jec·to·scope
sub·jee
sub·ju·gal
sub·la·bi·al
sub·la·tio
   s. retinae
sub·la·tion
sub·le·sion·al
sub·le·thal
sub·li·mate
   corrosive s.
sub·li·ma·tion
Sub·li·maze
sub·lime
sub·lim·i·nal
sub·li·mis
sub·line
sub·lin·gual
sub·lin·gui·tis
sub·lobe
sub·lob·u·lar
sub·lux·ate
sub·lux·a·tion
   atlantoaxial s.
   congenital s. of hip
   s. of lens
   Volkmann's s.
sub·lym·phe·mia
sub·mam·ma·ry
sub·man·dib·u·lar
sub·ma·nia
sub·mar·gi·nal
sub·max·il·la
sub·max·il·lar·itis
sub·max·il·lary
sub·me·di·al

sub·me·di·an
sub·mem·bra·nous
sub·me·nin·ge·al
sub·men·tal
sub·mer·sion
sub·meta·cen·tric
sub·mi·cro·scop·ic
sub·mi·cro·scop·i·cal
sub·mor·phous
sub·mu·co·sa
sub·mu·co·sal
sub·mu·cous
sub·nar·cot·ic
sub·na·sal
sub·na·sa·le
sub·na·sion
sub·na·tant
sub·neu·ral
sub·ni·trate
sub·nor·mal
sub·nor·mal·i·ty
   mental s.
sub·no·to·chor·dal
sub·nu·cle·us
sub·nu·tri·tion
sub·oc·cip·i·tal
sub·oper·cu·lum
sub·op·tic
sub·op·ti·mal
sub·or·bi·tal
sub·or·der
sub·ox·i·da·tion
sub·ox·ide
sub·pap·il·lary
sub·pap·u·lar
sub·par·a·lyt·ic
sub·pa·ri·e·tal
sub·pa·tel·lar
sub·pec·tor·al
sub·pe·dun·cu·lar
sub·pel·vi·peri·to·ne·al
sub·peri·car·di·al
sub·peri·os·te·al
sub·peri·os·teo·cap·su·lar
sub·peri·to·ne·al
sub·peri·to·neo·ab·dom·i·nal
sub·peri·to·neo·pel·vic
sub·pe·tro·sal

sub·pha·ryn·ge·al
sub·phren·ic
sub·phy·lum *pl.* sub·phy·la
sub·pi·al
sub·pi·tu·i·ta·rism
sub·pla·cen·ta
sub·pla·cen·tal
sub·pleu·ral
sub·pon·tine
sub·pop·u·la·tion
sub·pre·pu·tial
sub·pu·bic
sub·pul·mo·nary
sub·pul·pal
sub·py·ram·i·dal
sub·rec·tal
sub·ret·i·nal
sub·ros·tral
sub·scapho·ceph·a·ly
sub·scap·u·lar
sub·scle·ral
sub·scle·rot·ic
sub·scrip·tion
sub·se·ro·sa
sub·se·rous
sub·set
sub·sib·i·lant
sub·sig·moid
sub·son·ic
sub·spec·ial·ty
sub·spe·cies
sub·spi·na·le
sub·spi·nous
sub·sple·ni·al
sub·stage
sub·stance
    A s.
    α-s.
    acute phase s.
    ad s.
    adamantine s. of tooth
    agglutinating s.
    alpha s.
    anterior pituitary-like s.
    antidiuretic s.
    anti-immune s.
    arborescent white s. of
      cerebellum

sub·stance *(continued)*
    B s.
    β-s.
    beta s.
    black s.
    blood group s's
    blood grouping specific s's
    bony s. of tooth
    C s.
    cement s.
    cementing s.
    central gray s. of cerebrum
    central intermediate s. of
      spinal cord
    chromidial s.
    chromophil s.
    colloid s.
    compact s. of bones
    controlled s.
    cortical s. of bone
    cortical s. of kidney
    cortical s. of lens
    cortical s. of lymph nodes
    cortical s. of suprarenal
      gland
    depressor s.
    exophthalmos-producing s.
    external s. of suprarenal
      gland
    filar s.
    gelatinous s. of spinal cord
    glandular s. of prostate
    gray s.
    gray s. of cerebrum, central
    gray reticular s. of medulla
      oblongata
    gray s. of spinal cord
    ground s.
    H s.
    hyaline s.
    I s.
    interfibrillar s. of
      Flemming
    interfilar s.
    intermediate gray s. of
      spinal cord, central
    intermediate gray s. of
      spinal cord, lateral

sub·stance *(continued)*
  intermediate s. of
    suprarenal gland
  internal s. of suprarenal
    gland
  interpeduncular perforated
    s.
  interprismatic s.
  interspongioplastic s.
  interstitial s.
  intertubular s. of tooth
  ivory s. of tooth
  ketogenic s.
  s. of lens
  medullary s.
  medullary s. of bone
  medullary s. of bone, red
  medullary s. of bone,
    yellow
  medullary s. of kidney
  medullary s. of suprarenal
    gland
  metachromatic s.
  molecular s.
  müllerian inhibiting s.
  muscular s. of prostate
  neurosecretory s.
  s. of Nissl
  no-threshold s's
  onychogenic s.
  organ-forming s's
  s. P
  pellagra-preventing s.
  perforated s., anterior
  perforated s.,
    interpeduncular
  perforated s., posterior
  periventricular gray s.
  P.-P. s.
  prelipid s.
  pressor s.
  proper s. of choroid
  proper s. of cornea
  proper s. of sclera
  proper s. of tooth
  red s. of spleen
  reducing s.
  Reichert's s.

sub·stance *(continued)*
  released s.
  reticular s.
  reticular s. of medulla
    oblongata
  reticular s., white, of
    Arnold
  Rolando's gelatinous s.
  Rollett's secondary s.
  rostral perforated s.
  sarcous s.
  Schwann's white s.
  s. sensibilisatrice
  sensitizing s.
  slow-reacting s., of
    anaphylaxis
  specific soluble s. (SSS)
  spongy s. of bone
  threshold s's
  thromboplastic s.
  tigroid s.
  trabecular s. of bone
  transmitter s.
  white s.
  white reticular s.
  white s. of Schwann
  white s. of spinal cord
  zymoplastic s.
sub·stan·tia *pl.* sub·stan·tiae
  s. adamantina dentis
  s. alba
  s. cinerea
  s. compacta ossium
  s. corticalis
  s. eburnea dentis
  s. ferruginea
  s. gelatinosa
  s. glandularis prostatae
  s. gliosa centralis
  s. grisea
  s. hyalina
  s. innominata
  s. innominata of Reichert
  s. innominata of Reil
  s. intermedia
  s. intertubularis dentis
  s. lentis
  s. medullaris

sub·stan·tia *(continued)*
  s. metachromatico-
    granularis
  s. muscularis prostatae
  s. nigra
  s. opaca
  s. ossea dentis
  s. perforata anterior
  s. perforata
    interpeduncularis
  s. perforata posterior
  s. perforata rostralis
  s. propria choroideae
  s. propria corneae
  s. propria sclerae
  s. reticularis alba of Arnold
  s. reticularis alba gyri
    fornicati Arnoldi
  s. reticularis medullae
    oblongatae
  s. reticulofilamentosa
  s. Rolandi
  s. spongiosa
  s. spongiosa ossium
  s. trabecularis ossium
  s. visceralis secundaria
sub·ster·nal
sub·ster·no·mas·toid
sub·stit·u·ent
sub·sti·tute
  Biobrane synthetic skin s.
  blood s.
  plasma s.
sub·sti·tu·tion
  creeping s. of bone
  gene s.
sub·sti·tu·tive
sub·strain
sub·strate
  renin s.
sub·stra·tum
sub·struc·ture
  implant s.
sub·sul·cus
sub·sul·fate
sub·sul·tus
sub·syl·vi·an
sub·syn·ap·tic

sub·ta·lar
sub·tar·sal
sub·telo·cen·tric
sub·tem·por·al
sub·te·ni·al
sub·ten·to·ri·al
sub·ter·mi·nal
sub·ter·tian
sub·te·tan·ic
sub·tha·lam·ic
sub·thal·a·mus
sub·thresh·old
sub·thy·roid·ism
sub·tile
sub·til·in
sub·til·i·sin
sub·tle
sub·to·tal
sub·tra·pe·zi·al
sub·tribe
sub·trig·o·nal
sub·tro·chan·ter·ic
sub·troch·le·ar
sub·tu·ber·al
sub·tym·pan·ic
sub·typ·i·cal
sub·um·bil·i·cal
sub·un·gual
sub·unit
  catalytic s.
  regulatory s.
sub·ure·thral
sub·vag·i·nal
sub·ver·te·bral
sub·vi·ral
sub·vi·ta·min·o·sis
sub·vit·ri·nal
sub·vo·lu·tion
sub·wak·ing
sub·zo·nal
sub·zy·go·mat·ic
suc·ca·gogue
suc·ce·da·ne·ous
suc·ce·da·ne·um
suc·cen·tu·ri·ate
suc·ces·sion
suc·ci·nate
suc·ci·nate-CoA li·gase

suc·ci·nate de·hy·dro·gen·ase
suc·cin·ic acid
Suc·ci·ni·mo·nas
Suc·ci·ni·vib·rio
suc·ci·nyl
suc·ci·nyl·cho·line chlo·ride
suc·ci·nyl-CoA
suc·ci·nyl-CoA syn·the·tase
suc·ci·nyl·co·en·zyme A
suc·ci·nyl·sul·fa·thi·a·zole
suc·cor·rhea
suc·cu·lence
suc·cus *pl.* suc·ci
    s. cerasi
    s. entericus
    s. gastricus
    s. pancreaticus
    s. prostaticus
    s. rubi idaei
suc·cus·sion
    hippocratic s.
suck·le
suck·ling
Su·cos·trin
Suc·quet-Hoy·er anastomosis
Suc·quet-Hoy·er canal
su·cral·fate
su·crase
su·crate
su·cro·clas·tic
su·crose
    s. octaacetate
su·crose α-D-glu·co·hy·dro·lase
su·crose α-D-glu·co·si·dase
su·cros·emia
su·cros·uria
suc·tion
    DeLee s.
    post-tussive s.
    wall s.
    Wangensteen s.
suc·to·ri·al
Su·da·fed
su·da·men *pl.* su·da·mi·na
su·dam·i·na
su·dam·i·nal

Su·dan
    S. I
    S. II
    S. III
    S. IV
    S. black B
    S. G
    S. yellow G
su·dano·phil
su·dano·phil·ia
su·dano·phil·ic
su·dan·oph·i·lous
su·da·ri·um
su·da·tion
su·da·tory
Su·deck's atrophy
Su·deck's disease
Su·deck's point
Su·deck-Le·riche syndrome
su·do·gram
su·do·mo·tor
su·dor
su·do·ral
su·do·re·sis
su·do·rif·er·ous
su·do·rif·ic
su·do·rip·a·rous
su·do·rom·e·ter
su·dox·i·cam
SUDS — sudden unexplained
  death syndrome
su·et
    benzoinated s.
    prepared s.
Su·fen·ta
su·fen·ta·nil
suf·fo·cant
suf·fo·cate
suf·fo·ca·tion
suf·frag·i·nis
suf·fu·sion
sug·ar
    anhydrous s.
    barley s.
    beet s.
    blood s.
    burnt s.

sug·ar *(continued)*
   cane s.
   compressible s.
   confectioner's s.
   diabetic s.
   invert s.
   reducing s.
   simple s.
   starch s.
   threshold s.
sug·ges·ti·bil·i·ty
sug·ges·ti·ble
sug·ges·tion
   hypnotic s.
   posthypnotic s.
sug·gil·la·tion
Su·gi·u·ra procedure
su·i·cide
   immunologic s.
   psychic s.
su·i·ci·dol·o·gy
sui·gen·der·ism
suint
su·i·pes·ti·fer
suit
   antiblackout s.
   anti-G s.
   antishock s.
   G s.
   pressure s.
   space s.
Sul·am·yd
sul·a·ze·pam
sul·ben·ox
sul·cal
sul·cate
sul·ca·tion
sul·ci
sul·ci·form
sul·con·a·zole ni·trate
sul·cu·lus *pl.* sul·cu·li
sul·cus *pl.* sul·ci
   alveolabial s.
   alveolingual s.
   alveolobuccal s.
   s. ampullaris
   ampullary s.
   angular s.

sul·cus *(continued)*
   ansate s.
   anterolateral s.
   s. anterolateralis
   s. anthelicis transversus
   aortic s.
   s. aorticus
   s. arteriae occipitalis
   s. arteriae subclaviae
   s. arteriae temporalis
     mediae
   s. arteriae vertebralis
     atlantis
   sulci arteriales
   sulci arteriosi
   atrioventricular s.
   s. of auditory tube
   s. of auricle, posterior
   s. auriculae posterior
   basilar s. of occipital bone
   basilar s. of pons
   s. basilaris pontis
   bicipital s., lateral
   bicipital s., medial
   bicipital s., radial
   bicipital s., ulnar
   s. bicipitalis lateralis
   s. bicipitalis medialis
   s. bicipitalis radialis
   s. bicipitalis ulnaris
   s. brevis
   bulbopontine s.
   s. bulbopontinus
   bulboventricular s.
   calcaneal s.
   s. calcanei
   calcarine s.
   s. calcarinus
   callosal s.
   callosomarginal s.
   s. callosus
   s. canaliculi mastoidei
   s. canalis innominatus
   s. caroticus
   carotid s.
   carpal s.
   s. carpi
   central s. of cerebrum

sul·cus *(continued)*
  central s. of insula
  s. centralis cerebri
  s. centralis insulae
  cerebral s., lateral
  sulci cerebri
  sulci of cerebrum
  chiasmatic s.
  s. chiasmatis
  s. cingulatus
  s. cinguli
  s. of cingulum
  circular s. of insula
  s. circularis insulae
  collateral s.
  s. collateralis
  s. colli mandibulae
  s. coronarius cordis
  coronary s. of heart
  s. corporis callosi
  s. of corpus callosum
  s. costae
  costal s.
  costal s., inferior
  cruciate s.
  s. cruris helicis
  s. of crus of helix
  cuboid s.
  sulci cutis
  dorsolateral s.
  s. dorsolateralis
  ethmoidal s. of Gegenbaur
  ethmoidal s. of nasal bone
  s. ethmoidalis ossis nasalis
  s. of eustachian tube
  external spiral s.
  fimbriodentate s.
  frontal s., inferior
  frontal s., superior
  s. frontalis inferior
  s. frontalis superior
  gingival s.
  s. gingivalis
  gingivobuccal s.
  gingivolingual s.
  gluteal s.
  s. glutealis
  greater palatine s.

sul·cus *(continued)*
  s. of habenula
  s. habenulae
  habenular s.
  s. habenularis
  s. hamuli pterygoidei
  Harrison's s.
  hemispheric s.
  s. hippocampalis
  s. hippocampi
  s. horizontalis cerebelli
  hypothalamic s.
  s. hypothalamicus
  s. hypothalamicus [Monro]
  infraorbital s. of maxilla
  s. infraorbitalis maxillae
  infrapalpebral s.
  s. infrapalpebralis
  s. of innominate canal
  interarticular s. of
    calcaneus
  interarticular s. of talus
  interatrial s.
  intermediate s. of spinal
    cord, dorsal
  internal spiral s.
  interparietal s.
  s. interparietalis
  intertubercular s. of
    humerus
  s. intertubercularis humeri
  interventricular s.,
    anterior
  interventricular s., inferior
  interventricular s.,
    posterior
  interventricular s. of heart
  s. interventricularis
    anterior
  s. interventricularis cordis
  s. interventricularis
    inferior
  s. interventricularis
    posterior
  intraparietal s.
  s. intraparietalis
  Jacobson's s.
  labiodental s.

sul·cus *(continued)*
s. lacrimalis maxillae
s. lacrimalis ossis
lacrimalis
lacrimal s. of lacrimal bone
lacrimal s. of maxilla
lateral bicipital s.
lateral s. of medulla
oblongata, anterior
lateral s. of medulla
oblongata, posterior
lateral mesencephalic s.
lateral occipital s.
lateral s. of spinal cord,
anterior
lateral s. of spinal cord,
posterior
s. lateralis anterior
medullae oblongatae
s. lateralis anterior
medullae spinalis
s. lateralis cerebri
s. lateralis mesencephali
s. lateralis pedunculi
cerebri
s. lateralis posterior
medullae oblongatae
s. lateralis posterior
medullae spinalis
s. of lesser petrosal nerve
s. limitans
longitudinal s. of heart
lunate s.
s. lunatus
mallear s. of temporal bone
malleolar s. of fibula
malleolar s. of temporal
bone
malleolar s. of tibia
s. malleolaris fibulae
s. malleolaris tibiae
mandibular s.
marginal s.
s. of mastoid canaliculus
s. matricis unguis
s. of matrix of nail
medial bicipital s.
medial s. of crus cerebri

sul·cus *(continued)*
s. medialis cruris cerebri
median s. of fourth
ventricle
median s. of medulla
oblongata, dorsal
median s. of medulla
oblongata, posterior
median s. of spinal cord,
dorsal
median s. of spinal cord,
posterior
median s. of tongue
s. medianus dorsalis
medullae oblongatae
s. medianus dorsalis
medullae spinalis
s. medianus linguae
s. medianus posterior
medullae oblongatae
s. medianus posterior
medullae spinalis
s. medianus ventriculi
quarti
meningeal sulci
mentolabial s.
s. mentolabialis
s. mesencephali medialis
middle frontal s.
s. of middle temporal
artery
s. of Monro
muscular s. of tympanic
cavity
s. musculi flexoris hallucis
longi calcanei
s. musculi flexoris hallucis
longi tali
s. musculi peronaei
calcanei
s. musculi peronaei ossis
cuboidei
s. musculi subclavii
mylohyoid s. of mandible
s. mylohyoideus
mandibulae
nasal s., posterior

sul·cus *(continued)*
s. of nasal process of
maxilla
nasofrontal s.
nasolabial s.
s. nasolabialis
s. nervi oculomotorii
s. nervi petrosi majoris
s. nervi petrosi minoris
s. nervi petrosi superficialis
majoris
s. nervi petrosi superficialis
minoris
s. nervi radialis
s. nervi spinalis
s. nervi ulnaris
nymphocaruncular s.
nymphohymeneal s.
obturator s. of pubis
s. obturatorius ossis pubis
occipital sulci, lateral
occipital sulci, superior
occipital s., transverse
s. of occipital artery
s. occipitalis anterior
sulci occipitales laterales
sulci occipitales superiores
s. occipitalis transversus
occipitotemporal s.
s. occipitotemporalis
s. oculomotorius
s. olfactorius lobi frontalis
s. olfactorius nasi
olfactory s. of frontal lobe
olfactory s. of nose
optic s.
orbital sulci of frontal lobe
sulci orbitales lobi frontalis
palatine sulci of maxilla
sulci palatini maxillae
palatinovaginal s.
s. palatinovaginalis
s. palatinus major maxillae
s. palatinus major ossis
palatini
paracolic sulci
sulci paracolici

sul·cus *(continued)*
paraglenoid sulci of hip
bone
sulci paraglenoidales ossis
coxae
paramedial s.
paramedian s.
parasplenial s.
parietooccipital s.
s. parietooccipitalis
s. parolfactorius anterior
s. parolfactorius posterior
petrobasilar s.
petrosal s. of occipital bone,
inferior
petrosal s. of temporal
bone, inferior
petrosal s. of temporal
bone, posterior
petrosal s. of temporal
bone, superior
s. petrosus inferior ossis
occipitalis
s. petrosus inferior ossis
temporalis
s. petrosus superior ossis
temporalis
polar s.
pontobulbar s.
pontopeduncular s.
postcalcarine s.
postcentral s.
s. postcentralis
postclival s.
posterointermediate s. of
spinal cord
posterolateral s. of medulla
oblongata
posterolateral s. of spinal
cord
s. posterolateralis medullae
oblongatae
s. posterolateralis medullae
spinalis
postnodular s.
postolivary s.
postpyramidal s.
s. praecentralis

sul·cus *(continued)*
> preauricular s.
> precentral s.
> s. precentralis
> prechiasmatic s.
> s. prechiasmaticus
> s. prechiasmatis
> preclival s.
> prelunate s.
> prenodular s.
> prepyramidal s.
> prerolandic s.
> s. promontorii cavi
>   tympani
> s. of pterygoid hamulus
> pterygoid s. of pterygoid
>   process
> pterygopalatine s. of
>   palatine bone
> pterygopalatine s. of
>   pterygoid process
> s. pterygopalatinus ossis
>   palatini
> s. pterygopalatinus
>   processus pterygoidei
> s. pulmonalis thoracis
> pulmonary s. of thorax
> radial s. of humerus
> s. of radial nerve
> Reil's s.
> retrocentral s.
> rhinal s.
> s. rhinalis
> rolandic s.
> sagittal s.
> s. sclerae
> scleral s.
> sclercorneal s.
> s. of semicanal of humerus
> s. of semicanal of vidian
>   nerve
> semilunar s. of radius
> sigmoid s.
> s. sinus sagittalis
> s. sinus sagittalis superioris
> s. sinus sigmoidei
> s. sinus transversi
> sulci of skin

sul·cus *(continued)*
> sphenovomerian s.
> s. of spinal nerve
> spiral s.
> spiral s., external
> spiral s., internal
> spiral s. of humerus
> s. spiralis
> s. spiralis externus
> s. spiralis internus
> splenial s.
> s. subclaviae
> subclavian s.
> s. of subclavian artery
> subclavian s. of lung
> s. for subclavian muscle
> s. of subclavian vein
> s. subclavius
> s. subclavius pulmonis
> subparietal s.
> s. subparietalis
> s. of superior petrosal sinus
> supra-acetabular s.
> s. supra-acetabularis
> supraorbital s.
> suprasplenial s.
> suprasylvian s.
> s. Sylvii
> s. tali
> s. of talus
> temporal s., inferior
> temporal s., middle
> temporal s., superior
> temporal sulci, transverse
> temporal s. of temporal
>   bone
> s. temporalis inferior
> s. temporalis superior
> sulci temporales transversi
> terminal s. of right atrium
> terminal s. of thalamus
> terminal s. of tongue
> s. terminalis atrii dextri
> s. terminalis linguae
> s. of tongue
> transverse s. of anthelix
> transverse s. of heart

sul·cus *(continued)*
 transverse s. of occipital bone
 transverse s. of parietal bone
 s. of transverse sinus
 transverse s. of temporal bone
 s. transversus ossis occipitalis
 s. transversus ossis parietalis
 s. tubae auditivae
 s. tubae auditoriae
 Turner's s.
 tympanic s. of temporal bone
 s. tympanicus ossis temporalis
 s. of ulnar nerve
 s. of umbilical vein
 uvulonodular s.
 s. valleculae
 sulci for veins
 s. of vena cava
 s. venae cavae
 s. venae cavae cranialis
 s. venae subclaviae
 s. venae umbilicalis
 sulci venosi
 venous sulci
 s. ventralis medullae spinalis
 ventrolateral s. of spinal cord
 s. ventrolateralis medullae spinalis
 vermicular s.
 vertical s.
 vomeral s.
 s. vomeris
 vomerovaginal s.
 s. vomerovaginalis
 Waldeyer's s.
 s. of wrist
sul·fa·benz·a·mide
sul·fa·cet·a·mide
 s. sodium

sulf·a·ce·tic acid
sulf·ac·id
sul·fa·cy·tine
sul·fa·di·a·zine
 s. silver
 s. sodium
sul·fa·di·me·thox·ine
sul·fa·di·me·tine
sul·fa·di·mi·dine
sul·fa·dox·ine
sul·fa·eth·i·dole
sul·fa·fu·ra·zole
sul·fa·guan·i·dine
sul·fa·lene
sul·fa·mer·a·zine
sul·fa·me·ter
sul·fa·meth·a·zine
sul·fa·meth·i·zole
sul·fa·meth·ox·a·zole
sul·fa·meth·oxy·py·rid·a·zine
sul·fa·meth·yl·di·a·zine
sul·fa·meth·yl·thi·a·di·a·zole
Sul·fa·mez·a·thine
sul·fam·i·do
sul·fam·i·do·chry·soi·dine
sul·fam·ine
sul·fa·mono·me·thox·ine
sul·fa·mox·ole
Sul·fa·my·lon
sul·fan blue
sul·fa·nil·amide
sul·fan·i·late
sul·fa·nil·ic acid
sul·fa·nil·yl·sul·fa·nil·amide
sul·fa·ni·tran
sul·fa·nu·ria
sul·fa·pyr·i·dine
sul·fa·py·rim·i·dine
sul·fa·quin·ox·a·line
sul·fa·sal·a·zine
Sul·fa·sux·i·dine
sul·fa·tase
 multiple s. deficiency
sul·fate
 acid s.
 active s.
 s. adenylyltransferase
 basic s.

sul·fate *(continued)*
    chondroitin s.
    conjugated s's
    cupric s.
    dermatan s.
    ethereal s's
    hydrogen s.
    mineral s's
    neutral s.
    normal s.
    piperazine estrone s.
    preformed s's
sul·fat·emia
Sul·fa·thal·i·dine
sul·fa·thi·a·zole
sul·fa·ti·dase
sul·fa·tide
sul·fat·i·do·sis
sul·faz·a·met
sul·fen·ic acid
sulf·he·mo·glo·bin
sulf·he·mo·glo·bin·emia
sulf·hy·drate
sulf·hy·dric acid
sulf·hy·dryl
sul·fide
    mercuric s.
sul·fin
sul·fin·ic acid
sul·fin·ide
sul·fin·py·ra·zone
sul·fi·nyl
β-sul·fin·yl·py·ru·vic acid [beta-]
sul·fi·som·i·dine
sul·fi·sox·a·zole
    s. acetyl
    s. diolamine
sul·fite
sul·fite ox·i·dase
sulf·met·he·mo·glo·bin
sul·fo·ac·id
sul·fo·ami·no
sul·fo·bro·mo·phthal·e·in
sul·fo·con·ju·ga·tion
sul·fo·cy·a·nate
sul·fo·cy·an·ic acid
sul·fo·gel

N-sul·fo·glu·cos·amine sul·fo·hy·dro·lase
sul·fo·hy·drate
sul·fo·id·uron·ate sul·fa·tase
sul·fo·lip·id
sul·fo·litho·cho·lyl·gly·cine
sul·fo·litho·cho·lyl·tau·rine
sul·fol·y·sis
sul·fo·mu·cin
Sul·fo·nal
sul·fon·amide
sul·fon·am·i·de·mia
sul·fon·am·i·do·cho·lia
sul·fon·am·i·do·ther·a·py
sul·fon·am·i·du·ria
sul·fo·nate
sul·fone
sul·fon·eth·yl·meth·ane
sul·fon·ic
sul·fon·ic ac·id
sul·fo·ni·um
sul·fon·meth·ane
Sul·fon·sol
sul·fon·ter·ol hy·dro·chlo·ride
sul·fo·nyl
sul·fo·nyl·urea
sul·fo·pro·tein
sul·fo·sal·i·cyl·ic acid
sul·fo·salt
Sul·fose
sul·fo·sol
sul·fo·trans·fer·ase
sul·fox·ide
    methionine s.
sul·fox·ism
sul·fox·one so·di·um
sul·fur
    s. 35
    colloidal s.
    s. dioxide
    flower of s.
    s. hydride
    lac s.
    s. lotum
    s. monochloride
    precipitated s.
    radioactive s.
    roll s.

sul·fur *(continued)*
    sublimed s.
    washed s.
    wettable s.
sul·fu·rat·ed
sul·fu·ra·tor
sul·fu·ret·ed
sul·fur·ic acid
sul·fur·is
sul·fu·rize
sul·fur·ous acid
sul·fur·trans·fer·ase
sul·fu·ryl
sul·fy·dryl
sul·in·dac
sul·i·so·ben·zone
Sul·ko·witch's test
Sul·la
sul·lage
Sul·li·van's test
sul·nid·a·zole
sul·oc·ti·dil
sul·ox·i·fen ox·a·late
sul·pi·ride
sul·pros·tone
Sul-Span·sion
sul·thi·ame
Sulz·ber·ger-Gar·be syndrome
sum. — L. sumat (let him
  take)
    L. sumendum (to be taken)
su·mac
    poison s.
    swamp s.
sum·ma·tion
    central s.
    spatial s.
    temporal s.
sum·mit
    s. of bladder
    s. of nose
Sum·ner, James Batcheller
Sum·ner's method
Sum·ner's reagent
Sum·ner's sign
Su·my·cin
sun·burn
sun·cil·lin so·di·um

Sun·Dare
sun·spot
sun·stroke
su·per·ab·duc·tion
su·per·ac·id
su·per·acid·i·ty
su·per·acro·mi·al
su·per·ac·tiv·i·ty
su·per·acute
su·per·al·i·men·ta·tion
su·per·al·ka·lin·i·ty
su·per·an·ti·gen
su·per·au·ra·le
su·per·car·bon·ate
su·per·cen·tral
su·per·cil·ia
su·per·cil·i·ary
su·per·cil·i·um *pl.* su·per·cil·
  ia
su·per·class
su·per·coil
su·per·cooled
su·per·dis·ten·tion
su·per·duct
su·per·duc·tion
su·per·ego
su·per·ex·ci·ta·tion
su·per·ex·tend·ed
su·per·ex·ten·sion
su·per·fam·i·ly
su·per·fe·cun·da·tion
su·per·fe·ta·tion
su·per·fi·cial
su·per·fi·ci·a·lis
su·per·fi·ci·es
su·per·fis·sure
su·per·flex·ion
su·per·func·tion
su·per·gene
su·per·gen·u·al
su·per·gyre
su·per·he·lix
su·per·im·preg·na·tion
su·per·in·duce
su·per·in·fec·tion
su·per·in·vo·lu·tion
su·pe·ri·or
su·per·ja·cent

su·per·lac·ta·tion
su·per·le·thal
su·per·lig·a·men
su·per·me·di·al
su·per·mi·cro·scope
su·per·mo·til·i·ty
su·per·na·tant
su·per·nate
su·per·nor·mal
su·per·nu·mer·ary
su·per·nu·tri·tion
su·per·oc·cip·i·tal
su·pero·lat·er·al
su·pero·me·di·al
su·per·ov·u·la·tion
su·per·ox·ide
su·per·ox·ide dis·mu·tase
su·per·par·a·site
su·per·par·a·sit·ic
su·per·par·a·sit·ism
su·per·pe·tro·sal
su·per·phos·phate
su·per·re·gen·e·ra·tion
su·per·salt
su·per·sat·u·rate
su·per·scrip·tion
su·per·se·cre·tion
su·per·sen·si·tive
su·per·sen·si·tiv·i·ty
    disuse s.
su·per·sen·si·ti·za·tion
su·per·soft
su·per·son·ic
su·per·son·ics
su·per·spe·cies
su·per·sphe·noid
su·per·struc·ture
    implant s.
su·per·sul·cus
su·per·vas·cu·lar·iza·tion
su·per·ve·nos·i·ty
su·per·ven·tion
su·per·ver·sion
su·per·vis·or
su·per·vi·ta·min·o·sis
su·per·vol·tage
su·pi·nate
su·pi·na·tion

su·pi·na·tor
su·pine
sup·ple·men·tal
sup·ply
    extrinsic nerve s.
    intrinsic nerve s.
sup·port
    advanced cardiac life s.
    advanced life s. (ALS)
    advanced trauma life s.
    basic life s. (BLS)
    s. of the promontory
sup·port·ive
sup·pos·i·to·ry
    glycerin s.
sup·pres·sant
sup·pres·sion
    otoacoustic s.
    phenotypic s.
sup·pres·sor
    amber s.
    codon-specific s.
    crossover s.
    soluble immune response s.
sup·pu·rant
sup·pu·rate
sup·pu·ra·tion
    alveodental s.
sup·pu·ra·tive
su·pra-acro·mi·al
su·pra-anal
su·pra-aor·tic
su·pra-au·ric·u·lar
su·pra-ax·il·lary
su·pra·buc·cal
su·pra·bulge
su·pra·cal·lo·sal
su·pra·cer·e·bel·lar
su·pra·cer·e·bral
su·pra·cer·vi·cal
su·pra·cho·roid
su·pra·cho·roi·dea
su·pra·cil·i·ary
su·pra·cla·vic·u·lar
su·pra·cla·vic·u·la·ris
su·pra·cli·noid
su·pra·clu·sion
su·pra·con·dy·lar

su·pra·con·dy·loid
su·pra·cos·tal
su·pra·cot·y·loid
su·pra·cra·ni·al
su·pra·di·a·phrag·mat·ic
su·pra·duc·tion
su·pra·du·ral
su·pra·epi·con·dy·lar
su·pra·epi·troch·le·ar
su·pra·ge·nic·u·late
su·pra·gle·noid
su·pra·glot·tic
su·pra·gran·u·lar
su·pra·he·pat·ic
su·pra·hy·oid
su·pra·il·i·ac
su·pra·in·gui·nal
su·pra·in·tes·ti·nal
su·pra·le·thal
su·pra·lim·i·nal
su·pra·lum·bar
su·pra·mal·le·o·lar
su·pra·mam·il·lary
su·pra·mam·ma·ry
su·pra·man·dib·u·lar
su·pra·mar·gi·nal
su·pra·mas·toid
su·pra·max·il·lary
su·pra·max·i·mal
su·pra·me·a·tal
su·pra·men·tal
su·pra·men·ta·le
su·pra·na·sal
su·pra·nor·mal
su·pra·nu·cle·ar
su·pra·oc·cip·i·tal
su·pra·oc·clu·sion
su·pra·oc·u·lar
su·pra·omo·hy·oid
su·pra·op·tic
su·pra·op·ti·mal
su·pra·op·ti·mum
su·pra·or·bi·tal
su·pra·pa·tel·lar
su·pra·pel·vic
su·pra·phar·ma·co·log·ic
su·pra·pin·e·al
su·pra·pon·tine

su·pra·pro·mon·to·ri·al
su·pra·pu·bic
su·pra·re·nal
su·pra·re·nal·ec·to·my
su·pra·re·nal·ism
su·pra·re·nal·op·a·thy
Su·pra·ren·in
su·pra·re·no·gen·ic
su·pra·re·nop·a·thy
su·pra·re·no·trop·ic
su·pra·scap·u·la
su·pra·scap·u·lar
su·pra·scle·ral
su·pra·seg·men·tal
su·pra·sel·lar
su·pra·sep·tal
su·pra·spi·nal
su·pra·spi·nous
su·pra·sta·pe·di·al
su·pra·ster·nal
su·pra·ster·nale
su·pra·ster·ol
su·pra·syl·vi·an
su·pra·tem·po·ral
su·pra·ten·to·ri·al
su·pra·tho·rac·ic
su·pra·ton·sil·lar
su·pra·troch·le·ar
su·pra·tur·bi·nal
su·pra·tym·pan·ic
su·pra·um·bil·i·cal
su·pra·vag·i·nal
su·pra·val·vu·lar
su·pra·ven·tric·u·lar
su·pra·ver·gence
su·pra·ver·sion
su·pra·vi·tal
su·pra·xi·phoid
su·pro·fen
su·ra
Su·ra·gi·na
su·ral
sur·al·i·men·ta·tion
su·ra·min so·di·um
sur·cin·gle
sur·di·mute
sur·di·mu·tism

sur·di·tas
  s. congenita
sur·di·ty
sur·ex·ci·ta·tion
Sur·fa·caine
sur·face
  alveolar s.
  anterior s.
  anterior talar articular s.
  anteromedial s.
  approximal s.
  articular s.
  axial s.
  basal s.
  buccal s.
  carpal articular s.
  colic s.
  condyloid s.
  contact s.
  costal s.
  cuboid articular s.
  denture foundation s.
  denture impression s.
  diaphragmatic s.
  distal s.
  dorsal s.
  extensor s.
  facial s.
  flexor s.
  foundation s.
  gastric s.
  impression s.
  incisal s.
  inferior s.
  infratemporal s.
  interlobar s.
  isodose s.
  labial s.
  lateral s.
  left s. of heart
  lingual s.
  masticatory s.
  medial s.
  mediastinal s.
  mesial s.
  morsal s's
  occlusal s.
  oral s.

sur·face (continued)
  orbital s.
  polished s.
  posterior s.
  proximal s.
  proximate s.
  pulmonary s. of heart
  renal s.
  right s. of heart
  sacropelvic s.
  sternocostal s. of heart
  subocclusal s.
  superior s.
  symphysial s.
  temporal s.
  tentorial s.
  total body s.
  ventral s.
  vestibular s.
  visceral s.
sur·face-ac·tive
sur·fac·tant
  pulmonary s.
Sur·fak
sur·geon
  acting assistant s.
  assistant s.
  attending s.
  barber s.
  contract s.
  dental s.
  district s.
  s. general
  house s.
  oral s.
  orthopedic s.
  post s.
sur·gery
  abdominal s.
  ambulatory s.
  anaplastic s.
  antiseptic s.
  arthroscopic s.
  aseptic s.
  aural s.
  bench s.
  cardiac s.
  cardiovascular s.

sur·gery *(continued)*
   cineplastic s.
   clinical s.
   closed s.
   closed heart s.
   conservative s.
   cosmetic s.
   cryogenic s.
   day s.
   definitive s.
   dental s.
   dentofacial s.
   elective s.
   esthetic s.
   exploratory s.
   featural s.
   foot-plate s.
   general s.
   in-and-out s.
   laser s.
   major s.
   maxillofacial s.
   microvascular s.
   minor s.
   Mohs's.
   mucogingival s.
   open heart s.
   operative s.
   operative dental s.
   oral s.
   oral and maxillofacial s.
   orthopedic s.
   palliative s.
   peripheral vascular s.
   plastic s.
   psychiatric s.
   radical s.
   rapid in-and-out s.
   reconstructive s.
   sonic s.
   stapes s.
   stereotactic s.
   stereotaxic s.
   structural s.
   thoracic s.
   transsexual s.
   veterinary s.
sur·gi·cal

Sur·gi·cel
Sur·i·tal
sur·ma
sur·ro·gate
sur·sum·duc·tion
sur·sum·ver·gence
sur·sum·ver·sion
su·ruçu·cu
sur·veil·lance
   epidemiologic s.
   immune s.
   immunological s.
sur·vey·ing
sur·vey·or
sur·vi·val
   five-year s.
sur·vi·vor·ship
sus·cep·ti·bil·i·ty
   differential s.
   magnetic s.
sus·cep·ti·ble
sus·pect
sus·pen·op·sia
sus·pen·si·om·e·ter
sus·pen·sion
   alumina and magnesia oral s.
   ampicillin for oral s.
   betamethasone sodium phosphate and betamethasone acetate s., sterile
   chloramphenicol palmitate oral s.
   chlorothiazide oral s.
   cholestyramine for oral s.
   Coffey s.
   colistin sulfate for oral s.
   colloid s.
   corticotropin zinc hydroxide s., sterile
   cortisone acetate s., sterile
   cortisone acetate ophthalmic s.
   cuff s.
   demeclocycline oral s.
   desoxycorticosterone pivalate s., sterile

sus·pen·sion *(continued)*
    dicloxacillin sodium for oral s.
    diphenylhydantoin oral s.
    epinephrine oil s., sterile
    estradiol s., sterile
    extended insulin zinc s.
    hydrocortisone acetate s., sterile
    hydrocortisone acetate ophthalmic s.
    hydrocortisone cypionate oral s.
    hydroxyzine pamoate oral s.
    ipodate calcium for oral s.
    levopropoxyphene napsylate oral s.
    magaldrate oral s.
    magnesia and alumina oral s.
    medroxyprogesterone acetate s., sterile
    medrysone ophthalmic s.
    meprobamate oral s.
    methacycline hydrochloride oral s.
    methenamine mandelate oral s.
    methylprednisolone acetate s., sterile
    neomycin and polymyxin B sulfates and hydrocortisone otic s.
    nitrofurantoin oral s.
    novobiocin calcium oral s.
    oxytetracycline calcium oral s.
    penicillin G benzathine s., sterile
    penicillin G procaine s., sterile
    penicillin G procaine with aluminum stearate s., sterile
    penicillin V benzathine oral s.

sus·pen·sion *(continued)*
    penicillin V hydrabamine oral s.
    penicillin V for oral s.
    penicillin V potassium for oral s.
    phensuximide oral s.
    phenytoin oral s.
    prednisolone acetate s., sterile
    primidone oral s.
    progesterone s., sterile
    prompt insulin zinc s.
    propoxyphene napsylate oral s.
    propyliodone s., sterile
    propyliodone oil s., sterile
    protamine zinc insulin s.
    pyrantel pamoate oral s.
    pyrvinium pamoate oral s.
    salicylamide oral s.
    selenium sulfide detergent s.
    simethicone oral s.
    sitosterols s.
    sulfacetamide, sulfadiazine, and sulfamerazine oral s.
    sulfadimethoxine oral s.
    sulfamethizole oral s.
    sulfamethoxazole oral s.
    sulfisoxazole acetyl oral s.
    testolactone s., sterile
    testosterone s., sterile
    tetracycline hydrochloride ophthalmic s.
    tetracycline oral s.
    thiabendazole oral s.
    triamcinolone acetonide s., sterile
    triamcinolone diacetate s., sterile
    triamcinolone hexacetonide s., sterile
    trisulfapyrimidines oral s.
    troleandomycin oral s.
sus·pen·soid
sus·pen·so·ri·us

sus·pen·so·ry
Sus-Phrine
sus·pi·ri·ous
sus·ten·tac·u·lar
sus·ten·tac·u·lum *pl.* sus·ten·
  tac·u·la
    s. lienis
    s. tali
    s. of talus
sus·to
su·sur·ra·tion
su·sur·rus
su·ti·ka
su·ti·lains
Sut·ton's disease
Sut·ton's nevus
su·tu·ra *pl.* su·tu·rae
    s. coronalis
    suturae craniales
    suturae cranii
    s. dentata
    s. ethmoidolacrimalis
    s. ethmoidomaxillaris
    s. frontalis
    s. fronto-ethmoidalis
    s. frontolacrimalis
    s. frontomaxillaris
    s. frontonasalis
    s. frontozygomatica
    s. harmonia
    s. incisiva
    s. infraorbitalis
    s. intermaxillaris
    s. internasalis
    s. lacrimoconchalis
    s. lacrimomaxillaris
    s. lambdoidea
    s. limbosa
    s. metopica
    s. nasofrontalis
    s. nasomaxillaris
    s. occipitomastoidea
    s. palatina mediana
    s. palatina transversa
    s. palato-ethmoidalis
    s. palatomaxillaris
    s. parietomastoidea
    s. plana

su·tu·ra *(continued)*
    s. sagittalis
    s. serrata
    s. spheno-ethmoidalis
    s. sphenofrontalis
    s. sphenomaxillaris
    s. sphenoorbitalis
    s. sphenoparietalis
    s. sphenosquamosa
    s. sphenovomeriana
    s. sphenozygomatica
    s. squamosa
    s. squamosa cranii
    s. squamosomastoidea
    s. temporozygomatica
    s. vera
    s. zygomaticofrontalis
    s. zygomaticomaxillaris
    s. zygomaticotemporalis
su·tur·al
su·tur·a·tion
su·ture
    absorbable s.
    absorbable surgical s.
    Albert's s.
    s. of Albrecht
    Appolito's s.
    apposition s.
    approximation s.
    arcuate s.
    atraumatic s.
    baseball s.
    basilar s.
    bastard s.
    Bell's s.
    biparietal s.
    blanket s.
    bolster s.
    bony s.
    bregmatomastoid s.
    bridle s.
    Bunnell's s.
    buried s.
    button s.
    buttonhole s.
    catgut s.
    chain s.
    circular s.

su·ture *(continued)*
  coaptation s.
  cobblers' s.
  Connell s.
  continuous s.
  coronal s.
  cranial s's
  cruciform s.
  Cushing s.
  cutaneous s. of palate
  Czerny's s.
  Czerny-Lembert s.
  delayed s.
  delayed primary s.
  dentate s.
  denticulate s.
  dermal s.
  double-button s.
  doubly armed s.
  Dupuytren's s.
  endognathic s.
  endomesognathic s.
  end-on mattress s.
  epineural s.
  ethmoidolacrimal s.
  ethmoidomaxillary s.
  everting s.
  everting interrupted s.
  false s.
  far-and-near s.
  figure-of-eight s.
  flat s.
  frontal s.
  fronto-ethmoidal s.
  frontolacrimal s.
  frontomalar s.
  frontomaxillary s.
  frontonasal s.
  frontoparietal s.
  frontosphenoid s.
  frontozygomatic s.
  Frost s.
  furrier's s.
  Gaillard-Arlt s.
  Gély's s.
  glover's s.
  s. of Goethe
  Gussenbauer's s.

su·ture *(continued)*
  guy s.
  Halsted s.
  harelip s.
  hemostatic s's
  implanted s.
  incisive s.
  infolding s.
  infraorbital s.
  interendognathic s.
  intermaxillary s.
  internasal s.
  interpalatine s.
  interparietal s.
  interrupted s.
  intradermal mattress s.
  intradermic s.
  invaginating s.
  inverting s.
  jugal s.
  lacrimoconchal s.
  lacrimo-ethmoidal s.
  lacrimomaxillary s.
  lacrimoturbinal s.
  lambdoid s.
  Le Dentu's s.
  Le Fort's s.
  Lembert s.
  lens s's
  s. ligature
  limbous s.
  lock-stitch s.
  longitudinal s.
  longitudinal s. of palate
  loop s.
  loop-on mucosa s.
  malomaxillary s.
  mamillary s.
  mastoid s.
  mattress s., horizontal
  mattress s., right-angle
  mattress s., vertical
  Mersilene s.
  metopic s.
  nasal s.
  nasofrontal s.
  nasomaxillary s.
  nerve s.

su·ture *(continued)*
- nonabsorbable s.
- nonabsorbable surgical s.
- occipital s.
- occipitomastoid s.
- occipitoparietal s.
- occipitosphenoidal s.
- over-and-over s.
- overlapping s.
- palatine s., anterior
- palatine s., median
- palatine s., middle
- palatine s., posterior
- palatine s., transverse
- palato-ethmoidal s.
- palatomaxillary s.
- Pancoast's s.
- Paré's s.
- parietal s.
- parietomastoid s.
- parietooccipital s.
- parietotemporal s.
- Parker-Kerr s.
- peg-and-socket s.
- petrobasilar s.
- petrosphenobasilar s.
- petrosphenooccipital s. of Gruber
- petrosquamous s.
- plane s.
- plastic s.
- plicating s.
- premaxillary s.
- presection s.
- primary s.
- primary delayed s.
- primo-secondary s.
- pursestring s.
- quilt s.
- quilted s.
- relaxation s.
- retention s.
- rhabdoid s.
- Richter s.
- sagittal s.
- scaly s.
- secondary s.
- seroserous s.

su·ture *(continued)*
- serrate s.
- serrated s.
- shotted s.
- Sims' s.
- s's of skull
- spheno-ethmoidal s.
- sphenofrontal s.
- sphenomalar s.
- sphenomaxillary s.
- sphenooccipital s.
- sphenoorbital s.
- sphenoparietal s.
- sphenopetrosal s.
- sphenosquamous s.
- sphenotemporal s.
- sphenovomerine s.
- sphenozygomatic s.
- spiral s.
- squamosal s.
- squamosomastoid s.
- squamosoparietal s.
- squamososphenoid s.
- squamous s.
- squamous s. of cranium
- stay s.
- subcuticular s.
- superficial s.
- temporal s.
- temporomalar s.
- temporozygomatic s.
- tension s.
- through-and-through s.
- tongue-and-groove s.
- transfixion s.
- transverse s. of Krause
- transverse palatine s.
- true s.
- tympanomastoid s.
- uninterrupted s.
- zygomaticofrontal s.
- zygomaticomaxillary s.
- zygomaticosphenoid s.
- zygomaticotemporal s.

sux·a·me·tho·ni·um chlo·ride
Sux-Cert
sux·em·e·rid sul·fate
Su·zanne's gland

SV — simian virus
   sinus venosus
   stroke volume
SV40 — simian virus 40
Sv — sievert
SVC — superior vena cava
sved·berg
Sved·berg flotation unit
Sved·berg unit
swab
   NIH s.
swad·dler
   silver s.
swage
swag·er
swal·low
   barium s.
swal·low·ing
   air s.
   infantile s.
   tongue s.
swarm·ing
sway·back
swear·ing
   compulsive s.
sweat
   bloody s.
   blue s.
   fetid s.
   green s.
   night s.
   phosphorescent s.
sweat·ing
   insensible s.
   sensible s.
Swe·di·aur's disease
Sweet's syndrome
sweet·en·er
   artificial s.
sweet·gum
swell·ing
   albuminous s.
   arytenoid s.
   blennorrhagic s.
   brain s.
   bulbar s's
   Calabar s's
   capsular s.

swell·ing (continued)
   cloudy s.
   familial fibrous s. of jaws
   fugitive s.
   genital s.
   glassy s.
   hunger s.
   labial s.
   labioscrotal s.
   lateral lingual s's
   levator s.
   premenstrual s.
   scrotal s.
   Soemmering's crystalline s.
   tropical s's
   tubular cloudy s.
   tympanic s.
   white s.
Swen·son's operation
Swen·son's procedure
Swift's disease
swing
   mood s's
   torsion s.
switch
   class s.
   selector s.
swoon
SWS — slow wave sleep
Swy·er-James syndrome
Swy·er-James-Mac·leod
  syndrome
sy·ceph·a·lus
sych·nu·ria
sy·co·si·form
sy·co·sis
   s. barbae
   Brocq's lupoid s.
   coccogenic s.
   keloid s.
   lupoid s.
   s. nuchae
   s. tarsi
   s. vulgaris
Syd·en·ham's chorea
Syd·en·ham's cough
syl·vat·ic
Syl·vest's disease

syl·vi·an
syl·vi·duct
Syl·vi·us' angle
Syl·vi·us' aqueduct
Syl·vi·us' fissure
Syl·vi·us' fossa
Syl·vi·us' valve
sym·bal·lo·phone
sym·bi·ol·o·gy
sym·bi·on
sym·bi·on·ic
sym·bi·ont
sym·bi·o·sis
    antagonistic s.
    antipathetic s.
    conjunctive s.
    constructive s.
    disjunctive s.
sym·bi·ote
sym·bi·ot·ic
sym·bleph·a·ron
    anterior s.
    posterior s.
    total s.
sym·bleph·a·rop·ter·yg·i·um
sym·bol
    phallic s.
sym·bo·lia
sym·bol·ism
sym·bol·iza·tion
sym·brachy·dac·tyl·ia
sym·brachy·dac·tyl·ism
sym·brachy·dac·ty·ly
sym·clo·sene
Syme's amputation
sym·e·lus
Sy·ming·ton's body
sym·me·lia
sym·me·lus
Sym·mers' disease
Sym·mers fibrosis
Sym·me·trel
sym·met·ri·cal
sym·me·try
    bilateral s.
    inverse s.
    radial s.
sym·pa·thec·to·mize

sym·pa·thec·to·my
    cervical s.
    chemical s.
    lumbar s.
    lumbodorsal s.
    periarterial s.
sym·pa·the·tec·to·my
sym·pa·thet·ic
sym·pa·thet·i·co·mi·met·ic
sym·pa·thet·i·co·par·a·lyt·ic
sym·pa·thet·i·co·to·nia
sym·pa·thet·i·co·ton·ic
sym·pa·theto·blast
sym·path·ic
sym·path·i·cec·to·my
sym·path·i·co·blast
sym·path·i·co·blas·to·ma
sym·path·i·co·gen·ic
sym·path·i·co·go·ni·o·ma
sym·path·i·co·lyt·ic
sym·path·i·co·mi·met·ic
sym·path·i·cop·a·thy
sym·path·i·co·ther·a·py
sym·path·i·co·to·nia
sym·path·i·co·ton·ic
sym·path·i·co·trip·sy
sym·path·i·co·trope
sym·path·i·co·trop·ic
sym·path·i·cus
sym·pa·thism
sym·pa·thi·zer
sym·patho·adre·nal
sym·patho·blast
sym·patho·blas·to·ma
sym·patho·chro·maf·fin
sym·pa·tho·gone
sym·pa·tho·go·nia
sym·pa·tho·go·ni·o·ma
sym·pa·tho·go·ni·um
sym·pa·tho·lyt·ic
sym·pa·tho·mi·met·ic
sym·patho·par·a·lyt·ic
sym·pa·thy
sym·pec·to·thi·ene
sym·pec·to·thi·on
sym·peri·to·ne·al
sym·pex·ion *pl.* sym·pex·ia

sym·pha·lan·gia
sym·pha·lan·gism
sym·pha·lan·gy
sym·pha·lo·ceph·a·lus
sym·phor·i·car·pus
Sym·phor·o·my·ia
sym·phyo·ceph·a·lus
sym·phys·e·al
sym·phys·e·or·rha·phy
sym·phy·ses
sym·phys·i·al
sym·phys·ic
sym·phy·si·ec·to·my
sym·phys·i·ol·y·sis
sym·phys·i·or·rha·phy
sym·phys·io·tome
sym·phys·i·ot·o·my
sym·phy·sis *pl.* sym·phy·ses
    intervertebral s.
    s. intervertebralis
    s. ligamentosa
    s. mandibulae
    mandibular s.
    manubriosternal s.
    s. manubriosternalis
    s. mentalis
    s. menti
    s. ossium pubis
    pubic s.
    s. pubica
    s. pubis
    s. sacrococcygea
    sacrococcygeal s.
    sacroiliac s.
sym·phy·si·tis
sym·phy·so·dac·ty·ly
Sym·phy·tum
sym·phy·tum
sym·plasm
sym·plas·mat·ic
sym·plast
sym·plex
sym·po·dia
sym·port
symp·tom
    abstinence s's
    accessory s.
    Anton's s.

symp·tom *(continued)*
    assident s.
    Bárány's s.
    Béhier-Hardy s.
    Bekhterev's s.
    Berger's s.
    Bonhoeffer's s.
    Brauch-Romberg s.
    Buerger's s.
    Burghart's s.
    Capgras s.
    Cardarelli's s.
    cardinal s.
    Castellani-Low s.
    characteristic s.
    Chvostek's s.
    Colliver's s.
    concomitant s.
    consecutive s.
    constitutional s.
    crossbar s. of Fraenkel
    deficiency s.
    delayed s.
    direct s.
    dissociation s.
    endothelial s.
    Epstein's s.
    equivocal s.
    esophagosalivary s.
    Frenkel s.
    Froin s.
    fundamental s.
    Ganser s.
    general s.
    Goldthwait's s.
    gramophone s.
    Griesinger's s.
    guiding s.
    Haenel s.
    halo s.
    Huchard's s.
    incarceration s.
    indirect s.
    induced s.
    Jellinek's s.
    Jonas s.
    Kerandel's s.
    Kocher's s.

symp·tom *(continued)*
 Kussmaul s.
 labyrinthine s's
 Lade s.
 Liebreich's s.
 local s.
 localizing s's
 Loewi s.
 Magendie's s.
 Magnan's s.
 neighborhood s.
 nostril s.
 objective s.
 Oehler's s.
 passive s.
 pathognomonic s.
 Pel-Ebstein s.
 precursory s.
 premonitory s.
 presenting s.
 prodromal epileptic s.
 rainbow s.
 rational s.
 reflex s.
 Remak's s.
 Roger's s.
 Romberg-Howship s.
 Séguin's signal s.
 signal s.
 Skeer s.
 Sklowsky's s.
 static s.
 Stellwag's s.
 Stierlin's s.
 subjective s.
 sympathetic s.
 systemic s.
 Tar's s.
 Trendelenburg's s.
 Uhthoff s.
 Wartenberg's s.
 Weber's s.
 Wernicke's s.
 Westphal's s.
 withdrawal s's
symp·to·mat·ic
symp·tom·a·tol·o·gy
symp·to·ma·to·lyt·ic

symp·tome
symp·to·mo·lyt·ic
symp·to·sis
sym·pus
 s. apus
 s. dipus
 s. monopus
Syms's tractor
syn·a·del·phus
syn·ae·ti·on
Syn·a·lar
syn·al·bu·min
syn·al·gia
syn·al·gic
syn·anas·to·mo·sis
syn·an·che
syn·an·thrin
syn·an·throse
syn·aph·y·men·i·tis
syn·apse
 axoaxonic s.
 axodendritic s.
 axodendrosomatic s.
 axosomatic s.
 dendrodendritic s.
 electrogenic s.
 electrotonic s.
 en passant s.
 false s.
 loop s.
 neuromuscular s.
 pericorpuscular s.
syn·ap·sis
syn·ap·tene
syn·ap·tic
syn·ap·tol·o·gy
syn·ap·to·some
syn·ar·thro·dia
syn·ar·thro·di·al
syn·ar·thro·phy·sis
syn·ar·thro·ses
syn·ar·thro·sis *pl.* syn·ar·thro·ses
syn·ath·re·sis
syn·ath·roi·sis
syn·caine
syn·can·thus
syn·cary·on

syn·ce·lom
syn·ceph·a·lus
    s. asymmetros
syn·che·sis
syn·chi·lia
syn·chi·ria
syn·cho·lia
syn·chon·drec·to·my
syn·chon·dro·se·ot·o·my
syn·chon·dro·sis *pl.* syn·chon·
  dro·ses
    s. arycorniculata
    costoclavicular s.
    synchondroses craniales
    synchondroses cranii
    synchondroses of cranium
    intersphenoidal s.
    s. intersphenoidalis
    intraoccipital s., anterior
    intraoccipital s., posterior
    s. intra-occipitalis anterior
    s. intra-occipitalis posterior
    manubriosternal s.
    s. manubriosternalis
    petro-occipital s.
    s. petro-occipitalis
    pubic s.
    s. pubis
    sacrococcygeal s.
    synchondroses of skull
    sphenobasilar s.
    sphenoethmoidal s.
    s. spheno-ethmoidalis
    spheno-occipital s.
    s. spheno-occipitalis
    s. sphenopetrosa
    sphenopetrosal s.
    sternal s.
    s. sternalis
    s. xiphosternalis
syn·chon·drot·o·my
syn·cho·ri·al
syn·chro·nia
syn·chro·nism
syn·chro·ni·za·tion
    s. of potentials
syn·chro·nous
syn·chro·ny

syn·chro·ny
    bilateral s.
syn·chro·tron
syn·chy·sis
    s. scintillans
syn·ci·ne·sis
syn·ci·put
syn·cli·nal
syn·clit·ic
syn·clit·i·cism
syn·clit·ism
syn·clo·nus
    s. beriberica
syn·co·pal
syn·co·pe
    Adams-Stokes s.
    s. anginosa
    cardiac s.
    carotid sinus s.
    cough s.
    defecation s.
    digital s.
    heat s.
    laryngeal s.
    micturition s.
    orthostatic s.
    postural s.
    stretching s.
    swallow s.
    tussive s.
    vasodepressor s.
    vasovagal s.
syn·cop·ic
syn·cre·tio
Syn·cu·rine
syn·cy·tial
    respiratory s. virus (RSV)
syn·cyt·i·ol·y·sin
syn·cyt·i·o·ma
    s. malignum
syn·cyt·io·tox·in
syn·cyt·io·tropho·blast
syn·cy·ti·um
syn·cy·toid
syn·dac·tyl·ia
syn·dac·ty·lism
syn·dac·ty·lous
syn·dac·ty·lus

syn·dac·ty·ly
   complete s.
   complicated s.
   double s.
   partial s.
   simple s.
   single s.
   triple s.
syn·dec·to·my
syn·del·phus
syn·de·sine
syn·de·sis
syn·des·mec·to·my
syn·des·mec·to·pia
syn·des·mi·tis
   s. metatarsea
syn·des·mo·cho·ri·al
syn·des·mo·di·as·ta·sis
syn·des·mog·ra·phy
syn·des·mo·lo·gia
syn·des·mol·o·gy
syn·des·mo·ma
syn·des·mo-odon·toid
syn·des·mo·pexy
syn·des·mo·phyte
syn·des·mo·plas·ty
syn·des·mor·rha·phy
syn·des·mo·sis *pl.* syn·des·
  mo·ses
   radioulnar s.
   s. radio-ulnaris
   tibiofibular s.
   s. tibiofibularis
   s. tympanostapedia
   tympanostapedial s.
syn·des·mot·o·my
syn·drome
   Aarskog s.
   Aarskog-Scott s.
   Aase s.
   Abercrombie's s.
   abruptio placentae s.
   abstinence s.
   abused child s.
   accelerated conduction s.
   Achard s.
   Achard-Thiers s.

syn·drome *(continued)*
   acquired immune
     deficiency s. (AIDS)
   acquired immunodeficiency
     s. (AIDS)
   acute brain s.
   acute cervical
     centromedullary s.
   acute nephritic s.
   acute organic brain s.
   acute radiation s.
   acute retinal necrosis s.
   Adair-Dighton s.
   Adamantiades-Behçet s.
   Adams-Stokes s.
   addisonian s.
   adherence s.
   Adie's s.
   adiposogenital s.
   adrenal virilism s.
   adrenogenital s.
   Adson s.
   adult respiratory distress s.
     (ARDS)
   afferent loop s.
   aglossia-adactylia s.
   Ahumada-del Castillo s.
   Aicardi's s.
   akinetic-abulic s.
   Alajouanine's s.
   Albright's s.
   Albright-McCune-Sternberg-
     s.
   alcohol withdrawal s.
   Aldrich's s.
   Alezzandrini's s.
   "Alice in Wonderland" s.
   Allemann's s.
   Alport's s.
   Alström s.
   alveolar-capillary block s.
   alveolar hypoventilation s.
   amnesic s.
   amnestic s.
   amnestic-confabulatory s.
   amniotic band s.
   amniotic fluid s.

syn·drome *(continued)*

amniotic infection s. of Blane
amyostatic s.
Andersen's s.
androgen insensitivity s.
androgenital s.
Angelucci s.
angiectid s.
anginal s.
angular gyrus s.
aniridia-Wilms tumor s.
ankyloglossia superior s.
anorectal s.
anorexia-cachexia s.
anterior abdominal wall s.
anterior cerebral s.
anterior chamber cleavage s.
anterior choroidal artery s.
anterior compartment s.
anterior cord s.
anterior cornual s.
anterior spinal artery s.
anterior tibial compartment s.
anterior tibial nerve s.
anterolateral s.
anticholinergic s.
Anton's s.
Anton-Babinski s.
anxiety s.
aortic arch s.
aortoiliac steal s.
Apert's s.
aqueduct of Sylvius s.
argentaffinoma s.
Argonz-del Castillo s.
Arnold-Chiari s.
Arnold's nerve reflex cough s.
arthrogryposis s.
Ascher s.
Asherman's s.
Asherson's s.
asplenia s.
ataxia-telangiectasia s.
auriculotemporal s.

syn·drome *(continued)*

autoerythrocyte sensitization s.
autoimmune poly-endocrine-candidiasis s.
Avellis' s.
Avellis-Longhi s.
Axenfeld's s.
Ayerza's s.
Baastrup's s.
Babinski's s.
Babinski-Fröhlich s.
s. of Babinski-Nageotte
Babinski-Vaquez s.
bacterial overgrowth s.
BADS s.
Bäfverstedt's s.
Baillarger s.
Balint's s.
Ballantyne s.
Baller-Gerold s.
Bannwarth's s.
Banti's s.
Bard-Pick s.
Bardet-Biedl s.
Barlow s.
Barraquer-Simons' s.
Barré-Guillain s.
Barrett's s.
Barsony-Teschendof s.
Bart's s.
Bartter's s.
Bartter-Schwartz s.
basal cell nevus s.
Bassen-Kornzweig s.
Bastian s.
battered-child s.
Baumgarten's s.
Bazex's s.
BBB s.
Beals' s.
Bearn-Kunkel s.
Bearn-Kunkel-Slater s.
Beau's s.
Beckwith's s.
Beckwith-Wiedemann s.
Behçet's s.
s. of Benedikt

syn·drome *(continued)*
   Bennet s.
   Berardinelli s.
   Berardinelli-Seip s.
   Bernard's s.
   Bernard-Horner s.
   Bernard-Sergent s.
   Bernard-Soulier s. (BSS)
   Bernhardt-Roth s.
   Bernheim's s.
   Berry-Perkins-Young s.
   Bertolotti's s.
   Bianchi's s.
   Biedl s.
   Bielschowsky-Dollinger s.
   Biemond s., II
   Binder s.
   Bing-Neel s.
   Biörck s.
   Biörck-Thorson s.
   bisected brain s.
   Björnstad's s.
   Blackfan-Diamond s.
   Blatin's s.
   blind loop s.
   BLM (buccal-lingual-masticatory) s.
   Bloch-Sulzberger s.
   Bloom s.
   blue diaper s.
   blue sclera s.
   blue toe s.
   body of Luys s.
   Boerhaave's s.
   Bonnet sphenoidal foramen s.
   Bonnevie-Ullrich s.
   Bonnier's s.
   Böök's s.
   Börjeson's s.
   Börjeson-Forssman-Lehmann s.
   Bouillaud's s.
   Bourneville-Pelizzi s.
   Bourneville-Pringle s.
   Bouveret's s.
   bowel bypass s.
   brachial s.

syn·drome *(continued)*
   Brachmann-de Lange s.
   bradycardia-tachycardia s.
   Brennemann's s.
   Briquet's s.
   Brissaud-Marie s.
   Brissaud-Sicard s.
   Bristowe's s.
   brittle bone s.
   brittle cornea s.
   broad thumb-hallux s.
   Brock s.
   Brown sheath s.
   Brown's vertical retraction s.
   Brown-Séquard s.
   Bruns' s.
   Brunsting's s.
   Brushfield-Wyatt s.
   bubbly lung s.
   buccal-lingual-masticatory (BLM) s.
   Buckley's s.
   Budd-Chiari s.
   bulbar s.
   Bürger-Grütz s.
   Burnett's s.
   burning feet s.
   Buschke-Ollendorff s.
   Bywaters' s.
   Caffey's s.
   Caffey-Silverman s.
   Cairns s.
   calcarine artery s.
   callosal s.
   camptomelic s.
   Canada-Cronkhite s.
   Capgras' s.
   Caplan's s.
   capsular thrombosis s.
   capsulothalamic s.
   carcinoid s.
   cardioauditory s.
   cardiobulbar s.
   cardiofacial s.
   cardiopulmonary-obesity s.
   carotid sinus s.
   carpal tunnel s.

syn·drome *(continued)*

Carpenter's s.
cartilage-hair hypoplasia s.
Cassidy s.
Cassidy-Scholte s.
cat's cry s.
cat-eye s.
cat's eye s.
Cauchois-Eppinger-
   Frugoni s.
cauda equina s.
caudal dysplasia s.
caudal regression s.
cavernous sinus s.
celiac s.
celiac band s.
central cord s.
centroposterior s.
cerebellar s.
cerebellomedullary
   malformation s.
cerebellopontine angle s.
cerebellopyramidal s.
cerebellosympathetic s.
cerebellothalamic s.
cerebrocardiac s.
cerebrohepatorenal s.
cervical s.
cervical disk s.
cervical fusion s.
cervical radicular s.
cervical rib s.
cervical tension s.
cervicobrachial s.
cervicothoracic outlet s.
Cestan's s.
s. of Cestan-Chenais
Cestan-Raymond s.
chancriform s.
Charcot's s.
Charcot-Marie-Tooth-Hoffman s.
Charcot-Weiss-Baker s.
Charlin's s.
Chauffard's s.
Chauffard-Still s.
Chédiak-Higashi s.
Chiari's s.

syn·drome *(continued)*

Chiari-Arnold s.
Chiari-Frommel s.
chiasma s.
chiasmatic s.
Chilaiditi s.
Chinese restaurant s. (CRS)
Chotzen's s.
Christ-Siemens s.
Christ-Siemens-Touraine s.
Christian's s.
chromosome breakage s.
chronic brain s.
chronic organic brain s.
Churg-Strauss s.
Citelli's s.
Clarke-Hadefield s.
Claude's s.
Claude-Loyez s.
Claude's red nucleus s.
Claude Bernard–Horner s.
Clérambault-Kandinsky s.
click s.
closed head s.
Clough and Richter's s.
Clouston's s.
clumsy child s.
Cockayne's s.
Cogan's s.
cold agglutinin s.
Collet's s.
Collet-Sicard s.
combined
   immunodeficiency s.
compartmental s.
compression s.
concussion s.
Condorelli s.
congenital rubella s.
Conn's s.
Conradi's s.
Conradi-Hünermann s.
Conradi-Raap s.
contiguous gene s.
contracture s.
conus s.
Coote s.
Coote-Hunauld s.

syn·drome *(continued)*
  Cornelia de Lange's s.
  corpora quadrigeminal s.
  corpus callosum s.
  s. of corpus striatum
  Costen's s.
  costochondral s.
  costoclavicular s.
  costoclavicular
    compression s.
  Cotard's s.
  cough s.
  Courvoisier-Terrier s.
  couvade s.
  Cowden's s.
  CPD (chorioretinopathy
    and pituitary
    dysfunction) s.
  craniocarpotarsal s.
  craniosynostosis–radial
    aplasia s.
  CREST s.
  Creutzfeldt-Jakob s.
  cricopharyngeal achalasia
    s.
  cri du chat s.
  Crigler-Najjar s.
  s. of crocodile tears
  Cronkhite-Canada s.
  Cross s.
  Cross-McKusick-Breen s.
  CRST s.
  crus s.
  crush s.
  Cruveilhier-Baumgarten s.
  cryptophthalmia-syn-
    dactyly s.
  cryptophthalmos s.
  cubital s.
  cubital tunnel s.
  culture-specific s.
  Curtis and Fitz-Hugh s.
  Curtius' s.
  Cushing's s.
  Cushing's s. medicamen-
    tosus
  cutaneomucouveal s.
  Cyriax's s.

syn·drome *(continued)*
  cystic duct stump s.
  DaCosta's s.
  Danbolt-Closs s.
  dancing eye–dancing feet s.
  Dandy-Walker s.
  Danlos' s.
  dead fetus s.
  deafness-earpits s.
  Debré-de Toni-Fanconi s.
  Debré-Sémélaigne s.
  defibrination s.
  Degos' s.
  Dejerine's s.
  Dejerine's anterior bulbar
    s.
  Dejerine's interolivary s.
  Dejerine-Klumpke s.
  s. of Dejerine-Roussy
  Dejerine-Sottas s.
  de Lange's s.
  delayed stress s.
  del Castillo's s.
  de Morsier s.
  de Morsier-Gauthier s.
  dengue shock s.
  Dennie-Marfan s.
  Denny-Brown s.
  depersonalization s.
  depressive s.
  dermatostomato-ophthal-
    mic s.
  DES (diethylstilbestrol) s.
  De Sanctis-Cacchione s.
  de Toni-Debré-Fanconi s.
  de Toni-Fanconi s.
  dialysis disequilibrium s.
  Diamond-Blackfan s.
  diencephalic s.
  diencephalic s. of infancy
  DiGeorge s.
  Dighton-Adair s.
  Di Guglielmo s.
  DIMOAD s.
  Diogenes s.
  disk s.
  Donath-Landsteiner s.
  Donohue's s.

syn·drome *(continued)*

Down s.
Dresbach's s.
Dressler's s.
dry eye s.
Duane's s.
Dubin-Johnson s.
Dubin-Sprinz s.
Dubovitz s.
Dubreuil-Chambardel s.
Duchenne's s.
Duchenne-Erb s.
dumping s.
Duncan's s.
Dupré's s.
Dupuy s.
dwarfism-diabetes s.
Dyke-Davidoff s.
Dyke-Young s.
dysarthria–clumsy hand s.
dyscontrol s.
dysequilibrium s.
dysmnesic s.
dysplasia
   oculodentodigitalis s.
dysplastic nevus s.
dyssynchronous child s.
dystocia-dystrophia s.
Eagle-Barrett s.
Eaton-Lambert s.
ectopic ACTH s.
ectopic Cushing s.
ectopic-hypercalcemia s.
ectrodactyly-ectodermal
   dysplasia-clefting s.
Eddowes s.
Edwards's.
EEC s.
effort s.
egg-white s.
Ehlers-Danlos s.
Eisenmenger's s.
Ekbom s.
elbow pain s.
elfin facies s.
Ellis-van Creveld s.
embryonic testicular
   regression s.

syn·drome *(continued)*

EMG s.
emotional deprivation s.
empty nest s.
empty-sella s.
encephalotrigeminal
   vascular s.
endocrine polyglandular s.
eosinophilia-myalgia s.
eosinophilic s.
epiphyseal s.
Epstein's s.
Erb's s.
Erb-Oppenheim-Goldflam
   s.
Erdheim s.
Erdheim cystic medial s.
erythrocyte
   autosensitization s.
erythroderma-atopy-
   bamboo hair s.
Estren-Dameshek s.
E_1 trisomy s.
euthyroid sick s.
Evans's s.
exomphalos-macroglossia-gi-
   gantism s.
external carotid steal s.
extrapyramidal s.
Faber's s.
Fabry s.
facet s.
faciodigitogenital s.
Fallot's s.
Fanconi's s.
Farber s.
Farber-Uzman s.
Favre-Racouchot s.
Fazio-Londe s.
Fegeler s.
Felty's s.
feminizing testes s.
fertile eunuch s.
fetal alcohol s.
fetal aspiration s.
fetal distress s.
fetal face s.
fetal hydantoin s.

syn·drome *(continued)*
Fèvre-Languepin s.
fibrosing s.
Fiessinger-Leroy-Reiter s.
Fiessinger-Rendu s.
first arch s.
Fisher s.
Fitz s.
Fitz-Hugh–Curtis s.
Fitzgerald-Gardner s.
fleck s's
floppy infant s.
floppy valve s.
focal dermal hypoplasia s.
Foix paramedian s.
Foix-Alajouanine s.
Forbes-Albright s.
Forsius-Eriksson s.
Förster s.
Foster Kennedy s.
four-day s.
Foville's s.
Foville's median s.
Foville's peduncular s.
Foville's superior s.
fragile X s.
Franceschetti s.
Franceschetti-Jadassohn s.
François' s.
Fraser s.
Freeman-Sheldon s.
Frey's s.
Frey-Baillarger s.
Friderichsen-Waterhouse
　s.
Friedmann's vasomotor s.
Fröhlich's s.
Froin's s.
Frommel-Chiari s.
frontal lobe s.
Fuchs's s.
functional prepubertal
　castrate s.
G s.
Gailliard's s.
Gaisböck's s.
galactorrhea-amenorrhea
　s.

syn·drome *(continued)*
Ganser s.
Gardner's s.
Gardner-Diamond s.
Gasser's s.
gasserian s.
Gastaut s.
gay bowel s.
Gee-Herter-Heubner s.
Gélineau's s.
gender dysphoria s.
general adaptation s.
genital ulcer s.
Gerhardt's s.
Gerlier's s.
Gerstmann's s.
Gerstmann-Badal s.
Gianotti-Crosti s.
giant platelet s.
Gilbert s.,
Gilbert-Behçet s.
Gilles de la Tourette's s.
Gjessing s.
glioma-polyposis s.
s. of globus pallidus
glucagonoma s.
Goldenhar's s.
Goldstein-Reichmann s.
Goltz s.
Good's s.
Goodman s.
Goodpasture's s.
Gopalan's s.
Gordon s.
Gorlin-Goltz s.
Gorlin-Psaume s.
Gottron s.
Gougerot-Blum s.
Gougerot-Carteaud s.
Gougerot-Nulock-Houwer
　s.
Gowers' s.
gracilis s.
Gradenigo's s.
Gradenigo-Lannois s.
Graham Little s.
gray s.
gray baby s.

syn·drome *(continued)*
  gray platelet s.
  gray spinal s.
  Greig's s.
  Greither s.
  Griscelli s.
  Grisel-Bourgeois s.
  Grönblad-Strandberg s.
  Gruber's s.
  Guillain-Barré s.
  Gunn's s.
  gustatory sweating s.
  gynandrism s.
  gynecomastia-aspermatogen-
    esis s.
  Haber s.
  Hadefield-Clarke s.
  Hakim's s.
  Halbrecht s.
  Hallermann-Streiff s.
  Hallermann-Streiff-
    François s.
  Hallervorden-Spatz s.
  Hallgren s.
  Hallopeau-Siemens s.
  Hamman's s.
  Hamman-Rich s.
  hand-foot-and-mouth s.
  hand-foot-uterus s.
  Hand-Schüller-Christian s.
  hand-shoulder s.
  Hanhart's s.
  Hanot's s.
  Hanot-Chauffard s.
  happy-puppet s.
  Harada's s.
  Hare's s.
  Harris' s.
  Hartnup s.
  Haven s.
  Hawes-Pallister-Landor s.
  Hayem-Widal s.
  Head-Holmes s.
  heart-hand s.
  Hedinger s.
  Heerfordt's s.
  Heidenhaim's s.
  HELLP s.

syn·drome *(continued)*
  hemangioma-thrombocytope-
    nia s.
  hemohistioblastic s.
  hemolytic-uremic s.
  hemopleuropneumonic s.
  Hench-Rosenberg s.
  Henoch-Schönlein s.
  hepatocerebral s.
  hepatorenal s.
  hereditary benign
    intraepithelial
    dyskeratosis s.
  Hermansky-Pudlak s.
  herniated disk s.
  Hertwig-Magendie s.
  HHE (hemiplegia,
    hemiconvulsions, and
    epilepsy) s.
  high-pressure neurologic s.
    (HPNS)
  Hines-Bannick s.
  Hitzig s.
  Hoffmann s.
  Hoffmann-Werdnig s.
  holiday heart s.
  Holmes-Adie s.
  Holt-Oram s.
  Homén's s.
  Hoppe-Goldflam s.
  Horner's s.
  Horner-Bernard s.
  Horton's s.
  Houssay s.
  Houssay-Biasotti s.
  Howel-Evans' s.
  Hunt's s.
  Hunt striatal s.
  Hunter's s.
  Hunter-Hurler s.
  Hurler s.
  Hurler-Scheie s.
  Hutchinson's s.
  Hutchinson-Boeck s.
  Hutchinson-Gilford s.
  Hutchison s.
  hyaline membrane s.
  hydralazine lupus s.

syn·drome *(continued)*
17-hydroxylase deficiency s.
hyperabduction s.
hyperactive child s.
hypercalcemia s.
hypereosinophilic s.
hypergonadotropic s.
hyperimmunoglobulinemia E s.
hyperkinetic s.
hyperkinetic heart s.
hyperlucent lung s.
hyperophthalmopathic s.
hypersensitive xiphoid s.
hypersomnia-bulimia s.
hypertelorism-hypospadias s.
hyperventilation s.
hyperviscosity s.
hypoglossia-hypodactyly s.
hypo-osmolar s.
hypophysial s.
hypophysiodiencephalic s.
hypoplastic left-heart s.
hypospadias-dysphagia s.
hypothalamic s.
hypothalamic chiasmal s.
hypothalamic commissural s.
hypothalamohypophysial s.
ICE (irido-corneal-endothelial) s.
idiopathic postprandial s.
iliac compression s.
Imerslund s.
Imerslund-Graesbeck s.
Imerslund-Najman-Graesbeck s.
Imerslund immobilization s.
immotile-cilia s.
immunodeficiency s.
impingement s.
s. of inappropriate antidiuretic hormone (SIADH)

syn·drome *(continued)*
infantile cortical hyperostosis s.
infantile myxedema-muscular hypertrophy s.
inferior pontine s.
inferior s. of red nucleus
infraclinoid s.
infundibular s.
infundibulohypophysial s.
inhibitory s.
inspissated bile s.
internal capsule s.
internal carotid artery s.
intestinal polyposis-cutaneous pigmentation s.
intrauterine parabiotic s.
irido-corneal-endothelial (ICE) s.
irritable bowel s.
irritable colon s.
Irvine s.
Isaacs s.
Ivemark's s.
Jaccoud's s.
Jackson's s.
Jackson-Mackenzie s.
Jacod s.
Jacod-Negri s.
Jadassohn-Lewandowsky s.
Jaffe-Lichtenstein s.
Jahnke's s.
jaw-winking s.
Jefferson s.
jejunal s.
Jervell and Lange-Nielsen s.
Jeune's s.
Job s.
Jones-Nevin s.
Josephs-Blackfan-Diamond s.
jugular foramen s.
Kahlbaum s.
Kahlbaum-Wernicke s.
Kallmann's s.
Kanner's s.

syn·drome *(continued)*
- Karroo s.
- Kartagener's s.
- Kasabach-Merritt s.
- Kast's s.
- Kawasaki s.
- Kaznelson's s.
- Kearns-Sayre s.
- Kearns-Sayre-Shy s.
- Kehrer-Adie s.
- Kennedy's s.
- keratitis-ichthyosis-deafness-(KID) s.
- Kernohan s.
- Kestenbaum s.
- KID s.
- Kiloh-Nevin s.
- Kimmelstiel-Wilson s.
- kinky-hair s.
- Kinsbourne s.
- Klauder s.
- kleeblattschädel (cloverleaf skull) s.
- Klein-Waardenburg s.
- Kleine-Levin s.
- Klinefelter's s.
- Klippel-Feil s.
- Klippel-Trenaunay s.
- Klippel-Trenaunay-Weber s.
- Klumpke-Dejerine s.
- Klüver-Bucy s.
- Köbberling-Dunnigan s.
- Kocher-Debré-Sémélaigne s.
- Koerber-Salus-Elschnig s.
- König's s.
- Korsakoff's s.
- Kostmann's s.
- Krause's s.
- Kulenkampff-Tarnow s.
- Kunkel's s.
- lacunar s.
- Ladd's s.
- Lambert-Eaton s.
- Landry's s.
- Landry-Guillain-Barré s.
- Langer-Giedion s.

syn·drome *(continued)*
- Larsen's s.
- laryngeal-vertigo s.
- lateral bulbar s.
- lateral medullary s.
- lateral pontine s.
- Laubry-Soulle s.
- Launois' s.
- Launois-Cléret s.
- Laurence-Moon s.
- Laurence-Moon-Biedl s.
- Läwen-Roth s.
- Lawford's s.
- Lawrence-Seip s.
- lazy leukocyte s.
- left heart hypoplasia s.
- Legg-Calvé-Perthes s.
- Leigh s.
- Leitner s.
- Lejeune's s.
- Lennox s.
- Lennox-Gastaut s.
- Lenz's s.
- leopard s.
- Lépine-Froin s.
- Leredde's s.
- Léri-Weill s.
- Leriche's s.
- Lermoyez's s.
- Lesch-Nyhan s.
- levator s.
- Lévi-Lorain s.
- Lévy-Roussy s.
- Leyden-Moebius s.
- Lhermitte and McAlpine s.
- Libman-Sacks s.
- Lichtheim's s.
- Liddle s.
- Lightwood's s.
- Lignac's s.
- Lignac-Fanconi s.
- limp infant s.
- liver-kidney s.
- Lloyd s.
- Lobstein's s.
- "locked-in" s.
- loculation s.
- Löffler's s.

syn·drome *(continued)*
  Looser-Milkman s.
  Lorain-Lévi s.
  Louis-Bar s.
  Lowe s.
  Lowe-Terrey-MacLachlan
    s.
  lower radicular s.
  Lown-Ganong-Levine s.
  Lucey-Driscoll s.
  Luder-Sheldon s.
  lumbago-sciatica s.
  lupus-like s.
  Lutembacher's s.
  Lyell's s.
  lymphadenopathy s.
  lymphoproliferative s.
  lymphoreticular s's
  McArdle s.
  McCune-Albright s.
  Mackenzie's s.
  Macleod's s.
  Maffucci's s.
  malabsorption s.
  malarial hyperreactive
    spleen s.
  male Turner s.
  Malin's s.
  Mallory-Weiss s.
  mandibulo-oculofacial s.
  manic s.
  Marchesani's s.
  Marchiafava-Bignami s.
  Marchiafava-Micheli s.
  Marcus Gunn's s.
  Marcus Gunn inverse s.
  Marcus Gunn jaw-winking
    s.
  Marden-Walker s.
  Marfan s.
  Marie s.
  Marie-Bamberger s.
  Marin Amat s.
  Marinesco-Sjögren's s.
  Marinesco-Sjögren-
    Garland s.
  marker X s.
  Markus-Adie s.

syn·drome *(continued)*
  Maroteaux-Lamy s.
  Marshall's s.
  Martin-Bell s.
  Martorell's s.
  mastocytosis s.
  maternal deprivation s.
  Mauriac s.
  Mayer-Rokitansky-Küster-
    Hauser s
  Meckel's s.
  Meckel-Gruber s.
  meconium aspiration s.
  meconium blockage s.
  meconium plug s.
  medial longitudinal
    fasciculus s.
  median medullary s.
  megacystic s.
  megacystis-megaureter s.
  megacystis-microcolon
    intestinal hypoperistalsis
    s. (MMIHS)
  Meigs' s.
  Melkersson's s.
  Melkersson-Rosenthal s.
  Melnick-Needles s.
  Mendelson's s.
  Mengert's shock s.
  Meniere's s.
  meningeal s.
  meningococcic adrenal s.
  Menkes' s.
  metameric s.
  metastatic carcinoid s.
  methionine malabsorption
    s.
  Meyer-Schwickerath and
    Weyers s.
  Michel s.
  micrognathia-glossopthosis
    s.
  middle cerebral artery s.
  middle lobe s.
  midline s.
  Miege s.
  Miescher s.
  Mikulicz's s.

syn·drome *(continued)*
Mikulicz-Radecki s.
Mikulicz-Sjögren s.
milk-alkali s.
Milkman's s.
Millard-Gubler s.
Miller Fisher s.
minimal brain dysfunction s.
minimal chronic brain s.
Minkowski-Chauffard s.
minor contusion s.
Minot-von Willebrand s.
mitral valve prolapse s.
Möbius' s.
Moersch-Woltman s.
Mohr s.
Monakow's s.
monosomy s.
Moore's s.
morbid hunger s.
Morel's s.
Morel-Wildi s.
Morgagni's s.
Morgagni-Adams-Stokes s.
Morgagni-Stewart-Morel s.
morning glory s.
Morquio s.
Morquio-Brailsford s.
Morquio-Ullrich s.
Morris s.
Morton's s.
Morvan's s.
Mosse's s.
motor radicular s.
Mount s.
Mount-Reback s.
Moynahan s.
Muckle-Wells s.
mucocutaneous lymph node s. (MLNS)
mucosal neuroma s.
multiple glandular deficiency s.
multiple hamartoma s.
multiple lentigines s.
Munchausen s.
Munchausen s. by proxy

syn·drome *(continued)*
Münchmeyer s.
Murchison-Sanderson s.
myasthenia gravis s.
myasthenic s.
myasthenic-myopathic s.
myatonia congenita s.
myelofibrosis-osteosclerosis s.
myeloproliferative s.
myocardial postinfarction s.
myokymia-hyperhidrosis s.
myonephropathic metabolic s.
Naegeli s.
Naffziger's s.
Nager s.
nail-patella s.
Nelson's s.
neocerebellar s.
neonatal thymectomy s.
neostriatal s.
nephrotic s.
nerve compression s.
Netherton's s.
Neumann s.
neurocutaneous s.
neuroleptic malignant s.
nevoid basal cell carcinoma s.
nevoid basalioma s.
Nezelof s.
night-eating s.
nitritoid s.
Noack's s.
Nonne's s.
Nonne-Froin s.
Nonne-Marie s.
Nonne-Milroy-Meige s.
nonsense s.
Noonan's s.
Norman-Wood s.
Nothnagel's s.
OAV s.
ocular–mucous membrane s.
oculobuccogenital s.

syn·drome *(continued)*
  oculocerebral-hypopigmenta-
    tion s.
  oculocerebrorenal s.
  oculocutaneous s.
  oculodento-osseous s.
  oculoglandular s.
  oculomandibulofacial s.
  oculo-otocutaneous s. of
    Yuge
  oculopharyngeal s.
  oculovertebral s.
  oculovestibuloauditory s.
  ODD (oculodentodigital) s.
  odor-of-sweaty-feet s.
  OFD s.
  Ogilvie's s.
  Oldfield's s.
  olfactory groove s.
  OMM s.
  OPD (otopalatodigital) s.
  ophthalmoplegia-ataxia-
    areflexia s.
  opticopyramidal s.
  oral-facial-digital (OFD) s.,
    type I
  oral-facial-digital (OFD) s.,
    type II
  oral-facial-digital (OFD) s.,
    type III
  orbital apex s.
  organic anxiety s.
  organic brain s.
  organic delusional s.
  organic mental s.
  organic mood s.
  organic personality s.
  orofaciodigital (OFD) s.,
    type I
  orofaciodigital (OFD) s.,
    type II
  orogenital s.
  osteomyelofibrotic s.
  Ostrum-Furst s.
  otopalatodigital s.
  outlet s.
  ovarian-remnant s.
  ovarian vein s.

syn·drome *(continued)*
  oversuppression s.
  overwear s.
  Paget-von Schroetter s.
  pain dysfunction s.
  painful arc s.
  painful bruising s.
  paleocerebellar s.
  paleostriatal s.
  pallidal s.
  pallidomesencephalic s.
  Pancoast's s.
  pancreatic cholera s.
  pancreaticohepatic s.
  pancytopenia-dysmelia s.
  papillary muscle s.
  Papillon-Léage and
    Psaume s.
  Papillon-Lefèvre s.
  paramedian s.
  paramedian pontine s.
  paraneoplastic s.
  paratrigeminal s.
  parietal s.
  Parinaud's s.
  Parinaud's oculoglandular
    s.
  parkinsonian s.
  Parry-Romberg s.
  Parsonage-Turner s.
  Pasini-Pierini s.
  Patau's s.
  Paterson's s.
  Paterson-Brown-Kelly s.
  Paterson-Kelly s.
  Paxson s.
  peduncular s.
  Pellegrini-Stieda s.
  Pellizzi's s.
  pelvic congestion s.
  Pendred's s.
  Penfield s.
  penta-X s.
  Pepper s.
  pericolic-membrane s.
  periodic somnolence s.
  persistent müllerian duct s.
  pertussis s.

syn·drome *(continued)*

pertussis-like s.
Peters s.
petrosphenoid s.
Peutz-Jeghers s.
Pfeiffer's s.
pharyngeal pouch s.
PHC s.
phobic anxiety-
depersonalization s.
Picchini's s.
pickwickian s.
PIE (pulmonary
infiltration with
eosinophilia) s.
Pierre Robin s.
pineal s.
placental dysfunction s.
placental hemangioma s.
placental transfusion s.
pleurideficiency s.
pleuriglandular s.
Plummer-Vinson s.
Poland's s.
Polhemus-Schafer-Ivemark
s.
polyangiitis overlap s.
polycystic ovary s.
polyglandular s.
poly-X s.
pontine s.
pontocerebellar angle s.
popliteal entrapment s.
popliteal pterygium s.
popliteal web s.
postcardiac injury s.
postcardiotomy psychosis s.
postcholecystectomy s.
postcommissurotomy s.
postconcussional s.
posterior cerebral artery s.
posterior column s.
posterior cord s.
posterior cranial fossa s.
posterior lacertocondylar s.
posterolateral s.
postgastrectomy s.
postgonococcal urethritis s.

syn·drome *(continued)*

postinfarction s.
postirradiation s.
post–lumbar puncture s.
postmaturity s.
postmyocardial infarction
s.
postpartum
panhypopituitary s.
postpartum pituitary
necrosis s.
postperfusion s.
postpericardiotomy s.
postphlebitic s.
post-thrombotic s.
post-transfusion s.
post-traumatic brain s.
post-traumatic cervical s.
postvalvulotomy s.
Potter's s.
Pötzel's s.
P-pulmonale s.
Prader-Willi s.
preexcitation s.
prefrontal s.
premature senility s.
premenstrual s.
premotor s.
Profichet's s.
pronator s.
prune-belly s.
pseudo-Turner s.
pseudoclaudication s.
puffy hand s.
pulmonary acid aspiration
s.
pulmonary dysmaturity s.
pulmonary-renal s.
punch-drunk s.
Putnam-Dana s.
Putti s.
QT s.
Racine s.
radial s.
radiation s.
radicular s.
radiculoneuritic s.
Raeder s.

syn·drome *(continued)*
  Ramsay Hunt s.
  Raymond s.
  Raymond-Cestan s.
  Raynaud's s.
  red diaper s.
  Refsum's s.
  Reichmann's s.
  Reifenstein's s.
  Reiter's s.
  release s.
  Rendu-Osler-Weber s.
  residual ovary s.
  respiratory distress s. of
    newborn
  restless legs s.
  retraction s.
  retrolenticular s.
  s. of retroparotid space
  retrosubthalamic s.
  Rett s.
  Reye's s.
  Reynold-Revillod-Dejerine
    s.
  Rh-null s.
  rib-tip s.
  Richards-Rundle s.
  Richter's s.
  Rieder s.
  Rieger's s.
  Riley-Day s.
  Riley-Smith s.
  Robert's s.
  Robertson s.
  Robin s.
  Robinow's s.
  Rochan-Duvigneaud s.
  Roger's s.
  Rokitansky-Küster-Hauser
    s.
  rolandic vein s.
  Romano-Ward s.
  Romberg-Howship s.
  Rosenbach's s.
  Rosenberg-Chutorian s.
  Rosenthal s.
  Rosenthal-Kloepfer s.
  Rosewater's s.

syn·drome *(continued)*
  Rot's s.
  Rot-Bernhardt s.
  rotational shift s.
  Roth's s.
  Roth-Bernhardt s.
  Rothmann-Makai s.
  Rothmund s.
  Rothmund-Thomson s.
  Rotor's s.
  Roussy-Dejerine s.
  Roussy-Lévy s.
  Rovsing s.
  RSH s.
  rubella s.
  Rubinstein's s.
  Rubinstein-Taybi s.
  rubrospinal cerebellar
    peduncle s.
  Rud's s.
  rudimentary testis s.
  Rundles-Falls s.
  runting s.
  Russell's s.
  Rust's s.
  Ruvalcaba's s.
  Sabin-Feldman s.
  Sabinas s.
  Saethre-Chotzen s.
  sagittal imbalance s.
  Sakati-Nyhan s.
  salt-depletion s.
  salt-losing s.
  Sandifer's s.
  Sanfilippo's s.
  Sanger-Brown s.
  scalded skin s.,
    nonstaphylococcal
  scalded skin s.,
    staphylococcal
  scalenus s.
  scalenus anticus s.
  scapulocostal s.
  Schafer's s.
  Schanz's s.
  Schaumann's s.
  Scheie's s.
  Schirmer's s.

syn·drome *(continued)*
Schmid-Fraccaro s.
Schmidt's s.
Schönlein-Henoch s.
Schüller's s.
Schüller-Christian s.
Schultz s.
Schwachman s.
Schwartz-Bartter s.
Schwartz-Jampel s.
scimitar s.
s. of sea-blue histiocyte
Seabright bantam s.
Seckel's s.
segmentary s.
Seip s.
Seip-Lawrence s.
Selye s.
Senear-Usher s.
s. of sensory dissociation
  with brachial
  amyotrophy
Senter s.
Sertoli-cell–only s.
serum sickness-like s.
Sézary s.
Sheehan's s.
Sheehy s.
Shone's s.
short-bowel s.
short-gut s.
shoulder-hand s.
shoulder-neck s.
Shwachman s.
Shwachman-Diamond s.
Shy-Drager s.
Sicard's s.
Sicard's posterior condylar
  s.
sicca s.
sick sinus s.
Sidbury s.
sideropenic s.
Silver's s.
Silver-Russell s.
Silverskiöld's s.
Silvestrini-Corda s.
Simmonds' s.

syn·drome *(continued)*
Sipple's s.
Sjögren's s.
Sjögren-Larsson s.
sleep apnea s.
SLE-like s.
Sluder's s.
Sly s.
small meal s.
Smith-Lemli-Opitz s.
social breakdown s.
Sohval-Soffer s.
somnolence s.
Sorsby's s.
Sotos' s.
Sotos' s. of cerebral
  gigantism
space adaptation s.
Spens's s.
spherophakia-brachy-
  morphia s.
Spiller s.
spinal block s.
splenic flexure s.
split-brain s.
Sprinz-Dubin s.
Sprinz-Nelson s.
Spurway s.
stagnant loop s.
stasis s.
static cerebellar s.
Steele-Richardson-
  Olszewski s.
steely-hair s.
Stein-Leventhal s.
Steinbrocker's s.
Steiner's s.
steroid withdrawal s.
Stevens-Johnson s.
Stewart-Morel s.
Stewart-Treves s.
Stickler s.
"stiff heart" s.
stiff-man s.
Still-Chauffard s.
Stilling s.
Stilling-Turk-Duane s.
stippled epiphyses s.

syn·drome *(continued)*
 Stokes' s.
 Stokes-Adams s.
 Stokvis-Talma s.
 Strachan's s.
 Strachan-Scott s.
 straight back s.
 striatal s.
 striocortical s.
 striopallidal s.
 stroke s.
 Strudwick s.
 Stuart-Bras s.
 Sturge's s.
 Sturge-Kalischer-Weber s.
 Sturge-Weber s.
 subclavian steal s.
 subcoracoid-pectoralis
  minor s.
 substantia nigra s.
 subthalamic s.
 sudden infant death s.
 sudden unexplained death
  s.
 Sudeck-Leriche s.
 Sulzberger-Garbe s.
 superior caval s.
 superior cerebellar artery
  s.
 superior mesenteric artery
  s.
 superior midbrain s.
 superior orbital fissure s.
 superior pontine s.
 superior sulcus tumor s.
 superior vena cava s.
 supine hypotensive s.
 supraspinatus s.
 surdocardiac s.
 survivor s.
 swallowed blood s.
 sweat retention s.
 sweaty feet s.
 Sweet's s.
 Swyer-James s.
 Swyer-James-Macleod s.
 sylvian s.
 sylvian aqueduct s.

syn·drome *(continued)*
 sylvian artery s.
 syringomelic s.
 Takayasu's s.
 Tapia's s.
 tarsal tunnel s.
 Taussig-Bing s.
 tegmental s.
 telangiectasia-pigmenta-
  tion cataract s.
 temporomandibular
  dysfunction s.
 temporomandibular joint s.
 Terry's s.
 Terson's s.
 testicular dysgenesis s.
 testicular feminization s.
 tethered cord s.
 tetra-X s.
 thalamic s.
 thalidomide s.
 Thibierge-Weissenbach s.
 Thiele s.
 Thiemann's s.
 thoracic outlet s.
 Thorn's s.
 Thorn salt-depletion s.
 thrombocytopenia–absent
  radius (TAR) s.
 thromboembolic s.
 thrombopathic s.
 Tietze's s.
 tired housewife s.
 Tolosa-Hunt s.
 Tommaselli's s.
 TORCH (toxoplasmosis,
  rubella, cytomegalovirus,
  herpes) s.
 Torres' s.
 total allergy s.
 Touraine-Solente-Golé s.
 Tourette s.
 toxic fat s.
 toxic shock s.
 transcortical s.
 transfusion s.
 translocation Down s.
 transplant lung s.

syn·drome *(continued)*
- traumatic vasospastic s.
- Treacher Collins s.
- Treacher Collins-Franceschetti s.
- triad s.
- trichorhinophalangeal s.
- triparanol s.
- triple-X s.
- trisomy 8 s.
- trisomy 13 s.
- trisomy 18 s.
- trisomy 21 s.
- trisomy 22 s.
- trisomy C s.
- trisomy D s.
- trisomy E s.
- Troisier's s.
- tropical splenomegaly s.
- Trousseau's s.
- tuberohypophysial s.
- tuberoinfundibular s.
- tumor lysis s.
- Turcot s.
- Turner's s.
- Turner's s., male
- Turner-Keiser s.
- Ullrich s.
- Ullrich-Feichtiger s.
- Ullrich-Turner s.
- unilateral nevoid telangiectasia s.
- Unna-Thost s.
- Unverricht's s.
- urethral s.
- Usher s.
- uveoparotid s.
- vagoaccessory s.
- van Bogaert-Divry s.
- van Bogaert-Scherer-Epstein s.
- van Buchem's s.
- van der Hoeve's s.
- van der Hoeve-de Kleyn s.
- Van der Woude's s.
- vanishing testes s.
- vascular s.

syn·drome *(continued)*
- vasculitis-hypersensitivity s.
- velopalatine myoclonic s.
- Verbiest s.
- Verger-Dejerine s.
- vermis s.
- Verner-Morrison s.
- Vernet's s.
- vertebrobasilar s.
- vertical retraction s.
- Vieusseux-Wallenberg s.
- Villaret's s.
- Vinson's s.
- Vogt's s.
- Vogt-Koyanagi s.
- Vogt-Koyanagi-Harada s.
- Vohwinkel's s.
- Volkmann's s.
- von Hippel-Lindau s.
- von Mikulicz s.
- vulnerable child s.
- Waardenburg's s.
- WAGR s.
- Wallenberg's s.
- Ward-Romano s.
- Waterhouse-Friderichsen s.
- WDHA s.
- s. of Weber
- Weber-Christian s.
- Weber-Cockayne s.
- Weber-Dubler s.
- Weber-Leyden s.
- Wegener's s.
- Weil's s.
- Weill-Marchesani s.
- Weill-Reys s.
- Weill-Reys-Adie s.
- Weingarten's s.
- Wermer's s.
- Werner s.
- Wernicke's s.
- Wernicke-Korsakoff s.
- West s.
- Weyers' oligodactyly s.
- whiplash shake s.
- whistling face s.

syn·drome *(continued)*
    whistling face–windmill
      vane hand s.
    Widal s.
    Wildervanck s.
    Wilks s.
    Willebrand's s.
    Williams s.
    Williams-Campbell s.
    Wilson's s.
    Wilson-Mikity s.
    Winter's s.
    Wiskott-Aldrich s.
    Wissler-Fanconi s.
    withdrawal s.
    Wolf-Hirschhorn s.
    Wolff-Parkinson-White s.
    Wolfram s.
    Woltman-Kernohan s.
    Woringer-Kolopp s.
    Wright's s.
    X-linked
      lymphoproliferative s.
    XO s.
    XXXX s.
    XXXXY s.
    XXY s.
    yellow nail s.
    yellow vernix s.
    Young's s.
    Yuge s.
    ZE (Zollinger-Ellison) s.
    Zellweger s.
    Zieve s.
    Zinsser-Cole-Engman s.
    Zollinger-Ellison s.
syn·drom·ic
syn·dro·mol·o·gist
syn·drom·ol·o·gy
Syn·drox
syn·ech·ia *pl.* syn·ech·iae
    annular s.
    anterior s.
    circular s.
    s. pericardii
    posterior s.
    ring s.
    total anterior s.

syn·ech·ia *(continued)*
    total posterior s.
    s. vulvae
syn·ech·i·al·y·sis
syn·echo·tome
syn·echot·o·my
syn·ech·ten·ter·ot·o·my
syn·ecol·o·gy
Syn·e·mol
syn·en·ceph·a·lo·cele
syn·en·ceph·a·lus
syn·en·ceph·a·ly
syn·er·e·sis
syn·er·gen·e·sis
syn·er·get·ic
syn·er·gia
syn·er·gic
syn·er·gism
syn·er·gist
syn·er·gis·tic
syn·er·gy
syn·es·the·sia
    s. algica
syn·es·the·si·al·gia
syn·e·ze·sis
syn·ga·mous
syn·ga·my
syn·ge·ne·ic
syn·ge·ne·sio·graft
syn·ge·ne·sio·plas·tic
syn·ge·ne·sio·trans·plan·ta·
  tion
syn·gen·e·sis
syn·gna·thia
syn·gon·ic
syn·graft
syn·hex·yl
syn·hi·dro·sis
syn·i·ze·sis
    s. pupillae
syn·kary·on
Syn·kay·vite
syn·ki·ne·sia
syn·ki·ne·sis
    brachiobranchial s.
    contralateral s.
    coordination s.
    crurocrural s.

syn·ki·ne·sis *(continued)*
    imitative s.
    mouth-and-hand s.
    reflex s.
    spasmodic s.
syn·ki·net·ic
syn·ne·cro·sis
syn·ne·ma·tin
syn·neu·ro·sis
syn·o·cha
syn·o·chal
syn·onych·ia
syn·o·nym·ize
syn·oph·rid·ia
syn·oph·rys
syn·oph·thal·mia
syn·oph·thal·mus
Syn·o·phy·late
syn·op·to·phore
syn·or·chi·dism
syn·or·chism
syn·os·che·os
syn·os·te·ol·o·gy
syn·os·te·o·sis
syn·os·te·ot·ic
syn·os·te·ot·o·my
syn·os·to·sis *pl.* syn·os·to·ses
    cranial s.
    radioulnar s.
    sagittal s.
    tarsal s.
    transphalangeal s.
    tribasilar s.
syn·os·tot·ic
sy·no·tia
sy·no·tus
syn·o·vec·to·my
    radioisotope s.
sy·no·via
sy·no·vi·al
sy·no·vi·a·lis
sy·no·vi·a·lo·ma
sy·no·vi·anal·y·sis
sy·no·vin
sy·no·vio·blast
sy·no·vio·cyte
sy·no·vi·o·ma
    benign s.

sy·no·vi·o·ma *(continued)*
    malignant s.
sy·no·vi·or·these
sy·no·vi·or·the·sis
sy·no·vi·or·tho·sis
sy·no·vio·sar·co·ma
syn·o·vip·a·rous
syno·vi·tis
    bursal s.
    chronic purulent s.
    dendritic s.
    dry s.
    filiarial s.
    fungous s.
    s. hyperplastica
    localized nodular s.
    pigmented villonodular s.
    proliferative s.
    puerperal s.
    purulent s.
    scarlatinal s.
    serous s.
    s. sicca
    simple s.
    suppurative s.
    tendinous s.
    transient s.
    traumatic s.
    tuberculous s.
    vaginal s.
    vibration s.
    villonodular s.
syn·phal·an·gism
syn·pneu·mon·ic
syn·re·flex·ia
syn·tac·tic
syn·ta·sis
syn·tax·is
syn·tec·tic
syn·ten·ic
syn·te·no·sis
syn·te·ny
syn·ter·e·sis
syn·ter·et·ic
syn·tex·is
syn·thase
    lanosterol s.
    pantothenate s.

syn·ther·mal
syn·the·sis
    s. of continuity
    de novo s.
    distributive s.
    inducible enzyme s.
    morphologic s.
    unscheduled DNA s.
syn·the·size
syn·the·siz·er
    speech s.
syn·the·tase
    heme s.
syn·thet·ic
syn·the·tism
syn·tho·rax
Syn·throid
Syn·to·ci·non
syn·ton·ic
syn·to·nin
syn·to·pie
syn·to·py
syn·trip·sis
Syn·tro·pan
syn·troph·ism
syn·tropho·blast
syn·trop·ic
syn·tro·py
    inverse s.
syn·u·lo·sis
syn·u·lot·ic
Syn·u·ra
syn·xen·ic
syph·i·le·mia
syph·i·lid
    acuminate papular s.
    annular s.
    ecthymatous s.
    erythematous s.
    follicular s.
    macular s.
    papulosquamous s.
    pemphigoid s.
    pigmentary s.
    pustular s.
    roseolar s.
    secondary s.
    serpiginous s.

syph·i·lide *pl.* syph·i·lides
syph·i·lid·oph·thal·mia
syph·i·lis
    acquired s.
    cardiovascular s.
    cerebrospinal s.
    congenital s.
    early s.
    early latent s.
    s. d'emblée
    endemic s.
    equine s.
    gummatous s.
    s. hereditaria tarda
    horse s.
    late s.
    late benign s.
    late latent s.
    latent s.
    meningovascular s.
    noduloulcerative s.
    nonvenereal s.
    parenchymatous s.
    prenatal s.
    primary s.
    rabbit s.
    secondary s.
    tertiary s.
syph·i·lit·ic
syph·i·lol·o·gist
syph·i·lo·ma
syph·i·lo·ma·nia
syph·i·lom·a·tous
syph·i·lo·nech·ia
    s. sicca
    s. ulcerans
syph·i·lo·pho·bia
Syr. — L. syrupus (syrup)
syr·ig·mo·pho·nia
sy·rig·mus
syr·ing·ad·e·no·ma
    papillary s.
syr·ing·ad·e·no·sis
sy·ringe
    air s.
    Anel's s.
    aural s.
    chip s.

sy·ringe *(continued)*
    continuous-flow s.
    dental s.
    ear s.
    fountain s.
    hand air s.
    hypodermic s.
    Luer's s.
    Luer-Lok s.
    probe s.
    two-way s.
    water s.
    wound s.
syr·in·gec·to·my
syr·in·gi·tis
sy·rin·go·ad·e·no·ma
sy·rin·go·bul·bia
sy·rin·go·car·ci·no·ma
sy·rin·go·cele
sy·rin·go·coele
sy·rin·go·cys·tad·e·no·ma
    s. papilliferum
sy·rin·go·cys·to·ma
sy·rin·go·en·ce·pha·lia
sy·rin·go·en·ceph·a·lo·my·e·
    lia
sy·rin·goid
sy·rin·go·ma
    chondroid s.
sy·rin·go·me·nin·go·cele
sy·rin·go·my·e·lia
    traumatic s.
sy·rin·go·my·eli·tis
syr·in·go·my·elo·bul·bia
sy·rin·go·my·elo·cele
sy·rin·go·my·elus
sy·rin·go·pon·tia
sy·rin·go·tome
sy·rin·got·o·my
syr·inx *pl.* syr·in·ges
sy·ro·sin·go·pine
Syr·phi·dae
syr·up
    acacia s.
    amantadine hydrochloride
      s.
    aminocaproic acid s.
    aromatic eriodictyon s.

syr·up *(continued)*
    bromides s.
    cacao s.
    cherry s.
    chloral hydrate s.
    chlorpheniramine maleate
      s.
    chlorpromazine
      hydrochloride s.
    citric acid s.
    cocoa s.
    compound sarsaparilla s.
    corn s.
    cyproheptadine
      hydrochloride s.
    demethylchlortetracycline
      s.
    dexchlorpheniramine
      maleate s.
    dextromethorphan
      hydrobromide s.
    dicyclomine hydrochloride
      s.
    dihydrocodeinone
      bitartrate s.
    dimenhydrinate s.
    dimethindene maleate s.
    dioctyl sodium
      sulfosuccinate s.
    docusate sodium s.
    doxylamine succinate s.
    ephedrine sulfate s.
    eriodictyon s., aromatic
    ferrous iodide s.
    ferrous sulfate s.
    garlic s.
    ginger s.
    glyceryl guaiacolate s.
    glycyrrhiza s.
    guaifenesin s.
    hydriodic acid s.
    hydrocodone bitartrate s.
    hydroxyzine hydrochloride
      s.
    ipecac s.
    isoniazid s.
    lemon s.
    licorice s.

syr·up *(continued)*
  s. of liquid glucose
  medicated s.
  meperidine hydrochloride
    s.
  methapyrilene fumarate s.
  methdilazine hydrochloride
    s.
  orange s.
  phenindamine tartrate s.
  piperazine citrate s.
  prochlorperazine edisylate
    s.
  promazine hydrochloride s.
  promethazine
    hydrochloride s.
  pseudoephedrine
    hydrochloride s.
  pyridostigmine bromide s.
  raspberry s.
  senna s.
  simple s.
  s. of squills
  s. of tolu
  tolu balsam s.
  triamcinolone diacetate s.
  trifluoperazine
    hydrochloride s.
  trimeprazine tartrate s.
  triprolidine hydrochloride
    s.
  white pine s., compound
  white pine s., compound,
    with codeine
  wild cherry s.
  Yerba santa s., aromatic
sys·sar·co·sic
sys·sar·co·sis
sys·sar·cot·ic
sys·so·mus
sys·tal·tic
sys·tat·ic
sys·tem
  ABO blood group s.
  accessory portal s. of
    Sappey
  adipose s.
  adrenergic s.

sys·tem *(continued)*
  alimentary s.
  anesthesia-breathing s.
  arch-loop-whorl s.
  ascending reticular
    activating s.
  association s.
  autonomic nervous s.
  balanced lethal s.
  Batson's s.
  biliary s.
  biological s.
  blood group s.
  blood-vascular s.
  boarding-out s.
  body exhaust s.
  Boorman gastric cancer
    typing s. (I-IV)
  brain cooling s.
  brain stem activating s.
  breathing s.
  buffer s.
  bulbospiral s.
  cardiovascular s.
  case s.
  centimeter-gram-second s.
  central nervous s. (CNS)
  centrencephalic s.
  cerebellorubral s.
  cerebellorubrospinal s.
  cerebrospinal s.
  CGS (centimeter-gram-
    second) s.
  CGS electromagnetic s.
  chemoreceptor s.
  chromaffin s.
  circle absorption s.
  circulatory s.
  coherent s. of units
  complement s.
  complete nonrebreathing s.
  conducting s. of heart
  conduction s. of heart
  coordinate s.
  corticobulbar s.
  corticopontine projection s.
  corticopontocerebellar s.
  corticostrionigral s.

sys·tem *(continued)*
  craniosacral autonomic
    nervous s.
  cutaneous s.
  dentatorubral s.
  dentinal s.
  dermal s.
  dermoid s.
  digestive s.
  dioptric s.
  disperse s.
  dispersion s.
  dopaminergic s.
  dosimetric s.
  dual-probe s.
  duplex scanning s.
  ecological s.
  endocrine s.
  endothelial s.
  endovestibular s.
  exteroceptive nervous s.
  extracorticospinal s.
  extrapyramidal s.
  flush s.
  fusimotor s.
  Galton s. of classification of
    fingerprints
  gamma efferent s.
  gamma motor s.
  genital s.
  genitourinary s.
  glandular s.
  Grosse and Kempf locking
    nail s.
  haversian s.
  hematopoietic s.
  hemolytic s.
  Henry's s.
  Henry s. of classification of
    fingerprints
  hepatic duct s.
  hepatic portal s.
  heterogeneous s.
  hexaxial reference s.
  H-2 histocompatibility s.
  HLA histocompatibility s.
  homogeneous s.
  hormonopoietic s.

sys·tem *(continued)*
  humoral amplification s's
  hypophyseoportal s.
  hypophysioportal s.
  hypothalamoneurohypophy-
    sial s.
  hypothalmohypophysial s.
  hypoxia warning s.
  immune s.
  inducible s.
  integumentary s.
  interfusal motor s.
  International 10-20 s.
  International S. of Units
  interoceptive nervous s.
  interofective s.
  interrenal s.
  interstitial s.
  involuntary nervous s.
  kallikrein s.
  keratinizing s.
  kinesiodic s.
  kinety s.
  kinin s.
  labyrinthine s.
  limbic s.
  Luhr maxillofacial s.
  lymphatic s.
  lymphoid s.
  lymphoreticular s.
  McIntire
    aspiration-irrigation s.
  macrophage s.
  malpighian s.
  Manchester s.
  masticatory s.
  mastigont s.
  melanocyte s.
  metameric nervous s.
  metanephric excretory s.
  metanephric secretory s.
  meter-kilogram-second s.
  metric s.
  Meyer's s.
  microcirculatory s.
  MKS (meter-kilogram-
    second) s.

sys·tem *(continued)*
 mobile artery and vein
  imaging s. (MAVIS)
 mononuclear phagocyte s.
  (MPS)
 muscular s.
 musculoskeletal s.
 neokinetic s.
 nervous s.
 neuromuscular s.
 nonspecific s.
 oculomotor s.
 open s.
 pallidal s.
 palm-and-sole s. of
  identification
 parasympathetic nervous s.
 peripheral nervous s.
 periventricular s.
 phagocytic s.
 pigmentary s.
 pituitary portal s.
 plenum s.
 pneumatic s. of temporal
  bone
 portal s.
 pressoreceptor s.
 projection s.
 properdin s.
 proprioceptive nervous s.
 Purkinje s.
 pyramidal s.
 renin-angiotension-
  aldosterone s.
 reproductive s.
 resonating s.
 respiratory s.
 reticular activating s.
 reticuloendothelial s. (RES)
 rubrospinal s.
 schlieren s.
 self s.
 sensory storage s.
 SI s.
 sinospiral s.
 skeletal s.
 somatic nervous s.
 somesthetic s.

sys·tem *(continued)*
 stomatognathic s.
 supraopticohypophysial s.
 supraopticoneurohypophysi-
  al s.
 sympathetic nervous s.
 T s.
 thoracicolumbar
  autonomic nervous s.
 to-and-fro absorption s.
 triad s.
 urinary s.
 urogenital s.
 uropoietic s.
 vagal autonomic s.
 vascular s.
 vasomotor s.
 vegetative nervous s.
 vertebral-basilar s.
 vertebral-venous s.
 vestibular s.
 villa s.
 visceral nervous s.
 Waring's s.
sys·te·ma
 s. conducens cardiacum
 s. conducens cordis
 s. digestorium
 s. lymphaticum
 s. nervosum
 s. nervosum autonomicum
 s. nervosum autonomicum,
  pars parasympathetica
 s. nervosum autonomicum,
  pars sympathetica
 s. nervosum centrale
 s. nervosum periphericum
 s. nervosum
  sympatheticum
 s. respiratorium
 s. skeletale
 s. urogenitale
 s. vasorum
sys·te·mat·ic
sys·te·mat·ics
sys·tem·a·ti·za·tion
sys·te·ma·tol·o·gy

Sys·tème In·ter·na·tio·nal
  d'Uni·tés
sys·tème sé·cant
sys·tem·ic
  s. lupus erythematosus
    (SLE)
sys·te·moid
sys·to·le
  aborted s.
  atrial s.
  end s.
  extra s.
  frustrate s.
  premature s.

sys·to·le *(continued)*
  ventricular s.
sys·tol·ic
sys·to·lom·e·ter
sys·trem·ma
Sy·to·bex
sy·zyg·i·al
sy·zyg·i·ol·o·gy
sy·zyg·i·um
syz·y·gy
Sza·bo's test
Szent-Györ·gyi reaction
Szon·di's test
Szy·ma·now·ski's operation

T

T — intraocular tension
  temperature
  tera-
  tesla
  thoracic vertebrae
    (T1–T12)
  threonine
  thymidine
  thymine
  time
T^+ — increased intraocular
  tension
T^- — decreased intraocular
  tension
T — absolute temperature
  transmittance
$T_{1/2}$ — half-life
  half-time
T_3 — triiodothyronine
T_4 — thyroxine
T_m — melting temperature
  tubular maximum
t — translocation
t — time and temperature
$t_{1/2}$ — half-life

$t_{1/2}$ — half-life
  half-time
τ — mean life
  torque
TA — toxin-antitoxin
tab·a·cism
tab·a·co·sis
tab·a·cum
tab·a·gism
tab·a·nid
Ta·ba·nus
  T. atratus
  T. bovinus
  T. ditaeniatus
  T. fasciatus
  T. gratus
  T. lineola
  T. nigrovittatus
  T. punctifer
  T. quinquevittatus
  T. similis
  T. sulcifrons
tab·ar·di·llo
ta·ba·tière ana·to·mique
ta·be·fac·tion

ta·bel·la *pl.* ta·bel·lae
tab·er·nan·thine
ta·bes
    cerebral t.
    cervical t.
    diabetic t.
    t. dorsalis
    t. ergotica
    Friedreich's t.
    t. infantum
    t. mesaraica
    t. mesenterica
    peripheral t.
    t. spasmodica
    t. spinalis
    t. superior
ta·bes·cent
ta·bet·ic
ta·bet·i·form
tab·ic
tab·id
tab·i·fi·ca·tion
tab·la·ture
ta·ble
    abridged life t.
    Albee fracture t.
    Aub-Dubois t.
    Bull and Fischer mortality
      t's
    CHICK fracture t.
    cohort life t.
    complete life t.
    contingency t.
    demographic life t.
    Ely's t.
    fourfold t.
    Gaffky t.
    inner t. of frontal bone
    inner t. of skull
    life t.
    Mendeleev's t.
    mortality t.
    occlusal t.
    outer t. of frontal bone
    outer t. of skull
    periodic t.
    Reuss' t's
    Stintzing's t's

ta·ble *(continued)*
    vitreous t.
    water t.
ta·ble·spoon
tab·let
    buccal t.
    dispensing t.
    enteric-coated t.
    hypodermic t.
    sublingual t.
    t. triturate
ta·boo
ta·bo·pa·ral·y·sis
ta·bo·pa·re·sis
tab·u·la *pl.* tab·u·lae
    t. externa ossis cranii
    t. interna ossis cranii
    t. vitrea
tab·u·lar
Tac·a·ryl
TACE
tache
    t. blanche
    t's bleuâtres
    t. cérébrale
    t's laiteuses
    t. méningéale
    t. motrice
    t. noire
    t's noire sclérotiques
    t. spinale
ta·chis·to·scope
ta·chis·tos·co·py
tacho·gram
tach·og·ra·phy
tachy·al·i·men·ta·tion
tachy·ar·rhyth·mia
tachy·aux·e·sis
tachy·car·dia
    atrial t.
    bidirectional t.
    double t.
    ectopic t.
    fetal t.
    junctional t.
    nodal t.
    orthostatic t.
    paroxysmal t.

tachy·car·dia *(continued)*
   paroxysmal atrial t.
   paroxysmal nodal t.
   paroxysmal ventricular t.
   reflex t.
   sinus t.
   t. strumosa exophthalmica
   supranodal t.
   supraventricular t.
   ventricular t.
tachy·car·di·ac
tachy·car·dic
tachy·gen·e·sis
tachy·kin·in
ta·chym·e·ter
tachy·pha·gia
tachy·pnea
tachy·rhyth·mia
tach·ys·te·rol
tachy·tro·phism
tachy·zo·ite
ta·cla·mine hy·dro·chlo·ride
tac·tic
tac·tic·i·ty
tac·tile
tac·ti·log·i·cal
tac·tion
tac·tom·e·ter
tac·tor
tac·tu·al
tac·tus
   t. eruditus
   t. expertus
Tae·nia
   T. africana
   T. armata
   T. balaniceps
   T. brachysoma
   T. bremneri
   T. cervi
   T. confusa
   T. crassiceps
   T. crassicollis
   T. cucurbitina
   T. demarariensis
   T. dentata
   T. diminuta
   T. echinococcus

Tae·nia (continued)
   T. elliptica
   T. hydatigena
   T. krabbei
   T. madagascariensis
   T. marginata
   T. mediocanellata
   T. minima
   T. nana
   T. ovis
   T. philippina
   T. pisiformis
   T. saginata
   T. solium
   T. taeniaeformis
tae·nia *pl.* tae·niae
   taeniae acusticae
   t. choroidea
   t. cinerea
   taeniae coli
   t. fimbriae
   t. fornicis
   t. of fornix
   t. of fourth ventricle
   t. hippocampi
   t. libera
   t. medullaris thalami optici
   medullary t. of thalamus
   t. mesocolica
   t. omentalis
   t. pontis
   taeniae pylori
   Tarin's t.
   t. tectae
   t. telae
   t. terminalis
   t. thalami
   t. of thalamus
   t. of third ventricle
   t. tubae
   taeniae of Valsalva
   t. ventriculi quarti
   t. ventriculi tertii
tae·ni·a·cide
tae·niae
tae·ni·a·fu·gal
tae·ni·a·fuge
tae·ni·al

Tae·nia·rhyn·chus
   T. saginatus
tae·ni·a·sis
taen·i·form
tae·ni·id
Tae·ni·i·dae
tae·ni·oid
tae·ni·o·la
   t. cinerea
   t. corporis callosi of Reil
tag
   auricular t's
   cutaneous t.
   radioactive t.
   sentinel t.
   skin t.
Tag·a·met
ta·gli·a·co·tian operation
ta·gli·a·co·tian rhinoplasty
Ta·gli·a·coz·zi flap
Ta·gli·a·coz·zi rhinoplasty
tag·ma *pl.* tag·ma·ta
tail
   axillary t.
   t. of caudate nucleus
   t. of epididymis
   occult t.
   t. of pancreas
   polyadenylate (polyA) t.
   t. of Spence
   t. of spermatozoon
   t. of spleen
tail·gut
Tail·le·fer's valve
Ta·ka·di·as·tase
Ta·ka·ha·ra's disease
Tak·a·ta's reagent
Ta·ka·ya·su's arteritis
Ta·ka·ya·su's disease
Ta·ka·ya·su's syndrome
Tal. — L. talis (such a one)
tal·al·gia
tal·amp·i·cil·lin hy·dro·chlo·
   ride
tal·an·tro·pia
ta·lar
tal·bu·tal
talc

tal·co·sis
   pulmonary t.
tal·cum
tal·ec·to·my
ta·ler·a·nol
ta·li
tal·i·a·co·tian
tal·i·ped
tal·i·pe·dic
tal·i·pes
   t. adductus
   t. arcuatus
   t. calcaneocavus
   t. calcaneovalgocavus
   t. calcaneovalgus
   t. calcaneovarus
   t. calcaneus
   t. cavovalgus
   t. cavus
   t. equinocavus
   t. equinovalgus
   t. equinovarus
   t. equinus
   t. planovalgus
   t. plantaris
   t. planus
   spasmodic t. planus
   t. spasmodicus
   t. transversoplanus
   t. valgus
   t. varus
tal·i·pom·a·nus
Tal·ler·man's treatment
Tall·qvist's scale
Tal·ma's disease
Tal·ma's operation
ta·lo·cal·ca·ne·al
ta·lo·cal·ca·ne·an
ta·lo·cru·ral
ta·lo·fib·u·lar
tal·on
   t. noir
ta·lo·na·vic·u·lar
tal·o·nid
talo·pram hy·dro·chlo·ride
ta·lo·scaph·oid
ta·lo·tib·i·al

ta·lus *pl.* ta·li
Tal·win
Tam·bo·cor
tam·bour
Tamm-Hors·fall mucoprotein
Tamm-Hors·fall protein
ta·mox·i·fen cit·rate
tam·pan
tam·pon
    Corner's t.
    Trendelenburg's t.
    vaginal t.
tam·pon·ade
    balloon t.
    cardiac t.
    chronic t.
    esophagogastric t.
    heart t.
tam·pon·age
tam·pon·ing
tam·pon·ment
Ta·mus
ta·na·pox
tan·da·mine hy·dro·chlo·ride
Tan·de·a·ril
tan·gen·ti·al·i·ty
tan·ghin
Tan·gier disease
tan·gle
    intraneural fibrillary t.
    neurofibrillary t's
tan·go·re·cep·tor
tank
    activated sludge t.
    digestion t.
    Dortmund t.
    Emsher t.
    Hubbard t.
    Imhoff t.
    septic t.
    settling t.
tan·nase
tan·nate
Tan·ner developmental scale
Tan·ner's operation
Tan·ner's procedure
Tan·ner stages (I–V)
tan·nic acid

tan·nin
Tan·ret's reaction
Tan·ret's reagent
Tan·ret's test
Tan·si·ni's operation
tan·ta·lum
    t. 182
tan·trum
tan·y·cyte
tap
    bloody t.
    front t.
    heel t.
    mitral t.
    patellar t.
    spinal t.
    subdural t.
    tendon t.
Tap·a·zole
tape
    adhesive t.
    adhesive t., sterile
    dental t.
    Montgomery's t's
tap·ei·no·ce·phal·ic
tap·ei·no·ceph·a·ly
ta·pe·tal
ta·pe·tum *pl.* ta·pe·ta
    t. cellulosum
    t. choroideae
    t. corporis callosi
    t. fibrosum
    t. lucidum
    t. nigrum
    t. ventriculi
tape·worm
    African t.
    armed t.
    beef t.
    broad t.
    dog t.
    double-pored dog t.
    dwarf t.
    fish t.
    fringed t.
    heart-headed t.
    hydatid t.
    Madagascar t.

tape·worm *(continued)*
    Manson's larval t.
    measly t.
    pork t.
    rat t.
    Swiss t.
    unarmed t.
taph·e·pho·bia
Tap·ia's syndrome
tap·i·no·ce·phal·ic
tap·i·no·ceph·a·ly
tap·i·o·ca
ta·pi·roid
ta·po·tage
ta·pote·ment
TAR — thrombocytopenia-absent radius (syndrome)
tar
    coal t.
    gas t.
    juniper t.
    pine t.
Tar's symptom
Tar·ac·tan
ta·ran·tu·la
    American t.
    black t.
    European t.
tar·ba·dil·lo
tar·ba·gan
Tar·dieu's spots
Tar·dieu's test
tar·dive
tare
tar·get
    enriched t.
tar·get·ing
tar·ich·a·tox·in
Ta·rin (Ta·ri·ni, Ta·ri·nus), Pierre
Ta·rin's band
Ta·rin's fascia
Ta·rin's foramen
Ta·rin's plate
Ta·rin's recess
Ta·rin's space
Ta·rin's taenia
Ta·rin's valve

Tar·lov cyst
Tar·nier's forceps
tars·ad·e·ni·tis
tar·sal
tar·sal·gia
tar·sa·lia
tar·sa·lis
tar·sec·to·my
tar·sec·to·pia
tar·sen
tar·si·tis
tar·so·chei·lo·plas·ty
tar·soc·la·sis
tar·so·ma·la·cia
tar·so·meg·a·ly
tar·so·meta·tar·sal
tar·so-or·bi·tal
tar·so·pha·lan·ge·al
tar·so·pla·sia
tar·so·plas·ty
tar·sop·to·sis
tar·sor·rha·phy
tar·so·tar·sal
tar·so·tib·i·al
tar·sot·o·my
tar·sus
    bony t.
    t. inferior palpebrae
    t. osseus
    t. superior palpebrae
tar·tar
    borated t.
    cream of t.
tar·tar·at·ed
tar·tar·ic acid
tar·tar·ized
tar·trate
    acid t.
    morphine t.
    normal t.
    potassium acid t.
tar·trat·ed
task
    dichotic learning t's
tas·tant
taste
    color t.
    franklinic t.

taste-blind·ness
tast·er
TAT — thematic apperception
   test
      toxin-antitoxin
Tat·lock·ia mic·da·dei
tat·too
      accidental t.
      amalgam t.
      dirt t.
tat·too·ing
      t. of the cornea
Ta·tum, Edward Lawrie
Ta·tu·mel·la
tau
      Kendall's t.
tau·rine
tau·ro·che·no·de·oxy·cho·late
tau·ro·che·no·de·oxy·cho·lic
   acid
tau·ro·cho·lan·er·e·sis
tau·ro·cho·lano·poi·e·sis
tau·ro·cho·late
tau·ro·cho·le·mia
tau·ro·cho·lic acid
tau·ro·cy·amine
tau·ro·don·tism
Taus·sig-Bing syndrome
tau·to·me·ni·al
tau·to·mer
tau·tom·er·al
tau·tom·er·ase
tau·to·mer·ic
tau·tom·er·ism
      enol-keto t.
      proton t.
      ring-chain t.
Ta·wa·ra's node
taxa
tax·ine
tax·is
tax·ol·o·gy
tax·on *pl.* taxa
taxo·nom·ic
tax·on·o·mist
tax·on·o·my
      numerical t.
Tay's choroiditis

Tay's disease
Tay's sign
Tay's spot
Tay-Sachs disease
Tay·lor apparatus
Tay·lor splint
taz·et·tine
ta·zo·lol hy·dro·chlo·ride
TB — tubercle bacillus
      tuberculin
      tuberculosis
Tb — terbium
      tubercle bacillus
TBE — tuberculin bacillin
   emulsion
TBG — thyroxine-binding
   globulin
TBII — TSH-binding
   inhibitory immunoglobulins
TBPA — thyroxine-binding
   prealbumin
tbs — tablespoon
TBSA — total body surface
   area
tbsp — tablespoon
TC — to contain
      transcobalamin
      tuberculin, contagious
TCA — tricarboxylic acid
      trichloracetic acid
TCD_{50} — median tissue
   culture dose
TCDD — 2,3,7,8-tetrachlorodi-
   benzo-para-dioxin
TCi — tetracurie
$TCID_{50}$ — median tissue
   culture infective dose
TCMI — T cell–mediated
   immunity
TCP — tricresyl phosphate
TCR — T cell antigen receptor
TD — threshold of discomfort
      to deliver
TD_{50} — median toxic dose
Td — tetanus and diphtheria
   toxoids, adult type
TDA — TSH-displacing
   antibody

TDE — tetrachlorodiphenyleth-
ane (pesticide)
TDI — toluene diisocyanate
tDNA — transfer-DNA
t.d.s. — L. ter die sumendum
(to be taken three times a
day)
TdT — terminal
deoxynucleotidyl transferase
Te — tetanus
TEA — tetraethylammonium
Teale's amputation
Teale's operation
tear
    bucket-handle t.
    cemental t.
    cementum t.
    Mallory-Weiss t.
    retinal t.
tears
    crocodile t.
tease
tea·spoon
teat
TeBG — testosterone-estra-
diol–binding globulin
teb·u·tate
tech·ne·ti·um
    t. 99m
    t. Tc 99m aggregated
        albumin
    t. Tc 99m DTPA
    t. Tc 99m etidronate
    t. Tc 99m MDP
    t. Tc 99m methylene
        diphosphonate
    t. Tc 99m pentetate
    t. Tc 99m pentetate
        injection
    t.-99m pertechnetate
tech·ne·ti·um-sul·fur col·loid
tech·nic
tech·ni·cal
tech·ni·cian
    audiologic t.
    dental t.
    radiologic t.
    x-ray t.

tech·nique
    abrasion t.
    absorption-elution t.
    absorption-inhibition t.
    angle bisection t.
    atrial-wall t.
    Baermann funnel t.
    Begg t.
    bisection t.
    Brackin t.
    Brock t.
    Buerhenne t.
    cerebral flow image t.
    clamp t.
    clonogenic t.
    Coffey t.
    competitive binding t.
    Conway t.
    cross-fire t.
    Cutler-Beard t.
    dilution-filtration t.
    dip slide t.
    direct fluorescent antibody
        t.
    Dotter-Judkins t.
    double antibody t.
    Enzyme-Multiplied
        Immunoassay T.
    Farr t.
    Fernandez t.
    Ferris Smith t.
    fingerprinting t.
    fluorescent antibody t.
    flush t.
    Fones t.
    funicular suture t.
    hanging drop t.
    helium dilution t.
    hemolytic plaque t.
    Heyman's t.
    hybridoma t.
    immunoferritin t.
    immunoperoxidase t.
    indicator-dilution t.
    indirect fluorescent
        antibody t.
    inhibition t.

tech·nique *(continued)*
    intermediate gel t.
    inversion-recovery t.
    Jerne plaque t.
    Judkins t.
    Kleinschmidt t.
    Kristeller t.
    Lash t.
    Laurell t.
    Leboyer t.
    McGoon's t.
    Madden t.
    Maquet t.
    Merendino's t.
    microtiter t.
    Millen t.
    Mohs' t.
    multiple pressure t.
    Nars-Hunter t.
    Oakley-Fulthorpe t.
    opsonic t.
    Orr t.
    Orr-Loygue t.
    Ouchterlony t.
    Oudin t.
    parallel t.
    Paris t.
    peroxidase-antiperoxidase (PAP) t.
    plaque t.
    projective t.
    pulse echo t.
    push-back t.
    Q t.
    radioxenon t.
    Rebuck skin window t.
    Regaud and Lacassagne t.
    renal micropuncture t.
    right-angle t.
    rosette t.
    sandwich t.
    saturation recovery t.
    Schultz-Dale t.
    scintillation counting t.
    Seldinger t.
    single layer immunofluorescence t.
    skin window t.

tech·nique *(continued)*
    Sones t.
    Southern blot t.
    squash t.
    Stockholm t.
    Takatsy t.
    thermal expansion t.
    thermodilution t.
    time diffusion t.
    Trueta t.
    Warburg's t.
    wax expansion t.
    Weigert-Pal t.
    Western blot t.
    Yasargil t.
    Ziehl-Neelsen t.
tech·no·cau·sis
tech·nol·o·gist
    medical t.
    radiation therapy t.
    radiologic t.
tech·nol·o·gy
tec·lo·zan
tec·tal
tec·to·ce·phal·ic
tec·to·ceph·a·ly
tec·tol·o·gy
tec·to·ri·al
tec·to·ri·um *pl.* tec·to·ria
tec·to·spi·nal
tec·to·tha·lam·ic
tec·tum
    t. mesencephali
    t. of mesencephalon
    optic t.
TED — threshold erythema dose
TEE — transesophageal echocardiography
teeth
teeth·ing
Tee·van's law
Tef·lon
tef·lur·ane
teg·a·fur
teg·men *pl.* teg·mi·na
    t. antri
    t. cellulae

teg·men *(continued)*
  t. cranii
  t. cruris
  t. mastoideotympanicum
  t. mastoideum
  t. tympani
  t. ventriculi quarti
teg·men·tal
teg·men·tum *pl.* teg·men·ta
  t. auris
  hypothalamic t.
  t. mesencephali
  t. of mesencephalon
  t. of pons
  pontile t.
  t. pontis
  t. rhombencephali
  subthalamic t.
Teg·o·pen
Teg·re·tol
teg·u·ment
teg·u·men·tal
teg·u·men·ta·ry
Teich·mann's crystals
Teich·mann's test
tei·cho·ic acid
  membrane t. a.
  streptococcal t. a.
Tei·cholz ejection fraction
tei·chop·sia
tei·no·dyn·ia
tek·no·cyte
te·la *pl.* te·lae
  t. cellulosa
  t. choroidea inferior
  t. choroidea superior
  t. conjunctiva
  t. elastica
  t. subcutanea
  t. submucosa
  t. submucosa gastrica
  t. subserosa
  t. vasculosa
te·lae
tel·al·gia
tel·an·gi·ec·ta·sia
  ataxia-t.
  cephalo-oculocutaneous t.

tel·an·gi·ec·ta·sia *(continued)*
  familial t.
  generalized essential t.
  hereditary hemorrhagic t.
  lymphatic t.
  t. lymphatica
  t. macularis eruptiva
    perstans
  spider t.
  unilateral nevoid t.
tel·an·gi·ec·ta·sis *pl.* tel·an·gi·ec·ta·ses
  spider t.
  stellate t.
tel·an·gi·ec·tat·ic
tel·an·gi·ec·to·des
tel·an·gi·itis
tel·an·gi·on
tel·an·gi·o·sis
te·lar
te·lar·che
Tel·drin
tele·bi·noc·u·lar
tele·can·thus
tele·car·dio·gram
tele·car·di·og·ra·phy
tele·car·dio·phone
tele·cep·tive
tele·cep·tor
tele·co·balt
tele·cord
tele·cu·rie·ther·a·py
tel·e·den·drite
tel·e·den·dron
tele·di·ag·no·sis
tele·flu·o·ros·co·py
tele·gram·ma·tism
tele·ir·ra·di·a·tion
tele·ki·ne·sis
tele·ki·net·ic
tel·elec·tro·car·dio·gram
tel·elec·tro·car·dio·graph
tele·med·i·cine
te·lem·e·ter
tel·em·e·try
  cardiac t.
tele·mne·mon·i·ke
tel·en·ce·phal

tel·en·ce·phal·ic
tel·en·ceph·al·iza·tion
tel·en·ceph·a·lon
tele·neu·rite
tele·neu·ron
tel·eo·log·i·cal
tel·e·ol·o·gy
tel·eo·mi·to·sis
tel·eo·nom·ic
tele·on·o·my
tele·op·sia
tele·or·gan·ic
tel·eo·roent·geno·gram
tel·eo·roent·gen·og·ra·phy
tel·eo·ther·a·peu·tics
tele·paque
te·lep·a·thist
te·lep·a·thize
te·lep·a·thy
tele·ra·di·og·ra·phy
tele·ra·dio·ther·a·py
tele·ra·di·um
tele·re·cep·tor
tel·er·gic
tel·er·gy
tele·roent·geno·gram
tel·e·roent·ge·nog·ra·phy
tele·roent·gen·ther·a·py
    whole-body t.
tel·es·the·sia
tel·es·theto·scope
tele·tac·tor
tele·ther·a·py
tele·ther·mom·e·ter
tel·lu·ric
tel·lu·rism
tel·lu·ri·um
Tell·yes·nic·zky's fluid
Tell·yes·nic·zky's mixture
telo·bio·sis
telo·cen·tric
tel·o·ci·ne·sia
tel·o·ci·ne·sis
telo·coele
tel·o·den·dri·on *pl.* te·lo·den·
    dria
telo·den·dron
tel·o·gen

tel·og·lia
tel·og·no·sis
telo·ki·ne·sis
telo·lec·i·thal
telo·lem·ma
telo·mere
telo·pep·tide
telo·phase
telo·phrag·ma
telo·re·cep·tor
telo·sy·nap·sis
telo·tax·is
telo·tism
tel·son
Tem·a·ril
te·maz·e·pam
tem·e·fos
Te·min
tem·o·dex
temp. dext. — L. tempori
    dextro (to the right temple)
tem·per·a·ment
    choleric t.
    epileptic t.
    melancholic t.
    phlegmatic t.
    sanguine t.
tem·per·a·ture
    absolute t.
    basal body t.
    body t.
    body t., basal
    core t.
    critical t.
    maximum t.
    minimum t.
    normal t.
    optimum t.
    permissive t.
    restrictive t.
    room t.
    standard t. and pressure
        (STP)
    subnormal t.
tem·per·a·ture-sen·si·tive
tem·plate
    surgical t.
    wax t.

tem·ple
tem·po·la·bile
tem·po·ra
tem·po·ral
tem·po·ra·lis
tem·po·ro·au·ric·u·lar
tem·po·ro·fa·cial
tem·po·ro·fron·tal
tem·po·ro·hy·oid
tem·po·ro·ma·lar
tem·po·ro·man·dib·u·lar
tem·po·ro·max·il·lary
tem·po·ro-oc·cip·i·tal
tem·po·ro·pa·ri·e·tal
tem·po·ro·pon·tile
tem·po·ro·spa·tial
tem·po·ro·sphe·noid
tem·po·ro·zy·go·mat·ic
tem·po·sta·bile
temp. sinist. — L. tempori
  sinistro (to the left temple)
tem·pus *pl.* tem·po·ra
te·na·cious
te·nac·i·ty
  cellular t.
te·nac·u·lum
  t. tendinum
te·nal·gia
ten·der·ness
  pencil t.
  rebound t.
ten·di·nes
ten·di·ni·tis
  bicipital t.
  calcific t.
  t. of horse
  t. ossificans traumatica
  t. stenosans
  stenosing t.
ten·di·no·plas·ty
ten·di·no·su·ture
ten·di·nous
ten·do *pl.* ten·di·nes
  t. Achillis
  t. calcaneus
  t. conjunctivus
  t. cordiformis
  t. crico-esophageus

ten·do *(continued)*
  t. infundibuli
  t. oculi
  t. palpebrarum
ten·dol·y·sis
ten·do·mu·cin
ten·don
  Achilles t.
  calcaneal t.
  central t. of diaphragm
  central t. of perineum
  common t.
  conjoined t.
  conjoint t.
  t. of conus arteriosus
  cordiform t. of diaphragm
  coronary t's
  crico-esophageal t.
  Gerlach's annular t.
  hamstring t.
  t. of Hector
  heel t.
  t. of infundibulum
  intermediate t. of
    diaphragm
  membranaceous t.
  t. of origin
  patellar t., anterior
  patellar t., inferior
  pulled t.
  riders' t.
  slipped t.
  snapping t.
  trefoil t.
  t. of Zinn
ten·do·ni·tis
ten·do·plas·ty
ten·do·syn·o·vi·tis
ten·do·tome
ten·dot·o·my
ten·do·vag·i·nal
ten·do·vag·i·ni·tis
  t. granulosa
  t. stenosans
te·neb·ri·my·cin
te·ne·brio
te·nec·to·my
ten·e·my·cin

Ten·er·ic·u·tes
te·nes·mic
te·nes·mus
    rectal t.
    vesical t.
te·nia *pl.* te·ni·ae
te·ni·a·cide
ten·i·a·fu·gal
ten·i·a·fuge
te·ni·al
te·ni·a·my·ot·o·my
te·ni·a·sis
te·ni·o·la
te·nio·tox·in
ten·i·po·side
teno·de·sis
ten·odyn·ia
teno·fi·bril
te·nol·o·gy
ten·ol·y·sis
teno·myo·plas·ty
teno·my·ot·o·my
Te·non's capsule
Te·non's fascia
Te·non's membrane
Te·non's space
teno·nec·to·my
teno·ni·tis
teno·nom·e·ter
ten·on·os·to·sis
ten·on·ta·gra
ten·on·ti·tis
    t. prolifera calcarea
ten·on·to·dyn·ia
ten·on·tog·ra·phy
ten·on·to·lem·mi·tis
ten·on·tol·o·gy
ten·on·to·myo·plas·ty
ten·on·to·my·ot·o·my
ten·on·to·phy·ma
ten·on·to·plas·ty
ten·on·to·the·ci·tis
ten·on·tot·o·my
te·nop·a·thy
teno·phyte
teno·plas·tic
teno·plas·ty
teno·re·cep·tor

Ten·or·min
ten·or·rha·phy
teno·si·tis
ten·os·to·sis
teno·sus·pen·sion
teno·su·ture
teno·sy·ni·tis
teno·syn·o·vec·to·my
teno·syn·o·vi·o·ma
teno·syn·o·vi·tis
    t. acuta purulenta
    adhesive t.
    t. crepitans
    gonococcic t.
    gonorrheal t.
    granulomatous t.
    t. granulosa
    t. hypertrophica
    infectious t.
    nodular t.
    ossifying t.
    t. serosa chronica
    t. stenosans
    stenosing t.
    tuberculous t.
    villonodular t.
    villous t.
teno·tome
ten·ot·o·my
    curb t.
    fenestrated t.
    graduated t.
    stapedial t.
teno·vag·i·ni·tis
TENS — transcutaneous
electrical nerve stimulation
tense
Ten·si·lon
ten·sio-ac·tive
ten·si·om·e·ter
ten·sion
    arterial t.
    electric t.
    interfacial surface t.
    intraocular t.
    intravenous t.
    muscular t.
    oxygen t.

ten·sion *(continued)*
    premenstrual t.
    specific t.
    surface t.
    tissue t.
    wall t.
tens·om·e·ter
ten·sor
    t. fasciae latae
    t. ligamenti annularis
    t. tympani
    t. veli palatini
tent
    air flow t.
    oxygen t.
    sponge t.
    steam t.
ten·ta·cle
tent·ing
    t. of hemidiaphragm
ten·to·ria
ten·to·ri·al
ten·to·ri·um *pl.* ten·to·ria
    t. cerebelli
    t. of cerebellum
    t. of hypophysis
Ten·u·ate
ten·u·is
Tep·a·nil
teph·ro·ma·la·cia
teph·ro·my·eli·tis
tep·i·da·ri·um
te·por
tep·ro·tide
tera·curie (TCi)
te·ras *pl.* te·ra·ta
    terata anadidyma
    terata kata-anadidyma
    terata katadidyma
ter·a·ta
ter·at·ic
ter·a·tism
ter·a·to·blas·to·ma
ter·a·to·car·ci·no·gen·e·sis
ter·a·to·car·ci·no·ma
ter·a·to·gen
ter·a·to·gen·e·sis
ter·a·to·ge·net·ic

ter·a·to·gen·ic
ter·a·to·ge·ni·ci·ty
ter·a·tog·e·nous
ter·a·tog·e·ny
ter·a·toid
ter·a·to·log·ic
ter·a·to·log·i·cal
ter·a·tol·o·gist
ter·a·tol·o·gy
te·ra·to·ma *pl.* te·ra·to·mas,
  te·ra·to·ma·ta
    adult t.
    anaplastic malignant t.
    benign cystic t.
    cystic t.
    differentiated t.
    immature t.
    malignant t.
    mature t.
    monodermal t.
    t. orbitae
    sacrococcygeal t.
    solid t.
    tridermal t.
    triphyllomatous t.
    tropoblastic malignant t.
    undifferentiated malignant
      t.
ter·a·to·ma·ta
ter·a·to·ma·tous
ter·a·to·sis
ter·a·to·sper·mia
ter·bi·um
ter·bu·ta·line sul·fate
ter·chlo·ride
te·re
ter·e·bene
ter·e·ben·thene
ter·e·bin·thi·nate
ter·e·bin·thi·nism
ter·e·brant
ter·e·brat·ing
ter·e·bra·tion
te·res
ter·fen·a·dine
Ter·fo·nyl
ter·gal
ter in die

term
  ontogenetic t's
Ter·man test
ter·mi·nad
ter·mi·nai·son
  t's en grappe
  t. en ligne
  t's en panier
  t. en plaque
ter·mi·nal
  axion t.
  C t.
  en plaque t.
  grapelike t's
  N t.
  Wilson central t.
ter·mi·nal ad·di·tion en·zyme
ter·mi·nal de·oxy·nu·cleo·ti·
  dyl trans·fer·ase
ter·mi·nal de·oxy·ri·bo·nu·
  cleo·ti·dyl trans·fer·ase
ter·mi·na·le
  filum t.
ter·mi·nal·iza·tion
ter·mi·na·tio *pl.* ter·mi·na·ti·
  o·nes
  terminationes nervorum
    liberae
ter·mi·na·tion
ter·mi·na·ti·o·nes
ter·mi·nol·o·gy
ter·mi·nus *pl.* ter·mi·ni
ter·mo·lec·u·lar
ter·na·ry
ter·ni·trate
ter·o·di·line hy·dro·chlo·ride
ter·ox·ide
ter·pene
ter·pen·ism
ter·pin
  t. hydrate
Ter·pi·nol
ter·ra
  t. alba
  t. silicea purificata
Ter·ra·my·cin
ter·res·tric acid
Ter·ri·dens

Ter·ri·dens
  T. diminutus
Ter·ri·en's degeneration
Ter·ri·er's valve
ter·ri·to·ri·al·i·ty
ter·ror
  day t's
  night t's
Ter·ry syndrome
ter·sul·fide
ter·tian
  double t.
  malignant t.
ter·ti·ary
ter·ti·grav·i·da
ter·tip·a·ra
tes·i·cam
tes·i·mide
tes·la
Tes·lac
Tes·sa·lon
tes·sel·lat·ed
test
  ABLB (alternate binaural
    loudness balance) t.
  abortus Bang ring (ABR) t.
  ABR t.
  absorption elution t.
  acetoacetic acid t.
  acetone t.
  achievement t.
  acid elution t.
  acidified serum t.
  acid-lability t.
  acid phosphatase t.
  acoustic reflex t.
  ACTH-stimulation t.
  active rosette t.
  acute toxicity t.
  adaptation t. of Rademaker
    and Garcin
  Addis t.
  Adler's t.
  Adson's t.
  afterimage t.
  agglutination t.
  air conduction t.
  alkali denaturation t.

test *(continued)*
- allelism t.
- Allen's t.
- Allen-Doisy t.
- Almén's t.
- alpha t.
- alpha fetoprotein lab t.
- alternate binaural loudness balance (ABLB) t.
- alternate cover t.
- alternate loudness balance t.
- amebocyte lysate t.
- Ames t.
- amino acid t.
- Ammons Full-Range Picture Vocabulary t.
- Anderson and Goldberger t.
- anesthetic t.
- angular deviation t.
- antibiotic sensitivity t.
- antibody absorption t.
- antibody screening t.
- antiglobulin t. (AGT)
- antiglobulin consumption t.
- antiglobulin inhibition t.
- antihuman serum t.
- antimicrobial susceptibility t.
- antimony trichloride t.
- antistreptolysin O (ASO) t.
- antithrombin t.
- Apgar t.
- Apley's t.
- apprehension t.
- Apt t.
- aptitude t's
- arginine stimulation t.
- arginine tolerance t. (ATT)
- Army General Classification t.
- arylsulfatase t.
- Aschner's t.
- Aschner-Danini t.
- Ascoli's t.
- ascorbate cyanide t.

test *(continued)*
- ASO (antistreptolysin O) t.
- association t.
- atrial pacing t.
- auditory acuity t.
- augmented histamine t.
- autohemolysis t.
- automated reagin t. (ART)
- Ayer's t.
- Ayer-Tobey t.
- Babinski's t.
- Babinski-Weil t.
- Bachman's t.
- bacteriolytic t.
- bacteriophage neutralization t.
- Baermann t.
- balance t.
- Bang t.
- Bárány's t.
- Bárány's pointing t.
- bar-reading t.
- basophil degranulation t.
- Bass-Watkins t.
- battery of t's
- Becker's t.
- Bekhterev's t.
- Bender's t.
- Bender Gestalt t.
- Bender Visual-Motor Gestalt t.
- Benedict's t.
- Bennet and Cash t.
- Benton t. for visual retention
- bentonite flocculation t.
- benzidine t.
- Berens 3-character t.
- Bernard t.
- Bernstein t.
- beta t.
- BG (Bordet-Gengou) t.
- Bial's t.
- Bielschowsky head-tilting t.
- bile acid tolerance t.
- bile esculin t.
- bile solubility t.

test *(continued)*

bilirubin t.

binaural distorted speech t's

Binet's t.

Binet-Simon t.

Bing t.

Bischoff's t.

bithermal caloric t.

biuret t.

Blackberg and Wanger's t.

Block-Steiger t.

blocking t.

blood cholesterol t.

Bodal's t.

bone conduction t.

Boyden's t.

Bozicevich's t.

bracelet t.

breath analysis t.

breath-holding t.

Brenner's t.

Brieger's t.

Broadbent's t.

bromphenol t.

bromsulfophthalein (BSP) t.

Bromsulphalein t.

Burchard-Liebermann t.

butyric acid t.

Caille's t.

calcium t.

California mastitis t. (C.M.T.)

Callaway's t.

Calmette's t.

caloric t.

CAMP t.

capillary fragility t.

capillary resistance t.

carbohydrate t.

carbohydrate tolerance t.

carbohydrate utilization t.

carbon clearance t.

carbon monoxide t.

cardiolipin t.

carotid sinus t.

Carr-Price t.

test *(continued)*

Casoni's intradermal t.

catalase t.

catoptric t.

cervical posture t.

chemiluminescence t.

Chick-Martin t.

Children's Apperception t. (CAT)

Chimani-Moos t.

chi-squared (χ^2) t.

chlorpromazine stimulation t.

cholesterol t.

Chopra's antimony t.

Chrobak's t.

chromatin t.

chronic toxicity t.

Chvostek t.

cis-trans t.

citrate t.

Clark's t.

Clauberg's t.

clomiphene t.

coagulase t.

cocaine t.

coccidioidin t.

Cohn's t.

colchicin t.

cold agglutinin t.

cold pressor t.

coliform t.

collateral circulation t.

colloidal gold t.

color perception t.

complementation t.

complement fixation t.

concentrating ability t.

concentration t.

concentration-dilution t.

confrontation t.

conglutinating complement absorption t. (CCAT)

Congo red t.

conjunctival t.

Conn's t.

consumption t.

contact t.

test *(continued)*

contraction stress t. (CST)
contralateral straight leg
 raising t.
contrast t.
controlled association t.
Coombs' t.
copper t.
corneal t.
Corner-Allen t.
cortisone-glucose tolerance
 t.
cover t.
cover-uncover t.
Crafts' t.
Crampton's t.
creatinine t.
cross agglutination t.
crossed acoustic reflex t.
cuff t.
Cuignet's t.
culture-fair t.
curare t.
cyanide-nitroprusside t.
cysteine t.
cystine t.
cytosine t.
cytotoxicity t.
dark-adaptation t.
darkroom t.
Davidsohn's t.
Davidsohn differential
 absorption t.
decarboxylase t.
Dehio's t.
dehydration t's
dehydrocholate t.
delayed auditory feedback
 t.
Denes-Naunton t.
Denver Developmental
 Screening t.
deoxyribonuclease (DNase)
 t.
deoxyuridine suppression t.
dexamethasone
 suppression t.
dextrose t.

test *(continued)*

DFA (direct fluorescent
 antibody) t.
diabetes t.
diacetyl t.
Diagnex blue t.
Dick t.
differential t. for infectious
 mononucleosis
diffusion t.
dinitrophenylhydrazine t.
diphtheria t.
direct antiglobulin t.
direct Coombs' t.
direct fluorescent antibody
 (DFA) t.
direct immunofluorescence
 t.
disk diffusion t.
distribution-free t.
Dix-Hallpike t.
DNase (deoxyribonuclease)
 t.
Doerfler-Stewart t.
Dolman's t.
Donath's t.
Donath-Landsteiner t.
Donders' t.
L-dopa response t.
Dorn-Sugarman t.
double-blind t.
double diffusion t.
double glucagon t.
Draize t.
draw-a-bicycle t.
draw-a-family t.
draw-a-person t.
Dreyer's t.
drinking t.
Duane's t.
duck waddle t.
Dugas' t.
Duke's t.
Duke bleeding time t.
dye exclusion t.
early pregnancy t.
echinococcus skin t.
effort tolerance t.

test *(continued)*

Ehrlich's t.
Einhorn string t.
Elek t.
ELISA (enzyme-linked
  immunosorbent assay) t.
Ellsworth-Howard t.
Elsberg's t.
Ely's t.
epithyroid iodine uptake t.
Erhard's t.
Erichsen t.
E rosette t.
erythrocyte adherence t.
erythrocyte fragility t.
erythrocyte protoporphyrin
  (EP) t.
erythrocyte sedimentation
  t.
Escherich's t.
esophageal acid infusion t.
estrogen stimulation t.
estrogen suppression t.
euglobulin lysis t.
exercise t's
exercise tolerance t.
F t.
fabere t.
face-hand t.
facial nerve function t.
Fahraeus t.
Fajersztajn's t.
FANA (fluorescent
  antinuclear antibody) t.
Fantus t.
Farber's t.
Farr t.
fat t.
FE_{Na} t.
Fehling's t.
femoral nerve stretch t.
fermentation t.
fern t.
ferric chloride t.
fetal acoustic stimulation t.
  (for assessing fetal health
  in compromised
  pregnancies)

test *(continued)*

Feulgen's t.
FIGLU t.
Finckh's t.
finger-to-finger t.
finger-nose t.
fingerprint sweat t.
Finkelstein's t.
Fishberg concentration t.
Fisher exact t.
Fishman-Doubilet t.
fistula t.
fixation t.
Flack t.
flicker t.
flicking t.
flocculation t.
fluctuation t.
Fluhmann's t.
fluorescein t.
fluorescent antibody t.
fluorescent antinuclear
  antibody (FANA) t.
fluorescent treponemal
  antibody (FTA) t.
fluorescent treponemal
  antibody absorption
  (FTA-ABS) t.
Folin and Wu t.
forced duction t.
formaldehyde t.
Foshay's t.
Fouchet's t.
Fournier t.
Fowler's t.
fragility t.
Francis' t.
Fränkel's t.
free association t.
free urinary cortisol t.
Friderichsen's t.
Friedman's t.
Friedman-Lapham t.
friend t.
frog t.
Frostig Developmental T.
  of Visual Perception
fructose t.

test *(continued)*

FTA (fluorescent treponemal antibody) t.
FTA-ABS t.
fundus reflex t.
Funkenstein t.
furfurol t.
Gaenslen's t.
β-galactosidase t. [beta-]
gallbladder function t.
Galli Mainini t.
gastric function t.
Gault t.
gel diffusion t.
Gellé's t.
Gerhardt's t.
Gerrard's t.
Gesell t.
Gibbon and Landis t.
Gies' biuret t.
globulin t.
glucagon response t.
glucagon stimulation t.
glucose t.
glucose oxidase paper strip t.
glucose suppression t.
glucose tolerance t.
glutoid t.
Gluzinski's t.
glycerol t.
glycerophosphate t.
glycosylated hemoglobin t.
glycuronates t.
glycyltryptophan t.
glyoxylic acid t.
Gmelin's t.
Goetsch's t.
Gofman's t.
gold number t.
gold-sol t.
gonadotropin-releasing hormone stimulation t.
Goodenough draw-a-man t.
Goodenough draw-a-person t.
Goodenough-Harris drawing t.

test *(continued)*

Gordon's biological t.
Göthlin's t.
Graefe's t.
Graham's t.
Gregerson and Boas' t.
Griess t.
Grigg's t.
Gross' t.
group t.
Gruber-Widal t.
guaiac t.
Gunning's t.
Gunning-Lieben t.
Günzberg's t.
Guthrie t.
Gutzeit's t.
Haagensen t.
Haines' t.
Hallion's t.
Hallpike's t.
Halstead-Reitan t's
Ham t.
Hamburger's t.
Hamel's t.
Hamilton's t.
Hammarsten's t.
Hammerschlag's t.
Hamolsky's t.
Hanfmann-Kasanin t.
hanging drop t.
Hanke and Koessler's t.
hapten inhibition t.
Harding and Ruttan's t.
Harris and Ray t.
Harrison's t.
Harrison spot t.
Hart's t.
hatching t.
Hay's t.
Heaf t.
heat stability t.
heel-knee t.
heel-to-shin t.
heel-tap t.
Heinz body t.
Heller's t.
hemadsorption t.

test *(continued)*

- hemadsorption inhibition t.
- hemagglutination inhibition t. (HI, HAI)
- hematein t.
- hematin t.
- heme t.
- hemin t.
- Hemoccult t.
- hemoglobin t.
- hemolytic plaque t.
- hemosiderin t.
- Hench-Aldrich t.
- Hendler screening t.
- Henle-Coenen t.
- Hennebert's t.
- Henshaw t.
- hepatic function t.
- Hering's t.
- Herter's t.
- Herzberg's t.
- Hess capillary t.
- heterophile antibody t.
- Heynsius' t.
- Hickey-Hare t.
- Hildebrandt's t.
- Hindenlang's t.
- Hines and Brown t.
- hippuric acid t.
- Hirschberg's t. for strabismus
- Histalog t.
- histamine t.
- histamine flare t.
- histamine stimulation t.
- histidine loading t.
- histoplasmin t.
- Hitzig t.
- hock t.
- Hoffmann's t.
- Hofmeister's t.
- Hogben t.
- Hollander's t.
- Holmgren's t.
- Hopkins' thiophene t.
- Hopkins-Cole t.
- Hoppe-Seyler t.
- hormone t.

test *(continued)*

- horse cell t.
- Horsley's t.
- Hotis t.
- house-tree-person (HTP) t.
- Howard t.
- Howell's t.
- Huddleson's t.
- Huhner t.
- Huppert's t.
- Huppert-Cole t.
- Hurtley's t.
- hydrochloric acid t.
- hydrogen peroxide t.
- hydrostatic t.
- hydroxyaromatic acid t.
- 17-hydroxycorticosteroid t.
- hydroxylamine t.
- hyperemia t.
- hypochlorite-orcinol t.
- hypothesis t.
- hypoxanthine t.
- Ilimow's t.
- Ilosvay's t.
- imidazole t.
- immobilizaton t.
- immunodiffusion t.
- immunofluorescence t.
- IMViC t.
- incomplete sentences t.
- indican t.
- indigo carmine t.
- indigo red t.
- indirect antiglobulin t.
- indirect Coombs' t.
- indirect hemagglutination t.
- indirect immunofluorescence t.
- indocyanine green t.
- indole t.
- indophenol t.
- induced hypercalciuria t.
- induced hypoglycemia t.
- induced phosphaturia t.
- inhibition t.
- inkblot t.
- inoculation t.

test *(continued)*
- inosite t.
- insulin-glucose tolerance t.
- insulin hypoglycemia t.
- insulin tolerance t.
- intelligence t.
- interfacial precipitin t.
- intracutaneous t.
- intracutaneous tuberculin t.
- intradermal t.
- inulin clearance t.
- iodide-perchlorate discharge t.
- iodine t.
- iodoform t.
- ^{131}I-oleic acid t.
- Iowa pressure articulation t.
- irresistible impulse t.
- irrigation t.
- Ishihara's t.
- isopropanol precipitation t.
- Ito-Reenstierna t.
- ^{131}I uptake t. [131-I]
- Ivy bleeding time t.
- Jacoby's t.
- Jacquemin's t.
- Jadassohn's t.
- Jaffé's t.
- Jaksch's t.
- Janet's t.
- Jansen's t.
- Javorski's (Jaworski's) t.
- Jenning's t.
- jerk t.
- Johnson's t.
- Jolles' t.
- Jones and Cantarow t.
- Jorissen's t.
- Kantor and Gies' t.
- Kaplan's t.
- Kapsinow's t.
- Kashiwado's t.
- Kastle's t.
- Kastle-Meyer t.
- Katayama's t.
- Kathrein's t.

test *(continued)*
- Kato t.
- Kelling's t.
- Kentmann's t.
- Kerner's t.
- 17-ketogenic steroid t.
- kidney function t.
- Killian's t.
- Kinberg's t.
- Kjeldahl's t.
- Kleihauer t.
- Kleihauer-Betke t.
- Klimow's t.
- Knapp's t.
- knee dropping t.
- Knott t.
- Kober t.
- Kobert's t.
- Kolmer t.
- Komolgorov-Smirnov t.
- Kondo's t.
- Korotkoff's t.
- Kossel's t.
- Kowarsky's t.
- Krokiewicz's t.
- Kuhlmann's t.
- Külz's t.
- Kurzrok-Miller t.
- Kveim t.
- Kveim-Siltzbach t.
- labyrinthine t.
- lactic acid t.
- lactose t.
- Ladendorff's t.
- Lancefield precipitation t.
- Lang's t.
- Lange's t.
- lantern t.
- LAP (leucine aminopeptidase) t.
- laryngeal mirror t.
- Lasègue's t.
- latex agglutination t.
- latex fixation t.
- latex particle agglutination t.
- Laurell rocket t.

test *(continued)*
- LE (lupus erythematosus) cell t.
- Leach's t.
- Lebbin's t.
- Lechini's t.
- Lee's t.
- Legal's t.
- leishmanin t.
- Le Nobel's t.
- Leo's t.
- lepromin t.
- Lesser's t.
- leucine t.
- leucine aminopeptidase (LAP) t.
- leukocyte bactericidal t.
- leukocyte migration t.
- Levinson t.
- levulose t.
- levulose tolerance t.
- Lewis and Pickering t.
- Lezak's Malingering T.
- Lichtheim t.
- Lieben's t.
- Lieben-Ralfe t.
- Liebermann's t.
- Liebermann-Burchard t.
- Liebig's t.
- Ligat's t.
- limulus t.
- limulus lysate t.
- Lindemann's t.
- Lindner's t.
- Linzenmeier's t.
- lipase t.
- Lipps' t.
- litmus milk t.
- liver function t.
- Loewe's t.
- Loewi's t.
- logrank t.
- Lombard's t.
- long-term toxicity t.
- Löwenthal's t.
- Lücke's t.
- Luebert's t.
- Luenbach-Koeppe t.

test *(continued)*
- lupus band t.
- lupus erythematosus (LE) cell t.
- Lüttke's t.
- Lyle and Curtman's t.
- lymphocyte proliferation t.
- Macdonald's t.
- Machado t.
- Machado-Guerreiro t.
- Machover t.
- MacLean t.
- MacLean-de Wesselow t.
- MacMunn's t.
- McMurray's t.
- McNemar t.
- MacWilliams' t.
- magnesionitric t.
- Magpie's t.
- male frog t.
- male toad t.
- Malerba's t.
- mallein t.
- malonate t.
- Malot's t.
- maltose t.
- Maly's t.
- Mancini t.
- Mann-Whitney t.
- Mann-Whitney U t.
- Mann-Whitney-Wilcoxon t.
- manometric t.
- Mantoux t.
- Manzullo's t.
- Maréchal's t.
- Maréchal-Rosin t.
- Marlow's t.
- Marquis' t.
- Marshall's t.
- Maschke's t.
- Masset's t.
- Master "2-step" exercise t.
- Matas' t.
- match t.
- Mátéfy t.
- Mathews' t.
- Matzker t.
- Maumené t.

test *(continued)*

Mauthner's t.
Mayer's t.
Mayerhofer's t.
Mazzotti t.
mecalil provocation t.
mecholyl t.
Méhu's t.
Meigs' t.
melanin t.
Meltzer-Lyon t.
Mendel's t.
Mendelsohn's t.
meningitis t.
mercaptoethanol
    agglutination inhibition t.
mercury t.
Mester's t.
metabisulfate t.
methylene blue t.
methylphenylhydrazine t.
methyl red t.
metoclopramide
    stimulation t.
Mett's t.
metyrapone t.
Michailow's t.
microhemagglutination t.
    for *Treponema pallidum*
    (MHA-TP)
microprecipitation t.
MIF t.
migration inhibitory factor
    (MIF) t.
milk t.
milk ring t.
Millard's t.
Miller-Kurzrok t.
40 millimeter t.
Millon's t.
Mills' t.
Mingazzini's t.
minimal caloric t.
Minnesota Multiphasic
    Personality t.
mirror t.
Mitscherlich's t.
Mitsuda t.

test *(continued)*

Mittelmeyer's t.
mixed agglutination t.
mixed leukocyte culture t.
mixed lymphocyte culture
    t.
M'Naghten t.
Moerner-Sjöqvist t.
Mohr's t.
Molisch's t.
Moloney t.
Moloney-Underwood t.
monaural distorted speech
    t's
monaural loudness balance
    (MLB) t.
Monospot t.
Mono-Vac t.
Montenegro t.
Montigne's t.
Moore's t.
Morelli's t.
Moretti's t.
Moritz t.
Mörner's t.
Moro t.
morphine t.
Morton's t.
Moschcowitz t.
Mosenthal's t.
motility t.
Moynihan's t.
Mulder's t.
multiple-puncture t.
mumps sensitivity t.
mumps skin t.
murexide t.
Murphy's t.
mycobiologic t.
mycologic t.
Myers and Fine t.
Mylius' t.
Naffziger's t.
Nagel's t.
Nagler's t.
Nakayama's t.
Nardi t.
NBT t.

test *(continued)*
    Nencki's t.
    Nessler's t.
    Neubauer and Fischer's t.
    Neufeld's t.
    Neukomm's t.
    neuraminidase inhibition t.
    neutralization t.
    niacin t.
    Nickerson-Kveim t.
    nicotine t.
    Ninhydrin t.
    Nippe's t.
    nitrate reduction t.
    nitric acid t.
    nitric acid–magnesium sulfate t.
    nitrites t.
    nitroblue tetrazolium (NBT) t.
    nitrogenous compounds t.
    nitrogen partition t.
    nitrogen washout t.
    nitropropiol t.
    nitroprusside t.
    nitroso-indole-nitrate t.
    Nobel's t.
    Noguchi's t.
    Nonne's t.
    Nonne-Apelt t.
    nonparametric t.
    nonstress t. (NST)
    nonverbal intelligence t.
    nucleoalbumin t.
    Nyiri's t.
    nystagmus t.
    Oakley-Fulthorpe t.
    Ober's t.
    Obermayer's t.
    Obermüller's t.
    obturator t.
    occult blood t.
    octopus t.
    Oliver's t.
    one-stage prothrombin time t.
    one-tailed t.
    ONPG t.

test *(continued)*
    opsonocytophagic t.
    Optochin t.
    oral lactose tolerance t.
    orcinol t.
    organic acid t.
    orientation t.
    orthotoluidine t.
    osazone t.
    Osgood-Haskins t.
    Osterberg's t.
    Ott's t.
    Ouchterlony t.
    Oudin t.
    ovarian hyperemia t.
    ox cell hemolysin t.
    oxidase t.
    oxyphenylsulfonic acid t.
    oxytocin challenge t. (OCT)
    oxytocin sensitivity t.
    Pachon's t.
    Paget's t.
    palmin t.
    palmitin t.
    pancreatic function t.
    pancreozymin-secretin t.
    Pándy's t.
    p24 antigen t.
    Pap t.
    Papanicolaou t.
    paradimethylaminobenzaldehyde t.
    parallel swing t.
    parentage t.
    Parnum's t.
    partial thromboplastin time t.
    PAS (periodic acid–Schiff) t.
    passive agglutination t.
    passive cutaneous anaphylaxis t.
    passive protection t.
    passive transfer t.
    patch t's
    paternity t.
    Patrick's t.
    Patterson's t.

test (continued)
  patting t.
  Paul's t.
  Paul-Bunnell t.
  Paul-Bunnell-Davidsohn t.
  Pavy's t.
  PCA t.
  Pélouse-Moore t.
  pendular eye-tracking t.
    (PETT)
  pendulousness of legs t.
  pentose t.
  Penzoldt's t.
  Penzoldt-Fischer t.
  pepsin t.
  peptide t.
  peptone t.
  perchlorate discharge t.
  perchloride t.
  performance t.
  Peria's t.
  periodic acid–Schiff (PAS)
    t.
  Perls' t.
  permanganate t.
  peroxidase t.
  Perthes' t.
  Petri's t.
  Pettenkofer's t.
  Petzetaki's t.
  phage neutralization t.
  Phalen's t.
  phenacetin t.
  phenol t.
  phenolphthalein t.
  phenolsulfonphthalein t.
  phenoltetrachloro-
    phthalein t.
  phentolamine t.
  phenylalanine deaminase
    t.
  phenylhydrazine t.
  phlorhizin t.
  phlorizin t.
  phosphatase t.
  phosphoric acid t.
  photostress t.
  phthalein t.

test (continued)
  picrotoxin t.
  Pincus t.
  pineapple t.
  pine wood t.
  Piotrowski's t.
  Piria's t.
  Pirquet t.
  pivot shift t.
  P-K (Prausnitz-Küstner) t.
  plantar ischemia t.
  plasma ACTH t.
  plasma cortisol t.
  platelet aggregation t.
  Plesch's t.
  Plugge's t.
  pneumatic t.
  Pohl's t.
  pointing t.
  Politzer's t.
  Pollacci's t.
  polystyrene latex t.
  porphobilinogen t.
  Porter's t.
  Porter-Silber chromogens
    t.
  Porteus maze t.
  Posner's t.
  postauricular myogenic
    (PAM) reflex t.
  potassium cyanide t.
  potassium iodide t.
  P and P (prothrombin and
    proconvertin) t.
  Prausnitz-Küstner (P-K) t.
  precipitation t.
  precipitin t.
  Pregl's t.
  pregnancy t.
  Prendergast's t.
  Preyer's t.
  Proetz t.
  projective t.
  prolonged toxicity t.
  pronation-supination t.
  protection t.
  protein t.
  proteose t.

test *(continued)*
  prothrombin t.
  prothrombin consumption
    t.
  prothrombin-proconvertin
    t.
  proverbs t.
  provocative t.
  psoas t.
  psychological t.
  psychomotor t.
  pulp t.
  Purdy's t.
  purine bodies t.
  pus t.
  Pyramidon t.
  quadriceps t.
  quantitative gel diffusion t.
  Queckenstedt's t.
  Queckenstedt-Stookey t.
  quellung t.
  Quick's t.
  Quick tourniquet t.
  Quinlan's t.
  Raabe's t.
  Rabuteau's t.
  Race-Coombs t.
  radial diffusion t.
  radioactive iodine (RAI) t.
  radioactive renogram t.
  radioallergosorbent t.
    (RAST)
  radioimmunosorbent t.
    (RIST)
  radioisotope renal
    excretion t.
  Ralfe's t.
  Ramon flocculation t.
  Randolph's t.
  rank sum t.
  Rantzman's t.
  rapid plasma reagin (RPR)
    t's
  rapid serum amylase t.
  Raygat's t.
  Rebuck t.
  recruitment t.
  red t.

test *(continued)*
  red cell adherence t.
  red-glass t.
  Rees' t.
  Regitine t.
  Rehberg's t.
  Rehfuss' t.
  Reichl's t.
  Reinsch's t.
  Remont's t.
  renal function t.
  renin suppression t.
  rennin t.
  resorcinol t.
  resorcinol–hydrochloric
    acid t.
  Reuss' t.
  Reynold's t.
  rheumatoid arthritis t.
  rhubarb t.
  Rideal-Walker t.
  Riegel's t.
  Riegler's t.
  ring t.
  Rinne t.
  Rivalta's t.
  Roberts' t.
  Robinson-Kepler t.
  Robinson-Kepler-Power
    water t.
  Rocher's drawer t.
  rollover t.
  Romberg t.
  Ronchese t.
  Roos t.
  Rorschach t.
  Rose's t.
  Rose-Waaler t.
  rose bengal t.
  Rosenbach-Gmelin t.
  Rosenheim-Drummond t.
  Rosenthal's t.
  Rosenzweig picture
    frustration t.
  Rosin's t.
  Ross-Jones t.
  rotation t.
  Rothera's t.

test *(continued)*

Rotozyme t.
Rotter's t.
Rous t.
Roussin's t.
Rowntree and Geraghty's t.
RPR t.
Rubin's t.
Rubino's t.
Rubner's t.
Ruhemann's t.
ruler t.
Rumpel-Leede t.
Russo's t.
Ruttan and Hardisty's t.
Saathoff's t.
Sabin-Feldman dye t.
saccharimeter t.
Sachsse's t.
Sahli's t.
Sahli-Nencki t.
Sahli's glutoid t.
Sakaguchi t.
saline fragility t.
salicylic acid t.
Salkowski's t.
Salkowski-Ludwig t.
Salkowski and Schipper's t.
salol t.
Salomon's t.
sand t.
Sandrock t.
Sanford's t.
santonin t.
Saundby's t.
scarification t.
Schaffer's t.
Schalfijew's t.
Schalm t.
Scherer's t.
Schick t.
Schiff's t.
Schiller's t.
Schilling t.
Schirmer's t.
Schlesinger's t.
Schlichter t.
Schober t.

test *(continued)*

Schönbein's t.
Schroeder's t.
Schulte's t.
Schultz-Charlton t.
Schultze's t.
Schultze's indophenol
  oxydase t.
Schumm's t.
Schwabach t.
sciatic stretch t.
Scivoletto's t.
scleroscope t.
scratch t.
screen t.
screening t.
Seashore t.
secretin t.
sedimentation t.
Seidel's t.
Seidlitz powder t.
Selivanoff's (Seliwanow's) t.
semen t.
senna t.
sensitized sheep cell t.
Sereny t.
serologic t.
serologic t. for syphilis
  (STS)
serum bactericidal activity
  t.
serum neutralization t.
Sgambati's t.
shadow t.
Shear's t.
sheep cell agglutination t.
short increment sensitivity
  index (SISI) t.
short-term toxicity t.
Sia t.
Sia water t.
Sibley-Lehninger t.
Sicard-Cantelouble t.
sickling t.
Siebold and Bradbury's t.
sign t.
signed rank t.
silver t.

test *(continued)*

Simonelli's t.
Sims' t.
single-breath oxygen t.
single diffusion t.
single radial diffusion t.
single radial hemolysis t.
single-tail t.
SISI (short increment sensitivity index) t.
skatole t.
skin t.
skin-puncture t.
skin window t.
slide agglutination t.
slide flocculation t.
Slocum's t.
small increment sensitivity index t.
smear t.
Smith's t.
Snellen's t.
Snider match t.
sniff t.
Snyder's t.
Soldaini's t.
Solera's t.
solubility t.
Sonnenschein's t.
soy bean t.
spavin t.
specific gravity t.
spectroscopic t.
sphenopalatine t.
Spiegler's t.
Spiro's t.
split-renal function t.
sponge t.
squatting t.
Stamey's t.
standing plasma t.
Stanford-Binet t.
starch t.
starch hydrolysis t.
station t.
Staub-Traugott t.
Stein's t.
Stenger t.

test *(continued)*

stereognostic t.
Sterneedle t.
stiff wrist t.
Stock t.
Stokvis' t.
Stoll t.
Storck's t.
straight leg raising t. (SLRT)
Strassburg's t.
Straus' biological t.
streptolysin O t.
stress t's
string t.
Struve's t.
strychnine t.
Student's *t*-t.
Stypven time t.
subchronic toxicity t.
sucrose hemolysis t.
sucrose lysis t.
sucrose tolerance t.
sugar t.
sulfosalicylic acid t.
sulfur t.
Sulkowitch's t.
Sullivan's t.
susceptibility t.
syphilis t.
Szabo's t.
Szondi's t.
t-t.
tanned red cells (TRC) t.
tannic acid t.
Tanret's t.
Tardieu's t.
taurine t.
Taylor's t.
Teichmann's t.
tellurite t.
Tensilon t.
Terman t.
thalleioquin t.
thallium stress t.
thematic apperception t. (TAT)
thermal t.

test *(continued)*
thiamine t.
thiochrome t.
thiocyanate t.
Thomas t.
Thompson's t.
Thormählen's t.
threshold tone decay t.
thromboplastin generation
t.
Thudichum's t.
thumb-nail t.
thyroid function t.
thyroid suppression t.
thyrotropin-releasing
hormone stimulation t.
Tidy's t.
tine t.
Tinel t.
tine tuberculin t.
(Rosenthal)
Tizzoni's t.
toad t.
Tobey-Ayer t.
tolbutamide tolerance t.
tolerance t.
Tollens, Neuberg, and
Schwket's t.
tone decay t.
tongue t.
Töpfer's t's
Torquay's t.
tourniquet t.
toxigenicity t.
TPHA *(Treponema*
pallidum hemagglu-
tination) t.
TPI t.
traction t.
Trambusti t.
trapeze t.
Trendelenburg's t.
Treponema pallidum
complement fixation t's
Treponema pallidum
hemagglutination
(TPHA) t.

test *(continued)*
Treponema pallidum
immobilization (TPI) t.
treponemal antibody t.
treponemal hemmaglu-
tination (TPHA) t.
T_3 resin uptake t.
Tretop's t.
T_4 RIA t.
Triboulet's t.
trichophytin t.
tricresol peroxidase t.
triiodothyronine uptake t.
triketohydrindene hydrate
t.
Trommer's t.
Trousseau's t.
T_3 suppression t.
tuberculin t.
tuberculin t., Sterneedle
tuberculin patch t.
tuberculin titer t.
tuberculosis t.
tubular reabsorption of
phosphate t.
Tuffier's t.
two-glass t.
two-stage prothrombin t.
two-tailed t.
typhoid fever t.
tyrosine t.
Tyson's t.
Tzanck t.
U t.
Udránszky's t.
Uffelmann's t.
Ulrich's t.
Ultzmann's t.
Umber's t.
unheated serum reagin
(USR) t.
Unterberger's t.
uracil t.
urea t.
urea concentration t.
urease t.
Urecholine
supersensitivity t.

test *(continued)*
- uric acid t.
- urine concentration t.
- urobilin t.
- urochromogen t.
- urorosein t.
- urorrhodin t.
- USR t.
- vaginal cornification t.
- Valenta's t.
- Valsalva's t.
- van den Bergh t.
- van den Velden's t.
- vanillylmandelic acid (VMA) t.
- Van Slyke t.
- Van Slyke and Cullen's t.
- variance ratio t.
- Vaughan and Novy's t.
- VDRL [Venereal Disease Research Laboratory] t.
- ventilation t.
- virulence t.
- virus neutralization t.
- Visscher-Bowman t.
- visual field t.
- visual-motor gestalt t.
- Vitali's t.
- vitality t.
- vitamin t.
- vitamin K t.
- VMA (vanillylmandelic acid) t.
- Voelcker and Joseph's t.
- Vogel and Lee's t.
- Voges-Proskauer t.
- Vollmer's t.
- von Aldor's t.
- von Jaksch's t.
- von Maschke's t.
- von Pirquet t.
- von Recklinghausen's t.
- von Stein's t.
- von Zeynek and Mencki's t.
- Waaler-Rose t.
- Wada t.
- Wagner's t.

test *(continued)*
- WAIS (Wechsler Adult Intelligence Scale) t.
- Waldenström's t.
- Wang's t.
- Warren's t.
- Wassermann t.
- water deprivation t.
- water-gurgle t.
- water provocative t.
- Watson-Schwartz t.
- Weber's t.
- Weichbrodt's t.
- Weidel's t.
- Weigl-Goldstein-Scheerer t.
- Weil-Felix t.
- Weiss' t.
- Well-Cogen latex agglutination t.
- Welland's t.
- Wender's t.
- Wenzell's t.
- Weppen's t.
- Werner's t.
- Wernicke's t.
- Westergren sedimentation rate t.
- Western blot electrotransfer t.
- Wetzel's t.
- Weyl's t.
- Wheeler and Johnson's t.
- Whiteside t.
- Widal's t.
- Widal's serum t.
- Wideroe's t.
- Widmark's t.
- Wijs' t.
- Wilbrand's prism t.
- Wilcoxon's rank sum t.
- Wilcoxon's signed rank t.
- Wilkinson and Peter's t.
- Williamson's blood t.
- Winckler t.
- wipe t.
- Wishart t.
- Witz's t.

test *(continued)*
    Woldman's t.
    Wolff-Eisner t.
    Wolff-Junghans t.
    Woodbury's t.
    word association t.
    Worm-Müller t.
    Wormley's t.
    worsted t.
    Worth four-dot (W4D) t.
    Wright t.
    Wurster's t.
    X^2 t.
    xanthine t.
    xanthoproteic t.
    X-chromatin t.
    Xenopus t.
    xylidine t.
    D-xylose absorption t.
    xylose concentration t.
    D-xylose tolerance t.
    Y-chromatin t.
    Yergason t.
    Young's t.
    Zaleski's t.
    Zangemeister's t.
    Zappacosta's t.
    Zeisel's t.
    Zeller's t.
    zinc fluorescence t.
    zona hamster egg t.
    Zondek-Aschheim t.
    Zouchlos' t.
    Zsigmondy's gold number t.
    Zung depression scale t.
    Zwenger's t.
tes·ta *pl.* tes·tae
Tes·ta·cea
Tes·ta·ce·a·lo·bo·sia
tes·ta·ce·an
tes·ta·ceous
tes·tal·gia
Tes-Tape
test card
    stigmometric t. c.
test·cross
tes·tec·to·my

test·er
    pulp t.
tes·tes
tes·ti·cle
    retained t.
    undescended t.
tes·ti·cond
tes·tic·u·lar
tes·tic·u·li
tes·tic·u·lo·ma
    t. ovarii
tes·ti·cu·lus *pl.* tes·ti·cu·li
tes·ti·mo·ny
    expert t.
test·ing
    histocompatibility t.
    nondestructive t.
    reality t.
    visual field t.
tes·tis *pl.* tes·tes
    abdominal t.
    Cooper's irritable t.
    ectopic t.
    femoral t.
    inguinal t.
    inverted t.
    t. muliebris
    obstructed t.
    perineal t.
    pulpy t.
    t. redux
    retained t.
    retractile t.
    undescended t.
tes·ti·tis
test let·ter
test meal
    Boyden t. m.
    motor t. m.
test-ob·ject
tes·toid
tes·to·lac·tone
tes·top·a·thy
tes·tos·te·rone
    t. cyclopentylpropionate
    t. cypionate
    t. enanthate

tes·tos·te·rone *(continued)*
    ethinyl t.
    t. heptanoate
    t. ketolaurate
    methyl t.
    t. phenylacetate
    t. propionate
Tes·tryl
test type
    Jaeger's t. t.
    Landolt's t. t.
    Snellen's t. t.
te·tan·ic
te·tan·i·form
tet·a·nig·e·nous
tet·a·ni·za·tion
tet·a·nize
tet·a·no·can·na·bin
tet·a·node
tet·a·noid
tet·a·nol·y·sin
tet·a·nom·e·ter
tet·a·no·spas·min
tet·a·nus
    cephalic t.
    cerebral t.
    cryptogenic t.
    t. infantum
    Janin's t.
    Klemm's t.
    neonatal t.
    t. neonatorum
    t. paradoxus
    physiological t.
    Rose's t.
tet·a·ny
    duration t.
    epidemic t.
    gastric t.
    grass t.
    hyperventilation t.
    hypoparathyroid t.
    infantile t.
    lactation t.
    latent t.
    neonatal t.
    t. of newborn
    parathyroid t.

tet·a·ny *(continued)*
    parathyroprival t.
    phosphate t.
    postoperative t.
    transit t.
    transport t.
tet·ar·ta·nope
tet·ar·ta·no·pia
tet·ar·ta·nop·ic
tet·ar·ta·nop·sia
te·tar·to·cone
te·tar·to·co·nid
te·tio·thal·ein so·di·um
tetra-
tet·ra-ame·lia
tet·ra·ba·sic
tet·ra·blas·tic
tet·ra·bo·ric acid
tet·ra·bra·chi·us
tet·ra·bro·mo·flu·o·res·ce·in
tet·ra·bro·mo·phe·nol blue
tet·ra·bro·mo·phe·nol·
    phthal·ein
tet·ra·bro·mo·phthal·ein so·
    di·um
tet·rac
tet·ra·caine
    t. hydrochloride
tet·rac·e·tate
tet·ra·chi·rus
tet·ra·chlor·eth·ane
tet·ra·chlo·ride
tet·ra·chlor·meth·ane
2,3,7,8-tet·ra·chlo·ro·di·ben·
    zo-*para*-di·ox·in
tet·ra·chlo·ro·eth·ane
tet·ra·chlo·ro·eth·y·lene
tet·ra·chlor·phen·ox·ide
tet·ra·chro·mic
tet·rac·id
tet·ra·co·sa·no·ic acid
tet·ra·crot·ic
tet·ra·cy·cline
    t. hydrochloride
    t. phosphate complex
Tet·ra·cyn
tet·rad
    Fallot's t.

tet·ra·dac·ty·lous
tet·ra·dac·ty·ly
tet·ra·ene
tet·ra·er·y·thrin
tet·ra·eth·yl·am·mo·ni·um
tet·ra·eth·yl·mono·thio·no·
   py·ro·phos·phate
tet·ra·eth·yl·thi·uram di·sul·
   fide
tet·ra·fil·con A
tet·ra·gly·cine hy·dro·per·io·
   dide
tet·ra·go·num
   t. lumbale
tet·ra·go·nus
tet·ra·he·dron
tet·ra·hy·dric
tet·ra·hy·dro·can·nab·i·nol
tet·ra·hy·dro·fo·late
tet·ra·hy·dro·fo·late de·hy·
   dro·gen·ase
tet·ra·hy·dro·fo·lic acid
tet·ra·hy·dro·pal·ma·tine
tet·ra·hy·dro·pter·o·yl·glu·
   ta·mate meth·yl·trans·fer·
   ase
tet·ra·hy·dro·zo·line hy·dro·
   chlo·ride
Tet·ra·hy·me·na
   T. pyriformis
Tet·ra·hy·me·ni·na
tet·ra·iodo·phe·nol·phthal·
   ein
tet·ra·iodo·phthal·ein so·di·
   um
tet·ra·iodo·thy·ro·nine
te·tral·o·gy
   t. of Eisenmenger
   t. of Fallot
tet·ra·mas·tia
tet·ra·mas·ti·gote
tet·ra·ma·zia
te·tram·e·lus
Te·tram·er·es
   T. americana
tet·ra·mer·ic
tet·ra·mer·ism
tet·ra·meth·yl

tet·ra·meth·yl·am·mo·ni·um
   hy·drox·ide
tet·ra·meth·yl·am·mo·ni·um
   io·dide
tet·ra·meth·yl·benz·i·dine
tet·ra·meth·yl·ene·di·amine
tet·ra·meth·yl·pu·tres·cine
tet·ra·meth·yl·rho·da·mine
   iso·thio·cy·a·nate (TMRITC)
tet·ra·mine
te·tram·i·sole hy·dro·chlo·
   ride
tet·ra·mi·ti·a·sis
tet·ra·ni·trol
tet·ran·oph·thal·mos
tet·ran·op·sia
tet·ra·nu·cleo·tide
Tet·ran·y·chus
   T. autumnalis
   T. molestissimus
   T. montensis
   T. telarius
   T. urticae
Tet·ra·odon·toi·dea
tet·ra·odon·tox·in
tet·ra·odon·tox·ism
tet·ra·otus
tet·ra·pa·re·sis
tet·ra·pep·tide
tet·ra·pero·me·lia
tet·ra·pho·co·me·lia
tet·ra·ple·gia
tet·ra·ploid
tet·ra·ploi·dy
tet·ra·pod
tet·ra·pus
tet·ra·sac·cha·ride
tet·ras·ce·lus
tet·ra·som·ic
tet·ra·so·my
tet·ra·spore
tet·ras·ter
tet·ra·sti·chi·a·sis
tet·ra·thi·o·nate
tet·ra·tom·ic
tet·ra·va·lent
tet·ra·zo·li·um
   t. blue

te·tro·don·ic acid
tet·ro·do·tox·in
tet·ro·do·tox·ism
tet·ro·nal
tet·roph·thal·mos
tet·rose
tet·ro·tus
te·trox·ide
te·try·da·mine
tet·ryl
tet·ter
    honeycomb t.
    milky t.
Teut·le·ben's ligament
tex·ti·form
tex·to·blas·tic
tex·tur·al
tex·ture
tex·tus *pl.* tex·tus
    t. adiposus fuscus
    t. connectivus collagenosus
    t. connectivus elasticus
    t. connectivus fibrosus
      compactus
    t. connectivus fibrosus
      lamellaris
    t. connectivus pigmentosus
    t. connectivus reticularis
    t. muscularis
    t. muscularis nonstriatus
    t. muscularis striatus
    t. muscularis striatus
      cardiacus
    t. nervosus
TF — tetralogy of Fallot
    transfer factor
    tuberculin filtrate
T-group
TGA — transposition of the
  great arteries
TGC — time gain
  compensation
TGF — transforming growth
  factor
TG-globulin
TGT — thromboplastin
  generation test
thal·a·mec·to·my

thal·a·men·ce·phal·ic
thal·a·men·ceph·a·lon
thal·a·mi
tha·lam·ic
thal·a·mo·coele
thal·a·mo·cor·ti·cal
thal·a·mo·cru·ral
thal·a·mo·len·tic·u·lar
thal·a·mo·mam·il·lary
thal·a·mo·pa·ri·e·tal
thal·a·mo·pe·dun·cu·lar
thal·a·mo·teg·men·tal
thal·a·mot·o·my
    anterior t.
    dorsomedial t.
    parafascicular t. (PFT)
tha·la·mus *pl.* tha·la·mi
    dorsal t.
    t. dorsalis
    optic t.
    t. ventralis
tha·las·sa·ne·mia
thal·as·se·mia
    α-t.
    β-t.
    δ-t.
    $\delta\ \beta$-t.
    hemoglobin C–t.
    hemoglobin C-β-t.
    hemoglobin E–t.
    hemoglobin E-α-t.
    hemoglobin E-β-t.
    hemoglobin Lepore-β-t.
    hemoglobin S–t.
    hemoglobin S-α-t.
    hemoglobin S-β-t.
    t. intermedia
    t. major
    t. minor
    sickle cell–t.
tha·las·sin
tha·las·so·po·sia
tha·las·so·ther·a·py
tha·lid·o·mide
thal·lei·o·quin
thal·li·tox·i·co·sis
thal·li·um
    t.-201

Thal·lo·bac·te·ria
Thal·loph·y·ta
thal·lo·phyte
thal·lo·spore
thal·lo·tox·i·co·sis
thal·lous chlo·ride Tl 201
thal·lus
thal·po·sis
thal·pot·ic
Tham·nid·i·um
tham·uria
than·a·to·bi·o·log·ic
than·a·to·gno·mon·ic
than·a·toid
than·a·tol·o·gy
than·a·tom·e·ter
than·a·to·phid·ia
than·a·to·phid·i·al
than·a·to·pho·bia
than·a·to·pho·ric
than·a·top·sia
than·a·top·sy
than·a·to·sis
Thane's method
thau·mat·ro·py
Thay·er-Mar·tin culture
    medium
Thay·sen's disease
THC — tetrahydrocannabinol
thea·ism
the·ba·ic
the·baine
the·be·sian
The·be·si·us' valve
The·be·si·us' vein
the·ca *pl.* the·cae
    t. cordis
    t. externa
    t. of follicle
    t. of follicle of von Baer
    t. folliculi
    t. interna
    t. medullare spinalis
    t. tendinis
    t. vertebralis
the·cae
the·cal
the·ci·tis

the·co·dont
the·co·ma
the·co·ma·to·sis
the·co·steg·no·sis
The·den's bandage
Thee·lin
Theile's canal
Theile's glands
Thei·ler
Thei·ler's disease
Thei·ler's virus
Thei·le·ria
    T. annulata
    T. dispar
    T. hirci
    T. lawrencei
    T. mutans
    T. ovis
    T. parva
    T. tsutsugamushi
thei·le·ri·a·sis
    bovine t.
    tropical t.
thei·le·ri·o·sis
the·ine
the·in·ism
the·lal·gia
the·lar·che
    precocious t.
The·la·zia
the·la·zi·a·sis
thele
the·le·plas·ty
thel·er·e·thism
the·lio·lym·pho·cyte
the·li·tis
the·li·um *pl.* the·lia
The·lo·ha·nia
the·lor·rha·gia
the·lo·thism
the·lo·tism
thel·y·blast
thel·y·blas·tic
thel·y·gen·ic
thel·y·to·cia
the·lyto·cous
the·lyt·o·ky
the·nad

the·nal
the·nar
then·i·um clo·sy·late
then·yl·di·amine hy·dro·chlo·ride
Then·y·lene
then·yl·pyr·amine
The·o·bal·dia
The·o·bro·ma
the·o·bro·mine
The·o·gly·ci·nate
the·o·lin
the·oph·yl·line
    t. aminoisobutanol
    t. cholinate
    t. ethanolamine
    t. ethylenediamine
    t. methylglucamine
    t. monoethanolamine
    t. olamine
    t. sodium acetate
    t. sodium glycinate
The·o·rell, Axel Hugo Teodor
the·o·rem
    Bayes' t.
    central limit t.
    Gibbs' t.
the·o·ry
    Adami's t.
    Adler's t.
    aging t. of atherosclerosis
    Altmann's t.
    apposition t.
    Arrhenius' t.
    atomic t.
    avalanche t.
    behavior t.
    Bohr's t.
    Bolk's retardation t.
    Buergi's t.
    Burn and Rand t.
    Cannon's t.
    Cannon-Bard t.
    cell t.
    cell-chain t.
    cellular immunity t.
    t. of central analysis
    chemicoparasitic t.

the·o·ry *(continued)*
    clonal deletion t.
    clonal selection t.
    closed circulation t.
    closed-open circulation t.
    Cohnheim's t.
    t. of concrescence
    contractile ring t.
    convergence-projection t.
    core conductor t.
    Dalcq-Pasteels t.
    darwinian t.
    t. of demographic transition
    dimer t.
    drive-reduction t.
    dualistic t.
    duplicity t.
    ectopic focus t.
    Ehrlich's biochemical t.
    Ehrlich's side-chain t.
    electron t.
    electron-hole t.
    embryonal t.
    emergency t.
    emigration t.
    encrustation t.
    equilibrium t.
    expanding surface t.
    fast circulation t.
    fetal rest-cell t.
    frequency t.
    gametoid t.
    gate t.
    gate-control t.
    t. of gene-culture evolution
    germ t.
    germ layer t.
    gestalt t.
    Golgi's t.
    Goltz's t.
    group factor t.
    Helmholtz t.
    Hering's t.
    hit t.
    humoral t.
    hydrate microcrystal t.
    incasement t.

the·o·ry *(continued)*
    information t.
    inside-outside t.
    instructive t.
    ionic t.
    Jackson's t.
    James-Lange t.
    James-Lange-Sutherland t.
    Kern plasma relation t.
    Ladd-Franklin t.
    Lamarck's t.
    lateral chain t.
    Liebig's t.
    lipoid t. of narcosis
    local circuit t.
    lock and key t.
    Lumsden-Wilson t.
    malthusian t.
    mass action t.
    Melzack and Wall gate
      control t.
    membrane ionic t.
    mendelian t.
    metabolic t. of
      atherosclerosis
    Metchnikoff's
      (Mechnikov's) cellular
      immunity t.
    Meyer's t.
    Meyer-Overton t.
    miasma t.
    migration t.
    monophyletic t.
    Morawitz's t.
    myoelastic t.
    myogenic t.
    natural selection t.
    network t. of immunity
    neucleocytoplasmic
      relation t.
    neurochronaxic t.
    neurogenic t.
    neuron t.
    open circulation t.
    open-closed circulation t.
    operon t.
    opponent colors t.
    overflow t.

the·o·ry *(continued)*
    overproduction t.
    Papez t.
    paralytic t.
    Pasteur's t.
    perceptual defense t.
    phlogiston t.
    pithecoid t.
    place t.
    Planck's t.
    plasma relation t.
    polarization-membrane t.
    polychromatic t.
    polyphyletic t.
    population t.
    P. O. U. t.
    preformation t.
    proteomorphic t.
    quantum t.
    Ranke's t.
    recapitulation t.
    recombinational germline
      t.
    t. of reentry
    resonance t.
    Ribbert's t.
    t. of rotation
    Rutherford's t.
    t. of saltatory conduction
    Schiefferdecker's symbiosis
      t.
    Schön's t.
    shunt muscle t.
    side-chain t.
    signal detection t.
    single hit t.
    sliding filament t.
    slow circulation t.
    somatic mutation t.
    sound pattern t.
    spindle elongation t.
    Spitzer's t.
    structural t.
    target t.
    telephone t.
    template t.
    thermostat t.
    Traube's resonance t.

the·o·ry *(continued)*

trialistic t.
two-sympathin t.
underfilling t.
undulatory t.
unitarian t.
unitary t.
Warburg's t.
wave t.
Weismann's t.
Woods-Fildes t.
Young-Helmholtz t.
Yukawa t.
theo·ther·a·py
Theph·o·rin
theque
ther·a·peu·sis
ther·a·peu·tic
ther·a·peu·tics
ther·a·peu·tist
Ther·a·pho·si·dae
ther·a·pia
t. sterilisans magna
ther·a·pist
corrective t.
occupational t.
physical t.
radiation t.
respiratory t.
speech t.
ther·a·py
active t.
adjuvant t.
aerosol t.
alimentary t.
alkali t.
analytic t.
anticoagulant t.
anticonvulsant t.
antigametocyte t.
antiplatelet t.
art t.
autoserum t.
aversion t.
beam t.
behavior t.
Bernheim's t.

ther·a·py *(continued)*
bilateral electroconvulsive t.
biological t.
blunderbuss t.
brief stimulus t. (BST)
buffer t.
carbon dioxide t.
Chaoul t.
client-centered t.
cognitive t.
collapse t.
combined t.
conditioning t.
contact t.
contact radiation t.
convulsive t.
corrective t.
couples t.
deep roentgen-ray t.
deleading t.
diathermic t.
diet t.
duplex t.
electric convulsive t. (ECT)
electric shock t. (EST)
electroconvulsive t. (ECT)
electromagnetic field t.
electron beam t.
electroshock t. (EST)
electrotherapeutic sleep t.
endocrine ablative t.
family t.
fango t.
fever t.
gametocyte t.
gamma-ray t.
gene t.
gestalt t.
grid t.
group t.
heat t.
heterovaccine t.
high-voltage roentgen t.
humidification t.
hyperbaric oxygen t.
hypoglycemic t.
immunization t.

ther·a·py *(continued)*
  immunosuppressive t.
  Indoklon convulsive t.
  inhalation t.
  insulin coma t. (ICT)
  insulin shock t. (IST)
  interstitial radiation t.
  interstitial radium t.
  intraosseous t.
  intrathecal t.
  intravenous t.
  larval t.
  learning-theory t.
  light t.
  liquid air t.
  malaria t.
  manipulative t.
  marriage t.
  megavoltage t.
  metatrophic t.
  Metrazol shock t.
  milieu t.
  Morita t.
  multiple t.
  myofunctional t.
  narcosis t.
  nondirective t.
  nonspecific t.
  occupational t.
  organic t.
  orthomolecular t.
  oxygen t.
  paraspecific t.
  parenteral t.
  pharmacological convulsive
    t.
  photodynamic t.
  physical t.
  play t.
  primal t.
  protective t.
  psychoanalytic t.
  pulp canal t.
  PUVA t.
  radionuclide t.
  radium t.
  radium beam t.
  rational t.

ther·a·py *(continued)*
  reflex t.
  relaxation t.
  replacement t.
  rhythmic sensory
    bombardment t.
  root canal t.
  rotation t.
  sclerosing t.
  serum t.
  shock t.
  short wave t.
  sleep t.
  sleep-electroshock t.
  social t.
  solar t.
  somatic cell gene t.
  sparing t.
  specific t.
  speech t.
  subcoma insulin t.
  substitution t.
  substitutive t.
  suggestion t.
  supervoltage t.
  supplementary x-ray t.
  supportive t.
  telecobalt t.
  total-push t.
  ultrasonic t.
  unilateral
    electroconvulsive t.
  vaccine t.
  zone t.
The·ria
the·ri·a·ca
Ther·i·di·i·dae
the·rio·geno·log·ic
the·rio·geno·log·i·cal
the·rio·gen·ol·o·gist
the·rio·gen·ol·o·gy
therm
ther·ma·co·gen·e·sis
ther·mae
therm·aero·ther·a·py
ther·mal
ther·mal·ge·sia
ther·mal·gia

therm·an·al·ge·sia
therm·an·es·the·sia
ther·ma·tol·o·gy
ther·mel·om·e·ter
therm·es·the·sia
therm·es·the·si·om·e·ter
therm·hy·per·es·the·sia
therm·hy·pes·the·sia
ther·mic
ther·mi·on
ther·mi·on·ics
ther·mis·tor
Ther·mo·ac·ti·no·my·ces
    T. vulgaris
ther·mo·aes·the·sia
ther·mo·al·ge·sia
ther·mo·an·al·ge·sia
ther·mo·an·es·the·sia
ther·mo·cau·ter·ec·to·my
ther·mo·cau·tery
ther·mo·chem·is·try
ther·mo·chro·ic
ther·mo·chro·ism
ther·mo·chro·sis
ther·mo·co·ag·u·la·tion
ther·mo·cou·ple
ther·mo·cur·rent
ther·mo·dif·fu·sion
ther·mo·di·lu·tion
ther·mo·du·ric
ther·mo·dy·nam·ics
    equilibrium t.
    laws of t.
    nonequilibrium t.
ther·mo·elec·tric
ther·mo·elec·tric·i·ty
ther·mo·es·the·sia
ther·mo·es·the·si·om·e·ter
ther·mo·ex·ci·to·ry
ther·mo·gen·e·sis
    dietary induced t.
    nonshivering t.
    shivering t.
ther·mo·ge·net·ic
ther·mo·gen·ic
ther·mo·gen·ics
ther·mog·e·nous
ther·mo·gram

ther·mo·gram
    liquid crystal t.
ther·mo·graph
    continuous scan t.
ther·mo·graph·ic
ther·mog·ra·phy
    liquid crystal t. (LCT)
ther·mo·gra·vim·e·ter
ther·mo·hy·per·al·ge·sia
ther·mo·hy·per·es·the·sia
ther·mo·hy·pes·the·sia
ther·mo·hy·po·es·the·sia
ther·mo·in·ac·ti·va·tion
ther·mo·in·hib·i·to·ry
ther·mo·in·te·gra·tor
ther·mo·junc·tion
ther·mo·la·bile
ther·mo·lamp
ther·mol·o·gy
ther·mo·lu·mi·nes·cence
ther·mol·y·sis
ther·mo·lyt·ic
ther·mo·mas·sage
ther·mo·mas·tog·ra·phy
ther·mom·e·ter
    air t.
    alcohol t.
    axilla t.
    Beckmann t.
    bimetal t.
    Celsius t.
    centigrade t.
    clinical t.
    depth t.
    differential t.
    Fahrenheit t.
    fever t.
    gas t.
    half-minute t.
    kata t.
    Kelvin t.
    liquid-in-glass t.
    maximum t.
    mercurial t.
    metallic t.
    metastatic t.
    minimum t.
    oral t.

ther·mom·e·ter *(continued)*
    Rankine t.
    Réaumur t.
    recording t.
    rectal t.
    resistance t.
    self-registering t.
    surface t.
    thermocouple t.
ther·mo·met·ric
ther·mom·e·try
ther·mo·pal·pa·tion
ther·mo·pen·e·tra·tion
ther·mo·phile
ther·mo·phil·ic
ther·mo·phore
ther·mo·pile
ther·mo·plac·en·tog·ra·phy
ther·mo·plas·tic
ther·mo·ple·gia
ther·mo·pol·yp·nea
ther·mo·pol·yp·ne·ic
ther·mo·pre·cip·i·ta·tion
ther·mo·ra·dio·ther·a·py
ther·mo·re·cep·tor
ther·mo·reg·u·la·tion
ther·mo·reg·u·la·tor
ther·mo·re·sis·tance
ther·mo·re·sis·tant
ther·mo·scope
ther·mo·sta·bile
ther·mo·sta·bil·i·ty
ther·mo·sta·sis
ther·mo·stat
    hypothalamic t.
ther·mo·ste·re·sis
ther·mo·strom·uhr
ther·mo·sys·tal·tic
ther·mo·sys·tal·tism
ther·mo·tac·tic
ther·mo·tax·ic
ther·mo·tax·is
ther·mo·ther·a·py
ther·mot·ics
ther·mo·tol·er·ant
ther·mo·to·nom·e·ter
ther·mo·tox·in
ther·mo·trop·ic

ther·mot·ro·pism
the·ro·morph
the·ro·mor·phism
Ther·o·my·zon
the·ront
the·ve·tin
THF — tetrahydrofolate
thi·a·ben·da·zole
thi·a·cet·a·zone
thi·a·di·a·zide
thi·a·di·a·zine
thi·am·a·zole
thi·am·bu·to·sine
thi·am·i·nase
thi·a·mine
    t. hydrochloride
    t. mononitrate
    phosphorylated t.
    t. pyrophosphate
thi·am·phen·i·col
thi·am·y·lal so·di·um
Thi·a·ra
thi·a·sine
thi·a·zide
thi·a·zole
thi·a·zo·li·um
Thi·bi·erge-Weis·sen·bach
  syndrome
thick·ness
    half-value t.
    s-t. skin graft
Thiele's syndrome
Thie·mann disease
thi·emia
thi·ena·my·cin
Thiersch's graft operation
Thiersch-Du·play
  urethroplasty
thi·eth·yl·per·a·zine
    t. malate
    t. maleate
thigh
    cricket t.
    drivers' t.
    Heilbronner's t.
thigh-lift
thig·mes·the·sia
thig·mo·tac·tic

thig·mo·tax·is
thig·mo·trop·ic
thig·mot·ro·pism
thi·hex·i·nol meth·yl·bro·
    mide
thim·ble
thi·mero·sal
thi·meth·a·phan cam·phor·
    sul·fo·nate
think·ing
    autistic t.
    concrete t.
    dereistic t.
    preoperational t.
    pressured t.
thio-ac·id
thio·al·co·hol
thio·ar·se·nite
thio·bar·bi·tal
thio·bar·bit·u·rate
thio·bar·bi·tu·ric acid
thio·car·ba·mide
thio·chrome
thi·oc·tic acid
thio·cy·a·nate
thio·cy·an·ic acid
thio·cy·a·nide
thio·di·phen·yl·amine
thio·do·ther·a·py
thio·ether
thio·eth·yl·amine
thio·fla·vine
thio·ga·lac·to·side
    isopropyl t.
thio·glu·cose
thio·gly·co·late
thio·gly·col·ic acid
thio·gua·nine
thio·ki·nase
thi·ol
thi·o·lase
thi·o·late
thi·ol es·ter
thi·ol·his·ti·dine
thio·mer·sa·late
thio·ne·ine
thi·o·nin
thi·o·nyl

thio·pan·ic acid
thio·pec·tic
thio·pen·tal so·di·um
thio·pen·tone
thio·pro·pa·zate di·hy·dro·
    chlo·ride
thio·pro·pa·zate hy·dro·chlo·
    ride
thio·re·dox·in
thio·re·dox·in re·duc·tase
thio·rid·a·zine hy·dro·chlo·
    ride
thio·semi·car·ba·zone
thio·strep·ton
thio·sul·fate
    t. sulfurtransferase
Thio·sul·fil
thio·sul·fur·ic acid
thio·tepa
thio·thix·ene
    t. hydrochloride
thio·ura·cil
thio·urea
thio·xan·thene
thio·zine
thi·phen·a·mil hy·dro·chlo·
    ride
thi·ram
thirst
    insensible t.
    real t.
    subliminal t.
    true t.
    twilight t.
Thi·ry's fistula
Thi·ry-Vel·la fistula
thixo·la·bile
thix·o·trop·ic
thix·ot·ro·pism
thix·ot·ro·py
thlip·sen·ceph·a·lus
Tho·ma's ampulla
Tho·ma's fluid
Tho·ma-Zeiss cell
Tho·ma-Zeiss counting
    chamber
Thom·as pessary
Thom·as' splint

Thom·as' test
Thomp·son's test
Thom·sen's antibody
Thom·sen's disease
Thom·son's disease
Thom·son's poikiloderma
   congenitale
Thom·son scattering
Thom·son's sign
thon·zo·ni·um bro·mide
thon·zyl·amine hy·dro·chlo·
   ride
tho·ra·cal
tho·ra·cal·gia
tho·ra·cec·to·my
tho·ra·cen·te·sis
tho·ra·ces
tho·rac·ic
tho·rac·i·co·ab·dom·i·nal
tho·rac·i·co·hu·mer·al
tho·raci·spi·nal
tho·ra·co·ab·dom·i·nal
tho·ra·co·acro·mi·al
tho·ra·co·ce·los·chi·sis
tho·ra·co·cen·te·sis
tho·ra·co·cyl·lo·sis
tho·ra·co·cyr·to·sis
tho·ra·co·del·phus
tho·ra·co·did·y·mus
tho·ra·co·dor·sal
tho·ra·co·dyn·ia
tho·ra·co·gas·tro·did·y·mus
tho·ra·co·gas·trop·a·gus
tho·ra·co·gas·tros·chi·sis
tho·ra·co·graph
tho·ra·co·lap·a·rot·o·my
tho·ra·co·lum·bar
tho·ra·col·y·sis
tho·ra·com·e·lus
   t. parasiticus
tho·ra·com·e·ter
tho·ra·com·e·try
tho·ra·co·my·odyn·ia
tho·ra·co·om·pha·lop·a·gus
tho·ra·cop·a·gus
   t. epigastricus
   t. parasiticus
   tribrachial t.

tho·ra·co·para·ceph·a·lus
tho·ra·cop·a·thy
tho·ra·co·plas·ty
   costoversion t.
   lateral t.
tho·ra·co·pneu·mo·graph
tho·ra·cos·chi·sis
tho·ra·co·scope
tho·ra·cos·co·py
tho·ra·co·ste·no·sis
tho·ra·cos·to·my
   tube t.
tho·ra·cot·o·my
tho·ra·del·phus
Tho·rae·us filter
tho·rax pl. tho·ra·ces
   amazon t.
   barrel-shaped t.
   cholesterol t.
   Peyrot's t.
   pyriform t.
Thor·a·zine
Tho·rel's bundle
tho·ri·um
   t. dioxide
   radioactive t.
   sodium t. tartrate
Thor·mäh·len's test
Thorn salt-depletion syndrome
Thorn·ton's sign
Thorn·waldt
Tho·ro·trast
thor·ough·pin
thought broad·cast·ing
thought in·ser·tion
thought with·draw·al
tho·zal·i·none
Thr — threonine
thread
   t's of Golgi-Rezzonico
   Simonart's t.
thread·worm
thre·o·nine
   t. dehydratase
thre·o·nyl
thre·ose
threp·sis

thres·hold
- absolute t.
- achromatic t.
- alpha t.
- audiometric t.
- auditory t.
- chromatic t.
- colorless visual t.
- t. of consciousness
- convulsant t.
- difference t.
- differential t.
- differential light t.
- differential sensory t.
- t. of discomfort
- displacement t.
- double point t.
- epileptic t.
- erythema t.
- excretion t.
- flicker fusion t.
- galvanic t.
- light t.
- myoclonic t.
- neuron t.
- t. of nose
- olfactory t.
- pain t.
- relational t.
- renal t.
- renal t. for glucose
- resolution t.
- sensitivity t.
- speech reception t. (SRT)
- stimulus t.
- stretch t.
- swallowing t.
- t. for two-point discrimination
- t. of visual sensation

thrill
- aneurysmal t.
- aortic t.
- arterial t.
- arteriovenous t.
- diastolic t.
- fat t.
- hydatid t.

thrill (continued)
- presystolic t.
- purring t.
- systolic t.

thrix

throat
- septic sore t.
- sore t.
- streptococcal sore t.
- ulcerated sore t.
- ulceromembranous sore t.

throb

throb·bing

Throck·mor·ton's reflex

throe

throm·ba·phe·re·sis

throm·base

throm·bas·the·nia
- Glanzmann's t.

throm·bec·to·my

throm·bem·bo·lia

throm·bi

throm·bin
- topical t.

throm·bin·o·gen

throm·bo·ag·glu·ti·nin

throm·bo·an·gi·itis
- t. obliterans

throm·bo·ar·te·ri·tis
- t. purulenta

throm·bo·as·the·nia

throm·bo·cla·sis

throm·bo·clas·tic

throm·bo·cyst

throm·bo·cys·tis

throm·bo·cy·ta·phe·re·sis

throm·bo·cy·tas·the·nia

throm·bo·cyte

throm·bo·cy·the·mia
- essential t.
- hemorrhagic t.
- idiopathic t.
- primary t.

throm·bo·cyt·ic

throm·bo·cy·tin

throm·bo·cy·to·crit

throm·bo·cy·tol·y·sis

throm·bo·cy·to·path·ia

throm·bo·cy·to·path·ic
throm·bo·cy·top·a·thy
   constitutional t.
throm·bo·cy·to·pe·nia
   essential t.
   immune t.
   malignant t.
   secondary t.
throm·bo·cy·to·poi·e·sis
throm·bo·cy·to·poi·et·ic
throm·bo·cy·to·sis
throm·bo·elas·to·gram
throm·bo·elas·to·graph
throm·bo·elas·tog·ra·phy
throm·bo·em·bo·lec·to·my
throm·bo·em·bo·lia
throm·bo·em·bol·ic
throm·bo·em·bo·lism
throm·bo·end·ar·ter·ec·to·my
   coronary t.
throm·bo·end·ar·ter·itis
throm·bo·en·do·car·di·tis
throm·bo·gen·e·sis
throm·bo·gen·ic
β-throm·bo·glob·u·lin
throm·boid
throm·bo·ki·nase
throm·bo·ki·ne·sis
throm·bo·ki·net·ics
throm·bo·lym·phan·gi·tis
Throm·bol·y·sin
throm·bol·y·sis
throm·bo·lyt·ic
throm·bo·mod·u·lin
throm·bon
throm·bo·path·ia
throm·bop·a·thy
throm·bo·pe·nia
   essential t.
throm·bo·phil·ia
throm·bo·phle·bi·tis
   iliofemoral t.
   intracranial t.
   t. migrans
   postpartum t.
   t. purulenta
   septic t.
   spinal t.

throm·bo·phle·bi·tis
   (continued)
   suppurative t.
throm·bo·plas·tic
throm·bo·plas·tid
throm·bo·plas·tin
   extrinsic t.
   intrinsic t.
   tissue t.
throm·bo·plas·tin·o·gen
throm·bo·poi·e·sis
throm·bo·poi·et·ic
throm·bo·poi·e·tin
throm·bose
throm·bosed
throm·bo·si·nu·si·tis
throm·bo·sis
   agonal t.
   atrophic t.
   ball-valve t.
   calcarine t.
   cardiac t.
   cavernous sinus t.
   cerebellar t.
   cerebral t.
   coronary t.
   creeping t.
   deep venous t. (DVT)
   dilatation t.
   effort t.
   iliofemoral t.
   infective t.
   intracardiac t.
   intraventricular t.
   jumping t.
   marantic t.
   marasmic t.
   mesenteric t.
   migrating t.
   mural t.
   placental t.
   plate t.
   platelet t.
   propagating t.
   puerperal t.
   Ribbert's t.
   sinus t.
   suppurative venous t.

throm·bo·sis *(continued)*
    traumatic t.
    venous t.
throm·bos·ta·sis
throm·bo·sthe·nin
throm·bo·test
throm·bot·ic
throm·bo·to·nin
throm·box·ane
throm·bus *pl.* throm·bi
    agglutinative t.
    agonal t.
    agony t.
    annular t.
    antemortem t.
    ball t.
    ball-valve t.
    bile t.
    blood plate t.
    blood platelet t.
    calcified t.
    canalized t.
    coral t.
    coronary t.
    currant jelly t.
    fibrin t.
    hyaline t.
    infective t.
    laminated t.
    lateral t.
    marantic t.
    marasmic t.
    milk t.
    mixed t.
    mural t.
    obstructive t.
    occluding t.
    occlusive t.
    organized t.
    pale t.
    parasitic t.
    parietal t.
    phagocytic t.
    pigmentary t.
    plate t.
    platelet t.
    postmortem t.
    primary t.

throm·bus *(continued)*
    propagated t.
    red t.
    saddle t.
    septic t.
    stratified t.
    traumatic t.
    valvular t.
    white t.
thrush
thrust
    extensor t.
    paraspinal t.
    spinal t.
    tongue t.
thryp·sis
Thu·di·chum's test
Thu·ja
thu·ja
thu·jone
thu·li·um
thumb
    bifid t.
    cortical t.
    gamekeeper's t.
    tennis t.
    trigger t.
thumb·print·ing
thumb-suck·ing
thun·der·clap head·ache
thyme
    creeping t.
    wild t.
thy·mec·to·mize
thy·mec·to·my
thy·mel·co·sis
thy·mic
thy·mi·co·lym·phat·ic
thy·mi·dine
    t. kinase
thy·mi·dyl·ate
thy·mi·dyl·ate syn·thase
thy·mi·dyl·ic acid
thy·mi·dyl·yl
thy·min
thy·mine
thy·min·ic acid
thym·i·on

thym·i·o·sis
thy·mi·tis
    autoimmune t.
thy·mo·cyte
thy·mo·hy·dro·quin·one
thy·mo·ke·sis
thy·mo·ki·net·ic
thy·mol
    t. phthalein
thy·mo·lep·tic
thy·mol·ize
thy·mol·phthal·ein
thy·mol·sul·fon·phthal·ein
thy·mol·y·sis
thy·mo·lyt·ic
thy·mo·ma
thy·mo·me·tas·ta·sis
thy·mo·path·ic
thy·mop·a·thy
thy·mo·pen·tin
thy·mo·poi·e·tin
thy·mo·priv·ic
thy·mop·ri·vous
thy·mo·sin
thy·mo·tox·ic
thy·mo·tox·in
thy·mo·troph·ic
Thy·mus
thy·mus
    accessory t.
    t. persistens hyperplastica
    persistent t.
thy·mus-de·pen·dent
thy·mus·ec·to·my
thy·mus-in·de·pen·dent
Thy·rar
thy·ra·tron
thy·ro·ac·tive
thy·ro·ad·e·ni·tis
thy·ro·apla·sia
thy·ro·ar·y·te·noid
thy·ro·cal·ci·to·nin
thy·ro·car·di·ac
thy·ro·car·di·tis
thy·ro·cele
thy·ro·chon·drot·o·my
thy·ro·col·loid
thy·ro·cri·cot·o·my

thy·ro·epi·glot·tic
thy·ro·fis·sure
thy·ro·gen·ic
thy·rog·e·nous
thy·ro·glob·u·lin
thy·ro·glos·sal
thy·ro·hy·al
thy·ro·hy·oid
thy·roid
    aberrant t.
    accessory t.
    ectopic t.
    intrathoracic t.
    lingual t.
    retrosternal t.
    substernal t.
thy·roi·dea
    t. ima
thy·roid·ec·to·mize
thy·roid·ec·to·my
    medical t.
thy·roid·ism
thy·roid·itis
    acute t.
    acute nonsuppurative t.
    acute suppurative t.
    autoimmune t.
    chronic t.
    chronic atrophic t.
    chronic fibrous t.
    chronic lymphadenoid t.
    chronic lymphocytic t.
    de Quervain's t.
    focal lymphocytic t.
    giant cell t.
    giant follicular t.
    granulomatous t.
    Hashimoto's t.
    invasive t.
    ligneous t.
    lymphocytic t.
    lymphoid t.
    painless t.
    parasitic t.
    postpartum t.
    pseudotuberculous t.
    pyogenic t.
    Riedel's t.

thy·roid·itis *(continued)*
  silent t.
  subacute diffuse t.
  subacute granulomatous t.
  subacute lymphocytic t.
  woody t.
thy·roid·iza·tion
  de Quervain's t.
thy·roido·ther·a·py
thy·roid·ot·o·my
thy·roido·tox·in
thy·roid per·ox·i·dase
thy·ro·in·tox·i·ca·tion
Thy·ro·lar
thy·ro·la·ryn·ge·al
thy·ro·lin·gual
thy·ro·lyt·ic
thy·ro·meg·a·ly
thy·ro·mi·met·ic
thy·ro·nine
thy·ro·para·thy·roid·ec·to·my
thy·ro·para·thy·ro·priv·ic
thy·rop·a·thy
thy·ro·pe·nia
thy·ro·pha·ryn·ge·al
thy·ro·pri·val
thy·ro·priv·ia
thy·ro·priv·ic
thy·rop·ri·vous
thy·rop·to·sis
thy·ro·ther·a·py
thy·ro·tome
thy·rot·o·my
thy·ro·tox·emia
thy·ro·tox·ic
thy·ro·tox·i·co·sis
  t. factitia
thy·ro·trope
thy·ro·troph
thy·ro·troph·ic
thy·ro·troph·in
thy·ro·trop·ic
thy·rot·ro·pin
  human chorionic t.
thy·rox·in
thy·rox·ine
  levo t.

thy·rox·ine *(continued)*
  radioactive t.
thy·rox·in·ic
Thys·a·no·so·ma
  T. actinioides
Thy·tro·par
TIA — transient ischemic attack
ti·a·men·i·dine hy·dro·chlo·ride
ti·az·ur·il
TIBC — total iron-binding capacity
tib·ia
  saber t.
  saber-scabbard t.
  saber-shaped t.
  t. valga
  t. vara
tib·i·ad
tib·i·al
tib·i·a·le
  t. externum
  t. posticum
tib·i·al·gia
tib·i·a·lis
tib·io·cal·ca·ne·an
tib·io·fem·or·al
tib·io·fib·u·lar
tib·io·na·vic·u·lar
tib·io·per·o·ne·al
tib·io·scaph·oid
tib·io·tar·sal
ti·bo·lone
ti·bric acid
tic
  blinking t.
  bowing t.
  compulsive t.
  convulsive t.
  degenerative t.
  t. de pensée
  diaphragmatic t.
  t. douloureux
  facial t.
  gesticulatory t.
  t. de Guinon
  habit t.

tic *(continued)*
    laryngeal t.
    local t.
    mimic t.
    motor t.
    t. nondouloureux
    progressive choreic t.
    respiratory t.
    rocking t.
    rotatory t.
    saltatory t.
    t. de sommeil
    spasmodic t.
    wide-eyed t.
    winking t.
Ti·car
ti·car·bo·dine
ti·car·cil·lin
    t. cresyl sodium
    t. disodium
    t. sodium
tick
    adobe t.
    American dog t.
    bandicoot t.
    beady-legged winter horse t.
    black pitted t.
    bont t.
    British dog t.
    brown dog t.
    castor bean t.
    cattle t.
    dog t.
    ear t.
    Gulf Coast t.
    hard t.
    hard-bodied t.
    Kenya t.
    Lone Star t.
    miana t.
    Pacific coast dog t.
    pajaroello t.
    pigeon t.
    rabbit t.
    Rocky Mountain wood t.
    russet t.
    scrub t.

tick *(continued)*
    seed t.
    sheep t.
    soft t.
    soft-bodied t.
    spinous ear t.
    taiga t.
    tampan t.
    winter t.
    wood t.
tick·ling
tic·la·tone
ti·clo·pi·dine hy·dro·chlo·ride
tic·po·lon·ga
t.i.d. — L. ter in die (three times a day)
tide
    acid t.
    alkaline t.
    fat t.
    red t.
Ti·dy's test
Tie·de·mann's nerve
Tiet·ze's syndrome
Tiet·ze's disease
Ti·gan
ti·ges·tol
tig·lic acid
ti·groid
ti·grol·y·sis
ti·ki·ti·ki
ti·let·a·mine hy·dro·chlo·ride
til·i·dine hy·dro·chlo·ride
Til·laux's disease
Til·le·tia
Til·le·ti·a·ceae
til·mus
til·or·one
    t. hydrochloride
til·tom·e·ter
tim·bre
    t. métallique
time
    action t.
    activated partial thromboplastin t. (APTT, aPTT, PTT)

time *(continued)*
  adaptation t.
  apex t.
  aquisition t.
  arm-lung t.
  association t.
  biologic t.
  bleeding t.
  bleeding t., secondary
  blocking t.
  chromoscopy t.
  circulation t.
  clot retraction t.
  clotting t.
  coagulation t.
  conduction t.
  counter resolving t.
  dead t.
  decimal reduction t.
  deep tendon reflex
    relaxation t.
  delay t.
  dextrinizing t.
  doubling t.
  echo t. (TE)
  euglobulin clot lysis t.
  expiratory pause t.
  filter bleeding t.
  generation t.
  inertia t.
  insensitive t.
  inspiratory pause t.
  interpulse t.
  inversion t.
  Ivy bleeding t.
  lead t.
  longitudinal relaxation t.
  mean generation t.
  one-stage prothrombin t.
  partial thromboplastin t.
    (PTT)
  perception t.
  plasma clot t.
  prothrombin t.
  pulmonary circulation t.
  reaction t.
  real-t.
  recalcification t.

time *(continued)*
  recognition t.
  relaxation t.
  repetition t.
  resolving t.
  response t.
  retention t.
  retinocortical t.
  rise t.
  sedimentation t.
  serum prothrombin t.
  spin-lattice relaxation t.
  spin-spin relaxation t.
  survival t.
  synaptic transmission t.
  T_1 relaxation t.
  T_2 relaxation t.
  template bleeding t.
  thermal death t.
  thrombin t. (TT)
  tincture of t.
  transit t.
  transverse relaxation t.
  treadmill walking t.
  ventricular activation t.
tim·er
  electronic t.
  photoelectric t.
ti·mo·lol mal·e·ate
tin
  t. chloride
  t. oxide
tina
Tin·ac·tin
Tin·berg·en, Nikolaas
tinct. — tinctura
  tincture
tinc·ta·ble
tinc·tion
tinc·to·ri·al
tinc·tu·ra *pl.* tinc·tu·rae
tinc·tur·a·tion
tinc·ture
  belladonna t.
  benzethonium chloride t.
  benzoin t., compound
  capsicum t.
  cardamom t., compound

tinc·ture *(continued)*
    digitalis t.
    ferric citrochloride t.
    green soap t.
    iodine t.
    iodine t., strong
    lemon t.
    myrrh t.
    nitromersol t.
    opium t.
    opium t., camphorated
    opium t., deodorized
    rhubarb t., aromatic
    sweet orange peel t.
    thimerosal t.
    t. of time
    tolu balsam t.
    vanilla t.
Tin·dal
tin·ea
    t. amiantacea
    asbestos-like t.
    t. axillaris
    t. barbae
    t. capitis
    t. ciliorum
    t. circinata
    t. corporis
    t. cruris
    t. faciale
    t. faciei
    t. favosa
    t. galli
    t. glabrosa
    t. imbricata
    t. inguinalis
    t. interdigitalis
    t. kerion
    t. manus
    t. manuum
    t. nigra
    t. nodosa
    t. pedis
    t. profunda
    t. sycosis
    t. tarsi
    t. tondens
    t. tonsurans

tin·ea *(continued)*
    t. unguium
    t. versicolor
Tin·el's sign
tin·foil
tin·gi·bil·i·ty
tin·gi·ble
ting·ling
    distal t. on percussion
ti·nid·a·zole
tin·kle
    metallic t.
tin·ni·tus
    t. aurium
    t. cerebri
    clicking t.
    Leudet's t.
    nervous t.
    nonvibratory t.
    objective t.
    pulsatile t.
    subjective t.
    vibratory t.
tin·tom·e·ter
tin·to·met·ric
tin·tom·e·try
ti·o·do·ni·um chlo·ride
ti·o·per·i·done hy·dro·chlo·ride
ti·o·pi·nac
ti·ox·i·da·zole
tip
    t. of nose
    pinched nasal t.
    policeman's t.
    root t.
    t. of sacral bone
    t. of tongue
    Woolner's t.
tip·ping
ti·pren·o·lol hy·dro·chlo·ride
ti·queur
ti·quin·amide hy·dro·chlo·ride
tires
tir·ing
Ti·se·li·us apparatus

tis·sue
- accidental t.
- adenoid t.
- adipose t.
- adipose t., brown
- adipose t., white
- adipose t., yellow
- adrenogenic t.
- analogous t.
- aponeurotic t.
- areolar t.
- areolar connective t.
- basement t.
- bony t.
- brown fat t.
- bursa-equivalent t.
- bursal equivalent t.
- cancellous t.
- cartilaginous t.
- cavernous t.
- cellular t.
- chondroid t.
- chordal t.
- chromaffin t.
- cicatricial t.
- compact t.
- connective t.
- cribriform t.
- critical t.
- dartoid t.
- dense fibrous connective t.
- elastic t.
- elastic t., yellow
- embryonal connective t.
- endothelial t.
- episcleral t.
- epithelial t.
- epivaginal connective t.
- erectile t.
- erectile t. of penis
- extracellular t.
- extraperitoneal t.
- fatty t.
- fibroareolar t.
- fibrocellular t.
- fibroelastic t.
- fibrohyaline t.
- fibrous t.

tis·sue *(continued)*
- fibrous t., white
- Gamgee t.
- gelatiginous t.
- gelatinous t.
- glandular t.
- granulation t.
- gut-associated lymphoid t. (GALT)
- hematopoietic t.
- heterologous t.
- heterotopic t.
- homologous t.
- hyperplastic t.
- indifferent t.
- inflammatory t.
- interrenal t.
- interstitial t.
- junctional t.
- keratinized t.
- Kuhnt's intermediary t.
- laminated t.
- lardaceous t.
- loose connective t.
- lymphadenoid t.
- lymphatic t.
- lymphoid t.
- mesenchymal t.
- metanephrogenic t.
- mucoid t.
- mucous t.
- multilocular adipose t.
- muscular t.
- myeloid t.
- nephrogenic t.
- nerve t.
- nervous t.
- nodal t.
- osseous t.
- osteogenic t.
- osteoid t.
- parenchymatous t.
- periapical t.
- periodontal t.
- periosteal t.
- pigmented connective t.
- protochondral t.
- pseudoerectile t.

tis·sue *(continued)*
    reticular t.
    reticulated t.
    retroperitoneal t.
    rubber t.
    scar t.
    scleral t.
    sclerous t's
    shock t.
    skeletal t.
    splenic t.
    subcutaneous t.
    subcutaneous fatty t.
    sustentacular t.
    symplastic t.
    target t.
    tendinous t.
    tuberculosis granulation t.
    vesicular supporting t.
tis·sue-ac·tive
tis·sue-borne
tis·sul·ar
ti·ta·ni·um
    t. dioxide
ti·ter
    agglutination t.
    anti-hyaluronidase t.
    anti-RHO-D t.
    anti-teichoic acid t.
    CF antibody t.
    HI (hemagglutination
      inhibition) t.
    TORCH (toxoplasmosis,
      other, rubella, cytomega-
      lovirus, herpes) t.
    whole complement t.
tit·il·la·tion
ti·trant
ti·trate
ti·tra·tion
    colorimetric t.
    complexometric t.
    coulometric t.
    Dean and Webb t.
    formol t.
    potentiometric t.
ti·tre

tit·ri·met·ric
tit·rim·e·try
tit·u·bant
tit·u·ba·tion
    lingual t.
Tit·y·us ser·ru·la·tus
tix·a·nox
Tiz·zo·ni's test
TK — thymidine kinase
TKD — tokodynamometer
TKG — tokodynagraph
TL — temporal lobe
    total lipids
    tubal ligation
TLC — thin-layer
    chromatography
    total lung capacity
TLE — thin-layer
    electrophoresis
TLSO — thoracolumbosacral
    orthosis
Tm — transport maximum
TMI — transmandibular
    implant
TMIF — tumor cell migration
    inhibition factor
TMJ — temporomandibular
    joint
TMV — tobacco mosaic virus
Tn — normal intraocular
    tension
TNF — tumor necrosis factor
TNM — tumor-node-
    metastasis
TNS — transcutaneous nerve
    stimulation
TNT — trinitrotoluene
TO — tincture of opium
TOA — tubo-ovarian abscess
toad·skin
toad·stool
to·bac·co
    mountain t.
to·bac·co·ism
To·bey-Ay·er test
to·bra·my·cin
to·cai·nide
to·cam·phyl

To·clase
to·co·al·gog·ra·phy
to·co·dy·na·graph
to·co·dy·na·mom·e·ter
to·co·graph
to·cog·ra·phy
to·col
to·col·y·sis
to·com·e·ter
to·coph·er·ol
    α-t.
    alpha-t.
to·coph·er·ol·qui·none
to·co·pho·bia
To·da·ro's tendon
Todd bodies
Todd's cirrhosis
Todd's palsy
Todd's paralysis
Todd's process
Tod·dal·ia
toe
    curly t's
    down-going t's
    great t.
    hammer t.
    little t.
    mallet t.
    Morton's t.
    pigeon t.
    seedy t.
    stiff t.
    tennis t.
    up-going t.
    webbed t's
toe·nail
    ingrowing t.
Toep·fer
to·fen·a·cin hy·dro·chlo·ride
To·fra·nil
To·ga·vi·ri·dae
to·ga·vi·rus
toi·let
    pulmonary t.
Toi·son's fluid
Toi·son's solution
to·ke·lau
to·ko·dy·na·graph

to·ko·dy·na·mom·e·ter
to·la·mo·lol
tol·az·amide
tol·az·o·line hy·dro·chlo·ride
tol·bu·ta·mide
    t. sodium
tol·ci·clate
Tol·ec·tin
tol·er·ance
    acoustic t.
    acquired t.
    adaptation t.
    adoptive t.
    alkali t.
    crossed t.
    drug t.
    G t.
    glucose t.
    high-dose t.
    high-zone t.
    immune t.
    immunologic t.
    impaired glucose t. (IGT)
    low-dose t.
    low-zone t.
    self t.
    species t.
    split t.
tol·er·ant
tol·er·a·tion
tol·ero·gen
tol·ero·gen·e·sis
tol·er·o·gen·ic
to·li·dine
Tol·in·ase
to·lin·date
to·li·o·di·um chlo·ride
Tol·lens' test
tol·met·in so·di·um
tol·naf·tate
to·lo·ni·um chlo·ride
To·lo·sa-Hunt syndrome
Tol·ser·ol
tol·u·ene
    t. diisocyanate (TDI)
tol·u·i·dine
    t. blue O
tol·u·yl

tol·u·yl·ene
tol·yl
    t. hydroxide
to·ma·tin
to·men·tum
    t. cerebri
Tomes' fiber
Tomes' fibril
Tomes' layer
Tomes' process
to·mite
Tom·ma·sel·li's disease
Tom·ma·sel·li's syndrome
to·mo·gram
to·mo·graph
to·mog·ra·phy
    computed t.
    computerized axial t. (CAT)
    dynamic computerized t.
    focal plane t.
    high-resolution
      computerized t.
    hypocycloidal t.
    positron emission t. (PET)
    single photon emission
      computed t. (SPECT)
    ultrasonic t.
to·mo·lev·el
to·mont
ton·a·pha·sia
tone
    arterial t.
    feeling t.
    heart t's
    jecoral t.
    muscle t.
    myogenic t.
    nervous t.
    neurogenic t.
    peripheral vasomotor t.
    plastic t.
    Traube's double t.
    Williams' tracheal t.
tongs
    Crutchfield's t.
    skull t.
tongue
    adherent t.

tongue *(continued)*
    amyloid t.
    antibiotic t.
    baked t.
    bald t.
    beefy t.
    bifid t.
    black t.
    black hairy t.
    blue t.
    burning t.
    cardinal t.
    cerebriform t.
    choreic t.
    cleft t.
    coated t.
    cobble-stone t.
    crescent t.
    crocodile t.
    dotted t.
    double t.
    earthy t.
    encrusted t.
    fern leaf t.
    filmy t.
    fissured t.
    flat t.
    frog t.
    furred t.
    furrowed t.
    geographic t.
    glazed t.
    grooved t.
    hairy t.
    hobnail t.
    lobulated t.
    magenta t.
    mappy t.
    parrot t.
    plicated t.
    raspberry t.
    raw-beef t.
    Sandwith's bald t.
    scrotal t.
    smokers' t.
    smooth t.
    t. of sphenoid bone
    split t.

tongue *(continued)*
  sprue t.
  stippled t.
  strawberry t., red
  strawberry t., white
  sulcated t.
  timber t.
  trombone t.
  white t.
  wooden t.
  wrinkled t.
tongue-tie
ton·ic
  bitter t.
  cardiac t.
  digestive t.
  general t.
  intestinal t.
  stomachic t.
  vascular t.
ton·ic-clo·nic
to·nic·i·ty
ton·i·cize
ton·i·co·clon·ic
ton·ka bean
tono·clon·ic
tono·fi·bril
tono·fil·a·ment
tono·gram
tono·graph
to·nog·ra·phy
  carotid compression t.
to·nom·e·ter
  air-puff t.
  applanation t.
  electronic t.
  Gärtner's t.
  Goldmann's applanation t.
  impression t.
  indentation t.
  MacKay-Marg electronic t.
  McLean t.
  Musken's t.
  pneumatic t.
  Recklinghausen's t.
  Schiøtz t.

to·nom·e·try
  applanation t.
  digital t.
  impression t.
tono·plast
tono·scope
tono·top·ic
tono·top·ic·i·ty
ton·sil
  adenoid t.
  buried t.
  t. of cerebellum
  eustachian t.
  faucial t.
  Gerlach's t.
  intestinal t.
  lingual t.
  Luschka's t.
  nasopharyngeal t.
  palatine t.
  pharyngeal t.
  submerged t.
  third t.
  t. of torus tubarius
  tubal t's
ton·sil·la *pl.* ton·sil·lae
  t. adenoidea
  t. cerebelli
  t. of cerebellum
  t. intestinalis
  t. lingualis
  t. palatina
  t. pharyngea
  t. pharyngealis
    pharyngealis
  t. tubaria
ton·sil·lar
ton·sil·lec·tome
ton·sil·lec·to·my
  dissection t.
  guillotine t.
ton·sil·lith
ton·sil·lit·ic
ton·sil·li·tis
  caseous t.
  catarrhal t., acute
  catarrhal t., chronic

ton·sil·li·tis *(continued)*
    chronic t.
    diphtherial t.
    erythematous t.
    follicular t.
    herpetic t.
    lacunar t.
    t. lenta
    lingual t.
    mycotic t.
    parenchymatous t., acute
    phlegmonous t.
    preglottic t.
    pustular t.
    streptococcal t.
    superficial t.
    suppurative t.
    ulceromembranous t.
    Vincent's t.
ton·sil·lo·ad·e·noid·ec·to·my
ton·sil·lo·hemi·spo·ro·sis
ton·sil·lo·lith
ton·sil·lo·mo·ni·li·a·sis
ton·sil·lo·my·co·sis
ton·sil·lop·a·thy
ton·sil·lo·tome
ton·sil·lot·o·my
ton·sil·lo·ty·phoid
ton·so·lith
to·nus
    acerebral t.
    chemical t.
    myogenic t.
    neurogenic t.
tooth *pl.* teeth
    abutment t.
    accessional teeth
    accessory t.
    anatomic teeth
    anchor t.
    ankylosed t.
    anterior teeth
    artificial t.
    auditory teeth of Huschke
    t. of axis
    baby teeth
    bicuspid teeth
    buccal teeth

tooth *(continued)*
    canine teeth
    cheek teeth
    conical t.
    connate t.
    corner t.
    Corti's auditory t.
    cross-bite teeth
    cross-pin teeth
    cuspid teeth
    cuspless t.
    cutting t.
    dead t.
    deciduous teeth
    diatoric teeth
    drifting t.
    embedded t.
    t. of epistropheus
    eye t.
    Fournier teeth
    fused teeth
    geminate t.
    Goslee t.
    green t.
    hag teeth
    hereditary brown
      opalescent t.
    Horner's teeth
    Hutchinson's teeth
    hutchinsonian t.
    impacted t.
    incisor teeth
    labial teeth
    malacotic teeth
    malposed t.
    mandibular teeth
    maxillary teeth
    metal insert t.
    migrating t.
    milk t.
    molar teeth
    Moon's teeth
    morsal teeth
    mottled teeth
    mulberry t.
    multicuspid t.
    natal t.
    neonatal t.

tooth *(continued)*
    nonanatomic teeth
    nonvital t.
    notched t.
    peg t.
    peg-shaped t.
    pegtop t.
    permanent teeth
    pink t. of Mummery
    pinless teeth
    posterior teeth
    predeciduous t.
    premature teeth
    premolar teeth
    primary teeth
    pulpless t.
    rake teeth
    rootless teeth
    rotated t.
    sclerotic teeth
    screwdriver teeth
    shell t.
    snaggle t.
    stomach t.
    straight-pin teeth
    submerged t.
    succedaneous teeth
    successional teeth
    superior teeth
    supernumerary teeth
    supplemental teeth
    syphilitic t.
    temporary teeth
    tube teeth
    Turner's t.
    unerupted t.
    vital teeth
    wandering t.
    wisdom t.
    wolf t.
    zero degree teeth
Tooth's atrophy
Tooth's disease
Tooth's type
tooth·ache
tooth-borne
tooth·brush·ing
top·ag·no·sia

top·ag·no·sis
to·pal·gia
to·pec·to·my
top·es·the·sia
Töp·fer's test
to·pha·ceous
to·phi
topho·li·po·ma
to·phus *pl.* to·phi
    auricular t.
    dental t.
    t. of pinna
    t. syphiliticus
top·i·cal
Top·i·cort
Top·i·cy·cline
Top·i·nard's angle
Top·i·nard's line
topo·al·gia
topo·an·es·the·sia
topo·chem·is·try
topo·dys·es·the·sia
top·og·no·sis
topo·graph·ic
topo·graph·i·cal
to·pog·ra·phy
topo·isom·er·ase
to·pol·o·gy
topo·nar·co·sis
topo·nym
to·pon·y·my
topo·par·es·the·sia
topo·phy·lax·is
topo·therm·es·the·si·om·e·ter
Top·syn
top·te·rone
TOPV — poliovirus vaccine
    live oral trivalent
tor·cu·lar
    t. Herophili
Tor·e·can
To·rek operation
to·ri
to·ric
Tor·kild·sen's operation
tor·mi·na
tor·mi·nal

Torn·waldt's (Thorn·waldt's)
  bursa
Torn·waldt's bursitis
Torn·waldt's disease
to·rose
to·rous
tor·pent
tor·pid
tor·pid·i·ty
tor·por
    t. retinae
    summer t.
    winter t.
torque
torqu·ing
torr
tor·re·fac·tion
tor·re·fy
tor·ri·cel·li·an
tor·sades de pointes
tor·sion
    lateral t.
    negative t.
    positive t.
tor·sion·om·e·ter
tor·sive
tor·si·ver·sion
tor·so
tor·ti·col·lar
tor·ti·col·lis
    acute t.
    congenital t.
    dermatogenic t.
    fixed t.
    hysteric t.
    hysterical t.
    infantile t.
    intermittent t.
    labyrinthine t.
    mental t.
    myogenic t.
    nasopharyngeal t.
    neurogenic t.
    ocular t.
    paralytic t.
    reflex t.
    rheumatoid t.
    spasmodic t.

tor·ti·col·lis *(continued)*
    spastic t.
    spurious t.
    symptomatic t.
tor·ti·pel·vis
tor·tua
tor·tu·ous
tor·u·li
tor·u·loid
Tor·u·lop·sis
    T. glabrata
    T. histolytica
    T. pintolopesii
tor·u·lop·so·sis
tor·u·lo·sis
tor·u·lus *pl.* tor·u·li
    toruli tactiles
to·rus *pl.* to·ri
    buccal t.
    t. frontalis
    t. levatorius
    t. mandibulae
    t. mandibularis
    t. occipitalis
    palatine t.
    t. palatinus
    supraorbital t.
    t. tubarius
    t. uretericus
to·si·fen
to·sy·late
To·ta·cil·lin
To·ti's operation
to·ti·po·ten·cy
to·tip·o·tent
to·ti·po·ten·tial
to·ti·po·ten·ti·al·i·ty
touch
    abdominal t.
    double t.
    rectal t.
    royal t.
    vaginal t.
    vesical t.
Tou·raine's aphthosis
Tou·raine-So·lente-Go·lé
  syndrome
Tou·rette's disease

Tou·rette's syndrome
tour·ni·quet
    automatic rotating t.
    Esmarch's t.
    forceps t.
    garrote t.
    Lynn Thomas t.
    pneumatic t.
    scalp t.
    Spanish t.
    torcular t.
    windlass t.
Tour·tu·al's canal
Tou·ton giant cell
Towne projection radiograph
Town·send ionization
tox·ane·mia
tox·a·phene
Tox·as·ca·ris
    T. leonina
tox·emia
    eclamptic t.
    eclamptogenic t.
    hydatid t.
    preeclamptic t.
    t. of pregnancy
    pregnancy t. in ewes
tox·emic
tox·en·zyme
tox·ic
tox·i·cant
tox·i·ca·tion
tox·i·ce·mia
tox·i·cide
tox·ic·i·ty
    O_2 t.
    oxygen t.
tox·i·co·den·drol
tox·i·co·gen·ic
tox·i·co·he·mia
tox·i·coid
tox·i·co·ki·net·ics
tox·i·co·log·ic
tox·i·col·o·gist
tox·i·col·o·gy
    prospective t.
    predictive t.
tox·i·co·path·ic

tox·i·cop·a·thy
tox·i·co·pec·tic
tox·i·co·pex·ic
tox·i·co·pex·is
tox·i·co·pexy
tox·i·co·phid·ia
tox·i·co·pho·bia
tox·i·co·sis
    aspergillus t.
    endogenic t.
    exogenic t.
    gestational t.
    hemorrhagic capillary t.
    proteinogenous t.
    retention t.
    T_3 t.
toxi·cyst
toxi·fer·ine
tox·if·er·ous
tox·i·gen·ic
tox·i·ge·nic·i·ty
tox·ig·nom·ic
tox·im·e·try
tox·in
    amanita t.
    animal t.
    anthrax t.
    bacterial t's
    botulinus t.
    cholera t.
    clostridial t.
    dermonecrotic t.
    Dick t.
    dinoflagellate t.
    diphtheria t.
    diphtheria t., diagnostic
    diphtheria t., inactivated
      diagnostic
    diptheria t. for Schick test
    dysentery t.
    epidermolytic t.
    erythrogenic t.
    extracellular t.
    fatigue t.
    fugu t.
    fusarial t.
    gas gangrene t.
    gonococcal t.

tox·in *(continued)*
 intracellular t.
 labile t. (LT)
 meningococcal t.
 necrotizing t.
 perfringens alpha t.
 perfringens theta t.
 plague t.
 plant t.
 pseudomonal t.
 rickettsial t.
 scarlatinal t.
 scarlet fever erythrogenic
  t.
 Shiga t.
 soluble t.
 stable t. (ST)
 staphylococcal t.
 streptococcal t.
 streptococcus erythrogenic
  t.
 tetanus t.
 whooping cough t.
tox·in-an·ti·tox·in
tox·in·emia
tox·in·ol·o·gy
tox·in·o·sis
tox·ip·a·thy
toxi·pho·bia
toxi·res·in
tox·is·ter·ol
Tox·o·ca·ra
 T. canis
 T. cati
 T. mystax
tox·o·car·al
tox·o·car·i·a·sis
 human t.
tox·o·gen
toxo·glob·u·lin
tox·oid
 adsorbed t.
 bacterial t.
 diphtheria t.
 formol t.
 tetanus t.
tox·oid-an·ti·tox·oid
toxo·lec·i·thid

toxo·lec·i·thin
toxo·neme
toxo·no·sis
toxo·pex·ic
toxo·phil
toxo·phil·ic
tox·oph·i·lous
toxo·phore
tox·oph·o·rous
Tox·o·plas·ma
 T. cuniculi
 T. gondii
toxo·plas·mic
toxo·plas·min
tox·o·plas·mo·sis
 ocular t.
toxo·pro·tein
Toxo·rhyn·chi·tes
 T. rutilus
tox·uria
Toyn·bee's corpuscles
Toyn·bee's experiment
Toyn·bee's law
Toyn·bee's ligament
Toyn·bee's otoscope
TP — threshold potential
 tuberculin precipitation
t-PA — tissue plasminogen
 activator
TPC — thromboplastic plasma
 component
TPHA — *Treponema pallidum*
 hemagglutination assay
TPI — *Treponema pallidum*
 immobilization
TPN — total parenteral
 nutrition
  triphosphopyridine
   nucleotide
TPPN — total peripheral
 parenteral nutrition
TR — tricuspid regurgitation
 tuberculin residue
tra·bec·u·la *pl.* tra·bec·u·lae
 arachnoid trabeculae
 trabeculae of bone
 trabeculae carneae cordis
 trabeculae cordis

tra·bec·u·la *(continued)*
    trabeculae cranii
    fleshy trabeculae of heart
    trabeculae lienis
    Rathke's trabeculae
    septomarginal t.
    t. septomarginalis
    trabeculae of spleen
    trabeculae splenicae
tra·bec·u·lae
tra·bec·u·lar
tra·bec·u·lar·ism
tra·bec·u·late
tra·bec·u·la·tion
    t. of bladder dome
tra·bec·u·lec·to·my
tra·bec·u·lo·plas·ty
    laser t.
trabs *pl.* tra·bes
    contact t's
trac·er
    arrow-point t.
    Gothic arch t.
    needle-point t.
    radioactive t.
    stylus t.
tra·chea *pl.* tra·cheae
    cervical t.
    scabbard t.
tra·cheae
tra·chea·ec·ta·sy
tra·che·al
tra·che·al·gia
tra·che·itis
    t. sicca
tra·che·lec·to·my
tra·che·lem·a·to·ma
tra·che·lism
tra·che·lis·mus
tra·che·li·tis
tra·che·lo·cele
tra·che·lo·cyl·lo·sis
tra·che·lo·cyr·to·sis
tra·che·lo·cys·ti·tis
tra·che·lo·dyn·ia
tra·che·lo·ky·pho·sis
tra·che·lol·o·gist
tra·che·lol·o·gy

tra·che·lo·pexy
tra·che·lo·plas·ty
tra·che·lor·rha·phy
tra·che·los·chi·sis
tra·che·lo·syr·in·gor·rha·phy
tra·che·lot·o·my
tra·cheo·aero·cele
tra·cheo·bron·chi·al
tra·cheo·bron·chi·tis
tra·cheo·bron·cho·meg·a·ly
tra·cheo·bron·chos·co·py
tra·cheo·cele
tra·cheo·esoph·a·ge·al
tra·cheo·fis·tu·li·za·tion
tra·che·o·gen·ic
tra·che·og·ra·phy
tra·cheo·la·ryn·ge·al
tra·cheo·lar·yn·got·o·my
tra·che·ole
tra·cheo·ma·la·cia
tra·cheo·path·ia
    t. osteoplastica
tra·che·op·a·thy
tra·cheo·pha·ryn·ge·al
tra·cheo·pho·ne·sis
tra·che·oph·o·ny
tra·cheo·plas·ty
tra·cheo·py·o·sis
tra·che·or·rha·gia
tra·che·or·rha·phy
tra·che·os·chi·sis
tra·cheo·scope
tra·cheo·scop·ic
tra·che·os·co·py
    percervical t.
    peroral t.
tra·cheo·ste·no·sis
tra·che·os·to·ma
tra·che·os·tome
    end t.
tra·che·os·to·mize
tra·che·os·to·my
tra·cheo·tome
tra·che·ot·o·mize
tra·che·ot·o·my
    inferior t.
    superior t.
tra·chi·tis

tra·cho·ma *pl.* tra·cho·ma·ta
    Arlt's t.
    Türck's t.
    t. of vocal bands
tra·cho·ma·ta
tra·cho·ma·tous
tra·chy·chro·mat·ic
tra·chy·pho·nia
trac·ing
    arrow-point t.
    cephalometric t.
    contact t.
    extraoral t.
    Gothic arch t.
    intraoral t.
    flat t.
    needle-point t.
    pantographic t.
    stylus t.
track
    germ t.
    ionization t.
Tracrium
tract
    afferent t.
    alimentary t.
    anterior cerebrospinal t.
    arcuatofloccular t.
    ascending t.
    ascending t's of spinal cord
    association t.
    atrio-His t.
    Bekhterev's t.
    biliary t.
    Bruce's t.
    t. of Bruce and Muir
    bulbar t.
    bulbospinal t.
    Burdach's t.
    t. of Calza
    central t. of acoustic nerve
    central t. of auditory nerve
    central t. of cochlear nerve
    central t. of cranial nerves
    central t. of thymus
    central tegmental t.
    central t. of trigeminal
      nerve

tract *(continued)*
    cerebellobulbar t.
    cerebelloreticular t.
    cerebellorubral t.
    cerebellorubrospinal t.
    cerebellospinal t.
    cerebellotegmental t's of
      bulb
    cerebellothalamic t.
    cerebellovestibular t.
    colliculorubral t.
    Collier's t.
    comma t. of Schultze
    commissurospinal t.
    conariohypophyseal t.
    cornucommissural t.
    corticobulbar t.
    corticocerebellar t.
    corticocollicular t.
    corticogeniculate t.
    corticohypothalamic t's
    corticonigral t.
    corticonuclear t.
    corticopallidal t.
    corticopontile t.
    corticopontine t.
    corticopontocerebellar t's
    corticorubral t.
    corticospinal t., anterior
    corticospinal t., crossed
    corticospinal t., direct
    corticospinal t., lateral
    corticospinal t. of medulla
      oblongata
    corticospinal t's of spinal
      cord
    corticotectal t.
    corticothalamic t.
    dead t.
    Deiters' t.
    dentatothalamic t.
    descending t.
    descending t's of spinal
      cord
    descending vestibular t.
    digestive t.
    direct cerebellar t. of
      Flechsig

tract *(continued)*
    direct vestibulocerebellar t.
    dopaminergic t.
    dorsolateral t.
    efferent t.
    extracorticospinal t.
    extrapyramidal t.
    fastigiobulbar t's
    fastigiovestibular t.
    fiber t's of spinal cord
    Flechsig's t.
    flow t. of the heart
    foraminous spiral t.
    fronto-occipital t.
    frontopontile t.
    gastrointestinal t.
    generative t.
    geniculocalcarine t.
    geniculostriate t.
    geniculotemporal t.
    genital t.
    genitourinary t.
    Goll's t.
    Gowers' t.
    Gudden's t.
    habenular t.
    habenulodiencephalic t. of
        Edinger
    habenulointerpeduncular t.
    habenulopeduncular t.
    Helweg's t.
    Hoche's t.
    hypothalamohypophysial t.
    iliopubic t.
    iliotibial t.
    intermediolateral t.
    internuncial t.
    intersegmental t's of spinal
        cord, anterior
    intersegmental t's of spinal
        cord, dorsal
    intersegmental t's of spinal
        cord, lateral
    intersegmental t's of spinal
        cord, posterior
    intersegmental t's of spinal
        cord, ventral
    intestinal t.

tract *(continued)*
    lateral t. of isthmus
    lateral olfactory t.
    lenticulothalamic t.
    Lissauer's t.
    Löwenthal's t.
    lower respiratory t.
    Maissiat's t.
    mamillointerpeduncular t.
    mamillopeduncular t.
    mamillotegmental t.
    mamillothalamic t.
    Marchi's t.
    marginal t., crossed
    mesencephalic t. of
        trigeminal nerve
    Meynert's t.
    Monakow's t.
    motor t.
    nigrorubral t.
    nigrostriatal t.
    occipitopontile t.
    occipitopontine t.
    olfactohabenular t.
    olfactohypothalamic t.
    olfactory t.
    olivocerebellar t.
    olivospinal t.
    optic t.
    pallidoreticular t.
    pallidosubthalamic t.
    pallidotegmental t.
    pallidothalamic t.
    parietopontine t.
    peduncular t., transverse
    periependymal t.
    periventricular t.
    t. of Philippe-Gombault
    pontocerebellar t.
    portal t.
    predorsal t.
    prepyramidal t.
    projection t.
    pyramidal t.
    pyramidal t., anterior
    pyramidal t., crossed
    pyramidal t., direct
    pyramidal t., lateral

tract *(continued)*
  pyramidal t's of spinal cord
  pyramidoanterior t.
  pyramidolateral t.
  respiratory t.
  reticulobulbar t.
  reticulo-olivary t.
  reticuloreticular t.
  reticulospinal t.
  reticulospinal t., anterior
  reticulospinal t., ventral
  rubro-olivary t.
  rubroreticular t.
  rubroreticulospinal t.
  rubrospinal t.
  rubrothalamic t.
  Schultze's t.
  semilunar t.
  seminal t.
  sensory t.
  septohabenular t.
  septomarginal t.
  solitariospinal t.
  solitary t. of medulla
    oblongata
  spinal t. of trigeminal
    nerve
  spinal vestibular t.
  spinocerebellar t., anterior
  spinocerebellar t., direct
  spinocerebellar t., dorsal
  spinocerebellar t., posterior
  spinocervicothalamic t.
  spino-olivary t.
  spinospinal t.
  spinotectal t.
  spinothalamic t., anterior
  Spitzka's t.
  Spitzka-Lissauer t.
  Spitzka's marginal t.
  strionigral t.
  striorubral t.
  striothalamic t.
  sulcomarginal t.
  supraopticohypophysial t.
  tectobulbar t.
  tectocerebellar t.
  tectorubral t.

tract *(continued)*
  tectospinal t.
  tectotegmental t.
  tegmental t.
  tegmento-olivary t.
  tegmentospinal t.
  temporopontile t.
  temporopontine t.
  thalamocortical t.
  thalamohypothalamic t.
  thalamo-occipital t.
  thalamo-olivary t.
  tracheobronchial t.
  transverse peduncular t.
  triangular t.
  triangular t. of
    Philippe-Gombault
  trigeminothalamic t.
  tuberohypophysial t.
  tuberoinfundibular t.
  Türck's t.
  upper respiratory t.
  urinary t.
  urogenital t.
  uveal t.
  ventral corticospinal t.
  ventral pyramidal t.
  ventral spinocerebellar t.
  ventral spinothalamic t.
  vestibulocerebellar t.
  vestibulo-ocular t.
  vestibulospinal t.
  t. of Vicq d'Azyr
  vocal t.
  Waldeyer's t.
trac·tel·lum *pl.* trac·tel·la
trac·tion
  axis t.
  Bryant's t.
  Buck's t.
  cervical t.
  Crutchfield's skeletal t.
  elastic t.
  elastic finger t.
  external t.
  halo t.
  halo-pelvic t.
  halter t.

trac·tion *(continued)*
  intermaxillary t.
  internal t.
  intramaxillary t.
  intraoral elastic t.
  isometric t.
  lumbar t.
  maxillomandibular t.
  Russell t.
  skeletal t.
  skin t.
  tongue t.
  vertebral t.
  vitreous t.
  weight t.
  windlass t.
trac·tol·o·gy
trac·tor
  prostatic t.
  Syms' t.
  urethral t.
trac·tot·o·my
  descending root t.
  intramedullary t.
  mesencephalic t.
  pyramidal t.
  Sjöqvist t.
  spinothalamic t.
  trigeminal t.
trac·tus *pl.* trac·tus
  t. bulboreticulospinalis
  t. centralis thymi
  t. cerebellorubralis
  t. cerebellothalamicus
  t. corticobulbaris
  t. corticohypothalamici
  t. corticohypothalamicus
  t. corticonuclearis
  t. corticopontinus
  t. corticospinalis anterior
  t. corticospinalis lateralis
  t. corticospinalis ventralis
  t. dentatothalamicus
  t. dorsolateralis
  t. frontopontinus
  t. habenulo-
    interpeduncularis

trac·tus *(continued)*
  t. hypothalamohypo-
    physialis
  t. iliopubicus
  t. iliotibialis
  t. iliotibialis [Maissiati]
  t. mamillothalamicus
  t. mesencephalicus nervi
    trigemini
  t. occipitopontinus
  t. olfactorius
  t. olivocerebellaris
  t. olivocochlearis
  t. olivospinalis
  t. opticus
  t. paraventriculohypo-
    physialis
  t. parietopontinus
  t. pontoreticulospinalis
  t. pyramidalis
  t. pyramidalis anterior
  t. pyramidalis lateralis
  t. reticulospinalis
  t. reticulospinalis anterior
  t. reticulospinalis ventralis
  t. rubrospinalis
  t. solitarius medullae
    oblongatae
  t. spinalis nervi trigemini
  t. spinocerebellaris
    anterior
  t. spinocerebellaris dorsalis
  t. spinocerebellaris
    posterior
  t. spinocerebellaris
    ventralis
  t. spino-olivaris
  t. spinoreticularis
  t. spinotectalis
  t. spinothalamicus anterior
  t. spinothalamicus lateralis
  t. spinothalamicus
    ventralis
  t. spiralis foraminosus
  t. subarcuatus
  t. supraopticohypophysialis
  t. tectobulbaris
  t. tectospinalis

trac·tus *(continued)*
 t. tegmentalis centralis
 t. temporopontinus
 t. triangularis
 t. trigeminothalamicus
 t. tuberohypophysialis
 t. vestibulospinalis
trag·a·canth
 Indian t.
tra·gal
Tra·gia
trag·i·on
trag·o·mas·chal·ia
trag·o·pho·nia
tra·goph·o·ny
trag·o·po·dia
tra·gus *pl.* tra·gi
train
 t. of four
 t. of pulses
train·a·ble
train·ing
 assertiveness t.
 auditory t.
 bladder t.
 bowel t.
 expressive t.
 habit t.
 sensitivity t.
 toilet t.
trait
 dominant t.
 Hageman t.
 recessive t.
 secretor t.
 sickle cell t.
 single gene t.
 thalassemia t.
tra·jec·tor
Tral
tra·lo·nide
tra·ma·dol hy·dro·chlo·ride
tra·maz·o·line hy·dro·chlo·ride
Tram·bus·ti reaction
Tram·bus·ti test
tram·itis
 alcoholic t.

tram·itis *(continued)*
 induced t.
trance
 hypnotic t.
 somnambulistic t.
Tran·co·pal
Tran·date
tran·ex·am·ic acid
tran·qui·liz·er
 major t.
 minor t.
trans·ab·dom·i·nal
trans·ac·e·tyl·ase
trans·ac·e·tyl·a·tion
trans·ac·y·lase
trans·ac·y·la·tion
trans·al·do·lase
trans·am·i·da·tion
trans·am·i·din·ase
trans·am·i·nase
trans·am·i·na·tion
trans·an·i·ma·tion
trans·an·tral
trans·aor·tic
trans·atri·al
trans·au·di·ent
trans·ax·i·al
trans·ax·o·nal
trans·ba·sal
trans·ca·lent
trans·cal·var·i·al
trans·car·ba·mo·yl·ase
trans·car·boxy·lase
trans·cath·e·ter
trans·cav·i·tary
trans·cer·vi·cal
trans·clo·mi·phene
trans·co·bal·a·min
trans·con·dy·lar
trans·con·dy·loid
trans·cor·ti·cal
trans·cor·tin
trans·cri·co·thy·roid
trans·cript
 primary t.
trans·crip·tase
 reverse t.

trans·crip·tion
  complementary t.
  reverse t.
  symmetric t.
trans·cu·ta·ne·ous
trans·der·mal
trans·der·mic
trans·de·ter·mi·na·tion
trans·du·cer
  acoustic t.
  bone conduction t.
  electrochemical t.
  neuroendocrine t.
  piezoelectric t.
  pressure t.
  quarter-wave t.
  rotating t.
  ultrasound t.
trans·du·cin
trans·duc·tant
trans·duc·tion
  abortive t.
  vestibular t.
trans·du·o·de·nal
trans·du·ral
tran·sect
tran·sec·tion
trans·epi·der·mal
trans·eth·moi·dal
trans·fau·na·tion
trans·fec·tion
trans·fec·to·ma
trans·fer
  adoptive t.
  Bunnell tendon t.
  egg t.
  embryo t.
  group t.
  linear energy t.
  nuclear t.
  passive t.
  phosphate-group t.
  placental t.
  temporalis t.
  tendon t.
trans·fer·ase
trans·fer·ence
  counter t.

trans·fer·ence *(continued)*
  institutional t.
trans·fer·rin
trans·fix
trans·fix·ion
trans·for·ma·tion
  antigenic t.
  asbestos t.
  bacterial t.
  blast t.
  Bliss t.
  globular-fibrous t.
  lymphocyte t.
  membranous t.
trans·form·er
  filament t.
  resonance t.
  step-down t.
  step-up t.
trans·for·mim·i·nase
trans·fruc·to·syl·ase
trans·fuse
trans·fu·sion
  arterial t.
  autologous t.
  bone marrow t.
  cell saver t.
  direct t.
  drip t.
  exchange t.
  exsanguination t.
  fetomaternal t.
  granulocyte t.
  immediate t.
  indirect t.
  intra-arterial t.
  intraperitoneal t.
  intrauterine t.
  leukocyte t.
  mediate t.
  placental t.
  replacement t.
  substitution t.
  sternal t.
trans·fu·sion·al
trans·glu·co·syl·ase
trans·glu·tam·in·ase
trans·gly·co·si·da·tion

trans·gly·co·syl·ase
trans·he·mo·phil·in
trans·he·pat·ic
trans·hi·a·tal
trans·hy·dro·gen·ase
tran·sient
trans·il·i·ac
tran·sil·i·ent
trans·il·lu·mi·na·tion
trans·in·su·lar
trans·is·chi·ac
trans·isth·mi·an
trans·is·tor
    field-effect t.
tran·si·tion
    cervicothoracic t.
    forbidden t.
    isomeric t.
tran·si·tion·al
trans·ke·to·lase
trans·lat·er·al
trans·la·tion
    nick t.
trans·lo·case
trans·lo·ca·tion
    balanced t.
    group t.
    insertional t.
    nonreciprocal t.
    reciprocal t.
    robertsonian t.
    unbalanced t.
trans·lu·cent
trans·lu·mi·nal
trans·me·a·tal
trans·meth·y·lase
trans·meth·y·la·tion
trans·mi·gra·tion
    external t.
    internal t.
trans·mis·si·bil·i·ty
trans·mis·si·ble
trans·mis·sion
    arthropod t.
    cochlear t.
    cyclical t.
    direct t.
    duplex t.

trans·mis·sion *(continued)*
    ephaptic t.
    hereditary arthropod t.
    horizontal t.
    humoral t.
    insect t.
    neurochemical t.
    neurohumoral t.
    neuromuscular t.
    placental t.
    synaptic t.
    vertical t.
trans·mit·tance
trans·mit·ter
trans·mu·ral
trans·mu·ta·tion
trans·oc·u·lar
tran·so·nance
tran·son·ic
trans·or·bi·tal
trans·ovar·i·al
trans·ovar·i·an
trans·pal·a·tal
trans·par·ent
trans·pa·ri·e·tal
trans·pep·ti·da·tion
trans·peri·to·ne·al
trans·phos·phor·y·lase
trans·phos·phor·y·la·tion
tran·spi·ra·tion
    pulmonary t.
tran·spire
trans·pla·cen·tal
trans·plant
    Gallie t.
trans·plan·tar
trans·plan·ta·tion
    allogeneic t.
    corneal t.
    heart t.
    heterotopic t.
    homotopic t.
    liver t.
    lung t.
    orthotopic t.
    pancreatic t.
    pancreaticoduodenal t.
    renal t.

trans·plan·ta·tion *(continued)*
    syngeneic t.
    syngenesioplastic t.
    tendon t.
    tooth t.
trans·pleu·ral
trans·port
    active t.
    active renal tubular t.
    bulk t.
    competitive t.
    membrane t.
    passive t.
    tubal t.
trans·po·sase
trans·po·si·tion
    corrected t. of great vessels
    t. of the great arteries
      (TGA)
    t. of great vessels
    partial t. of great vessels
trans·po·son
trans·pu·bic
trans·sa·cral
trans·scle·ral
trans·sec·tion
trans·seg·men·tal
trans·sep·tal
trans·sex·u·al
trans·sex·u·al·ism
trans·sphe·noi·dal
trans·ster·nal
trans·suc·ci·ny·lase
trans·syn·ap·tic
tran·sta·di·al
trans·tem·po·ral
trans·ten·to·ri·al
trans·tha·lam·ic
trans·ther·mia
trans·tho·rac·ic
trans·thy·re·tin
trans·tra·che·al
trans·tym·pan·ic
tran·su·date
    pleural t.
tran·su·da·tion
trans·ura·ni·um

trans·ure·tero·ure·ter·os·to·my
trans·ure·thral
trans·vag·i·nal
trans·va·te·ri·an
trans·vec·tor
trans·ve·nous
trans·ven·tric·u·lar
trans·ver·sa·lis
trans·verse
trans·ver·sec·to·my
trans·ver·sion
trans·ver·so·cos·tal
trans·ver·sot·o·my
trans·ver·so·ure·thral·is
trans·ver·sus
trans·ves·i·cal
trans·ves·tism
trans·ves·tite
trans·ves·ti·tism
Tran·tas' dots
Tran·xene
tran·yl·cy·pro·mine sul·fate
tra·pe·zi·al
tra·pez·i·form
tra·pe·zio·meta·car·pal
tra·pe·zi·um
trap·e·zoid
Trapp's coefficient
Trapp's formula
Tras·en·tine
Tras·y·lol
Traube's curves
Traube's dyspnea
Traube's heart
Traube's membrane
Traube's space
Traube-Her·ing curves
Traube-Her·ing waves
trau·ma *pl.* trau·mas, trau·ma·ta
    acoustic t.
    birth t.
    occlusal t.
    perinatal t.
    periodontal t.
    potential t.
    psychic t.

trau·ma·ta
trau·ma·ther·a·py
trau·mat·ic
trau·ma·tism
    occlusal t.
    periodontal t.
trau·ma·tize
trau·ma·to·gen·ic
trau·ma·tol·o·gist
trau·ma·tol·o·gy
trau·ma·top·a·thy
trau·ma·to·phil·ia
trau·ma·top·nea
trau·ma·to·sis
trau·ma·to·ther·a·py
trau·mat·ro·pism
Traut·mann triangle
Trav·ase
Trav·a·sol
tray
    acrylic resin t.
    impression t.
tra·zo·done hy·dro·chlo·ride
TRBF — total renal blood flow
TRC — tanned red cells
Trea·cher Col·lins syndrome
Trea·cher Col·lins-Fran·ce·
  schet·ti syndrome
tread
treat·ment
    active t.
    Ascoli's t.
    Beard's t.
    Bell t.
    Bier's t.
    Bird's t.
    Bouchardat's t.
    Brandt t.
    Brehmer's t.
    Brown-Séquard t.
    Calot's t.
    carbon dioxide t.
    Carrel's t.
    Carrel-Dakin t.
    Castellani's t.
    causal t.
    Chervin's t.
    choline t.

treat·ment *(continued)*
    Coffey-Humber t.
    conservative t.
    continuous sleep t.
    Cox's t.
    cross-fire t.
    curative t.
    Dancel's t.
    dietetic t.
    drip t.
    drug t.
    electroconvulsive t.
    electroshock t.
    empiric t.
    eventration t.
    expectant t.
    fever t.
    Fichera's t.
    Fitz Gerald t.
    fractionated t.
    Fränkel's t.
    Frenkel's t.
    Girard's t.
    Goeckerman t.
    Guinard's t.
    Hartel's t.
    high-frequency t.
    hygienic t.
    hyperbaric oxygen t.
    hypoglycemic shock t.
    insulin coma t.
    insulin shock t.
    isoserum t.
    Jacquet's biokinetic t.
    Keating-Hart t.
    Kenny t.
    Killgren t.
    Kittel's t.
    Klapp's creeping t.
    Koga t.
    Lambotte's t.
    Lerich's t.
    light t.
    McPheeters' t.
    Matas' t.
    medicinal t.
    Minot-Murphy t.
    Murphy's t.

treat·ment *(continued)*
 Noorden t.
 Nordach t.
 oatmeal t.
 Orr t.
 palliative t.
 Pasteur t.
 Paul's t.
 Plummer's t.
 Politzer's t.
 Potter t.
 preventive t.
 Proetz t.
 prolonged sleep t.
 prophylactic t.
 rational t.
 Rollier t.
 salicyl t.
 Schlösser's t.
 sewage t.
 shock t.
 Sippy t.
 slush t.
 solar t.
 specific t.
 Stoker's t.
 subcoma insulin t.
 supporting t.
 surgical t.
 symptomatic t.
 Tallerman's t.
 teleradium t.
 total-push t.
 Trueta t.
 underwater t.
 venous heart t.
 Weir Mitchell t.
 Yeo's t.
tre·ben·zo·mine hy·dro·chlo·ride
tree
 arterial t.
 bronchial t.
 laryngotracheobronchial t.
 tracheobronchial t.
 vascular t.
 venous t.
tre·ha·la

tre·ha·lose
Treitz's arch
Treitz's fossa
Treitz's hernia
Treitz's ligament
Treitz's muscle
tre·lox·i·nate
Trem·a·to·da
trem·a·tode
trem·a·to·di·a·sis
trem·a·toid
trem·el·loid
tre·mel·lose
trem·ens
 delirium t.
trem·e·tol
trem·e·tone
Trem·in
tre·mo·gram
tre·mo·graph
tre·mo·la·bile
tre·mom·e·ter
trem·or
 action t.
 alternating t.
 arsenic t.
 asynergic family t.
 attitudinal t.
 benign familial t.
 bread-crumbling t.
 coarse t.
 coin-counting t.
 continuous t.
 convulsive t.
 t. cordis
 darkness t.
 effort t.
 epidemic t.
 epileptoid t.
 essential t.
 familial t.
 fibrillary t.
 fine t.
 flapping t.
 forced t.
 hereditary essential t.
 heredofamilial t.
 Hunt's t.

trem·or *(continued)*
    intention t.
    intermittent t.
    kinetic t.
    lenticulostriate t.
    t. linguae
    t. mercurialis
    metallic t.
    motofacient t.
    motor t.
    muscular t.
    nonintention t.
    t. opiophagorum
    passive t.
    persistent t.
    pill-rolling t.
    postural t.
    t. potatorum
    progressive cerebellar t.
    purring t.
    rest t.
    saturnine t.
    t. saturninus
    senile t.
    static t.
    striocerebellar t.
    t. tendinum
    titubating t.
    toxic t.
    trombone t. of tongue
    volitional t.
trem·or·gram
trem·or·ine
tre·mo·sta·ble
trem·u·lor
trem·u·lous
Tren·del·en·burg operation
Tren·del·en·burg position
Tren·del·en·burg symptom
Tren·del·en·burg tests
trend·scrib·er
trend·scrip·tion
tre·pan
trep·a·na·tion
tre·pan·ner
treph·i·na·tion
    corneoscleral t.
    dental t.

tre·phine
tre·phine·ment
tre·phin·er
trepho·cyte
trep·i·dant
trep·i·da·tio
    t. cordis
trep·i·da·tion
Trep·o·mo·nas
Trep·o·ne·ma
    T. buccale
    T. calligyrum
    T. carateum
    T. cuniculi
    T. denticola
    T. genitalis
    T. herrejoni
    T. hyodysenteriae
    T. macrodentium
    T. microdentium
    T. mucosum
    T. pallidum
    T. pallidum subsp.
     pertenue
    T. paraluiscuniculi
    T. pertenue
    T. phagedenis
    T. refringens
    T. reiteri
    T. vincentii
trep·o·ne·ma
trep·o·ne·mal
Trep·o·ne·ma·ta·ceae
trep·o·ne·ma·to·sis
trep·o·neme
trep·o·ne·mi·a·sis
trep·o·ne·mi·ci·dal
tre·pop·nea
trep·pe
Tre·sil·i·an's sign
Trest
tres·to·lone ac·e·tate
tret·amine
tret·i·no·in
Treves fold
Tre·vor's disease

TRF — thyrotropin releasing
  factor
    T-cell replacing factor
TRH — thyrotropin releasing
  hormone
tri·ac
tri·acan·thine
tri·ac·e·tate
tri·ac·e·tin
tri·ac·e·tyl·o·le·an·do·my·
  cin
tri·ac·id
tri·ac·yl·glyc·er·ol
tri·ac·yl·glyc·er·ol li·pase
tri·ad
    acute compression t.
    adrenomedullary t.
    AGR t.
    anal t.
    Andersen's t.
    Beck's t.
    Bezold's t.
    Charcot's t.
    Dieulafoy's t.
    Gougerot's t.
    Grancher's t.
    hepatic t's
    Hutchinson's t.
    Kartagener's t.
    t. of Luciani
    Marburg's t.
    meningitic t.
    Oppenheim's t.
    Osler's t.
    portal t's
    t. of retinal cone
    Saint's t.
    t. of Schultz
    t. of skeletal muscle
    Whipple's t.
tri·ad·i·tis
    portal t.
tria·fun·gin
tri·age
tri·al
    Bernoulli t's
    clinical t.
    crossover t.

tri·al (continued)
    double-blind t.
    t. of labor
    phase I t.
    phase II t.
    phase III t.
    preventive t.
    randomized controlled t.
tri·al·ism
tri·al·lyl·am·ine
tri·am·cin·o·lone
    t. acetonide
    t. acetonide sodium
      phosphate
    t. diacetate
    t. hexacetonide
tria·me·lia
tri·am·ine
tri·am·ter·ene
tri·am·y·lose
tri·an·gle
    Alsberg's t.
    anal t.
    anterior t. of neck
    aortic t.
    Assézat's t.
    auditory t.
    auricular t.
    t. of auscultation
    axillary t.
    Béclard's t.
    Bolton t.
    Bonwill t.
    brachial t.
    Bryant's t.
    t. of Budde
    Burger's scalene t.
    Burow's t.
    Calot's t.
    cardiohepatic t.
    carotid t.
    carotid t., inferior
    carotid t., superior
    cephalic t.
    cervical t.
    clavipectoral t.
    Codman's t.
    color t.

tri·an·gle *(continued)*
  crural t.
  cystohepatic t.
  digastric t.
  Dunham's t's
  Einthoven's t.
  Elaut's t.
  t. of elbow
  t. of election
  extravesical t.
  facial t.
  Farabeuf's t.
  femoral t.
  fetal t.
  frontal t.
  Garland's t.
  Gerhardt's t.
  Gombault-Philippe t.
  Grocco's t.
  Grynfeltt's t.
  t. of Grynfeltt and Lesgaft
  Henke's t.
  Hesselbach's t.
  hypoglossal t.
  hypoglossohyoid t.
  iliofemoral t.
  infraclavicular t.
  inguinal t.
  Jackson's safety t.
  Kanavel's t.
  Korányi-Grocco t.
  Labbé's t.
  Langenbeck's t.
  Lesgaft's t.
  Lesser's t.
  Lieutaud's t.
  Livingston's t.
  lumbar t.
  lumbocostoabdominal t.
  lymphoid t.
  Macewen's t.
  Malgaigne's t.
  mesenteric t.
  Minor's t.
  Mohrenheim's t.
  muscular t.
  t. of necessity
  t's of neck

tri·an·gle *(continued)*
  nodal t.
  occipital t.
  occipital t., inferior
  omoclavicular t.
  omotracheal t.
  palatal t.
  paravertebral t.
  Pawlik's t.
  Petit's t.
  Petit's lumbar t.
  Pinaud's t.
  Pirogoff's t.
  popliteal t. of femur
  posterior t. of neck
  pubourethral t.
  Rauchfuss' t.
  reactive t.
  rectal t.
  Reil's t.
  retromandibular t.
  retromolar t.
  sacral t.
  t. of safety
  Scarpa's t.
  Sherren's t.
  sternocostal t.
  subclavian t.
  subinguinal t.
  submandibular t.
  submaxillary t.
  submental t.
  suboccipital t.
  superior lumbar t.
  suprameatal t.
  surgical t.
  surgical lumbar t.
  tracheal t.
  Trautmann's t.
  Tweed t.
  umbilicomammillary t.
  urogenital t.
  vaginal t.
  vesical t.
  von Weber's t.
  Ward's t.
  Weber's t.
  Wernicke's t.

tri·an·gu·lar
tri·an·gu·la·ris
tri·an·te·bra·chia
Tri·at·o·ma
    T. megista
    T. sanguisuga
tri·atom·ic
tri·atri·al
tri·atri·a·tum
    cor t.
tri·a·zene
tri·a·zo·lam
tri·az·o·lo·gua·nine
trib·a·dism
tri·ba·sic
tribe
tri·ben·o·side
Tri·bo·li·um
tri·bol·o·gy
tri·bo·lu·mi·nes·cence
tri·bra·chia
tri·bra·chi·us
tri·brom·eth·a·nol
tri·bro·mide
tri·bro·mo·eth·a·nol
tri·brom·sa·lan
trib·u·lo·sis
Trib·u·ron
tri·bu·tyr·in
tri·bu·tyr·i·nase
TRIC — trachoma inclusion
  conjunctivitis (group of
  organisms)
tri·cal·cic
tri·car·box·yl·ic acid
tri·cel·lu·lar
tri·ceph·a·lus
tri·ceps
    t. surae
tri·cep·tor
tri·chei·ria
trich·es·the·sia
tri·chi·a·sis
trich·i·lem·mo·ma
tri·chi·na *pl.* tri·chi·nae
Trich·i·nel·la
    T. spiralis
trich·i·nel·li·a·sis

trich·i·nel·loi·dea
trich·i·nel·lo·sis
trich·i·ni·a·sis
trich·i·nif·er·ous
trich·i·ni·za·tion
trich·i·no·scope
trich·i·nosed
trich·i·no·sis
trich·i·not·ic
trich·i·nous
trich·i·on *pl.* trich·ia
tri·chite
tri·chlor·fon
tri·chlo·ride
tri·chlor·me·thi·a·zide
tri·chlo·ro·ac·et·al·de·hyde
tri·chlo·ro·ace·tic acid
tri·chlo·ro·eth·y·lene
tri·chlo·ro·meth·ane
tri·chlo·ro·meth·yl·chlo·ro·
  for·mate
tri·chlo·ro·mono·flu·o·ro·
  meth·ane
tri·chlo·ro·phe·nol
2,4,5-tri·chlo·ro·phen·oxy·
  ace·tic acid
tri·chlo·ro·tri·vi·nyl·ar·sine
tri·chlor·phon
tricho·aes·the·sia
tricho·an·es·the·sia
tricho·bac·te·ria
tricho·ba·sal·i·o·ma hy·a·lin·
  i·cum
tricho·be·zoar
Trich·o·bil·har·zia
    T. ocellata
tricho·car·dia
tricho·ceph·a·li·a·sis
tricho·ceph·a·lo·sis
tricho·cla·sia
trich·oc·la·sis
tricho·cyst
Trich·o·dec·tes
    T. canis
    T. climax
    T. equi
    T. hermsi
    T. latus

Trich·o·dec·tes (continued)
   T. pilosus
   T. retusis
   T. sphaerocephalus
Trich·o·der·ma
tricho·epi·the·li·o·ma
   t. papillosum multiplex
tricho·es·the·sia
tricho·es·the·si·om·e·ter
tricho·fol·lic·u·lo·ma
tricho·glos·sia
tricho·graph·ism
tricho·hy·a·lin
trich·oid
tricho·lem·mo·ma
tricho·leu·ko·cyte
tricho·lith
tricho·lo·gia
trich·ol·o·gy
tri·cho·ma
tricho·ma·la·cia
tricho·ma·nia
tri·chom·a·tous
tri·chome
tricho·meg·a·ly
tricho·mo·na·ci·dal
tricho·mo·na·cide
tricho·mo·nad
Tricho·mo·nad·i·da
tricho·mo·nal
Trich·o·mo·nas
   T. buccalis
   T. elongata
   T. foetus
   T. gallinae
   T. gallinarum
   T. hominis
   T. intestinalis
   T. tenax
   T. vaginalis
tricho·mo·ni·a·sis
   urogenital t.
   t. vaginalis
tricho·my·co·sis
   t. axillaris
   t. chromatica
   t. nodosa
   pubic t.

tricho·my·co·sis *(continued)*
   t. pustulosa
trich·on
tricho·no·car·di·o·sis
   t. axillaris
tricho·no·do·sis
tricho·path·ic
trich·op·a·thy
tricho·pha·gia
trich·oph·a·gy
tricho·phyt·ic
tri·choph·y·tid
tri·choph·y·tin
tricho·phy·to·be·zoar
Tri·choph·y·ton
   T. acuminatum
   T. arloingi
   T. asteroides
   T. ceratophagus
   T. ectothrix
   T. endothrix
   T. epilans
   T. flavum
   T. gypseum
   T. interdigitale
   T. mentagrophytes
   T. niveum
   T. purpureum
   T. quinckeanum
   T. rubrum
   T. sabouraudi
   T. schoenleinii
   T. tonsurans
tricho·phy·to·sis
   t. cruris
Tri·chop·tera
trich·op·ti·lo·sis
trich·or·rhex·is
   t. invaginata
   t. nodosa
trich·os·chi·sis
tri·chos·co·py
tricho·sid·er·in
tri·cho·sis
   t. carunculae
Trich·o·so·moi·des
   T. crassicauda

Tri·chos·po·ron
  T. *beigelii*
  T. *cutaneum*
  T. *giganteum*
  T. *pedrosianum*
tricho·spo·ro·sis
tri·chos·ta·sis spin·u·lo·sa
Tricho·sto·mat·i·da
Tricho·sto·ma·ti·na
tricho·stron·gyle
tricho·stron·gy·li·a·sis
Tricho·stron·gyl·i·dae
tricho·stron·gy·lo·sis
Trich·o·stron·gy·lus
  T. *capricola*
  T. *colubriformis*
  T. *instabilis*
  T. *orientalis*
  T. *probolurus*
  T. *vitrinus*
Trich·o·the·ci·um
  T. *roseum*
tricho·thio·dys·tro·phy
tricho·til·lo·ma·nia
tri·chot·o·mous
tri·chot·o·my
tri·cho·tox·in
tri·chro·ic
tri·chro·ism
tri·chro·ma·sy
  anomalous t.
tri·chro·mat
tri·chro·mat·ic
tri·chro·ma·tism
  anomalous t.
tri·chro·ma·top·sia
tri·chro·mic
trich·ter·brust
trich·u·ri·a·sis
Trich·u·ris
  T. *trichiura*
Trich·u·roi·dea
tri·cip·i·tal
tri·clo·bi·so·ni·um chlo·ride
tri·clo·car·ban
tri·clo·fen·ol pi·per·a·zine
tri·clo·fos so·di·um
tri·clo·nide

Tri·clos
tri·clo·san
Tri·co·fu·ron
Tri·co·loid
tri·corn
tri·cor·nute
tri·cre·sol
tri·cre·syl phos·phate (TCP)
tri·crot·ic
tri·cro·tism
tri·cus·pid
tri·cy·cla·mol chlo·ride
tri·cyc·lic
Trid. — L. triduum (three
  days)
tri·dac·ty·lism
tri·dac·ty·lous
tri·dent
tri·den·tate
tri·der·mic
tri·der·mo·gen·e·sis
tri·der·mo·ma
Tri·des·i·lon
tri·dig·i·tate
tri·di·hex·eth·yl chlo·ride
Tri·di·one
trid·y·mite
trid·y·mus
tri·en·ceph·a·lus
tri·es·ter
tri·eth·a·nol·amine
tri·eth·yl·amine
tri·eth·yl·ene·mel·amine
tri·eth·yl·ene·phos·pho·ra·
  mide
tri·eth·yl·ene·thio·phos·pho·
  ra·mide
tri·fa·cial
tri·fid
tri·flo·cin
tri·flu·mi·date
tri·flu·o·per·a·zine hy·dro·
  chlo·ride
5-tri·flu·o·ro·meth·yl·de·oxy·
  uri·dine
tri·flu·per·i·dol
tri·flu·pro·ma·zine
  t. hydrochloride

tri·flur·i·dine
tri·flu·ro·meth·yl·thi·a·zide
tri·fo·cal
tri·fo·li·o·sis
tri·fur·cate
tri·fur·ca·tion
tri·gas·tric
tri·gas·tri·cus
tri·gem·i·nal
tri·gem·i·nus
tri·gem·i·ny
tri·glyc·er·ide
tri·go·ceph·a·lus
tri·go·na
tri·go·nal
tri·gone
   t. of bladder
   carotid t.
   cerebral t.
   collateral t. of fourth
    ventricle
   femoral t.
   fibrous t. of heart, left
   fibrous t. of heart, right
   t. of habenula
   habenular t.
   Henke's t.
   hypoglossal t.
   t. of hypoglossal nerve
   iliopectineal t.
   inguinal t.
   interpeduncular t.
   Lieutaud's t.
   lumbar t.
   olfactory t.
   omoclavicular t.
   Pawlik's t.
   t. of Reil
   submandibular t.
   urogenital t.
   vagal t.
   t. of vagus nerve
   vesical t.
tri·go·nec·to·my
trig·o·nel·line
tri·gon·id
trig·o·ni·tis
trig·o·no·ce·pha·lia

trig·o·no·ce·phal·ic
trig·o·no·ceph·a·lus
trig·o·no·ceph·a·ly
tri·go·num *pl.* tri·go·na
   t. acustici
   t. caroticum
   t. cerebrale
   t. cervicale
   t. cervicale anterius
   t. cervicale posterius
   t. clavipectorale
   t. collaterale ventriculi
    laterale
   t. collaterale ventriculi
    quarti
   t. colli laterale
   t. coracoacromiale
   t. deltoideopectorale
   t. femorale
   t. fibrosum dextrum cordis
   t. fibrosum sinistrum
    cordis
   t. habenulae
   t. habenularis
   t. hypoglossale
   t. hypoglossi
   t. inguinale
   t. interpedunculare
   t. lemnisci
   t. lumbale
   t. lumbare
   t. lumbare [Petiti]
   t. lumbocostale
   t. musculare
   t. nervi hypoglossi
   t. nervi vagi
   t. olfactorium
   t. omoclaviculare
   t. omotracheale
   t. pontocerebellare
   t. sternocostale
   t. submandibulare
   t. submentale
   t. urogenitale
   t. vagale
   t. vagi
   t. ventriculi lateralis
   t. vesicae

tri·go·num *(continued)*
    t. vesicae [Lieutaudi]
tri·hex·o·syl·cer·a·mide ga·lac·to·syl·hy·dro·lase
tri·hex·y·phen·i·dyl hy·dro·chlo·ride
tri·hy·brid
tri·hy·drate
tri·hy·dric
tri·hy·drol
tri·hy·drox·ide
tri·hy·droxy·es·trin
tri-in·i·od·y·mus
tri·io·dide
tri·io·do·eth·i·on·ic acid
tri·io·do·meth·ane
tri·io·do·thy·ro·nine
    reverse t. (rT₃)
tri·ke·to·hy·drin·dene hy·drate
tri·ke·to·pu·rine
tri·labe
Tri·la·fon
tri·lam·i·nar
tri·lat·er·al
tri·lau·rin
tri·lin·o·le·in
Tril·i·sate
tri·lo·bate
tri·lobed
tri·loc·u·lar
tril·o·gy
    t. of Fallot
tri·lo·stane
tri·mag·ne·si·um phos·phate
tri·mas·ti·gote
tri·ma·zo·sin hy·dro·chlo·ride
tri·me·dox·ime
tri·men·su·al
tri·mep·ra·zine tar·trate
tri·mer
tri·mer·cu·ric
Trim·e·re·su·rus
tri·mer·ic
tri·mes·ter
tri·meth·a·di·one
tri·meth·a·phan cam·sy·late

tri·meth·i·din·i·um meth·o·sul·fate
tri·meth·o·ben·za·mide hy·dro·chlo·ride
tri·meth·o·prim
    t.-sulfamethoxazole
tri·meth·y·lene
tri·meth·yl·xan·thine
tri·met·o·zine
tri·mip·ra·mine
    t. maleate
tri·mo·pam mal·e·ate
tri·mor·phism
tri·mor·phous
tri·neg·a·tive
tri·neu·ral
tri·neu·ric
tri·ni·trate
tri·ni·trin
tri·ni·tro·cel·lu·lose
tri·ni·tro·glyc·er·in
tri·ni·tro·glyc·er·ol
tri·ni·tro·phe·nol
tri·ni·tro·tol·u·ene
tri·no·mi·al
tri·nu·cle·ate
tri·nu·cleo·tide
trio·ceph·a·lus
tri·o·le·in
trio·lism
tri·oph·thal·mos
tri·o·pod·y·mus
tri·or·chid
tri·or·chi·dism
tri·or·chis
tri·or·chism
tri·ose
tri·ose ki·nase
tri·ose·phos·phate de·hy·dro·gen·ase
tri·ose·phos·phate isom·er·ase
tri·otus
tri·ox·ide
tri·ox·sa·len
tri·oxy·pu·rine
tri·pal·mi·tin
trip·a·ra
tri·par·tite

tri·pe·len·na·mine
    t. citrate
    t. hydrochloride
tri·pep·tide
Tri·per·i·dol
tri·pha·lan·ge·al
tri·pha·lan·gia
tri·pha·lan·gism
tri·phar·ma·con
tri·pha·sic
tri·phen·yl·chlor·eth·y·lene
tri·phen·yl·eth·y·lene
tri·phen·yl·meth·ane
tri·phos·phate
tri·phos·pho·pyr·i·dine nu·cle·o·tide
tri·phos·phor·ic acid
Trip·ier's amputation
trip·le-an·gle
trip·le blind
trip·le·gia
trip·let
tri·plex
trip·lo·blas·tic
trip·loid
trip·loi·dy
trip·lo·ko·ria
trip·lo·pia
tri·pod
    Haller's t.
    t. of life
    vital t.
tri·po·dia
tri·pod·ing
trip·o·li
tri·pos·i·tive
tri·pro·li·dine hy·dro·chlo·ride
tri·pro·so·pus
trip·sis
trip·to·ko·ria
tri·pus
    t. halleri
tri·que·tral
tri·que·trous
tri·que·trum
tri·ra·di·al
tri·ra·di·ate

tri·ra·di·a·tion
tri·ra·di·us
tri·sac·cha·ride
tris(hy·droxy·meth·yl)·am·i·no·meth·ane
tris·mic
tris·moid
tris·mus
    t. cynicus
    t. dolorificus
    t. neonatorum
    t. sardonicus
tri·so·mia
tri·so·mic
tri·so·my
Tri·sor·a·len
tri·splanch·nic
tri·spor·ic acids
tri·stea·rin
tri·stich·ia
tris·ti·ma·nia
tri·sub·sti·tut·ed
tri·sul·cate
tri·sul·fa·py·rim·i·dines
tri·sul·fate
tri·sul·fide
Trit. — L. tritura (triturate)
tri·tan
tri·ta·nom·al
tri·ta·nom·a·lous
tri·ta·nom·a·ly
tri·ta·nope
tri·ta·no·pia
tri·ta·nop·ic
tri·ta·nop·sia
trit·i·ate
tri·ti·ceous
tri·tic·e·um
trit·i·um
trit·o·cone
trit·o·co·nid
tri·ton
Tri·trich·o·mo·nas
tri·tu·ber·cu·lar
trit·ur·a·ble
trit·ur·ate
    tablet t.
trit·ur·a·tion

trit·ur·a·tor
tri·va·lence
tri·va·lent
tri·valve
tri·zo·nal
tRNA — transfer RNA
Tro·bi·cin
tro·car
    Durham's t.
    Lichtwicz t.
    piloting t.
    rectal t.
troch. — trochiscus
tro·chan·ter
    greater t.
    lesser t.
    t. major
    t. minor
    rudimentary t.
    small t.
    t. tertius
    third t.
tro·chan·ter·i·an
tro·chan·ter·ic
tro·chan·ter·itis
tro·chan·ter·plas·ty
tro·chan·tin
tro·chan·tin·i·an
tro·che
tro·chin·i·an
tro·chis·ca·tion
tro·chis·cus *pl.* tro·chis·ci
troch·i·ter
troch·i·te·ri·an
troch·lea *pl.* troch·leae
    t. fibularis calcanei
    t. humeri
    t. of humerus
    t. labyrinthi
    muscular t.
    t. muscularis
    t. musculi obliqui
      superioris bulbi
    t. musculi obliqui
      superioris oculi
    peroneal t. of calcaneus
    t. peronealis calcanei

troch·lea *(continued)*
    t. phalangis digitorum
      manus
    t. phalangis digitorum
      pedis
    t. of superior oblique
      muscle
    t. tali
    t. of talus
troch·le·ar
troch·le·ar·i·form
troch·le·a·ris
tro·cho·ce·pha·lia
tro·cho·ceph·a·ly
tro·choid
tro·choi·des
Tro·ci·nate
Trog·lo·tre·ma
    T. salmincola
troi·lism
Troi·sier's ganglion
Troi·sier's node
Troi·sier's sign
Troi·sier's syndrome
tro·la·mine
tro·land
Tro·lard's net
Tro·lard's plexus
Tro·lard's vein
tro·le·an·do·my·cin
trol·ni·trate phos·phate
Tröltsch's corpuscles
Tröltsch's recesses
Tröltsch's spaces
Trom·bic·u·la
    T. akamushi
    T. alfreddugèsi
    T. autumnalis
    T. deliensis
    T. fletcheri
    T. holosericeum
    T. intermedia
    T. irritans
    T. muscae domesticae
    T. muscarum
    T. pallida
    T. scutellaris
    T. tsalsahuatl

trom·bic·u·li·a·sis
trom·bic·u·lid
Trom·bic·u·li·dae
trom·bid·i·i·a·sis
trom·bid·i·o·sis
tro·meth·amine
Trom·mer's test
Tröm·ner's sign
tromo·pho·nia
tron·cha·do
Tron·o·thane
tro·pae·o·lin
    t. D
    t. G
tro·pate
tro·pe·ine
tro·pe·in·ism
troph·ec·to·derm
troph·ede·ma
    congenital t.
    hereditary t.
troph·ic
tro·phic·i·ty
troph·ism
tropho·blast
tropho·blas·tic
tropho·blas·to·ma
tropho·cyte
tropho·derm
tropho·der·ma·to·neu·ro·sis
tropho·dy·nam·ics
tropho·ede·ma
tropho·lec·i·thal
tropho·lec·i·thus
tro·phol·o·gy
tropho·neu·ro·sis
    disseminated t.
    facial t.
    lingual t.
    muscular t.
    t. of Romberg
tropho·neu·rot·ic
troph·o·no·sis
tro·phont
tropho·nu·cle·us
tropho·path·ia
tro·phop·a·thy
tropho·plast

tro·pho·spon·gi·um *pl.* tro·pho·spon·gia
tropho·tax·is
tropho·ther·a·py
tro·pho·trop·ic
tropho·tro·pism
tropho·zo·ite
tro·pia
tro·pic acid
trop·i·cal
tro·pic·a·mide
trop·i·dine
tro·pin
tro·pine
tro·pism
tro·po·chrome
tro·po·col·la·gen
tro·po·elas·tin
tro·pom·e·ter
tro·po·my·o·sin
    t. A
tro·po·nin
tro·tyl
trough
    gingival t.
    Langmuir t.
    synaptic t's
    vestibular t.
trousers
    military (medical) antishock t. (MAST)
Trous·seau's phenomenon
Trous·seau's sign
Trous·seau's spot
Trous·seau's twitching
Trous·seau-Lal·le·mand bodies
trox·i·done
troy
Trp — tryptophan
TRU — turbidity reducing unit
Tru·e·ta method
Tru·e·ta technique
Tru·e·ta treatment
trun·cal
trun·cate
trun·co·co·nal
trun·cus *pl.* trun·ci
    t. arteriosus

trun·cus *(continued)*
   t. arteriosus, persistent
   t. arteriosus communis
   t. brachiocephalicus
   t. bronchomediastinalis
     dexter/sinister
   t. coeliacus
   t. corporis callosi
   t. costocervicalis
   t. encephalicus
   t. fasciculi
     atrioventricularis
   t. inferior plexus brachialis
   trunci intestinales
   t. jugularis dexter/sinister
   t. linguofacialis
   trunci lumbales
   t. lumbaris dexter/sinister
   t. lumbosacralis
   trunci lymphatici
   t. medius plexus brachialis
   t. nervi accessorii
   t. nervi spinalis
   trunci plexus brachialis
   t. pulmonalis
   t. subclavius
     dexter/sinister
   t. superior plexus
     brachialis
   t. sympatheticus
   t. sympathicus
   t. thyreocervicalis
   t. thyrocervicalis
   t. transversus
   t. vagalis anterior
   t. vagalis posterior
trunk
   anterior gastric t.
   t. of atrioventricular
     bundle
   basilar t.
   t's of brachial plexus
   brachiocephalic t.
   bronchomediastinal t.
   t. of bundle of His
   celiac t.
   t. of corpus callosum
   costocervical t.

trunk *(continued)*
   inferior t. of brachial
     plexus
   intestinal t's
   intestinal lymphatic t's
   jugular t.
   left bronchomediastinal t.
   linguofacial t.
   lumbar t.
   lumbosacral t.
   lymphatic t's
   middle t. of brachial plexus
   nerve t.
   posterior gastric t.
   pulmonary t.
   right bronchomediastinal t.
   subclavian t.
   superior t. of brachial
     plexus
   sympathetic t.
   sympathetic ganglionated
     t.
   thyrocervical t.
tru·sion
truss
   nasal t.
   yarn t.
try-in
try·pan·id
try·pano·ci·dal
try·pano·cide
try·pan·ol·y·sis
try·pano·lyt·ic
Try·pan·o·so·ma
   T. brucei
   T. brucei brucei
   T. brucei gambiense
   T. brucei rhodesiense
   T. congolense
   T. cruzi
   T. dimorphon
   T. equinum
   T. equiperdum
   T. escomili
   T. evansi
   T. gambiense
   T. guatemalensis
   T. hippicum

Try·pan·o·so·ma (continued)
   T. hominis
   T. lewisi
   T. melophagium
   T. nanum
   T. neotomae
   T. nigeriense
   T. pecaudi
   T. rangeli
   T. rhodesiense
   T. rotatorium
   T. rougeti
   T. simiae
   T. theileri
   T. theodori
   T. triatomae
   T. ugandense
   T. uniforme
   T. vivax
try·pano·so·mal
try·pano·so·mat·ic
try·pano·so·ma·tid
try·pano·so·mat·i·dae
Try·pano·so·ma·ti·na
try·pano·so·ma·to·trop·ic
try·pano·some
try·pano·so·mi·a·sis
   acute t.
   African t.
   American t.
   Brazilian t.
   chronic t.
   Congo t.
   Cruz t.
   t. cruzi
   East African t.
   Gambian t.
   Rhodesian t.
   South American t.
   West African t.
try·pano·som·ic
try·pano·so·mi·ci·dal
try·pano·so·mi·cide
try·pano·so·mid
try·pano·so·mo·sis
Try·pan·o·zo·on
try·par·o·san
tryp·ar·sa·mide

try·pe·sis
try·po·che·tes
try·po·mas·ti·gote
try·po·nar·syl
try·po·tan
tryp·sin
   crystallized t.
tryp·sin·ize
tryp·sin·o·gen
tryp·ta·mine
Tryp·tar
tryp·tic
tryp·tone
tryp·to·phan
tryp·to·phan·ase
tryp·to·phan 2,3-di·oxy·gen·ase
tryp·to·phan·uria
tryp·to·phyl
TS — test solution
   tricuspid stenosis
TSA — tumor-specific antigen
tset·se
TSF — triceps skinfold
TSH — thyroid-stimulating hormone
tsp — teaspoon
TSTA — tumor-specific transplantation antigen
Tsu·ga
   T. canadensis
tsu·tsu·ga·mu·shi
TT — thrombin time
TU — tuberculin unit
Tu·a·mine
tu·am·i·no·hep·tane
   t. sulfate
tu·ba *pl.* tu·bae
   t. acustica
   t. auditiva
   t. auditoria
   t. uterina
   t. uterina [Falloppii]
Tu·ba·dil
tu·bae
tu·bal
Tu·ba·rine
tu·ba·tor·sion

tube
    Abbott-Miller t.
    Abbott-Rawson t.
    Aberdeen t.
    Adson suction t.
    air t.
    Alder Hey t.
    Argyle-Salem sump t.
    auditory t.
    auscultation t.
    Ayre's t.
    Bellocq's t.
    Blakemore-Sengstaken t.
    Bouchut's t's
    Bowman's t's
    breathing t.
    bronchial t.
    buccal t.
    Cantor t.
    capillary t.
    cardiac t.
    Carlens t.
    cathode-ray t.
    Celestin's t.
    cerebromedullary t.
    Chaoul t.
    chest t.
    collecting t's
    Coolidge t.
    corneal t's
    Craigies t.
    Crookes t.
    cuffed t.
    Diamond's t.
    digestive t.
    discharge t.
    Dobbhoff feeding t.
    drainage t.
    drawing t.
    Durham's t.
    electron multiplier t.
    embryonic fallopian t.
    empyema t.
    end t.
    endobronchial t.
    endocardial t's
    endotracheal t.
    esophageal t.

tube *(continued)*
    eustachian t.
    Ewald t.
    fallopian t.
    feeding t.
    fermentation t.
    Ferrein's t's
    Fuller t.
    fusion t's
    Geiger-Müller t.
    grenz-ray t.
    Harris t.
    horizontal t.
    hot-cathode t.
    image intensifier t.
    intestinal t.
    Jackson t.
    Jackson-Pratt t.
    KCH (King's College
      Hospital) t.
    Killian's t's
    Kobelt's t's
    Kuhn's t.
    laryngostomy t.
    laryngotomy t.
    Lepley-Ernst t.
    Levin t.
    Linton t.
    lobster-tail t.
    malpighian t's
    medullary t.
    Mett's t's
    Miescher's t.
    Miller-Abbott t.
    Minnesota t.
    Montgomery T t.
    nasogastric t.
    nasopharyngeal t.
    nasotracheal t.
    Negus t.
    nephrostomy t.
    neural t.
    observation t.
    Olshevsky t.
    orotracheal t.
    otopharyngeal t.
    ovarian t's
    Parker t.

tube *(continued)*
- Paul-Mixter t.
- Pflüger's t's
- pharyngotympanic t.
- photomultiplier t.
- polar t.
- pus t.
- Rainey's t.
- Rehfuss' t.
- Robertshaw t.
- roentgen t.
- Roida's t.
- roll t.
- rotating anode t.
- Ruysch's t.
- Ryle's t.
- Schachowa's spiral t's
- sediment t.
- sedimentation t.
- Sengstaken-Blakemore t.
- Shiner's t.
- Souttar's t.
- speaking t.
- sputum t.
- stomach t.
- sump t.
- T t.
- tampon t.
- test t.
- thoracostomy t.
- Thunberg t.
- tracheal t.
- tracheostomy t.
- tracheotomy t.
- Tucker t's
- tympanostomy t.
- uterine t.
- vacuum t.
- valve t.
- Veillon t.
- ventilation t.
- Venturi t.
- vertical t.
- Voltolini's t.
- Wangensteen t.
- Wintrobe t.
- x-ray t.

tu·bec·to·my

tu·ber *pl.* tu·bers, tu·be·ra
- t. anterius hypothalami
- t. calcanei
- t. cinereum
- t. cochleae
- t. corporis callosi
- t. dorsale
- eustachian t.
- external t. of Henle
- frontal t.
- t. frontale
- iliopubic t.
- t. ischiadicum
- t. ischiale
- t. maxillae
- t. maxillare
- maxillary t.
- mental t.
- t. omentale hepatis
- t. omentale pancreatis
- omental t. of liver
- omental t. of pancreas
- papillary t. of liver
- parietal t.
- t. parietale
- t. radii
- t. of radius
- sciatic t.
- t. valvulae cerebelli
- t. vermis
- t. zygomaticum

tu·bera

tu·ber·cle
- accessory t.
- acoustic t.
- adductor t. of femur
- amygdaloid t. of Schwalbe
- anal t.
- anatomical t.
- t. of anterior scalene muscle
- articular t. of temporal bone
- t. of atlas, anterior
- t. of atlas, posterior
- auditory t.
- auricular t.

tu·ber·cle *(continued)*
Babès' t's
brachial t. of humerus
calcaneal t.
Carabelli t.
carotid t.
caseous t.
caudal t. of liver
cervical t's
t. of cervical vertebrae, anterior
t. of cervical vertebrae, posterior
Chassaignac's t.
condyloid t.
conglomerate t.
conoid t.
corniculate t.
costal t.
crude t.
t. of cuneate nucleus
cuneiform t.
t. of Czermak
darwinian t.
deltoid t.
dental t.
dissection t.
dorsal t. of radius
ear t.
epiglottic t.
Farre's t's
fibrous t.
t. of fibula, posterior
genial t.
genital t.
Gerdy's t.
Ghon t.
gracile t.
gray t.
greater t. of calcaneus
t. of greater multangular bone
hard t.
hepatic t.
hippocampal t.
His' t.
t. of humerus

tu·ber·cle *(continued)*
t. of humerus, anterior, of Meckel
t. of humerus, anterior, of Weber
t. of humerus, external
t. of humerus, greater
t. of humerus, internal
t. of humerus, lesser
t. of humerus, posterior
iliac t.
iliopectineal t.
iliopubic t.
inferior genial t.
inferior t. of Humphrey
infraglenoid t.
intercolumnar t.
intercondylar t.
intercondylar t., lateral
intercondylar t., medial
intervenous t.
intravascular t.
jugular t. of occipital bone
labial t.
lacrimal t.
lateral orbital t.
lateral palpebral t.
lesser t. of calcaneus
Lisfranc's t.
Lister's t.
Lower's t.
Luschka's t.
lymphoid t.
mamillary t.
mamillary t. of hypothalamus
marginal t. of zygomatic bone
mental t.
mental t., external
mental t. of mandible
miliary t.
Montgomery's t's
Morgagni's t.
Müller's t.
müllerian t.
muscular t. of atlas
naked t.

tu·ber·cle *(continued)*
t. of navicular bone
necrogenic t.
nuchal t.
t. of nucleus cuneatus
t. of nucleus gracilis
obturator t., anterior
obturator t., posterior
olfactory t.
orbital t.
palpebral t.
papillary t.
paramolar t.
peroneal t.
pharyngeal t.
plantar t.
t. of posterior process of
   talus, lateral
t. of posterior process of
   talus, medial
postglenoid t.
postmortem t.
preglenoid t.
prosector's t.
pterygoid t.
pubic t. of pubic bone
rabic t's
t. of rib
t. of Rolando
t. of root of zygoma
t. of Santorini
scalene t.
t. of scaphoid bone
sebaceous t.
t. of sella turcica
t. of sixth cervical vertebra,
   anterior
t. of sixth cervical vertebra,
   carotid
t. of sixth cervical vertebra,
   posterior
spinous t.
superior genial t.
superior t. of Henle
superior t. of Humphrey
supraglenoid t.
supratragic t.
t. of thalamus, anterior

tu·ber·cle *(continued)*
t. of thalamus, posterior
thyroid t., inferior
thyroid t., superior
t. of tibia
transverse t. of fourth
   tarsal bone
t. of trapezium
trochanteric t.
trochlear t.
t. of ulna
t. of upper lip
t's of vertebra
Whitnall's t.
Wrisberg's t.
yellow t.
t. of zygoma
zygomatic t.
tu·ber·cu·la
tu·ber·cu·lar
Tu·ber·cu·lar·i·a·ceae
tu·ber·cu·lase
tu·ber·cu·late
tu·ber·cu·lat·ed
tu·ber·cu·la·tion
tu·ber·cu·lid
micronodular t.
papular t.
papulonecrotic t.
rosacea-like t.
tu·ber·cu·lin
alkaline t.
autogenous t.
Behring's t.
Béraneck's t.
Buchner's t.
Calmette's t.
Dixon's t.
endotin t.
Klemperer's t.
Koch's t.
Landmann's t.
Maragliano's t.
Maréchal's t.
Moro's t.
Old t. (O.T.)
original t.
perlsucht t. original

tu·ber·cu·lin *(continued)*
    perlsucht t. rest
    purified t.
    purified protein derivative
    (PPD) t.
    Ruck's t.
    Seibert's t.
    Spengler's t.
    Vaudremer's t.
tu·ber·cu·lin·iza·tion
tu·ber·cu·lin·um
tu·ber·cu·li·tis
tu·ber·cu·li·za·tion
tu·ber·cu·lo·cele
tu·ber·cu·lo·ci·dal
tu·ber·cu·lo·cide
tu·ber·cu·lo·derm
tu·ber·cu·lo·der·ma
tu·ber·cu·lo·fi·broid
tu·ber·cu·loid
tu·ber·cu·loi·din
tu·ber·cu·lo·ma
    t. en plaque
tu·ber·cu·lo·sil·i·co·sis
tu·ber·cu·lo·sis
    active t.
    adrenal t.
    adult t.
    aerogenic t.
    anthracotic t.
    attenuated t.
    atypical t.
    basal t.
    bronchogenic t.
    bronchopneumonic t.
    caseous t.
    cerebral t.
    cestodic t.
    childhood t.
    chronic fibroid t.
    chronic ulcerative t.
    t. colliquativa cutis
    cutaneous t.
    t. cutis
    t. cutis indurativa
    t. cutis lichenoides
    t. cutis miliaris
      disseminata

tu·ber·cu·lo·sis *(continued)*
    t. cutis orificialis
    t. cutis verrucosa
    cystic t. of bones
    disseminated t.
    endogenous t.
    endothelial t.
    extrapulmonary t.
    exudative t.
    fibrocaseous t.
    fibrosing t.
    t. fungosa cutis
    genital t.
    genitourinary t.
    glandular t.
    hematogenous t.
    hilus t.
    ileocecal t.
    t. indurativa
    inhalation t.
    t. of intestines
    laryngeal t.
    t. of larynx
    latent t.
    t. lichenoides
    t. of lungs
    t. luposa
    lymphogenous t.
    lymphoid t.
    meningeal t.
    t. miliaris cutis
    t. miliaris disseminata
    miliary t.
    open t.
    oral t.
    orificial t.
    t. orificialis
    papulonecrotic t.
    t. papulonecrotica
    postprimary t.
    primary t.
    primary inoculation t.
    productive t.
    pulmonary t.
    reinfection t.
    renal t.
    t. of serous membranes
    skeletal t.

tu·ber·cu·lo·sis *(continued)*
 t. of skin
 spinal t.
 t. of spine
 surgical t.
 tracheobronchial t.
 t. ulcerosa
 t. verrucosa cutis
 warty t.
tu·ber·cu·lo·stat·ic
tu·ber·cu·lot·ic
tu·ber·cu·lo·tox·in
tu·ber·cu·lous
tu·ber·cu·lum *pl.* tu·ber·cu·la
 t. acusticum
 t. adductorium femoris
 t. anterius
 t. arthriticum
 t. articulare
 t. auriculae
 t. auriculae [Darwini]
 Béraneck's t.
 t. calcanei
 t. caroticum
 t. cinereum
 t. conoideum
 t. corniculatum
 t. corniculatum [Santorini]
 t. coronae
 t. costae
 t. cuneatum
 t. cuneiforme
 t. cuneiforme [Wrisbergi]
 t. dentale
 t. dolorosum
 t. dorsale radii
 t. epiglotticum
 t. geniale
 t. gracile
 t. hypoglossi
 t. iliacum
 t. impar
 t. infraglenoidale
 t. intercondylare
 t. intercondyloideum
 t. intervenosum
 t. intervenosum [Loweri]
 t. jugulare ossis

tu·ber·cu·lum *(continued)*
 t. labii superioris
 t. laterale
 t. Loweri
 t. majus humeri
 t. marginale
 t. mediale
 t. mentale mandibulae
 t. minus humeri
 t. nuclei cuneati
 t. nuclei gracilis
 t. of nucleus gracilis
 t. obturatorium anterius
 t. obturatorium posterius
 t. olfactorium
 t. ossis multanguli majoris
 t. ossis navicularis
 t. ossis scaphoidei
 t. ossis trapezii
 t. pharyngeum
 t. posterius
 t. pubicum
 t. retrolobare
 t. Santorini
 t. scaleni [Lisfranci]
 t. sellae ossis sphenoidalis
 t. sellae turcicae
 t. septi
 t. supraglenoidale
 t. supratragicum
 t. thyreoideum inferius
 t. thyreoideum superius
 t. thyroideum inferius
 t. thyroideum superius
 t. trigeminale
tu·ber·o·sis
tu·be·ros·i·tas *pl.* tu·be·ro·si·
 ta·tes
 t. coracoidea
 t. costae II
 t. costalis claviculae
 t. deltoidea humeri
 t. femoris externa
 t. femoris interna
 t. glutea femoris
 t. glutea ossis femoris
 t. iliaca
 t. infraglenoidalis

tu·be·ros·i·tas *(continued)*
  t. masseterica
  t. musculi serrati
    anterioris
  t. ossis cuboidei
  t. ossis metatarsalis primi
  t. ossis metatarsalis quinti
  t. ossis navicularis
  t. patellaris
  t. phalangis distalis manus
  t. phalangis distalis pedis
  t. pterygoidea mandibulae
  t. radii
  t. sacralis
  t. supraglenoidalis
    scapulae
  t. tibiae
  t. tibiae externa
  t. tibiae interna
  t. ulnae
  t. unguicularis manus
  t. unguicularis pedis
tu·be·ros·i·ta·tes
tu·be·ros·i·ty
  t. for anterior serratus
    muscle
  bicipital t.
  t. of calcaneus
  t. of clavicle
  coracoid t.
  costal t. of clavicle
  t. of cuboid bone
  deltoid t. of humerus
  distal t. of fingers
  distal t. of toes
  t. of femur, external
  t. of femur, internal
  t. of femur, lateral
  t. of femur, medial
  t. of fifth metatarsal
  t. of first carpal bone
  t. of first metatarsal
  t. of fourth tarsal bone
  frontal t.
  gluteal t. of femur
  greater t. of humerus
  t. of greater multangular
    bone

tu·be·ros·i·ty *(continued)*
  t's of humerus
  iliac t.
  infraglenoid t.
  ischial t.
  t. of ischium
  lesser t. of humerus
  malar t.
  masseteric t.
  t. of maxilla
  maxillary t.
  t. of navicular bone
  omental t.
  parietal t.
  patellar t.
  pterygoid t. of mandible
  t. of pubic bone
  pyramidal t. of palatine
    bone
  radial t.
  t. of radius
  sacral t.
  t. of scaphoid bone
  scapular t. of Henle
  t. of second rib
  t. for serratus anterior
    muscle
  supraglenoid t.
  t. of tibia
  t. of tibia, external
  t. of tibia, internal
  t. of trapezium
  t. of ulna
  ungual t.
  unguicular t.
tu·ber·ous
tu·bi
tu·bif·er·ous
tu·bo·ab·dom·i·nal
tu·bo·ad·nexo·pexy
tu·bo·cu·ra·rine
  t. chloride
  dimethyl t. iodide
tu·bo·gas·tros·to·my
tu·bo·lig·a·men·tous
tu·bo-ovar·i·an
tu·bo-ovar·i·ec·to·my
tu·bo-ovar·i·ot·o·my

tu·bo-ova·ri·tis
tu·bo·peri·to·ne·al
tu·bo·plas·ty
    balloon t.
    eustachian t.
tu·bor·rhea
tu·bo·tor·sion
tu·bo·tym·pa·nal
tu·bo·tym·pan·ic
tu·bo·tym·pa·num
tu·bo·uter·ine
tu·bo·vag·i·nal
tub·u·lar
tu·bule
    Albarrán's t's
    Bellini's t's
    biliferous t.
    caroticotympanic t's
    collecting t's
    connecting t's
    convoluted t's
    convoluted t., distal
    convoluted t., proximal
    convoluted seminiferous t's
    dental t's
    dentinal t's
    discharging t's
    Ferrein's t's
    galactophorous t's
    Henle's t's
    Kobelt's t's
    lactiferous t's
    malpighian t.
    mesonephric t's
    metanephric t's
    Miescher's t.
    paraurethral t's
    pronephric t's
    Rainey's t.
    renal t's
    renal t's, convoluted
    renal t's, straight
    segmental t's
    seminiferous t's
    seminiferous t's,
      convoluted
    seminiferous t's, straight
    Skene's t's

tu·bule *(continued)*
    spiral t's
    straight t's
    subtracheal t.
    T t's
    tracheal t.
    transverse t.
    uriniferous t's
    uriniparous t's
    vertical t's
tu·bu·li
tu·bu·li·form
tu·bu·lin
Tu·bu·li·na
tu·bu·li·za·tion
tu·bu·lo·ac·i·nar
tu·bu·lo·ac·i·nous
tu·bu·lo·cyst
tu·bu·lo·rac·e·mose
tu·bu·lor·rhex·is
    ischemic t.
tu·bu·lo·sac·cu·lar
tu·bu·lous
tu·bu·lo·ves·i·cle
tu·bu·lo·ve·sic·u·lar
tu·bu·lo·vil·lous
tu·bu·lus *pl.* tu·bu·li
    t. biliferus
    tubuli contorti
    t. epoophori
    tubuli recti
    t. rectus
    tubuli renales
    tubuli renales contorti
    tubuli renales recti
    tubuli seminiferi contorti
    tubuli seminiferi recti
tu·bus *pl.* tu·bi
    t. digestorius
    t. vertebralis
Tuck·er-Mc·Lean forceps
Tuf·fier's method
Tuf·fier's test
tuft
    enamel t's
    hair t's
    synovial t's
    ungual t.

tuft·sin
  tracheal t.
tug·ging
  tracheal t.
tu·la·re·mia
  gastrointestinal t.
  glandular t.
  oculoglandular t.
  oropharyngeal t.
  pneumonic t.
  pulmonary t.
  pulmonic t.
  typhoidal t.
  ulceroglandular t.
tu·la·rine
tulle gras
Tul·lio phenomenon
Tul·pi·us' valve
tu·me·fa·cient
tu·me·fac·tion
tu·me·fy
tu·men·tia
  vasomotor t.
tu·mes·cence
tu·mes·cent
tu·meur
    t. perlée
    t. pileuse
tu·mid
tu·mor
  Abrikosov's (Abrikossoff's)
    t.
  Ackerman's t.
  acoustic nerve t.
  acute splenic t.
  adenoid t.
  adenomatoid t.
  adenomatoid odontogenic t.
  adipose t.
  adrenal rest t.
  t. albus
  alpha cell t.
  alveolar t.
  ameloblastic adenomatoid
    t.
  aneurysmal giant cell t.
  angiomatoid t.
  angle t.

tu·mor *(continued)*
  aniline t.
  aortic body t.
  argentaffin carcinoid t.
  ascites t.
  benign t.
  benign mixed t.
  benign triton t.
  Brenner t.
  Brodie's t.
  Brooke's t.
  brown t.
  brown fat t.
  Brown-Pearce t.
  Burkitt's t.
  Buschke-Löwenstein t.
  butyroid t.
  calcifying epithelial
    odontogenic t.
  carcinoid t. of bronchus
  carotid body t.
  cartilaginous t.
  cavernous t.
  cellular t.
  cerebellopontine angle t.
  chemoreceptor t.
  chromaffin-cell t.
  chromophil t.
  clear cell t.
  Cock's t.
  Codman's t.
  t. colli
  collision t.
  colloid t.
  colloid ovarian t.
  connective-tissue t.
  craniopharyngeal duct t.
  cystic t.
  dermoid t.
  desmoid t.
  dumb-bell t.
  dysontogenetic t.
  Ehrlich's t.
  eighth-nerve t.
  eiloid t.
  embryonal t.
  embryoplastic t.
  encysted t.

tu·mor *(continued)*
eosinophilic t.
epithelial t.
erectile t.
extramedullary
  hematopoietic t.
Ewing's t.
false t.
fatty t.
fecal t.
fibrocellular t.
fibroid t.
fibroplastic t.
fibrous t.
fungating t.
Furth's t.
ganglion nodosum t.
G-cell t.
gelatinous t.
germinal t.
giant cell t. of bone
giant cell t. of tendon
  sheath
glomus t.
glomus jugulare t.
granular cell t.
granulation t.
granulosa t.
granulosa cell t.
granulosa-theca cell t.
Grawitz's t's
Gubler's t.
gummy t.
heterologous t.
heterotypic t.
hilar cell t.
histioid t.
homoiotypic t.
homologous t.
Hortega cell t.
hourglass t.
Hürthle cell t.
infiltrating t.
innocent t.
interstitial cell t.
iron-hard t.
islet cell t.
ivory-like t.

tu·mor *(continued)*
Jensen's t.
juxtaglomerular t.
Koenen's t.
Krompecher's t.
Krukenberg's t.
lacteal t.
Leydig cell t.
t. lienis
lipoid cell t. of ovary
luteinized granulosa-theca
  cell t.
Malherbe's t.
malignant t.
malignant triton t.
march t.
margaroid t.
mast cell t.
melanotic neuroectodermal
  t.
Merkel cell t.
metastatic t.
migrated t.
migratory t.
mixed t.
mucoepidermoid t.
mucous t.
muscular t.
Nélaton's t.
neuroepithelial t.
nonencapsulated sclerosing
  t.
odontogenic t.
oozing t.
organoid t.
oxyphil cell t.
pacinian t.
Pancoast's t.
papillary t.
paraffin t.
parvilocular pseudo-
  mucinous t.
pearl t.
pearly t.
Perlmann's t.
phantom t.
phyllodes t.
Pindborg t.

tu·mor *(continued)*
  pineal t.
  plasma cell t.
  polypoid t.
  pontine angle t.
  potato t.
  Pott's puffy t.
  Pott's t.
  pregnancy t.
  premalignant fibro-
    epithelial t.
  pseudointraligamentous t.
  pulmonary sulcus t.
  ranine t.
  Rathke's t.
  Rathke's pouch t.
  Recklinghausen's t.
  recurring digital fibrous t's
    of childhood
  retinal anlage t.
  Ringertz t.
  sacrococcygeal t.
  salivary mixed cutaneous t.
  sand t.
  Schmincke t.
  Schwann-cell t.
  sentinel t.
  Sertoli's t.
  Sertoli cell t.
  Sertoli-Leydig cell t.
  sheath t.
  Spiegler's t's
  Steiner's t's
  stercoral t.
  superior sulcus t.
  teratoid t.
  theca cell t.
  thoracic inlet t.
  transition t.
  tridermic t.
  true t.
  turban t.
  varicose t.
  vascular t.
  villous t.
  Warthin's t.
  white t.
  Wilms' t.

tu·mor *(continued)*
  yolk sac t.
  Yoshida's t.
  Zollinger-Ellison (ZE) t.
tu·mor·af·fin
tu·mor·i·ci·dal
tu·mor·i·gen·e·sis
tu·mor·i·gen·ic
tu·mor·let
tu·mor·ous
tu·mul·tus
  t. cordis
Tun·ga
  T. penetrans
tun·gi·a·sis
tung·sten
tu·nic
  Bichat's t.
  Brücke's t.
  fibrous t. of eyeball
  fibrous t. of liver
  mucous t.
  muscular t.
  pharyngeal t.
  pharyngobasilar t.
  proper t.
  Ruysch's t.
  t's of spermatic cord
tu·ni·ca *pl.* tu·ni·cae
  t. abdominalis
  t. adnata oculi
  t. adnata testis
  t. adventitia
  t. albuginea
  t. conjunctiva
  t. dartos
  t. decidua
  t. elastica interna
  t. fibrosa
  t. interna bulbi
  t. interna thecae folliculi
  t. intima
  t. media
  t. mucosa
  t. muscularis
  t. nervea of Brücke
  t. propria
  t. ruyschiana

tu·ni·ca *(continued)*
   t. sclerotica
   t. sensoria bulbi
   t. serosa
   t. spongiosa
   t. submucosa
   tunicae testis
   t. uvea
   t. vaginalis testis
   t. vasculosa
tu·ni·cary
Tu·ni·ca·ta
tu·ni·cate
tu·ni·cin
tun·ing fork
tun·nel
   aortico-left ventricular t.
   carpal t.
   cervical t's
   Corti's t.
   cubital t.
   flexor t.
   inner t.
   outer t.
   tarsal t.
   Witzel t.
TUR — transurethral resection
tu·ra·nose
Tur·ba·trix
   T. aceti
tur·bid
tur·bi·dim·e·ter
tur·bid·i·met·ric
tur·bi·dim·e·try
tur·bid·i·ty
tur·bi·nal
tur·bi·nate
   inferior t.
   nasal t.
   t. of Santorini
   sphenoid t.
   t. of Zuckerkandl
tur·bi·nat·ed
tur·bi·nec·to·my
tur·bino·tome
tur·bi·not·o·my
Türck's bundle

Türck's cell
Türck's column
Türck's degeneration
Türck's fasciculus
Türck's trachoma
Turck's zone
Tur·cot syndrome
tur·ges·cence
tur·ges·cent
tur·gid
tur·gid·iza·tion
tur·gom·e·ter
tur·gor
   t. vitalis
tu·ris·ta
Türk's cell
Türk's irradiation leukocyte
tur·mer·ic
turm·scha·del
Tur·ner's cerate
Tur·ner hypoplasia
Tur·ner's sign
Tur·ner's sulcus
Tur·ner's syndrome
Tur·ner tooth
Tur·ner-Kei·ser syndrome
Tur·ner-War·wick urethroplasty
tur·nera
turn·over
   erythrocyte iron t. (EIT)
   plasma iron t. (PIT)
   red blood cell iron t. (RBC IT)
turn·sick
turn·sick·ness
turn·sol
TURP — transurethral prostatic resection
tur·pen·tine
tur·ri·ceph·a·ly
tu·run·da
Tu·ryn's sign
tus. — L. tussis (a cough)
tus·sal
tus·sic·u·la
tus·sic·u·lar
tus·sic·u·la·tion

tus·si·gen·ic
tus·sis
    t. convulsiva
    t. stomachalis
tus·sive
tu·ta·men *pl.* tu·ta·mi·na
    t. cerebri
    tutamina oculi
Tut·tle's proctoscope
Tween
tweez·ers
t_1-weight·ed
t_2-weight·ed
twig
twin
    acardiac t.
    allantoidoangiopagous t's
    binovular t's
    conjoined t's
    conjoined t's, asymmetrical
    conjoined t's, equal
    conjoined t's, symmetrical
    conjoined t's, unequal
    dichorial t's
    dichorionic t's
    dissimilar t's
    dizygotic t's
    enzygotic t's
    false t's
    fraternal t's
    heterologous t's
    hetero-ovular t's
    identical t's
    impacted t's
    monoamniotic t's
    monochorial t's
    monochorionic t's
    mono-ovular t's
    monovular t's
    monozygotic t's
    omphaloangiopagous t's
    one-egg t's
    parabiotic t's
    parasitic t.
    placental parasitic t.
    Siamese t's
    similar t's
    true t's

twin *(continued)*
    two-egg t's
    uniovular t's
    unlike t's
twinge
twin·ning
    experimental t.
    spontaneous t.
twin·ship
Twis·ton
twitch
    fast t.
    skin t.
    slow t.
twitch·ing
    fascicular t.
    fibrillar t.
    Trousseau's t.
two-di·men·sion·al
Twort-d'He·relle phenomenon
TXA_2 — thromboxane A_2
TXB_2 — thromboxane B_2
ty·ba·mate
ty·lec·to·my
Ty·le·nol
tyl·i·on
ty·lo·ma
ty·lo·sis
    t. ciliaris
    t. palmaris et plantaris
ty·lot·ic
ty·lox·a·pol
tym·pa·nal
tym·pa·nec·to·my
tym·pan·ia
tym·pan·ic
tym·pani·chord
tym·pa·nic·i·ty
tym·pa·nism
tym·pa·ni·tes
    false t.
    uterine t.
tym·pa·nit·ic
tym·pa·ni·tis
tym·pa·no·cen·te·sis
tym·pa·no·eu·sta·chi·an
tym·pa·no·gen·ic
tym·pa·no·gram

tym·pa·no·hy·al
tym·pa·no·lab·y·rin·tho·pexy
tym·pa·no·mal·le·al
tym·pa·no·mas·toid
tym·pa·no·mas·toid·itis
tym·pa·no·met·ric
tym·pa·nom·e·try
tym·pa·no·plas·tic
tym·pa·no·plas·ty
    combined approach t.
    intact canal-wall t.
tym·pa·no·scle·ro·sis
tym·pa·no·sis
tym·pa·no·squa·mo·sal
tym·pa·no·sta·pe·di·al
tym·pa·no·sym·pa·thec·to·
  my
tym·pa·no·tem·po·ral
tym·pa·not·o·my
    posterior t.
    transmeatal t.
tym·pa·nous
tym·pa·num
tym·pa·ny
    bell t.
    Skoda's t.
    skodaic t.
    t. of the stomach
Tyn·dall effect
Tyn·dall light
Tyn·dall phenomenon
tyn·dal·li·za·tion
type
    amyostatic-kinetic t.
    asthenic t.
    athletic t.
    Aztec t.
    basic personality t.
    bird's head t.
    blood t's
    body t.
    buffalo t.
    Charcot-Marie t.
    Charcot-Marie-Tooth t.
    constitutional t.
    cycloid t.
    Dejerine t.
    Dejerine-Landouzy t.

type *(continued)*
    Duchenne's t.
    Duchenne-Aran t.
    Duchenne-Landouzy t.
    Duffy blood antibody t.
    dysplastic t.
    Eichhorst's t.
    Erb-Zimmerlin t.
    Fazio-Londe t.
    Hutchison t.
    Kalmuk t.
    Kell blood antibody t.
    Kidd blood antibody t.
    Kretschmer t's
    Landouzy's t.
    Landouzy-Dejerine t.
    leg t.
    Leichtenstern's t.
    Levi-Lorain t.
    Leyden-Möbius t.
    Lorain t.
    mating t.
    Nothnagel's t.
    personality t.
    phage t.
    Putnam's t.
    pyknic t.
    Raymond's t. of apoplexy
    Remak's t.
    scapulohumeral t.
    schizoid t.
    Schultze's t.
    Simmerlin t.
    Strümpell's t.
    sympatheticotonic t.
    test t.
    Tooth's t.
    Werdnig-Hoffmann t.
    Wernicke-Mann t.
    wild t.
    Zimmerlin's t.
type-spe·cif·ic
ty·phe·mia
ty·phin·ia
typh·lec·ta·sis
typh·lec·to·my
typh·lo·ap·pen·di·ci·tis
Typh·lo·coe·lum

Typh·lo·coe·lum
    T. cucumerinum
typh·lo·dic·li·di·tis
typh·lo·lex·ia
typh·lol·o·gy
typh·lo·meg·a·ly
typh·lo·pexy
typh·lo·sis
typh·los·to·my
typh·lot·o·my
typh·lo·ure·ter·os·to·my
ty·pho·bac·ter·in
ty·phoid
    ambulatory t.
    fowl t.
    latent t.
    provocation t.
ty·phoi·dal
ty·pho·ma·nia
Ty·pho·ni·um tril·o·ba·tum
    (L.) Schott. (Araceae)
ty·phous
ty·phus
    African tick t.
    Australian tick t.
    benign t.
    chigger-borne t.
    classic t.
    collapsing t.
    endemic t.
    epidemic t.
    epidemic louse-borne t.
    European t.
    exanthematic t. of São
        Paulo
    t. exanthematique
    exanthematous t.
    flea-borne t.
    Gubler-Robin t.
    Hildenbrand's t.
    Indian tick t.
    t. inversus
    Kenya tick t.
    latent t.
    louse-borne t.
    Manchurian t.
    Mexican t.
    mite-borne t.

ty·phus *(continued)*
    t. mitior
    Moscow t.
    murine t.
    North Asian tick t.
    North Queensland tick t.
    petechial t.
    Queensland tick t.
    rat t.
    recrudescent t.
    rural t.
    São Paulo t.
    scrub t.
    shop t.
    Siberian tick t.
    sporadic t.
    tick t.
    tickborne t.
    Toulon t.
    tropical t.
    urban t.
typ·i·cal
typ·ing
    t. of blood
    colicin t.
    HLA t.
    phage t.
    primed lymphocyte t. (PLT)
    tissue t.
ty·po·dont
ty·pol·o·gy
ty·po·scope
ty·pus
    t. degenerativus
        amstelodamensis
Tyr — tyrosine
ty·ra·mine
ty·ra·mine ox·i·dase
tyr·an·nism
ty·re·in
ty·re·sin
ty·ro·ci·din
ty·ro·ci·dine
Ty·rode's solution
ty·rode-B
ty·rog·e·nous
Ty·rog·ly·phus
    T. castellani

Ty·rog·ly·phus (continued)
  T. farinae
  T. longior
  T. siro
ty·roid
ty·ro·ma·to·sis
ty·ro·pa·no·ate so·di·um
Ty·roph·a·gus
  T. castellani
  T. farinae
  T. longior
  T. siro
ty·ros·amine
ty·ro·sin·ase
ty·ro·sine
ty·ro·sine am·i·no·trans·fer·ase
ty·ro·sin·emia
  neonatal t.
ty·ro·sin·o·sis

ty·ro·sin·uria
ty·ro·sis
ty·ro·syl
ty·ro·syl·uria
ty·ro·thri·cin
ty·ro·tox·i·con
ty·ro·tox·i·co·sis
ty·ro·tox·ism
Tyr·rell's fascia
Tyr·rell's hook
Ty·son's crypts
Ty·son's glands
ty·so·ni·an
ty·so·ni·tis
ty·vel·ose
Ty·zine
Tyz·ze·ria
Tzanck cell
Tzanck test
tzet·ze

U — international unit (of enzyme activity)
  unit
  uracil
  uranium
  uridine
u — atomic mass unit
uar·thri·tis
UBC (University of British Columbia) brace
uber·ous
uber·ty
ubiq·ui·nol
ubiq·ui·nol-cy·to·chrome c re·duc·tase
ubiq·ui·nol de·hy·dro·gen·ase
ubiq·ui·none
ubiq·ui·tin
UDP — uridine diphosphate

UDP-*N*-ac·e·tyl·glu·co·sa·mine-ly·so·so·mal-en·zyme *N*-ac·e·tyl·glu·co·sa·mine·phos·pho·trans·fer·ase
UDPG — uridine diphosphate glucose
UDPga·lac·tose 4-epim·er·ase
UDPglu·cose 4-epim·er·ase
UDPglu·cose-hex·ose-1-phos·phate uri·dyl·yl·trans·fer·ase
UDPglu·cose py·ro·phos·pho·ry·lase
UDPglu·cu·ro·nate-bil·i·ru·bin-glu·co·ro·no·syl·trans·fer·ase
Udrán·szky's test
UFA — unesterified fatty acids

Uf·fel·mann's reagent
Uf·fel·mann's test
Uht·hoff's sign
UK — urokinase
Ula·cort
ula·ga·nac·te·sis
ulal·gia
ulat·ro·phy
    afunctional u.
    atrophic u.
    calcic u.
    ischemic u.
    traumatic u.
ul·cer
    Aden u.
    Allingham's u.
    amebic u.
    amputating u.
    anastomotic u.
    aphthous u.
    arteriosclerotic u.
    atheromatous u.
    atonic u.
    Barrett's u.
    Bazin's u.
    Bouveret-Duguet u.
    burrowing phagedenic u.
    Buruli u.
    catarrhal corneal u.
    chicle u.
    chiclero u.
    chrome u.
    cold u.
    concealed u.
    contact u. of larynx
    corneal u.
    creeping u.
    Cruveilhier's u.
    Cushing's u.
    Cushing-Rokitansky u.
    decubital u.
    decubitus u.
    dendriform u.
    dendritic u.
    diabetic u.
    diphtheritic u.
    duodenal u.
    elusive u.

ul·cer *(continued)*
    exuberant u.
    Fenwick-Hunner u.
    fissured u.
    fistulous u.
    flask u.
    follicular u.
    frenal u.
    gastric u.
    gastroduodenal u.
    giant peptic u's
    girdle u.
    gouty u.
    gravitational u.
    groin u.
    gummatous u.
    herpetic u.
    Hunner's u.
    hyperkeratotic u.
    hypertensive ischemic u.
    hypopyon u.
    hypostatic u.
    indolent u.
    Jacob's u.
    jejunal u.
    kissing u's
    Kocher's dilatation u.
    Lipschütz u.
    lupoid u.
    Mann-Williamson u.
    marginal u.
    Marjolin's u.
    Meleney's u.
    Meleney's chronic
      undermining u.
    mercurial u.
    Mooren's u.
    mycotic u.
    neurogenic u.
    neurotrophic u.
    Parrot's u.
    penetrating u.
    peptic u.
    perambulating u.
    perforating u.
    phagedenic u.
    plantar neurotrophic u.
    pneumococcus u.

ul·cer *(continued)*
    post-thrombotic u.
    pudendal u.
    radiation u.
    ring u.
    rodent u.
    Rokitansky-Cushing u's
    round u.
    Saemisch's u.
    scorbutic u.
    sea anemone u.
    secondary jejunal u.
    serpiginous corneal u.
    serpiginous u.
    simple u.
    sloughing u.
    soft u.
    stasis u.
    stercoraceous u.
    stercoral u.
    stoma u.
    stomal u.
    stress u.
    sublingual u.
    submucous u.
    symptomatic u.
    syphilitic u.
    tanner's u.
    transparent u. of cornea
    trophic u.
    trophoneurotic u.
    tropical u.
    tropical phagedenic u.
    undermining burrowing u.
    varicose u.
    venereal u.
    venous stasis u.
    warty u.
ul·cera
ul·cer·ate
ul·cer·a·tion
    u. of Daguet
    ischemic u.
    tracheal u.
ul·cer·a·tive
ul·cero·gan·gre·nous
ul·cer·o·gen·ic
ul·cero·glan·du·lar

ul·cero·gran·u·lo·ma
ul·cero·mem·bra·nous
ul·cer·ous
ul·cus *pl.* ul·ce·ra
    u. ambulans
    u. grave
    u. hypostaticum
    u. interdigitale
    u. penetrans
    u. scorbuticum
    u. serpens corneae
    u. simplex vesicae
    u. tropicum
    u. tuberculosum
    u. venereum
    u. ventriculi
    u. vulvae acutum
ul·da·ze·pam
ulec·to·my
ule·gy·ria
ulem·or·rha·gia
uler·y·the·ma
    u. ophryogenes
ulex·ine
ulig·i·nous
uli·tis
Ull·mann's line
Ull·rich syndrome
Ull·rich-Feich·ti·ger syndrome
Ull·rich-Tur·ner syndrome
Ul·mus
    U. fulva
ul·na *pl.* ul·nae
ul·nad
ul·nar
ul·na·re
ul·na·ris
ul·nen
ul·no·car·pal
ul·no·ra·di·al
uloc·a·ce
ulo·car·ci·no·ma
ulo·glos·si·tis
ulor·rha·gia
ulor·rhea
ulose
ulo·sis
ulot·o·my

ulo·trip·sis
ul·ti·mate
ul·ti·mi·ster·nal
ul·ti·mum mo·ri·ens
ult. praes. — L. ultimum
    praescriptus (last prescribed)
ul·tra·brachy·ce·phal·ic
ul·tra·cen·trif·u·ga·tion
ul·tra·cen·tri·fuge
ul·tra·di·an
ul·tra·dol·i·co·ce·phal·ic
ul·tra·fil·ter
ul·tra·fil·trate
ul·tra·fil·tra·tion
    sequential u.-hemodialysis
ul·tra·gas·e·ous
ul·tra·li·ga·tion
ul·tra·mi·cro·chem·is·try
ul·tra·mi·cron
ul·tra·mi·cro·pi·pet
ul·tra·mi·cro·scope
ul·tra·mi·cro·scop·ic
ul·tra·mi·cros·co·py
ul·tra·mi·cro·tome
Ul·tran
ul·tra·phago·cy·to·sis
ul·tra·pro·phy·lax·is
ul·tra·son·ic
ul·tra·son·ics
ul·tra·sono·gram
ul·tra·sono·graph
ul·tra·sono·graph·ic
ul·tra·so·nog·ra·phy
    Doppler u.
    endoscopic u.
    gray-scale u.
ul·tra·so·nom·e·try
ul·tra·sono·scope
ul·tra·sound
    Doppler u.
ul·tra·struc·ture
Ul·tra·tard
ul·tra·vi·o·let
    u. A (UVA)
    u. B (UVB)
    u. C (UVC)
    far u.
    near u.

ul·tra·vi·rus
ul·tra·vis·i·ble
ul·tro·mo·tiv·i·ty
Ultz·mann's test
um·bau·zo·nen
um·bel·lif·er·one
um·ber
Um·ber's test
um·bil·i·cal
um·bil·i·cate
um·bil·i·cat·ed
um·bil·i·ca·tion
um·bil·i·cus
    amniotic u.
    decidual u.
    posterior u.
um·bo pl. um·bo·nes
    u. membranae tympani
    u. of tympanic membrane
um·bo·nate
um·bo·nes
um·bra
um·bras·co·py
um·brel·la
    Mobin-Uddin u.
UMP — uridine
    monophosphate
un·azo·tized
un·bal·ance
un·cal
Un·car·ia
    U. gambier
un·car·thro·sis
un·ci
un·cia pl. un·ciae
un·ci·form
un·ci·for·me
un·ci·nal
Un·ci·nar·ia
    U. americana
    U. duodenalis
    U. stenocephala
un·cin·a·ri·a·sis
un·cin·a·ri·at·ic
un·ci·nate
un·ci·na·tum
un·ci·pres·sure
un·com·pen·sat·ed

un·com·ple·ment·ed
un·con·di·tioned
un·con·scious
    collective u.
un·co-os·si·fied
un·cot·o·my
un·coup·ling
un·co·ver·te·bral
un·crossed
unc·tion
unc·tu·ous
un·cus
    u. corporis
    u. of hamate bone
    neomycin u.
un·dec·e·no·ic acid
    neomycin u.
un·de·cyl·en·ic acid
un·der·cut
un·der·horn
un·der·nu·tri·tion
un·der·stain
un·der·toe
Un·der·wood's disease
un·dif·fer·en·ti·a·tion
un·dine
un·din·ism
un·du·lant
un·du·late
un·du·la·tion
    jugular u.
    respiratory u.
ung. — L. unguentum
  (ointment)
un·gual
un·guent
un·guen·tum *pl.* un·guen·ta
un·gues
un·guic·u·late
un·guic·u·lus
un·guis *pl.* un·gues
    u. avis
    u. incarnatus
    u. ventriculi lateralis
      cerebri
uni·ar·tic·u·lar
uni·ar·tic·u·late
uni·au·ral

uni·ax·i·al
uni·ba·sal
uni·cam·er·al
uni·cel·lu·lar
uni·cen·tral
uni·cen·tric
uni·ceps
uni·col·lis
uni·cor·nous
uni·cus·pid
uni·cus·pi·date
uni·di·rec·tion·al
uni·flag·el·late
uni·fo·cal
uni·fo·rate
Uni·form An·a·tom·i·cal Gift
  Act
uni·gem·i·nal
uni·ger·mi·nal
uni·glan·du·lar
uni·grav·i·da
uni·lam·i·nar
uni·lat·er·al
uni·lo·bar
uni·loc·u·lar
uni·mo·dal
uni·nu·cle·ar
uni·nu·cle·at·ed
uni·oc·u·lar
un·ion
    faulty u.
    immediate u.
    primary u.
    syngamic nuclear u.
    vicious u.
uni·ov·u·lar
unip·a·ra
uni·pa·ren·tal
unip·a·rous
Uni·pen
uni·pen·nate
uni·po·lar
uni·po·ten·cy
uni·po·tent
uni·po·ten·tial
un·ir·ri·ta·ble
uni·sep·tate
uni·sex·u·al

unit
  absolute u.
  Allen-Doisy u.
  alpha u's
  amboceptor u.
  American Drug
    Manufacturers'
    Association u.
  androgen u.
  Angström u.
  Ansbacher u.
  antigen u.
  antitoxic u.
  antivenene u.
  atomic mass u.
  atomic weight u.
  base u.
  Behnken's u.
  Bethesda u.
  Bodansky u.
  British thermal u.
  burn u.
  C. G. S. u.
  CH_{50} (CH50) u.
  clinical u.
  cobalt 60 beam therapy u.
  coherent u.
  coincidence u.
  Collip u.
  colony-forming u.
  complement u.
  Corner-Allen u.
  coronary care u.
  corpus luteum hormone u.
  dental u.
  derived u.
  digitalis u.
  electromagnetic u's
  electrostatic u's
  enzyme u.
  estrone u.
  Felton's u.
  flotation u.
  Hampson u.
  hemolytic u.
  hemorrhagin u.
  Hounsfield u.
  insulin u.

unit *(continued)*
  intensive care u.
  international androgen u.
  International u.
  international u. of enzyme
    activity (IU)
  international u. of
    estrogenic activity
  international estrone u.
  international u. of
    gonadotrophic activity
  international u. of
    immunological activity
  international insulin u.
  international u. of
    luteinizing activity
  international u. of male
    hormone
  international u. of
    penicillin
  international u. of
    progestational activity
  international progesterone
    u.
  international prolactin u.
  international u. of vitamin
    A
  international u. of vitamin
    D
  Kienböck u.
  King u.
  King-Armstrong u.
  Lf u.
  lung u.
  Mache u.
  map u.
  minimal hemolytic u.
  Montevideo u's
  motor u.
  mouse u.
  muscle u.
  nerve u.
  Noon pollen u.
  parathyroid u.
  pepsin u.
  peripheral resistance u.
    (PRU)
  pilosebaceous u.

unit *(continued)*
    progesterone u.
    prolactin u.
    psychiatric u.
    quantum u.
    rat u.
    sensation u.
    SI u.
    Siegbahn u.
    skin test u.
    slow motor u.
    Somogyi u.
    specific smell u.
    Steenbock u. of vitamin D
    sudanophobic u.
    supplementary u.
    Svedberg u.
    Svedberg flotation u.
    terminal airway u.
    Thayer-Doisy u.
    Todd u.
    toxic u.
    toxin u.
    tuberculin u. (TU)
    turbidity reducing u.
    unified atomic mass u.
    U.S.P. u.
    vitamin A u.
    u. of vitamin B_1
    vitamin D u.
    Voegtlin u.
    x-ray u.
unit·age
uni·tary
Unit·ed States Adopt·ed
  Names (USAN)
Unit·ed States Phar·ma·co·
  peia
Uni·ten·sen
uni·ter·mi·nal
uni·va·lence
uni·va·lent
uni·vi·tel·line
un·med·ul·lat·ed
un·my·eli·nat·ed
Un·na's boot
Un·na's cell
Un·na's dermatosis

Un·na-Pap·pen·heim stain
Un·na-Thost disease
Un·na-Thost syndrome
un·or·ga·nized
un·phys·i·o·log·ic
un·primed
un·rest
    peristaltic u.
un·sat·u·rat·ed
Un·schuld's sign
un·sex
un·stri·at·ed
Un·ver·richt's disease
Un·ver·richt's syndrome
up·gaze
up·right·ing
up·si·loid
up·si·lon
up·take
    absolute iodine u. (AIU)
    iodine-131 u.
UR — unconditioned response
ura·chal
ura·cho·ves·i·cal
ura·chus
    patent u.
ura·cil
    5-methyl u.
ura·cra·sia
ura·cra·tia
ura·gogue
ura·nis·co·chas·ma
ura·nis·co·la·lia
ura·nis·co·plas·ty
ura·nis·cor·rha·phy
ura·nis·cus
ura·ni·um
ura·no·plas·ty
ura·no·ple·gia
ura·nor·rha·phy
ura·nos·chi·sis
ura·nos·chism
ura·no·staph·y·lo·plas·ty
ura·no·staph·y·lor·rha·phy
ura·no·staph·y·los·chi·sis
ura·nos·teo·plas·ty
Ura·no·tae·nia
    U. sapparinus

ura·no·ve·los·chi·sis
ura·nyl
ura·pos·te·ma
urar·thri·tis
urate
urate ox·i·dase
ura·te·mia
urate·ri·bo·nu·cleo·ti·dase
  phos·pho·ryl·ase
urat·ic
ura·to·his·tech·ia
ura·to·ma
ura·to·sis
ura·tu·ria
ura·zin
ura·zine
Ur·bach-Op·pen·heim disease
Ur·bach-Wiethe disease
ur·ce·i·form
ur·ce·o·late
ur-de·fense
urea
  u. nitrogen
  plasma u.
  sterile u.
  u. stibamine
urea·ge·net·ic
ure·al
ure·am·e·try
Urea·phil
Ure·a·plas·ma
urea·poi·e·sis
ure·ase
urec·chy·sis
Urech·i·tes
  U. suberecta
urech·i·tin
urech·i·tox·in
Ure·cho·line
ure·de·ma
ure·do·fos
ure·ide
urel·co·sis
ure·mia
  prerenal u.
ure·mic
ure·mi·gen·ic
ure·ol·y·sis

ureo·lyt·ic
ure·om·e·try
ureo·tel·ic
ure·si·es·the·sis
ure·sis
ure·tal
ure·ter
  aberrant u.
  circumcaval u.
  double u.
  ectopic u.
  postcaval u.
  retrocaval u.
  retroiliac u.
ure·ter·al
ure·ter·al·gia
ure·ter·ec·ta·sis
ure·ter·ec·to·my
ure·ter·ic
ure·ter·itis
  u. cystica
  u. glandularis
ure·tero·cele
  ectopic u.
ure·tero·ce·lec·to·my
ure·tero·cer·vi·cal
ure·tero·co·los·to·my
ure·tero·cu·ta·ne·os·to·my
ure·tero·cys·ta·nas·to·mo·sis
ure·tero·cys·to·ne·os·to·my
ure·tero·cys·to·scope
ure·tero·cys·tos·to·my
ure·tero·di·al·y·sis
ure·tero·du·o·de·nal
ure·tero·en·ter·ic
ure·tero·en·tero·anas·to·mo·
  sis
ure·tero·en·ter·os·to·my
ure·tero·gram
ure·ter·og·ra·phy
ure·tero·hemi·ne·phrec·to·
  my
ure·tero·il·e·os·to·my
ure·tero·in·tes·ti·nal
ure·tero·lith
ure·tero·li·thi·a·sis
ure·tero·li·thot·o·my
ure·ter·ol·y·sis

ure·tero·me·a·tot·o·my
ure·tero·neo·cys·tos·to·my
ure·tero·neo·py·elos·to·my
ure·tero·ne·phrec·to·my
ure·ter·op·a·thy
ure·tero·pel·vic
ure·tero·pel·vio·ne·os·to·my
ure·tero·pel·vio·plas·ty
    Culp-DeWeerd u.
    Foley Y-V u.
    Scardino's u.
    Scardino-Prince u.
ure·tero·phleg·ma
ure·tero·plas·ty
ure·tero·proc·tos·to·my
ure·tero·py·eli·tis
ure·tero·py·elog·ra·phy
ure·tero·py·elo·ne·os·to·my
ure·tero·py·elo·ne·phri·tis
ure·tero·py·elo·ne·phros·to·
  my
ure·tero·py·elo·plas·ty
ure·tero·py·elos·to·my
ure·tero·py·o·sis
ure·tero·rec·tal
ure·tero·rec·to·ne·os·to·my
ure·tero·rec·tos·to·my
ure·tero·re·no·scope
ure·tero·re·nos·co·py
ure·ter·or·rha·gia
ure·ter·or·rha·phy
ure·tero·scope
ure·ter·os·copy
ure·tero·sig·moi·dos·to·my
ure·tero·steg·no·sis
ure·tero·ste·no·ma
ure·tero·ste·no·sis
ure·tero·sto·ma
ure·ter·os·to·my
    cutaneous u.
ure·ter·ot·o·my
ure·tero·tri·go·no·en·ter·os·
  to·my
ure·tero·tri·go·no·sig·moi·
  dos·to·my
ure·tero·ure·ter·al
ure·tero·ure·ter·os·to·my
ure·tero·uter·ine

ure·tero·vag·i·nal
ure·tero·ves·i·cal
ure·tero·ves·i·co·plas·ty
    Leadbetter-Politano u.
ure·tero·ves·i·cos·to·my
ure·thane
ure·thra
    anterior u.
    cavernous u.
    double u.
    female u.
    u. feminina
    imperforate u.
    male u.
    u. masculina
    membranous u.
    u. muliebris
    penile u.
    posterior u.
    primary u.
    prostatic u.
    spongy u.
    u. virilis
ure·thral
ure·thral·gia
ure·thra·scope
ure·thra·tre·sia
ure·threc·to·my
ure·threm·phrax·is
ureth·reu·ryn·ter
ure·thrism
ure·thri·tis
    atrophic u.
    u. cystica
    u. glandularis
    gonococcal u.
    gonorrheal u.
    gouty u.
    u. granulosa
    nongonococcal u.
    nonspecific u.
    u. orificii externi
    u. petrificans
    polypoid u.
    prophylactic u.
    senile u.
    simple u.
    specific u.

ure·thri·tis *(continued)*
   u. venerea
ure·thro·blen·nor·rhea
ure·thro·bul·bar
ure·thro·cele
ure·thro·cys·ti·tis
ure·thro·cys·to·cele
ure·thro·cys·to·gram
ure·thro·cys·tog·ra·phy
ure·thro·cys·tom·e·try
ure·thro·cys·to·pexy
ure·thro·dyn·ia
ure·thro·graph
ure·throg·ra·phy
ure·throm·e·ter
ure·throm·e·try
ure·thro·pe·nile
ure·thro·peri·ne·al
ure·thro·peri·neo·scro·tal
ure·thro·pexy
ure·thro·phrax·is
ure·thro·phy·ma
ure·thro·plas·ty
   Thiersch-Duplay u.
ure·thro·pros·tat·ic
ure·thro·rec·tal
ure·thror·rha·gia
ure·thror·rha·phy
ure·thror·rhea
ure·thro·scope
ure·thro·scop·ic
ure·thros·co·py
ure·thro·scro·tal
ure·thro·spasm
ure·thro·stax·is
ure·thro·ste·no·sis
ure·thros·to·my
ure·thro·tome
   dilating u.
   Maisonneuve's u.
ure·throt·o·my
   external u.
   internal u.
ure·thro·tri·go·ni·tis
ure·thro·vag·i·nal
ure·thro·ves·i·cal
uret·ic
Urex

URF — unidentified reading frame
ur·gen·cy
Ur·gin·ea
ur·hi·dro·sis
   u. crystallina
URI — upper respiratory infection
uri·an
uric
uric acid
uric·ac·i·de·mia
uric·ac·i·du·ria
uri·case
uri·ce·mia
uri·co·cho·lia
uri·col·y·sis
uri·co·lyt·ic
uri·com·e·ter
   Ruhemann's u.
uri·co·poi·e·sis
uri·co·su·ria
uri·co·su·ric
uri·co·tel·ic
uri·co·tel·ism
Uri·cult
uri·dine
   u. diphosphate (UDP)
   u. diphosphate acetylgalactosamine
   u. diphosphate acetylglucosamine
   u. diphosphate galactose
   u. diphosphate glucose
   u. diphosphoglucose
   u. diphosphoglucuronate
   u. monophosphate
   u. 5′-phosphate
   u. triphosphate (UTP)
uri·dine di·phos·pho·ga·lac·tose-4-epim·er·ase
uri·dine di·phos·pho·glu·cose de·hy·dro·gen·ase
uri·dro·sis
uri·dyl·ate
uri·cyl·ic acid
uri·dyl trans·fer·ase
uri·dyl·yl

uri·es·the·sis
urin·a·ble
urin·ac·cel·er·a·tor
urin·ac·i·dom·e·ter
uri·nae·mia
uri·nal
   condom u.
uri·nal·y·sis
uri·nary
uri·nate
uri·na·tion
   precipitant u.
   stuttering u.
uri·na·tive
urine
   Bence Jones u.
   black u.
   chylous u.
   cloudy u.
   crude u.
   diabetic u.
   dyspeptic u.
   febrile u.
   gouty u.
   milky u.
   nebulous u.
   residual u.
uri·ne·mia
urine-mu·coid
urin·i·dro·sis
uri·nif·er·ous
uri·nif·ic
uri·nip·a·rous
uri·no·cry·os·co·py
uri·no·gen·i·tal
uri·nog·e·nous
uri·no·glu·co·som·e·ter
uri·nol·o·gist
uri·nol·o·gy
uri·no·ma
uri·nom·e·ter
uri·nom·e·try
uri·noph·i·lous
uri·nos·co·py
uri·no·sex·u·al
uri·nous
uri·po·sia
urish·i·ol

Uri·spas
Uri·tone
uro·ac·i·dim·e·ter
uro·am·mo·ni·ac
uro·an·the·lone
uro·az·o·tom·e·ter
uro·ben·zo·ic acid
uro·bi·lin
uro·bil·in·emia
uro·bi·lino·gen
uro·bi·lino·gen·emia
uro·bi·lino·gen·uria
uro·bil·i·noid
uro·bil·i·noi·den
uro·bil·in·uria
uro·can·ase
uro·can·ate
uro·can·ate hy·dra·tase
uro·can·ic acid
uro·cele
uroch·er·as
uro·che·zia
Uro·chor·da·ta
uro·chor·date
uro·chrome
uro·chro·mo·gen
uro·ci·net·ic
uro·clep·sia
uro·co·pro·por·phyr·ia
uro·cris·ia
uro·cri·te·ri·on
Uro·cys·tis
   U. tritici
uro·cys·ti·tis
uro·di·al·y·sis
uro·do·chi·um
uro·dy·nam·ic
uro·dy·nam·ics
uro·dyn·ia
uro·dys·func·tion
uro·ede·ma
uro·en·ter·one
uro·er·y·thrin
uro·fla·vin
uro·flo·me·ter
uro·flow·me·ter
uro·fus·cin
uro·fus·co·hem·a·tin

uro·gas·ter
uro·gas·trone
uro·gen·i·tal
urog·e·nous
uro·gram
urog·ra·phy
    ascending u.
    cystoscopic u.
    descending u.
    excretion u.
    excretory u.
    intravenous u.
    oral u.
    retrograde u.
uro·gra·vim·e·ter
uro·hem·a·tin
uro·hem·a·to·ne·phro·sis
uro·hem·a·to·por·phy·rin
uro·ki·nase
uro·ki·net·ic
uro·ky·mog·ra·phy
uro·lag·nia
uro·lith
uro·li·thi·a·sis
uro·lith·ic
uro·li·thol·o·gy
uro·li·thot·o·my
uro·log·ic
uro·log·i·cal
urol·o·gist
urol·o·gy
uro·lyt·ic
uro·man·cy
uro·mel·a·nin
urom·e·lus
urom·e·ter
uro·met·ric
urom·e·try
uro·nate
uron·cus
uro·ne·phro·sis
ur·on·ic acid
uro·nol·o·gy
uron·on·com·e·try
uro·patho·gen
urop·a·thy
    obstructive u.
uro·pe·nia

uro·pep·sin·o·gen
uro·phan
uro·phan·ic
uro·phe·in
uro·phil·ia
uro·pho·bia
uro·phos·phom·e·ter
uro·pit·tin
uro·pla·nia
uro·pod
uro·poi·e·sis
uro·poi·et·ic
uro·por·phyr·ia
    erythropoietic u.
uro·por·phy·rin
uro·por·phy·rin·o·gen
uro·por·phy·rin·o·gen de·car·
    boxy·lase
uro·por·phy·rin·o·gen III syn·
    thase
uro·psam·mus
urop·ter·in
uro·pyo·ne·phro·sis
uro·pyo·ure·ter
uro·ra·di·ol·o·gy
uro·rhyth·mog·ra·phy
uro·ro·se·in
uro·ro·se·in·o·gen
uror·rho·din
uror·rho·din·o·gen
uro·ru·bin
uro·ru·bin·o·gen
uro·sac·cha·rom·e·try
uro·sa·cin
uros·cheo·cele
uros·che·sis
uro·scop·ic
uros·co·py
uro·sem·i·ol·o·gy
uro·sep·sis
uro·sep·tic
uro·sis
uro·spec·trin
uro·stal·ag·mom·e·try
uro·ste·a·lith
uro·the·li·al
uro·the·li·um
uro·tox·ia

uro·tox·ic
uro·tox·ic·i·ty
uro·tox·in
Urot·ro·pin
uro·ure·ter
urox·in
ur·rho·din
ur·so·de·oxy·cho·late
ur·so·de·oxy·cho·lic acid
ur·so·de·oxy·cho·lyl·gly·cine
ur·so·de·oxy·cho·lyl·tau·rine
Ur·ti·ca
   U. dioica
ur·ti·cant
ur·ti·car·ia
   acute u.
   aquagenic u.
   u. bullosa
   bullous u.
   cholinergic u.
   chronic u.
   cold u.
   contact u.
   factitious u.
   u. febrilis
   giant u.
   heat u.
   hemorrhagic u.
   heredofamilial u.
   light u.
   u. maritima
   u. medicamentosa
   u. multiformis endemica
   papular u.
   u. perstans
   u. petechialis
   u. photogenica
   physical u.
   u. pigmentosa
   pressure u.
   solar u.
   u. solaris
ur·ti·car·i·al
ur·ti·car·i·o·gen·ic
ur·ti·car·i·ous
ur·ti·cate
ur·ti·ca·tion
uru·shi·ol

US — ultrasound
USDA — United States
   Department of Agriculture
Ush·er syndrome
Us·nea bar·ba·ta
us·ne·in
USPHS — United States
   Public Health Service
USR — unheated serum
   reagin (test)
Us·ti·lag·i·na·les
us·ti·lag·i·nism
Us·ti·la·go
   U. maydis
us·tion
us·tu·la·tion
usu·sta·tus
uta
Ut dict. — L. ut dictum (as
   directed)
Utend. — L. utendus (to be
   used)
uter·al·gia
uter·cys·tos·to·my
uteri
uter·ine
utero·ab·dom·i·nal
utero·cer·vi·cal
uter·odyn·ia
utero·fix·a·tion
uter·o·gen·ic
utero·ges·ta·tion
utero·glob·u·lin
uter·og·ra·phy
utero·lith
uter·om·e·ter
uter·om·e·try
utero-ovar·i·an
utero·pexy
utero·pla·cen·tal
utero·plas·ty
utero·rec·tal
utero·sa·cral
utero·sal·pin·gog·ra·phy
utero·scle·ro·sis
utero·scope
utero·ther·mom·e·try
uter·ot·o·my

utero·ton·ic
uter·o·trop·ic
utero·tu·bal
utero·tu·bog·ra·phy
uter·o·vag·i·nal
utero·ven·tral
uter·o·ves·i·cal
uter·us *pl.* uteri
   u. acollis
   arcuate u.
   u. arcuatus
   u. bicameratus vetularum
   u. bicornis
   u. bicornis bicollis
   u. bicornis unicollis
   bicornuate u.
   u. biforis
   u. bilocularis
   bipartite u.
   u. bipartitus
   boggy u.
   cochleate u.
   u. cordiformis
   Couvelaire u.
   u. didelphys
   double-mouthed u.
   duplex u.
   u. duplex
   embryonic u.
   fetal u.
   fibroid u.
   gravid u.
   u. incudiformis
   infantile u.
   u. masculinus
   ovoid u.
   u. parvicollis
   Piskacek u.
   u. planifundalis
   pubescent u.
   ribbon u.
   u. rudimentarius
   sacculated u.
   saddle-shaped u.
   u. septus
   u. simplex
   u. subseptus
   u. triangularis

uter·us *(continued)*
   u. unicornis
Uti·bid
Uti·cil·lin
util·iza·tion
   red cell u. (RCU)
UTP — uridine triphosphate
UTP–ga·lac·tose-1-phos·phate
   uri·dyl·yl·trans·fer·ase
UTP–glu·cose-1-phos·phate
   uri·dyl·yl·trans·fer·ase
utri·cle
   prostatic u.
   urethral u.
utric·u·lar
utric·u·li
utric·u·li·tis
utric·u·lo·sac·cu·lar
utri·cu·lus *pl.* utri·cu·li
   u. masculinus
   u. prostaticus
   u. vestibuli
utri·form
UVA — ultraviolet A
uva *pl.* uvae
   u. ursi
Uval
UVB — ultraviolet B
UVC — ultraviolet C
uvea
uve·al
uve·it·ic
uve·itis
   anterior u.
   Förster's u.
   granulomatous u.
   heterochromic u.
   lens-induced u.
   nongranulomatous u.
   phacoanaphylactic u.
   phacoantigenic u.
   phacotoxic u.
   posterior u.
   sympathetic u.
   toxoplasmic u.
   tuberculous u.
uveo·lab·y·rin·thi·tis
uveo·me·nin·gi·tis

uveo·me·nin·go·en·ceph·a·li·
    tis
uveo·neur·ax·itis
uveo·pa·rot·id
uveo·par·o·ti·tis
uveo·scle·ri·tis
uvi·form
uvio·fast
uvi·ol
uvio·re·sis·tant
uvio·sen·si·tive
uvu·la *pl.* uvu·lae
    bifid u.
    u. of bladder
    u. cerebelli
    u. of cerebellum
    cleft u.

uvu·la *(continued)*
    u. fissura
    forked u.
    Lieutaud's u.
    u. palatina
    palatine u.
    split u.
    u. vermis
    u. vesicae
uvu·lar
uvu·la·ris
uvu·lec·to·my
uvu·li·tis
uvu·lond·u·lar
uvu·lop·to·sis
uvu·lo·tome
uvu·lot·o·my

V

V — valine
    vanadium
    velocity
    volt
    voltage
    volume
V — voltage
    volume
V_{max} — maximum velocity of
    an enzyme-catalyzed reaction
V_T — tidal volume
v. — L. vena (vein)
v — velocity
    voltage
VA — Veterans
    Administration
    visual acuity
vac·cin·a·ble
vac·ci·nal
vac·ci·nate
vac·ci·na·tion
    autogenous v.

vac·ci·na·tion *(continued)*
    booster v.
vac·ci·na·tor
vac·cine
    adjuvant v.
    adsorbed diphtheria and
        tetanus toxoids and
        pertussis v.
    anaplasmosis v.
    anthrax v.
    anthrax spore v.
    attenuated v.
    autogenous v.
    bacterial v.
    BCG v.
    bronchitis v.
    Brucella abortus v.
    Castañeda's v.
    Castellani's v.
    cholera v.
    coccidiosis v.
    cowpox v.

vac·cine *(continued)*

Cox v.
Danysz v.
DPT (diphtheria, pertussis, and tetanus toxoids) v.
duck embryo v.
Durand's v.
Durand and Giroud v.
encephalomyelitis v.
epidemic typhus v.
Erysipelothrix rhusiopathiae v.
Felix v.
Fermi's v.
Haffkine's v.
hepatitis B v.
heterologous v.
heterotypic v.
HIB polysaccharide v.
human diploid cell v.
humanized v.
Idanov and Fadeewa v.
influenza virus v.
Kelev's v.
Kolle's v.
Lépine's v.
live v.
Lustig-Galeotti v.
Marek's disease v.
measles v.
measles virus v. live
meningococcal polysaccharide v.
mixed v.
MMR (measles, mumps, and rubella) v.
monovalent v.
multivalent v.
mumps virus v. live
Newcastle disease v.
paratyphoid v.
Pasteur v.
Pasteurella multocida v.
pertussis v.
plague v.
pneumococcal polysaccharide v.
poliomyelitis v.

vac·cine *(continued)*

poliovirus v. inactivated (IPV)
poliovirus v. live oral (OPV)
poliovirus v. live oral trivalent (TOPV)
polyvalent v.
pseudorabies v.
rabies v.
reo-corona viral calf diarrhea v.
replicative v.
Rocky Mountain spotted fever v.
rubella virus v. live
Sabin v.
Salk v.
Sauer's v.
smallpox v.
Spencer-Parker v.
split-virus v.
streptococcus v.
streptococcus group E v.
Strong's v.
subunit v.
subvirion v.
TAB v.
tenosynovitis v.
tetanus v.
transmissible gastroenteritis v.
triple v.
trivalent v.
tuberculosis v.
tularemia v.
typhoid v.
typhoid-paratyphoid A and B, and cholera v.
typhus v.
univalent v.
varicella v.
Weigl's v.
whooping cough v.
yellow fever v.
ZIG (zoster immune globulin) v.
Zinsser-Castañeda v.

vac·cin·ia
   chronic progressive v.
   fetal v.
   v. gangrenosa
   generalized v.
   v. progressiva
   progressive v.
vac·cin·i·al
vac·cin·id
vac·cin·i·form
vac·cino·gen
vac·ci·nog·e·nous
vac·ci·noid
vac·cin·o·la
vac·cino·style
vac·ci·no·ther·a·py
vac·u·o·lar
vac·u·o·late
vac·u·o·lat·ed
vac·u·o·la·tion
vac·u·ole
   autophagic v.
   condensing v's
   contractile v.
   digestive v.
   food v.
   heterophagic v.
   plasmocrine v.
   rhagiocrine v.
   secretory v.
   water v.
vac·u·o·li·za·tion
vac·u·ome
vac·u·um
   high v.
   torricellian v.
vac·u·um·iz·ing
va·dum
va·gal
va·gec·to·my
va·gi
va·gi·na *pl.* va·gi·nae
   bipartite v.
   v. bulbi
   v. carotica fasciae
    cervicalis
   v. cellulosa

va·gi·na *(continued)*
   v. communis musculorum
    flexorum
   v. cordis
   embryonic v.
   v. externa nervi optici
   v. femoris
   v. fibrosa tendinis
   v. interna nervi optici
   v. masculina
   vaginae mucosae
   v. mucosa tendinis
   v. muliebris
   vaginae nervi optici
   v. oculi
   v. processus styloidei
   vaginae synoviales
   v. tendinis
   v. vasorum
va·gi·nae
vag·i·nal
vag·i·na·lec·to·my
vag·i·na·li·tis
   plastic v.
vag·i·na·pexy
vag·i·nate
vag·i·nec·to·my
vag·i·ni·peri·ne·ot·o·my
vag·i·nis·mus
   perineal v.
   posterior v.
   superficial v.
   vulvar v.
vag·i·ni·tis
   v. adhaesiva
   adhesive v.
   atrophic v.
   v. cystica
   desquamative
    inflammatory v.
   diphtheritic v.
   v. emphysematosa
   emphysematous v.
   exfoliative v.
   gonococcal v.
   granular v.
   mucous v.
   pneumocystic v.

vag·i·ni·tis *(continued)*
  postmenstrual v.
  senile v.
  v. testis
  trichomonas v.
vag·i·no·ab·dom·i·nal
vag·i·no·cele
vag·i·no·cu·ta·ne·ous
vag·i·no·dyn·ia
vag·i·no·fix·a·tion
vag·i·no·gram
vag·i·nog·ra·phy
vag·i·no·la·bi·al
vag·i·nom·e·ter
vag·i·no·my·co·sis
vag·i·nop·a·thy
vag·i·no·per·i·ne·al
vag·i·no·peri·neo·plas·ty
vag·i·no·peri·ne·or·rha·phy
vag·i·no·peri·ne·ot·o·my
vag·i·no·peri·to·ne·al
vag·i·no·pexy
vag·i·no·plas·ty
vag·i·no·scope
vag·i·nos·co·py
vag·i·no·sis
  bacterial v.
vag·i·not·o·my
vag·i·no·ves·i·cal
vag·i·no·vul·var
va·gi·tus
  v. uterinus
  v. vaginalis
va·go·ac·ces·so·ri·us
va·go·glos·so·pha·ryn·ge·al
va·go·gram
va·gol·y·sis
va·go·lyt·ic
va·go·mi·met·ic
va·go·splanch·nic
va·go·sym·pa·thet·ic
va·got·o·my
  bilateral v.
  highly selective v.
  medical v.
  parietal cell v.
  selective v.
  surgical v.

va·got·o·my *(continued)*
  truncal v.
va·go·to·nia
va·go·ton·ic
va·go·to·nin
va·got·o·ny
va·go·trope
va·go·trop·ic
va·got·ro·pism
va·go·va·gal
va·gus *pl.* va·gi
Vahl·kamp·fia
Val — valine
va·lence
Val·en·tin's corpuscles
Val·en·tin's ganglion
Val·en·tin's pseudoganglion
Val·en·tine's position
va·le·ri·an
  Greek v.
val·eth·a·mate bro·mide
val·e·tu·di·nar·i·an
val·e·tu·di·nar·i·an·ism
val·gus
val·i·da·tion
  consensual v.
va·lid·i·ty
  face v.
val·ine
val·in·emia
val·i·no·my·cin
Val·i·sone
Val·i·um
val·late
val·le·cu·la *pl.* val·le·cu·lae
  v. cerebelli
  v. cerebri lateralis
  v. epiglottica
  v. fossa sylvii
  v. ovata
  v. for petrosal ganglion
  v. sylvii
  v. unguis
val·lec·u·lar
Val·leix's points
Val·les·tril
val·ley
  v. of cerebellum

val·li
val·lic·e·po·bu·fa·gin
Val·li-Rit·ter law
val·lis
val·lum *pl.* val·la
    v. unguis
Val·mid
val·noc·ta·mide
Val·pin
val·pro·ate so·di·um
Val·sal·va's experiment
Val·sal·va's ligaments
Val·sal·va's maneuver
Val·sal·va's sinus
Val·sal·va's zone
val·ue
    acetyl v.
    acid v.
    adaptive v.
    biological v.
    buffer v.
    cot v.
    cryocrit v.
    D v.
    fuel v.
    Hehner's v.
    iodine v.
    lethal equivalent v.
    liminal v.
    mean clinical v.
    normal v's
    normothetic v.
    P v.
    predictive v.
    reference v's
    relative v.
    saponification v.
    survival v.
    threshold v.
    valence v.
val·va *pl.* val·vae
    v. aortae
    v. aortica
    v. atrioventricularis dextra
    v. atrioventricularis
      sinistra
    v. ilealis
    v. ileocaecalis

val·va *(continued)*
    v. mitralis
    v. pulmonaria
    v. sinus venosi
    v. tricuspidalis
    v. trunci pulmonalis
val·val
val·var
val·vate
valve
    anal v's
    anterior urethral v's
    v. of aorta
    aortic v.
    artificial v.
    atrioventricular v., left
    atrioventricular v., right
    auriculoventricular v., left
    auriculoventricular v.,
      right
    Ball's v's
    ball v.
    Bauhin's v.
    Béraud's v.
    Bianchi's v.
    bicuspid v.
    bicuspid aortic v.
    bicuspid pulmonary v.
    Bjork-Shiley v.
    Blom-Singer v.
    Bochdalek's v.
    caged-ball v.
    cardiac v's
    cardiac v., artificial
    Carpentier-Edwards v.
    caval v.
    congenital ureteric v's
    congenital urethral v.
    coronary v.
    v. of coronary sinus
    directional v.
    duckbill v.
    escape v.
    eustachian v.
    expiratory v.
    fallopian v.
    flair v.
    flow-control v.

valve *(continued)*
  Foltz's v.
  v. of foramen ovale
  Gerlach's v.
  glutaraldehyde-tanned
    porcine heart v.
  Guérin's v.
  Hancock v.
  Hasner's v.
  heart v's
  heart v., artificial
  Heister's v.
  Heyer v.
  Hoboken's v's
  hot cathode v.
  Houston's v's
  Huschke's v.
  hymenal v. of male urethra
  ileocecal v.
  ileocolic v.
  v. of inferior vena cava
  inspiratory v.
  interauricular v.
  Ionescu v.
  Kerckring's v's
  Kohlrausch's v's
  Krause's v.
  LeVeen peritoneal v.
  lymphatic v.
  v. of Macalister
  Mercier's v.
  mitral v.
  monocuspid aortic v.
  Morgagni's v's
  v. of navicular fossa
  nonrebreathing v.
  O'Beirne's v.
  oxygen flush v.
  parachute mitral v.
  popoff v.
  porcine v.
  posterior urethral v's
  pressure-limiting v.
  Pudenz-Heyer v.
  pulmonary v.
  pulmonary trunk v.
  v. of pulmonary trunk
  pyloric v.

valve *(continued)*
  quadricuspid v.
  relief v.
  Rosenmüller's v.
  semilunar v.
  semilunar v's of colon
  semilunar v's of Morgagni
  semilunar v's of rectum
  sigmoid v's of colon
  speaking v.
  spiral v. of cystic duct
  spiral v. of Heister
  Spitz-Holter v.
  Starr-Edwards v.
  v. of Sylvius
  Taillefer's v.
  Tarin's v.
  Tarinus'v.
  Terrier's v.
  thebesian v.
  Thebesius' v.
  thermionic v.
  tilting-disk v.
  tracheostoma v.
  tricuspid v.
  v. of Tulpius
  unidirectional v.
  ureteral v.
  urethral v's
  v. of Varolius
  v. of veins
  v. of vermiform appendix
  v. of Vieussens
  Willis' v·
val·vec·to·my
valved
val·vi·form
val·vo·plas·ty
val·vo·tome
val·vot·o·my
  mitral v.
  pulmonary v.
  rectal v.
  transventricular closed v.
  transventricular
    pulmonary v.
val·vu·la *pl.* val·vu·lae
  Amussat's v.

val·vu·la *(continued)*
  valvulae anales
  v. biscuspidalis [mitralis]
  valvulae conniventes
  v. foraminis ovalis
  v. fossae navicularis
  Gerlach's v.
  v. hobokenii
  v. ileocolica
  v. lymphaticum
  v. mitralis
  v. processus vermiformis
  v. prostatica
  v. pylori
  v. semilunaris
  v. sinus coronarii
  v. sinus coronarii [Thebesii]
  v. spiralis [Heisteri]
  v. tricuspidalis
  v. venae cavae inferioris
  v. venae cavae inferioris
    [Eustachii]
  v. venosa
  v. vestibuli
val·vu·lae
val·vu·lar
val·vu·late
val·vule
  v. of Béraud
  v. of Bochdalek
  v. of Foltz
  v. of Guérin
val·vu·lec·to·my
val·vu·li·tis
  rheumatic v.
  uricemic v.
val·vu·lo·plas·ty
val·vu·lo·tome
val·vu·lot·o·my
val·yl
van·a·date
va·nad·ic acid
va·na·di·um
va·na·di·um·ism
van Bo·gaert's encephalitis
van Bo·gaert's sclerosing
  leukoencephalitis
van Bo·gaert-Ber·trand disease

van Bo·gaert-Div·ry syndrome
van Bo·gaert-Nys·sen-Peif·fer
  disease
van Bo·gaert-Scher·er-Ep·
  stein syndrome
van Bu·chem's disease
van Bu·chem's syndrome
van Bu·ren's disease
Van·co·cin
van·co·my·cin hy·dro·chlo·
  ride
Van de Graaff machine
van den Bergh's disease
van den Bergh's test
van der Hoeve syndrome
van der Hoeve-de Kleyn
  syndrome
van der Vel·den's test
van der Waals radius
Vane, John Robert
van Ge·huch·ten's cells
van Ge·huch·ten's method
Van·ghet·ti's prosthesis
van Gie·son's stain
van Hel·mont's mirror
van Hook's operation
van Hoorne's canal
Va·nil·la
va·nil·la
va·nil·lal
va·nil·lic acid
  v. a. diethylamide
va·nil·lin
  ethyl v.
va·nil·lism
va·nil·lyl·man·del·ic acid
Van·o·gel
Van·sil
Van Slyke's formula
Van Slyke's method
Van Slyke's tests
Van Slyke-Cul·len method
Van Slyke-Cul·len test
Van Slyke-Fitz method
Van Slyke and Neill method
van't Hoff's law
van't Hoff's rule
Van·zet·ti's sign

va·po·cau·ter·iza·tion
va·po-cool·ant
va·por *pl.* va·po·res, va·pors
   quenching v.
va·po·rar·i·um
va·por·iza·tion
va·por·ize
va·por·iz·er
   anesthetic v.
   Copper Kettle v.
   Fluotec v.
   Vernitrol v.
va·pors
va·po·ther·a·py
Va·quez's disease
var. — variety
var·i·a·bil·i·ty
var·i·a·ble
   acoustic v.
   confounding v.
   continuous v.
   dependent v.
   discrete v.
   dummy v.
   explanatory v.
   independent v.
   intervening v.
   predictor v.
   random v.
var·i·ance
   environmental v.
   genetic v.
var·i·ant
   alpha v.
   Haenel's v.
   L-phase v.
var·i·ate
   binary v.
   continuous v.
   discrete v.
var·i·a·tion
   allotypic v.
   antigenic v.
   continuous v.
   discontinuous v.
   genetic v.
   genotypic v.
   idiotypic v.

var·i·a·tion *(continued)*
   impressed v.
   inborn v.
   isotypic v.
   meristic v.
   microbial v.
   phase v.
   phenotypic v.
   quasicontinuous v.
   saltatory v.
   sampling v.
   smooth-rough (S-R) v.
vari·cat·ed
var·i·ca·tion
var·i·ce·al
var·i·cec·to·my
var·i·cel·la
   v. bullosa
   v. gangrenosa
   v. inoculata
   pustular v.
   v. pustulosa
   vaccination v.
var·i·cel·la·tion
var·i·cel·li·form
var·i·cel·loid
var·i·ces
var·ic·i·form
var·i·co·bleph·a·ron
var·i·co·cele
   ovarian v.
   pelvic v.
   utero-ovarian v.
var·i·co·ce·lec·to·my
var·i·cog·ra·phy
var·i·coid
var·i·cole
var·i·com·pha·lus
var·i·co·phle·bi·tis
var·i·cose
var·i·co·sis
var·i·cos·i·ty
var·i·cot·o·my
va·ric·u·la
Var·i·dase
va·ri·e·ty
va·ri·o·la
   v. major

va·ri·o·la *(continued)*
  v. minor
va·ri·o·lar
va·ri·o·late
va·ri·o·la·tion
var·i·ol·ic
va·ri·ol·i·form
va·ri·o·li·za·tion
va·ri·o·loid
va·ri·o·lous
va·ris·tor
var·ix *pl.* var·i·ces
  v. afferens arteriae
    interlobularis
  anastomotic v.
  aneurysmal v.
  aneurysmoid v.
  arterial v.
  chyle v.
  cirsoid v.
  v. corona
  v. efferens arteriae
    interlobularis
  esophageal v.
  Ferrein's v. aberrantia
  gelatinous v.
  lymph v.
  v. lymphaticus
  papillary v's
var·nish
  cavity v.
va·ro·li·an
Va·ro·li·us' bridge
Va·ro·li·us' valve
var·us
vas *pl.* va·sa
  v. aberrans
  v. aberrans of Roth
  vasa aberrantis hepatis
  v. afferens glomeruli
  vasa afferentia
  vasa afferentia
    lymphoglandulae
  vasa afferentia nodi
    lymphatici
  v. anastomoticum
  vasa auris internae
  vasa brevia

vas *(continued)*
  v. capillare
  v. collaterale
  v. deferens
  v. efferens glomeruli
  vasa efferentia
  vasa efferentia
    lymphoglandulae
  vasa efferentia nodi
    lymphatici
  v. epididymidis
  vasa intestini tenuis
  vasa lymphatica
  v. lymphaticum
  v. lymphaticum profundum
  v. lymphaticum
    superficiale
  v. lymphocapillare
  vasa nervorum
  vasa nutritia
  vasa praevia
  v. prominens ductus
    cochlearis
  vasa propria of Jungbluth
  vasa recta
  vasa sanguinea retinae
  v. sinusoideum
  v. spirale
  vasa vasorum
  vasa vorticosa
va·sa
Vas·al
va·sal
va·sal·gia
va·sa·li·um
Vas·co·ray
vas·cu·lar
vas·cu·lar·i·ty
vas·cu·lar·iza·tion
vas·cu·lar·ize
vas·cu·la·ture
vas·cu·lit·ic
vas·cu·li·tis
  allergic v.
  hypersensitivity v.
  leukocytoclastic v.
  livedo v.
  necrotizing v.

vas·cu·li·tis *(continued)*
   nodular v.
   overlap v.
   retinal v.
   segmented hyalinizing v.
vas·cu·lo·car·di·ac
vas·cu·lo·gen·e·sis
vas·cu·lo·gen·ic
vas·cu·lo·lym·phat·ic
vas·cu·lo·mo·tor
vas·cu·lop·a·thy
vas·cu·lo·tox·ic
vas·cu·lum *pl.* vas·cu·la
   v. aberrans
va·sec·to·mized
va·sec·to·my
   cross-over v.
vasi·fac·tion
vas·i·fac·tive
vas·i·form
va·si·tis
   v. nodosa
vaso·ac·tive
vaso·con·stric·tion
   active v.
   passive v.
vaso·con·stric·tive
vaso·con·stric·tor
vaso·co·ro·na
vaso·de·pres·sion
vaso·de·pres·sor
Vaso·di·lan
vaso·di·la·ta·tion
   active v.
   passive v.
vaso·di·la·tion
   reflex v.
vaso·di·la·tive
vaso·di·la·tor
vaso·epi·did·y·mog·ra·phy
vaso·epi·did·y·mos·to·my
vaso·fac·tive
vaso·for·ma·tive
vaso·gan·gli·on
va·sog·ra·phy
vaso·hy·per·ton·ic
vaso·hy·po·ton·ic
vaso·in·ert

vaso·in·hib·i·tor
vaso·in·hib·i·to·ry
vaso·la·bile
vaso·li·ga·tion
vaso·lig·a·ture
vaso·mo·tion
vaso·mo·tor
vaso·mo·to·ri·al
vaso·mo·tor·ic·i·ty
vaso·mo·to·ri·um
vaso·mo·to·ry
vaso·neu·rop·a·thy
vaso·neu·ro·sis
vaso-or·chid·os·to·my
vaso·pa·ral·y·sis
vaso·pa·re·sis
vaso·per·me·a·bil·i·ty
vaso·pres·sin
   arginine v. (AVP)
   lysine v.
   v. 8-lysine
   v. tannate
vaso·pres·sin·ase
vaso·pres·sor
vaso·punc·ture
vaso·re·flex
vaso·re·lax·a·tion
vaso·re·sec·tion
vas·or·rha·phy
vaso·sec·tion
vaso·sen·so·ry
vaso·spasm
vaso·spas·mo·lyt·ic
vaso·spas·tic
vaso·stim·u·lant
va·sos·to·my
vaso·to·cin
   arginine v.
va·sot·o·my
vaso·to·nia
vaso·ton·ic
vaso·tribe
vaso·trip·sy
vaso·troph·ic
vaso·trop·ic
vaso·va·gal
vaso·va·sos·to·my
vaso·ve·sic·u·lec·to·my

vaso·ve·sic·u·li·tis
Vas·ox·yl
vas·tus
    v. lateralis
Va·ter's ampulla
Va·ter's corpuscles
Va·ter's duct
Va·ter's papilla
Va·ter-Pa·ci·ni corpuscles
Vaughan-No·vy's test
vault
    cranial v.
    v. of pharynx
VC — vital capacity
VCE — vagina ectocervix and
    endocervix (smear)
VCG — vectorcardiogram
V-Cil·lin
VD — venereal disease
VDEL — Venereal Disease
    Experimental Laboratory
VDH — vascular disease of
    the heart
VDRL — Venereal Disease
    Research Laboratories
vec·tion
vec·tis
vec·tor
    biological v.
    cardiac v.
    cloning v.
    instantaneous v.
    manifest v.
    macroscopic magnetization
        v.
    mechanical v.
    recombinant v.
    spatial v.
vec·tor-borne
vec·tor·car·dio·gram
vec·tor·car·dio·graph
vec·tor·car·di·og·ra·phy
    spatial v.
vec·to·ri·al
vec·tor·scope
Vec·trin
ve·cu·ro·ni·um bro·mide
Ved·der's agar

Ved·der's culture medium
Ved·der's sign
VEE — Venezuelan equine
    encephalomyelitis
Vee·tids
veg·an
veg·a·nism
veg·e·ta·ble
veg·e·tal
veg·e·tal·i·ty
veg·e·tar·i·an
veg·e·tar·i·an·ism
veg·e·ta·tion
    adenoid v.
    bacterial v's
    dendritic v.
    verrucous v's
veg·e·ta·tive
veg·e·to·an·i·mal
ve·hi·cle
veil
    Fick's v.
    Jackson's v.
    Sattler's v.
    vitreous v's
Veil·lon tube
Veil·lon·el·la
Veil·lon·el·la·ceae
vein
    accompanying v.
    adrenal v's
    afferent v's
    allantoic v's
    anastomotic v., inferior
    anastomotic v., superior
    angular v.
    anonymous v's
    antebrachial v., median
    anticlinal v.
    appendicular v.
    aqueous v's
    arciform v's
    arcuate v's of kidney
    arterial v.
    arterial v. of Soemmering
    articular v's
    ascending v's of Rosenthal
    atrial v's of heart

vein *(continued)*
- atrial v., lateral
- atrial v., medial
- atrioventricular v's of heart
- auditory v's, internal
- auricular v's, anterior
- auricular v., posterior
- avalvular v's
- axillary v.
- azygos v.
- azygos v., left
- azygos v., lesser superior
- basal v.
- basilic v.
- basilic v., median
- basivertebral v's
- brachial v's
- brachiocephalic v's
- Braune's v.
- Breschet's v's
- bronchial v's
- Browning's v.
- buccal v's
- Burow's v.
- capillary v.
- capsular v.
- cardiac v's
- cardiac v's, anterior
- cardiac v., great
- cardiac v., middle
- cardiac v., small
- cardiac v's, smallest
- cardinal v's
- carotid v., external
- cavernous v's of penis
- central v.
- cephalic v.
- cephalic v., accessory
- cephalic v., median
- cerebellar v's
- cerebellar v's, inferior
- cerebellar v's, superior
- cerebral v's
- cerebral v's, anterior
- cerebral v's, deep
- cerebral v., great
- cerebral v's, inferior

vein *(continued)*
- cerebral v's, internal
- cerebral v., middle, deep
- cerebral v., middle, superficial
- cerebral v's, superficial
- cerebral v's, superior
- cervical v., deep
- cervical v's, transverse
- choroid v., inferior
- choroid v., superior
- ciliary v's
- ciliary v's, anterior
- ciliary v's, posterior
- circumflex femoral v's, lateral
- circumflex femoral v's, medial
- circumflex iliac v., deep
- circumflex iliac v., superficial
- v. of cochlear canaliculus
- colic v., left
- colic v., middle
- colic v., right
- communicating v's
- companion v.
- conjunctival v's
- coronary v., left
- v. of corpus callosum, dorsal
- v. of corpus callosum, posterior
- costoaxillary v's
- cubital v., median
- cutaneous v.
- cutaneous v., ulnar
- cystic v.
- deep v.
- digital v's, palmar
- digital v's, plantar
- digital v's of foot, common
- digital v's of foot, dorsal
- diploic v's
- diploic v., frontal
- diploic v., occipital
- diploic v., temporal, anterior

vein *(continued)*

diploic v., temporal,
posterior
dorsal v. of clitoris, deep
dorsal v's of clitoris,
superficial
dorsal v. of penis, deep
dorsal v's of penis,
superficial
dorsal v's of tongue
dorsispinal v's
emissary v.
emissary v., condylar
emissary v., mastoid
emissary v., occipital
emissary v., parietal
emulgent v.
epigastric v., inferior
epigastric v., superficial
epigastric v's, superior
epiploic v., left
epiploic v., right
episcleral v's
esophageal v's
ethmoidal v's
facial v.
facial v., anterior
facial v., common
facial v., deep
facial v., posterior
facial v., transverse
femoral v.
femoral v., deep
femoropopliteal v.
fibular v's
frontal v's
Galen's v's
gastric v., left
gastric v., right
gastric v's, short
gastroepiploic v., left
gastroepiploic v., right
gastro-omental v., left
gastro-omental v., right
genicular v's
gluteal v's, inferior
gluteal v's, superior
hemiazygos v.

vein *(continued)*

hemiazygos v., accessory
hemorrhoidal v's, inferior
hemorrhoidal v's, middle
hemorrhoidal v., superior
hepatic v's
hepatic v's, intermediate
hepatic v's, middle
hypogastric v.
hypophyseoportal v's
ileal v's
ileocolic v.
iliac v., common
iliac v., external
iliac v., internal
iliolumbar v.
infralobar v.
infrasegmental v.
innominate v's
insular v's
intercalated v.
intercapital v's
intercapitular v's of foot
intercapitular v's of hand
intercostal v's, anterior
intercostal v., highest
intercostal v's, posterior
intercostal v., superior, left
intercostal v., superior,
right
interlobar v's of kidney
interlobular v's of kidney
interlobular v's of liver
intermediate v.
interosseous v's of foot,
dorsal
interosseous metacarpal
v's, dorsal
intersegmental v.
intervertebral v.
intrasegmental v.
jejunal v's
jugular v., anterior
jugular v., anterior
horizontal
jugular v., external
jugular v., internal
v's of kidney

vein *(continued)*

Kohlrausch v's
Krukenberg's v's
Kuhnt's postcentral v.
Labbé's v.
labial v's, anterior
labial v's, inferior
labial v's, posterior
labial v., superior
v's of labyrinth
lacrimal v.
laryngeal v., inferior
laryngeal v., superior
Latarjet's v.
lateral direct v's
v. of lateral ventricle, lateral
v. of lateral ventricle, medial
levoatriocardinal v.
lingual v.
lingual v., deep
lingual v's, dorsal
v's of lower member, deep
v's of lower member, superficial
lumbar v's
lumbar v., ascending
mammary v's, external
mammary v., internal
v. of Marshall
Marshall's oblique v.
masseteric v's
maxillary v's
Mayo's v.
median v. of elbow
median v. of forearm
median v. of neck
mediastinal v's
v's of medulla oblongata
meningeal v's
meningeal v's, middle
mesencephalic v's
mesenteric v., inferior
mesenteric v., superior
metacarpal v's, dorsal
metacarpal v's, palmar
metatarsal v's, dorsal

vein *(continued)*

metatarsal v's, plantar
muscular v's
musculophrenic v's
nasal v's, external
nasofrontal v.
oblique v. of left atrium
obturator v's
occipital v.
v. of olfactory gyrus
omphalomesenteric v's
ophthalmic v., inferior
ophthalmic v., superior
ophthalmomeningeal v.
ovarian v., left
ovarian v., right
palatine v.
palatine v., external
palpebral v's
palpebral v's, inferior
palpebral v's, superior
pancreatic v's
pancreaticoduodenal v's
paraumbilical v's
paraureteric v's
parietal v's
parietal v. of Santorini
parotid v's
parotid v's, anterior
parotid v's, posterior
parumbilical v's
peduncular v's
perforating v's
pericardiac v's
pericardiacophrenic v's
pericardial v's
pericorneal v's
peroneal v's
petrosal v.
pharyngeal v's
phrenic v's, inferior
phrenic v's, superior
pontomesencephalic v., anterior
popliteal v.
portal v.
postcardinal v's
posterior v. of left ventricle

vein *(continued)*

precardinal v's
precentral v. of cerebellum
prefrontal v's
prepyloric v.
primary head v's
pudendal v's, external
pudendal v., internal
pulmonary v's
pulmonary v., left inferior
pulmonary v., right inferior
pulmonary v., left superior
pulmonary v., right superior
pulp v's
pyloric v.
radial v's
radial v., external, of Soemmering
ranine v.
rectal v's, inferior
rectal v's, middle
rectal v., superior
renal v's
retromandibular v.
retroperitoneal v.
Retzius's v's
revehent v.
Rosenthal's v.
Ruysch's v's
sacral v's, lateral
sacral v., middle
salvatella v.
saphenous v., accessory
saphenous v., great
saphenous v., small
v's of Sappey
scleral v's
scrotal v's, anterior
scrotal v's, posterior
v. of septum pellucidum, anterior
v. of septum pellucidum, posterior
sigmoid v's
small v. of heart
spermatic v.

vein *(continued)*

sphenopalatine v.
spinal v's, anterior and posterior
spiral v. of modiolus
splenic v.
stellate v's of kidney
Stensen's v's
sternocleidomastoid v.
striate v's
stylomastoid v.
subcardinal v's
subclavian v.
subcostal v.
sublingual v.
sublobular v's
submental v.
superficial v.
supracardinal v's
supraorbital v.
suprarenal v., left
suprarenal v., right
suprascapular v.
supratrochlear v's
sylvian v.
v. of sylvian fossa
systemic v.
temporal v's, deep
temporal v., middle
temporal v's, superficial
temporomandibular articular v's
terminal v.
testicular v., left
testicular v., right
thalamostriate v's, inferior
thalamostriate v., superior
thebesian v's
v's of Thebesius
thoracic v's, internal
thoracic v., lateral
thoracoacromial v.
thoracoepigastric v's
thymic v's
thyroid v., inferior
thyroid v's, middle
thyroid v., superior
tibial v's, anterior

vein *(continued)*
    tibial v's, posterior
    tonsillar v.
    trabecular v's
    tracheal v's
    transverse v. of face
    transverse v's of neck
    Trolard's v.
    tympanic v's
    ulnar v's
    umbilical v.
    umbilical v., left
    v. of uncus
    uterine v's
    varicose v.
    ventricular v's of heart
    ventricular v., inferior
    v. of vermis, inferior
    v. of vermis, superior
    vertebral v.
    vertebral v., accessory
    vertebral v., anterior
    vertebral v's, superficial
    vesalian v.
    vesical v's
    vestibular v's
    vidian v's
    v's of Vieussens
    vitelline v's
    vorticose v's
Vein·a·mine
vein·let
Ve·jo·vis
    V. carolinianus
    V. flavus
    V. spinigerus
ve·la
Vel·a·cy·cline
ve·la·men *pl.* ve·la·mi·na
    v. vulvae
vel·a·men·ta
vel·a·men·tous
vel·a·men·tum *pl.* vel·a·men·ta
    velamenta cerebri
ve·lar
Vel·ban
vel·i·form

Vel·la's fistula
vel·lo·sine
vel·lus
    v. olivae
ve·lo·cim·e·try
    laser-Doppler v.
ve·loc·i·ty
    conduction v.
    limiting v.
    propagation v.
    sedimentation v.
    sensory conduction v.
ve·lo·no·ski·as·co·py
ve·lo·pha·ryn·ge·al
ve·lo·plas·ty
Vel·o·sef
Ve·lo·su·lin
ve·lour
Vel·peau's bandage
Vel·peau's deformity
Vel·peau's hernia
ve·lum *pl.* ve·la
    artificial v.
    Baker's v.
    v. interpositum cerebri
    v. interpositum
      rhombencephali
    v. medullare anterius
    v. medullare caudale
    v. medullare inferius
    v. medullare posterius
    v. medullare rostralis
    v. medullare superius
    medullary v., anterior
    medullary v., cranial
    medullary v., inferior
    medullary v., posterior
    medullary v., rostral
    medullary v., superior
    nursing v.
    v. palati
    v. palatinum
    v. semilunare
    v. of Tarinus
    v. transversum
    v. triangulare
ve·na *pl.* ve·nae
    venae advehentes

ve·na *(continued)*

- v. anastomotica inferior
- v. anastomotica superior
- v. angularis
- venae anonymae [dextra et sinistra]
- venae anteriores cerebri
- v. anterior septi pellucidi
- v. appendicularis
- v. aqueductus cochleae
- v. aqueductus vestibuli
- venae arciformes renis
- venae arcuatae renis
- venae articulares
- venae articulares temporomandibulae
- venae atriales cordis
- v. atrii lateralis
- v. atrii medialis
- venae atrioventriculares cordis
- venae auditivae internae
- venae auriculares anteriores
- v. auricularis posterior
- v. axillaris
- v. azygos
- v. basalis
- v. basalis [Rosenthali]
- v. basilica
- venae basivertebrales
- venae brachiales
- venae brachiocephalicae (dextra/sinistra)
- venae bronchiales
- venae bronchiales anteriores
- venae bronchiales posteriores
- v. canaliculi cochleae
- v. canalis pterygoidei
- v. canalis pterygoidei [Vidii]
- venae cardiacae anteriores
- v. cardiaca magna
- v. cardiaca media
- venae cardiacae minimae
- v. cardiaca parva

ve·na *(continued)*

- venae cavae
- v. cava inferior
- v. cava superior
- v. cava superior, persistent left
- venae cavernosae penis
- v. centralis glandulae suprarenalis
- venae centrales hepatis
- v. centralis retinae
- v. cephalica
- v. cephalica accessoria
- venae cerebelli
- venae cerebri
- venae cerebri anteriores
- venae cerebri inferiores
- venae cerebri internae
- v. cerebri magna
- v. cerebri media profunda
- venae cerebri mediae superficiales
- venae cerebri profundae
- venae cerebri superficiales
- venae cerebri superiores
- v. cervicalis profunda
- v. choroidea inferior
- venae choroideae oculi
- v. choroidea superior
- venae ciliares
- venae circumflexae femoris laterales
- venae circumflexae femoris mediales
- v. circumflexa iliaca profunda
- v. circumflexa ilium profunda
- v. circumflexa ilium superficialis
- venae circumflexae laterales femoris
- venae circumflexae mediales femoris
- v. circumflexa superficialis ilium
- v. colica dextra
- v. colica intermedia

ve·na *(continued)*
- v. colica media
- v. colica sinistra
- venae columnae vertebralis
- v. comitans
- venae conjunctivales
- venae cordis
- venae cordis anteriores
- v. cordis magna
- v. cordis media
- venae cordis minimae
- v. cordis parva
- venae costoaxillares
- v. cutanea
- v. cystica
- venae digitales communes pedis
- venae digitales dorsales pedis
- venae digitales palmares
- venae digitales pedis dorsales
- venae digitales plantares
- venae digitales volares communes
- venae digitales volares propriae
- venae diploicae
- v. diploica frontalis
- v. diploica occipitalis
- v. diploica temporalis anterior
- v. diploica temporalis posterior
- venae directae laterales
- v. dorsalis clitoridis profunda
- venae dorsales clitoridis superficiales
- v. dorsalis corporis callosi
- venae dorsales linguae
- v. dorsalis penis profunda
- venae dorsales penis superficiales
- v. dorsalis profunda clitoridis
- v. dorsalis profunda penis

ve·na *(continued)*
- venae dorsales superficiales clitoridis
- venae dorsales superficiales penis
- v. emissaria
- v. emissaria condylaris
- v. emissaria condyloidea
- v. emissaria mastoidea
- v. emissaria occipitalis
- v. emissaria parietalis
- v. epigastrica inferior
- v. epigastrica superficialis
- venae epigastricae superiores
- v. epiploica dextra
- v. epiploica sinistra
- venae episclerales
- venae esophageae
- venae esophageales
- venae ethmoidales
- v. ethmoidalis anterior
- v. ethmoidalis posterior
- v. facialis
- v. facialis anterior
- v. facialis communis
- v. facialis posterior
- v. faciei profunda
- v. femoralis
- v. femoropoplitea
- venae fibulares
- venae frontales
- venae gastricae breves
- v. gastrica dextra
- v. gastrica sinistra
- v. gastroepiploica dextra
- v. gastroepiploica sinistra
- v. gastro-omentalis dextra
- v. gastro-omentalis sinistra
- venae geniculares
- venae genus
- venae gluteae inferiores
- venae gluteae superiores
- v. gyri olfactorii
- venae haemorrhoidales inferiores
- v. haemorrhoidalis media

ve·na *(continued)*
v. haemorrhoidalis
superior
v. hemiazygos
v. hemiazygos accessoria
venae hepaticae
venae hepaticae dextrae
venae hepaticae
intermediae
venae hepaticae mediae
venae hepaticae sinistrae
v. hypogastrica
venae ileales
v. ileocolica
v. iliaca communis
v. iliaca externa
v. iliaca interna
v. iliolumbalis
inferior v. cava
v. inferior vermis
venae insulares
venae intercapitales
venae intercapitales manus
venae intercapitulares
manus
venae intercapitulares
pedis
venae intercostales
venae intercostales
anteriores
venae intercostales
posteriores
v. intercostalis superior
dextra
v. intercostalis superior
sinistra
v. intercostalis suprema
venae interlobares renis
venae interlobulares
hepatis
venae interlobulares renis
v. intermedia antebrachii
v. intermedia basilica
v. intermedia cephalica
v. intermedia cubiti
venae internae cerebri
vena intervertebralis
venae jejunales

ve·na *(continued)*
v. jugularis anterior
v. jugularis externa
v. jugularis interna
venae labiales anteriores
venae labiales inferiores
venae labiales posteriores
v. labialis superior
venae labyrinthi
v. lacrimalis
v. laryngea inferior
v. laryngea superior
v. lateralis atrii
v. lienalis
v. lingualis
venae lumbales
v. lumbalis ascendens
v. magna cerebri
v. mammaria interna
venae massetericae
venae maxillares
v. medialis atrii
v. mediana antebrachii
v. mediana basilica
v. mediana cephalica
v. mediana colli
v. mediana cubiti
v. media profunda cerebri
venae mediastinales
venae mediastinales
anteriores
venae medullae oblongatae
venae meningeae
venae meningeae mediae
venae mesencephalicae
v. mesenterica inferior
v. mesenterica superior
venae metacarpales
dorsales
venae metacarpales
palmares
venae metacarpeae
dorsales
venae metacarpeae
palmares
venae metatarsales
dorsales

ve·na *(continued)*
venae metatarsales
  plantares
venae metatarseae dorsales
venae metatarseae
  plantares
venae musculares
venae musculophrenicae
venae nasales externae
v. nasofrontalis
venae nuclei caudati
v. obliqua atrii sinistri
v. obliqua atrii sinistri
  [Marshalli]
venae obturatoriae
venae occipitales
v. occipitalis
venae oesophageales
v. ophthalmica inferior
v. ophthalmica superior
v. ophthalmomeningea
v. ovarica
v. ovarica dextra
v. ovarica sinistra
v. palatina
v. palatina externa
venae palpebrales
venae palpebrales
  inferiores
venae palpebrales
  superiores
venae pancreaticae
venae pancreatico-
  duodenales
venae paraumbilicales
venae parietales
venae parotideae
venae parotideae
  anteriores
venae parotideae
  posteriores
venae parumbilicales
  [Sappeyi]
venae pectorales
venae pedunculares
venae perforantes
venae pericardiacae

ve·na *(continued)*
venae pericardiaco-
  phrenicae
venae pericardiales
venae peroneae
v. petrosa
venae pharyngeae
venae pharyngeales
venae phrenicae inferiores
venae phrenicae superiores
v. pontomesencephalica
  anterior
v. poplitea
v. portae hepatis
v. portalis hepatis
v. posterior corporis callosi
v. posterior septi pellucidi
v. posterior ventriculi
  sinistri cordis
v. precentralis cerebelli
venae prefrontales
v. prepylorica
vena profunda
venae profundae cerebri
venae profundae clitoridis
v. profunda facialis
v. profunda faciei
v. profunda femoris
v. profunda linguae
venae profundae penis
venae pudendae externae
v. pudenda interna
venae pulmonales
venae pulmonales dextrae
v. pulmonalis dextra
  inferior
v. pulmonalis dextra
  superior
v. pulmonalis inferior
  dextra
v. pulmonalis inferior
  sinistra
venae pulmonales sinistrae
v. pulmonalis sinistra
  inferior
v. pulmonalis sinistra
  superior

ve·na *(continued)*

- v. pulmonalis superior dextra
- v. pulmonalis superior sinistra
- venae radiales
- v. recessus lateralis ventriculi quarti
- venae rectales inferiores
- venae rectales mediae
- v. rectalis superior
- venae renales
- venae renis
- v. retromandibularis
- venae revehentes
- venae sacrales laterales
- v. sacralis media
- v. sacralis mediana
- v. saphena accessoria
- v. saphena magna
- v. saphena parva
- v. scapularis dorsalis
- venae sclerales
- venae scrotales anteriores
- venae scrotales posteriores
- v. septi pellucidi anterior
- v. septi pellucidi posterior
- venae sigmoideae
- v. spermatica
- venae spinales anteriores/posteriores
- venae spinales externae anteriores
- venae spinales externae posteriores
- venae spinales internae
- v. spiralis modioli
- v. splenica
- venae stellatae renis
- v. sternocleidomastoidea
- venae striatae
- v. stylomastoidea
- v. subclavia
- v. subcostalis
- venae subcutaneae abdominis
- v. sublingualis
- v. submentalis

ve·na *(continued)*

- v. superficialis
- superior v. cava
- v. supraorbitalis
- venae suprarenales
- v. suprarenalis dextra
- v. suprarenalis sinistra
- v. suprascapularis
- venae supratrochleares
- v. temporalis media
- venae temporales profundae
- venae temporales superficiales
- v. terminalis
- v. testicularis
- v. testicularis dextra
- v. testicularis sinistra
- venae thalamostriatae inferiores
- v. thalamostriata superior
- v. thoracalis lateralis
- venae thoracicae internae
- v. thoracica lateralis
- v. thoracoacromialis
- venae thoracoepigastricae
- venae thymicae
- v. thyreoidea ima
- venae thyreoideae inferiores
- venae thyreoideae superiores
- v. thyroidea inferior
- venae thyroideae mediae
- v. thyroidea superior
- venae tibiales anteriores
- venae tibiales posteriores
- venae tracheales
- venae transversae cervicis
- venae transversae colli
- v. transversa facialis
- v. transversa faciei
- v. transversa scapulae
- venae trunci encephalici
- venae tympanicae
- venae ulnares
- v. umbilicalis
- v. umbilicalis sinistra

ve·na *(continued)*
    v. unci
    venae uterinae
    venae vasorum
    venae ventriculares cordis
    v. ventricularis inferior
    v. ventriculi lateralis
      lateralis
    v. ventriculi lateralis
      medialis
    v. vermis inferior
    v. vermis superior
    v. vertebralis
    v. vertebralis accessoria
    v. vertebralis anterior
    venae vesicales
    venae vestibulares
    venae vorticosae
ve·na·ca·vo·gram
ve·na·ca·vog·ra·phy
ve·nae
Ve·na med·i·nen·sis
ve·na·tion
ve·nec·ta·sia
ve·nec·to·my
ve·neer
    full v.
ven·e·na·tion
ve·nene
ven·e·nif·er·ous
ven·e·nif·ic
ven·e·no·sal·i·vary
ven·e·nos·i·ty
ven·e·nous
vene·punc·ture
ve·ne·re·al
ve·ne·re·ol·o·gist
ve·ne·re·ol·o·gy
vene·sec·tion
vene·su·ture
veni·punc·ture
veni·sec·tion
veni·su·ture
ve·no·at·ri·al
ve·no·au·ric·u·lar
ve·noc·ly·sis
ve·no·fi·bro·sis
ve·no·gram

ve·nog·ra·phy
    ascending v.
    descending v.
    extradural v.
    impedance v.
    intraosseous v.
    portal v.
    radionuclide v.
    splenic v.
    uterine v.
    vertebral v.
ven·om
    bee v.
    cobra v.
    kokoi v.
    moccasin v.
    rattlesnake v.
    Russell's viper v.
    snake v.
    spider v.
    toad v.
    viper v.
ven·om·iza·tion
ven·o·mo·sal·i·vary
ve·no·mo·tor
ven·o·mous
ve·no-oc·clu·sive
ve·no·peri·to·ne·os·to·my
ve·no·pres·sor
ve·no·scle·ro·sis
ve·nose
ve·no·si·nal
ve·nos·i·ty
ve·no·sta·sis
ve·not·o·my
ve·nous
ve·no·ve·nos·to·my
vent
    pulmonic alveolar v's
Ven·taire
ven·ter *pl.* ven·tres
    v. anterior musculi
      digastrici
    v. frontalis musculi
      occipitofrontalis
    v. ilii
    v. imus

ven·ter *(continued)*
    v. inferior musculi
      omohyoidei
    v. medius
    v. musculi
    v. occipitalis musculi
      occipitofrontalis
    v. posterior musculi
      digastrici
    v. propendens
    v. scapulae
    v. superior musculi
      omohyoidei
    v. supremus
ven·ti·late
ven·ti·la·tion
    alveolar v.
    artificial v.
    assist/control mode v.
    assisted v.
    control-mode v.
    dead space v.
    downward v.
    exhausting v.
    expired air v.
    intermittent demand v.
    intermittent mandatory v.
      (IMV)
    intermittent positive
      pressure v.
    maximum voluntary v.
      (MVV)
    mechanical v.
    middle ear v.
    minute v.
    natural v.
    negative pressure v.
    plenum v.
    synchronized intermittent
      mandatory v. (SIMV)
    total v.
    upward v.
    vacuum v.
    walking v.
ven·ti·la·tor
    mechanical v.
    pressure-cycled v.
    tank v.

ven·ti·la·tor *(continued)*
    time-cycled v.
    volume-cycled v.
ven·ti·lom·e·ter
ven·ti·lom·e·try
vent·plant
ven·trad
ven·tral
ven·tra·lis
ven·tral·ward
ven·tri·cle
    aortic v. of heart
    v. of Arantius
    auxiliary v.
    v's of the brain
    cerebral v.
    v. of cord
    double-inlet v.
    double-outlet right v.
    Duncan's v.
    fifth v.
    first v. of cerebrum
    fourth v. of cerebrum
    Galen's v.
    v. of heart
    v. of larynx
    lateral v. of cerebrum
    left v. of heart
    Morgagni's v.
    optic v.
    pineal v.
    primitive v.
    right v. of heart
    second v. of cerebrum
    single v.
    sixth v.
    v. of Sylvius
    terminal v. of spinal cord
    third v. of cerebrum
    Verga's v.
    Vieussen's v.
ven·tri·cor·nu
ven·tri·cor·nu·al
ven·tri·cose
ven·tric·u·lar
ven·tric·u·li
ven·tric·u·li·tis
ven·tric·u·lo·atri·os·to·my

ven·tric·u·lo·cis·ter·nos·to·
　my
　　third v.
ven·tric·u·lo·gram
ven·tric·u·log·ra·phy
　　isotope v.
ven·tric·u·lom·e·try
ven·tric·u·lo·my·ot·o·my
ven·tric·u·lo·nec·tor
ven·tric·u·lo·pha·sic
ven·tric·u·lo·plas·ty
ven·tric·u·lo·punc·ture
ven·tric·u·lo·scope
ven·tric·u·los·co·py
ven·tric·u·los·ti·um
ven·tric·u·los·to·my
　　third v.
ven·tric·u·lo·sub·arach·noid
ven·tric·u·lot·o·my
ven·tric·u·lo·ve·nos·to·my
ven·tric·u·lus *pl.* ven·tric·u·li
　　v. cordis
　　v. dexter cerebri
　　v. dexter cordis
　　v. laryngis
　　v. laryngis [Morgagnii]
　　v. lateralis cerebri
　　v. medius
　　v. quartus cerebri
　　v. quintus
　　v. sinister cerebri
　　v. sinister cordis
　　v. terminalis medullae
　　　spinalis
　　v. tertius cerebri
ven·tri·cum·bent
ven·tri·duct
ven·tri·duc·tion
ven·tri·flex·ion
ven·tri·me·sal
ven·trim·e·son
ven·tro·cys·tor·rha·phy
ven·tro·dor·sad
ven·tro·dor·sal
ven·tro·fix·a·tion
ven·tro·hys·tero·pexy
ven·tro·in·gui·nal
ven·tro·lat·er·al

ven·tro·me·di·an
ven·tro·pos·te·ri·or
ven·trop·to·sia
ven·trop·to·sis
ven·tros·co·py
ven·trose
ven·tro·sus·pen·sion
ven·trot·o·my
Ven·tu·ri effect
Ven·tu·ri principle
Ven·tu·ri tube
ven·tu·rim·e·ter
ven·u·la *pl.* ven·u·lae
　　v. macularis inferior
　　v. macularis superior
　　v. medialis retinae
　　v. nasalis retinae inferior
　　v. nasalis retinae superior
　　v. postcapillaris
　　venulae rectae renis
　　v. retinae medialis
　　venulae stellatae renis
　　v. temporalis retinae
　　　inferior
　　v. temporalis retinae
　　　superior
ven·u·lae
ven·u·lar
ven·ule
　　high endothelial v's
　　inferior macular v.
　　inferior nasal v. of retina
　　inferior temporal v. of
　　　retina
　　medial v. of retina
　　postcapillary v's
　　stellate v's of kidney
　　straight v's of kidney
　　superior macular v.
　　superior nasal v. of retina
　　superior temporal v. of
　　　retina
ven·u·li·tis
　　cutaneous necrotizing v.
VEP — visual evoked
　potential
Ve·Pe·sid
Ver·a·cil·lin

Ve·ra·guth's fold
Ver·al·ba
ver·ap·a·mil
Ve·ra·trum
ver·bal
ver·be·none
Ver·biest syndrome
ver·big·er·a·tion
ver·bo·ma·nia
Ver·cyte
ver·do·he·min
ver·do·he·mo·chro·mo·gen
ver·do·he·mo·glo·bin
ver·do·per·ox·i·dase
Ver·ga's lacrimal groove
Ver·ga's ventricle
verge
    anal v.
ver·gence
ver·gen·cy
Ver·hey·en's stars
Ver·hoeff's operation
Ver·hoeff's stain
Ver·i·loid
ver·mes
ver·me·toid
ver·mi·an
Ver·mi·cel·la
ver·mi·ci·dal
ver·mi·cide
ver·mic·u·lar
ver·mic·u·la·tion
ver·mi·cule
    traveling v.
ver·mic·u·lose
ver·mic·u·lous
ver·mi·form
ver·mif·u·gal
ver·mi·fuge
ver·mil·ion·ec·to·my
ver·min
ver·mi·nal
ver·mi·na·tion
ver·mi·no·sis
ver·mi·not·ic
ver·mi·nous
ver·mis
    v. cerebelli

ver·mis *(continued)*
    inferior v.
    superior v.
ver·mix
ver·mog·ra·phy
Ver·mox
ver·nal
Ver·ner-Mor·ri·son syndrome
Ver·net's syndrome
Ver·neuil's canals
Ver·neuil's disease
Ver·neuil's neuroma
ver·ni·er
ver·nix
    v. caseosa
Ver·o·cay bodies
Ve·ron·i·cel·la
    V. leydigi
ver·ru·ca *pl.* ver·ru·cae
    v. acuminata
    v. digitata
    v. filiformis
    v. mollusciformis
    v. necrogenica
    v. peruana
    v. peruviana
    v. plana
    v. plana juvenilis
    v. plantaris
    v. seborrheica
    v. vulgaris
ver·ru·cae
ver·ru·ci·form
ver·ru·cose
ver·ru·co·sis
    lymphostatic v.
ver·ru·cos·i·ty
ver·ru·cous
ver·ru·ga
    v. peruana
Ver·sa·pen
Ver·sene
ver·si·co·lor
    tinea v.
ver·sion
    abdominal v.
    bimanual v.
    bipolar v.

ver·sion *(continued)*
   Braxton Hicks v.
   cephalic v.
   combined v.
   Denman's spontaneous v.
   external v.
   Hicks v.
   internal v.
   pelvic v.
   podalic v.
   Potter v.
   spontaneous v.
   Wigand's v.
ver·te·bra *pl.* ver·te·brae
   abdominal vertebrae
   basilar v.
   butterfly v.
   caudal vertebrae
   caudate vertebrae
   cervical vertebrae
   vertebrae cervicales
   cleft v.
   vertebrae coccygeae
   coccygeal vertebrae
   vertebrae colli
   cranial v.
   v. dentata
   dorsal vertebrae
   false vertebrae
   vertebrae lumbales
   lumbar vertebrae
   v. magnum
   movable v.
   odontoid v.
   v. plana
   primitive v.
   v. prominens
   prominent v.
   sacral vertebrae
   vertebrae sacrales
   sternal v.
   terminal v., great
   vertebrae thoracales
   thoracic vertebrae
   vertebrae thoracicae
   tricuspid v.
   true vertebrae
ver·te·brae

ver·te·bral
ver·te·brar·i·um
ver·te·brar·te·ri·al
Ver·te·bra·ta
ver·te·brate
ver·te·brate col·la·gen·ase
ver·te·brat·ed
ver·te·brec·to·my
ver·te·bro·ar·te·ri·al
ver·te·bro·bas·i·lar
ver·te·bro·chon·dral
ver·te·bro·cos·tal
ver·te·bro·did·y·mus
ver·te·brod·y·mus
ver·te·bro·fem·or·al
ver·te·bro·gen·ic
ver·te·bro·il·i·ac
ver·te·bro·mam·ma·ry
ver·te·bro·sa·cral
ver·te·bro·ster·nal
ver·tex *pl.* ver·ti·ces
   v. of bony cranium
   v. cordis
   v. of cornea
   v. corneae
   v. cranii
   v. cranii ossei
ver·ti·cal
ver·ti·ca·lis
ver·tic·il·late
Ver·ti·cil·li·um
   V. graphii
ver·ti·co·men·tal
ver·tig·i·nous
ver·ti·go
   alternobaric v.
   angiopathic v.
   apoplectic v.
   arteriosclerotic v.
   auditory v.
   aural v.
   benign paroxysmal
     positional (or postural) v.
   cardiac v.
   cardiovascular v.
   central v.
   cerebral v.
   disabling positional v.

ver·ti·go *(continued)*
    disorientation v.
    encephalic v.
    endemic paralytic v.
    epidemic v.
    epileptic v.
    essential v.
    galvanic v.
    gastric v.
    height v.
    horizontal v.
    hysterical v.
    labyrinthine v.
    laryngeal v.
    lateral v.
    lithemic v.
    mechanical v.
    nocturnal v.
    objective v.
    ocular v.
    organic v.
    paralytic v.
    paralyzing v.
    peripheral v.
    pilot's v.
    positional v.
    post-traumatic v.
    postural v.
    pressure v.
    primary v.
    residual v.
    riders'v.
    rotary v.
    rotatory v.
    sham-movement v.
    special sense v.
    stomachal v.
    v. ab stomacho laeso
    subjective v.
    systematic v.
    tenebric v.
    toxemic v.
    toxic v.
    vertical v.
    vestibular v.
    voltaic v.
ver·tig·ra·phy
ve·ru·mon·ta·ni·tis

ve·ru·mon·ta·num
ve·sa·li·an
ve·sa·li·a·num
Ve·sa·li·us
Ve·sa·li·us' foramen
Ve·sa·li·us' ligament
Vesic. — L. vesicatorium (a
    blister)
    L. vesicula (a blister)
ve·si·ca *pl.* ve·si·cae
    v. biliaris
    v. fellea
    v. prostatica
    v. urinaria
ve·si·cae
ves·i·cal
ves·i·cant
ves·i·cate
ves·i·ca·tion
ves·i·ca·to·ry
ves·i·cle
    acoustic v.
    acrosomal v.
    air v.
    allantoic v.
    amniocardiac v's
    anhidrotic v.
    archoplasmic v.
    auditory v.
    Baer's v.
    blastodermic v.
    brain v's
    brain v's, primary
    brain v's, secondary
    cephalic v's
    cerebral v's
    cervical v.
    chorionic v.
    coated v.
    compound v.
    concentrating v's
    encephalic v's
    endocytic v's
    germinal v.
    graafian v's
    intermediate v's
    lens v.
    lung v's

ves·i·cle *(continued)*
    Malpighi's v's
    matrix v's
    medullary coccygeal v.
    micropinocytotic v.
    midbrain v.
    multilocular v.
    Naboth's v's
    ocular v.
    olfactory v.
    ophthalmic v.
    optic v.
    otic v.
    phagocytotic v.
    pinocytotic v.
    pituitary v.
    plasmalemmal v.
    primitive brain v.
    prostatic v.
    pulmonary v's
    Purkinje's v.
    secretory v's
    seminal v.
    sense v.
    spermatic v., false
    synaptic v's
    telencephalic v's
    transfer v's
    transitional v's
    transport v's
    umbilical v.
    Unna's v.
    water expulsion v.
ves·i·co·ab·dom·i·nal
ves·i·co·bul·lous
ves·i·co·cav·er·nous
ves·i·co·cele
ves·i·co·cer·vi·cal
ves·i·coc·ly·sis
ves·i·co·col·ic
ves·i·co·co·lon·ic
ves·i·co·en·ter·ic
ves·i·co·fix·a·tion
ves·i·co·in·tes·ti·nal
ves·i·co·per·i·ne·al
ves·i·co·pros·tat·ic
ves·i·co·pu·bic
ves·i·co·pus·tule

ves·i·co·rec·tal
ves·i·co·rec·tos·to·my
ves·i·co·re·nal
ves·i·co·sig·moid
ves·i·co·sig·moid·os·to·my
ves·i·co·spi·nal
ves·i·cos·to·my
    cutaneous v.
ves·i·cot·o·my
ves·i·co·um·bil·i·cal
ves·i·co·ura·chal
ves·i·co·ure·ter·al
ves·i·co·ure·ter·ic
ves·i·co·ure·thral
ves·i·co·uter·ine
ves·i·co·uter·o·vag·i·nal
ves·i·co·vag·i·nal
ves·i·co·vag·i·no·rec·tal
ve·sic·u·la *pl.* ve·sic·u·lae
    v. bilis
    v. fellea
    v. germinativa
    vesiculae graafianae
    vesiculae nabothi
    v. ophthalmica
    v. prostatica
    v. seminalis
    v. serosa
ve·sic·u·lae
ve·sic·u·lar
ve·sic·u·late
ve·sic·u·lat·ed
ve·sic·u·la·tion
ve·sic·u·lec·to·my
ve·sic·u·li·form
ve·sic·u·li·tis
    seminal v.
ve·sic·u·lo·bron·chi·al
ve·sic·u·lo·cav·er·nous
ve·sic·u·lo·gram
ve·sic·u·log·ra·phy
ve·sic·u·lo·pap·u·lar
ve·sic·u·lo·pros·ta·ti·tis
ve·sic·u·lo·pus·tu·lar
ve·sic·u·lot·o·my
    seminal v.
ve·sic·u·lo·tu·bu·lar
ve·sic·u·lo·tym·pan·ic

Ves·lin·gi·us line
ves·per·al
Ves·prin
ves·sel
    absorbent v's
    afferent v. of glomerulus
    afferent v's of lymph node
    anastomotic v.
    arterioluminal v's
    arteriosinusoidal v's
    bile v.
    blood v.
    chyliferous v's
    collateral v.
    efferent v. of glomerulus
    efferent v's of lymph node
    ghost v.
    great v's
    hemorrhoidal v's
    Jungbluth's v's
    lacteal v's
    lymphatic v.
    lymphatic v., deep
    lymphatic v., superficial
    lymphocapillary v.
    nutrient v's
    sinusoidal v.
    Warburg v.
ves·tib·u·la
ves·tib·u·lar
ves·ti·bule
    v. of aorta
    buccal v.
    v. of ear
    Gibson's v.
    labial v.
    v. of larynx
    v. of mouth
    nasal v.
    v. of nose
    v. of omental bursa
    v. of oral cavity
    v. of pharynx
    Sibson's v.
    v. of vagina
    v. of vulva
ves·tib·u·lec·to·my
Ves·ti·bu·li·fer·ia

ves·tib·u·lo·cer·e·bel·lar
ves·tib·u·lo·cer·e·bel·lum
ves·tib·u·lo·coch·le·ar
ves·tib·u·lo·gen·ic
ves·tib·u·lo-oc·u·lar
ves·tib·u·lo·plas·ty
ves·tib·u·lo·spi·nal
ves·tib·u·lot·o·my
ves·tib·u·lo·ure·thral
ves·tib·u·lum *pl.* ves·tib·u·la
    v. auris
    v. bursae omentalis
    v. glottidis
    v. laryngis
    v. nasi
    v. oris
    v. vaginae
ves·tige
    caudal medullary v.
    coccygeal v.
    v. of vaginal process
    wolffian v's
ves·tig·ia
ves·tig·i·al
ves·tig·i·um *pl.* ves·tig·ia
    v. processus vaginalis
ve·su·vin
vet·er·i·nar·i·an
vet·er·i·nary
VF — ventricular fibrillation
    visual field
    vocal fremitus
vf — field of vision
    visual field
vi·a·bil·i·ty
vi·a·ble
Vi·a·dril
vi·al
vi·be·sate
vi·bex *pl.* vi·bi·ces
vi·bi·ces
Vi·bra·my·cin
vi·bra·tile
vi·bra·tion
    bone conduction v.
    chest wall v.
vi·bra·tive
vi·bra·tode

vi·bra·tor
vi·bra·to·ry
Vib·rio
    V. alginolyticus
    V. anguillarum
    V. cholerae
    V. cholerae biotype
      albensis
    V. cholerae biotype
      cholerae
    V. cholerae biotype *eltor*
    V. cholerae biotype *proteus*
    V. coli
    V. comma
    V. damsela
    V. danubicus
    V. eltor
    V. fetus
    V. fluvialis
    V. ghinda
    V. harveyi
    V. hollisae
    V. jejuni
    V. leonardii
    V. massauah
    V. metschnikovii
    V. mimicus
    V. parahaemolyticus
    V. phosphorescens
    V. piscium
    V. proteus
    V. septicus
    V. succinogenes
    V. vulnificus
vib·rio *pl.* vib·rios or vib·ri·o·
nes
    Celebes v.
    cholera v.
    El Tor v.
    v. group EF-6
    v. group F
    NAG v's
    nonagglutinating v's
    noncholera v's
    paracholera v's
vib·rio·ci·dal
vib·ri·ol·y·sis
Vib·rio·na·ceae

vib·ri·o·nes
vib·ri·o·sis
    bovine genital v.
    ovine genital v.
vi·bris·sa *pl.* vi·bris·sae
vi·bris·sae
vi·bro·acous·tic
vi·bro·car·dio·gram
vi·bro·car·di·og·ra·phy
vi·bro·lode
vi·bro·mas·sage
vi·bro·pho·no·car·dio·graph
vi·bro·ther·a·peu·tics
Vi·bur·num
    V. opulus
    V. prunifolium
vi·car·i·ous
Vic·ia
    V. faba (fava)
vi·cin·al
vi·cine
Vicq d'Azyr's band
Vicq d'Azyr's body
Vicq d'Azyr's fasciculus
Vicq d'Azyr's foramen
Vicq d'Azyr's stripe
Vi·cryl
Vi·dal's disease
vi·dar·a·bine
vid·e·og·no·sis
vid·eo·mi·cros·co·py
vid·i·an artery
vid·i·an canal
vid·i·an nerve
Vieth-Mül·ler horopter
Vie·us·sens' ansa
Vie·us·sens' foramen
Vie·us·sens' limbus
Vie·us·sens' valve
Vie·us·sens' vein
Vie·us·sens' ventricle
    apical lordotic v.
    Arcelin's v's
    coned-down v.
    Law's v's
    parasternal long axis v.
    tunnel v.
    Waters v.

VIG — vaccinia immune
  globulin
vig·il·am·bu·lism
vig·i·lance
vi·gin·ti·nor·mal
Vig·nal's cells
vig·or
    hybrid v.
Vil·lar·et's syndrome
vil·li
vil·lif·er·ous
vil·li·ki·nin
vil·li·tis
vil·lo·ma
vil·lo·nod·u·lar
vil·lose
vil·lo·si·tis
vil·los·i·ty
vil·lous
vil·lus *pl.* vil·li
    amniotic v.
    anchoring v.
    arachnoid villi
    chorionic v.
    v. of choroid plexus
    floating v.
    free v.
    intestinal villi
    villi intestinales
    labial v.
    lingual villi
    pericardial v.
    pleural villi
    villi pleurales
    primary v.
    secondary v.
    villi of small intestine
    synovial villi
    villi synoviales
    tertiary v.
    zonary v.
vil·lus·ec·to·my
vi·lox·a·zine hy·dro·chlo·ride
vi·men·tin
vin·bar·bi·tal
    sodium v.
vin·blas·tine sul·fate
Vin·ca

vin·ca·leu·ko·blas·tine
vin·ca·mine
Vin·cent's angina
Vin·cent's gingivitis
Vin·cent's infection
Vin·cent's spirillum
vin·co·fos
vin·cris·tine sul·fate
vin·cu·lum *pl.* vin·cu·la
    v. breve
    v. linguae
    vincula lingulae cerebelli
    v. longum
    vincula tendinum
      digitorum manus
    vincula tendinum
      digitorum pedis
    vincula of tendons of
      fingers
    vincula of tendons of toes
vin·de·sine
Vine·berg operation
vin·e·gar
vin·e·ga·roon
Vin·son's syndrome
vi·nyl
    v. acetate
    v. chloride
    v. ether
vio·cid
Vi·o·cin
Vi·o·form
Vi·o·kase
vi·o·la·ce·in
vi·o·la·ceous
vi·o·les·cent
vi·o·let
    amethyst v.
    ammonium oxalate crystal
      v.
    aniline gentian v.
    v. 7 B or C
    bismuth v.
    bismuth crystal v.
    cresyl v.
    cresyl v. acetate
    cresylecht v.
    crystal v.

vi·o·let *(continued)*
    v. G
    gentian v.
    hexamethyl v.
    Hofmann's v.
    iodine v.
    iris v.
    Lauth's v.
    methyl v.
    methylene v.
    neutral v.
    Paris v.
    pentamethyl v.
    visual v.
vi·o·my·cin sul·fate
vi·os·ter·ol
VIP — vasoactive intestinal
  polypeptide
vi·per
    European v.
    Gaboon v.
    nose-horned v.
    palm v.
    pit v.
    rhinoceros v.
    Russell's v.
    sand v.
    true v.
Vi·pera
vi·per·id
Vi·per·i·dae
Vi·per·i·nae
vi·per·ine
vi·po·ma
vi·pry·ni·um em·bo·nate
vi·ra·gin·i·ty
vi·ral
Vir·chow, Rudolf Ludwig Karl
Vir·chow's angle
Vir·chow's cell
Vir·chow's corpuscle
Vir·chow's crystal
Vir·chow's degeneration
Vir·chow's granulation
Vir·chow's line
Vir·chow's node
Vir·chow-Has·sall body
Vir·chow-Rob·in spaces

vi·re·mia
vir·gin
vir·gin·al
vir·gin·ia·my·cin
vir·gin·i·ty
vir·i·ci·dal
vir·i·cide
vi·rid·in
vir·i·do·bu·fa·gin
vir·ile
vir·i·les·cence
vi·ril·ia
vir·i·lism
    adrenal v.
vir·il·i·ty
vir·il·iza·tion
vir·i·lize
vir·i·liz·ing
vi·ri·on
vi·rip·o·tent
vi·ro·cyte
vi·ro·gene
vi·ro·ge·net·ic
vi·roid
vi·ro·lac·tia
vi·rol·o·gist
vi·rol·o·gy
vi·ro·mi·cro·some
vi·ro·pex·is
vi·ro·plasm
vi·rose
vi·ro·sis *pl.* vi·ro·ses
vi·ro·stat·ic
vi·ru·ci·dal
vi·ru·cide
vir·u·lence
vir·u·lent
vir·u·lic·i·dal
vir·u·lif·er·ous
vir·uria
vi·rus
    2060 v.
    acute laryngotracheo-
      bronchitis v.
    adeno-associated v.
    Amapari v.
    animal v's
    Apeú v.

vi·rus *(continued)*
    Apoi v.
    arbor v's
    Argentine hemorrhagic
      fever v.
    arthropod-borne v.
    attenuated v.
    Australian X disease v.
    avian leukosis v.
    B v.
    bacterial v.
    Bangui v.
    Banzi v.
    Batai v.
    Bhanja v.
    Bittner v.
    Bolivian hemorrhagic fever
      v.
    Brunhilde v.
    Bunyamwera v.
    Bwamba fever v.
    C v.
    CA v.
    Cache Valley v.
    California v.
    California encephalitis v.
    California myxoma v.
    Calovo v.
    cancer-inducing v.
    Candiru v.
    Carparu v.
    Catu v.
    CCA v. (chimpanzee coryza
      agent)
    CELO (chicken-embryo-
      *l*ethalorphan) v.
    central European
      tick-borne encephalitis v.
    Chagres v.
    Chandipura v.
    Changuinola v.
    Chenuda v.
    chikungunya v.
    Coe v.
    Colorado tick fever v.
    Columbia SK v.
    common cold v's
    Congo v.

vi·rus *(continued)*
    contagious pustular
      dermatitis v.
    coryza v.
    cowpox v.
    Coxsackie v.
    Crimean hemorrhagic
      fever v.
    croup-associated v.
    CTF (Colorado tick fever) v.
    cytomegalic inclusion
      disease v.
    defective v.
    dengue v.
    DNA v's
    Dugbe v.
    Duvenhaga v.
    EB v.
    Ebola v.
    ECBO v.
    ECDO v.
    ECHO v.
    ECHO 28 v.
    ECMO v.
    ECSO v.
    EEE v.
    EMC v.
    encephalomyocarditis v.
    enteric v.
    enteric cytopathogenic
      human orphan (ECHO) v.
    enteric orphan v's
    epidemic
      keratoconjunctivitis v.
    epidemic pleurodynia v.
    Epstein-Barr v. (EB v.,
      EBV)
    equine encephalomyelitis
      v.
    equine influenza v.
    Everglades v.
    exanthematous disease v.
    FA v.
    filamentous bacterial v.
    filterable v.
    filtrable v.
    v. fixé
    fixed v.

vi·rus *(continued)*

foamy v.
fowl plague v.
Friend v.
Ganjam v.
Germistan v.
Graffi v.
granulosis v.
Gross v.
Guama v.
Guaroa v.
Hantaan (Hataan) v.
Hazara v.
helper v.
hemadsorption v., type 1 (HA1)
hemadsorption v., type 2 (HA2)
hemagglutinating v. of Japan
hepadna v.
hepatitis A v. (HAV)
hepatitis B v. (HBV)
hepatitis C v.
hepatitis delta v.
herpangina v.
herpes v.
herpes B v.
herpes simplex v.
human immunodeficiency v. (HIV)
human T-cell leukemia/lymphoma v.
human T-cell lymphotrophic v., (HTLV)
Ilesha v.
Ilheus v.
inclusion v.
infectious porcine encephalomyelitis v.
infectious wart v.
influenza v.
Ingwavuma v.
iridescent v.
Itaqui v.
Japanese B encephalitis v.
JC v.
JH v.

vi·rus *(continued)*

Junin v.
K v.
Karimabad v.
Kemerova v.
Korean hemorrhagic fever v.
Kumba v.
Kyasanur Forest disease v.
Langat v.
Lansing v.
Lassa fever v.
latent v.
Latino v.
LCM v.
Lenny v.
Leon v.
leukemia v.
leukemia-sarcoma v.
Lokern v.
Lunyo v.
lymphadenopathy-associated v. (LAV)
lymphocytic choriomeningitis (LCM) v.
lysogenic v.
lytic v.
M-25 v.
Machupo v.
McKrae herpes v.
Madrid v.
Makonde v.
mammary tumor v.
Marburg v.
Marcy v.
Marituba v.
masked v.
Mayaro v.
measles v.
Mengo v.
milker's node v.
MM v.
molluscum contagiosum v.
Moloney v.
monkeypox v.
Mossuril v.
mouse mammary tumor v.
Mucambo v.

vi·rus *(continued)*
- mumps v.
- murine leukemia v.
- Murray Valley encephalitis v.
- Murutucu v.
- myxoma v.
- myxomatosis v.
- Nakiwogo v.
- Negishi v.
- Nepuyo v.
- neurotropic v.
- newborn pneumonitis v.
- Newcastle disease v.
- non-A, non B-hepatitis v.
- nononcogenic v.
- Norwalk v.
- Ntaya v.
- Nyando v.
- Omsk hemorrhagic fever v.
- oncogenic v.
- O'nyong-nyong v.
- Oriboca v.
- Oropouche v.
- orphan v's
- Ossa v.
- pantropic v.
- papilloma v.
- pappataci fever v.
- parainfluenza v.
- Parana v.
- paravaccinia v.
- pharyngoconjunctival fever v.
- phlebotomus fever v.
- Pichinde v.
- Piry v.
- poliomyelitis v.
- polyoma v.
- Pongola v.
- Powassan v.
- pox v.
- pseudocowpox v.
- Punta Toro v.
- Quaranfil v.
- rabies v.
- Rauscher leukemia v.
- respiratory syncytial v.

vi·rus *(continued)*
- Restan v.
- Rift Valley fever v.
- RNA v.
- Ross River v.
- Rous-associated v. (RAV)
- Rous sarcoma v.
- RS v.
- rubella v.
- Russian autumn encephalitis v.
- Russian spring-summer encephalitis v.
- SA v.
- St. Louis encephalitis v.
- salivary gland v.
- satellite v.
- Schwartz leukemia v.
- Semliki Forest v.
- Semunya v.
- Sendai v.
- sigma v.
- Simbu v.
- Sindbis v.
- slow v.
- smallpox v.
- Spondweni v.
- street v.
- Tacaribe v.
- Tahyna v.
- Tamiami v.
- Tataguine v.
- temperate v.
- Tensaw v.
- Teschen v.
- Theiler's v.
- Thogoto v.
- tickborne v's
- tobacco mosaic v.
- trivittatus v.
- tumor v.
- Turlock v.
- type C v.
- U v.
- Uganda S v.
- Uppsala v.
- Uruma v.
- vaccinia v.

vi·rus *(continued)*
  vacuolating v.
  varicella-zoster v.
  variola v.
  VEE v.
  vesicular stomatitis v.
  wart v.
  WEE v.
  Wesselsbron v.
  West Nile v.
  Wyeomyia v.
  Yaba v.
  yabalike disease v.
  Yale SK v.
  yellow fever v.
  Zika v.
  Zimmermann v.
vi·rus·emia
viru·stat·ic
vis·ce·ra
vis·cer·ad
vis·cer·al
vis·cer·al·gia
vis·cer·al·ism
vis·ceri·mo·tor
vis·cero·cra·ni·um
vis·cero·gen·ic
vis·cer·og·ra·phy
vis·cero·in·hib·i·to·ry
vis·cero·meg·a·ly
vis·cero·mo·tor
vis·cero·pa·ri·e·tal
vis·cero·peri·to·ne·al
vis·cero·pleu·ral
vis·cer·op·to·sis
vis·cero·sen·so·ry
vis·cero·skel·e·tal
vis·cero·skel·e·ton
vis·cero·so·mat·ic
vis·cero·tome
vis·cer·ot·o·my
vis·cero·to·nia
vis·cero·troph·ic
vis·cer·o·trop·ic
vis·cid
vis·cid·i·ty
vis·co·elas·tic·i·ty
vis·co·gel

vis·com·e·ter
vis·com·e·try
vis·cose
vis·co·sim·e·ter
  monolayer v.
  Ostwald v.
  Stormer v.
vis·co·sim·e·try
vis·cos·i·ty
  absolute v.
  dynamic v.
  kinematic v.
vis·cous
vis·cus *pl.* vis·ce·ra
  cervical v.
vis·ile
Vi·sine
vi·sion
  achromatic v.
  binocular v.
  central v.
  chromatic v.
  color v.
  day v.
  dichromatic v.
  direct v.
  double v.
  epileptic panoramic v.
  facial v.
  foveal v.
  gun-barrel v.
  half v.
  halo v.
  haploscopic v.
  indirect v.
  low v.
  monocular v.
  multiple v.
  night v.
  v. null
  v. obscure
  oscillating v.
  peripheral v.
  photopic v.
  Pick's v.
  pseudoscopic v.
  rainbow v.
  rod v.

vi·sion *(continued)*
    scotopic v.
    shaft v.
    solid v.
    stereoscopic v.
    triple v.
    tubular v.
    tunnel v.
    twilight v.
    violet v.
    word v.
    yellow v.
vis·na
Vis·ta·ril
vis·u·al
vis·u·al·iza·tion
    double contrast v.
vis·u·al·ize
vis·uo·au·di·to·ry
visu·og·no·sis
vis·uo·psy·chic
vis·uo·sen·so·ry
vi·su·scope
vi·tag·o·nist
vi·tal
Vi·tali's test
vi·ta·lism
vi·tal·i·ty
    pulp v.
Vi·tal·li·um
vi·ta·mer
vi·ta·min
    v. A
    v. A_1
    v. A_2
    v. A esters
    anticanitic v.
    antihemorrhagic v.
    anti-infection v.
    antineuritic v.
    antipellagra v.
    antirachitic v.
    antiscorbutic v.
    antisterility v.
    antixerophthalmic v.
    v. B
    v. B complex
    v. B_1

vi·ta·min *(continued)*
    v. B_2
    v. B_6
    v. B_{12}
    v. B_{12b}
    v. B_{17}
    v. B_c
    v. B_c conjugate
    v. B_2 phosphate
    v. B_t
    v. C
    v. D
    v. D_2
    v. D_3
    v. D_4
    v. E
    fat-soluble v's
    v. G
    v. H
    v. K
    v. K_1
    v. K_2
    v. K_3
    v. L
    v. M
    v. P
    permeability v.
    therapeutic v's
    water-soluble v's
vi·ta·min A acid
vi·tam·i·no·gen·ic
vi·tam·i·noid
vi·ta·min·ol·o·gy
vi·tan·i·tion
vit·el·lar·i·um
vit·el·lary
vi·tel·li·cle
vi·tel·lin
vi·tel·line
vi·tel·lo·gen·e·sis
vi·tel·lo·lu·te·in
vi·tel·lo·mes·en·ter·ic
vi·tel·lo·ru·bin
vi·tel·lose
vi·tel·lus
    v. ovi
vi·ti·a·tin
vi·ti·a·tion

vit·i·lig·i·nes
vit·i·lig·i·nous
vit·i·li·go
   v. capitis
   Cazenave's v.
   v. iridis
Vi·tis
   V. vinifera
vit·i·um *pl.* vit·ia
   v. conformationis
   v. cordis
   v. primae formationis
vi·to·dy·nam·ics
vit. ov. sol. — L. vitello ovi
solutus (dissolved in yolk of
egg)
vi·trec·to·my
vit·reo·cap·su·li·tis
vit·reo·ret·i·nal
vit·reo·ret·i·nop·a·thy
vit·re·ous
   anterior v.
   detached v.
   primary v.
   primary persistent
    hyperplastic v.
   secondary v.
   tertiary v.
vit·re·um
vi·tri·na
   corpus v.
vit·ri·ol
   blue v.
vit·ro·pres·sure
Vi·vac·til
vivi·di·al·y·sis
vivi·dif·fu·sion
vivi·par·i·ty
vi·vip·a·rous
Vi·vip·a·rus
   V. javanicus
vivi·pa·tion
vivi·sec·tion
vivi·sec·tion·ist
Vlad·i·mir·off-Mik·u·licz
amputation
Vlad·i·mir·off's operation

VLBW — very low birth
weight
VLDL — very low-density
lipoprotein
VMA — vanillylmandelic acid
VMD — L. Veterinariae
Medicinae Doctor (Doctor of
Veterinary Medicine)
vo·cal
vo·ca·li·za·tion
   epileptic v.
   iterative v.
Voegt·lin unit
Vo·ges-Pros·kau·er reaction
Vo·ges-Pros·kau·er test
Vogt's angle
Vogt's disease
Vogt's point
Vogt's syndrome
Vogt-Hue·ter point
Vogt-Ko·ya·na·gi syndrome
Vogt-Spiel·mey·er disease
Voh·win·kel's syndrome
voice
   amphoric v.
   bronchial v.
   cavernous v.
   double v.
   eunuchoid v.
   myxedema v.
   whispered v.
voice·print
void
Voigt's boundary lines
Voille·mier's point
Voit's nucleus
voix
   v. de polichinelle
vo·la *pl.* vo·lae
   v. manus
   v. pedis
vo·lar
vo·lar·dor·sal
vo·la·ris
vol·a·tile
vol·a·til·iza·tion
vol·a·til·ize
vol·a·til·iz·er

vo·len·ti non fit in·ju·ria
Vol·hard's test
vo·li·tion
vo·li·tion·al
Volk·mann's canal
Volk·mann's contracture
Volk·mann's disease
Volk·mann's membrane
Volk·mann's paralysis
Volk·mann's spoon
vol·ley
    antidromic v.
Voll·mer's test
vol·sel·la
volt
    electron v., (eV, ev)
vol·tage
    effective v.
    inverse v.
    peak v.
    pulsating v.
    ripple v.
vol·ta·ic
vol·ta·ism
vol·tam·me·ter
volt·am·pere
volt·me·ter
    electrostatic v.
    sphere gap v.
Vol·to·li·ni's disease
Vol·to·li·ni's tube
vol·ume
    alveolar v.
    alveolar dead-space v.
    atomic v.
    blood v.
    circulation v.
    v. of circulation
    v. of distribution
    end-diastolic v.
    end-systolic v.
    expiratory reserve v.
    forced expiratory v. (FEV)
    gram-molecular v.
    inspiratory reserve v.
    inspiratory triggering v.
    maximal expiratory v.
    mean corpuscular v.

vol·ume *(continued)*
    minute v.
    normal v.
    packed-cell v. (PCV)
    v. of packed red cells
      (VPRC)
    partial v.
    plasma v.
    red cell v.
    residual v.
    standard v.
    stroke v.
    target v.
    tidal v.
vol·u·men·om·e·ter
vol·u·met·ric
vol·u·mette
vol·u·mom·e·ter
vol·un·tary
vo·lun·to·mo·to·ry
vo·lute
vo·lu·tin
    v. granules
vol·vu·late
vol·vu·lo·sis
vol·vu·lus
    v. of colon
    gastric v.
    v. neonatorum
vo·mer
vo·mer·ine
vo·mero·bas·i·lar
vo·mero·na·sal
vom·it
    Barcoo v.
    bilious v.
    black v.
    coffee-ground v.
vom·it·ing
    cerebral v.
    cyclic v.
    dry v.
    explosive v.
    fecal v.
    hysterical v.
    morning v.
    periodic v.
    pernicious v.

vom·it·ing *(continued)*
    v. of pregnancy
    projectile v.
    recurrent v.
    stercoraceous v.
vom·i·tive
vom·i·to
    v. negro
vom·i·to·ry
vom·it·u·ri·tion
vom·i·tus
    v. cruentus
    v. gravidarum
    v. matutinus
von Kos·sa stain
Von·trol
Voor·hees' bag
Vor·a·nil
Vo·ro·noff's operation
vor·tex *pl.* vor·ti·ces
    coccygeal v.
    v. coccygeus
    v. cordis
    Fleischer's v.
    v. of heart
    v. lentis
    vortices pilorum
vor·ti·ces
vor·ti·cose
v. o. s. — L. vitello ovi solutus
  (dissolved in yolk of egg)
Vos·si·us lenticular ring
vous·sure
vox *pl.* vo·ces
    v. cholerica
vo·yeur
vo·yeur·ism
VPC — volume of packed cells
VPF — vascular permeability
  factor
V-plas·ty
VPRC — volume of packed
  red cells
VR — vocal resonance
Vrolik's disease
VS — ventricular septum
    volumetric solution

VSD — ventricular septal
  defect
VSG — variable surface
  glycoprotein
VT — tidal volume
    vacuum tuberculin
    ventricular tachycardia
vu·er·om·e·ter
vul·ca·nize
vul·ga·ris
    acne v.
    verruca v.
vul·ga·ro·bu·fo·tox·in
vul·ner·a·bil·i·ty
vul·ner·ant
vul·ner·ary
vul·ner·ate
vul·nus *pl.* vul·ne·ra
Vul·pi·an's atrophy
vul·sel·la
vul·sel·lum
vul·va
    fused v.
vul·val
vul·var
vul·vec·to·my
vul·vis·mus
vul·vi·tis
    adhesive v.
    diabetic v.
    eczematiform v.
    erosive v.
    intertriginous v.
    leukoplakic v.
    phlegmonous v.
    plasma cell v.
    v. plasmocellularis
    pseudoleukoplakic v.
    ulcerative v.
vul·vo·cru·ral
vul·vop·a·thy
vul·vo·rec·tal
vul·vo·uter·ine
vul·vo·vag·i·nal
vul·vo·vag·i·ni·tis
    infectious pustular v.
    mycotic v.
    senile v.

vv. — L. venae (veins)
v/v — volume (of solute) per volume (of solvent)
VW — vessel wall

V-Y plas·ty
VZIG — varicella-zoster immune globulin

W — tungsten
   watt
W — work
Waal·er-Rose reaction
Waal·er-Rose test
Waar·den·burg's syndrome
Wach·en·dorf's membrane
wad·ding
Wag·ner's corpuscles
Wag·ner's disease
Wag·ner's hammer
Wag·ner's line
Wag·ner's spot
Wag·ner's theory
Wag·ner-Jau·regg treatment
Wag·staffe's fracture
WAIS — Wechsler Adult Intelligence Scale
waist
wake·ful·ness
Waks·man, Selman Abraham
Wald, George
Wal·den·burg's apparatus
Wal·den·ström's disease
Wal·den·ström's macroglobulinemia
Wal·dey·er's fluid
Wal·dey·er's fossa
Wal·dey·er's gland
Wal·dey·er's layer
Wal·dey·er's ring
Wal·dey·er's sulcus
walk·ing
   chromosome w.
   heel w.

walk·ing *(continued)*
   reflex w.
   sleep w.
wall
   axial w.
   capillary w. of glomerulus
   cavity w.
   cell w.
   germ w.
   gingival w.
   inferior w. of tympanic cavity
   jugular w. of tympanic cavity
   labyrinthine w. of middle ear
   medial w. of middle ear
   nail w.
   parietal w.
   periotic w.
   pulpal w.
   splanchnic w.
   subpulpal w.
   superior w. of orbit
   tegmental w. of middle ear
   tympanic w. of cochlear duct
   vestibular w. of cochlear duct
   visceral w.
Wal·len·berg's syndrome
Wal·ler's law
wal·le·ri·an degeneration
wal·le·ri·an law
wall·eye

Wall·gren's aseptic meningitis
Wall·hau·ser-White·head
   method
Wal·ter's bromide test
Wal·thard's cell rests
Wal·thard's inclusions
Wal·thard's islets
Wal·ther's ducts
Wal·ther's oblique ligament
wan·der·ing
    pathologic tooth w.
Wang's test
Wan·gen·steen apparatus
Wan·gen·steen drainage
Wan·gen·steen suction
Wan·gen·steen tube
Wan·scher's mask
War·burg's apparatus
War·burg's technique
War·burg's theory
War·burg's vessel
ward
    isolation w.
War·dill's method
war·fare
    biological w.
    chemical w.
war·fa·rin
    w. potassium
    sodium w.
War·ing's method
War·ing's system
War·ren's incision
War·ren shunt
wart
    acuminate w.
    anatomical w.
    cattle w.
    common w.
    digitate w.
    flat w.
    filiform w.
    fugitive w.
    genital w.
    Hassall-Henle w's
    juvenile w.
    juvenile plane w.
    moist w.

wart (continued)
    mosaic w.
    mother w.
    mucocutaneous w.
    necrogenic w.
    pathologist's w.
    periungual w.
    peruvian w.
    pitch w's
    plane w.
    plantar w.
    pointed w.
    postmortem w.
    prosector's w.
    seborrheic w.
    seed w.
    soft w.
    soot w.
    telangiectatic w.
    tuberculous w.
    venereal w.
War·ten·berg's disease
War·ten·berg's sign
War·ten·berg's symptom
War·thin's tumor
War·thin-Fin·kel·dey cell
War·thin-Star·ry silver stain
wash
    eye w.
    jet w.
    mouth w.
Wash·am forceps
wash·out
    nitrogen w.
Was·mann's gland
wasp
was·ser·hel·le
Was·ser·mann reaction
Was·ser·mann test
Was·ser·mann-fast
Was·si·lieff's disease
wast·age
    birth w.
    pregnancy w.
    reproductive w.
waste
    phonetic w. of the breath
wast·ing

wa·ter
  w. of adhesion
  ammonia w.
  ammonia w., stronger
  aromatic w.
  bag of w's
  body w.
  bound w.
  capillary w.
  chlorine w.
  cinnamon w.
  w. of combustion
  w. of crystallization
  deionized w.
  distilled w.
  egg w.
  false w's
  free w.
  Goulard's w.
  ground w.
  hamamelis w.
  hard w.
  heavy w.
  w. of hydration
  w. for injection
  w. for injection,
    bacteriostatic
  w. for injection, sterile
  lead w.
  lime w.
  metabolic w.
  mineral w.
  orange flower w.
  peppermint w.
  potable w.
  purified w.
  rose w.
  rose w., stronger
  saline w.
  soft w.
  witch-hazel w.
wa·ter-borne
wa·ter brash
Wa·ter·house-Fri·der·ich·sen
  syndrome
wa·ters
Wa·ters projection
Wa·ters view

wa·ter·shed
  abdominal w's
Wat·kins' operation
Wat·son, James Dewey
Wat·son-Crick helix
Wat·son-Schwartz test
watt
watt·age
watt-hour
watt·me·ter
wave
  a w.
  activation w.
  afterpotential w.
  alpha w's
  anacrotic w.
  anadicrotic w.
  arterial w.
  beta w's
  brain w's
  c w.
  cannon w.
  catacrotic w.
  catadicrotic w.
  complex w's
  continuous w. (CW)
  contraction w.
  cove-plane T w.
  delta w's
  dicrotic w.
  electroencephalographic
    w's
  electromagnetic w's
  Erb's w's
  excitation w.
  F w's
  ff w's
  fibrillary w's
  fibrillation w's
  flat-top w's
  fluid w.
  flutter w.
  gamma w.
  glottal w.
  h w.
  in phase w's
  kappa w's

wave *(continued)*
   lambda w's
   Liesegang's w's
   light w's
   longitudinal w.
   microelectric w.
   monomorphic w.
   monorhythmic w's
   P w.
   P mitrale w.
   papillary w.
   percussion w.
   peristaltic w.
   phrenic w.
   polymorphic w's
   polyrhythmic w's
   postextrasystolic T w.
   P pulmonale w.
   pulse w.
   Q w.
   QS w.
   R w.
   radio w's
   random w's
   recoil w.
   S w.
   sharp w.
   shear w.
   short w.
   sine w.
   slow occipital w's
   slow posterior w's
   sonic w's
   standing w's
   Stephenson's w.
   stimulus w.
   supersonic w's
   T w.
   theta w's
   tidal w.
   transverse w.
   Traube-Hering w's
   traveling w.
   tricrotic w.
   U w.
   ultrashort w.
   ultrasonic w's
   V_1 (V1) w.

wave *(continued)*
   V_2 (V2) w.
   v w.
   ventricular w.
   x w.
   y w.
wave·form
wave·length
   effective w.
   equivalent w.
   minimum w.
wave·me·ter
wax
   baseplate w.
   blockout w.
   bone w.
   boxing w.
   candelilla w.
   carding w.
   carnauba w.
   casting w.
   cetyl esters w.
   dental w.
   dental inlay casting w.
   ear w.
   emulsifying w.
   grave w.
   Horsley's w.
   inlay casting w.
   inlay pattern w.
   palm w.
   set-up w.
   sticky w.
   try-in w.
   tubercle bacillus w.
   utility w.
   vegetable w.
   white w.
   yellow w.
wax·ing
wax·ing up
Wb — weber
WBC — white blood cell
      white blood (cell) count
W4D — Worth four-dot (test)
WDLL — well-differentiated
   lymphocytic lymphoma
wean

wear
   interproximal w.
   occlusal w.
web
   w. of duodenum
   esophageal w.
   laryngeal w.
   subsynaptic w.
   terminal w.
webbed
web·bing
   congenital w. of neck
   skin w.
web·er
Web·er's corpuscle
Web·er's disease
Web·er's glands
Web·er's law
Web·er's organ
Web·er's paradox
Web·er's paralysis
Web·er's point
Web·er's sign
Web·er's symptom
Web·er's syndrome
Web·er's test
Web·er's triangle
Web·er's zone
Web·er-Chris·tian disease
Web·er-Chris·tian panniculitis
Web·er-Chris·tian syndrome
Web·er-Coc·kayne syndrome
Web·er-Fech·ner law
web-fin·gered
Web·ster's operation
Web·ster's test
Wechs·ler's Adult In·tel·li·
   gence Scale (WAIS)
Wechs·ler's In·tel·li·gence
   Scale for Chil·dren (WISC)
wedge
   dental w.
   step w.
WEE — western equine
   encephalomyelitis
weed
   jimson w.
Weeks' bacillus

weep
We·ge·ner's granulomatosis
Weg·ner's disease
Weg·ner's sign
Wei·chardt's antikenotoxin
Weich·brodt's reaction
Weich·brodt's test
Weich·sel·baum's diplococcus
Wei·del's test
Wei·gert's law
Wei·gert's method
Wei·gert's stain
Wei·gert-Pal method
Wei·gert-Pal technique
weight
   apothecaries' w.
   atomic w.
   avoirdupois w.
   birth w.
   combining w.
   equivalent w.
   gram-atomic w.
   gram molecular w.
   molecular w.
Weigl-Gold·stein-Scheer·er
   test
Weil's basal layer
Weil's disease
Weil's stain
Weil's syndrome
Weil's zone
Weil-Fe·lix reaction
Weil-Fe·lix test
Weill's sign
Weill-Mar·che·sa·ni syndrome
Wein·gar·ten syndrome
Weir Mitch·ell treatment
Weis·bach's angle
Weis·mann's theory
weis·mann·ism
Weiss' reflex
Weiss' sign
Weiss' test
Weit·brecht's cord
Weit·brecht's foramen
Weit·brecht's ligament
Welch's bacillus
Welck·er's method

well-be·ing
Wel·ler, Thomas Huckle
well·ness
welt
wen
Wen·cke·bach's disease
Wen·cke·bach's period
Wen·der's test
Wen·zell's test
Wep·fer's glands
Werd·nig-Hoff·mann atrophy
Werd·nig-Hoff·mann disease
Werd·nig-Hoff·mann paralysis
Werd·nig-Hoff·mann
  syndrome
Werd·nig-Hoff·mann type
Werl·hof's disease
Wer·mer syndrome
Wer·ner's syndrome
Wer·ner's test
Wer·ner-His disease
Wer·ni·cke's aphasia
Wer·ni·cke's campus
Wer·ni·cke's disease
Wer·ni·cke's encephalopathy
Wer·ni·cke's reaction
Wer·ni·cke's syndrome
Wer·ni·cke-Kor·sa·koff
  syndrome
Wer·ni·cke-Mann hemiplegia
Wer·ni·cke-Mann type
Wert·heim's operation
Wert·heim-Schau·ta operation
West·berg's space
Wes·ter·gren method
Wes·ter·mark's sign
Wes·tern blot
West Nile encephalitis
West Nile fever
West Nile virus
West·phal's nucleus
West·phal's phenomenon
West·phal's pupillary reflex
West·phal's sign
West·phal's symptom
West·phal-Piltz phenomenon
West·phal-Piltz reflex
West·phal-Strüm·pell disease

West·phal-Strüm·pell
  pseudosclerosis
wet-nurse
wet·pox
wet-scald
Wet·zel's grid
Wet·zel's test
We·ver-Bray effect
We·ver-Bray phenomenon
Weyl's test
Whar·ton's duct
Whar·ton's gelatin
Whar·ton's jelly
wheal
wheel
    Burlew w.
    Carborundum w.
    rag w.
Wheel·er and John·son test
wheeze
    asthmatoid w.
whelp
whip·lash
Whip·ple, George Hoyt
Whip·ple's disease
Whip·ple's operation
Whip·ple's tests
Whip·ple's triad
whip·worm
whis·per
whis·tle
    Galton's w.
White, Charles
White's operation
white
    visual w.
White·head's operation
white·head
White·horn's method
white·leg
white·pox
Whit·field's ointment
whit·low
    herpetic w.
    melanotic w.
    painless w.
    perionychial w.
    thecal w.

Whit·man's operation
Whit·more's bacillus
Whit·more's disease
Whit·more's fever
Whitnall's tubercle
whoop
whoop·ing cough
whorl
    bone w.
    coccygeal w.
    lens w.
Whytt's disease
Wich·mann's asthma
Wick·er·shei·mer's fluid
Wick·er·shei·mer's medium
Wick·ham's striae
    iris w.
Wi·dal's reaction
Wi·dal's serum test
Wi·dal's syndrome
Wi·dal's test
Wi·dal-Abra·mi disease
Wid·mark's conjunctivitis
width
    line w.
    pulse w.
    window w.
Wie·sel, Tolsten Nils
Wi·gand's maneuver
Wi·gand's version
Wil·bur-Ad·dis test
Wil·cox·on's rank sum test
Wil·cox·on's signed rank test
Wild·bolz reaction
Wild·bolz test
Wilde's cords
Wil·der's diet
Wil·der's law of initial value
Wil·der's sign
Wil·der·muth's ear
Wil·der·vanck syndrome
Wil·kins, Maurice Hugh
  Frederick
will
    living w.
Wil·lan's lepra
Wil·le·brand disease
Wil·le·brand factor

Wil·lett clamp
Wil·lett forceps
Wil·liams' sign
Wil·liams syndrome
Wil·liams' tracheal tone
Wil·liam·son's blood test
Wil·liam·son's sign
Wil·lis' antrum
Wil·lis' circle
Wil·lis' cords
Wil·lis' nerve
Wil·lis' paracusis
Wilms' tumor
Wil·son's block
Wil·son's degeneration
Wil·son's disease
Wil·son's muscle
Wil·son's pronator sign
Wil·son's syndrome
Wil·son-Mik·i·ty syndrome
Wims·hurst machine
Win·ckel's disease
wind·burn
wind·chill
win·di·go
wind·kes·sel
wind·lass, Spanish
win·dow
    acoustic w.
    aortic w.
    aorticopulmonary w.
    beryllium w.
    cochlear w.
    energy w.
    oval w.
    Rebuck skin w.
    round w.
    skin w.
    vestibular w.
win·dow·ing
wind·pipe
wind-suck·ing
wing
    ash-like w.
    external white w.
    great w. of sphenoid bone
    greater w. of sphenoid bone
    w. of ilium

wing *(continued)*
    w's of Ingrassias
    internal white w.
    lateral w. of sacrum
    lateral w. of sphenoid bone
    lesser w. of sphenoid bone
    major w. of sphenoid bone
    minor w. of sphenoid bone
    w. of nose
    orbital w. of sphenoid bone
    small w. of sphenoid bone
    w's of sphenoid bone
    superior w. of sphenoid
      bone
    temporal w. of sphenoid
      bone
    w. of vomer
Win·Gel
wink
    anal w.
Win·kel·man's disease
Win·kel·man's paralysis
wink·ing
    jaw w.
Wink·ler's disease
Wins·low's foramen
Wins·low's ligament
Wins·low's pancreas
Wins·low's star
Win·strol
Win·ter·bot·tom's sign
win·ter·green
Win·ter·nitz's sound
Win·ter·stei·ner's rosette
Win·trich's sign
Win·trobe hematocrit
Win·trobe method
Win·trobe and Lands·berg
  method
wire
    alignment w.
    alveolar w.
    arch w.
    arch w., ideal
    diagnostic w.
    guide w.
    Kirschner w.
    ligature w.

wire *(continued)*
    measuring w.
    olive w.
    orthodontic w.
    separating w.
    tantalum w.
    twin w.
wire·worm
wir·ing
    aortic aneurysm w.
    circumferential w.
    continuous loop w.
    craniofacial suspension w.
    eyelet w.
    Gilmer w.
    interdental w.
    Ivy's w.
    Ivy loop w.
    multiple loop w.
    perialveolar w.
    piriform aperture w.
    single loop w.
    Stout w.
Wir·sung's canal
Wir·sung's duct
WISC — Wechsler
  Intelligence Scale for
  Children
Wish·art test
Wis·kott-Al·drich syndrome
Wis·sler-Fan·co·ni syndrome
witch ha·zel
with·draw·al
    thought w.
wi·ti·go
wit·kop
Wit·kop-Von Sall·man disease
Wit·zel gastrostomy
Wit·zel operation
wit·zel·sucht
WMA — World Medical
  Association
wob·ble
Wohl·fahr·tia
    W. magnifica
    W. opaca
    W. vigil
Wold·man's test

Wolfe's graft
Wolfe-Krause graft
Wol·fen·den's position
Wolff's duct
Wolff's law
Wolff-Eis·ner reaction
Wolff-Eis·ner test
Wolff-Par·kin·son-White syndrome
wolf·fi·an
Wölf·ler's operation
wol·fram
Wolf·ring's glands
wolfs·bane
Wo·li·nel·la
    W. recta
    W. succinogenes
Woll·as·ton's doublet
womb
Wong's method
Wood's filter
Wood's glass
Wood's light
Wood's sign
wool
    collodion w.
    cotton w.
    lumpy w.
Wool·ner's tip
word sal·ad
work·ing through
work-up
World Health Or·ga·ni·za·tion (WHO)
worm
    African eye w.
    bilharzia w.
    bladder w.
    blinding w.
    caddis w.
    case w.
    cayor w.
    dragon w.
    eel w.
    eye w.
    flat w.
    fluke w.
    guinea w.

worm *(continued)*
    heart w.
    horsehair w.
    kidney w.
    lung w.
    maw w.
    meal w.
    Medina w.
    palisade w.
    pork w.
    screw w.
    seat w.
    serpent w.
    spinyheaded w.
    stomach w.
    thorny-headed w.
    tongue w.
    trichina w.
Worm-Mül·ler's test
wor·mi·an bones
Worm·ley's test
worm·seed
worm·wood
Woulfe's bottle
wound
    aseptic w.
    avulsion w.
    blowing w.
    contused w.
    defense w's
    entrance w.
    exit w.
    hesitation w's
    incised w.
    lacerated w.
    nonpenetrating w.
    open w.
    penetrating w.
    perforating w.
    puncture w.
    septic w.
    seton w.
    stab w.
    subcutaneous w.
    sucking w.
    summer w's
    tangential w.
    tetanus-prone w.

wound *(continued)*
    traumatopneic w.
W-plas·ty
WPW — Wolff-Parkinson-
  White (syndrome)
WR — Wassermann reaction
wrapping
    fundic w.
Wre·den's sign
Wright's stain
Wright's syndrome
Wris·berg's cartilage
Wris·berg's ganglion
Wris·berg's ligament
Wris·berg's line
Wris·berg's nerve
Wris·berg's tubercle
wrist
    tennis w.
wrist·drop

writ·ing
  mirror w.
  specular w.
wry·neck
wt — weight
Wu·cher·e·ria
    W. bancrofti
    W. malayi
wu·cher·e·ri·a·sis
Wun·der·lich's curve
Wundt's tetanus
Wur·ster's test
w/v — weight (of solute) per
  volume (of solvent)
Wy·a·mine
Wy·cil·lin
Wy·dase
Wye·o·my·ia
Wynn method

X

X — Kienbock's unit
  xanthine
  xanthosine
X — reactance
x — abscissa
Xan·ax
xan·chro·mat·ic
xan·ox·ate so·di·um
xan·thel·as·ma
  generalized x.
xan·thel·as·ma·to·sis
xan·them·a·tin
xan·the·mia
xan·thene
xan·thic
xan·thin
xan·thine
xan·thine de·hy·dro·gen·ase
xan·thine ox·i·dase

xan·thin·ox·i·dase
xan·thin·uria
xan·thin·uric
xan·thism
xan·thi·uria
xan·tho·chro·mat·ic
xan·tho·chro·mia
  x. striata palmaris
xan·tho·chro·mic
xan·tho·cy·a·nop·sia
xan·tho·cyte
xan·tho·der·ma
xan·tho·eryth·ro·der·mia
  x. perstans
xan·tho·fi·bro·ma the·co·cel·
  lu·la·re
xan·tho·gran·u·lo·ma
  juvenile x.
xan·tho·ky·an·o·py

xan·tho·ma
  craniohypophyseal x.
  diabetic x.
  x. diabeticorum
  disseminated x.
  x. disseminatum
  eruptive x.
  x. eruptivum
  generalized plane x.
  juvenile x.
  x. multiplex
  x. palpebrarum
  planar x.
  plane x.
  x. planum
  x. striatum palmare
  synovial x.
  x. tendinosum
  tendinous x.
  tuberoeruptive x.
  x. tuberosum
  x. tuberosum multiplex
  tuberous x.
xan·tho·ma·to·sis
  biliary
    hypercholesterolemic x.
  x. bulbi
  cerebrotendinous x.
  chronic idiopathic x.
  x. corneae
  x. generalisata ossium
  x. iridis
  normocholesterolemic x.
  primary familial x.
  Wolman x.
xan·tho·ma·tous
xan·thone
xan·thop·a·thy
xan·tho·phane
xan·tho·phore
xan·tho·phose
xan·tho·phyll
xan·tho·pia
xan·tho·pro·te·ic
xan·tho·pro·te·ic acid
xan·tho·pro·tein
xan·thop·sia
xan·thop·sin

xan·thop·sis
xan·thop·ter·in
xan·thor·rhea
xan·tho·ru·bin
xan·tho·sar·co·ma
xan·tho·sine
  x. monophosphate (XMP)
xan·tho·sis
  x. diabetica
  x. diabeticorum
  x. of septum nasi
xan·tho·tox·in
xan·thous
xanth·u·ren·ic acid
xan·thu·ria
xan·thyl
xan·thyl·ic
xan·thyl·ic acid
X-bite
xe·nia
xeno·an·ti·gen
xeno·bi·ot·ic
xeno·cy·to·phil·ic
xeno·di·ag·no·sis
xeno·di·ag·nos·tic
xeno·ge·ne·ic
xeno·gen·e·sis
xen·og·e·nous
xeno·graft
  Hancock porcine x.
  Ionescu-Shiley pericardial
    x.
  porcine x.
xen·ol·o·gy
xeno·me·nia
xe·non
  x. 133
xeno·para·site
xeno·pho·bia
xeno·pho·nia
xen·oph·thal·mia
xeno·plas·ty
Xen·op·syl·la
  X. astia
  X. brasiliensis
  X. cheopis
  X. hawaiiensis
  X. vexabilis

Xen·o·pus
    X. laevis
xeno·rex·ia
xeno·tope
xen·yl
xe·ro·che·lia
xe·ro·col·lyr·i·um
xe·ro·der·ma
    x. of Kaposi
    x. pigmentosum
xe·ro·der·mat·ic
xe·ro·der·mia
xe·ro·der·moid
    pigmented x.
Xe·ro·form
xe·ro·gel
xe·rog·ra·phy
xe·ro·ma
xe·ro·mam·mog·ra·phy
xe·ro·me·nia
xe·ro·myc·te·ria
xe·ro·pha·gia
xe·roph·thal·mia
xe·roph·thal·mus
xe·ro·ra·di·og·ra·phy
xe·ro·si·a·log·ra·phy
xe·ro·sis
    x. conjunctivae
    conjunctival x.
    x. corneae
    corneal x.
    x. cutis
    x. parenchymatosa
    x. superficialis
xe·ro·sto·mia
xe·rot·ic
xe·ro·to·cia
xe·ro·to·mog·ra·phy
xe·ro·trip·sis
xi·lo·bam
xip·amide
xiphi·ster·nal
xiphi·ster·num
xipho·cos·tal
xipho·did·y·mus
xi·phod·y·mus

xiph·odyn·ia
xiph·oid
xiph·oi·di·tis
xi·pho·om·pha·lo·isch·i·op·a·gus
xi·phop·a·gus
xipho·pha·got·o·my
X-linked
XMP — xanthosine monophosphate
XOAN — X-linked (Nettleship) ocular albinism
X-Prep
x-ra·di·a·tion
x-ray
    hard x-r.
    soft x-r.
    spark x-r's
xy·lan
xy·la·zine hy·dro·chlo·ride
xy·lem
xy·lene
xy·li·dine
xy·li·tol
xy·li·tol de·hy·dro·gen·ase
Xy·lo·caine
xy·lo·ke·tose
xy·lo·ke·tos·uria
xy·lol
xy·lo·met·a·zo·line hy·dro·chlo·ride
xy·lo·py·ra·nose
xy·lo·sa·zone
xy·lose
xy·lo·side
xy·los·uria
xy·lu·lose
    x. 5-phosphate
xy·lu·lose re·duc·tase
L-xy·lu·los·uria
xy·lyl
xy·phoid
xy·ro·spasm
xys·ma
xys·ter

y — ordinate
Yal·ow, Rosalyn Sussman
yard
yaw
    guinea corn y.
    mother y.
    ringworm y.
yawn·ing
yaws
    crab y.
    forest y.
year
    y's of potential life lost
        (YPLL)
yeast
    bakers' y.
    brewers' y.
    dried y.
    false y.
    imperfect y.
    perfect y.
    sporogenous y.
    true y.
yel·low
    acid y.
    alizarin y.
    brilliant y.
    butter y.
    canary y.
    corallin y.
    fast y.
    imperial y.
    Manchester y.
    Martius y.
    metanil y.
    metaniline y. (extra)
    naphthol y.
    naphthol y. S
    Philadelphia y.
    rhubarb y.
    visual y.
Yeo's treatment
yer·ba
    y. santa

Yer·ga·son test
Yer·kes discrimination box
Yer·sin serum
Yer·sin·ia
    Y. enterocolitica
    Y. frederiksenii
    Y. intermedia
    Y. kristensenii
    Y. pestis
    Y. pseudotuberculosis
    Y. ruckeri
Yer·sin·i·eae
yer·sin·i·o·sis
yo·chu·bio
Yo·dox·in
yo·him·bine
yoke
    aleolar y's of mandible
    alveolar y's of maxilla
    cerebral y's of bone of
        cranium
    sphenoidal y.
yolk
    accessory y.
    egg y.
    formative y.
    nutritive y.
Yo·me·san
Yorke-Ma·son incision
Yo·shi·da's tumor
Young's operation
Young's rule
Young-Helm·holtz theory
yper·ite
Y-plas·ty
    Foley Y-p.
    Schweizer-Foley Y-p.
YPLL — years of potential life
    lost
yp·sil·i·form
yp·si·loid
yt·ter·bi·um
yt·tri·um
Yu·to·par

Z — atomic number
  impedance
Zac·tane
Zahn's lines
Zahn's ribs
Za·hor·sky's disease
Zan·col·li procedure
Zan·der apparatus
Zang's space
Zange·mei·ster's test
Zan·o·sar
Zan·tac
Zap·pert's chamber
Za·ron·tin
Za·rox·o·lyn
Zau·fal's sign
ZE (Zol·lin·ger-El·li·son)
  syndrome
Zea
ze·a·tin
zed·o·ary
Zee·man effect
zein
zei·o·sis
Zeis's glands
zei·si·an gland
zei·si·an stye
ze·ism
ze·is·mus
Zeiss counting cell
ze·is·tic
Zel·ler's test
Zell·weg·er syndrome
Zen·ker's crystals
Zen·ker's degeneration
Zen·ker's diverticulum
Zen·ker's fixative
Zen·ker's fluid
Zen·ker's necrosis
Zen·ker's solution
zen·ker·ism
zen·ker·ize
ze·o·lite
zeo·scope
Zeph·i·ran
zer·a·nol

ze·ro
  absolute z.
  audiometric z.
  limes z.
  physiologic z.
ze·ta
ze·ta·crit
Ze·ta·fuge
zeug·ma·tog·ra·phy
zeu·go·po·di·um
Zick·el nail fixation
zi·do·met·a·cin
zi·do·vu·dine
Zie·gler's operation
Zie·hen's test
Zie·hen-Op·pen·heim disease
Ziehl's carbolfuchsin stain
Ziehl's solution
Ziehl-Neel·sen carbolfuchsin
  method
Ziehl-Neel·sen stain
Ziems·sen's motor points
Zieve syndrome
ZIG — zoster immune
  globulin (vaccine)
zig·zag·plas·ty
zil·an·tel
zi·mel·i·dine hy·dro·chlo·ride
Zim·mer·lin's atrophy
Zim·mer·lin's type
Zim·mer·mann's arch
Zim·mer·mann's corpuscle
Zim·mer·mann's pericyte
zinc
  z. 65
  z. acetate
  z. bacitracin
  z. caprylate
  z. carbonate
  z. chloride
  z. hydroxide
  z. oxide
  z. permanganate
  z. peroxide
  z. peroxide, medicinal

zinc *(continued)*
    z. pyrithione
    z. salicylate
    z. stearate
    z. sulfanilate
    z. sulfate
    z. undecylenate
    white z.
zinc·al·ism
zin·cif·er·ous
zin·coid
Zinn's annulus
Zinn's arteria
Zinn's artery
Zinn's cap
Zinn's circulus
Zinn's fibra
Zinn's zonula
Zins·ser-Cole-Eng·man
    syndrome
zin·te·rol hy·dro·chlo·ride
zipp
zir·co·ni·um
zisp
zo·ac·an·tho·sis
zo·an·throp·ic
zo·an·thro·py
zoe·scope
zo·ic
zo·ite
Zol·lin·ger-El·li·son syndrome
Zöll·ner's figures
Zöll·ner's lines
Zo·max
zo·me·pir·ac so·di·um
zo·met·a·pine
zo·na *pl.* zo·nae
    z. arcuata
    z. cartilaginea
    z. ciliaris
    z. denticulata
    z. dermatica
    z. epithelioserosa
    z. fasciculata
    z. ganglionaris
    z. glomerulosa
    z. granulosa
    z. hemorrhoidalis

zo·na *(continued)*
    z. incerta
    z. ignea
    z. ophthalmica
    z. orbicularis articulationis
      coxae
    z. pectinata
    z. pellucida
    z. perforata
    z. radiata
    z. reticularis
    z. rolandica
    z. serpiginosa
    z. spongiosa
    z. striata
    z. tecta
    zonae tendinosae cordis
    z. transformans
    z. Valsalvae
    z. vasculosa
    z. vasculosa of Waldeyer
    z. Weberi
zo·nae
zo·nal
zo·na·ry
zo·nate
Zon·dek-Asch·heim test
zone
    abdominal z's
    z. of adhesion
    algogenic z.
    analgesic z.
    androgenic z.
    anelectrotonic z.
    z. of antemortem wound
    z. of antibody excess
    z. of antigen excess
    apical z.
    arcuate z.
    Barnes z.
    biokinetic z.
    border z.
    cervical z.
    chondrogenic z.
    ciliary z.
    z. of coagulation
    comfort z.
    contact area z.

zone *(continued)*
>   cornuradicular z.
>   coronal z.
>   Cozzolino's z.
>   dead z.
>   dendritic z.
>   denticulate z.
>   dentofacial z.
>   z's of discontinuity
>   dolorogenic z.
>   dorsal z. of His
>   ectopic z. of Schulte
>   entry z.
>   ependymal z.
>   epigastric z.
>   epileptogenic z.
>   epileptogenous z.
>   z. of equivalence
>   ergotropic z.
>   erogenous z.
>   erotogenic z.
>   z. of exclusion
>   extravisual z's
>   fascicular z.
>   fetal z.
>   Flechsig's primordial z's
>   focal z.
>   Fraunhofer z.
>   Fresnel z.
>   glomerular z.
>   Golgi z.
>   H z.
>   Head's z's
>   hemorrhoidal z.
>   Hess z.
>   His' z's
>   z's of hyperalgesia
>   z. of hyperemia
>   hyperesthetic z.
>   hypnogenic z.
>   hypogastric z.
>   hysterogenic z.
>   hysterogenous z.
>   inhibition z.
>   interpalpebral z.
>   keratogenous z.
>   language z.
>   Lissauer's marginal z.

zone *(continued)*
>   Looser's transformation z's
>   mantle z.
>   Marchant's detachable z.
>   marginal z.
>   maturation z.
>   median root z.
>   medullary z.
>   mesogastric z.
>   motor z.
>   near z.
>   nephrogenic z.
>   neutral z.
>   neutral z. of His
>   Nitabuch z.
>   notogenetic z.
>   nuclear z.
>   occlusal z.
>   z. of optimal proportions
>   orbicular z. of hip joint
>   organizer z.
>   z. of oval nuclei
>   papillary z.
>   pectinate z.
>   pellucid z.
>   perifollicular z.
>   peripolar z.
>   placental z.
>   z. of plateaus and furrows
>   polar z.
>   pupillary z.
>   z. of rarefaction
>   reticular z.
>   Rolando's z.
>   root z.
>   z. of round nuclei
>   rugae z.
>   z's of Schreger
>   sclerotic z.
>   segmental z.
>   Spitzka's marginal z.
>   subcostal z.
>   sudanophobic z.
>   tendinous z's of heart
>   thymus-dependent z.
>   thymus-independent z.
>   transformation z.
>   transition z.

zone *(continued)*
    transitional z.
    trigger z.
    Turck's z.
    umbau z's
    Valsalva's z.
    vascular z.
    ventral z. of His
    vermilion z.
    vermilion transitional z.
    visual z.
    Weber's z.
    Weil's basal z.
    Wernicke's z.
    Westphal's z.
    X z.
    z. of Zinn
zo·nes·the·sia
zo·nif·u·gal
zon·ing
zo·nip·e·tal
zo·no·skel·e·ton
zo·nu·la *pl.* zo·nu·lae
    z. adherens
    z. ciliaris
    z. ciliaris [Zinnii]
    z. occludens
zon·u·lar
zon·ule
    ciliary z.
    lens z.
    z. of Zinn
zon·u·li·tis
zon·u·lol·y·sis
zon·u·lot·o·my
zo·nu·ly·sis
zoo-ag·glu·ti·nin
zoo·an·thro·po·no·sis
zoo·bi·ol·o·gy
zoo·bio·tism
zoo·blast
zoo·chem·i·cal
zoo·chem·is·try
zoo·der·mic
zoo·de·tri·tus
zoo·dy·nam·ic
zoo·dy·nam·ics
zoo·eras·tia

zoo·flag·el·late
zoo·gen·e·sis
zo·og·e·nous
zo·og·e·ny
zoo·ge·og·ra·phy
zoo·glea *pl.* zoo·gleae
zoo·gle·al
Zo·o·gloea
zo·og·o·nous
zo·og·o·ny
zoo·graft
zoo·graft·ing
zo·og·ra·phy
zoo·hor·mone
zo·oid
zoo·lag·nia
zo·ol·o·gy
    experimental z.
zoo·ma·nia
Zoo·mas·ti·goph·o·ra
Zoo·mas·ti·go·pho·rea
zoo·mas·ti·go·pho·re·an
Zoon's erythroplasia
zo·on·er·y·thrin
zoo·nite
zo·on·o·my
zoo·no·ses
zoo·no·sis *pl.* zoo·no·ses
zoo·no·sol·o·gy
zoo·not·ic
zoo·para·site
zoo·para·sit·ic
zoo·pa·thol·o·gy
zo·op·er·al
zo·op·ery
zoo·phag·ic
zo·oph·a·gous
zoo·phar·ma·col·o·gy
zoo·phar·ma·cy
zoo·pher·in
zoo·phile
zoo·phil·ia
zoo·phil·ic
zoo·phil·ism
    erotic z.
zo·oph·i·lous
zoo·pho·bia
zoo·phys·i·ol·o·gy

zoo·phyte
zoo·plank·ton
zoo·plas·ty
zoo·pre·cip·i·tin
zoo·pro·phy·lax·is
zo·op·sia
zoo·psy·chol·o·gy
zoo·sa·dism
zo·o·sis
zoo·sperm
zoo·sper·mia
zoo·spo·ran·gia
zoo·spo·ran·gi·um *pl.* zoo·spo·
  ran·gia
zoo·spore
zoo·ste·roid
zoo·ste·rol
zoo·tech·nics
zo·ot·ic
zo·ot·o·mist
zo·ot·o·my
zoo·tox·in
zoo·troph·ic
zoo·tropho·tox·ism
Zop·fi·us
zor·ba·my·cin
zo·ru·bi·cin hy·dro·chlo·ride
zos·ter
    z. auricularis
    z. facialis
    z. femoralis
    ophthalmic z.
    z. ophthalmicus
    z. oticus
    z. sine eruptione
    z. sine herpete
zos·ter·i·form
zos·ter·oid
Zo·vir·ax
Z-plas·ty
Zsig·mon·dy's gold number
  method
Zsig·mon·dy's test
ZSR — zeta sedimentation
  rate
Zu·ber·el·la
zuck·er·guss
~~zuck~~·er·guss·darm

zuck·er·guss·le·ber
Zuck·er·kan·dl's body
Zuck·er·kan·dl's convolution
Zuck·er·kan·dl's gland
Zuck·er·kan·dl's organs
zu·clo·mi·phene
Zum·busch's psoriasis
Zuntz's theory
Zwaarde·ma·ker's
  olfactometer
zwit·ter·ion
zy·gal
zy·ga·po·phys·e·al
zy·ga·poph·y·sis *pl.* zy·ga·
  poph·y·ses
zyg·ia
zyg·i·on *pl.* zyg·ia
zy·go·dac·ty·ly
zy·go·ma
zy·go·mat·ic
zy·go·mat·i·co·au·ric·u·lar
zy·go·mat·i·co·fa·cial
zy·go·mat·i·co·fron·tal
zy·go·mat·i·co·max·il·lary
zy·go·mat·i·co-or·bi·tal
zy·go·mat·i·co·sphe·noid
zy·go·mat·i·co·tem·po·ral
zy·go·max·il·la·re
zy·go·max·il·lary
Zy·go·my·ce·tes
zy·gon
zy·go·ne·ma
zy·go·po·di·um
zy·go·sis
zy·gos·i·ty
zy·go·sperm
zy·go·sphere
zy·go·spore
zy·go·style
zy·gote
    duplex z.
zy·go·tene
zy·got·ic
Zy·lo·prim
zy·mo·chem·is·try
zy·mo·gen
zy·mo·gen·e·sis
zy·mo·gen·ic

zy·mog·e·nous

zy·mog·ic

zy·mo·gram

Zy·mo·mo·nas

zy·mo·san

zy·mos·ter·ol

Zz. — L. zingiber (ginger)

ISBN 0-7216-3599-7

90016

0721 635996